Perinatal and Pediatric Pathophysiology

PERINATAL AND PEDIATRIC PATHOPHYSIOLOGY: A CLINICAL PERSPECTIVE

First Edition

EDITED BY

Peter D Gluckman

Professor of Pediatrics, University of Auckland School of Medicine, New Zealand

and

Michael A Heymann

Professor of Pediatrics, University of California, San Francisco, California, USA

ASSOCIATE EDITORS

H Lagercrantz

Professor of Pediatrics and Neonatology, Department of Pediatrics, Karolinska Institute, Stockholm, Sweden

R D G Milner

Chairman of Pediatrics, King Faisal Specialist Hospital and Research Center, Riyadh, Saudi Arabia

J A Whitsett

Professor of Pediatrics, Pulmonary Biology Division, University of Cincinnati College of Medicine, Cincinnati, USA

ASSISTANT EDITORS

Paul D Sagan and Christine Thomas

Edward Arnold

A division of Hodder & Stoughton

LONDON BOSTON MELBOURNE AUCKLAND

First published in Great Britain 1993

Distributed in the Americas by Little, Brown and Company
34 Beacon Street, Boston, MA 02108

British Library Cataloguing in Publication Data

Gluckman, Peter
Perinatal and Pediatric Pathophysiology:
Clinical Perspective
I. Title II. Heymann, Michael
612

ISBN 0-340-55268-9

Whilst the advice and information in this book is believed to be true and accurate at the date of going to press, neither the author nor the publisher can accept any legal responsibility or liability for any errors or omissions that may be made. In particular (but without limiting the generality of the preceding disclaimer) every effort has been made to check drug dosages; however, it is still possible that errors have been missed. Furthermore, dosage schedules are constantly being revised and new side effects recognised. For these reasons the reader is strongly urged to consult the drug companies' printed instructions before administering any of the drugs recommended in this book.

Typeset in 10/13pt Linotron Clearface by
Rowland Phototypesetting Limited, Bury St Edmunds, Suffolk.
Printed in Great Britain for Edward Arnold,
a division of Hodder and Stoughton Limited, Mill Road,
Dunton Green, Sevenoaks, Kent TN13 2YA by
St Edmundsbury Press Limited, Bury St Edmunds, Suffolk
and bound by Hunter and Foulis Ltd, Edinburgh.

◆ Preface

Clinical pediatrics presents many exciting challenges because of both the interaction between the doctor, child and family and the intellectual perspective. The latter reflects the remarkable changes in physiology consequent to passage from fetus to neonate to infant to child to adolescent. The major changes in normal body function apparent throughout this period are reflected in the patterns and processes of disease observed. Further these disease processes themselves alter the pattern of development. Thus the competent pediatrician must be fully aware of the processes of regulation of development and of how physiological, biochemical and molecular and cellular processes mature and alter from fetus to adulthood. The rapidity of the knowledge explosion in cell biology, molecular biology, biochemistry and physiology increases the imperative that the practising pediatrician understand developmental biology to fully advance his/her clinical understanding. Conversely the experimentalist must look for clinical relevance to his/her studies, and the gap between clinical practice and the cutting edge of biology must be minimized.

There are many textbooks in pediatrics and many in physiology, biochemistry and cellular biology. However, it has been distressing to see the trend of an increasingly synoptic approach to the scientific basis of clinical science in pediatric textbooks. Most basic science textbooks place minimal emphasis on the developmental perspective and examples are rarely orientated towards the pediatrician. We have undertaken the development of this book in the strong belief that clinical pediatrics must be closely linked to its scientific base and that developmental biology can be placed in clinical perspective.

Our philosophy has been to select contributors at the cutting edge of their fields. We have demanded that the emphasis be placed on new knowledge and have been richly rewarded. We have asked that the book be written to a standard such that the pediatrician in training can expect to find in it the resources in the fields of molecular biology, cellular biology, biochemistry and physiology needed to fully complement clinical study. The majority of authors work in clinical departments but have a strong reputation in basic science research. It is hoped that this volume can provide the depth of knowledge that clinicians require. It should prove particularly attractive to residents and fellows in training. Equally, we hope that experimentalists seeking an understanding of the developmental perspective will find that each section provides a comprehensive review of the developmental aspects of biology and physiology.

P D GLUCKMAN
M A HEYMANN
November 1992

Contents

List of Contributors

S L Adamson, PhD
Assistant Professor of Obstetrics, Gynaecology and Physiology, University of Toronto, Mount Sinai Hospital, Toronto, Ontario M5G 1X5, Canada

J W Adelson, MD PhD
Professor of Pediatrics and Physiology, Director, Division of Pediatric Gastroenterology and Nutrition, Brown University/Rhode Island Hospital, Providence, RI 02903, USA

T E Adrian, PhD MRCPath
Professor and Head of Physiology, Department of Biomedical Services, Creighton University School of Medicine, Omaha, NE 68178, USA

R A Akeson, MD
Professor of Pediatrics, Division of Basic Science Research, Children's Hospital Medical Center, Cincinnati, OH 45229, USA

G R Ambler
Department of Paediatrics, School of Medicine, University of Auckland, New Zealand

A J Ammann, MD
Genentech Inc., South San Francisco, CA 94080, USA

M Andrew, MD
Professor of Paediatrics and Pathology, McMaster University Medical Centre, Hamilton, Ontario L8N 3Z5, Canada

M Y Anthony
Academic Unit of Paediatrics, Department of Clinical Medicine, University of Leeds, Leeds LS2 9NS, UK

A Aperia, MD
Professor of Pediatrics, Department of Pediatrics, Karolinska Institute, St Göran's Children's Hospital, Stockholm, Sweden

J Atkinson
University of Cambridge, Visual Development Unit, Cambridge CB2 1QA, UK

D Aviles, MD
Fellow, Pediatric Nephrology, Georgetown University Children's Medical Center, Washington, DC 20007, USA

E Birk, MD
Anshey Bereshit Street, Hod-Hasharon, Israel

W F Blum, MD PhD
Section of Pediatric Endocrinology, University Children's Hospital D-7400 Tübingen, Germany

J Bristow, MD
Associate Professor of Pediatrics, Department of Pediatrics, University of California San Francisco, CA 94143-0544, USA

G M Buga, PhD
Department of Pharmacology, UCLA School of Medicine Center for the Health Sciences, Los Angeles, CA 90024, USA

S K Burchett, MD
Assistant Professor of Pediatrics, University of Washington, Division of Infectious Disease, Children's Hospital, Seattle, WA 98105-0371, USA

W E Cameron, PhD
Assistant Professor of Behavioral Neuroscience and Psychiatry, Department of Behavioral Neuroscience, University of Pittsburgh, PA 15260, USA

B Cannon, MD
Professor, Wenner-Gren Institute, The Arrhenius Laboratories, Stockholm University, S-106 91 Stockholm, Sweden

D P Carlton, MD
Neonatal Division, Department of Pediatrics, University of Utah, Salt Lake City, UT 84132, USA

D Chapman, MD
Neonatal Division, Department of Pediatrics, University of Utah, Salt Lake City, UT 84132, USA

R D Christensen, MD
Professor of Pediatrics, Divisions of Neonatology and Human Development and Aging, University of Utah School of Medicine, Salt Lake City, UT 84132, USA

D S Chudwin, MD
Lincolnshire, IL 60069, USA

R I Clyman, MD
Professor of Pediatrics, Cardiovascular Research Institute, Department of Pediatrics, University of California San Francisco, CA 94143-0544, USA

M B Cohen, MD
Associate Professor of Pediatrics, Children's Hospital Research Foundation and University of Cincinnati, OH 45229, USA

C L Cook, MD
Fellow, Division of Critical Care Medicine, University of Colorado Health Sciences Center, Developmental Lung Biology, Denver, CO 80262, USA

K D Crissinger, MD PhD
Associate Professor of Pediatrics and Physiology, Department of Pediatrics, Louisiana State University Medical Center, Shreveport, LA 71130, USA

S Cullheim
Department of Anatomy, Karolinska Institute, S-104 01 Stockholm, Sweden

W S Cutfield
Senior Lecturer in Paediatrics, Department of Paediatrics, School of Medicine, University of Auckland, New Zealand

S L Davis, MB BCh NCHRF
Senior Research Fellow, Department of Paediatrics, University of Auckland School of Medicine, New Zealand

T Ebendal, PhD
Department of Developmental Biology, Biomedical Center, Uppsala University, Uppsala, Sweden

L Edström, MD
Associate Professor of Neurology, Karolinska Institute, S-104 01 Stockholm, Sweden

M L Epstein, PhD
Associate Professor of Anatomy, University of Wisconsin Medical School, Madison, WI 53706, USA

A R Euler, MD
Director, Gastrointestinal Clinical Development, Glaxo Inc. Research Institute, Research Triangle Park, NC 27709, USA

J R Fineman, MD
Assistant Professor of Pediatrics, University of California San Francisco, CA 94143-0106, USA

M Fitzgerald
Department of Anatomy and Developmental Biology, University College London, London WC1E 6BT, UK

H Forssberg
Department of Pediatrics, Karolinska Hospital, S-104 01 Stockholm, Sweden

P D Gluckman, MD
Professor and Chairman, Department of Paediatrics, University of Auckland, Private Bag, Auckland, New Zealand

M S Golbus, MD
Professor of Obstetrics, Gynecology and Reproductive Sciences and of Pediatrics, University of California San Francisco, CA 94143, USA

G R Gourley, MD
Associate Professor, Department of Pediatrics, University of Wisconsin School of Medicine and Waisman Center on Mental Retardation and Human Development, Madison, WI 53706, USA

J M Greenberg, MD
Associate Professor of Pediatrics, University of Cincinnati College of Medicine, Children's Hospital Medical Center, Division of Pulmonary Biology, Cincinnati, OH 45229-2899, USA

T R Gunn, MD FRCPC
Associate Professor, Department of Paediatrics, School of Medicine, University of Auckland, New Zealand

B L Hamilton, MD PhD
Children's Hospital and Medical Center, Oakland, CA 94609, USA

V K M Han, MD
MRC Group in Fetal and Neonatal Health and Development, University of Western Ontario, Lawson Research Institute, London, Ontario 6A 4V2, Canada

M A Hanson, MD DPhil CertEd
Reader in Fetal and Neonatal Physiology, Department of Obstetrics and Gynaecology, University College and Middlesex School of Medicine, University College London, London WC1E 6HX, UK

A Haramati, PhD
Professor, Department of Physiology and Biophysics and Medicine, Georgetown University School of Medicine, Washington, DC 20007, USA

J E Harding, MB ChB FRACP DPhil
Senior Lecturer in Paediatrics, Department of Paediatrics, University of Auckland, New Zealand

S Hawgood, MB BS
Associate Professor of Pediatrics, Department of Pediatrics and Cardiovascular Research Institute, University of California San Francisco, CA 94143, USA

M Heimann, PhD
Associate Professor, Department of Psychology, University of Göteborg, S-413 33 Göteborg, Sweden

D J Henderson-Smart, MB BS PhD FRACP
Professor of Perinatal Medicine, King George V Memorial Hospital, Camperdown, NSW 2050, Australia

J E Heubi, MD
Professor of Pediatrics, University of Cincinnati College of Medicine, Children's Hospital Research Foundation, Cincinnati, OH 45229, USA

M A Heymann, MD
Professor of Pediatrics, Obstetrics, Gynecology and Reproductive Sciences, Cardiovascular Research Institute, Department of Pediatrics, University of California San Francisco, CA 94143-0544, USA

D J Hill
MRC Group in Fetal and Neonatal Health and Development, University of Western Ontario, Lawson Research Institute, London, Ontario 6A 4V2, Canada

J I E Hoffman, MD
Professor of Pediatrics, Cardiovascular Research Institute, Department of Pediatrics, University of California San Francisco, CA 94143-0544, USA

B M Holland, MB FRCP(Glas)
Consultant Neonatologist, Queen Mother's Hospital, University of Glasgow, UK

D Hull, FRCP
Professor, Department of Child Health, University of Nottingham, Nottingham NG7 2UH, UK

L J Ignarro, PhD
Professor and Associate Dean, Department of Pharmacology, UCLA School of Medicine Center for the Health Sciences, Los Angeles, CA 90024, USA

O G P Isaksson, MD
Department of Internal Medicine, Endocrine Division, Sahlgren's Hospital, Göteborg, Sweden

J Isgaard, MD PhD
Department of Internal Medicine, Endocrine Division, Sahlgren's Hospital, Göteborg, Sweden

H S Iwamoto, PhD
Associate Professor of Pediatrics, Physiology and Biophysics, Children's Hospital Research Foundation and University of Cincinnati Children's Hospital Medical Center, Cincinnati, OH 45229-2899, USA

B M Johnston, BSc DPhil
HRC Senior Fellow, Department of Paediatrics, University of Auckland, New Zealand

C H Joiner, MD PhD
Associate Professor of Pediatrics, Physiology and Biophysics, Division of Neonatology, Department of Pediatrics, University of Cincinnati College of Medicine, Children's Hospital Medical Center, Cincinnati, OH 45229, USA

J G Jones, BPharm PhD
Senior Lecturer in Biochemistry, Department of Biochemistry, University of Wales College of Cardiff, Cardiff CF1 1ST, UK

P A Jose, MD PhD
Vice Chairman, Department of Pediatrics, Professor of Pediatrics and Physiology and Biophysics, Georgetown University Children's Medical Center, Washington, DC 20007, USA

N Josso, MD
Directeur de Recherches à l'INSERM, Unité de Recherches sur l'Endocrinologie du Développement (INSERM), Département de Biologie, Ecole Normale Supérieure, 921120 Montrouge, France

D M Katz
Department of Neurosciences, Case Western Reserve University, School of Medicine, Cleveland, OH 44106, USA

S S Kaufman, MD
Associate Professor of Pediatrics, Section of Gastroenterology and Nutrition, Department of Pediatrics, University of Nebraska Medical Center, Omaha, NE 68198-5160, USA

G Koren, MD ABMT FRCP(C)
Director of the Motherisk Program, Clinical Pharmacology and Toxicology, Hospital for Sick Children, Toronto, Ontario M5G 1X8, Canada

J A Kuller, MD
Fellow, Reproductive Genetics, Department of Obstetrics, Gynecology and Reproductive Sciences, University of California San Francisco, CA 94143, USA

H Lagercrantz, MD PhD
Professor of Pediatrics and Neonatology, Department of Pediatrics, Karolinska Institute, S-104 01 Stockholm, Sweden

G Lennerstrand, MD PhD
Department of Ophthalmology, Karolinska Institute, Huddinge University Hospital, S-141 86 Huddinge, Sweden

M I Levene
Academic Unit of Paediatrics, Department of Clinical Medicine, University of Leeds, Leeds LS2 9NS, UK

G C Liggins, CBE FRCS FRACS MRCOG
Emeritus Professor, University of Auckland, National Women's Hospital, Auckland, New Zealand

G Lister, MD
Professor of Pediatrics and Anesthesiology, Department of Pediatrics, Yale University School of Medicine, New Haven, CT 06510, USA

R R Magness, PhD
Associate Professor of Pediatrics and Obstetrics/Gynecology, Department of Pediatrics, The University of Texas Southwestern Medical Center at Dallas, TX 75235-9063, USA

R A Majack, MD
Assistant Professor of Pediatrics, Division of Critical Care Medicine, University of Colorado Health Sciences Center, Developmental Lung Biology, Denver, CO 80262, USA

P M Martha Jr, MD
Assistant Professor of Pediatrics, Section of Pediatric Endocrinology and Diabetes, Department of Pediatrics, Baystate Medical Center and Tufts University School of Medicine, Springfield, MA 01199, USA

D Matsui, MD FRCP(C)
Clinical Pharmacology Fellow, Division of Clinical Pharmacology and Toxicology, Hospital for Sick Children, Toronto, Ontario M5G 1X8, Canada

J McIntyre, MRCP
Research Fellow, Department of Child Health, University of Nottingham, Nottingham NG7 2UH, UK

I C McMillen
Department of Physiology, The University of Adelaide, Adelaide, SA 5001, Australia

R L Meyers, MD
San Francisco, CA 94122, USA

J Milerad, MD PhD
Department of Pediatrics KS, Karolinska Institute, S-104 01 Stockholm, Sweden

R D G Milner, ScD MD FRCP
Chairman of Pediatrics, King Faisal Specialist Hospital and Research Center, PO Box 3354, Riyadh 1121, Saudi Arabia

M D Mitchell, PhD
Professor and Director, Division of Reproductive Sciences, Department of Obstetrics and Gynecology, University of Utah Medical Center, Salt Lake City, UT 84132, USA

K Møllgård
Medicinsk Anatomisk Institut, A. Panum Institutet, Köpenhavns Universitet, 2200 Köpenhavn N, Denmark

S E Mulroney, PhD
Research Associate Professor, Department of Physiology and Biophysics, Georgetown University School of Medicine, Washington, DC 20007, USA

R D Murray, MD
Assistant Professor of Pediatrics, Division of Gastroenterology and Nutrition, Department of Pediatrics, Ohio State University, Children's Hospital, Columbus, OH 43205, USA

L Myatt, PhD
Associate Professor of Obstetrics and Gynecology, Pediatrics, Physiology and Biophysics, The Perinatal Research Institute, University of Cincinnati College of Medicine, Cincinnati, OH 45267-0526, USA

J Nedergaard, MD
Associate Professor, The Wenner-Gren Institute, Stockholm University, S-106 91 Stockholm, Sweden

M I New, MD
Professor and Chairman, Department of Pediatrics, New York Hospital-Cornell Medical Center, New York, NY 10021, USA

J G Nijhuis, MD PhD
Department of Obstetrics and Gynecology, University Hospital Nijmegen, PO Box 9101, 6500 HB Nijmegen, The Netherlands

A Nilsson, MD PhD
Department of Physiology, University of Göteborg, Sweden

R S Nowakowski, PhD
Department of Neuroscience and Cell Biology, UMDNJ-Robert Wood Johnson Medical School, Piscataway, NJ 08854, USA

H D Ochs, MD
Professor of Pediatrics, Division of Immunology and Rheumatology, Department of Pediatrics, University of Washington School of Medicine, Seattle, WA 98195, USA

J F Padbury, MD
Professor of Pediatrics, UCLA School of Medicine, Perinatal Research Laboratories, Harbor-UCLA Medical Center, Torrance, CA 90509, USA

R P Paulick, MD
D-8202 Bad Aibling, Germany

W J Pearce, PhD
Associate Professor of Physiology and Pediatrics, Division of Perinatal Biology, Loma Linda University School of Medicine, Loma Linda, CA 92350, USA

J J Pérez Fontán, MD
Associate Professor of Pediatrics, Department of Pediatrics, Section of Pediatric Critical Care, Yale University School of Medicine, New Haven, CT 06510, USA

A G Pettigrew, BSc PhD(Syd)
Professor of Veterinary Physiology, University of Sydney, NSW 2006, Australia

M Post, PhD
Division of Neonatology, Hospital for Sick Children, Toronto, Ontario M5G 1X8, Canada

B Quistorff
Biological Institute MN, The Royal Danish School of Pharmacy and NMR-Center, Department of Biochemistry, University of Copenhagen, 2100 Copenhagen Ö, Denmark

E O Reiter, MD
Professor of Pediatrics, Section of Pediatric Endocrinology and Diabetes, Department of Pediatrics, Baystoke Medical Center, and Tufts University School of Medicine, Springfield, MA 01199, USA

G E Richards, MD
Division Head, Division of Pediatric Endocrinology, Children's Memorial Hospital, Chicago, IL 60614, USA

J M Roberts, MD
Professor of Obstetrics, Gynecology and Reproductive Sciences, Director, Magee Women's Research Institute, Department of Obstetrics, Gynecology and Reproductive Sciences, University of Pittsburgh, Pittsburgh, PA 15213, USA

J E Robillard, MD
Professor of Pediatrics, Director of Pediatrics, Nephrology Division, Department of Pediatrics and Cardiovascular Center, University of Iowa Hospital and Clinics, IA 52242, USA

C R Rosenfeld, MD
Professor of Pediatrics and Obstetrics/Gynecology, Department of Pediatrics, University of Texas Southwestern Medical Center at Dallas, TX 75235-9063, USA

C D Rudolph, MD PhD
Assistant Professor of Pediatrics, University of Cincinnati College of Medicine, Children's Hospital Research Foundation, Cincinnati, OH 45229, USA

M Rundgren, MD PhD
Department of Physiology, Karolinska Institute, S-104 01 Stockholm, Sweden

J P Ryan, PhD
Professor and Deputy Chairman, Department of Physiology, Temple University School of Medicine, Philadelphia, PA 19140, USA

J Sack, MD
Professor of Pediatrics and Endocrinology, Sackler School of Medicine, Tel-Aviv University, Israel

Y Sadovsky, MD
Postdoctoral Fellow, Department of Obstetrics, Gynecology and Reproductive Sciences and Cardiovascular Research Institute, University of California San Francisco, CA 94143, USA

L M Satlin, MD
Associate Professor of Pediatrics, Division of Pediatric Nephrology, Albert Einstein College of Medicine, Bronx, NY 10461, USA

K R Schibler, MD
Instructor of Pediatrics, Divisions of Neonatology and Human Development and Aging, University of Utah School of Medicine, Salt Lake City, UT 84132, USA

A Schousboe
Biological Institute MN, The Royal Danish School of Pharmacy and NMR-Center, Department of Biochemistry, University of Copenhagen, 2100 Copenhagen Ö, Denmark

D Scolnik, MB ChB
Clinical Pharmacology Fellow, Division of Clinical Pharmacology and Toxicology, Hospital for Sick Children, Toronto, Ontario M5G 1X8, Canada

R J Shulman, MD
Associate Professor of Pediatrics, Section of Nutrition and Gastroenterology, Director Nutritional Support Team, Children's Nutrition Research Center, Texas Children's Hospital, Baylor College of Medicine, Houston, TX, USA

S J Soifer, MD
Associate Professor of Pediatrics, Director, Division of Pediatric Critical Care Medicine, Cardiovascular Research Institute, University of California San Francisco, CA 94143-0106, USA

B Specker, PhD
Division of Neonatology, Children's Hospital Research Foundation, Cincinnati, OH 45229, USA

K R Stenmark, MD
Associate Professor of Pediatrics, Head, Division of Critical Care Medicine, University of Colorado Health Sciences Center and the Children's Hospital, Developmental Lung Biology, Denver, CO 80262, USA

D F Teitel, MD
Associate Professor of Pediatrics, Department of Pediatrics, University of California San Francisco, CA 94143-0544, USA

G N Thompson, MD PhD FRACP
Metabolic Paediatrician and Senior Lecturer, The Murdoch Institute, Department of Paediatrics, University of Melbourne, Royal Children's Hospital, Parkville, Victoria 3052, Australia

L-E Thornell, MD
Professor of Anatomy, University of Umeå, Umeå, Sweden

M S Trautman, MD
Department of Obstetrics and Gynecology, University of Utah Medical Center, Salt Lake City, UT 84132, USA

B Ulfhake
Department of Anatomy, Karolinska Institute, S-104 01 Stockholm, Sweden

G F Van Hare, MD
Assistant Professor of Pediatrics, Cardiology Division, Department of Pediatrics, University of California San Francisco, CA 94143, USA

O R Velasquez, MD
Department of Physiology, Louisiana State University Medical Center, Shreveport, LA 71130, USA

D Walker, PhD
Department of Physiology, Monash University, Melbourne, Australia

C A J Wardrop, MB FRCPE FRCPath
Senior Lecturer and Honorary Consultant in Haematology, Department of Haematology, University of Wales College of Medicine, Cardiff CF4 4XN, UK

T E Weaver, PhD
Assistant Professor of Pediatrics and Anatomy, University of Cincinnati College of Medicine, Children's Hospital Medical Center, Division of Pulmonary Biology, Cincinnati, OH 45229-2899, USA

B K Wershil, MD
Instructor in Pediatrics, Harvard Medical School, Research Associate in Pathology, Department of Pathology, Beth Israel Hospital, Boston, MA 02215, USA

J A Whitsett, MD
Department of Pediatrics, Pulmonary Biology Division, University of Cincinnati College of Medicine, Cincinnati, OH 45229, USA

C C Winterbourn, PhD
Professorial Research Fellow, Department of Pathology, The Christchurch School of Medicine, University of Otago, Christchurch, New Zealand

J R Wispé, MD
Pulmonary Biology, Department of Pediatrics, Children's Hospital of Cincinnati, OH 45267, USA

J Ygge, MD PhD
Department of Ophthalmology, Karolinska Institute, Huddinge University Hospital, S-141 86 Huddinge, Sweden

F de Zegher
Department of Pediatrics, University Hospital, Gasthuisberg, University of Leuven, Belgium

E Zeisberger
Professor, Physiological Institute, Justus Liebig University, D-6300 Giessen, Germany

1 • *Membrane physiology*

Editor: Jeffrey A Whitsett

A. Membrane Transport and Cellular Ion Regulation

C H Joiner

The cell membrane functions primarily as a barrier, separating the cellular interior from the extracellular milieu or compartmentalizing one region of the cell from another. The movements across cell membranes of most materials (salts, water, and substrates) are mediated by specialized proteins and are intricately controlled by the cell's regulatory machinery. Transport processes may be divided into two major functional classes: those pertaining to the maintenance of cellular homeostasis and those mediating the bulk transfer of material across epithelia. Cellular ion homeostasis involves volume regulation, control of intracellular pH, maintenance of Ca^{2+} ion concentration in the nanomolar range, and creation of monovalent cation gradients to support a variety of cellular functions, including electrical activity, secondary active transport processes, and the movement of metabolic substrates and waste products across the cell membrane. Epithelial transport is responsible for secretion and absorption of salt and water, and of the nutrients and waste products in the gut, kidneys, respiratory tract, and other tissues. Virtually all transport systems are subject to cellular regulatory control, and many exhibit physiologically important changes during development.

Types of transport mechanisms

The mechanisms that mediate the movement of substances across cell membranes can be divided into **active** and **passive** transport processes on the basis of whether the substance in question moves up or down its electrochemical gradient. Active transport of molecules against an electrochemical gradient requires energy, either from the hydrolysis of ATP (**primary active transport**) or from the downhill movement of another substance (**secondary active transport**). The Na^+-K^+-ATPase, Ca^{2+}-ATPase, and H^+-K^+-ATPase are members of a family of transport ATPases, which mediate active ion transport in many tissues and which have close structural homologies and functional similarities. A variety of secondary active transport processes are responsible for the transmembrane movement of many organic substances, as well as cations and anions. Most of these transporters utilize the energy stored in the transmembrane Na^+ gradient to drive the movement of another substance against its electrochemical gradient. Systems that move substances in the same direction as Na^+, i.e. into the cell, are called **symporters** and are exemplified by the Na^+-K^+-Cl^- cotransporter and Na^+-coupled transporters for sugars and amino acids. **Antiporters** couple the downhill movement of Na^+ to the uphill transport of another ion in the opposite direction, i.e. out of the cell. Physiologically important antiport systems include Na^+-H^+ and Na^+-Ca^{2+} exchangers. Such carriers may also function to regulate the movement of ions down their electrochemical gradients. Such is the case of the KCl cotransporter mediating K^+ loss to control cell volume or the Na^+-H^+ exchanger catalyzing H^+ loss from an acidified cell. Likewise, the anion exchanger, another physiologically important antiporter, exchanges HCO_3^- for Cl^- to dissipate the transmembrane gradients of these ions.

Passive movements of hydrophilic organic compounds are mediated by transporters that catalyze and regulate their passage through the hydrophobic lipid bilayer. The **facilitated diffusion** of certain sugars, amino acids, and other organic compounds is mediated by 'carrier' molecules, which have binding sites with discrete affinities for transported substrates and maximal velocities of transport and which exhibit saturation kinetics. Diffusional movement of ions generally is mediated by **channels** that are specific for certain ions, exhibit characteristic, discrete electrical conductances, and exist in either an open or closed state, subject to cellular regulatory control. Ion movements through channels are always driven by the electrochemical gradient of the transported ion. Ion channel function and its appropriate regulation are central to the function of excitable cells and epithelial tissues. In most cells, the transmembrane movement of water is also controlled by specialized channels, the regulation of which is best exemplified by the modulation of water permeability of the collecting duct of the kidney by vasopressin. Transport via channels is very fast (typically one million molecules per second per channel), while transmembrane movement via facilitated diffusion carriers, symporters, antiporters, and ATPases is generally much slower (around 1000 molecules per second per carrier). A notable exception is the anion exchanger which can catalyze Cl^--HCO_3^- exchange at a rate of one million ions per second.

Lipid-soluble substances, such as gases (O_2, CO_2, and N_2), hydrocarbons, protonated organic acids, and anesthetic gases, pass through the lipid bilayer by simple diffusion, without mediation by protein carriers or channels.

Cellular ion homeostasis

The Na^+-K^+-ATPase

Transmembrane ionic gradients

Maintenance of the intracellular ionic milieu is one of the most basic cellular functions. Intracellular Na^+ and K^+, as well as water, behave as if in free solution in most cells, i.e. the amount of ion or water bound to cellular proteins and lipids is relatively small. In most animal cells, water is at osmotic equilibrium across the membrane, and there is no hydrostatic pressure gradient across the cell membrane. Cellular K^+ is maintained at 90–120 mmol/l cell water, while Na^+ varies from 5 to 50 mmol/l cell water, depending on cell type and functional mode. These concentrations are the result of the activity of the Na^+-K^+-ATPase, which couples the energy of ATP hydrolysis to the movement of ions across the membrane against their electrochemical gradient. The potential energy of these gradients is used by the cell to perform a variety of vital functions including regulation of cellular volume and pH, electrical activity in excitable cells, modulation of cell Ca^{2+}, and membrane transport of organic compounds. Accordingly, the Na^+-K^+-ATPase is vital to cellular homeostasis and is found in virtually all cells. Its biochemistry, physiology, and molecular biology are better understood than any other transport protein and serve as a paradigm of this important class of membrane proteins.

Na^+-K^+-ATPase structure

The Na^+-K^+-ATPase comprises two protein polypeptides (referred to as the α and β chains), which are present in a heterodimer ($\alpha\beta$) in the membrane. The α chain mediates the catalytic/transport functions of the complex, although the β-subunit is necessary for activity and seems to be required for the proper insertion of the newly synthesized α-subunit into the membrane. Although relative transcription rates for the α and β chain mRNAs vary considerably among different cells and tissues, the two polypeptide chains are always found in a 1:1 ratio in the membrane. Three isotypes of the α chain have been identified ($\alpha1$, $\alpha2$, and $\alpha3$) and possess characteristic tissue specificities and functional differences. The isotypes exhibit greater homology across species lines than they do with each other, i.e. rat $\alpha1$ is more like human $\alpha1$ than like rat $\alpha2$. The $\alpha1$ isoform predominates in kidney, lung, and stomach but is detectable in virtually all tissues and cells. Cardiac and skeletal muscle contain appreciable amounts of $\alpha2$ mRNA, and neuronal tissue contains all three isoforms. Currently, information about the physiological differences among the different isoforms is sketchy, but evidence indicates that the kinetic characteristics and responses to cellular regulatory processes differ among the isoforms. For example, the Na^+ affinity of the $\alpha2$ isoform found in muscle is considerably lower than that of $\alpha1$ and is altered by insulin stimulation (see below). Cell- and tissue-specific patterns of Na^+-K^+-ATPase isoform expression and developmental changes in those patterns likely have important physiological correlates in enzyme function and its regulation.

The α chain is approximately 1000 amino acids in length with a molecular weight of 100 kDa, and contains the ATP hydrolysis site, cation, and cardiac glycoside-binding sites, as well as cytoplasmic domains that interact with the regulatory machinery of the cell to modulate Na^+-K^+-ATPase activity. The molecule (Fig. 1.1) has 6–10 membrane-spanning α-helical domains (depending on isotype and species) and several small extracellular domains, one of which binds inhibitory cardiac glycosides. Isotype and species differences in primary sequence in a small segment of one of the extracellular domains are associated with differences in cardiac glycoside-binding affinity. Several of the transmembrane domains of the protein have clusters of anionic amino acids, which are thought to be involved in the binding and translocation of

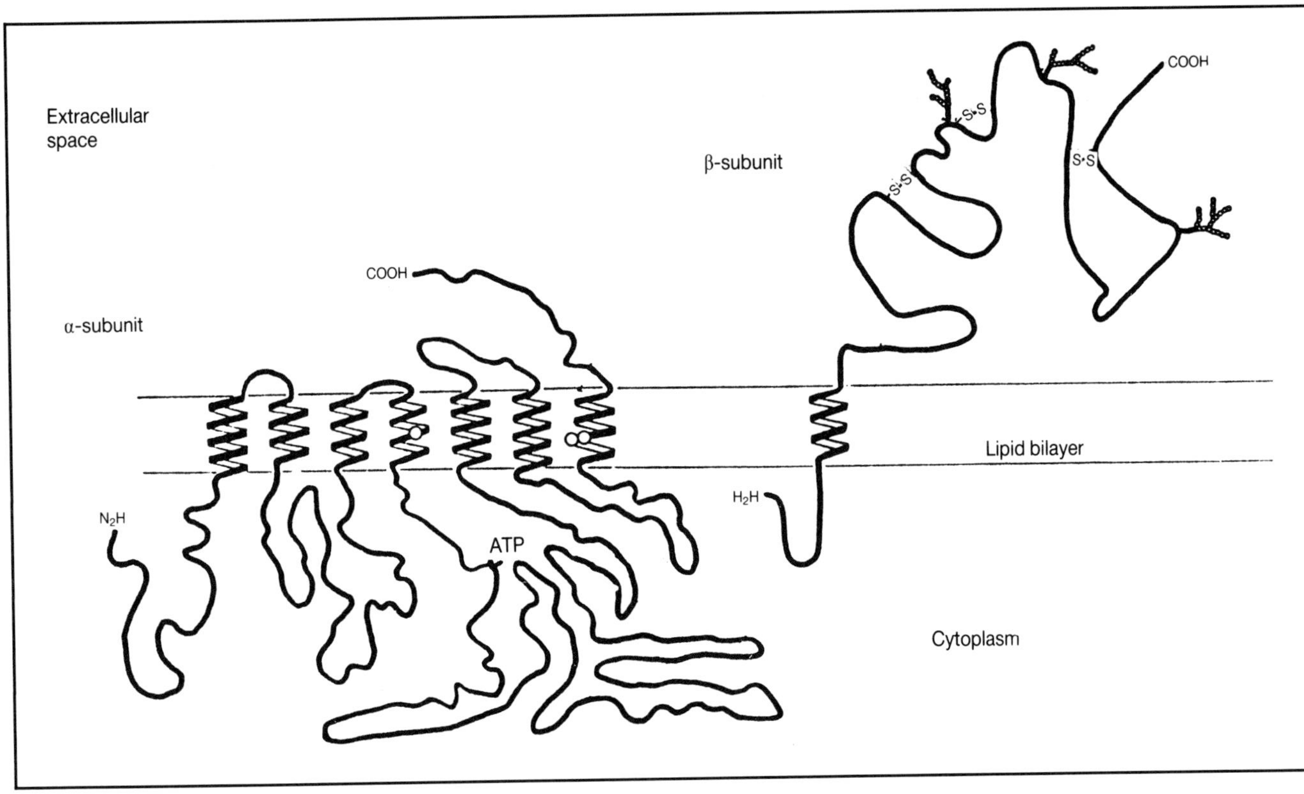

Fig. 1.1. Structure of the Na^+-K^+-ATPase. Seven membrane-spanning segments are shown for the α-subunit; the location of its –COOH terminus (extracellular vs cytoplasmic) is debated. The ATP-binding site, which is phosphorylated during the catalytic cycle, is indicated. (Modified from Pedemonte CH, Kaplan JH. *Am J Physiol* 1990; **258**: C1, with permission.)

cations across the membrane. Located at the cytoplasmic surface is a binding domain for ATP, which is highly conserved across species and isotype lines and which is shared by other members of the P-type ATPase class of enzymes, including the ubiquitous Ca^{2+}-ATPases and the H^+-K^+-ATPase responsible for acid secretion in lysosomes and gastric parietal cells.

The β-subunit of the Na^+-K^+-ATPase is a 35-kDa polypeptide that traverses the membrane once. The cytoplasmic domain is small, and the extracellular region has three sites bearing oligosaccharides, giving this glycoprotein a molecular weight of 53 kDa. Glycosylation has no effect on enzyme activity. Although the β-subunit has no intrinsic catalytic or transport function, its presence is required for the α-subunit to function. Furthermore, the β-subunit appears to play an important role in the insertion of newly synthesized polypeptide into the endoplasmic reticulum membrane and its transfer to the plasma membrane.

The catalytic cycle

The catalytic cycle of the Na^+-K^+-ATPase begins with the interaction of the cytoplasmic domain with Na^+, which promotes the phosphorylation of the protein by ATP at a specific aspartyl residue on the α chain, producing ADP at the cytoplasmic surface. In association with the phosphorylated enzyme, three Na^+ ions are then translocated across the membrane. Next, two external K^+ ions bind to the enzyme and induce the hydrolysis of the phosphoprotein, releasing the inorganic phosphate at the cytoplasmic surface. Subsequently, the K^+–enzyme complex reorients to the interior of the membrane, and the K^+ ions are released when the complex binds Mg^{2+}-ATP. The enzyme is then poised to interact with Na^+ to begin the cycle again. These events are associated with discrete conformation changes in the protein, which are detectable by physicochemical techniques such as changes in its susceptibility to proteolysis, binding of certain ligands, and spectrophotometric methods. Rather than gross movements of large segments of the protein across the membrane, these conformational changes are thought to represent small alterations in the relative positions of various domains in the protein, such as two adjacent α-helical transmembrane domains.

Na^+-K^+-ATPase regulation

The activity of Na^+-K^+-ATPase in the cell is subject to at least four types of physiological regulation: acute modulation of activity by changes in Na^+ and K^+ concentrations, modification by cellular regulatory processes, mobilization of enzyme from storage pools to the plasma membrane, and control of Na^+-K^+-ATPase gene expression. The first and last of these mechanisms are the most important. Short-term control of Na^+-K^+-ATPase activity represents a kinetic response to demand. The affinity (K_m) of the ATPase for internal Na^+ is around 20 mM in most cases, so that under steady-state conditions with intracellular Na^+ of about 10 mM, the pump operates well below its maximal capacity. If cellular Na^+ concentrations rise, Na^+-K^+-ATPase activity increases on the basis of substrate (Na^+) availability. Because of the kinetic characteristics of the system, relatively small changes in cellular Na^+ concentration can result in large increases in pump activity. Once the perturbation of membrane permeability has subsided and cellular Na^+ levels are brought back to normal by the Na^+-K^+-ATPase, its activity returns to normal. Most examples of acute stimulation of Na^+-K^+-ATPase activity by hormones or drugs involve this secondary reaction to increased intracellular Na^+, which results from the primary action of the stimulant to increased Na^+ influx into the cell by activation of Na^+-H^+ exchange or opening of Na^+ channels. The K_m of the pump for external K^+ is 1 mM, so that alterations of K^+ within the physiological range (3–5 mM) have little effect on Na^+-K^+-ATPase function.

An important example of a direct regulatory effect on Na^+-K^+-ATPase activity is the action of insulin on skeletal muscle. In the resting state, the majority of Na^+-K^+-ATPase molecules (about 75 percent) in this tissue are composed of α2 isoform. This isoform has low affinity for internal Na^+ in the resting state, so that the turnover of these pumps is quite low. Insulin acts via a tissue-specific membrane receptor to increase the affinity of the Na^+-K^+ pump for internal Na^+, thereby increasing the pumping rate appreciably. Although the mechanistic details of this phenomenon are not entirely clear, it is known to the clinician because it manifests as a reduction in serum K^+ following insulin infusion.

Several factors influence the number of Na^+-K^+-ATPase molecules in the plasma membrane of a cell. A number of hormones, notably mineralocorticoids and thyroid hormone, increase Na^+-K^+-ATPase gene expression, thereby increasing the number of pump sites on cells containing their respective receptors. In addition, prolonged elevation of intracellular Na^+ enhances expression of both α and β chains, which represents a response of the cell to added demand for Na^+ pumping. Experimentally, this is manifest as an increase in mRNA levels for the α and β genes and an increase in Na^+-K^+-ATPase activity assayed immunochemically or by ^3H-ouabain-binding sites within several hours of incubation of cells in the presence of low external K^+ or cardiac glycosides, both of which inhibit the pump and cause cellular Na^+ to rise. Biologically, this means that stimulation of Na^+ entry into the cell, e.g. by activation of Na^+ channels or Na^+-H^+ exchange or by damage to the cell membrane, results in a compensatory increase in Na^+ pumping capacity. This must be borne in mind when examining the physiological or developmental changes in Na^+-K^+-ATPase expression, because, as discussed above for acute modulation of Na^+-K^+-ATPase activity by physiological stimuli, some of the changes in gene expression may be secondary to an increase in cellular Na^+ induced by the primary event.

Cell volume regulation

Water occupies 70–90 percent of the volume of an animal cell, most of the remainder representing the volume of solutes, mostly protein. Because the membrane of most cells is highly permeable to water, no osmotic gradient exists between the intracellular and extracellular space in the steady state. This means that the water content of most cells is strictly a function of the osmotically active species of cell, and that the **control of cell volume hinges on the regulation of cation content**. The presence of negatively charged, membrane-impermeant proteins and organic phosphates in high concentrations in the cell creates electrical and colloid osmotic driving forces for cations and water to enter the cell (known as the Donnan effect). In the steady state, the cell uses the energy of the cation gradients established by the Na^+-K^+-ATPase, combined with tightly regulated passive permeabilities of the ions, to offset the tendency of the cell to gain cation and swell.

Note that the capacity of the Na^+-K^+-ATPase to carry out net extrusion of cations is not essential to this mechanism, only that it function to exchange Na^+ for K^+. The steady-state cation content and therefore cell volume is a function of Na^+-K^+ pump activity and its coupling ratio (Na^+ extruded:K^+ taken in) and the passive permeabilities of the membrane to Na^+ and K^+. This model, formulated for the mammalian red blood cell by Tosteson and Hoffman in 1960, also applies to nucleated cells, with the additional complexity that such cells are capable of rapidly altering passive cation permeabilities in response to changes in cell volume.

Cell volume regulation has been studied extensively in the nucleated red blood cells of fish, amphibians, and birds, as well as in the human reticulocyte, and there is evidence that other human somatic cells have similar mechanisms. Cell swelling (by reduction in medium osmolarity) elicits a volume regulatory decrease in which cation and water are lost by the cell to return it to its original volume. In the human reticulocyte, a KCl cotransport system performs this function. A brief review of this system illustrates the principle of downward volume regulation (Fig. 1.2). Upon acute reduction of extracellular osmolarity, a transient osmotic gradient is created across the membrane, causing water to move into the cell with resultant increase in volume; in reticulocytes, such osmotically driven water movements are complete within seconds. This swelling of the cell activates the KCl transporter, which moves K^+ out of the cell down its electrochemical gradient, coupled with the movement of Cl^- and carrying with it osmotically obliged water. The reticulocyte returns to its original volume within minutes. The mechanism of activation of the KCl cotransporter by cell swelling is not certain, but evidence suggests that sulfhydryl groups are involved in the volume-sensing mechanism and regulation of protein phosphorylation–dephosphorylation controls in the activity of the cotransporter.

Two distinct mechanisms have been described for volume regulatory increase in response to shrinkage in red cells. One system (Fig. 1.3), modeled in avian erythrocytes, involves a Na^+-K^+-Cl^- cotransporter stimulated by catecholamines via a cAMP-dependent mechanism and inhibited by loop diuretics such as furosemide, which moves salt into the cell to restore volume. A different system is found in fish red cells,

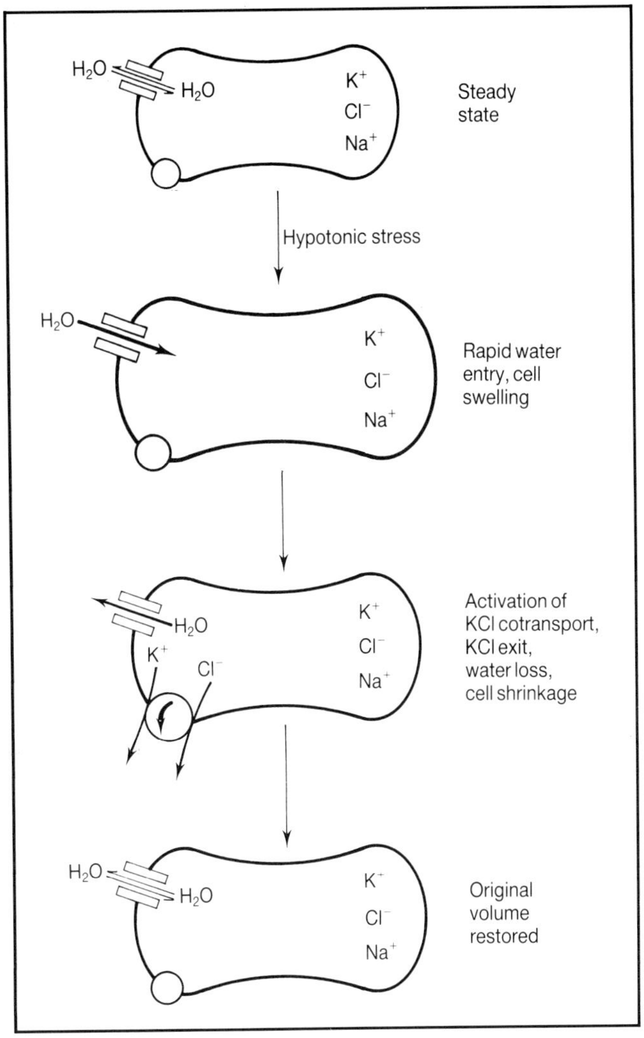

Fig. 1.2. Volume regulatory decrease in the red cell.*

which respond to cell shrinkage by activating a Na^+-H^+ exchanger that moves Na^+ into the cell in exchange for H^+; the resultant alkalinization of the cell interior increases the concentration of HCO_3^-, which is exchanged for extracellular Cl^- by the anion exchanger (Fig. 1.4). The net result is the uptake of NaCl and osmotically obliged water. Na^+-H^+ exchange is activated by a variety of tissue-specific receptors coupled to protein phosphorylation mechanisms. The response to changes in osmolality is demanded of cells in the gut and kidney, and volume control is also required of other epithelial cells in which the transcellular movement of large amounts of solute may perturb cell volume.

Both Na^+-H^+ exchange and Na^+-K^+-Cl^- cotransport systems are known to exist in a variety of cell types in

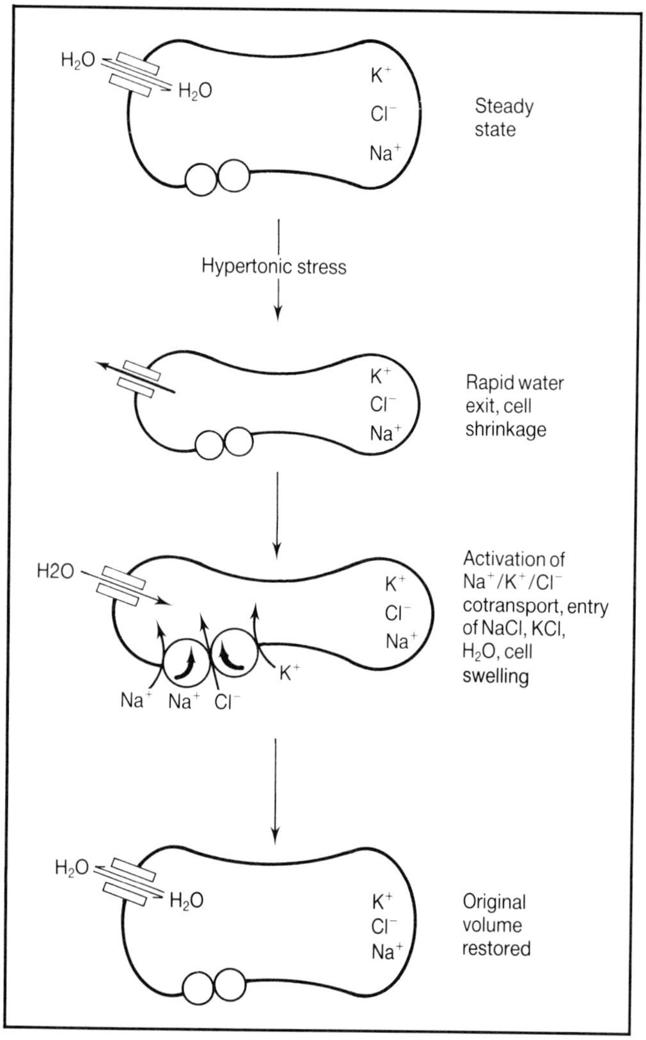

Fig. 1.3. Volume regulatory increase via Na+-K+-Cl cotransport.

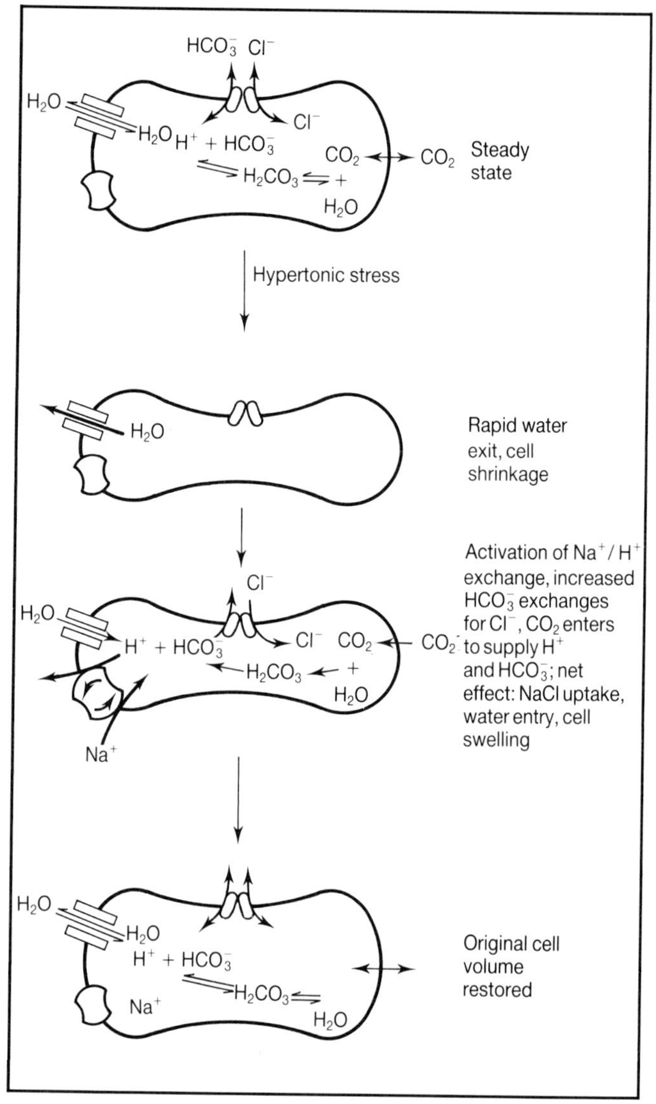

Fig. 1.4. Volume regulatory increase via Na+-H+ exchange functionally coupled to Cl−-HCO$_3$− exchange.

mammals and are likely to participate in volume regulation of these cells. In addition, certain K+ and Cl− channels appear to be opened in some cells by swelling, permitting electrically coupled KCl efflux from the cell.

Cellular pH regulation

Intracellular pH is normally slightly more acidic (by 0.1–0.3 pH units) than the extracellular compartment, reflecting the Donnan distribution of protons and the production by cellular metabolism of acidic compounds such as lactic acid and CO_2. Cellular pH is often perturbed by a number of physiological processes, including environmental pH changes, increased cellular metabolism, and hypoxemia–ischemia. Intracellular buffers, including HCO_3^-, phosphates, and proteins, absorb some of the protons produced by these processes, but the cell also has mechanisms to remove excess H^+, the two most important being Na^+-H^+ exchange and Cl^--HCO_3^- exchange.

Na^+-H^+ exchange functions as an antiporter to move Na^+ into the cell and H^+ outward, and is stimulated by increased intracellular H^+ concentration (decreased pH) (Fig. 1.5). The excess cellular Na^+ must be removed from the cell by the Na^+-K^+-ATPase. Under hypoxic–ischemic stress, when the cell's ATP supply falls below the level that

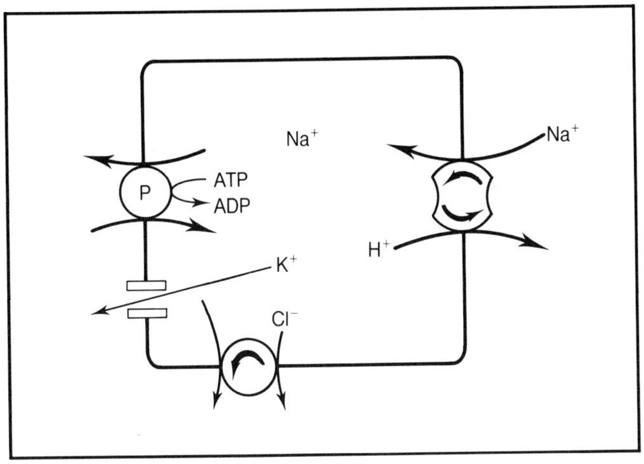

Fig. 1.5. Recovery from acid load via Na^+-H^+ exchange. Cellular acidification activates Na^+/H^+ exchange, extruding H^+; increased Na^+ stimulates Na^+/K^+ pump. Excess K^+ is recycled via K^+ channel and/or KCl cotransporter.

can sustain ATPase activity, cell Na^+ may rise, causing cell swelling and tissue edema. This mechanism may underlie the cerebral edema associated with hypoxic–ischemic brain injury. In certain cells, neurohumoral stimuli activate Na^+-H^+ exchange via cAMP-mediated protein phosphorylation, and the resultant alkalinization may trigger other cellular responses.

Under steady-state conditions, Cl^--HCO_3^- exchange tends to remove HCO_3^- from the cell as a consequence of the transmembrane gradients of the transport ions (Fig. 1.6). However, under conditions of acid stress, Cl^--HCO_3^- exchange can also function to maintain cellular pH. When cells experience intracellular acidification, H^+ reacts with HCO_3^-, and the resultant H_2CO_3 is converted to water and CO_2, which diffuses from the cell; the cell's HCO_3^- supply is then replenished by exchange of internal Cl^- for extracellular HCO_3^-, permitting ongoing H^+ buffering. The anion exchanger is therefore essential to the efficient functioning of the CO_2-HCO_3^- buffer system.

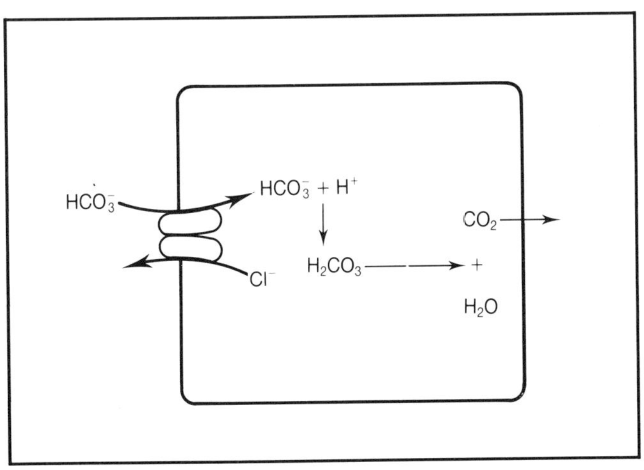

Fig. 1.6. Recovery from acid load via Cl^--HCO_3^- exchange.

Cl^--HCO_3^- exchange is also crucial to the respiratory function of the erythrocyte. As the red cell traverses the capillary, CO_2 diffuses into the cell, where it is converted into carbonic acid (H_2CO_3) by carbonic anhydrase. H_2CO_3 dissociates to form H^+, which is absorbed by intracellular buffers (mainly hemoglobin and phosphates), and HCO_3^-, which leaves the cell in exchange for Cl^-. This process, known as the Hamburger shift after the nineteenth-century physiologist who described it, is reversed in the lung and increases the blood's CO_2-carrying capacity by minimizing the perturbation of plasma and red cell pH.

Ca^{2+} homeostasis

The control of ionized Ca^{2+} concentration is another vital cellular function that depends primarily on ion transport and regulated membrane permeability. The precise regulation of Ca^{2+} is mandated in all cells by its universal role as a second messenger governing multiple cellular processes, and by its toxicity to the cell when concentrations rise above micromolar levels. In addition, in both smooth and striated muscle cells, Ca^{2+} is the primary determinant of contractile protein function. In the steady state in most cells and the resting state in contractile cells, intracellular ionized Ca^{2+} is maintained at 10–100 nM; with an extracellular concentration of 1–2 mM, a 10 000–100 000-fold transmembrane concentration gradient exists for Ca^{2+}, one of the largest of any physiologically relevant compound. This gradient is maintained by the Ca^{2+}-ATPase, which exists in several isoforms in different tissues and is a member of the common transport ATPase family. The high affinity of this enzyme for Ca^{2+} and ATP, its rapid reaction rate, and relatively high abundance contribute to its ability to keep intracellular Ca^{2+} concentrations low and to respond to the rapid changes in Ca^{2+} levels associated with stimulus secretion or excitation–contraction coupling. In skeletal and cardiac muscle, large amounts of Ca^{2+}-ATPase are found in the endoplasmic reticulum into which Ca^{2+} is pumped and sequestered after contraction occurs. In other cells, the enzyme is located in the plasma membrane and functions to extrude Ca^{2+} from the cell.

In addition to the Ca^{2+}-ATPase, Ca^{2+} is removed from some cells via a Na^{+}-Ca^{2+} exchanger; the inward movement of three Na^{+} ions energizes the outward movement of one Ca^{2+} ion against its large electrochemical gradient. The mechanism of cardiac glycoside inotropy is thought to involve this transporter: glycoside inhibition of the Na^{+}-K^{+}-ATPase leads to increased cellular Na^{+}, which diminishes the driving force of the Na^{+}-Ca^{2+} exchanger, an important regulator of Ca^{2+} concentration in cardiac muscle. This raises steady-state cellular Ca^{2+} levels, thereby augmenting the contractile function of the muscle.

Ca^{2+} entry into the cytoplasmic space, from either the extracellular space or endoplasmic reticulum, is mediated by a variety of intricately regulated channels. In cardiac and skeletal muscle, voltage-gated Ca^{2+} channels in the plasma membrane and sarcoplasmic reticulum are opened when an action potential depolarizes the membrane in which they reside. After a brief period in the open state, during which Ca^{2+} flows into the cytoplasm, the channel closes; the duration of the open state may be modulated by regulatory processes, mediated by receptor-linked protein kinases. This family of channels is blocked by compounds such as verapamil, nifedipine, and diltiazem. In neurons, arrival of the action potential at the presynaptic membrane opens a voltage-dependent Ca^{2+} channel, and the resultant Ca^{2+} influx triggers neurotransmitter release. In some nonexcitable cell types, the occupation of membrane receptors by a variety of hormones, growth factors, secretagogues, etc. increases cytoplasmic Ca^{2+} by activation of Ca^{2+} channels. In some cells, Ca^{2+} channels in the plasma membrane are activated by receptor-linked protein kinases. In other cells, receptor-linked activation of phospholipase C increases hydrolysis of inositol phospholipids to produce inositol-1,4,5-triphosphate (ITP), which activates an ITP-specific Ca^{2+} channel in the endoplasmic reticulum membrane, releasing Ca^{2+} into the cytoplasm. As a second messenger, Ca^{2+} may affect many cellular functions, by activating or inhibiting channels for other ions, specific protein kinases, proteases, or other enzymes.

Ca^{2+} movements across the apical membrane of certain epithelia in the gut, kidney and placenta associated with transepithelial Ca^{2+} movement appear to be mediated by carrier proteins, rather than channels, based on the physiological characteristics of Ca^{2+} transport in these tissues. The molecules associated with these functions have not yet been characterized.

Electrical activity

The membrane potential (E_m) of all cells is a function of the transmembrane gradients of charged species and their respective permeabilities, expressed in the Goldman equation, shown below. In most cells, Na^{+}, K^{+}, and Cl^{-} (HCO_3^{-}) are the ions which determine E_m.

In excitable cells, such as nerve and muscle, the action potential results from the coordinated opening and closing of Na^{+} and K^{+} channels. In the resting state, both Na^{+} and K^{+} channels are closed, and because the resting permeability of the membrane for K^{+} is high relative to that of Na^{+} and Cl^{-}, the membrane potential approximates the K^{+} equilibrium potential, around 90 mV interior negative. As the action potential approaches an area of membrane, it begins to depolarize due to current flowing across the membrane nearby; this depolarization activates the Na^{+} channel. The rapid increase in Na^{+} permeability causes the membrane potential in that area of the membrane to approach the Na^{+} potential (+40 mV). This strong depolarization opens K^{+} channels, which returns the membrane voltage toward the K^{+} potential. After a discrete period of time, both Na^{+} and K^{+} channels close to return the membrane permeability of both ions to resting values, and the action potential has passed. The Na^{+}-K^{+}-ATPase plays a crucial secondary role in these cells to maintain the transmembrane gradients of Na^{+} and K^{+}. Neurotransmitters interact with specific receptors on target neurons to activate or inhibit certain

$$E_m = -61 \log \frac{(P_{Na}[Na]_i + P_K[K]_i + P_{Cl}[Cl]_o + P_{HCO3}[HCO_3]_o + P_{Ca}[Ca]_i^2 + P_{Mg}[Mg]_i^2)}{(P_{Na}[Na]_o + P_K[K]_o + P_{Cl}[Cl]_i + P_{HCO3}[HCO_3]_i + P_{Ca}[Ca]_o^2 + P_{Mg}[Mg]_o^2)}$$

Goldman equation

ion channels. Transmitters that activate Na^+ channels depolarize the membrane to initiate an action potential, and therefore are stimulatory. Transmitters that activate K^+ channels inhibit neuronal activity by hyperpolarizing the membrane.

In striated muscle cells, the acetylcholine receptor is itself a subunit of a nonspecific Na^+ and K^+ channel at the motor end plate. Binding of acetylcholine to the receptor opens these channels, depolarizing the plasma membrane and propagating an action potential in the muscle cell membrane. The arrival of this action potential via transverse tubules depolarizes the endoplasmic reticulum membrane, activating a voltage-dependent Ca^{2+} channel and causing the release of Ca^{2+} into the cytoplasm, which initiates muscle contraction. The tonic contraction of smooth muscle is a function of intracellular Ca^{2+} levels, in turn a function of membrane potential determined by Na^+ and K^+ permeabilities of the plasma membrane, which can be modulated by neurohumoral influences.

Cells other than nerve or muscle may also exhibit physiologically important changes in membrane potential, either primarily or secondarily associated with cellular functions. Stimulus-secretion coupling involves changes in membrane potential or activation of specific ion channels. For example, the coupling of insulin secretion to serum glucose levels involves the regulation of several ion channels in the β cell of the pancreas (Fig. 1.7): glucose availability modulates ATP levels in the β cell; high ATP levels associated with high glucose concentrations close a specific K^+ channel, which depolarizes the membrane; in response to this change in membrane potential, a voltage-dependent Ca^{2+} channel is opened, permitting Ca^{2+} influx and increasing cytoplasmic Ca^{2+} concentration; this triggers Ca^{2+}-dependent protein phosphorylation responsible for exocytosis and insulin release; meanwhile, Ca^{2+} activation of a second K^+ channel allows repolarization of the membrane, damping and controlling the response.

Even in cells that do not undergo large changes in membrane potential, activation of Ca^{2+} channels by certain stimuli underlies the mechanism by which Ca^{2+} acts as a second messenger of hormone action. In transporting epithelia, changes in the membrane potential caused by the opening of one ion channel may alter the properties of other channels or transport proteins to maintain the functional activity of the cell. Virtually all of the regulated ion channels are susceptible to protein phosphorylation, and there are many examples in which hormones that may not have a primary regulatory action on a cellular process can modulate that process by affecting the activity of an ion channel via kinase–phosphatase interactions, thereby fine-tuning the cell's response to its primary stimulus.

Epithelial transport

Fluid movements into and out of the various luminal cavities of the body are controlled by transport of salt across epithelia. Epithelial cells of the kidney, of the respiratory, gastrointestinal, and genital tracts, of the exocrine, mucous, and sweat glands, and of the choroid plexus all perform important secretory and/or absorptive functions. Neurohumoral stimulation or inhibition of these processes modulates tissue functions to meet physiological needs.

Although tissue- or cell-specific mechanisms exist for movement of H^+, K^+, Ca^{2+}, and other substances, the regulation of **water** movements generally involves the active absorption of **Na^+** (lumen to blood) and the secretion of **Cl^-** (blood to lumen). The basic mechanisms underlying these processes will be detailed here, with specific examples of physiological regulation for individual tissues.

Sodium absorption

The absorption of Na^+ is driven by the Na^+-K^+-ATPase located in the basolateral membrane of the epithelial cell. The energy derived from the hydrolysis of ATP is used to pump Na^+ against its electrochemical gradient out of the cell (where Na^+ concentration is low) into the interstitial space (where it is high). Na^+ enters the cell's apical (luminal) membrane through a specific mechanism, usually either a regulated Na^+ channel or a Na^+-H^+ exchanger. In some cells in the renal tubule, Na^+-Cl^- or Na^+-K^+-Cl^- cotransport is responsible for transepithelial NaCl absorption, and the inhibition of this type of transporter by furosemide (Lasix®) accounts for the powerful diuretic effect of this drug. Channel-mediated Na^+ absorption is pictured in Fig. 1.8 and will be considered first. The function of an apical Na^+-H^+ exchanger will be considered below.

Under quiescent conditions, the Na^+ channel remains

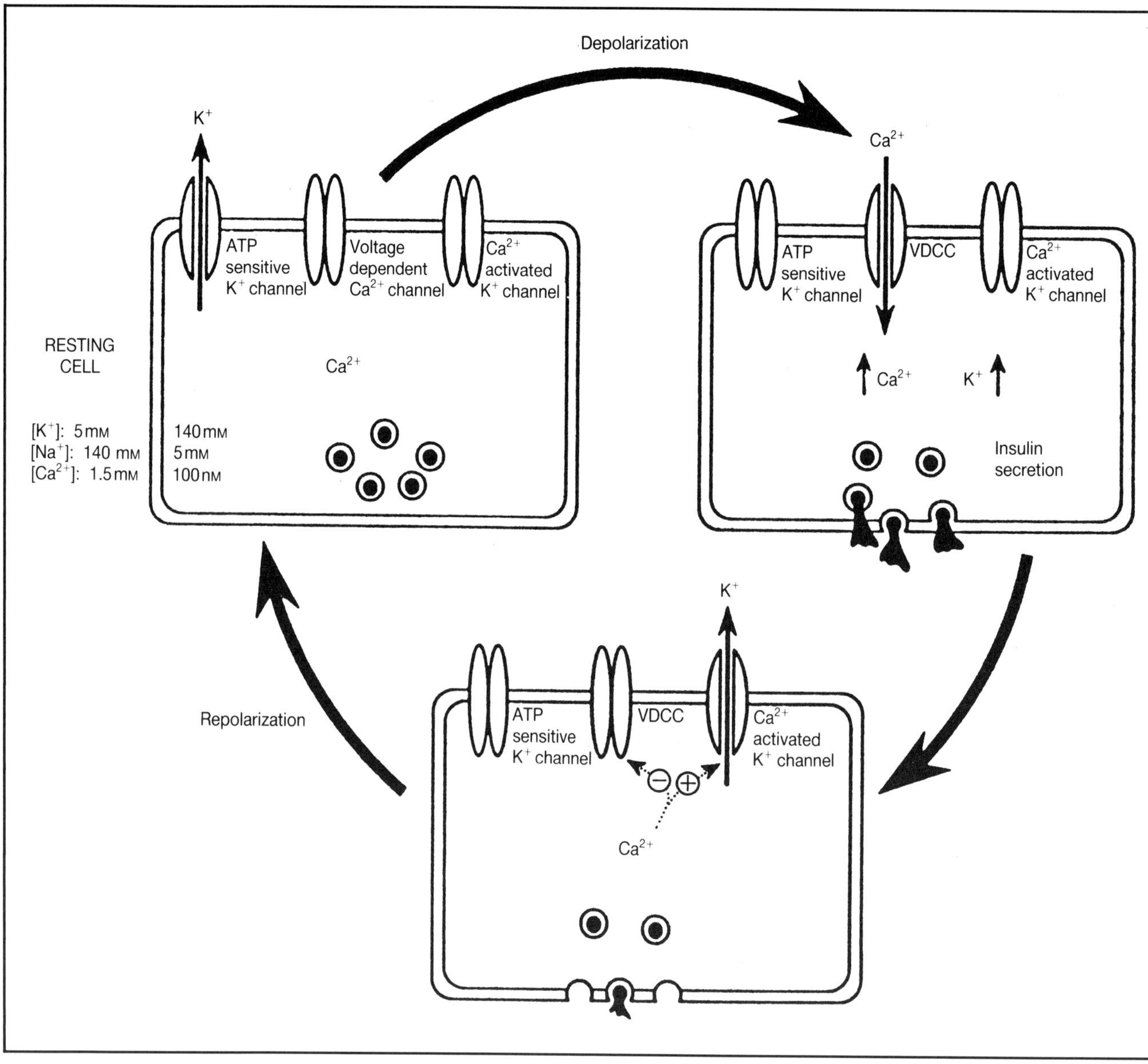

Fig. 1.7. Ion-channel modulation of insulin secretion. Resting membrane potential in pancreatic β cells is governed by K^+ conductance through ATP-sensitive K^+ channels. Closure of these channels leads to cell depolarization and Ca^{2+} influx through voltage-dependent Ca^{2+} channels (VDCC). Rise in free cytosolic Ca^{2+} triggers insulin secretion. In addition, rise in cytosolic Ca^{2+} activates Ca^{2+}-activated K^+ channels to enhance K^+ efflux and inactivate Ca^{2+} channels. This results in cell repolarization and reversion to resting state. (Reprinted with permission from Rajan AS *et al. Diabetes Care* 1990; **13**(3):341. Copyright © 1990 by the American Diabetes Association, Inc.)

closed and little Na^+ entry occurs. Upon stimulation, the channel opens and Na^+ enters the cell by diffusion down its electrochemical gradient. Intracellular Na^+ rises and stimulates the Na^+-K^+-ATPase to pump at a faster rate. A basolateral K^+ channel is also opened by the same initial stimulus or by the depolarization of the membrane, which accompanies the opening of the Na^+ channel and functions to permit exit of K^+ brought into the cell by the pump in exchange for Na^+. The movement of Na^+ across the epithelium causes an electrical potential difference to develop across the cell layer (lumen negative relative to interstitial space), which drives the movement of Cl^-. Chloride enters the interstitium either transcellularly by means of Cl^- channels in both apical and basolateral

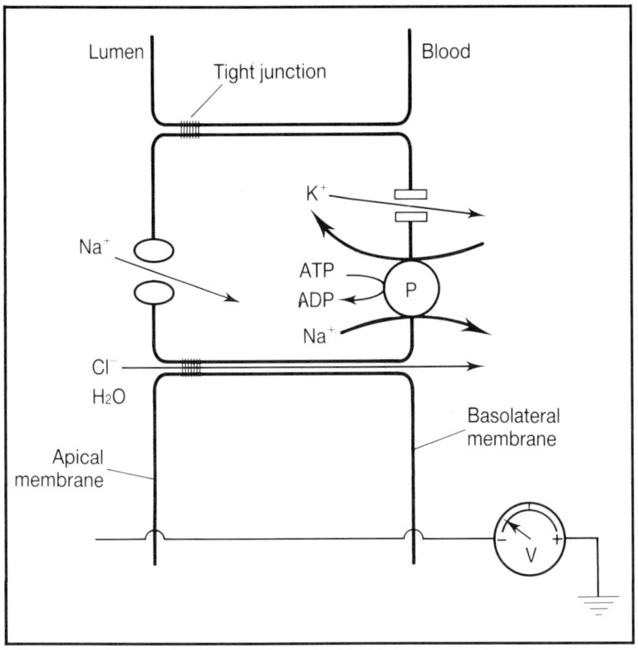

Fig. 1.8. Epithelial Na^+ absorption via the apical Na^+ channel.

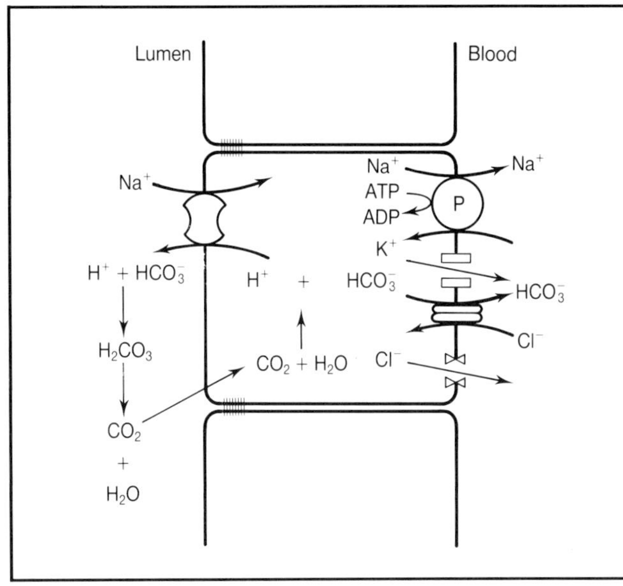

Fig. 1.9. Absorption of $NaHCO_3$ via coupling of Na^+-H^+ exchange and Cl^--HCO_3^- exchange.

membranes, or via a paracellular route through the tight junctions that join the epithelial cells together. Water follows the movements of Na^+ and Cl^-, driven by osmotic forces and moving across the cell membrane and through the paracellular pathway. In certain regions of the kidney tubule where passage of water is restricted, luminal fluid becomes hypotonic upon absorption of NaCl; but in most epithelia, isotonic conditions prevail on both sides of the cell and water moves along with salt.

In some epithelia, notably in the kidney and intestine, the primary entry step for Na^+ at the apical membrane is not a Na^+ channel, but rather a Na^+-H^+ exchange system (Fig. 1.9), and in this case the epithelium functions to excrete H^+ and absorb HCO_3^-. The intracellular proton secreted in exchange for luminal Na^+ reacts with luminal HCO_3^- to produce H_2CO_3. Luminal carbonic anhydrase catalyses the production of H_2O and CO_2, which diffuses back into the cell and forms H^+ and HCO_3^-. The H^+ is available for exchange with Na^+, and the HCO_3^- is extruded to the interstitium by a Cl^--HCO_3^- exchanger located on the basolateral membrane. The net result is $NaHCO_3$ absorption. This mechanism occurs in the intestine and is a predominant mode of Na^+ and HCO_3^- absorption in the kidney proximal tubule. The diuretic actions of amiloride and acetazolamide result from inhibition of Na^+-H^+ exchange and carbonic anhydrase, respectively. Amiloride also blocks the Na^+ channel. In addition, the dependence of Na^+ and water absorption on Na^+-K^+-ATPase activity renders the process susceptible to inhibition by hypokalemia, metabolic depletion and the cardiac glycoside, ouabain.

To stimulate salt and water absorption, a variety of neurohumoral agents activate the Na^+-H^+ exchanger or apical Na^+ channels in absorptive epithelia. Most responses are mediated by cAMP and activation of protein kinase A. Phosphorylation of the channel increases the time it spends in the open state and activation of the exchanger changes its affinity for Na^+ and/or H^+.

Na^+ channel activity is also affected by aldosterone. Acutely, this hormone increases Na^+ channel activity by stimulating methylation of the channel or its regulating subunits. Aldosterone may also have a long-term effect of increasing the number of Na^+ channels in the membrane. Such mechanisms may play a role in regulating renal Na^+ absorption.

Na^+ channels have been purified or cloned from several tissues in various species and differ considerably in molecular weight and protein subunit type and number. Nevertheless, the membrane-spanning domains, which are thought to form the actual channel structures, exhibit considerable homology among proteins derived from different tissues and species. These domains conform to the general motif of membrane transport proteins, with multiple hydrophobic α-helical sequences. The cytoplasmic domains, which interact with cellular regulatory mechanisms to modulate channel activity, are often quite different among tissues and species. Some of the components of multi-subunit channels may have primarily regulatory functions. There are striking sequence and structural homologies among Na^+, K^+, and Ca^{2+} channels within functional subclasses, such as voltage-gate channels, particularly in the membrane-spanning domains. This suggests that some of these families of channel proteins diverged from a common ancestral membrane protein.

Chloride secretion

Fluid secretion by epithelial tissues also depends on energy derived from ATP hydrolysis by the Na^+-K^+-ATPase, because Cl^- movements are driven by the Na^+ gradient. This is accomplished by a Na^+-K^+-Cl^- cotransport system (possibly a Na^+-Cl^- cotransporter) located on the basolateral membrane (Fig. 1.10).

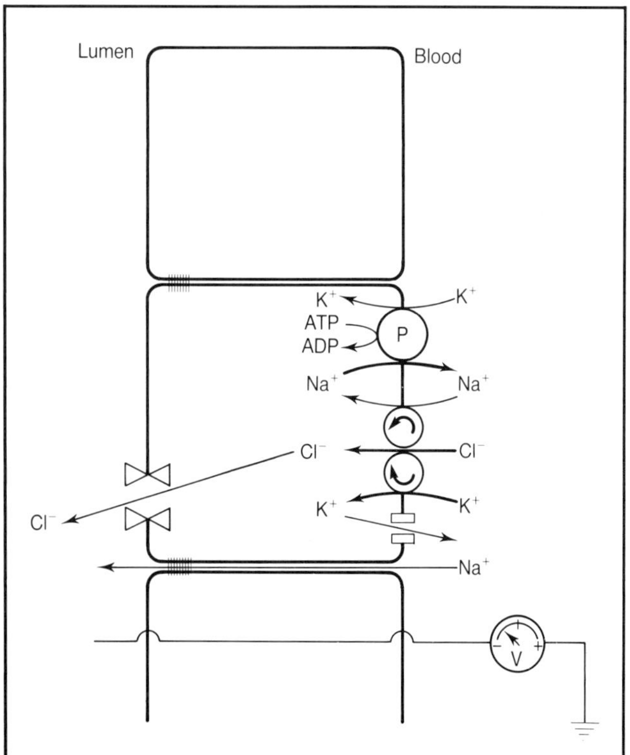

Fig. 1.10. Epithelial Cl^- secretion.

Although intracellular Cl^- concentration may be lower than external Cl^-, the resting membrane potential is negative, so that the electrochemical driving force (the algebraic sum of electrical and chemical forces) favors Cl^- exit in the steady state; thus, net movement of Cl^- from the interstitial space into the cell is **uphill** and requires energy, which is supplied via the cotransporter as Na^+ moves into the cell down its electrochemical gradient. Na^+ is pumped out again by the Na^+-K^+-ATPase and cellular K^+ is **recycled** by specific channels located at the basolateral membrane, as in Na^+-absorbing epithelia. Secretion of Cl^- is accomplished by opening of Cl^--specific channels at the apical surface of the cell. Chloride then moves down its electrochemical gradient into the lumen, creating an electrical potential across the membrane (lumen negative) that causes Na^+ and osmotically obliged water to move via paracellular pathways. Because of the transport systems involved, Cl^- secretion is susceptible to inhibition by ouabain and by the loop diuretics (furosemide), which inhibit Na^+-K^+-Cl^- cotransport.

As with Na^+ channels, Cl^- channels exhibit tissue-specific regulation by a variety of neurohumoral agents coupled to various second messengers. For example, Cl^- secretion in the trachea is stimulated by catecholamines and mediated by the cAMP-dependent protein kinase A, which apparently phosphorylates and activates the Cl^- channel. In the intestine the Cl^- channel associated with secretion is also activated by a cAMP-mediated kinase. Cholera toxin activates a G-protein leading to uncontrolled stimulation of adenylyl cyclase and producing high levels of cAMP. This results in maximal opening of this Cl^- channel and produces the secretory diarrhea characteristic of cholera. Some Cl^- channels are also activated by Ca^{2+}, and some are voltage dependent.

Several different Cl^- channels have been identified physiologically and characterized molecularly. These molecules exhibit the channel motif described above for Na^+ channels, with helical and hydrophobic transmembrane segments and cytoplasmic domains that interact with cellular regulatory machinery. Of considerable interest is the Cl^- channel defect associated with cystic fibrosis. In this disorder, the response of Cl^- channel function to β-adrenergic stimulation is abnormal in a number of tissues, although basal (i.e. unstimulated) Cl^- channel function may be normal. The protein affected by the gene defect in cystic fibrosis (dubbed the Cystic Fibrosis Transport Regulatory [CFTR] protein) resembles the family of proteins known as multiple drug resistance proteins, associated with extrusion of xenobiotics from cells. Recent research indicates that the CFTR is in fact a Cl^- channel that is either abnormally regulated by cellular protein kinases and consequently does not open under physiological conditions, or is improperly processed upon synthesis and is therefore degraded before reaching the plasma membrane. In either event, the result is a Cl^--secretion abnormality, which manifests as dehydration of pulmonary secretions and abnormal exocrine and sweat gland function.

The asymmetric distribution of channels and transporters between the apical and basolateral membranes of the epithelial cell is a key determinant of the physiological capabilities of the epithelium. For example, in the case of the Cl^--secreting cell described above, if the locations of the Cl^- channel and NaCl cotransporter are reversed so that the channel is basolateral and the cotransporter apical, the epithelium can now function as absorptive surface, carrying out the transcellular movement of Cl^- again driven by the Na^+ gradient. This mechanism has in fact been verified in certain tissues. In the distal tubule of the kidney, which regulates K^+ secretion, K^+ channels are located in both apical and basolateral membranes and are independently regulated, so the cell can control whether K^+ is secreted into the lumen or cycled to the interstitial space for reabsorption. The specific function of an epithelial cell, therefore, depends on the types of ion channels and transporters present, their polarized location on the cell membrane, and the nature of the cytokine or hormone receptors and associated regulatory mechanisms present in the cell.

Developmental aspects

Placental transport

One fundamental purpose of the placenta is to mediate the transport of nutrients to the developing fetus. Unfortunately, this process has proved difficult to study, and knowledge of placental transport is incomplete. This is due in part to the remarkable differences in placental anatomy and physiology among different species. Nevertheless, several generalizations are possible about transport of certain substances across the hemochorial placenta of humans.

Water, gases, and lipophilic substances diffuse freely across the placenta. Permeability to ions and even large polar solutes and proteins is quite high and has prompted speculation that relatively large pores exist in the syncytiotrophoblast, although no such pores have been demonstrated anatomically. This suggests that many high-capacity mechanisms exist for the transport of nonlipophilic substances. Transport systems known to exist in syncytiotrophoblast membranes include Na^+-K^+-ATPase, Ca^{2+}-ATPase, Cl^--HCO_3^- and Na^+-H^+ exchange, Na-dependent and independent glucose carriers, a variety of amino acid transporters, and other transport proteins. Active, uphill transport of Ca^{2+}, Mg^{2+}, and possibly K^+ have been demonstrated across the placenta, but the details of these processes are not known. As suitable trophoblast culture systems are developed and molecular biological techniques are applied to the study of placental transport, new insights into this important area of fetal physiology are likely to emerge.

Fetal life and perinatal changes in transport functions

The association between ion transport regulation and cell differentiation and development is illustrated by the fact that within minutes of fertilization, Na^+-H^+ exchange is activated in the zygote. The resulting alkalinization of the cell interior is thought to trigger increases in DNA synthesis and protein translation, formation of microtubules and microfilaments, and increased K^+ conductance. Similarly, activation of Na^+-H^+ exchange is one of the early events in a number of receptor- or chemical-induced differentiation of cultured cells. It is likely, though unproved, that many of the cellular differentiation processes that occur during fetal development involve changes in cellular ion homeostasis, and the function and regulation of specific ion channels and transporters. The differentiation of epithelial cells and establishment of transport function involve the translation and transcription of transport protein genes, modification of the protein and its insertion into the appropriate membrane, and the presence of appropriate regulatory mechanisms. Because epithelial transport involves multiple channels and transporters located at different membranes, any one component might be rate-limiting to the establishment of transport function. Very little is currently known about these processes in development, which constitute a fertile area for future research.

The development of ion transport capacity of the pulmonary epithelia involves changes in fluid secretion, which are important to the crucial transition from fluid-filled to air-filled lung. In fetal life, the lung secretes fluid, producing up to 500 ml per day in the late-gestation sheep fetus, in which most experimental work has been done. This fluid contributes to amniotic fluid volume, and the distension of the lung produced by the constant flow of fluid has an important effect on pulmonary development. Fluid is produced by proximal and distal airway epithelial cells by means of a Cl^--secretion mechanism similar to that described above. This mechanism persists in the adult trachea and is stimulated by adrenergic agents. Late in gestation, however, an absorptive mechanism appears, which is also sensitive to adrenergic stimulation. This mechanism may be similar to the Na^+ absorption system found in adult bronchi, which features an apical Na^+ channel (see Fig. 1.8), or may involve the Na^+-H^+ exchange system known to be present in alveolar type II cells. Regardless of the mechanism involved, late in gestation adrenergic stimulation results in a reversal of tracheal fluid flow, so that net secretion changes to net absorption. This suggests that the absorption by the airway epithelium can override the secretion of fluid under the influence of catecholamine near term. An increase in Na^+-K^+-ATPase gene expression (mRNA levels) in lung late in gestation in the rat also supports the notion that the capacity for ion transport increases in the perinatal period.

Studies in rabbit lung indicate that total lung water diminishes near term, and morphological studies demonstrate that a portion of the fluid filling the alveoli is absorbed before birth. Immediately after birth, fluid collects in the peribronchial space, presumably transported across the airway epithelium, before being removed by the pulmonary circulation and lymphatics. The maturation of the surfactant system also plays an important role in the ability of the newborn to maintain a 'dry' airway. Once the alveoli are air-filled, surface tension represents a significant hydraulic driving force for water entry into the alveoli from the interstitial space, which must be offset by other mechanisms of fluid removal, including active Na^+ transport. Reduction of surface tension by surfactant diminishes this driving force, thereby hastening fluid removal and lessening the tendency for pulmonary edema.

As in lung, many of the epithelial transport functions of the gut, kidney, and other organs mature in late fetal or neonatal life to the level characteristic of the adult animal. For example, the fetal proximal tubule of the kidney exhibits less than one-half the rate of Na^+-H^+ exchange as the adult kidney; this changes rapidly over the neonatal period, and reaches adult levels by 6 weeks of age. This relative deficiency of Na^+-H^+ exchange accounts for the poor handling of Na^+ and HCO_3^- by preterm kidney, which is often apparent clinically, and may relate to low levels of expression of the Na^+-H^+ exchanger in the tubular epithelial cells. Na^+-K^+-ATPase expression also increases in the kidney during the late fetal and neonatal period. A similar pattern of perinatal development of Na^+-H^+ exchange capacity is also observed in the small intestine.

Conclusion

Regulation of membrane permeability and ion transport is a vital cellular function, central to the maintenance of cell volume and pH; many cellular functions are primarily or secondarily affected by the intracellular ionic milieu. The transmembrane Na^+ gradient, maintained by the Na^+-K^+-ATPase, is important in many of these processes and also represents an energy source for the transport of other ions and substrates. Many pathological processes and pharmacological actions can be traced to effects of an injury or drug on a transport process.

Membrane transport of most ions and compounds is mediated by specific transport proteins. These ATPases, carriers, and channels share many common structural features, especially within functional classes. Species, tissue, and cell specificity often reside in the regulatory components of these membrane protein complexes. Intricate cellular regulation of transport protein activity is accomplished by a variety of acute and long-term mechanisms. These include substrate availability, phosphorylation–dephosphorylation mechanisms, sulfhydryl oxidation, Ca^{2+} activation, voltage sensitivity, and regulation of transcription, translation, and membrane insertion of transport protein.

Changes in ion transport occur during development from the zygote to the postnatal period. Some of these changes affect differentiation of cells, while others reflect the development of specific transport capacities in tissue such as renal tubule and intestinal epithelia. Much more information about the molecular biology, biochemistry, and physiology of these processes is required to build a coherent picture of this important component of developmental physiology.

Selected reading

Benos DJ, Sorcher EJ. Ion channels. In Seldin DW, Geibish G, eds. *The kidney: physiology and pathophysiology.* Vol. I. New York: Raven Press, 1992: 587.

Boron WF. Control of intracellular pH. In Seldin DW, Geibish G, eds. *The kidney: physiology and pathophysiology.* Vol. I. New York: Raven Press, 1992: 219.

Lingrell JB, Orlowski J, Shull MM, Price EM. Molecular genetics of Na,K-ATPase. *Nucleic Acid Res Mol Biol* 1990; **38**: 37.

Spring KR, Hoffman EK. Cellular volume control. In Seldin DW, Geibish G, eds. *The kidney: physiology and pathophysiology.* Vol. I. New York: Raven Press, 1992: 147.

Thorens B, Charron MJ, Lodish HF. Molecular physiology of glucose transporters. *Diabetes Care* 1990; **13**: 209.

Welsh MJ. Electrolyte transport in airway epithelia. *Physiol Rev* 1987; **67**: 1143.

B. Receptors

Y Sadovsky and J M Roberts

Survival of unicellular organisms depends on their ability to respond to extracellular signals. Coordinated function of multicellular organisms requires not only response to environmental signals, but also communication with neighboring and remote cells. To allow transfer of information into the cell, a signal must gain access across the cell membrane. Although lipid-soluble ligands, such as steroids, may enter the cell directly, the hydrophobic nature of the cell membrane prohibits entry of many signaling ligands, such as amines and peptides, into cells, and they require the presence of a transmembrane communication system. Receptors are specialized structures, designed to transmit signals between ligands and target molecules. Membrane receptors allow transmission across the phospholipid cell membrane, while intracellular receptors initiate signal transduction by lipophilic agents. To allow coordinated function, intracellular enzymes detect the transmitted stimulus and generate signaling molecules called 'second messengers', which lead to an orchestrated and reversible cell response (Fig. 1.11).

Recent progress in understanding cell signaling stems primarily from improved isolation and purification techniques, along with the ability to sequence, clone, and express the receptors in host cells. These techniques have allowed determination of the sequences that confer ligand and effector specificity, and insight into conformational changes that trigger transmembrane signaling. These approaches have also identified structural 'families' of receptors, some even functionally unrelated, yet with a high degree of similarity (homology) in portions of the amino acid sequences. Important portions of these molecules are identified by the fact that their sequences are virtually unchanged (conserved) across a wide range of species.

Receptors contain two functional domains: a ligand-binding domain, which determines initial interaction with the ligand, and a catalytic domain, which interacts with effectors for further signal processing and response. Membrane receptors also contain a transmembrane anchoring domain. In addition, a regulatory domain is present in many receptors. This domain contains phosphorylation sites, which provide targets for homologous regulation, induced in a receptor by its own specific ligand (e.g. tachyphylaxis), and heterologous regulation by other effectors (e.g. estrogen-induced up-regulation of progesterone receptors). This complex signal transmission machinery of sensors, modulators, and effectors determines the specificity of response, conferred by expression of different receptors among various cell types, and is capable of signal sorting and amplification of the message.

This section describes receptor systems that illustrate these principles. These systems (Fig. 1.12) include G-protein coupled receptors, tyrosine kinase receptors, endocytosis associated receptors, membrane-bound and cytosolic guanylyl cyclase, cell adhesion receptors, and the steroid receptor superfamily.

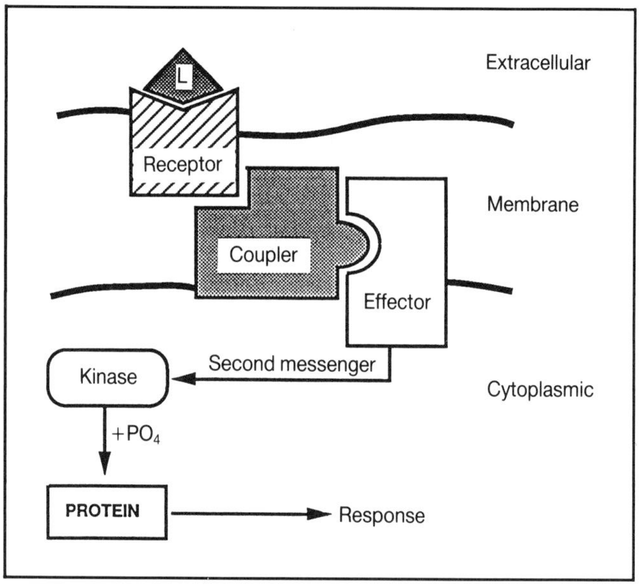

Fig. 1.11. Diagrammatic overview of a ligand (e.g. β-adrenergic agonist) stimulated response. Ligand (L) binding to the receptor activates a coupling protein (e.g. G-protein), which stimulates an effector (e.g. adenylyl cyclase) to generate a second messenger (e.g. cAMP). The second messenger activates a protein kinase (e.g. kinase A) which phosphorylates a target protein leading to a cellular response (e.g. ion channel activation, muscle contraction, and DNA synthesis). For other receptors (e.g. tyrosine kinase receptors) this system is combined in one membrane-spanning protein which includes the ligand recognition site, coupler, and the kinase.

Cell membrane receptors

Receptors in the cell membrane utilize several strategies to transfer information from hydrophilic ligands across the hydrophobic cell membrane. In some cases (e.g. G-protein linked receptors) these receptors interact with proteins on the cytosolic face of the membrane to access intracellular targets, while in others (e.g. tyrosine kinase receptors) the receptor itself interacts with the effectors. Still others (e.g. LDL receptors) carry the ligand into the cell.

G-protein linked receptors

The activation of cellular signaling mechanisms by many ligands is mediated by receptors that interact with a special group of GTP binding 'coupling' proteins termed 'G-proteins'. Examples include receptors for adrenergic, muscarinic, and dopaminergic activators, somatostatin, opiates, serotonin, adenosine and rhodopsin. All transmembrane receptors linked to G-proteins have a similar structure (Fig. 1.13). Seven transmembrane domains (M-I through M-VII) span the bilayer, with extracellular amino terminus and intracellular carboxy terminus. The hydrophilic domains include the extracellular (E-I through E-III) and cytoplasmic (C-I through C-III) loops. Disulfide bonds within cysteine-rich residues in the ligand-binding domain stabilize ligand-binding pockets. The transmembrane region, which includes segments of 20–28 amino acids, contains conserved regions also crucial for ligand binding. The cytoplasmic domain is involved in coupling with G-proteins, and specificity of this interaction is determined by the C-III loop.

Adrenergic receptor coupling to G-proteins is the most completely elucidated model of receptor and G-protein interaction (see Fig. 1.18). There are several distinct types of adrenergic receptors, defined by physiological action, pharmacological specificity, and deduced amino acid

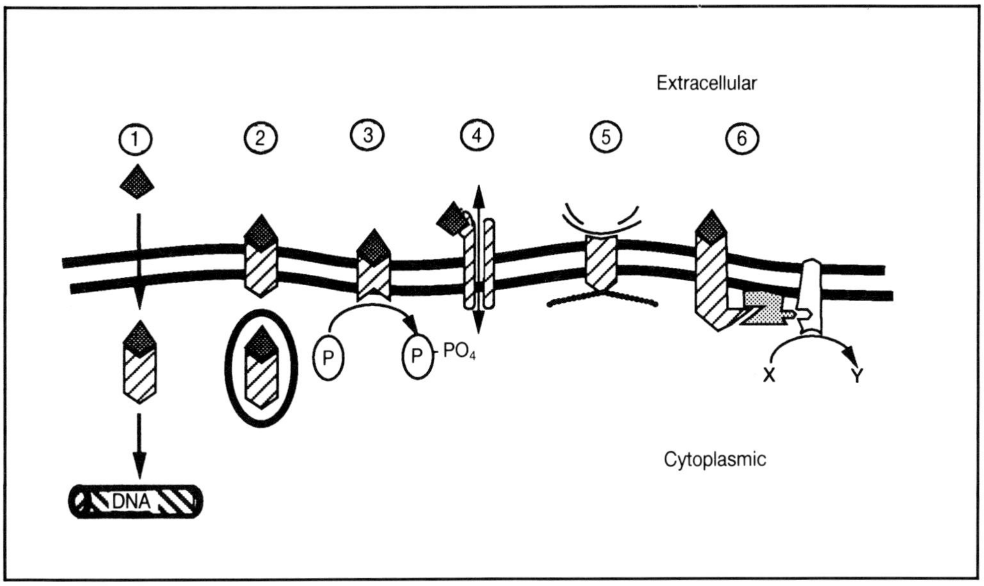

Fig. 1.12. Diagrammatic representation of receptor-mediated transmembrane signaling. 1, Lipid-soluble ligands, capable of crossing the lipid bilayer, interact with intracellular receptors (e.g. steroids) and regulate gene expression. 2, Ligands are transported across the membrane via receptor-mediated endocytosis (e.g. low-density lipoproteins). 3, Ligands bind to the extracellular region of the receptor (e.g. epidermal growth factor), resulting in allosteric changes that activate cytoplasmic catalytic domain, which phosphorylates (PO_4) cytoplasmic proteins (P). 4, Ligands (e.g. acetylcholine) bind to a receptor, which includes an ion channel, and open the channel to ion flux into the cells. 5, Ligands which are a component of the extracellular matrix, bind to a receptor (e.g. integrin) that interacts with cytoskeleton. 6, Ligands bind to receptors (e.g. β-adrenergic receptors) that span the membrane, causing activation of G-protein on the cytoplasmic side of the membrane, which converts inactive enzyme (X) to an active effector (Y).

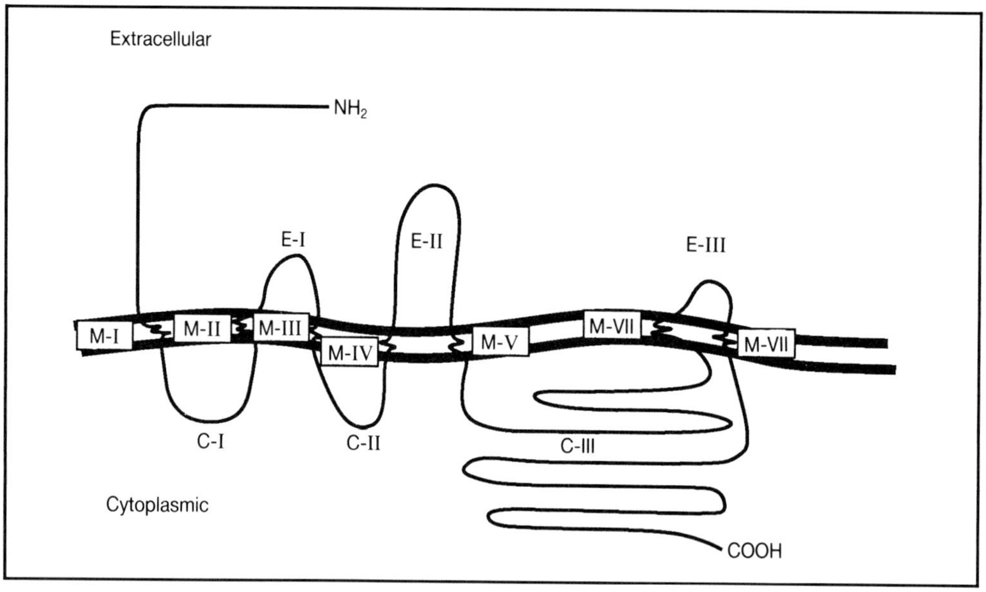

Fig. 1.13. Diagrammatic representation of G-protein linked receptors. The receptor is composed of seven α helices, which span the membrane bilayer. Stimulatory ligands interact with extracellular loops (E-I to E-III) and transmembrane helices (M-I to M-VII). G-protein interacts with cytoplasmic loops (C-I to C-III). The carboxy terminus and C-III contain multiple serine and threonine residues, target for phosphorylation, which induces receptor desensitization.

sequence. β-Receptors activate the enzyme adenylyl cyclase to stimulate cAMP generation. This effect is mediated by G_s-protein. α_2-Receptors are coupled by G_i-protein to inhibit adenylyl cyclase. In recent years the subtypes were further divided (e.g. α_{2a}, α_{2b}, and α_{2c}) and selective expression of these subtypes may explain tissue specific response. α_1-Receptors are coupled by G-proteins (e.g. G_q) to phospholipase C.

Characteristic of these receptors is their ability to undergo regulatory modifications. For the β-adrenergic receptors, for example, phosphorylation of the receptor protein results in alteration of interaction between the cytoplasmic domain and G-protein, sequestration of the receptor into membrane vesicles, internalization into the cytoplasm, and consequent receptor degradation. Phosphorylation of specific serine and threonine residues in the C-III loop produces the pharmacological phenomenon of desensitization by several independently regulated processes. These regulatory steps may be affected by the native ligand (homologous desensitization). The β-adrenergic receptor kinase, which phosphorylates agonist-occupied receptors, reduces the ability of agonists to activate β-adrenergic receptors. The phosphorylated receptor also has increased affinity for another regulatory protein, β-arrestin, which binds to the receptor and prevents its interaction with $G_{s\alpha}$ thus impeding activation of the second messenger cascade. Ligands that stimulate cAMP generation through other receptors can also reduce receptor function (heterologous desensitization) by phosphorylation through cAMP-dependent protein kinase (kinase A). The precise mechanisms of receptor regulation are currently under investigation. Because G-proteins are activated by synthetic peptides composed of the receptor domain that interacts with G-proteins, agonist binding likely results in an allosteric change of the receptor, allowing this portion to interact with G-protein. This disinhibition of the receptor by an agonist seems to be a common theme of activation (see The steroid receptor superfamily, below).

Tyrosine kinase receptors

This group of receptors binds growth factors, such as epidermal growth factor (EGF), platelet derived growth factor (PDGF), fibroblast growth factor (FGF), insulin-like growth factor (IGF), and insulin. The structure of tyrosine kinase receptors includes an extracellular ligand-binding domain, a transmembrane region, and a cytoplasmic catalytic domain that contains the tyrosine kinase active site. The composition of the extracellular and intracellular domains defines the several subclasses of tyrosine kinase receptors. The extracellular glycosylated ligand-binding domain consists of cysteine-rich repetitive sequences (Fig. 1.14), which in some cases (e.g. PDGF receptor) resemble immunoglobulin structure. The hydrophobic transmembrane region anchors the receptor to the plasma membrane and plays a passive role in signal transduction. The cytoplasmic portion of the receptor is composed of three domains: (1) the juxtamembrane domain, which is thought to be a target for modulation by heterologous stimuli; (2) the highly conserved tyrosine kinase domain, required for phosphorylation of tyrosine residues in intracellular target proteins and modulation of interactions with different second messengers; (3) the carboxy terminal tail, which exerts a negative control on receptor signaling functions.

There are three subclasses of tyrosine kinase receptors. Receptor activation by a ligand such as EGF results in a conformational change of the extracellular domain and dimer formation (subclass I). Alternatively, type-1 IGF and insulin receptors (subclass II) exist as a dimer even prior to ligand binding, while PDGF receptors (subclass III) undergo dimerization after binding a dimeric ligand to the receptors. Activation of the receptor leads to signal transduction by phosphorylating tyrosine residues of cytosolic targets. The tyrosine kinase receptor also phosphorylates its own tyrosine residues, leading to modification of the receptor conformation, which enhances the kinase activity. Activation is followed by aggregation at specialized membrane regions, which on electron microscopy appear as depressions coated with 'fuzzy' material. These 'coated pits' are characterized by constitutive invagination activity. Following aggregation, the receptor–ligand complex undergoes internalization and intracellular degradation, and provides a down-regulation mechanism to decrease receptor concentration. The signal is terminated by hydrolytic action of specific phosphatases.

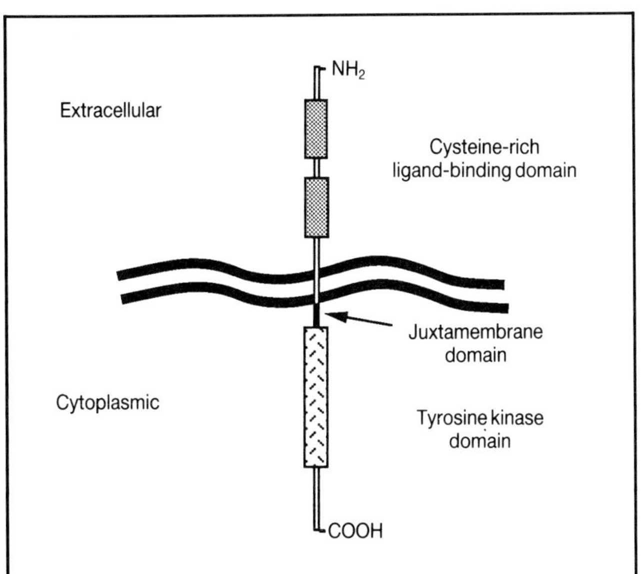

Fig. 1.14. Illustration of the epidermal growth factor receptor as a representative of the tyrosine kinase receptor family. The extracellular ligand-binding domain undergoes dimerization after ligand binding. The cytoplasmic region is composed of a regulatory juxtaglomerular domain, a conserved catalytic tyrosine kinase domain, and a carboxy terminal tail (COOH), which modulates the action of the tyrosine kinase domain.

Several signaling pathways are modulated by tyrosine kinase receptors. Many actions of growth factors are secondary to receptor mediated phospholipase C-induced inositol phosphate turnover; however, other signaling systems such as Ca^{2+} influx, sodium/hydrogen exchange, glucose, and amino acid transport are also enhanced by tyrosine kinase receptor activation. Thus these diverse pathways regulate growth as well as differentiated functions.

Receptors mediating endocytosis

Many large macromolecules enter the cell via receptor-mediated endocytosis (Fig. 1.15). Examples include low-density lipoproteins (LDL), transferrin, transcobalamin, and immune complexes. LDL receptors, which regulate plasma clearance of these lipoproteins, serve as a model for this receptor's mechanism of action.

The LDL receptor is a highly conserved membrane glycoprotein composed of five domains. The ligand-binding domain at the amino terminus mediates interaction of the receptor with the lipoproteins apo B and apo E. The transmembrane domain serves to anchor the receptor to the membrane. The cytoplasmic domain contains an O-linked carbohydrate chain domain and an EGF-like domain, the function of which remains unclear. LDL receptor concentration is regulated by the availability of its ligand, with cholesterol intake down-regulating LDL receptor synthesis.

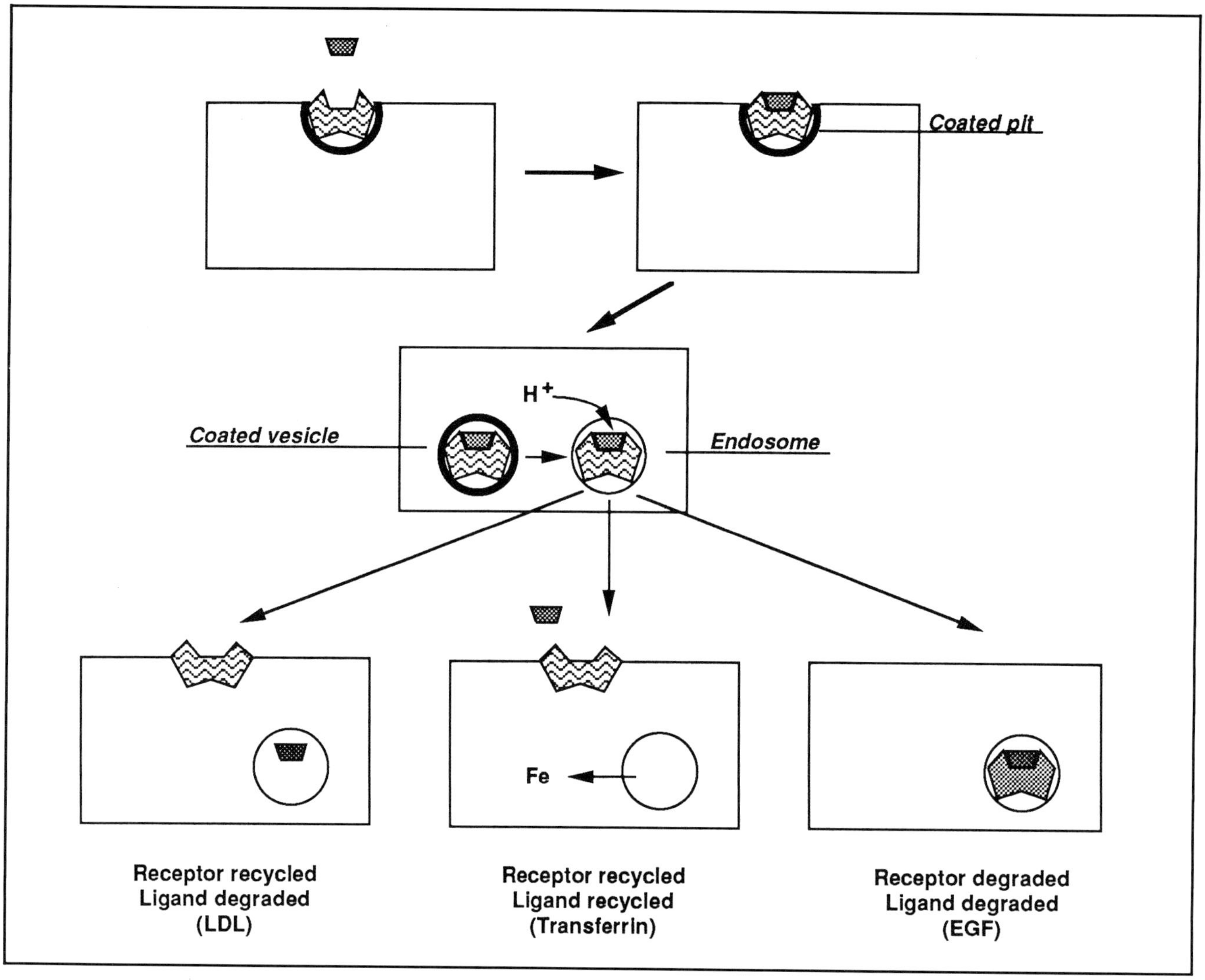

Fig. 1.15. Diagrammatic representation of receptor-mediated endocytosis. Ligand binds to receptors clustered in coated pits. The coated pits undergo internalization and form coated vesicles, becoming endosomes following acidification (H^+). Low-density lipoprotein (LDL) receptors recycle to the cell membrane while the LDL is degraded in lysosomes. For transferrin, both receptor and ligand recycle after iron (Fe) release in the cell. Epidermal growth factor (EGF) and its receptors are both degraded in the lysosomes.

As described for tyrosine kinase receptors, LDL receptors also aggregate at coated pits. In general, the internalization of the receptor–ligand complex of receptors mediating endocytosis results in recycling or degradation of the two components (see Fig. 1.15). Following internalization and endosome formation, the LDL receptor dissociates and free LDL is delivered to lysosomes and is degraded, while the unliganded receptor recycles to the cell membrane. This outcome is different among receptors. As described for EGF, both the ligand and receptor may be degraded. Alternatively, when the internalized iron–transferrin receptor complex dissociates, both transferrin and its receptor recycle to the plasma membrane where free transferrin is available for iron binding.

IGF-2/mannose 6-phosphate receptors

Although type-2 IGF receptors (which closely resemble mannose 6-phosphate receptors) share many features with receptors for other growth factors, this receptor type is distinguished by the lack of tyrosine kinase activity in its cytoplasmic region. Similarly, nerve growth factor (NGF) receptors also lack intrinsic tyrosine kinase activity. The mechanism of signal transduction by growth factors that lack kinase activity is not yet identified. Possibly, the major role of these receptors is transport of the ligand into the cells, as described above for LDL receptors, with subsequent, as yet undefined mechanisms resulting in intracellular signaling.

Membrane-bound guanylyl cyclase

Membrane-bound guanylyl cyclases are structurally similar to tyrosine kinase receptors. They consist of an extracellular ligand-binding domain at the amino terminus, a transmembrane domain, and a highly conserved cytosolic domain that includes the catalytic site. The catalytic domain contains sequences homologous to the catalytic domain of tyrosine kinase receptors.

There are several isoforms of membrane-bound guanylyl cyclase, each responsive to specific ligands. Not surprisingly, the major heterogeneity of these receptor subtypes is in the ligand-binding domain. At present a few endogenous ligands have been identified, all small peptides. Examples include atrial natriuretic hormone and heat stable enterotoxin of *E. coli*.

Receptors that include ion channels

The most direct receptor–ion channel interaction is found in receptors such as the nicotinic acetylcholine receptor, which is included as an integral part of the channel structure (single element signaling). The receptor is a pentamer made up of five polypeptide subunits. These polypeptides, all of which cross the lipid bilayer more than once, form a cylindrical structure 8 nm in diameter. Acetylcholine binding induces a conformational change which results in transient opening of a central aqueous pore through which extracellular Na^+ ions penetrate into the cell. Other examples of this type of receptor are the $GABA_A$, glutamate and glycine receptors.

Cell adhesion receptors

Virtually all cells contain adhesion receptors, mediating cell–cell and cell–extracellular matrix interactions. These receptors are divided into two major types (Fig. 1.16): the

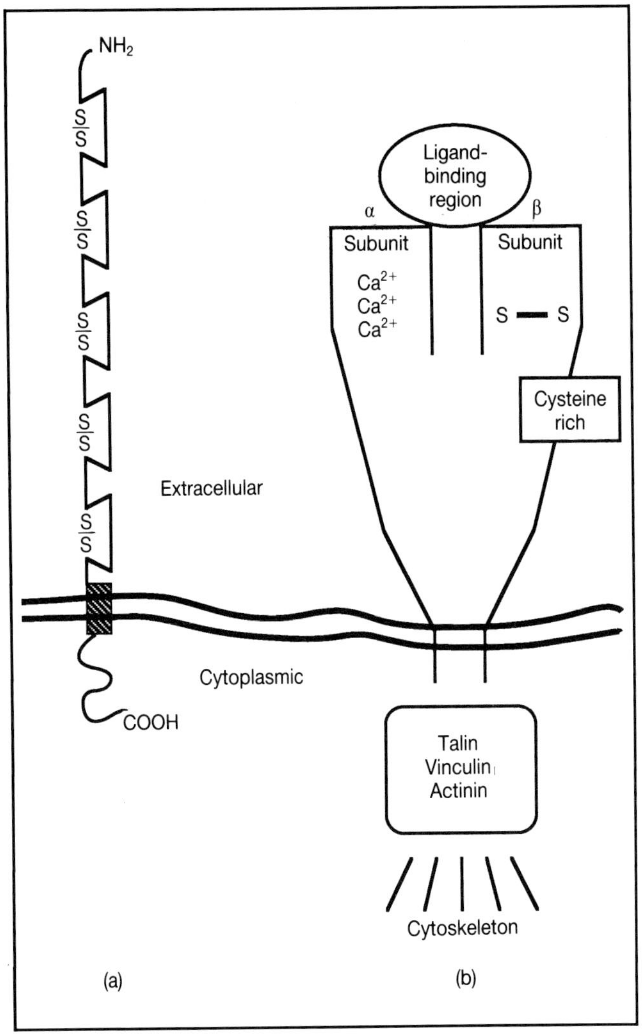

Fig. 1.16. Diagrammatic representation of cell adhesion receptors. (a) Cadherin contains an extracellular domain folded into five immunoglobulin-like regions, with disulfide bonds (SS) connecting the ends of each loop. (b) Integrin, composed of two noncovalently associated subunits: α, which contains areas thought to bind Ca^{2+}, and β, which contains four cysteine-rich repeats, and is characterized by disulfide bonds (S-S). The small cytoplasmic domain binds cytoskeleton elements.

immunoglobulin superfamily (e.g. cadherins), which bind to their identical molecules (homophilic binding), and the integrin superfamily, which can bind to nonidentical adhesion receptors (heterophilic binding).

Cadherins are Ca^{2+}-dependent adhesion molecules and have a structure characteristic of the immunoglobulin type of adhesion molecule. The extracellular amino terminus determines interaction specificity. The intracellular domain is a conserved region, and determines the adhesive properties of the receptor. This domain is associated with actin-binding cytoplasmic proteins called catenins. By contrast, the ligand-binding domain of the integrins contains two noncovalently associated subunits: the α-subunit, which has multiple Ca^{2+} binding residues, and a highly conserved β-subunit, folded into a loop stabilized by disulfide bonds. Several forms of both α- and β-subunits have been identified, and the specificity of ligand binding (e.g. fibronectin, laminin) is determined by the combination of these subunits. The interaction of the cytoplasmic domain with actin filaments is mediated by additional cytoskeleton molecules. This domain also contains a tyrosine phosphorylation site, a possible target for regulation.

Cell adhesion receptors also have a role in selective interactions among cells during morphogenesis. Cadherins are found on presumptive neural crest cells. When these cells convert from an ectoderm form to a migratory form they lose detectable cadherins. It has also been suggested that adhesion molecules have a role in cell signaling, mediated by the cytoplasmic domain.

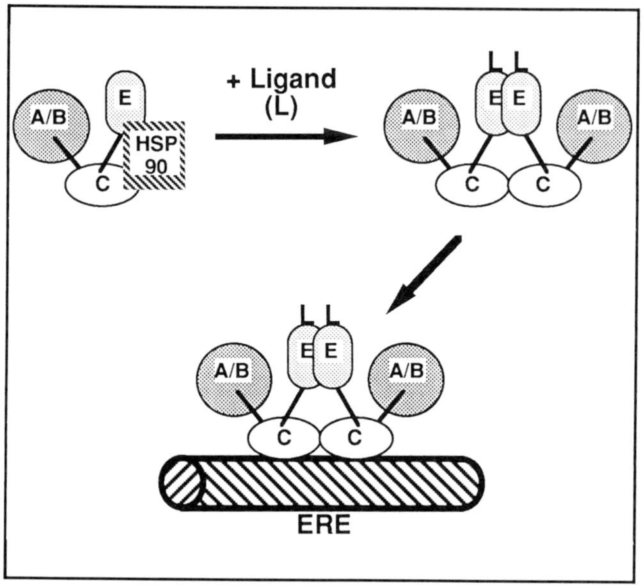

Fig. 1.17. Illustration of signal transduction by estrogen receptors as representatives of steroid-binding receptors. The lipophilic estrogen (L) crosses the lipid bilayer and binds to the intracellular receptor–heat shock protein 90 (HSP90) complex. This binding causes the release of HSP90, allowing dimerization of the bound receptor. The dimeric receptor can now bind to the DNA estrogen response element (ERE) to alter gene transcription. A/B represents the amino terminus region of the receptor, C the DNA-binding domain, and E the ligand-binding domain.

Intracellular receptors

The steroid receptor superfamily

This superfamily includes receptors for steroids and other lipid-soluble agonists, such as thyroid hormone, retinoic acid, and vitamin D. These hormones regulate development, cellular proliferation, and differentiation by crossing the hydrophobic cell membrane and binding to specific cytosolic (e.g. glucocorticoids) or nuclear (e.g. estrogen, thyroid) receptors. Cloning of these receptors and deducing their amino acid sequences reveals a high degree of similarity, leading to their classification as a 'superfamily'. In addition, several similar proteins, likely to be receptors, but for which there is as yet no known ligand, constitute an interesting subset of 'orphan receptors'.

The structure of members in this superfamily can be divided to several regions (A–E, Fig. 1.17). The conserved ligand-binding domain (E) confers ligand specificity. This domain also contains a region necessary for the receptor dimerization, which in the absence of agonist binding is occluded by an inhibitory protein called heat shock protein. Binding to DNA is at the cysteine-rich DNA-binding domain of the receptor (C), characterized by cysteine residues folded around a zinc ion to form 'zinc fingers'. It has recently been suggested that the amino acid sequence of the first zinc finger determines the DNA-binding site of the receptor, and that specific mutations in this region lead to alteration of DNA-binding properties. The variable amino terminus region contains a gene activation domain.

Hormone binding to the receptor induces allosteric alteration, which enables the receptor to dissociate from the heat shock protein (Fig. 1.17). The receptor then dimerizes and binds to a palindromic sequence ('inverted repeat') at the hormone response element in the promoter region of the target gene. Receptor binding to DNA alters the expression of the target gene, causing stimulation or inhibition of protein synthesis. Interestingly, deleting the ligand-binding domain of the glucocorticoid receptor results in constitutively active receptor, indicating that this domain inhibits receptor activation, and hormone binding relieves this inhibition.

Cytosolic guanylyl cyclase

In addition to a membrane-bound form, guanylyl cyclase is also present as a soluble intracellular enzyme. Unlike the former, the cytosolic form is a heterodimer, composed of two subunits the assembly of which is determined by the specific tissue in which the enzyme is localized. The carboxy terminus is homologous to the cytosolic domain of the membrane-bound enzyme and also to the cytosolic portion of adenylyl cyclase.

The primary agonist for this receptor is nitric oxide (NO). Interestingly, this lipid-soluble agonist, which was originally characterized as endothelial derived relaxing factor (EDRF), has also been shown to be a chemotactic agent, a cytotoxic agent, a mitogen and a neurotransmitter.

Selected reading

Albeda SM, Buck CA. Integrins and other cell adhesion molecules. *FASEB J* 1990; **4**: 2868.

Hollenberg MD. Structure-activity relationship for transmembrane signaling: the receptor's turn. *FASEB J* 1991; **5**: 178.

O'Malley B. The steroid receptor superfamily: more excitement predicted for the future. *Mol Endocrinol* 1990; **4**: 363.

Schneider WJ. The low density lipoprotein receptor. *Biochim Biophys Acta* 1989; **988**: 303.

Ullrich A, Schlessinger J. Signal transduction by receptors with tyrosine kinase activity. *Cell* 1990; **61**: 203.

C. Postreceptor Mechanisms

Y Sadovsky and J M Roberts

Intracellular signaling molecules that couple membrane events to intracellular effector systems are called 'second messengers'. To define a molecule as a second messenger, its concentration should be modified by a ligand-stimulated receptor system and lead to a parallel change in the cellular response. The second messenger also should elicit an appropriate response when applied, even in the absence of the receptor or its ligand. These molecules participate in the processing, sorting, amplification, and targeting of the initial signal. This section describes the major postreceptor messengers and pathways mediating intracellular signal transduction and integrated response.

G-proteins

The G-proteins are a subset of a larger family of GTP-binding proteins that also includes ribosomal protein synthesis components and $p21^{ras}$ protein. These proteins have GTPase activity, and their function is regulated by bound guanyl nucleotide (i.e. GTP or GDP). G-proteins are located on the cytoplasmic surface of cell membranes. They sort, amplify, and relay signals from membrane receptors to proteins that generate intracellular second messengers (e.g. inositol phosphates, cAMP, and Ca^{2+}).

At least 16 G-proteins have been characterized. They mediate diverse effects, but share a common general structure and mechanism of activation (Fig. 1.18). G-proteins are heterotrimeric, consisting of α-, β-, and γ-subunits. Specificity is conferred by the α-subunit. The β- and γ-subunits, usually associated as a tight complex, are highly conserved and functionally interchangeable. The βγ complex anchors the protein to the cytoplasmic aspect of the cell membrane and modulates the inhibitory or stimulatory signal originating in the α-subunit. In the heterotrimeric form, GDP is bound to G_α and stabilizes the complex (Fig. 1.18). Agonist binding facilitates interaction of the receptor with G-protein, causing allosteric alteration of G_α leading to the dissociation of GDP, which is replaced by GTP, present in excess intracellularly. GTP destabilizes the complex, and the βγ complex dissociates. The α-subunit is then free to bind and activate effector proteins. Effector molecule activation is terminated by GTPase-induced hydrolysis of GTP to GDP and subsequent reassociation of the heterotrimer complex. This cycle demonstrates one of the principles of signal amplification. A receptor's signal of a few milliseconds is converted by the G-protein into several seconds of effector activation, dictated by the timing of the 'turn off' signal by GTPase. Thus one receptor can activate many cytoplasmic messengers.

The identity and mechanism of action of several G-proteins were determined originally by the effect of specific bacterial toxins, and more recently by using mutated G-proteins. The first G-protein identified, G_s, was found to be irreversibly activated by cholera toxin, which inhibits the GTPase 'turn off' reaction. Several G-proteins are substrates for another bacterial toxin, pertussis toxin, which prevents receptor activation by interfering with the release of GDP. Using these approaches it was found that G_s activates not only adenylyl cyclase but also cardiac Ca^{2+} channels. Three inhibitory G-proteins (G_i) have been identified, which were found to suppress adenylyl cyclase action in response to adrenergic, muscarinic, or opioid ligands. The mechanism of inhibition appears to be partially explained by liberation of βγ complex, which binds to $G_{s\alpha}$ and inhibits adenylyl cyclase. Whether the dissociation is in fact the principal action of these heterotrimers or merely a minor effect is not clearly established. The unliganded $G_{i\alpha}$ can, for example, activate phosphatidylinositol-phospholipase C, phosphatidylcholine-phospholipase C, phospholipase A_2 as well as K^+ channels (Fig. 1.19). Other forms of G-proteins have also been identified. G_q-protein activates the phosphatidylinositol-phospholipase C pathway (Fig. 1.20), and is neither a target for cholera nor pertussis toxin. G_t links photoreceptors in the retina to cGMP phosphodiesterase, while G_{olf} couples olfactory receptors to adenylyl cyclase activation in the olfactory epithelium. The function of further members of the G-protein family is yet to be determined.

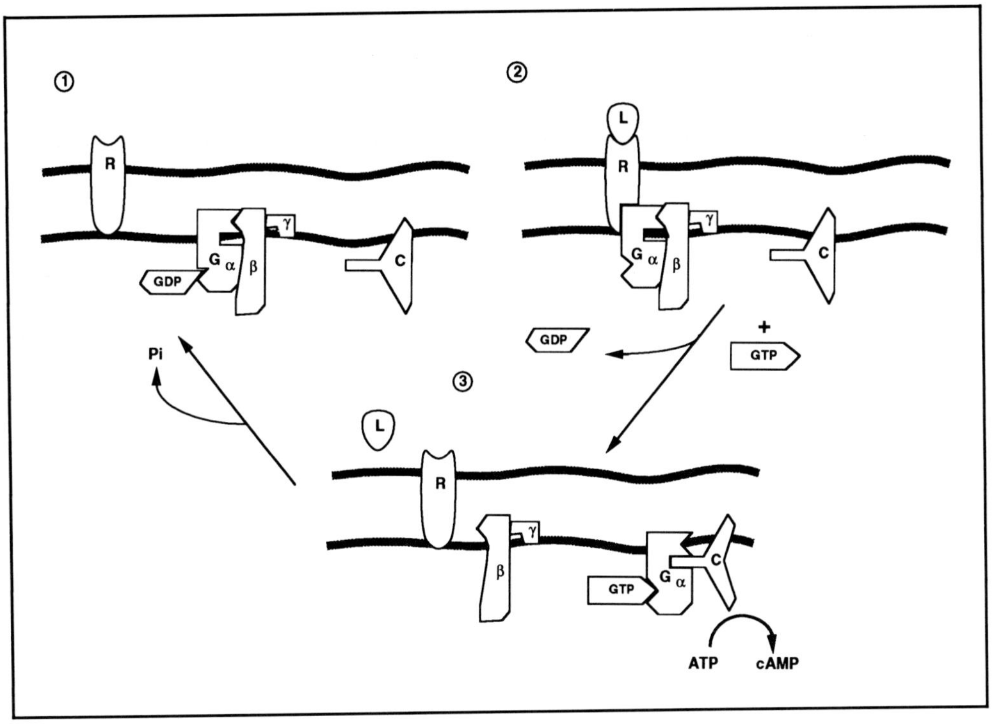

Fig. 1.18. Diagrammatic representation of receptor-mediated activation of adenylyl cyclase as an example of G-protein function. 1, In the resting state, $G_{s\alpha}$ is bound to βγ complex, and this heterotrimer binds to GDP. 2, Ligand (L) activation of the receptor (R) facilitates GDP dissociation from $G_{s\alpha}$, and replacement by GTP. 3, GTP binding reduces the affinity of $G_{s\alpha}$ for βγ complex, and the dissociation of this complex allows $G_{s\alpha}$ stimulation of adenylyl cyclase (C) activity. GTP hydrolysis by intrinsic $G_{s\alpha}$-GTPase action returns $G_{s\alpha}$ to the GDP-bound state, which then recycles to form the heterotrimer with βγ complex.

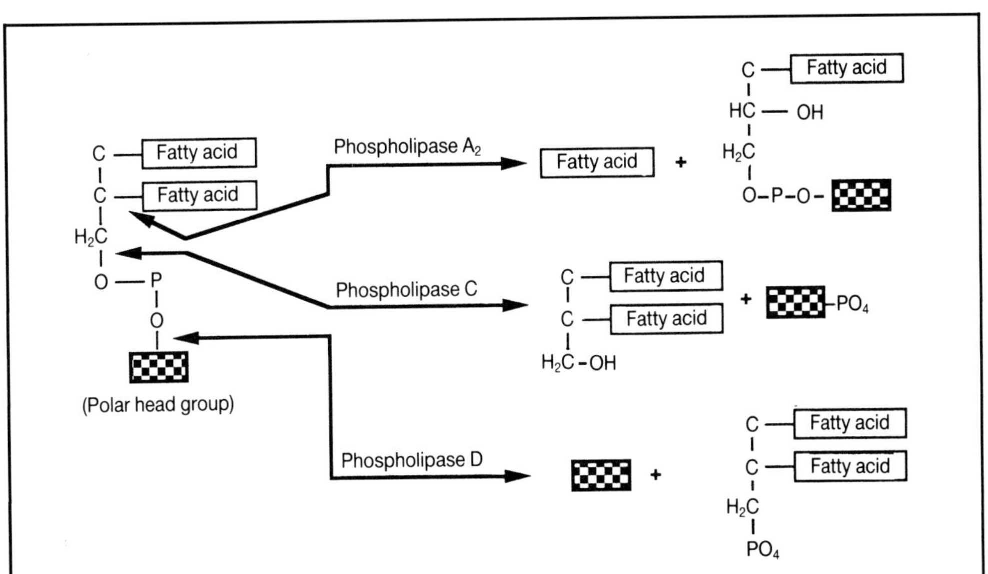

Fig. 1.19. Diagrammatic representation of phospholipid hydrolysis by phospholipases. Two fatty acids and a polar head group (e.g. choline, inositol, ethanolamine) are bound to the glycerol backbone. Phospholipase A_2 hydrolyzes the fatty acid (e.g. arachidonic acid) at the second position, yielding fatty acid and a lysophosphatide. Phospholipase C generates diacylglycerol and a phosphorylated head group, such as inositol phosphate. Phospholipase D generates a free polar head group and phosphatidic acid. Not illustrated: phospholipase D also catalyzes the transphosphatidylation of phospholipids (see text).

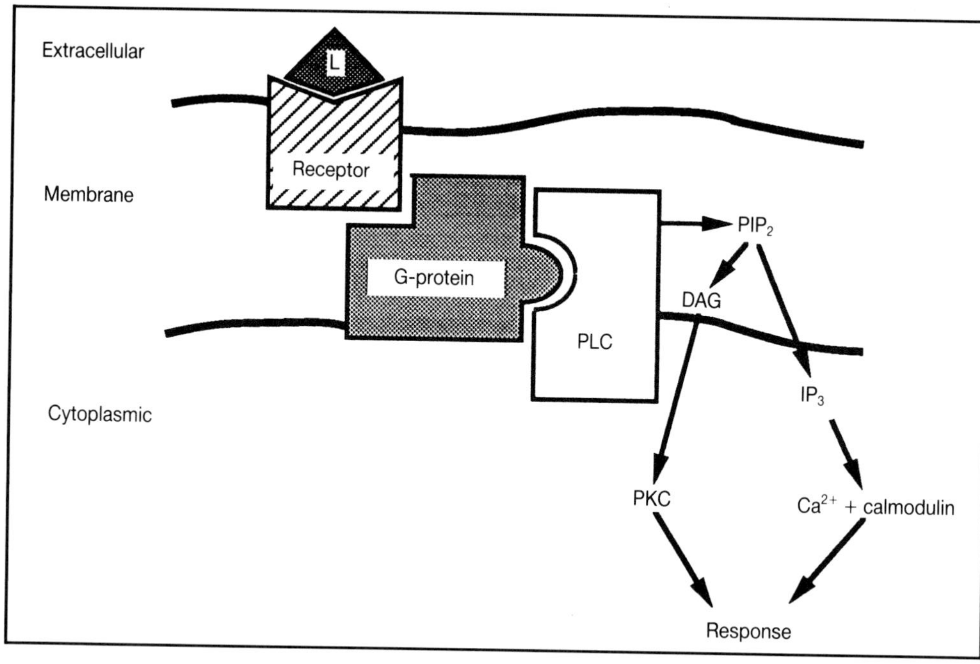

Fig. 1.20. Schematic representation of phospholipase C (PLC) mediated response. Receptor activation (e.g. α_1- receptor) by a ligand (L) activates a G-protein (e.g. G_q), which stimulates PLC hydrolysis of phosphatidyl-4,5-bisphosphate (PIP_2), releasing inositol-1,4,5-trisphosphate (IP_3) and diacylglycerol (DAG). IP_3 enhances the release of Ca^{2+}, which binds to calmodulin and stimulates cellular response (e.g. smooth muscle contraction). Diacylglycerol activates intracellular protein kinase C (PKC), which stimulates response by phosphorylation of specific cytoplasmic proteins.

Ion channel signaling pathways

Ion channels play a vital role in the maintenance and modulation of the electrochemical gradient across the cell membrane. These structures allow the flux of channel specific ions down a concentration gradient, and thus have lower energy requirements than ion pumps, which are responsible for maintenance of the concentration gradient. The dependence of enzymes involved in signal transduction on the cytoplasmic electrochemical milieu explains the ability of ion channels to effect signal transduction.

Ion channels are characterized by their ion specificity, the ligand that activates the channel (e.g. glycine, acetylcholine), and the tissue type. The ion channels are coupled to signaling pathways at several levels:

1. Direct coupling at the cell membrane. While some ion channels contain a receptor within the channel structure (single-element signaling, described in the previous section), the regulation of ion channels found in the brain, peripheral neurons, skeletal muscle, smooth muscle, epithelial cells, and many other tissues is mediated through G-proteins (multi-element signaling). In the cardiac muscle, for example, muscarinic m2 acetylcholine receptors activate G_i-proteins, which are coupled to inward K^+ channels. G-proteins including G_i and G_z mediate Ca^{2+} channel inhibition induced by several ligands, such as somatostatin, $GABA_B$, dopamine, enkephalins, adenosine and atrial natriuretic protein. Although response time is slower in a multi-element signaling system (500 ms for m2 acetylcholine receptor vs 1 ms for single-element nicotinic end-plate receptor), more complex regulation is possible than in a single-element system.
2. Indirect coupling via second messengers. These pathways utilize intracellular effectors, and commonly include at least four components. In ventricular myocytes, for example, norepinephrine binding to β-adrenergic receptors activates G_s, leading to adenylyl cyclase-mediated cAMP production, which permits protein kinase A phosphorylation of an intracellular regulatory site within the Ca^{2+} channel. Interestingly,

the same channels can be directly regulated by G_s, bypassing intracellular components. Other ion channels (e.g. K^+ channels) are activated through the phospholipase A_2 pathway or phospholipase C-mediated inositol phosphate generation. This pathway is the slowest, but also the most amenable to modulation.

Second messengers

Cyclic adenosine monophosphate (cAMP)

The formation of cAMP is catalyzed by the enzyme adenylyl cyclase, which is regulated by G_s and G_i-proteins. cAMP effects are extensive and include positive chronotropic and inotropic effects in the myocardium, mediation of β-adrenergic enhancement of glycogenolysis and lipolysis, vasopressin-induced renal water retention, and hormonal steroid production and secretion.

cAMP acts primarily by activation of the specific cAMP-dependent kinase, kinase A. Kinase A is a tetramer with two regulatory and two catalytic subunits. The regulatory subunits inhibit the catalytic subunits. Binding of cAMP to the regulatory subunit causes tetramer dissociation, allowing the catalytic subunit to phosphorylate target proteins. The signal generated by this phosphorylation can be reversed only by a specific phosphatase. Covalent modification by phosphorylation amplifies the receptor stimulus because it confers 'memory' to the system which persists long after the dissociation of the hormone–receptor complex. It also provides an additional site of regulation, determined by the 'turn off' action of the phosphatases.

Kinase A is structurally similar to a family of intracellular enzymes (kinases) that catalyze protein phosphorylation. Although subunit structure and regulatory regions vary, the catalytic core is conserved among all of these proteins.

Cyclic guanosine monophosphate (cGMP)

Cyclic GMP formation is through the enzyme guanylyl cyclase. In many respects the actions of cGMP are mediated in a manner similar to cAMP, through activation of an intracellular kinase (G-kinase). Unlike the ubiquitous cAMP, cGMP action has been demonstrated in only a few cell types. For example, cGMP mediates vascular smooth muscle relaxation induced by nitric oxide. In the intestinal mucosa, cGMP mediates water and electrolyte secretion by *E. coli* endotoxin. In contrast, high concentrations of cGMP in the retinal rods characterize the inactive dark state. Photons activate cGMP hydrolysis by cGMP phosphodiesterase, resulting in decreased cGMP levels and membrane hyperpolarization, which lead to visual signal transmission.

Phospholipid hydrolysis products

Stimulation of surface receptors coupled to specific G-proteins leads to the activation of several phospholipases (see Fig. 1.19). The hydrolysis products can act directly as second messengers or serve as precursors for other second messengers.

Phospholipase C (PLC) hydrolysis results in the release of phosphorylated sugars and diacylglycerols (see Fig. 1.20). The most extensively characterized form of this enzyme is the phosphatidyl-4,5-bisphosphate (PIP_2)-specific PLC. The products of PIP_2 hydrolysis are inositol-1,4,5-trisphosphate (IP_3) and diacylglycerol. Both of these products act as second messengers. IP_3 acts on intracellular organelles to stimulate Ca^{2+} release, while diacylglycerol activates the intracellular enzyme kinase C. Several PLC isoenzymes have been characterized and cloned; most are membrane-bound, although a few are cytoplasmic. Proteolytic cleavage of the membrane-anchoring domain and cytosolic enzyme release appear to play a role in signal transduction.

IP_3 is subject to extensive further metabolism, resulting in the formation of a myriad of phosphorylated inositols, some of which may also be biologically active. IP_3 is inactivated primarily by phosphorylation to inositol-1,3,4,5-tetrakisphosphate, with subsequent sequential dephosphorylation to free inositol.

Diacylglycerol allosterically activates the cytosolic enzyme protein kinase C, which catalyzes phosphorylation of many cellular proteins with diverse intracellular effects, such as smooth muscle contraction and gene transcription. In addition to stimulatory activities, it is a mediator of negative feedback systems. Thus kinase C-stimulated phosphorylation inhibits PLC activity, decreases IP_3 generation, enhances phosphatidylinositol degradation, and decreases the affinity of EGF for its receptor. Diacylglycerols formed from PIP_2 are a rich source of arachidonic acid. Over 60 percent of diacylglycerols from PIP_2 contain arachidonic acid, and their hydrolysis by diglyceride lipase results in the release of arachidonic acid, the precursor for the synthesis of prostaglandins and other eicosanoids (see p. 104).

Another species of PLC has phosphatidylcholine as a preferred substrate, resulting in the release of diacylglycerol and phosphorylated choline, which has yet to be established as a second messenger. The diacylglycerol formed from phosphatidylcholine is slowly metabolized to phosphatidic acid by diglyceride kinase. The reduced rate of recycling is apparently related to the low content of arachidonic acid of diacylglycerol in phosphatidylcholine, because diacylglycerols that originate from PIP_2, which are rich in arachidonic acid, are rapidly degraded. Thus it appears that the important consequence of phosphatidylcholine hydrolysis by PLC is a sustained elevation of diacylglycerol concentration.

Phospholipase D (PLD) hydrolyzes the polar head group of phosphatidylcholine, phosphatidylinositol, and phosphatidylethanolamine (see Fig. 1.19), with preferred substrate determined by the cell type. The active products include phosphatidic acid or phosphatidylated compounds, which result from the exchange of the polar head group for hydroxyl groups of intracellular molecules (transphosphatidylation). Although the understanding of the regulation and consequences of PLD activity is still incomplete, G-proteins, Ca^{2+}, and kinase C appear to be involved. Phosphatidic acid and the transphosphatidylation product phosphatidylethanol can, for example, modify Ca^{2+} channel activation. Phosphatidic acid has also been suggested to act as an intracellular signal. Transphosphatidylation of nucleotides also occurs, and may alter response by modifying the intracellular nucleotide concentration; alternatively, phosphatidylnucleotides themselves might serve as second messengers. Phosphatidic acid is also a source of diacylglycerols through hydrolysis by phosphohydrolase. PLC and PLD are closely linked. In several systems PLC activation precedes PLD, yet this is not the case for all tissues, and this temporal relationship may be secondary to differential activation by the same stimulator (e.g. G-protein).

Phospholipase A_2 hydrolysis of phospholipids liberates arachidonic acid (5,8,11,14-*cis*-eicosatetraenoic acid), which serves as a precursor for biologically active eicosanoids (Fig. 1.21). The specific eicosanoid produced is determined by three major enzymatic pathways: the cyclooxygenase pathway produces prostaglandins and leukotrienes; the lipoxygenase pathway forms leukotrienes, lipoxins, hydroxyeicosatetraenoic acids (HETE), and hydroxyperoxyeicosatetraenoic acids (HPETE); and the epoxygenase pathway forms epoxyeicosatrienoic acids (EET). These eicosanoids play an important modulatory role in tissue development and functions, e.g. chemotaxis, smooth muscle contraction, hormone release, and modulation of voltage-gated K^+ channels in the cardiac atrium. Unlike other second messengers, the eicosanoids also serve as primary ligands

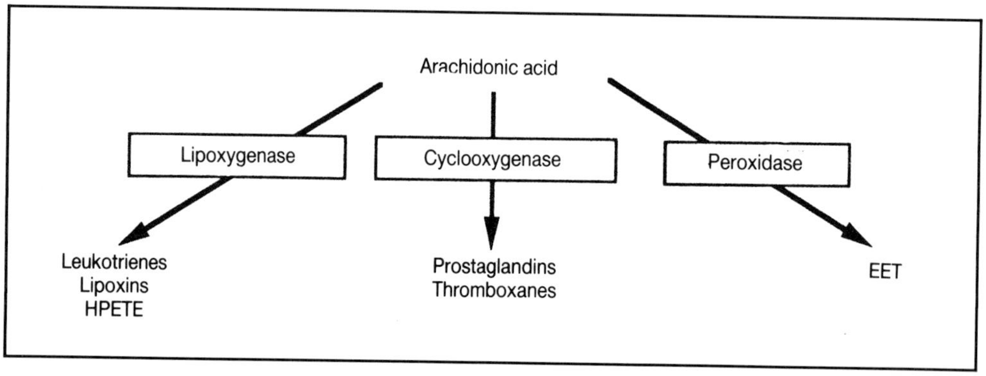

Fig. 1.21. Illustration of the major eicosanoid pathways. Arachidonic acid is converted by cyclooxygenase to prostaglandins and thromboxanes. Metabolism by lipoxygenase yields leukotrienes and lipoxins and stimulates hydroxyperoxyeicosatetraenoic acid (HPETE) production. Arachidonic acid can also undergo autooxidation to HPETE. Peroxidase (cytochrome P-450 enzyme) converts arachidonic acid to epoxyeicosatetraenoic acid (EET).

and affect neighboring cells either by binding to membrane receptors or, due to their lipid solubility, by direct intracellular actions.

Calcium

The intracellular concentration of free Ca^{2+} ion regulates a myriad of enzymes involved in vital cell functions, such as contractile protein action, secretory mechanisms, and transcellular communication via gap junctions or synaptic transmission. Many signaling systems converge on the regulation of the cytoplasmic concentration of unbound Ca^{2+} ion (approximately 100 nM), which is 10 000-fold lower than Ca^{2+} concentrations in the extracellular or intracellular Ca^{2+}-sequestering compartments. Cytoplasmic free Ca^{2+} concentration is determined by both transmembrane channel-mediated Ca^{2+} influx and second messenger-induced Ca^{2+} release from intracellular compartments, both leading to a transient 10-fold increase in cytoplasmic Ca^{2+} ion concentration. The resting Ca^{2+} concentration is restored by Ca^{2+}-ATPase pumps and Ca^{2+}-Na^{+} exchangers, which couple Ca^{2+} efflux with Na^{+} influx. The actions of intracellular Ca^{2+}, in many cases, are secondary to the kinase C-mediated phosphorylation previously described. At least as important are interactions with another ubiquitous intracellular signaling protein, calmodulin. Calmodulin is an intracellular Ca^{2+}-binding protein composed of a single polypeptide chain that contains four Ca^{2+}-binding sites. Ca^{2+} binding to calmodulin activates the protein with subsequent calmodulin binding to target proteins or activation of Ca^{2+}-calmodulin-dependent kinases.

Recent studies suggest that Ca^{2+} release from discrete intracellular stores may lead to an oscillating Ca^{2+} signal. Direct measurements of intracellular Ca^{2+} indicate that Ca^{2+} concentration spikes periodically above a constant baseline, with spike frequency being cell-type-dependent. Ca^{2+} spikes depend on the size of the intracellular pool, the rapidity of Ca^{2+} sequestration to the pools, and its extrusion to the extracellular space. The oscillating Ca^{2+} signal may be explained by Ca^{2+}-induced positive feedback on IP_3-mediated Ca^{2+} release. PIP_2 hydrolysis is negatively regulated by diacylglycerol activation of kinase C. Thus either increase in diacylglycerol or depletion of Ca^{2+} terminates the IP_3 signal.

Increased Ca^{2+} concentration triggers Ca^{2+} release from adjacent Ca^{2+} pools, leading to intracellular signal propagation. The propagating signal originates at the location of stimulated receptors. For example, the receptors at the site of egg–sperm fusion dictate the origin of Ca^{2+} signal propagation in the egg.

Summary

In a simplified model, a signal presented to a cell directly generates a response proportional to the original signal. However, the complex cellular communication system described allows processing, sorting, and amplification of the transmitted stimulus. This complexity is achieved by supplementing direct ligand–effector coupling with multi-junctional pathways, capable of vertical and horizontal regulation. Temporal regulation is conferred via covalent modification of target molecules by phosphorylation, allowing the signal to persist after dissociation of receptor and agonist. The signal is terminated by dephosphorylation of the target molecule by phosphatases, which themselves are subject to activation–inactivation by external signals. Integration of these converging and diverging signals forms the basis of coordinated cellular functions.

Selected reading

Berridge MJ, Irvine RF. Inositol phosphates and cell signalling. *Nature* 1989; **341**: 197.

Bourne HR, DeFranco AL. Signal transduction and intracellular messengers. In Winberg RA, ed. *Oncogenes and molecular origins of cancer*. Cold Spring Harbor: Cold Spring Harbor Laboratory Press, 1989: 97.

Koesling D, Bohme E, Schultz G. Guanylyl cyclase, a growing family of signal-transducing enzymes. *FASEB J* 1991; **5**: 2785.

Krueger BK. Toward an understanding of structure and function of ion channels. *FASEB J* 1989; **3**: 1906.

Shimizu T, Wolfe LS. Arachidonic acid cascade and signal transduction. *J Neurochem* 1990; **55**: 1.

2 • *Cellular physiology*

Editor: Jeffrey A Whitsett

A. DNA Replication, Chromatin Structure and the Cell Cycle

J M Greenberg and T E Weaver

Structural genes

Genetic heritage is contained in a polymer known as deoxyribonucleic acid, or **DNA**. In a mammalian somatic cell, the DNA polymer is composed of approximately six billion purine and pyrimidine bases linked to a backbone of phosphate and deoxyribose. The nucleus of a diploid somatic cell contains two copies of the DNA polymer arranged as an antiparallel **alpha helix**. DNA contains two purine bases, adenine (A) and guanine (G), and two pyrimidine bases, thymine (T) and cytosine (C). The two strands of the double helix associate via hydrogen bonding. Adenine from one DNA strand pairs with thymine from the other strand. Likewise, guanine pairs with cytosine. The precise sequence of these four bases within the DNA polymer ultimately dictates the nature of all structural and enzymatic proteins in an intact organism. The double-stranded structure of DNA with its specific base pairing allows for its faithful reproduction during cell division and provides for permanence of the species through inheritance.

Organization of genes and chromosomes

A typical DNA molecule stretched end to end would measure more than 1.5 meters. Because it is a highly charged polymer, DNA is also extremely viscous in aqueous solution. Thus it is of considerable interest to understand how DNA can be packaged in a nucleus measuring a few micrometers in diameter and still permit access to its genetic information to control gene expression and allow accurate replication during cell division. Nature has solved the problem of DNA packaging through a nuclear protein infrastructure. The DNA polymer associates with these nuclear proteins to form **chromatin** in a specific fashion described below.

At certain times during the cell cycle, individual DNA molecules within the cell are visible as **chromosomes**. Human somatic cells have 22 pairs of chromosomes plus 2 sex chromosomes for a total of 46. Individual chromosomes can be identified by differences in their staining by chemical dyes. The staining patterns are a function of how the DNA and protein interact to produce chromatin.

The fundamental protein components of chromatin are the **histones**. Five histones have been described: H1, H2A, H2B, H3, and H4. All are extremely basic with substantial lysine and/or arginine content. Their net positive charge at physiological pH may be important for interaction with the negatively charged phosphate backbone of DNA. Other **nonhistone** proteins are also found in chromatin. These include enzymes responsible for DNA replication and transcription as well as other protein factors that regulate these processes. Some of these proteins are discussed in additional detail in Section 2B.

Chromatin is organized into subunits called **nucleosomes**. An individual nucleosome contains a core complex of eight histone proteins: one pair each of H2A, H2B, H3, and H4. Approximately 200 base pairs of DNA are associated with each histone octomer. This includes 146 base pairs of DNA wrapped around the octomer core and variable lengths (8–114 base pairs) of free DNA that link one core to the next. Electron micrographs of intact nucleosomes suggest that their structure is analogous to beads on a string. A single H1 histone associates with the outer region of the DNA–histone octomer complex. The function of H1 may be to mediate organization of the nucleosome chain into a supercoiled chromatin fiber. The chromatin fiber in turn is supercoiled to achieve the density of DNA necessary to package it into the nucleus. Nucleosome structure is summarized in Fig. 2.1.

Successful gene transcription requires that regions of DNA containing genes be accessible to the appropriate enzymes and accessory factors that will produce a complementary copy of messenger RNA capable of being translated into a protein product. It has been shown that

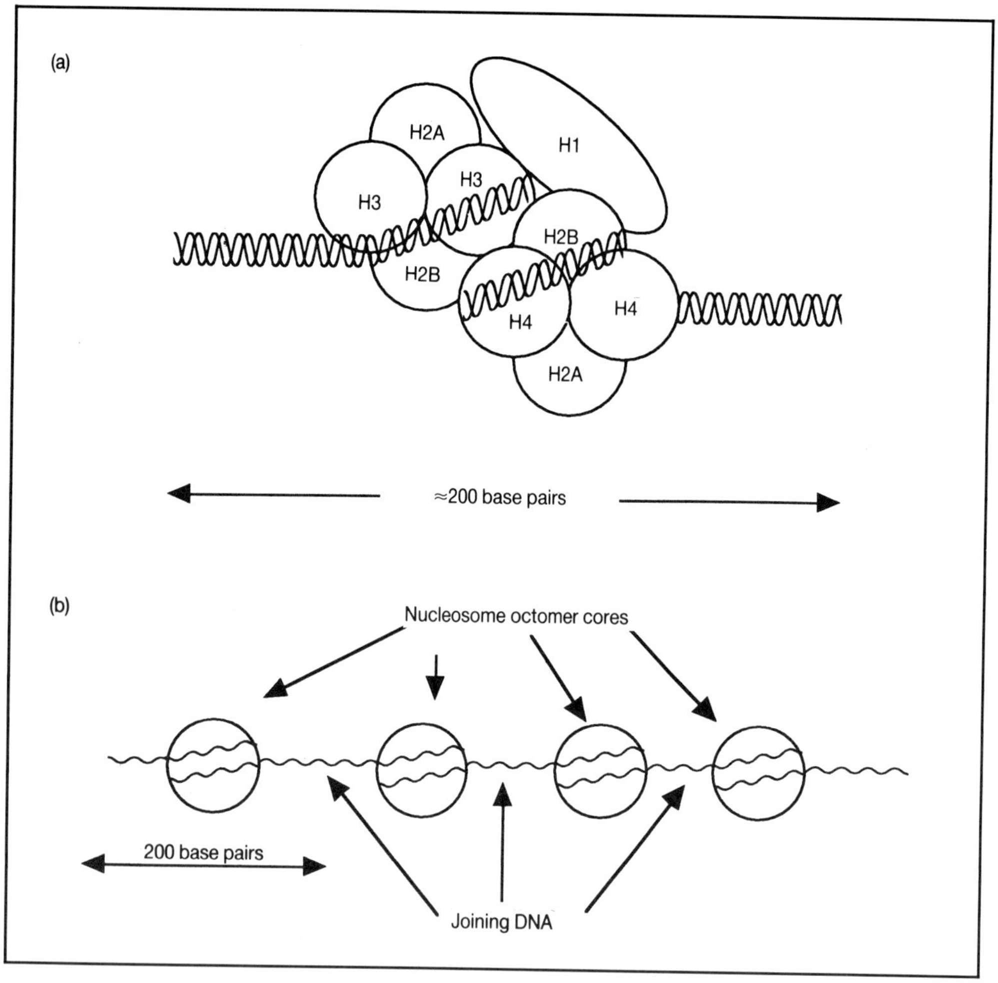

Fig. 2.1. An idealized scheme of DNA packaging in chromatin. (a) Organization of the histone proteins that make up the nucleosome core. DNA wraps twice around the core before proceeding to the nucleosome. The H1 histone binds to the outer region of the core. (b) The structure of several nucleosomes are shown, demonstrating their 'beads on a string' morphology. The DNA linking each nucleosome core is more susceptible to digestion by nucleases than the DNA associated with the histone proteins. Actively transcribed genes frequently may be located within joining DNA because these regions are more accessible to a variety of general and specific transcription factors required for gene transcription. The average length of DNA associated with a single nucleosome following digestion with a nonspecific nuclease is 200 base pairs.

many actively transcribed genes in chromatin contain regions that are hypersensitive to DNase I digestion. In certain instances, these **DNase hypersensitive sites** have been localized along the free DNA that links one nucleosome to another in chromatin. Enzymes involved in the transcription process such as RNA polymerase may preferentially bind to these sites, resulting in activation of transcription. Undermethylation of the DNA in these regions may also influence transcription activity. Chromatin structure appears to be modified in different tissues reflecting the need for varied gene transcription. A further discussion of chromatin structure and gene transcription is found in Section 2B.

DNA replication also requires modifications of chromatin structure. The process of mitosis requires access to DNA by enzymes such as DNA polymerase and DNA topoisomerase. The former enzyme catalyzes the complementary synthesis of DNA during mitosis and 'proof-reads' the newly synthesized DNA strand to make certain that it is an accurate copy. Topoisomerases are necessary to relax the supercoiled structure of packaged DNA, allowing DNA synthesis to take place. DNA strands synthesized during replication are almost immediately packaged into nucleosomes. Transient modification of histones during the cell cycle (see below) may mediate the formation of the DNA replication fork required for mitosis.

Cell cycle

The time required to accomplish cell division varies among cell types, and the phases of replication are termed the cell cycle (Fig. 2.2). The cell cycle can be divided temporally into four phases: G_1 (first gap), S (DNA synthesis), G_2 (second gap), and M (mitosis). The S phase

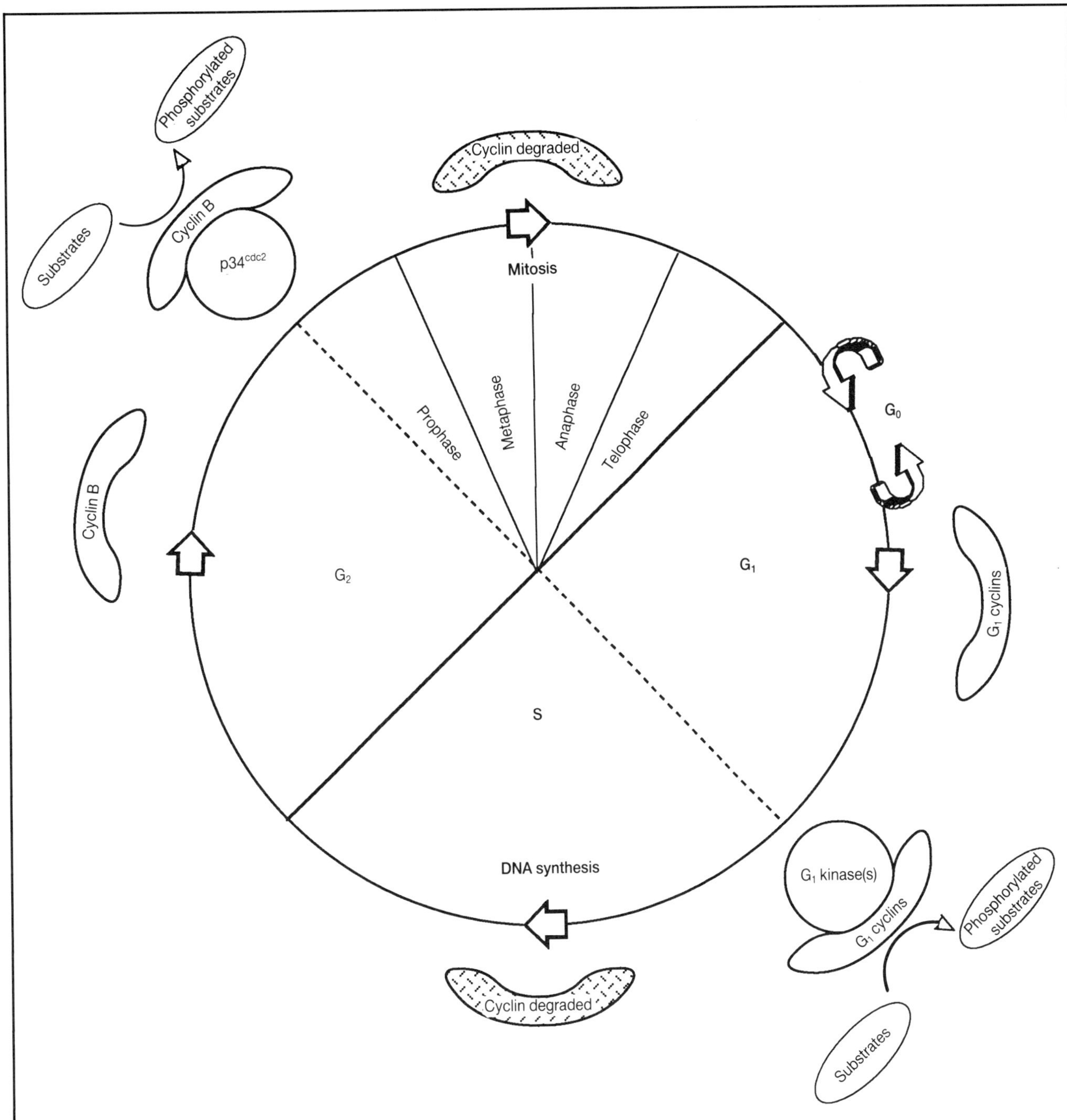

Fig. 2.2. The cell cycle. Resting cells (G_0) enter the cell cycle at the first gap (G_1) phase following growth factor stimulation. Continued stimulation promotes the accumulation of G_1 cyclins, which activate serine/threonine kinase(s) (G_1 kinases) involved in the initiation of DNA synthesis (the identification of proteins controlling the G_1/S phase transition is currently an active area of research). DNA duplication in S phase is followed by a second gap phase (G_2); collectively, the G_1, S, and G_2 phases are referred to as interphase. The transition from interphase to prophase of mitosis (G_2/M phase transition) is regulated by the serine/threonine kinase $p34^{cdc2}$. The accumulation of cyclin B during G_2 results in the activation of $p34^{cdc2}$ kinase and the phosphorylation of key proteins involved in the onset of mitosis. Destruction of cyclin B at the metaphase/anaphase transition results in the inactivation of $p34^{cdc2}$ and the completion of cell division to form independent daughter cells. Daughter cells may enter G_1 for another round of cell division or withdraw from the cell cycle into the resting phase (G_0).

is the period during which DNA is duplicated in preparation for nuclear division. The M phase is the portion of the cell cycle in which duplicated DNA is equally divided to form two nuclei followed division of the cytoplasm to produce independent daughter cells. The S and M phases are preceded by G_1 and G_2, respectively, during which the cell prepares for the events of DNA synthesis and mitosis.

DNA synthesis (S phase)

Somatic cells contain 23 chromosomes donated by the male parent and a homologous set donated by the female parent. Each set of 23 chromosomes is referred to as the 'n' (haploid) number of chromosomes; the somatic cell is therefore a 2n (diploid) cell. During the S phase DNA is replicated in a semi-conservative fashion, so that each daughter molecule (referred to as a chromatid in M phase) contains one newly synthesized and one parental strand of DNA, resulting in a 4n (tetraploid) cell. Individual chromosomes cannot be distinguished in S, G_1, or G_2 phases (collectively referred to as interphase) because the DNA is loosely organized in the form of chromatin (DNA/ protein complexes); however, chromosomes are readily detected and identified by histological stains following condensation in the M phase.

Mitosis (M phase)

Mitosis can be divided into four sequential stages, each of which is characterized by discrete morphological changes.

Prophase

The transition from G_2 to prophase of mitosis is marked by changes in the structure of centrioles, chromosomes, and the nuclear membrane. Centrioles are duplicated in interphase and play an important role in organizing the microtubular network (spindle) involved in orientation of chromosomes. In early prophase the centrioles are segregated toward opposite ends (poles) of the cell. By late prophase, 'spindle fibers' radiate from each pole and project to the centromeres of the chromosomes. Chromosomes first became morphologically detectable during prophase as condensation of DNA transforms dispersed chromatin into compacted duplicated chromosomes, each consisting of two chromatids (sister chromatids) associated at their centromeres. The end of prophase is marked by complete dissolution of the nuclear membrane.

Metaphase

During metaphase the chromosomes line up at the midline of the cell (equatorial plane). Sister chromatids are connected to opposite poles of the cell by microtubules emanating from the centriolar regions.

Anaphase

Anaphase commences with the separation of sister chromatids (now independent chromosomes) followed by their migration toward opposite poles to form daughter nuclei.

Telophase

In many ways telophase is a reversal of the events of prophase. A new nuclear membrane forms around each daughter nucleus, the chromosomes begin to uncoil, and the microtubular spindle is disassembled. In addition, the cytoplasm is equally divided (cytokinesis), resulting in independent daughter cells, each with an identical genetic complement.

Regulation of cell cycle progression

Resting cells (cells that are no longer dividing) withdraw from the cell cycle into a phase referred to as G_0 (quiescence). Many G_0 cells can be induced to resume cell division by exposure to specific polypeptide growth factors referred to as 'competent factors'. G_0 fibroblasts can be made competent by treatment with platelet derived growth factor (PDGF), which causes the cells to enter the G_1 phase of the cell cycle. In order to traverse G_1 and enter S phase, however, fibroblasts must be further treated with the 'progression factors' epidermal growth factor (EGF) and insulin-like growth factor-1 (IGF-1). In contrast to fibroblasts, macrophages require only colony stimulating factor-1 (CSF-1) to progress from G_0/G_1 to S phase. Although the requirement for specific competent and progression factors varies among cell types, their function is similar in that they all promote the accumulation of proteins that regulate transition to S phase, beyond which cells are irreversibly committed to DNA synthesis. Proteins that control the G_1/S phase transition (sometimes referred to as 'start' or the 'restriction point') are the primary regulators of cell division, and in their absence, cells become arrested in the G_1 phase of the cell cycle. Thus the identification of these molecules is critical for understanding the regulation of cell division during normal fetal growth and the changes that lead to uncontrolled cell division (*cancer*) and cessation of division (aging).

In addition to stringent controls at the G_1/S phase transition (initiation of DNA synthesis), progression through the cell cycle is also regulated at the G_2/M phase transition (initiation of mitosis). The control of the onset of mitosis has been extensively studied in yeast and has provided important insights into the regulation of both the G_1/S and G_2/M phase transitions. The central protein involved in the initiation of mitosis is a 34 000 Da serine/threonine kinase (an enzyme that catalyzes the addition of phosphate to serine or threonine in the substrate molecule); this protein is the product of the cell division cycle 2 (cdc2) gene and is therefore referred to as $p34^{cdc2}$. Depletion of $p34^{cdc2}$ or inactivation of the cdc2 gene results in G_2 arrest, so that cells are able to duplicate their DNA (in S phase) but are unable to initiate mitosis. $p34^{cdc2}$ kinase activity increases 10–20 fold at the G_2/M phase transition, resulting in the phosphorylation of substrates involved in chromosome condensation, mitotic spindle assembly, and nuclear membrane dissolution (the major events of prophase). The temporal activation of $p34^{cdc2}$ is the result of its association with cyclin B. Cyclin B, as its name implies, is a protein that accumulates in a cell cycle-dependent manner so that levels peak at the G_2/M phase transition, thereby leading to activation of $p34^{cdc2}$. Recently it has become evident that other kinases and phosphatases play critical roles in the precise timing of $p34^{cdc2}$/cyclin B activation. The abrupt degradation of cyclin B at the metaphase/anaphase transition of mitosis results in the inactivation of $p34^{cdc2}$ and the eventual exit of the cell from mitosis. Control of the G_1/S phase transition is mechanistically similar to G_2/M phase transition and involves both serine/threonine kinase(s) and cyclin-like proteins (G_1 cyclins). At least four G_1 cyclins have been identified (cyclins A, C, D, E), two of which associate with a serine/threonine kinase referred to as $p33^{cdk2}$ (a 33 000 Da protein that is the product of the cdk2 gene). Depletion of $p33^{cdk2}$ has been shown to delay the onset of DNA synthesis or to arrest cells in the G_1 phase of the cell cycle. The recent identification of novel genes encoding other serine/threonine kinases, with striking homology to $p33^{cdk2}$ and $p34^{cdc2}$, and the presence of multiple cyclins in the G_1 phase suggest that there may be several levels of regulation at the G_1/S phase transition. The substrates phosphorylated by $p33^{cdk2}$-like kinases and the role(s) of these phosphoproteins in facilitating G_1 progression remain to be elucidated.

Summary

Cell cycle progression is regulated at two critical phase transitions corresponding to the initiation of DNA synthesis (G_1/S) and mitosis (G_2/M). The key proteins controlling these two phase transitions are serine/threonine kinases the activity of which is activated in a cell cycle-dependent manner. The timing of kinase activation is due to association with labile cyclin proteins, which are expressed in a phase-specific manner.

Selected reading

Alberts B, Bray D, Lewis J, Raff M, Roberts K, Watson JD. *Molecular biology of the cell.* New York: Garland Publishing, Inc., 1983.

Darnell J, Lodish H, Baltimore D. *Molecular cell biology.* New York: WH Freeman and Company, 1986.

B. Gene Transcription

J M Greenberg

With rare exception, all somatic cells in a living organism contain the same genetic information as DNA within their nuclei. Normal development of a tissue or cell type from a fertilized ovum therefore depends upon when and where gene expression takes place.

Eukaryotic cells express three types of genes. The expression of genes that code for proteins, so-called **class II genes**, requires the production of an intermediate molecule known as **messenger RNA** (mRNA). Class I genes code for ribosomal RNA, and class III genes for transfer RNA and other small RNA molecules. These RNA molecules are the end product of class I or III gene expression. No protein product is generated. This discussion will not address transcription of class I or III genes because of their limited application to our understanding of developmental physiology and pathogenesis of disease.

In eukaryotic cells, mRNA synthesis is catalyzed by **RNA polymerase II**. The mRNA molecule includes the corresponding nucleotide sequences from the expressed gene required for subsequent generation of the protein product. The process of producing mRNA from the DNA in a structural gene is known as transcription. We now know that regulation of gene transcription is the primary means by which cells ultimately determine their phenotype.

The transcription unit

The initiation of transcription begins with the binding of RNA polymerase II to a specific region of DNA called the **promoter**. After binding, the synthesis of the primary mRNA transcript proceeds until the polymerase reaches a **termination** signal. The DNA spanned by the promoter and terminator defines a **transcription unit**. Promoter activity can be affected by other sequences contained within the transcription unit known as **enhancers**. While a promoter can function only if it is located at a specific place near the transcription start site, enhancers can exert their effect independent of their position and orientation relative to the promoter. Most eukaryotic transcription units contain one gene, but some can contain more than one. In either case, a transcription unit includes a promoter, multiple **exons** and **introns**, and a termination signal. Some transcription units also contain **enhancers** and **repressors**. The promoter is the site on the DNA molecule where transcription begins. RNA polymerase and its associated cofactors bind to the promoter through recognition of its nucleotide sequence (Figs 2.3, 2.4). The promoter region is a primary location for regulation of transcriptional activity (see below). Exons are regions of a gene that are contained in the mature, spliced mRNA. Exonic sequences include those that code for the protein product as well as sequences responsible for appropriate post-transcriptional processing of the mRNA. **Coding exons** include nucleotide sequences that will be translated into an amino acid sequence. **Noncoding exons** are spliced and included in the mature mRNA but do not code for an amino acid sequence. Intronic sequences are transcribed into the primary mRNA transcript but subsequently are removed by splicing together adjoining exonic sequences. Introns may contain sequences that are associated with dramatic increases (enhancers) or decreases (repressors) in transcriptional activity in specific cell types. The transcription process and the general structure of the transcription unit are summarized in Fig. 2.3.

Regulation of transcription and post-transcriptional modification—an overview

Regulation of gene transcription occurs at many levels. The manner in which DNA is packaged in the nucleus as well as its degree of methylation can affect transcriptional activity. Nucleotide sequences contained within the structural gene (***cis***-acting sequences) can determine the timing and site of transcription within developing and mature tissues. Transcription is also affected by regulatory proteins known as transcription factors. These proteins modulate transcriptional activity by binding to *cis*-acting sequences, and are therefore said to act in ***trans***. Certain

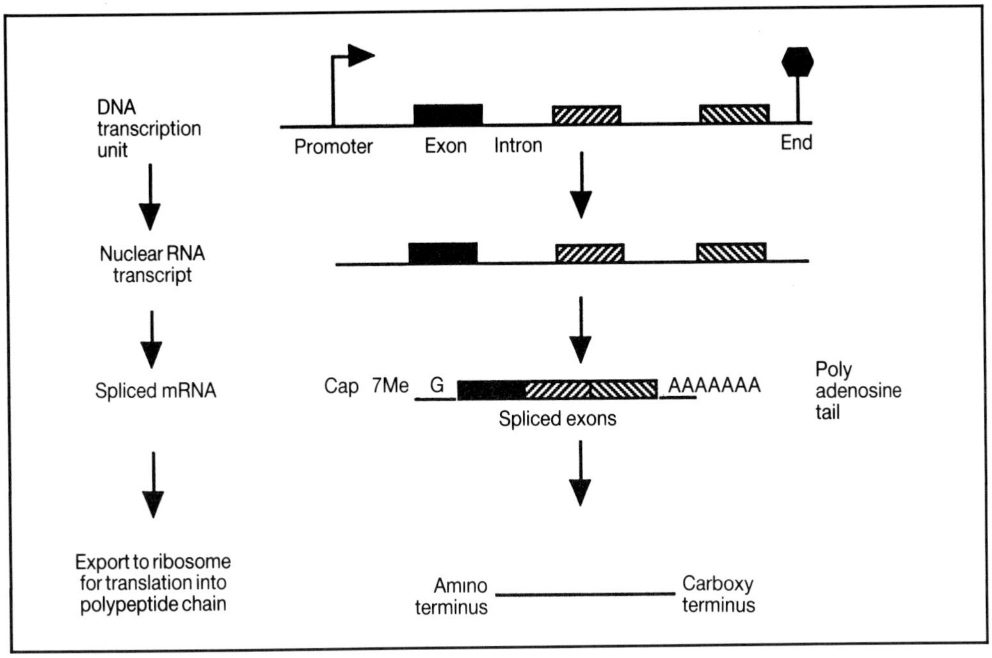

Fig. 2.3. Class II genes are transcribed from DNA by RNA polymerase II. The region from the beginning to the termination of transcription is designated a transcription unit. The primary or nuclear mRNA transcript corresponds to the DNA nucleotide sequence of the transcription unit. The primary transcript is processed to achieve a mature mRNA transcript that is ready for export to the ribosome for translation into a polypeptide chain. Messenger RNA processing may include, but is not limited to modifications such as splicing, capping, and polyadenylation.

cis- and *trans*-acting factors are found in virtually all expressed genes. These **general** factors are found in association with all protein-expressing genes and are necessary for efficient activity of RNA polymerase II, which catalyzes the synthesis of mRNA molecules. Conversely, **specific** *cis*- and *trans*-acting factors function as 'switches', activating or silencing gene transcription as required for appropriate cellular development and function.

Once the primary mRNA transcript is synthesized, sequences corresponding to noncoding introns in the structural gene are removed by splicing, allowing coding exons and regulatory regions of the mRNA to be joined together. In certain instances, alternative forms of spliced mRNA are produced by the use of certain exons and the deletion of other exons. Thus **alternative splicing** provides another means by which cells can alter the nature of the protein products produced by a given structural gene. Finally, transcriptional activity can be affected by the stability of the spliced mRNA. Sequences included within noncoding exons determine the rate at which an mRNA molecule is degraded, with direct consequences for the amount of protein that can be translated.

Figure 2.4 shows a summary of transcription and its regulation. It is not known whether all genes utilize all of the modalities depicted. One may reasonably assume that housekeeping genes, those that encode proteins involved in routine cellular physiology, such as actin, must be constantly expressed. Their transcription would require the presence of general *trans*- and *cis*-acting transcriptional factors but might not be affected by specific factors. In contrast, the gene coding for the immunoglobulin kappa light chain is likely to be under the control of specific transcriptional factors that permit transcription only in the appropriate tissue: B lymphocytes and plasma cells. In the subsequent discussion each component of transcriptional regulation will be considered separately. However, it is important to remember that the control of transcription involves multiple mechanisms acting in concert to achieve appropriate gene expression.

Chromatin structure

If extended as a linear molecule, the length of DNA from a single cell would vastly exceed its diameter. In order for DNA to fit into the nucleus, it is tightly packaged within a protein scaffold to form **chromatin**. The proteins of chromatin include a group of basic proteins known as histones, which bind tightly to the negatively charged phosphate backbone of the DNA double helix. The packaging of DNA within chromatin usually prevents the access of *trans*-acting transcriptional factors such as RNA

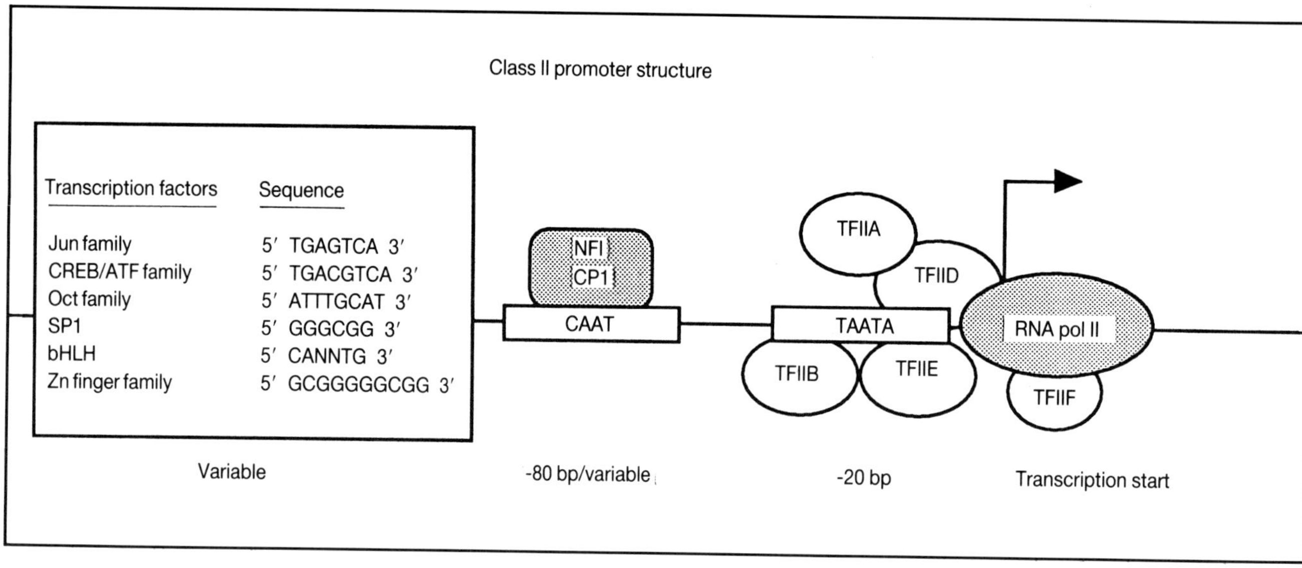

Fig. 2.4. An idealized eukaryotic class II promoter. A requisite TAATA motif is present approximately 20 base pairs before the actual transcription start site where RNA polymerase II attaches to the DNA template and gets oriented in the proper direction. A CAAT motif, also associated with proper RNA polymerase II function, is frequently located 80 base pairs in front of the transcription start site, although this can vary. Some promoters have more than one CAAT motif. General *trans*-acting factors that have been described in association with the TATA and CAAT sequences are depicted. The box contains examples of specific *trans*-acting transcription factors with their reported DNA binding sequences. The location of the binding sites for these transcription factors varies from gene to gene. Some are located near promoters while others may reside far from the promoter in an enhancer region. In this case, interaction with the promoter may require bending or looping of the genomic DNA.

polymerase II that are necessary for transcription. Active gene transcription requires that the structure of chromatin change to an 'open' configuration. This then allows access by transcriptional factors with subsequent interaction with the promoter of the transcriptional unit. The location of open chromatin regions can be established by treatment of nuclei with deoxyribonuclease I (DNase I). This enzyme promotes the nonspecific hydrolysis of DNA into deoxyribonucleotides. The DNA in intact nuclei is ordinarily resistant to digestion by DNase I because it is protected by the protein components of chromatin. However, DNA in regions of open chromatin is digested by DNase I. These sites are known as DNase I hypersensitive sites. They frequently correspond to promoter and enhancer sites. Presumably the same open structure responsible for access and subsequent digestion by DNase I allows access of transcriptional factors required for gene transcription. The mechanisms of chromatin opening are not well understood. Some have suggested that variations in histone production or modification of histone structure may be involved. Our future understanding of transcription factor access to DNA within chromatin will be facilitated by understanding the submicroscopic structure of chromatin.

Methylation

The bases of the DNA double helix can exist in methylated forms. In general, methylated DNA is not transcribed, presumably because the methyl groups cause stearic hindrance, preventing the binding of transcription factors. Thus the transcriptional activity of a given gene can be significantly affected by the methylation status of the promoter. Indeed, the promoters of most actively transcribed genes in a given tissue are hypomethylated relative to the remainder of the genome.

As with chromatin structure, the mechanism and control of gene methylation are not understood. However, the significance of methylation as a transcriptional control mechanism can be appreciated by considering the phenomenon of **CpG islands**. The deoxynucleotide 5′ CpG 3′ occurs five times less frequently than expected on a statistical basis in mammalian DNA. The majority of the C residues are methylated as 5-methylcytosine. Rather than being scattered randomly throughout the genome, CpG dinucleotides usually are found in clusters or islands near the 5′ portion of transcriptional units where promoters and enhancers are located. In actively transcribed genes, these CpG islands are hypomethylated. The identification of hypomethylated CpG islands has been used by investigators to identify the location of putative transcription units within a mammalian genome.

General transcription

Certain components of the transcriptional apparatus are common to genes transcribed by RNA polymerase II. These include *cis*- and *trans*-acting factors shown in Fig. 2.4 and summarized below.

General *cis*-acting sequences

Certain sequences frequently are found associated with the promoter regions of transcribed genes. Although the exact nucleotide sequence in these regions may vary from one gene to the next, general similarities have been defined in the form of **consensus sequences**, also referred to as **core, motif,** or **box sequences**. General *cis*-acting sequences that have been well characterized include the **TATA box** (consensus sequence 5′ TATAAAA 3′), **CAAT box** (consensus sequence 5′ GGCCAATCT 3′), **GC box** (consensus sequence 5′ GGGCGG 3′), and the **octamer motif** (consensus sequence 5′ ATGCAAAT 3′). While none of these sequence modules is absolutely required for transcription, two or more have been identified in association with nearly every RNA polymerase II promoter. The CAAT and GC boxes may mediate initial binding of the transcriptional apparatus to the DNA, while the TATA box may determine the transcription start site. The function of the octamer motif is not clear. Its presence is associated with general transcription as well as tissue-specific gene expression depending upon which *trans*-acting factors bind to it.

General *trans*-acting factors

All messenger RNA is transcribed by RNA polymerase II. In eukaryotic cells, this enzyme consists of several subunits that function to synthesize mRNA only if allowed to associate with at least five accessory proteins. Those characterized to date include **transcription factors (TF) IIA, IIB, IID, IIE,** and **IIF**. The accessory factors seem to stabilize the association of RNA polymerase II with the promoter and are required for accurate and efficient transcription. TFIID binds to the TATA box. TFIIA may be involved in stabilizing the TFIID–TATA box interaction. TFIIB and TFIIE may stabilize RNA polymerase II during the promoter binding process. More than one protein may be capable of binding the CAAT box. NF1 and CP1 are two described CAAT box-binding proteins that are associated with active transcription. Although the CAAT box is a common component of RNA polymerase II promoters, there appear to be *trans*-acting factors, so-called CAAT-displacement proteins, that prevent transcription factor binding (e.g. CP1) and subsequent transcription.

Specific transcription factors

While the general transcription factors described above are required for mRNA synthesis, the regulation of specific gene expression permits normal development to occur. Aberrant gene expression, either in an inappropriate tissue or at an inappropriate time during development, can result in deleterious consequences such as neoplasia or a congenital anomaly. The number of known *cis*- and *trans*-acting factors associated with tissue-specific gene expression has grown at a rapid rate. The box in Fig. 2.4 includes an abridged listing of some well described families of transcription factors. For each factor, the regulatory *cis*-acting DNA element is noted with a core or consensus sequence.

Within the diversity of specific transcription factors, some characteristics in common have emerged. Most have a region predominantly composed of basic amino acids such as arginine and lysine that comes into direct contact with DNA. The DNA sequence in this region likely determines the specific sequence recognized by the transcription factor. Most (if not all) transcription factors will only bind DNA (and activate transcription) as dimers with like or related members of the same family (homo- or heterodimers). Thus members of the basic helix-loop helix family of transcriptional regulatory proteins will activate transcription through direct contact with DNA at the basic region. DNA binding will occur only if preceded by dimerization mediated via the helix-loop helix structures. Members of the leucine zipper family, which include the *fos* and *jun* proto-oncogenes and CREB/ATF,

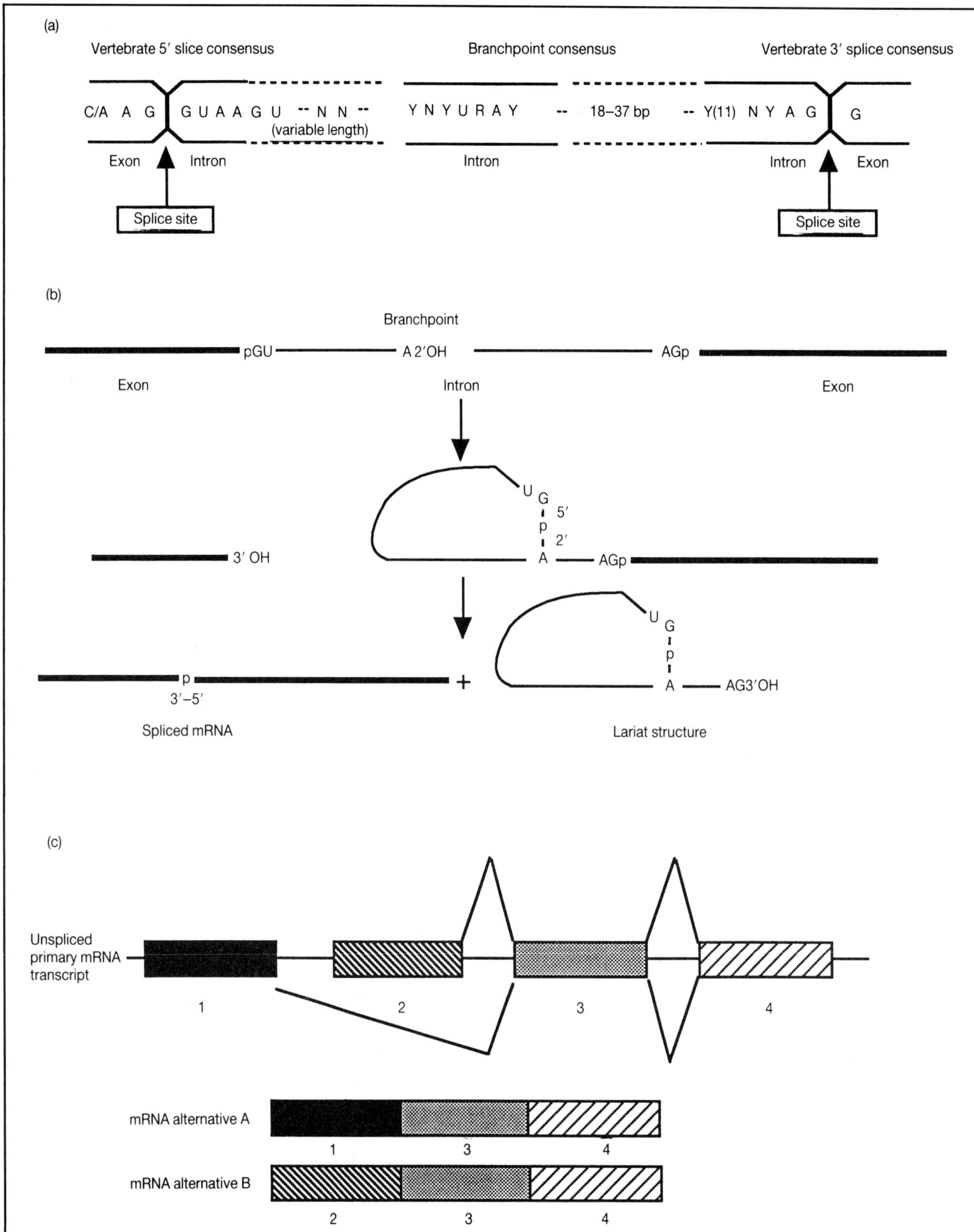
(a)
Vertebrate 5′ slice consensus
Branchpoint consensus
Vertebrate 3′ splice consensus
C/A A G
G U A A G U -- N N --
(variable length)
Y N Y U R A Y
-- 18–37 bp
-- Y(11) N Y A G
G
Exon
Intron
Intron
Intron
Exon
Splice site
Splice site
(b)
Branchpoint
pGU
A 2′OH
AGp
Exon
Intron
Exon
U
G
5′
p
2′
A
AGp
3′ OH
U
G
p
A
AG3′OH
p
3′–5′
+
Spliced mRNA
Lariat structure
(c)
Unspliced primary mRNA transcript
1
2
3
4
mRNA alternative A
1
3
4
mRNA alternative B
2
3
4

the cyclic AMP response element binding/activating transcription factor (see Fig. 2.4), also must form dimers before binding to DNA. Dimer formation, especially heterodimer formation, affords the cell with multiple mechanisms of transcriptional regulation, especially given the observation that different dimer combinations may have different transcription-stimulating activities. Another layer of transcriptional control (and complexity) is provided by related transcription factors that incorporate dimerization motifs but do not contain any sequences with abundant basic amino acid residues. Thus these transcription factors can form dimers with other members of their transcription factor family but actually prevent DNA binding by that dimer complex. Transcription factors that prevent DNA binding and consequently inhibit transcription are termed **dominant negative**. The number of permutations generated by dimerization of specific transcription factors and their dominant negative counterparts provides a developing cell with exquisite control over the transcriptional activity of its genetic complement. Regulation does not end with the generation of the primary transcript. In the next section, cellular options for post-transcriptional modification of mRNA and its consequences for gene expression will be discussed.

Splicing of mRNA

The primary mRNA transcript is synthesized within the nucleus and includes introns and exons covering the entire transcriptional unit. In order for the nuclear mRNA to be transcribed into a polypeptide, the noncoding intronic sequences must be removed. The cell accomplishes this by **splicing** out the intronic sequences from the nuclear mRNA, just as a movie editor splices film to produce a final cinematic production. Nuclear mRNA splicing is a remarkable process given the precision with which it typically occurs.

General principles of mRNA splicing

In mammalian genes, the number of introns may range from zero to 20 or more. Intron length also varies dramatically from a few dozen base pairs to more that 6 kilobases (6000 base pairs). Figure 2.5 depicts a simplified, general summary of nuclear mRNA splicing. Specific consensus sequences identify the 5′ and 3′ boundaries of an intron–exon junction. A consensus branchpoint sequence located near the 3′ splice boundary has also been described (Fig. 2.5). The splicing process requires many additional *trans*-acting protein and RNA-containing factors.

Alternative splicing

Splicing of mRNA can afford the cell another opportunity for transcriptional regulation. Many examples now exist of two or more different transcripts derived from the same transcription unit. The transcripts differ in exon content, and thus are said to have been generated by alternative splicing. Each transcript may contain common as well as alternate exons, resulting in the translation of proteins with identical carboxy termini but different amino termini. This may in turn result in differences in processing and compartmentalization between transcript products, i.e. secreted versus membrane-bound versions of a particular protein. An example of alternative splicing is shown in Fig. 2.5.

RNA processing

In addition to splicing, mRNA experiences other modifications before its export from the nucleus. In a modification known as **capping**, a guanosine residue methylated at its N7 position is added to the 5′ end of the

Fig. 2.5. A summary of mRNA splicing. (a) The consensus RNA sequences corresponding to splice sites in eukaryotic RNA transcripts. Much of this work is derived from studies of yeast and metazoans. While several of the nucleotide designations vary between species and genes, the **G U** at the exon/intron boundary of the 5′ splice consensus and the **A G** at the intron/exon boundary of the 3′ splice consensus appear to be invariable. The branchpoint consensus is based upon analysis of a limited number of genes. For the consensus sequences shown: A = adenine, C = cytosine, G = guanine, U = uracil, Y = C or U, N = any nucleotide. (b) The mechanism of mRNA splicing. This appears to be a two-step process. The first event is hydrolysis at the 5′ splice junction with the formation of a looped or lariat structure at an adenosine residue at the branchpoint within the intron. The second step is hydrolysis at the 3′ splice junction with removal of the intronic lariat structure and joining (also called ligation) of the two exons. (c) An example of alternative splicing. A primary mRNA transcript is produced containing four exons. However, exons 1 and 2 cannot be spliced because the appropriate splicing signals are not present in the sequence. Two processed mRNA molecules are generated, one containing exons 1, 3, and 4 (alternative A) and another containing exons 2, 3, and 4 (alternative B).

mRNA through its 5′ phosphate. This results in an unusual 5′–5′ triphosphate linkage between the cap and the first base of the mRNA transcript that may render it more resistant to degradation by endogenous nucleases. The 3′ end of the mRNA is also modified by the addition of a **polyadenosine (polyA) tail** of up to 200 residues in length. The polyA tail is synthesized in a nontemplate-dependent fashion after transcription has taken place. A consensus sequence signaling the end of transcription and the addition of the polyA tail is defined as 5′ AAUAAA 3′. The polyA tail appears to be required for efficient export of the mRNA from the nucleus and, like the 5′ cap, prevents enzymatic degradation during that process. The 3′ region of the mRNA molecule also contains other sequences that influence mRNA stability during transport from the nucleus to the ribosome where translation will take place.

Regulation of globin gene expression

The genes coding for the embryonic, fetal, and adult globins that form the protein component of hemoglobin have long been a paradigm for studies of regulated gene expression. Distinct globin genes are expressed at specific stages of embryonic, fetal, and postnatal life. In the human, the ζ, ε, γ, and α globins are expressed until up to eight weeks of gestation. During the remainder of fetal life, the α and γ globins are expressed, while the ζ and ε genes are silenced. In adults, the α, β , and δ genes are expressed. At any given point in development, globin expression is limited to cells of the erythroid lineage. The precise developmental and tissue-specific expression of the globin genes implies that they are controlled by specific *cis*- and *trans*-acting transcription factors. Although our understanding of the regulation of globin gene expression is far from complete, remarkable progress has been made since the first described cloning of a β globin gene in 1976. As discussed below, many of the previously described principles of transcriptional regulation apply to the globin gene locus.

The globin genes are derived from a single ancestral gene that has undergone duplication and modification over evolutionary time. The evidence for this is based upon similarities in sequence and structure. In higher vertebrates, the α and β genes exist as separate clusters. The human α locus resides on chromosome 16, and the β cluster on chromosome 11. Globin expression during development is recapitulated by their physical location within the α or β cluster. The earliest expressed globin genes are found in the 5′ region of the locus, while those expressed later during development are found at the 3′ end.

All expressed globin genes contain three exons separated by two introns belying their common evolutionary origins. Like the vast majority of genes transcribed by RNA polymerase II, the typical globin gene promoter includes a TATA box and a CCAAT box among its general *cis*-acting transcriptional factors. A CACCC sequence motif has also been identified as a common *cis*-acting sequence in β-globin promoters. Several DNase I hypersensitive sites have been identified within the β- and α-globin clusters. Many of these sites correspond to sequence elements that influence globin gene expression. These include promoter components as well as enhancer sequences. Some of these regions correspond to general *cis*- and *trans*-acting transcription factors, while other regions appear responsible for tissue-specific and developmental regulation of globin gene expression. Of particular interest are so-called DNase super-hypersensitive regions that flank the entire β-globin locus. These sequences, located approximately 6–20 kb 5′ of the ε gene and 20 kb 3′ of the β-globin gene activate expression of all genes within the locus. Because these sequences influence gene expression over a large distance of genomic DNA, they are defined as having enhancer activity and have been termed **dominant control regions (DCR)**. The mechanisms by which these enhancers function are not known. It has been suggested that these sequences may alter chromatin structure over the entire locus to allow the access of *trans*-acting transcription factors. The DCR is clearly required for high-level globin gene expression in erythroid cells. When it is absent, mRNA levels are only approximately 1 percent of normal. The DCR is not sufficient for the developmental regulation of globin gene expression within the α or β loci. However, changes in levels of globin gene expression may be mediated by the DCR. Local promoters for each globin gene may compete for interactions with the DCR allowing expression. Success in such a competition may depend on the expression of other *trans*-acting factors associated with a specific stage or hematopoietic lineage. An erythroid-specific *trans*-activating factor, GF-1, has been identified recently by several laboratories. The factor interacts with the conserved DNA sequence A/T **G A T A**/T A/G. Binding sites for GF-1 are found in the promoter regions of globin genes as well as other nonglobin, erythroid-specific genes such as the erythropoietin receptor gene. GF-1 does not appear specifically to direct the differentiation of erythroid cells. It has also been detected in cells of the megakaryocytic and mast cell lineages. Another factor distinct from GF-1, known as NF-E2, has also been described. This factor recognizes a distinct promoter sequence motif similar to that recognized by the *jun* oncogene. GF-1, NF-E2, and other *trans*-acting factors may mediate interactions with the DCR to produce stage-specific globin gene expression.

Although our understanding of globin gene expression is not complete, it should be evident that the long observed phenomenon of precise, sequential globin chain expression during development is a direct consequence of the regulation of globin gene transcription by the developing erythroid cell. Transcriptional regulation in turn is directly related to the structure and organization of the globin gene loci. This paradigm, that regulation follows from structure, is likely applicable to many (if not all) developmentally regulated genes.

The typical life span of an mRNA molecule is quite brief relative to other cellular components such as DNA and protein. Indeed, one might wonder why living things bother with the synthesis of an intermediate molecule between DNA and protein. The likely explanation is inherent in the very transience of mRNA. This property allows for the exquisite level of regulation of gene transcription we have described. This ultimately provides the cell with an appropriate complement of enzymatic and structural components to function properly. During dynamic processes such as development or differentiation, regulation at the transcriptional level, i.e. regulation of the quantity and quality of an mRNA transcript, becomes even more crucial. Thus the rapid phenotypic changes that occur as an organism develops are predominantly a function of transcriptional regulation. Continued progress in our understanding of the molecular basis of developmental biology will be based in large part upon our understanding of how gene transcription is regulated.

Selected reading

Evans T, Felsenfeld G, Reitman M. Control of globin gene expression. *Annu Rev Cell Biol* 1990; **6**: 95.

Faisst S, Meyer S. Compilation of vertebrate-encoded transcription factors. *Nucleic Acids Res* 1992; **20**: 3.

Heintz N. Transcriptional regulation. *Trends Biochem Sci* 1991; **16**: 393 (see other articles in this issue on selected topics on transcriptional regulation).

Tazi J, Bird A. Alternative chromatin structure at CpG islands. *Cell* 1990; **60**: 909.

C. Protein Synthesis, Sorting, Secretion and Degradation

T E Weaver

Genetic information stored in the form of nuclear DNA is sequentially disseminated in the form of RNA and protein. The transcription of DNA into RNA and the subsequent modifications that convert the primary transcript into a suitable template for protein synthesis are discussed earlier in this chapter. In this section, we focus on the synthesis of the polypeptide chain (protein translation) and the directed movement of newly synthesized proteins among cellular compartments.

Protein synthesis

The synthetic apparatus

The complexity of protein synthesis is related, in part, to the large number of components involved in the assembly of the polypeptide chain. The structure of each of these components is discussed individually and then in the context of its function.

Messenger RNA (mRNA)

Genetic information is transferred from the nucleus to the cytoplasm (the site of protein synthesis) in the form of mRNA. The protein sequence is encoded in the RNA molecule by triplet nucleotides (three nucleotides = one codon), which specify individual amino acids. Combinations of the four nucleotides (A, U, G, C) allow for 64 possible codons; three of these codons (UAA, UAG, UGA) do not encode an amino acid but signal the translation machinery to terminate synthesis, and are therefore referred to as STOP codons. Because only 20 amino acids are involved in the synthesis of eukaryotic proteins, the remaining 61 codons include many redundancies; for example, leucine is specified by six codons (CUU, CUC, CUA, CUG, UUA, UUG), whereas tryptophan (UGG) and methionine (AUG) are each specified by one codon (Table 2.1). Protein synthesis is initiated at the AUG codon closest to the 5′ end of the mRNA, thereby ensuring that all eukaryotic proteins begin with methionine. Decoding of the mRNA proceeds in a 5′ to 3′ direction, as codons are selected by the ribosome for translation, until a STOP codon (UAA, UAG, or UGA) is encountered.

Table 2.1. Codon dictionary

	Position of base in colon				
1	2				3
	U	C	A	G	
U	Phe	Ser	Tyr	Cys	U
	Phe	Ser	Tyr	Cys	C
	Leu	Ser	STOP	STOP	A
	Leu	Ser	STOP	Trp	G
C	Leu	Pro	His	Arg	U
	Leu	Pro	His	Arg	C
	Leu	Pro	Gln	Arg	A
	Leu	Pro	Gln	Arg	G
A	Ile	Thr	Asn	Ser	U
	Ile	Thr	Asn	Ser	C
	Ile	Thr	Lys	Arg	A
	Met (START)	Thr	Lys	Arg	G
G	Val	Ala	Asp	Gly	U
	Val	Ala	Asp	Gly	C
	Val	Ala	Glu	Gly	A
	Val	Ala	Glu	Gly	G

Ribosomes

The eukaryotic ribosome consists of two subunits that exist free in the cytosol: a large subunit (60S), composed of three ribosomal RNA molecules (28S, 5.8S, and 5S) and approximately 45 proteins, and a small subunit (40S), composed of one ribosomal RNA molecule (18S) and approximately 30 proteins. The 40S subunit binds to the 5′ end of the mRNA and moves toward the 3′ end of the molecule until it encounters an initiation (AUG) codon. The 60S subunit is then bound to form a functional (80S) ribosomal unit. Two binding sites on the 60S subunit are involved in assembly of amino acids into a polypeptide chain: The A-site (aminoacyl-tRNA binding site) is located over the codon to be translated and positions the appropriate incoming amino acid for attachment to the end of the growing polypeptide positioned in the neighboring P-site; the P-site (peptidyl-tRNA binding site) aligns the carboxyl-terminal amino acid of the nascent polypeptide chain with the amino acid positioned by the A-site. Correct alignment of the incoming amino acid with the growing polypeptide chain is achieved by the binding of tRNA molecules to the A- and P-sites.

Transfer RNA (tRNA)

Transfer RNA molecules are approximately 80 nucleotides in length and contain the sequence CCA at their 3′ end to which a specific amino acid can be covalently attached. There is at least one unique tRNA for each of the 20 amino acids, including an initiator Met-tRNA that is involved in the initiation of polypeptide synthesis. The codon positioned at the A-site of the 60S ribosomal subunit determines which tRNA and its attached amino acid will be bound to the A-site. Each tRNA contains an anticodon consisting of three nucleotides that are complementary to and form hydrogen bonds with the codon to be translated. Transfer RNA molecules are therefore molecular adapters that decode the mRNA molecule on the ribosomal scaffolding and mediate the transfer of the appropriate amino acid to the growing polypeptide chain.

Aminoacyl-tRNA synthetases

Attachment of the carboxyl-terminus of the amino acid to the CCA sequence at the 3′ end of the tRNA is catalyzed by an aminoacyl-tRNA synthetase. There is at least one aminoacyl-tRNA synthetase for each amino acid, which covalently links the appropriate amino acid to its corresponding tRNA.

The process of protein synthesis

Synthesis of the polypeptide chain can be divided into three discrete phases: initiation, elongation, and termination.

Initiation (Fig. 2.6)

At least 10 initiation factors, comprising as many as 25 different proteins, are necessary to initiate protein synthesis in eukaryotes. The initial step involves the formation of a complex consisting of the initiator Met-tRNA, GTP, and eukaryotic initiation factor-2 (eIF-2); this complex binds to the 40S ribosomal subunit, an association enhanced by eIF-3 and eIF-4C. The 40S subunit then binds to the 5′ end of the mRNA and moves in a 5′ to 3′ direction until it encounters the first AUG codon. This process involves the recognition and binding of the 5′ end of the mRNA (facilitated by initiation factors eIF-4E and eIF-4F) and removal of any secondary structure in the mRNA molecule in an energy-dependent process involving two separate initiation factors (eIF-4A and eIF-4B). Identification of the START codon (AUG) is accompanied by binding of the 60S subunit to form a functional (80S) ribosomal unit, a process that requires the participation of yet another initiation factor (eIF-5). This series of events establishes the reading frame of the mRNA by placing the initiator Met-tRNA in the P-site and positioning the ribosome so that the codon following the first AUG occupies the A-site. Thus every eukaryotic protein is translated with methionine as the first residue; for the majority of proteins, however, this methionine is subsequently removed by a cytoplasmic methionine aminopeptidase.

Elongation (Fig. 2.7)

The polypeptide chain is lengthened by the sequential addition of amino acids to the initiator methionine at the P-site. A complex, composed of the appropriate amino acid tRNA, GTP, and eukaryotic elongation factor-1α (eEF-1α), binds to the empty A-site. A peptide bond is then formed between the amino-terminus of the amino acid at the A-site and the carboxyl-terminus of the methionine at the P-site. The tRNA occupying the A-site (peptidyl-tRNA) is then translocated to the P-site, while the deacylated tRNA in the P-site is removed. This process is catalyzed by eEF-2 and results in movement of the ribosome exactly three bases in the 5′-to-3′ direction so that the next codon to be translated now occupies the empty A-site. This cycle is repeated for each amino acid and results in an average elongation rate of approximately five amino acids/second.

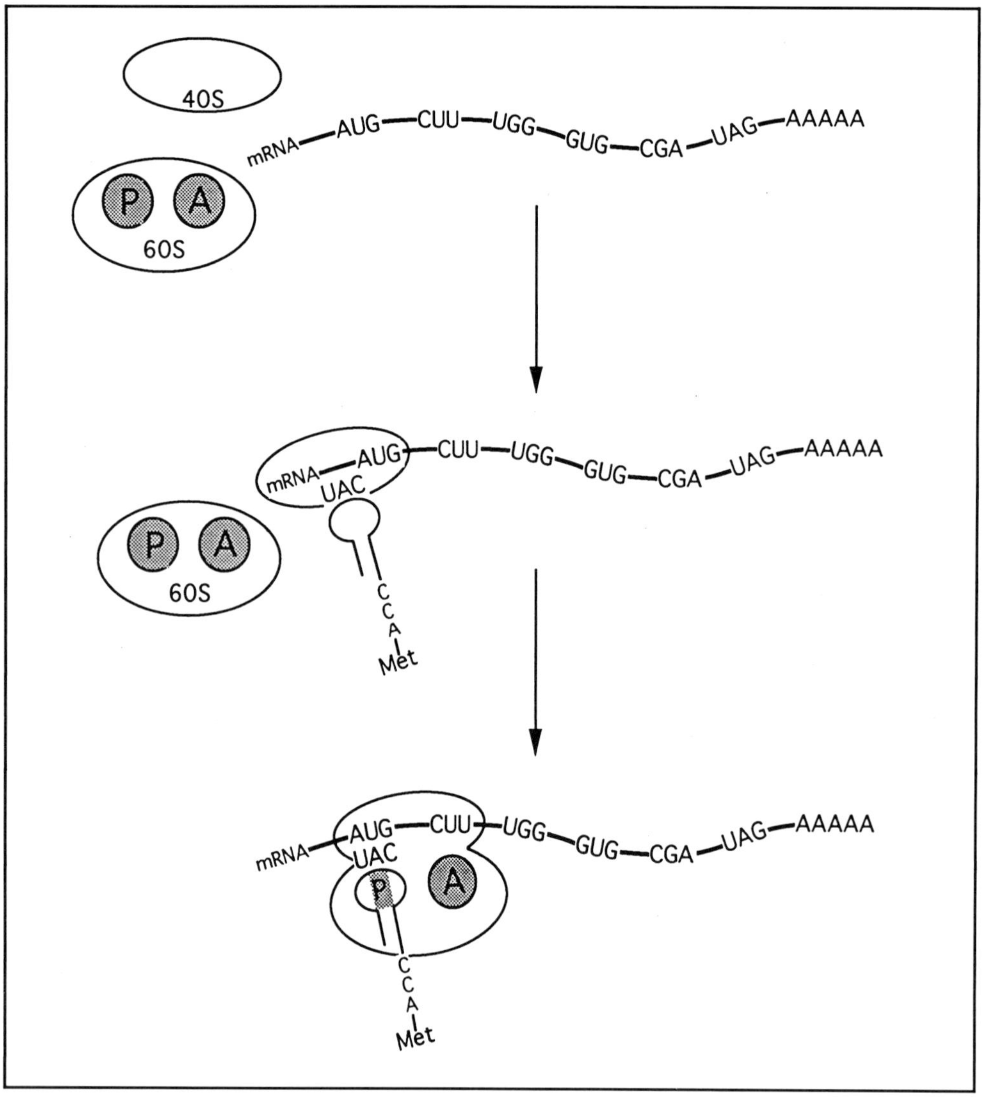

Fig. 2.6. Protein synthesis: initiation. See text for details.

Termination (Fig. 2.8)

Elongation of the polypeptide chain proceeds until a STOP codon (UAA, UAG, or UGA) is translocated into the A-site. No tRNA molecules recognize these codons; rather, these sequences are recognized by a protein referred to as eukaryotic release factor (RF). Binding of RF to the A-site blocks elongation and results in release of the polypeptide from the ribosome, which subsequently dissociates into 40S and 60S subunits.

Regulation of protein synthesis

Protein synthesis is expensive in terms of energy consumption. The formation of each peptide bond during elongation requires the hydrolysis of four GTP molecules. In addition, initiation and termination are energy-dependent processes. It is therefore critical that protein synthesis be tightly regulated. The rate-limiting step in protein synthesis is generally considered to be the initiation phase. Regulation at this level involves limiting the availability of initiation factors by reducing abundance or covalent modification (e.g. phosphorylation) of the factor. Polio virus infection reduces the rate of initiation by promoting the degradation of an eIF-4F subunit, thereby resulting in less efficient binding of the mRNA molecule by the 40S ribosomal subunit. The rate of initiation is also decreased by phosphorylation of eIF-2. Regulation of protein synthesis may also occur during the elongation phase, resulting in alteration of the rate of

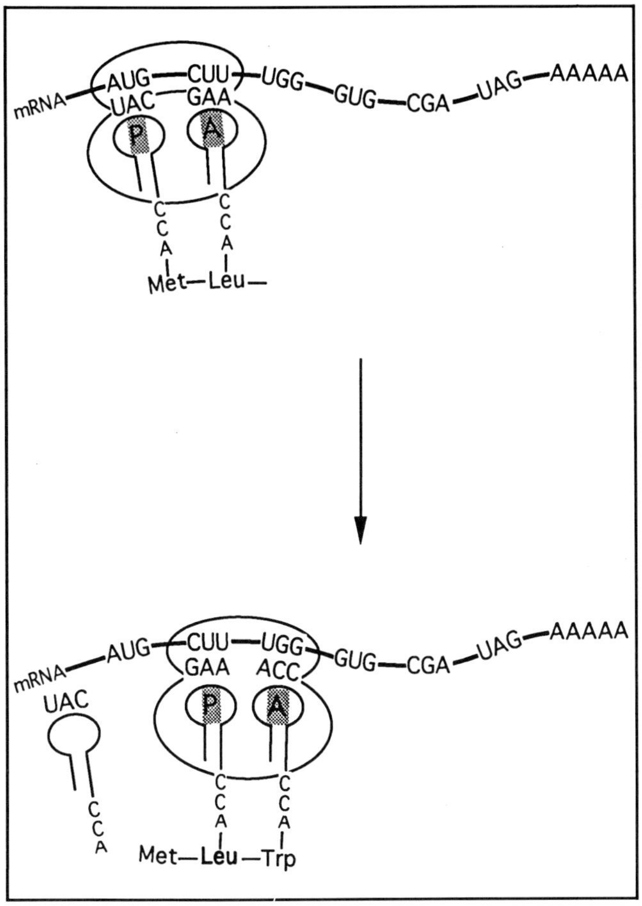

Fig. 2.7. Protein synthesis: elongation. See text for details.

elongation, e.g. phosphorylation of eEF-2 prevents it from catalyzing ribosome translocation, thereby decreasing the elongation rate.

Use of antibiotics to inhibit protein synthesis

The process of protein synthesis in prokaryotes is very similar to that for eukaryotes; however, many of the protein factors are different and not interchangeable, thus providing the opportunity for selective inhibition of bacterial protein synthesis. Tetracyclines, chloramphenicol, and erythromycin inhibit elongation, whereas streptomycin inhibits both initiation and elongation. Elongation is also inhibited by cycloheximide, which blocks peptide-bond formation, and puromycin, which displaces the mRNA from the ribosome. The latter two antibiotics have proved useful molecular tools for testing whether a particular event depends upon continued protein synthesis. For example, secretion via the regulated secretory pathway is blocked when protein synthesis is inhibited, while constitutive secretion continues unabated, indicating that newly synthesized protein(s) is necessary for regulated secretion.

Protein targeting

Newly synthesized proteins are directed to a particular destination by virtue of specific targeting signals encoded within the primary sequence. This section focuses on the identification of targeting signals and the cellular machinery that recognizes and decodes these signals. In most cases, the identity of the targeting signal has been examined by attaching the putative targeting sequence to a heterologous protein and determining whether the protein is redirected to a new cellular compartment specified by the signal.

Targeting to organelles

In the absence of targeting information, the default destination for newly synthesized proteins is the cytoplasm. These proteins make up approximately 20 percent of total cell protein and include proteins involved in glycolysis, cell division, protein synthesis, and the cytoskeleton. In contrast to these cytosolic proteins, proteins the location and function of which are restricted to the lumen or membrane of an intracellular organelle, are directed to their final destination by information encoded in the primary sequence.

Nucleus

Because all proteins are synthesized in the cytoplasm, proteins the function of which resides in the nucleus must be imported into this compartment. Communication between the cytoplasm and nucleus is mediated by the nuclear pore complex of the nuclear envelope. Targeting to the nucleus is mediated by a sequence referred to as the nuclear location sequence (NLS), which is typically characterized by the presence of three to five basic residues, e.g. lysine$_1$-(arginine/lysine)$_2$-X$_3$-(arginine/lysine)$_4$ (where X is any amino acid and either arginine or lysine will suffice at positions 2 and 4).

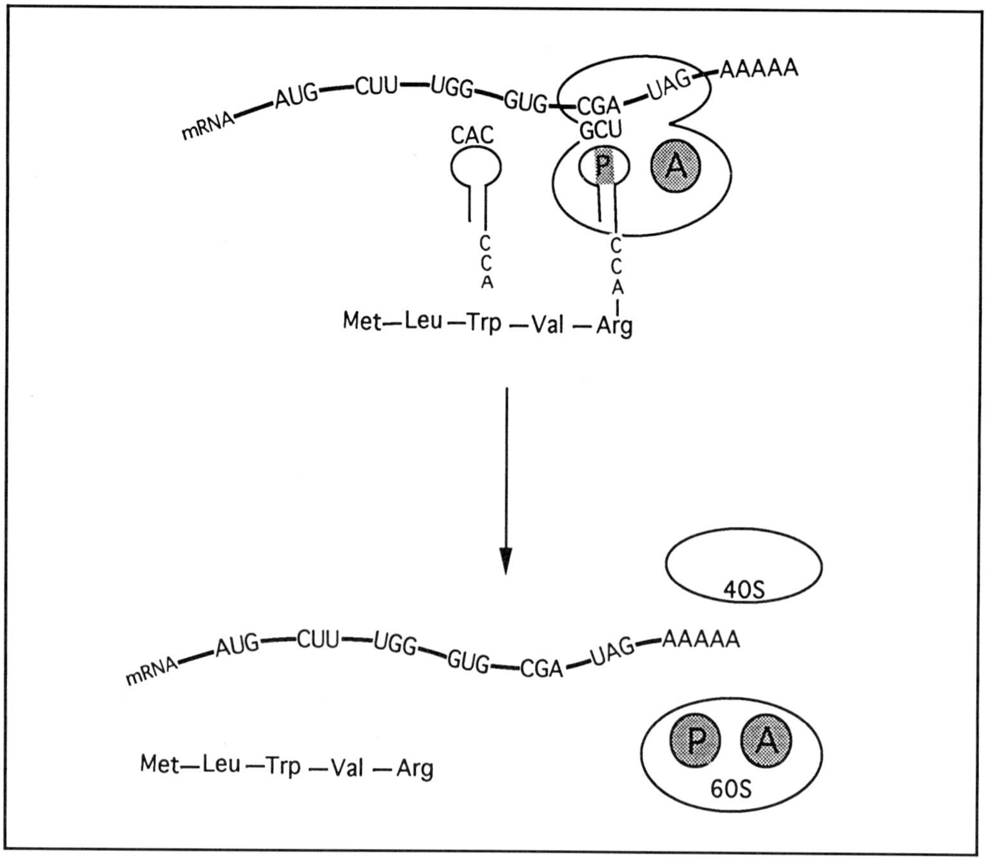

Fig. 2.8. Protein synthesis: termination. See text for details.

Recent evidence suggests that nuclear import occurs in three stages: (1) binding of proteins with an NLS to soluble cytoplasmic proteins (receptors); (2) NLS-dependent binding of the nuclear protein–receptor complex to the cytoplasmic face of the nuclear pore; and (3) ATP-dependent translocation through the nuclear pore. We emphasize that our current understanding of this process is very rudimentary and that this model does not readily account for proteins that are located in both the cytoplasm and the nucleus (e.g. actin).

Mitochondria

Mitochondria represent the principal site of cellular respiration. Although a very few proteins are encoded by mitochondrial DNA, most mitochondrial enzymes are encoded in the nucleus and must therefore be imported from the cytoplasm. The targeting signal for mitochondrial proteins is composed of 20–70 amino acids at the NH_2-terminus of the protein. This sequence, which is rich in basic and hydroxylated amino acids but contains very few acidic residues, is frequently cleaved during or after import. In addition to targeting the protein to the mitochondria, the presequence contains information for sorting the protein to the appropriate mitochondrial compartment, i.e. matrix, inner membrane, intermembrane space, or outer mitochondrial membrane.

Peroxisomes

Peroxisomes are cytoplasmic organelles involved in the β-oxidation of long-chain fatty acids and the metabolism of hydrogen peroxide. Import of proteins into this compartment is directed by the sequence serine-lysine-leucine (SKL), which is located at the carboxyl-terminus of peroxisomal enzymes.

Targeting to the secretory pathway

Proteins targeted to the secretory pathway have an NH_2-terminal targeting sequence referred to as the signal peptide. As for sequences that specify nuclear or mitochondrial destinations, the signal peptide is not conserved with respect to amino acid identity but rather in its composition, i.e. it consists of a core of approximately 7–16 hydrophobic amino acids, generally within five residues of the NH_2-terminus, and is flanked by charged residues. During translation, the signal recognition particle (SRP) binds the signal peptide as it emerges from the ribosome. Binding of SRP temporarily halts translation (translational pausing) as the SRP binds to a docking protein on the surface of the endoplasmic reticulum (ER), thereby bringing the translation apparatus into contact with the secretory pathway. The signal peptide is subsequently transferred from the SRP to the signal sequence receptor, an integral ER membrane protein. Translocation into the lumen of the ER is accompanied by cleavage of the signal peptide in most, but not all, cases. Membrane proteins represent a special situation in which translocation of the protein into the lumen of the ER is halted by a stop transfer sequence, a stretch of approximately 20 hydrophobic amino acids that anchor the protein in the membrane. Membrane proteins in which the NH_2-terminus of the protein is in the ER lumen while the carboxyl-terminus is located in the cytoplasm are referred to as type I integral membrane proteins (e.g. mannose-6-phosphate receptor, Fig. 2.9). When the orientation is reversed, the protein is referred to as a type II integral membrane protein. A number of proteins have multiple stop-transfer sequences and therefore span the membrane many times. Charged residues flanking the hydrophobic transmembrane domain likely help to establish the orientation (topography) of the protein in the membrane.

Protein secretion

Translocation into the ER effectively places a protein in the secretory pathway. Proteins within the secretory pathway can be divided into two groups: proteins 'in transit' and 'resident' proteins. Proteins in transit, such as those destined for secretion, integration into the plasma membrane (e.g. a cell-surface receptor), or lysosomes, are targeted to their final destination by sorting signals that are recognized by resident proteins (receptors) in the membranes of secretory pathway organelles (ER, Golgi, secretory vesicles). Resident proteins, which may be either soluble (i.e. located within the lumen of the secretory pathway organelle) or membrane-associated, are involved in the processing of secretory pathway proteins. Structural changes arising from processing may define a sorting signal or may affect the function of the modified protein. A brief overview of processing and sorting events in the secretory pathway is presented here.

Protein processing in the secretory pathway

Folding

Many proteins are modified during transit through the secretory pathway. During, or shortly after, translocation into the ER, proteins acquire their tertiary structure (conformation) in a process referred to as folding. Folding is facilitated by chaperonins, resident ER proteins that bind to, but are not included in, the final structure of the protein, e.g. heat shock protein (HSP) 70 is a family of proteins that function as chaperones in most compartments of eukaryotic cells. In addition to their role in facilitating folding, chaperones are believed to maintain the cytoplasmic polypeptide chain in the unfolded state, which assists translocation through the ER membrane. Incorrectly folded proteins tend to form aggregates, which are degraded rather than transported to the Golgi compartment. Many proteins will not be transported out of the ER until they attain their final conformation; therefore, folding may affect the rate of transport of some proteins from the ER to the Golgi. Folding may also bring noncontiguous regions of a protein into closer proximity, thereby forming a sorting signal that is dependent upon the tertiary structure of the protein.

Glycosylation

Proteins containing the sequence asparagine-X-threonine/serine (NXT/S), where X is any amino acid except proline, may be modified by the covalent addition of a carbohydrate side-chain to form a glycoprotein. An ènzyme (oligosaccharidyl transferase) on the luminal side of the ER membrane recognizes the NXT/S sequence and catalyzes the transfer of an oligosaccharide tree, consisting of two *N*-acetylglucosamine, nine mannose, and three glucose residues, to asparagine. This modification is referred to as asparagine-linked (N-linked) glycosylation. As the glycoprotein is transported through

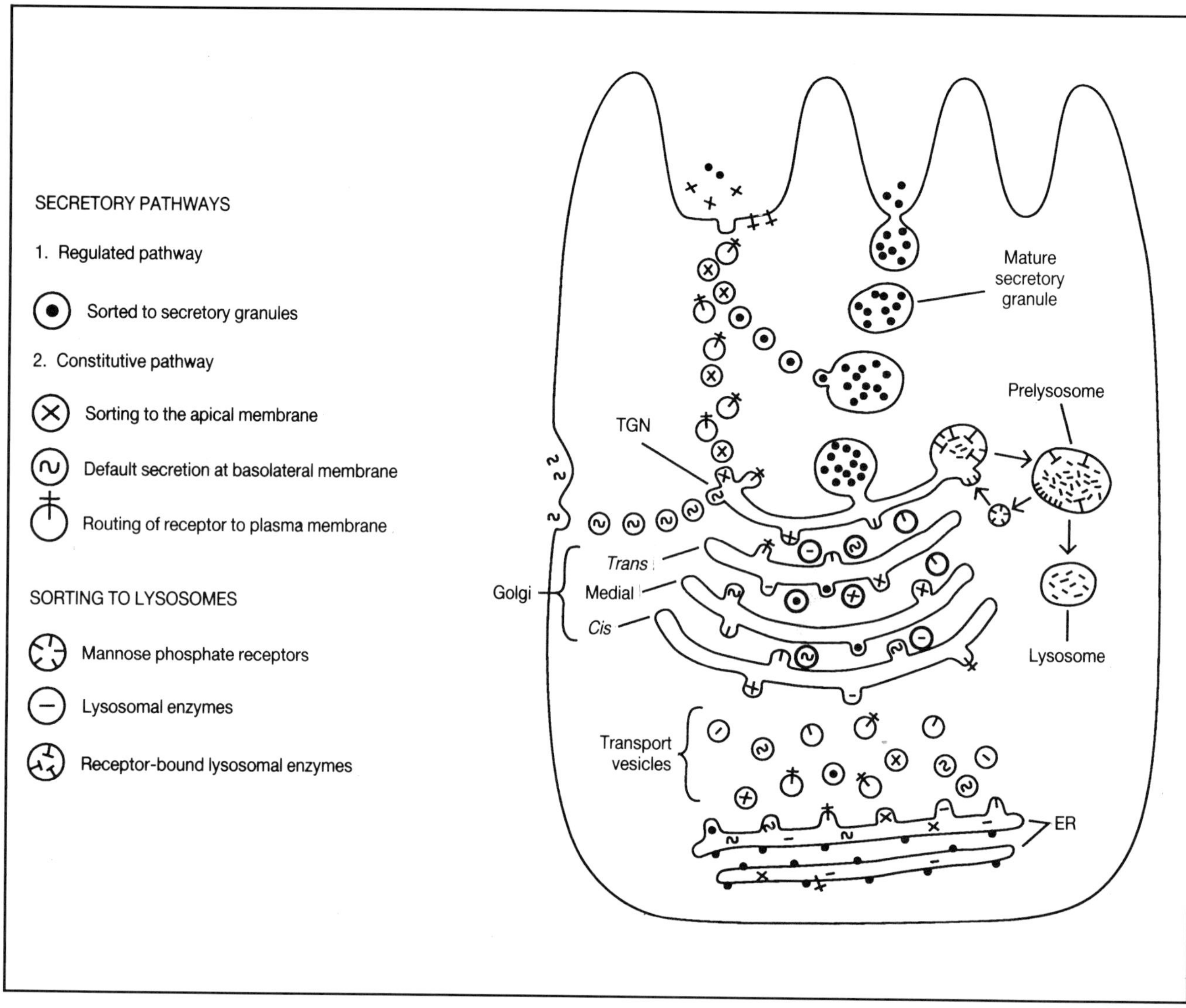

Fig. 2.9. Protein transport, sorting, and secretion in the polarized epithelial cell. The secretory pathway is involved in the routing of proteins to lysosomes and the plasma membrane as well as to the exterior of the cell. Proteins spanning the endoplasmic reticulum (ER) membrane are destined for incorporation into the plasma membrane or the limiting membrane of a secretory pathway organelle (ER, Golgi, lysosome); proteins within the lumen of the ER are destined for the lysosome or for secretion. Transport through the secretory pathway is accomplished by unidirectional budding and fusion of vesicles. Sorting of proteins for secretion or for routing to lysosomes occurs in the *trans*-Golgi network (TGN). All cells contain a constitutive secretory pathway in which proteins are released from the cell without prior concentration and in the absence of an extracellular stimulus. Constitutive secretion in polarized epithelial cells can occur at the basolateral membrane or at the apical membrane; secretion from the apical cell surface (i.e. into the lumen) probably requires a sorting signal that is recognized in the TGN. In addition to the constitutive secretory pathway, exocrine and endocrine cells contain a regulated secretory pathway in which selected proteins are concentrated within secretory granules that are released in response to an extracellular stimulus. See text for additional details.

the secretory pathway, the high-mannose oligosaccharide tree is modified by sequential trimming and addition of sugar residues to form a complex-type glycan. Glucosidases and mannosidases located in the ER remove the terminal glucose residues and four mannose residues; mannosidase in the Golgi removes two more mannose residues, while other Golgi enzymes catalyze the addition of sugars (*N*-acetylglucosamine, galactose, sialic acid, fucose) to form the complex-type glycan. The addition of phosphate to terminal mannose residues of certain glycoproteins tags these proteins for delivery to the lysosome (see below). Other than lysosomal enzymes, however, N-linked glycosylation does not appear to play a significant role in the routing of proteins in the secretory pathway.

Other post-translational modifications

Carbohydrate may also be covalently linked to proteins through serine or threonine residues (O-linked glycosylation). The addition of N- or O-linked carbohydrate has been shown to contribute to the formation of blood group antigens on some proteins and to affect the rate of internalization and degradation of other proteins; however, for many glycoproteins, the function of the carbohydrate moiety is not known. In addition to carbohydrate modification, it is becoming increasingly apparent that many proteins are modified by the covalent addition of lipid (acylation). The addition of myristic acid (myristoylation), which occurs only at an NH_2-terminal glycine, is essential for targeting of a p60 viral protein to the plasma membrane and for its transforming property. Palmitoylation (the addition of palmitic acid to cysteine, serine, or threonine) of specific proteins is essential for intracellular vesicular transport. Myristoylation, palmitoylation, and other newly uncovered lipid modifications of proteins therefore may play important roles in regulating diverse cellular functions. In addition to acylation, post-translational modifications such as phosphorylation, amidation, carboxylation, and proteolytic cleavage are well documented. For each post-translational event, corresponding information must be encoded within the protein structure that allows specific enzymes to recognize the signal and catalyze the modification. These covalent modifications in turn may direct the localization of proteins or alter the biological activity of the molecule.

Protein sorting in the secretory pathway (Fig. 2.9)

In the absence of sorting signals, proteins translocated into the ER are transported by bulk flow to the Golgi and from there to the plasma membrane for secretion. This is referred to as the default (constitutive) secretory pathway. Diversion from the default pathway requires recognition by sorting signals encoded within the protein structure.

Sorting in the endoplasmic reticulum

The ER is a membrane-limited tubular sac that forms an extensive network within the cytoplasm of the cell. This is the most proximal part of the secretory pathway, and proteins enter this compartment by virtue of an NH_2-terminal signal peptide (in most cases). In addition to secretory and membrane proteins that are in transit, the ER also contains proteins involved in post-translational processing and phospholipid synthesis that must be retained within this compartment. The soluble (cisternal) ER proteins BiP (binding protein, a member of the heat shock protein 70 family) and protein disulfide isomerase (PDI), which facilitate protein folding and assembly, contain the sequence lysine-aspartic acid-glutamic acid-leucine (KDEL) at their carboxyl termini. BiP and PDI enter the default secretory pathway, but are recovered in a post-ER compartment, by binding to a receptor recognizing the KDEL tag, and returned to the ER. Integral membrane proteins of the ER have a transmembrane domain that confers ER residency.

Sorting in the Golgi

The Golgi apparatus consists of a series of stacked membranes that can be divided functionally into the *cis*-, medial-, *trans*-Golgi and *trans*-Golgi network (TGN); some evidence indicates that the TGN may in fact be a discrete organelle. The most extensively characterized function of the Golgi is the modification of asparagine-linked oligosaccharide chain of glycoproteins, which are destined for integration into the plasma membrane or secretion. Oligosaccharide processing involves the sequential removal of mannose residues and the addition of specific sugar molecules (e.g. *N*-acetylglucosamine, galactose, and sialic acid). In the case of lysosomal proteins, mannose residues are not removed and phosphate is added as the terminal moiety. This mannose-phosphate structure serves as a sorting signal that diverts the protein from the secretory pathway to the lysosome. The machinery for protein sorting appears to be located primarily in the TGN; within this compartment, proteins targeted to lysosomes are separated from those destined for secretion. Secretory proteins are also sorted in the TGN so that those proteins containing sorting signals are diverted from the constitutive (default) secretory pathway into the regulated secretory pathway (see below). Finally, the TGN is also the site of sorting for membrane proteins in polarized epithelial cells, which have distinct apical and basolateral membranes (see below). Relatively little is known about the sorting signals or the machinery involved in the recognition of these signals, with the notable exception of lysosomal enzymes. Likewise, little is known about signals involved in the retention of resident Golgi proteins involved in glycoprotein processing.

Sorting to lysosomes

Lysosomes are acidic vacuoles that serve as the major site of intracellular degradation. Unlike other organelles (nucleus, mitochondria, peroxisomes), lysosomes import their proteins (hydrolytic enzymes, e.g. cathepsin D) through the secretory pathway rather than the cytoplasm. Lysosomal enzymes therefore must contain at least two targeting signals, i.e. a signal peptide for translocation into the ER lumen and a modified N-linked oligosaccharide chain that diverts the enzyme away from the constitutive secretory pathway and to the lysosome. The tag that directs specific glycoproteins to the lysosome is the addition of phosphate to terminal mannose residues, an event that occurs in the *cis*-Golgi compartment. Because many proteins contain N-linked oligosaccharide, the phosphorylating enzyme must recognize a structural determinant unique to all lysosomal enzymes. Mannosylphosphate residues are bound by mannose phosphate receptors (MPR) in the TGN. Receptor-bound lysosomal enzymes are transferred to an acidic prelysosomal compartment where dissociation of receptor and ligand is facilitated by the low pH. The soluble enzymes are then transferred to the lysosome, while the membrane-bound receptor is recycled to the Golgi.

Sorting into the regulated secretory pathway

The constitutive secretory pathway is common to all cell types and involves the continual release of secretory vesicle contents without prior concentration of the protein and in the absence of any extracellular stimulus. In addition to this pathway, exocrine and endocrine cells concentrate and store selected proteins in secretory granules that are released in response to an extracellular stimulus (regulation of secretion in this pathway is not absolute, and low-level basal secretion occurs in the absence of external cues). This pathway, referred to as the regulated secretory pathway, requires the presence of a sorting signal that allows diversion of the protein away from the constitutive secretory pathway. Sorting of proteins into the regulated secretory pathway occurs in the TGN and may occur by a receptor-mediated process similar to that described for lysosomal enzymes. Alternatively, the sorting signal may promote selective association of proteins bound for the same secretory granule leading to aggregation, condensation, and consequently, diversion from the constitutive pathway. The latter model has the advantage of explaining both the selective routing and concentration of proteins targeted to the regulated secretory pathway.

Epithelial cells represent a special situation in which the apical surface of the cell is opposed to a lumen whereas the basolateral cell surface is in contact with neighboring cells. The apical and basolateral domains established by epithelial cell polarity have distinct protein-lipid compositions. Fusion of secretory vesicles with the apical membrane results in the addition of integral membrane proteins to this domain of the plasma membrane and the release of secretory vesicle contents into the lumen. The current model of secretion by polarized cells proposes that secretion from the apical surface requires a sorting signal that is recognized in the TGN; secretory vesicle fusion with the basolateral membrane is the default pathway that does not require a sorting signal.

Protein transport (Figs 2.9, 2.10)

Transport in the biosynthetic pathway

Endoplasmic reticulum-to-Golgi transport

The analysis of protein transport within the secretory pathway has been greatly facilitated by the identification of yeast mutants in which transport can be selectively arrested at different points in the pathway. These studies indicate that as many as 25 distinct gene products are necessary for transport from the ER to the cell surface. Although the elucidation of the function of each of these proteins is ongoing, it is now evident that at least 10 of these proteins are involved in ER-to-Golgi transport.

Proteins leave the ER in transport vesicles that bud and pinch off from ribosome-free regions of the ER. Transport vesicles fuse with the *cis*-Golgi, thereby delivering their

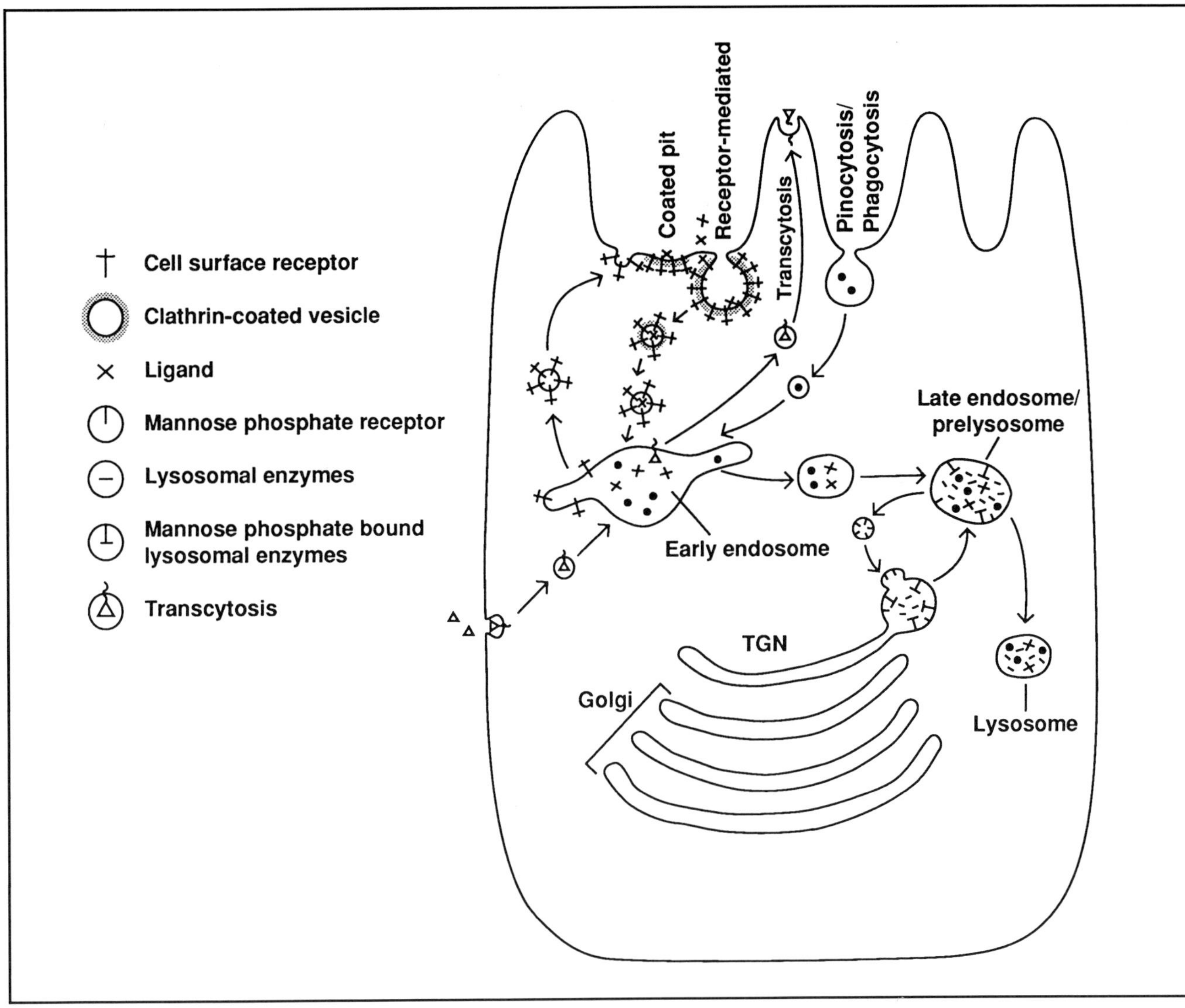

Fig. 2.10. The endocytic pathway. Proteins may be taken up by the cell in a nonspecific manner (pinocytosis or phagocytosis) or selectively (receptor-mediated internalization). Transport from the cell surface to the endosome occurs in endocytic vesicles; vesicles in the receptor-mediated pathway are distinguished by a clathrin coat (stippled vesicles), which is removed prior to fusion with the endosome. The lower pH in the endosome facilitates uncoupling of the receptor and ligand. The receptor may be recycled back to the cell surface or routed to the lysosome with the ligand for degradation. In polarized epithelial cells, the ligand and its receptors may be internalized at one surface and released at the opposing cell surface, a process referred to as transcytosis. Sorting of receptor and ligand for degradation, recycling, or transcytosis probably occurs in the endosome. See text for additional details.

contents and membrane to this organelle. Proteins involved in the transport process are required for vesicle budding, targeting of the vesicles to the *cis*-Golgi face, and fusion of transport vesicles with the Golgi membrane. GTP-binding proteins, GTP hydrolysis, and Ca^{2+} play a critical role in this process and likely contribute to the unidirectional flow of proteins from the ER to Golgi.

The rate of transport for a specific protein from the ER may be largely dependent upon the extent of interaction with the resident ER proteins. Proteins with complex structures interact extensively with resident proteins such as BiP and PDI, which promote correct folding and assembly. Incorrectly folded proteins are retained within the ER and selectively degraded. The half-time for transit in the secretory pathway therefore varies from as little as 20 minutes to as much as 3 hours.

Golgi-to-cell surface

The mechanism of transport through the Golgi cisternae and to the cell surface is similar to protein transport from the ER: transport vesicles bud and pinch off from the Golgi cisternae and are transferred to the target membrane with which they fuse. However, unlike ER-derived vesicles, Golgi-derived transport vesicles are covered by a protein coat that is distinguished from the protein coat of endocytic vesicles (see below) by the absence of the protein clathrin. This protein coat must be removed from the transport vesicle prior to fusion. Therefore, in addition to proteins involved in transport and targeting, Golgi-derived vesicles require coating and uncoating proteins.

The progression of secretory proteins from the *cis*-Golgi through the medial and *trans*-cisternae to the TGN depends upon the sequential budding and fusion of transport vesicles. Transport from the TGN varies depending upon the secretory pathway for which the protein is destined. Proteins following the constitutive secretory pathway are transported to the cell surface in vesicles similar to those involved in intra-Golgi transport. Transport vesicles in the regulated secretory pathway also serve as storage granules. These vesicles, referred to as secretory granules, arise as proteins are sorted away from the constitutive secretory pathway and begin to condense in the TGN. Secretory granules are released at the cell surface in response to an extracellular stimulus (secretagogue). There is evidence that elements of the cytoskeleton may play an important role in the transport of secretory granules and other transport vesicles bound for the cell surface.

Uptake of proteins (Fig. 2.10)

Exocytosis results in the incorporation of the membrane surrounding the transport vesicle into the plasma membrane. Membrane is returned to the cell interior by the process of endocytosis. The process of endocytosis involves the infolding of the plasma membrane to form an endocytic vesicle: when particulates are trapped in the vesicle, the process is referred to as phagocytosis; the uptake of soluble molecules is referred to as pinocytosis. Endocytosis is also the primary pathway for the internalization of proteins that bind to cell-surface receptors, a process referred to as receptor-mediated endocytosis. Internalization is preceded by clustering of receptors into coated pits (so called because of the clathrin protein coat) in the plasma membrane. Coated pits invaginate and pinch off to form coated vesicles (endocytic vesicles), which subsequently lose their clathrin coats before fusing with endosomes. The lower pH in the endosomal compartment results in the uncoupling of receptor and ligand followed by routing of the receptor back to the plasma membrane and the ligand to the lysosome. While this is a common pathway for many internalized receptor ligand complexes, alternate sorting pathways clearly are also present in the cell. The receptor and ligand may be individually or collectively sorted to the lysosome, the cytoplasm, or another plasma-membrane domain, a process referred to as transcytosis. The signals that define the destinations of the receptor and ligand and the cellular machinery involved in recognition and sorting are currently active areas of investigation. Recent studies suggest that the cytoplasmic domain of cell-surface receptors contain signals involved in internalization and targeting of many receptor–ligand complexes.

Protein degradation

In order to maintain a steady state, synthesis of new protein must be offset by the degradation of existing protein, a process referred to as protein turnover. The rate of protein degradation varies widely among proteins, and there is an absolute requirement for energy expenditure consistent with a highly selective process. Most proteins internalized by the endocytic pathway are degraded in the lysosome. Recent evidence suggests that specific cytoplasmic proteins may also be selectively targeted to the lysosomes for degradation by the sequence lysine-phenylalanine-glutamic acid-arginine-glutamine (KFERQ). Cytoplasmic proteins may also be targeted for degradation by covalent conjugation to the 76-amino acid polypeptide ubiquitin. Ubiquitin-conjugated proteins are selectively broken down in an ATP-dependent fashion by specific cytoplasmic proteases. In addition to these more extensively characterized pathways, evidence increases for a separate proteolytic pathway in the ER that is involved in the hydrolysis of incorrectly folded or assembled polypeptides. It seems increasingly likely that other pathways involved in selective protein degradation will be uncovered.

Summary

Cell types differ by expression of a unique subset of proteins that contribute to their specialized structure and/or function. Coordinated regulation of expression of these proteins during development is essential for the organization of specialized cells into tissues. Appropriate selection of specific proteins for expression, restriction of their expression to specific cell types, and timing of their expression during development are crucial for normal growth and differentiation. The basic machinery involved in protein expression is common to most cell types. Information encoded within the structure of the newly synthesized protein directs its movement among cellular compartments, regulates its function, and determines its fate. The decoding of this information by the cellular machinery plays an important role in integrating fundamental biological processes such as gene expression, proliferation, differentiation, metabolism, locomotion, and cell–cell communication.

Selected reading

Castle JD. Sorting and secretory pathways in exocrine cells. *Am J Respir Cell Mol Biol* 1990; **2**: 119.

Nygård O, Nilsson L. Translational dynamics. Interactions between the translational factors, tRNA and ribosomes during eukaryotic protein synthesis. *Eur J Biochem* 1987; **191**: 1.

Pfeffer SR, Rothman JE. Biosynthetic protein transport and sorting by the endoplasmic reticulum and Golgi. *Annu Rev Biochem* 1987; **56**: 829.

Schwartz AL. Cell biology of intracellular protein trafficking. *Annu Rev Immunol* 1990; **8**: 195.

D. Cell Interaction with the Microenvironment

R A Akeson

Interactions with the microenvironment are essential in the regulation of normal development and cell function. During development, cells proliferate as uncommitted precursors, often migrate to distinct locations, and after migration, differentiate to form mature populations of neuronal cells, lymphocytes, epithelial cells, etc. These combined processes underlie the morphogenesis that achieves the ultimate forms of cells, organs, and finally organisms. In multicellular organisms, individual cells do not develop into their mature shape and function autonomously, but are guided and regulated by complex series of interactions among molecules and cells. The genome contains the complete potential complement of gene products that constitute an organism. However, interactions between cells and their environment restrict the set of gene products that are expressed, creating cells of distinct phenotypes found in brain, bone marrow, lung, etc.

Cell proliferation is regulated by interactions with soluble growth factors and by interactions among adjacent cells. While many growth factors circulate in classical endocrine fashion, some growth factors are actually displayed on the surfaces of adjacent cells or sequestered from extracellular fluids by components of the microenvironment. The term paracrine refers to growth factors mediating interactions among neighboring cells. Autocrine interactions are those in which the cell produces and releases factors modulating its own growth. Thus the local environment plays two roles in cell division, and the combination of circulating and local factors is critical in regulating cell division.

Cell migration is fundamentally dependent on cell–environment interactions because, with the exception of sperm, vertebrate cells cannot swim in an oriented fashion. Cells that move in a directed fashion must do so in contact with a solid substrate. Even lymphoid cells which circulate must interact with solid tissue components of the vasculature in order to enter or leave the circulation. Furthermore the solid substrate is not simply a passive component in the migration process. Cells attach to and move on solid substrates via specific interactions with the polypeptide and carbohydrate containing constituents of the substrate. Thus in order for a cell to migrate it must display receptors appropriate for the substrate it encounters.

During development, cells migrate in distinct directions based on the composition of the substrate in different locations, along with the repertoire of receptors for that substrate that the cells express. Likewise, differentiation of a cell to the mature phenotype generally is not autonomous, but rather depends on mutual interactions between sets of cells and between cells and their environment. A classic example may be found in the interactions between developing epithelia and underlying mesenchyme. In general, the overlying epithelium will form a differentiated structure such as a hair follicle, sweat gland, feather, or tooth only in the presence of instructive signals from the underlying mesenchyme. While the epithelium forms the structure, the mesenchyme determines the type of structure formed. A remarkable model of such interaction is the experimental recombination of jaw mesenchyme from a mouse with epithelium from a chick. The epithelium differentiates to form a tooth of chick origin. Thus chick epithelium has the capability to form a tooth (despite the fact that birds and their ancestors have not formed teeth for 100 million years) and expresses this capability when in close contact with the appropriate mesenchyme. This epithelial–mesenchymal interaction is representative of similar interactions that mediate the development of all body organs. Local interactions combine with broader endocrine signaling to mediate development. Another familiar example of this phenomenon is the requirement for immature lymphocytes to migrate to the thymus and interact directly with thymic epithelial cells in order to become mature T cells or thymocytes. The structural development of the neural crest shows the most dramatic requirement for migration and tissue interaction. Neural crest cells originate and undergo initial cell divisions in contact with the neural tube. Some leave the neural tube and migrate under the skin to give rise to melanocytes. Others migrate in the body cavity and give rise to the sympathetic and sensory ganglia. Grafting experiments have shown that the premigratory crest cells are largely identical, and that the cell types and structures to which they give rise are determined by their migratory path and final environment.

Conceptually, cell microenvironment interactions can be divided into interactions among cells and interactions between cells and the extracellular matrix (ECM). This conceptual difference is applicable at the molecular level as well, because cells use distinct sets of cell-surface components for these two forms of interaction. This section first outlines the constituents of the ECM and the receptors used by cells to interact with both the ECM and other cells. Specific developmental and clinical examples follow to illustrate the role of these interactions in cellular physiology.

Extracellular matrix

The ECM comprises the scaffolding that helps to organize cells into discrete structures and organs. Together with the bony skeleton, it gives form to the body. The ECM is particularly prominent in relatively acellular structures such as cartilage and tendon, but also plays a major role in the formation of epithelial structures through the actions of basement membranes, and generally represents the major limiting structure dividing organs and body compartments. Thus with the exception of brain, all tissues contain significant amounts of ECM. The three major structural components of the ECM are the **collagens**, the **noncollagenous proteins**, and the complex carbohydrates of the ECM, the **glycosaminoglycans**.

Collagens

Collagens represent the single most abundant polypeptides in vertebrates. More than a dozen collagen genes have been identified to date. All have distinct patterns of expression in developing tissues. Collagen types I and III are the most abundant collagens in most connective tissues. These are synthesized as single procollagen chains, which are assembled through proteolytic processing and covalent modification of the procollagen monomers to form three-chain triple-helical structures called tropocollagens. The high proportion of glycine and proline or hydroxyproline residues, which are often found in repeating triplets of glycine-proline-X (where X = any amino acid), allows the collagens to form tight helices. Stretching of these helices is a major factor contributing to the elasticity of connective tissues. While collagens I and III are primarily triple-helical structures, many of the other collagens have both triple-helical and nonhelical globular regions. The globular regions appear to have more specialized functions, including formation of more complex structures. Collagen type IV, the major constituent of basement membranes, forms a mesh-like structure that represents the major element in the formation of these critical limiting membranes. In addition to underlying both epithelial and endothelial cell layers, basement membranes define structures including kidney glomeruli and the capsule of the lens. Collagens interact with glycosaminoglycans and the noncollagenous ECM components to give the ECM both its form and many of its physical characteristics of elasticity and resistance to tearing.

Defects in collagen synthesis and assembly during development contribute to a number of disease conditions. For example, some forms of *osteogenesis imperfecta,* a heterogeneous group of disorders characterized by abnormal bone formation, are due to mutations in the pro-α_1(I) collagen gene. Defects in a collagen-processing peptidase result in the soft, deformable skin and tendons observed in *Ehlers–Danlos syndrome.* A number of genetic conditions including *chondrodysplasia punctata* and *Marfan syndrome* appear to be due to unknown ECM defects. It is instructive to compare Marfan syndrome, which produces a substantially increased risk of aneurysms in adults, with a mouse model in which there is a total loss of collagen type I genes. Mice homozygous for this gene defect die *in utero* from internal hemorrhages at the age at which significant blood pressure develops. While the defect in Marfan syndrome is not a simple collagen defect, the requirement for ECM integrity in development and maintenance of the vascular and other systems is clear.

Glycosaminoglycans

The glycosaminoglycans (GAGs) are long, linear structures made up of repeating units of a dimer of two distinct hexasaccharides. Each GAG type has a unique dimer repeat. The sugars of GAGs are generally distinct from those found on glycoproteins and are often sulfated.

These long, linear chains are covalently attached to core proteins, the proteoglycans, which may be closely or loosely associated with the cell membrane. One exception to this generalization is hyaluronic acid, in which the repeating disaccharide lacks sulfate and which is not attached to a core protein. Hyaluronic acid is a major constituent of most ECM, particularly early in development, and the water-binding and viscoelastic characteristics of hyaluronic acid gels are major factors in the resilience and lubricating qualities of cartilage and joints. The sulfated GAGs, including chondroitin, dermatan, keratan, and heparan sulfate, are expressed by more specialized tissues and are implicated in a variety of functions including cell–ECM interaction and growth factor binding.

One category of defects in glycosaminoglycan metabolism deserves special mention, namely defects caused by failures in the ability to degrade the complex GAGs and glycolipids of the cell surface. These lysosomal storage diseases, often called the *mucopolysaccharidoses,* result in the formation of large secondary lysosomes filled with partially degraded carbohydrates. These lysosomes can inhibit cell function, causing a variety of symptoms among the conditions, the most universal symptom being mental retardation.

Noncollagenous proteins

Several large noncollagenous polypeptide components of the ECM have dramatic effects on cell behavior. These peptides, including fibronectin, laminin, and vitronectin, seem to comprise a number of independent peptide domains that have been recombined through evolution to create multifunctional proteins. Individual cell types have receptors that interact with one or often several of these proteins. Furthermore, cells may interact with multiple individual domains within a single protein. For example, fibronectin has domains that bind to cell-surface integrin receptors (below), to heparan sulfate-like carbohydrates found in cell-surface proteoglycans, and to the ECM components collagen and hyaluronic acid (Fig. 2.11). By binding through multiple interactions both to cells and to the ECM, fibronectin and the other members of this group serve as major mediators of cell–ECM adhesion and interaction. These polypeptides are particularly prominent in basement membranes, where they mediate adhesion and migration, but are found in other ECM-rich areas as well. Other noncollagenous components of the ECM, such as the multi-domain protein cytotactin, are thought to be antiadhesive. Soluble cytotactin inhibits adhesion of cultured cells to ECM. Such factors could serve to create boundaries limiting cell migration during development. These boundaries may help to create the major divisions between body structures. For example, migrating neural crest cells avoid regions of the somite rich in cytotactin. This avoidance forces the crest cells to migrate to more discrete regions of the embryo, and this is one factor in the later coalescence of these cells to form individual ganglia of the peripheral nervous system. In addition to their simple adhesive and antiadhesive functions, the noncollagenous ECM proteins also have been shown to promote cell differentiation. Thus this group of proteins plays a fundamental role in development.

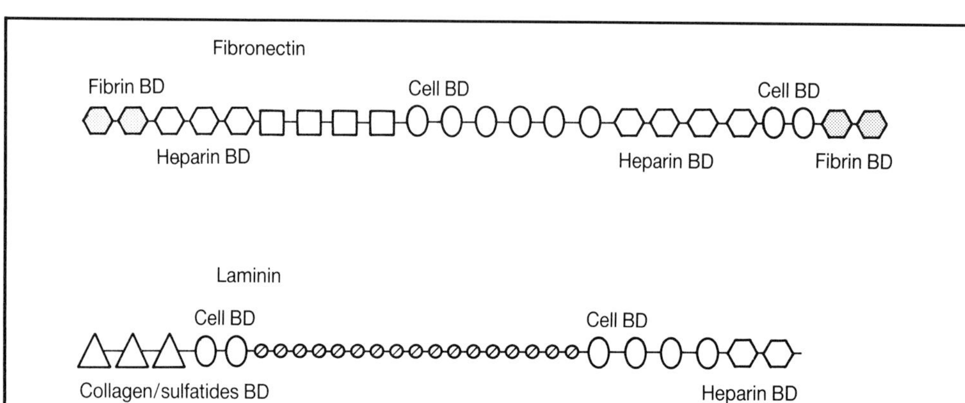

Fig. 2.11. The modular nature of the ECM noncollagenous proteins, fibronectin and laminin, is shown in these cartoons of single chains. Binding domains for cells (indicated as Cell BD) and for other ECM constituents are found at distinct sites in the linear polypeptide sequences. Although only single chains are schematically illustrated, fibronectin in ECM exists as disulfide-linked dimers and laminin exists as a trimer of nonidentical chains.

Cellular receptors for the microenvironment

Cellular receptors for the microenvironment can be divided into two groups: those that interact primarily or exclusively with components of the ECM, and those that interact with other cells (Table 2.2). The major receptor family that interacts with the ECM is the integrins, which are receptors composed of two polypeptide chains. Individual cells may express multiple α and β chains, which themselves can be combined variously to create receptors for fibronectin, laminin, collagen, and other ECM components. Some cells express receptors constitutively, while in others, particularly lymphocytes and monocytes, expression is induced by cytokines or other stimuli. Modulation of integrin expression is critical to normal development as well as to other events including tissue inflammation and wound healing.

Three major families of cellular receptors interact with other cells: the immunoglobulin supergene family, the cadherin family, and the selectin family. Members of the immunoglobulin supergene family are so named because, although entirely independent genes, they share a fundamental protein structural motif—the immunoglobulin domain—with true immunoglobulin molecules. Over 30 members of this group have been identified, and they are particularly prominent on cells of neural and lymphoid lineages. For example, I-CAM (immune-cell adhesion molecule), which has five immunoglobulin-like domains, is expressed on many lymphocyte subpopulations and mediates lymphocyte–lymphocyte interactions. Curiously, it also is the cell attachment site for the rhinovirus, the agent that mediates the common cold. Immunoglobulin supergene family members may bind to identical or distinct molecules on adjacent cells.

Cadherins require external calcium in order to mediate cell–cell adhesion. Members of this family tend to be tissue-specific (N- or neural cadherin, E- or epithelial cadherin, etc.) and are essential in establishing and maintaining tissue integrity. Cadherins on one cell bind to identical cadherins on adjacent cells. All cadherins studied to date bind only to themselves, e.g. N-cadherin-expressing cells bind to other N-cadherin-expressing cells, but not to E-cadherin-expressing cells.

The selectins are polypeptide receptors that bind to carbohydrate-containing glycoproteins or glycolipids on adjacent cells. This family, discovered more recently, has been found primarily on lymphoid and endothelial cells, although the full extent of its distribution is unknown. One notable example is the ELAM-1 receptor, which is expressed by cytokine-activated endothelium and mediates initial binding of granulocytes to endothelial cells. This binding is an early step in the extravasation of granulocytes during inflammation.

Individual cells interact with the ECM via integrins, proteoglycans, and other molecules. They interact simultaneously with adjacent cells via one or more of the cell–cell adhesion systems. The number and type of these interactions represent major regulatory points in controlling cell development and function (Fig. 2.12).

Cell–cell and cell–ECM interactions regulate cell division in development

Cell proliferation is regulated by both hormonal signals and local cell–cell interactions during development. The

Table 2.2. Categories of cell-adhesion systems

	Integrins	Immunoglobin supergene	Calcium-dependent	Selectins
Examples	Fn R (VLA-3) Fn R CSIII (VLA-4) Ln R (VLA-1) LFA-1 VnR	CEA L1/Ng-CAM DCC ICAM NCAM	N-cadherin P-cadherin E-cadherin T-cadherin R-cadherin	CD44/Hermes GMP-140 ELAM-1 LECAM-1
Polypeptide	Two chain	One chain	One chain	One chain
Distribution	Most cells	Many cells especially neurons + lymphocytes	On most cells—one cadherin only	Lymphocytes/endothelial

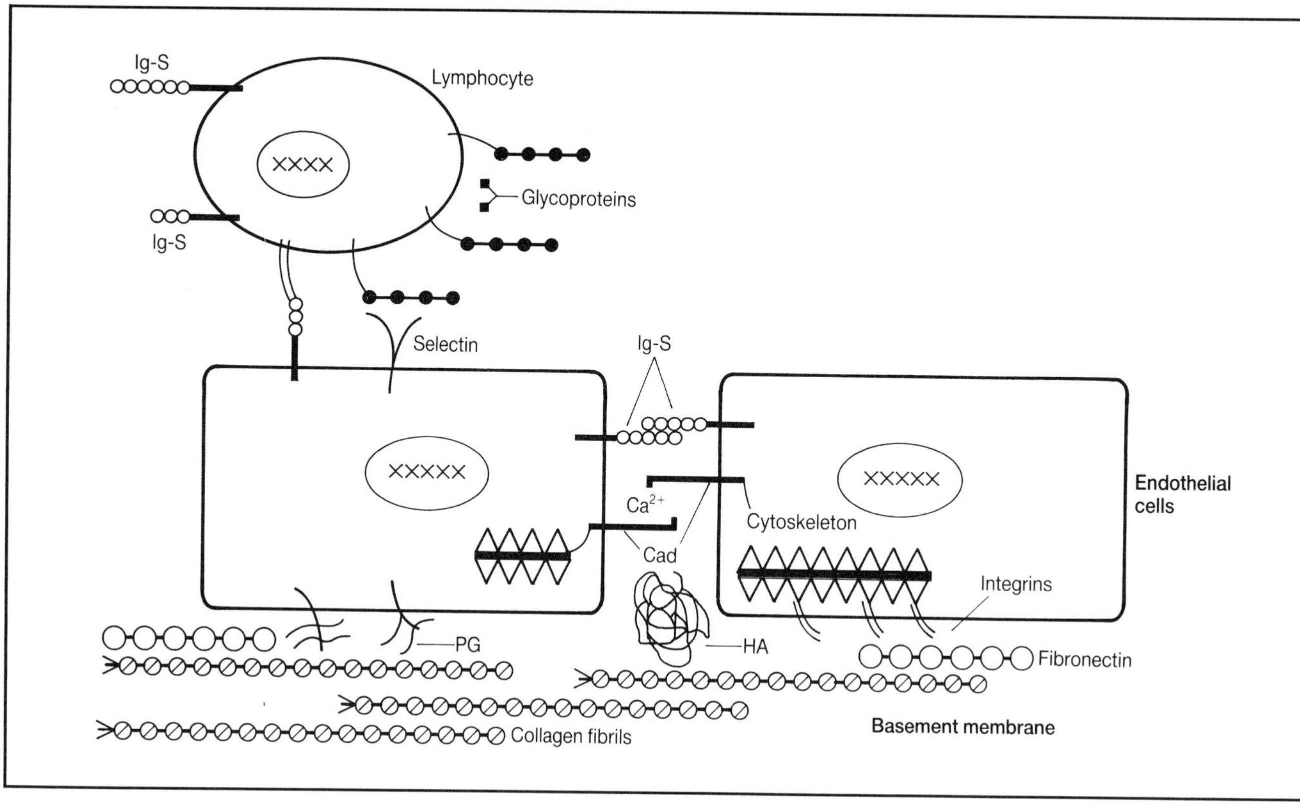

Fig. 2.12. Two endothelial cells are shown interacting with the collagen and fibronectin components of the basement membrane via cell-surface proteoglycan (PG) and integrin receptors. Hyaluronic acid (HA) in the ECM regulates physical properties of the matrix. The cells adhere to each other via both immunoglobulin superfamily class adhesion molecules (Ig-S) and also the calcium-dependent cadherin receptors (Cad). Both cadherins and integrins interact with cytoskeletal elements to stabilize their interactions. One of the cells interacts via the selectin class of receptors with carbohydrate-containing components of a lymphocyte. The lymphocyte and this cell also interact via integrin to immunoglobulin superfamily receptor binding. Distinct members of the immunoglobulin supergene family have varying numbers of immunoglobulin-like domains as indicated by the number of open circles in the cartoon representation.

white spotting (W) and steel mutant mice illustrate a unique system of interaction between these two regulatory systems. Mutant W and steel mice have defects in melanocyte migration (hence the name), the proliferation and/or migration of primitive germ cells, and aspects of hematopoiesis. Recent genetic analyses have demonstrated that steel mice lack a previously undiscovered growth factor now named stem cell growth factor or mast cell growth factor. W mice lack the receptor for this growth factor. Detailed analysis of the murine genes demonstrated that cells express this growth factor both by secretion as a diffusible hormone, and as a part of a larger polypeptide present at the cell surface. Initial evidence suggests that the cell-surface form is critical in regulating aspects of development and mediates both cell adhesion and cell proliferation. The soluble form may be more important in hematopoiesis and is currently in clinical trials. Thus analysis of these mouse mutations not only illustrates the intricacy with which cell–cell contact regulates cell division, but also has permitted the discovery of an entirely new growth factor.

The notch gene of *Drosophila* encodes a very large transmembrane protein that mediates cell adhesion in a calcium-dependent fashion, and so is by definition a cell-adhesion molecule. Notch is identified as a neurogenic gene based on the fact that *Drosophila* notch-deletion mutants undergo hyperplasia of neural cells with a consequent deficit of epithelial cells within the neuroepithelial region of the embryo. Genetic evidence suggests that notch mediates an inhibitory signal, passed from cell to cell by direct contact, which regulates the proportion of epithelial cells that undergo differentiation to neuroepithelial cells. Thus notch-mediated cell–cell communication regulates both cell division and differentiation at this point in development. In completely independent experiments, workers characterizing genes at the breakpoints of chromosomal locations characteristic of human T-cell lymphoblastic leukemias identified a human homolog of the notch gene. In many neoplasms, evidence indicates that altered expression of genes at or near characteristic chromosomal breakpoints plays a direct role in neoplastic transformation. The implication of a notch-like gene in T-cell transformation suggests that altered cell–cell interaction plays a role in the induction of this leukemia. Furthermore, it illustrates the diverse uses to which cell-surface signaling molecules can be utilized by different species during evolution. The *Drosophila* notch gene is expressed primarily by neural tissue, while the human (and mouse) notch homologue is expressed in many adult tissues, but most strongly in lymphoid tissues.

Improper regulation of epithelial proliferation is also observed in the gastrointestinal tract in familial syndromes of intestinal polyps. Most pediatric polyps are isolated and of acquired inflammatory origin. *Juvenile polyposis* syndromes are characterized by multiple polyps, which usually are not adenomatous in the pediatric period (except in Gardner syndrome), but generally indicate substantial risk of adenoma development in adult years. A variety of gene defects have been observed in adult colonic adenomas, some related to adhesion molecules. These include alterations in two members of the immunoglobulin supergene family. DCC (for deleted in colon cancer) levels are much reduced in at least some adenomas, and CEA (carcinoembryonic antigen) levels are elevated to the extent that CEA is often used as a serum marker for proliferative diseases of the colon of both inflammatory and neoplastic origin.

Disorders in the regulation of cell division are the hallmark of *neoplasia.* Studies of the interaction of normal and malignantly transformed cells with fibronectin have been particularly illustrative of the potential role of ECM components in regulating cell division. In comparisons of normal and transformed cells during the 1970s, a number of experimenters found that transformed cells lacked a large cell-surface constituent, which ultimately was purified and named fibronectin. In many cell lines, this absence was traced to a deficit in the integrin receptor for fibronectin. Further studies of the relationship between cell transformation and cell adhesion to the ECM demonstrated that for many tumors of solid-tissue origin, oncogenic transformation causes down-regulation of integrin expression and subsequent loss of adhesive capability. This loss may contribute to the potential of transformed cells to metastasize to distant sites in the body. In experimental models, artificial restoration of integrin levels by transfection of malignant cells with expression vectors containing integrin-encoding cDNAs for a fibronectin receptor resulted in loss of tumorigenicity *in vivo*. This loss of tumorigenicity was observed despite continued expression of oncogenes by the cells. These results indicate the key role that cell–ECM interactions play in regulating the behavior of malignant as well as normal cells.

Inhibition of cell migration alters development

Detailed analyses of the portion of the fibronectin to which most integrins bind have demonstrated that within this large molecule of over 2000 amino acids, the simple tripeptide arginine-glycine-aspartate (RGD in single letter abbreviations) represents the integrin-binding site. Added soluble peptides containing RGD inhibit cell–fibronectin adhesion *in vitro* and alter cell migration *in vivo*. For example, injection of such peptides into developing chick embryos can inhibit the migration of neural crest cells. The resultant embryos lack or have greatly reduced peripheral ganglia. This experiment demonstrates that the cell migration essential for development is mediated via cell adhesion to the RGD sequence of fibronectin (and other ECM components). While neural crest cells present a dramatic example, most cells express receptors with RGD affinity; thus many additional developmental events are mediated by this interaction. RGD-containing peptides are easily synthesized and can be incorporated into a variety of artificial matrices. Current clinical trials are evaluating the potential of such matrices to enhance wound repair. These agents also have potential value in other systems requiring restoration of normal ECM or manipulation of cell–ECM interaction.

Neural crest cells also give rise to the enteric neurons responsible for the innervation and coordinated function of the intestine and colon. In *Hirschprung disease* or aganglionic megacolon, the typical newborn presentation is failure to pass meconium. Rectal biopsy indicates an absence of neural tissue in the distal colon. The available evidence indicates that this deficit is due to failure of migration of the neural crest cells, and animal models reproducing this migration failure have been developed. Surgical resection is the current treatment for this defect in cell migration.

Kallman syndrome is an X-linked disease characterized by the unusual primary combination of hypogonadotropic hypogonadism and anosmia (inability to smell), with frequently observed neurological, eye, and kidney defects. The cause of the hypogonadism was defined decades ago as a hypothalamic inability to synthesize gonadotropin-releasing hormone (LHRH or GnRH), but the relationship between this deficit and the anosmia was unclear. Combined recent observations clearly indicate that Kallman syndrome is a disease of cell migration. The first set of observations came from embryological analyses of the origin of the hypothalamic LHRH-releasing cells. Unlike most cells of the midbrain and forebrain, these cells do not derive from the neurectoderm/neural tube, but instead are derived from the olfactory placode, an embryonic ectodermal thickening, which gives rise primarily to the cells of the nasal epithelium. A subset of olfactory placode cells migrate in development into the forebrain and become the LHRH-releasing cells. In Kallman syndrome, these cells are born but apparently fail to migrate. Recent molecular cloning of a gene product absent in Kallman syndrome has identified a new molecule, the predicted structure of which has some similarities to those of neural cell-adhesion molecules of the immunoglobulin supergene family. In the absence of this adhesion molecule, olfactory placode cells apparently cannot migrate to the hypothalamus and differentiate there, thus giving rise to the syndrome.

Deficits in cell adhesion molecules alter the functions of differentiated cells

One dramatic role of integrins in development is exemplified by the *Drosophila* 'lethal myospheroid' mutation. *Drosophila* embryos with this mutation develop normally until late stages. At this time, during which spontaneous muscle activity is initiated, the embryonic muscles pull loose from the tendons and ball up, forming 'myospheroids'. These embryos then die. Cloning of the mutated gene illustrated that it was a β_1-like integrin, which therefore appears to be critical for the normal interaction of muscle and connective tissue.

A clinically illustrative example of the effects of deficits in integrin-mediated cell adhesion comes not from cells adherent in solid tissues, but from leukocytes. Patients with *leukocyte adhesion deficiency,* a relatively rare syndrome, present as infants with recurrent bacterial infections that can be fatal. Although humoral immunity and T- and B-cell numbers are relatively normal, granulocytes from these patients show impaired chemotaxis, adherence to plastic, and phagocytosis *in vitro*. Analysis of cell-surface components of these granulocytes demonstrated the absence of a high molecular weight polypeptide, which ultimately was identified as the leukocyte adhesion molecule LFA-1, also known as Leu-CAM and integrin $\alpha_L\beta_2$. In granulocytes LFA-1 is a major mediator of phagocytosis, and deficits in LFA-1 result in the observed inability to clear bacterial infections. This deficiency thus presents a very clear example of the relationship between a molecular deficiency in a cellular receptor, a consequent change in cellular physiology, and human pathology.

Members of the calcium-dependent cadherin family of cell adhesion molecules are differentially expressed among tissues. A new member of this family has been identified through the identification of antigens reactive with autoantibodies from patients with *pemphigus vulgaris (PV),* an autoimmune disease of the skin in which loss of cell–cell adhesion of skin keratinocytes results in life-threatening blister formation. Screening of expression libraries with autoantibodies identified a target antigen having a sequence similar to previously identified cadherins. This target antigen is thus a new epithelial-specific cadherin. The symptoms of autoimmune disease are believed to be caused by competitive inhibition of cell–cell interaction by circulating antibody. This disease thus illustrates the potential consequences of alterations in cell–cell interaction and may be representative of a broader range of defects, the molecular bases of which are currently not understood. In this regard, it is interesting to note that the PV antigen is most closely related in sequence to the cadherin-related desmosome component desmoglein. Desmoglein is expressed by all desmosome-containing tissues, while the PV antigen is limited to stratified squamous epithelia. Autoantibodies to desmoglein are observed in another blistering disease, *pemphigus foliaceus,* in which blisters are found more superficially, in the epithelium above the squamous layer. This observation is consistent both with the tissue distributions of these antigens and with the hypothesis that other cell–cell interaction molecules may represent disease targets.

Summary

The development, structure, and functional integrity of organs is maintained by receptor-mediated interactions between adjacent cells and between cells and the extracellular matrix. Lymphoid cells also interact with each other and bind to and penetrate solid tissue through receptor-mediated events. Genetic deficits in the expression of matrix component or cellular receptors as well as extragenetic events that interfere with receptor function all can compromise cellular or organ function to cause developmental or functional pathology. At the same time, these processes represent target points at which pathological events can be understood, approached, and treated.

Selected reading

Albelda SM, Buck CA. Integrins and other cell adhesion molecules. *FASEB J* 1990; **4**: 2868.

Hay E, ed. *The cell biology of the extracellular matrix*. 2nd ed. New York: Plenum Press, 1991.

Labat-Robert J, Bihari-Varga M, Robert L. Extracellular matrix. *FEBS Lett* 1990; **268**: 386.

McDonald JA, Mecham RP, eds. *Receptors for extracellular matrix*. San Diego, California: Academic Press, 1991.

Ruoslahti E. Fibronectin and its receptors. *Annu Rev Biochem* 1988; **57**: 375.

3 ◆ *Developmental biochemistry and metabolism*

Editor: R D G Milner

A. Protein and Amino Acid Metabolism

R D G Milner

Protein requirements

Dietary protein provides all the amino acids necessary for the biosynthesis of tissue proteins and nonprotein nitrogenous compounds such as nucleic acids. Each day more amino acids are degraded and resynthesized in the body than are ordinarily consumed in the diet. Dietary amino acids are required for the synthesis of new tissue constituents at all ages but particularly during growth. Amino acids consumed in excess of these needs are not stored but are degraded, the nitrogen being excreted and the carbon skeleton recycled. All 20 amino acids must be present for protein synthesis to occur. Nine amino acids, histidine, isoleucine, leucine, lysine, methionine, phenylalanine, threonine, tryptophan and valine, are not synthesized in the body and are therefore **essential** for wellbeing. Arginine is essential in infancy and in the preterm infant there is a transient need for dietary tyrosine and cysteine.

Dietary protein requirements to maintain health are modest judged by Western intakes: an adult needs no more than 1 g protein/kg body weight and a baby no more than 3 g/kg each day, but dietary protein deficiency remains the most serious nutritional problem in the world and causes *kwashiorkor* in toddlers. A balanced shortage of all nutrients due to starvation results in *marasmus*.

Protein digestion and absorption

(see also Chapter 9)

Dietary protein is digested by proteolytic enzymes and peptidases in the gut. Proteolytic enzymes are secreted as large precursors called zymogens. Pepsinogen (a 40.4 kDa peptide) is secreted from the chief cells in the wall of the stomach under the stimulation of gastrin. Gastrin simultaneously stimulates the release of HCl from the parietal cells causing the pH of the stomach contents to drop and pepsinogen to be autocatalytically cleaved into pepsin (32.7 kDa) and inert peptides. Pepsin itself then causes the further activation of pepsinogen as well as cleaving dietary proteins into large peptides. Gastric protein hydrolysis is important but not essential in protein digestion. Passage of the stomach contents (chyme) into the duodenum stimulates the release of the hormones secretin and pancreozymin from the duodenal mucosa which in turn cause the secretion of pancreatic juice that is both alkaline and rich in digestive enzymes. Secretin alone causes the secretion of an alkaline protein-poor pancreatic juice, whereas pancreozymin causes the secretion of an enzyme-rich juice. There is a family of pancreatic proteolytic enzymes. Some, such as trypsin, chymotrypsin and elastase, split proteins and polypeptides at specific internal sites in contrast to carboxypeptidases that cleave individual amino acids from the carboxyl ends of polypeptide chains. The end products of pancreatic digestion are free amino acids, dipeptides and small peptides. Further amino acid hydrolysis takes place in intestinal mucosal cells by aminopeptidases and dipeptidases.

Both amino acids and small peptides are absorbed by stereospecific transport systems located in the membrane of the intestinal mucosal cell. There are at least five specific transport systems: one each for small neutral amino acids, large neutral and aromatic amino acids, basic amino acids, proline and glycine, and acidic amino acids (Table 3.1). Most of the transport mechanisms are coupled to Na^+ ion transport. Many if not all the transport mechanisms participate in the γ-glutamyl cycle immediately after the stereospecific uptake step. This involves the tripeptide glutathione serving as a donor of a γ-glutamyl group to form a dipeptide with the absorbed amino acid. Once in the cell the dipeptide is cleaved and the glutamyl group resynthesized in a five-step cycle. One turn of the wheel costs 3 ATP. Proline is not transported via the γ-glutamyl cycle. Any absorbed peptides are hydrolyzed in the mucosal cell and only amino acids are released into the portal blood. Inherited defects of an amino acid transport system in both the gut and the kidney may result in conditions such as *cystinuria, glycinuria,* or *Hartnup disease* (Table 3.1). Despite the inability of the intestine to transport large neutral and aromatic amino acids in *Hartnup disease* the patient faces

Table 3.1. Specific intestinal transport systems for amino acids and diseases associated with transport defects

Amino acid group	Examples of amino acids transported	Disease
Acidic	Aspartic and glutamic acids	
Basic	Arginine, lysine, ornithine, cystine	Cystinuria
Small neutral	Alanine, serine, threonine	
Large neutral and aromatic	Isoleucine, leucine, valine, tyrosine, tryptophan, phenylalanine	Hartnup disease
Glycine, proline		Glycinuria

few problems because essential amino acids bypass the block by being absorbed as peptides.

Amino acid catabolism

Deamination

Following absorption amino acids pass via the portal circulation to the liver to enter the metabolic pool of the body where they may undergo transamination or oxidative deamination (Fig. 3.1). Both processes produce keto acids, but oxidative deamination produces ammonium ions directly whereas in transamination the amino group passes to another keto acid. The coupling of the glutamate dehydrogenase reaction, in which the amino group is split from glutamate to produce α-ketoglutarate and ammonium, to a glutamate-requiring transaminase reaction produces a system capable of making ammonium from almost all amino acids. Aspartate aminotransferase is of particular significance because it contributes an amino group to oxaloacetate to make aspartate and aspartate is the donor of one of the two nitrogen atoms in urea. The deamination of amino acids by the L-amino acid oxidases of the liver and kidney is of lesser importance. These enzymes have a broad specificity but a slow rate of oxidation. The fate of amino acid nitrogen is dealt with on p. 79.

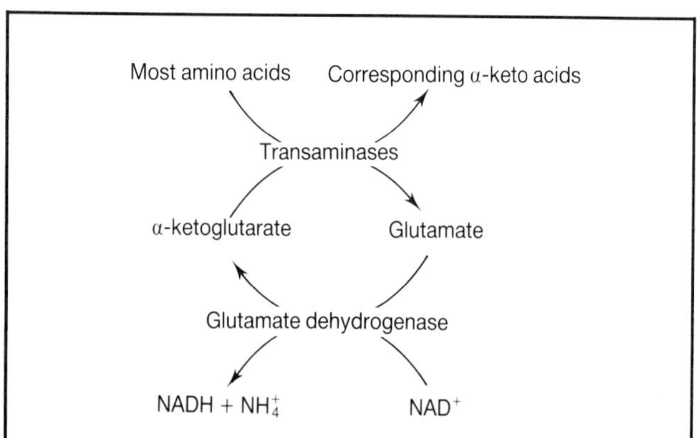

Fig. 3.1. Schematic representation of transamination and oxidative deamination.

Fate of the carbon skeleton

The fate of the amino acid carbon skeleton is particularly important during fasting when gluconeogenesis is essential in maintaining substrate delivery. Most of the amino acids utilized come from muscle. A certain degree of amino acid catabolism takes place *in situ* to cater to muscle energy needs, but a problem arises because the nitrogen generated from transamination and deamination can only be converted to urea in the liver. This is resolved by the synthesis of alanine from pyruvate which then acts as the nitrogen transporter to the liver where transamination yields glucose for the return journey. This is referred to as the 'glucose alanine cycle' (Fig. 3.2). Another mechanism for exporting nitrogen from muscle is by the synthesis of glutamine from glutamate. Glutamine can release its amine in both the intestine and kidney. The kidney uses serine as a nitrogen transporter to the liver.

The carbon skeletons provide energy via conversion into ketones, glucose, or both. Most amino acids are glycogenic. Only leucine is completely ketogenic. Isoleucine, lysine, phenylalanine, tyrosine and tryptophan are both ketogenic and glycogenic. The entry points of the amino acid skeletons into the metabolic pool and Krebs cycle are summarized in Fig. 3.3. More important than learning details of the pool is the appreciation that both types of precursor are energy sources and that certain

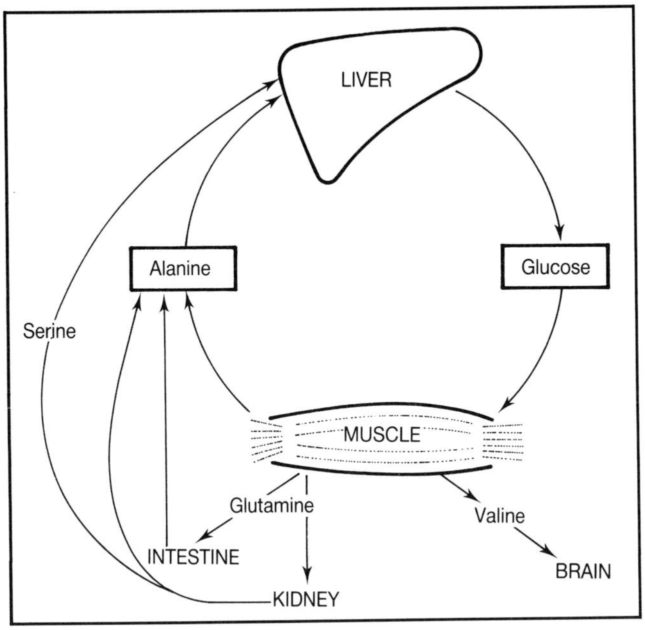

Fig. 3.2. The glucose–alanine cycle.

enzyme deficiencies in amino acid catabolism result in inborn metabolic errors which are clinically important. The reader should consult a reference text on inborn metabolic errors for information on specifics.

Amino acid synthesis

General principles

The mix of amino acids present in the diet is not in the proportions needed by the body and must be modified. Changes take place in the gut mucosa and the amino acid spectrum in the portal blood differs from that of the food ingested with alanine levels being higher and glutamate and aspartate being lower. Alanine is the principal transporter of nitrogen to the liver from both ingested food or from muscle during fasting.

Nonessential amino acids can be made by

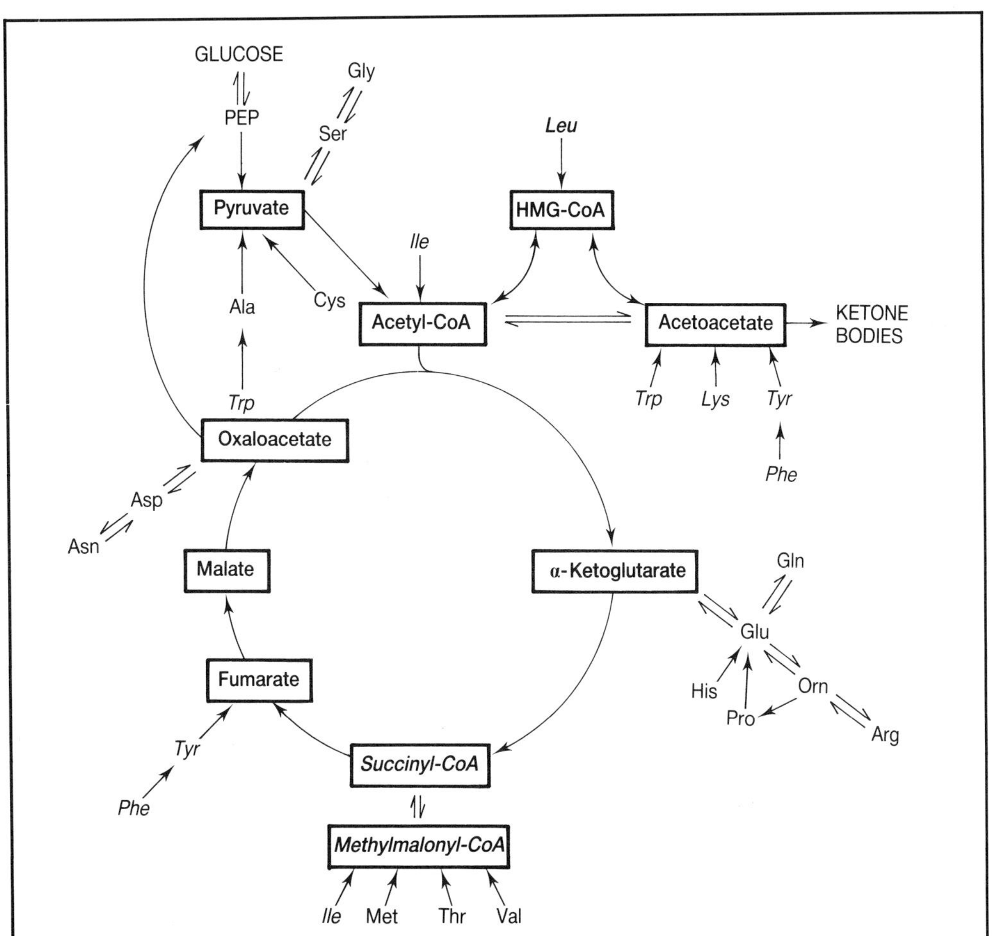

Fig. 3.3. The metabolic fates of the amino acid carbon skeletons. Amino acids shown in italics may be ketogenic. Only leucine and lysine must be ketogenic.

transamination of the carbon skeletons of intermediates of the glycolytic pathway and Krebs cycle. Glutamate is the commonest amino donor in all transamination reactions. Within the Krebs cycle glutamate and aspartate act as reciprocal amino donors in the transamination couplings glutamate/α-ketoglutarate and aspartate/oxaloacetate (see Fig. 3.1). Glutamate provides the amino acid for the transamination pairs: pyruvate/alanine and 3-phosphoglycerate/serine which occur in the glycolytic pathway. Serine is the precursor of glycine which is formed by transfer of the serine hydroxymethyl group to tetrahydrofolate.

Both aspartate and glutamate can be converted to their respective amides, asparagine and glutamine. Glutamine is formed by the direct linking of glutamate and ammonium under the influence of glutamine synthetase. Asparagine is formed by the donation of an amino group from glutamine to aspartate under the influence of asparagine synthetase. In each case ATP is consumed.

Methyl group transfer is biologically important and can be conveniently illustrated by the biosynthesis of cysteine from methionine. Hepatic methionine adenosyl transferase catalyzes the formation of *S*-adenosyl-methionine (SAM) from methionine and ATP. SAM is the principal methyl donor in the body and examples of the end products include: creatine, phosphatidylcholine, methylated RNA, methylated DNA and epinephrine. In yielding up the methyl group SAM becomes *S*-adenosyl-homocysteine which is then split by a hydrolase to homocysteine and adenosine. Homocysteine can be metabolized back to methionine by two routes. In one transmethylation reaction, betaine, derived from the oxidation of choline, is the donor. The other mechanism is important in folate and vitamin B_{12} metabolism and involves donation of a methyl group by 5-methyl tetrahydrofolate.

Specific amino acids

Cysteine

Cysteine is made up of a sulfhydryl derived from homocysteine and a carbon skeleton from serine. The two amino acids condense under the influence of cystathionine synthetase to form cystathionine which is then split by cystathionase to give homoserine and cysteine. *Homocystinuria* is due to a deficiency of cystathionine synthetase and *cystathioninuria* to a defective cystathionase that will not bind to the coenzyme pyridoxal phosphate. In addition to being required for protein synthesis, cysteine is also used to make the tripeptide glutathione and the amine taurine.

Tyrosine

If enough phenylalanine is available adequate amounts of tyrosine can be synthesized. The enzyme involved is phenylalanine hydroxylase and tetrahydrobiopterin is involved as a coenzyme. Deficiency of the enzyme results in *phenylketonuria*, an autosomal recessive condition characterized by mental retardation and underpigmentation. Tyrosine has a number of biosynthetic roles; it acts as a precursor for thyroxine, melanin pigments and catecholamines. Elevated blood concentrations of tyrosine may be found in all forms of *liver failure*, but are characteristic in *hepatorenal tyrosinemia (tyrosinemia type 1)* due to fumaryl acetoacetase deficiency which presents as *infantile cirrhosis* and *renal Fanconi syndrome*. *Tyrosine aminotransferase (TAT) deficiency (Richner–Hanhart syndrome* or *tyrosinemia type 2)* also causes high tyrosine concentrations and is characterized by keratosis and corneal dystrophy.

Proline

Proline is synthesized from arginine via a series of reactions. In the first arginase splits arginine to ornithine and urea. The ornithine is then transaminated to yield glutamate-γ-semialdehyde which, by closure of the Schiff base to form a ring and by subsequent reduction, is converted to proline.

Arginine and histidine

While both arginine and histidine are nonessential for the adult they may be needed in the diet of infants who cannot synthesize adequate amounts for growth. Arginine is made from ornithine in the urea cycle (see p. 80). The status of histidine as an essential/nonessential amino acid is not clear as deprivation experiments in man have been short term and under these conditions histidine shortage can be made good by conversion of the related molecule carnosine.

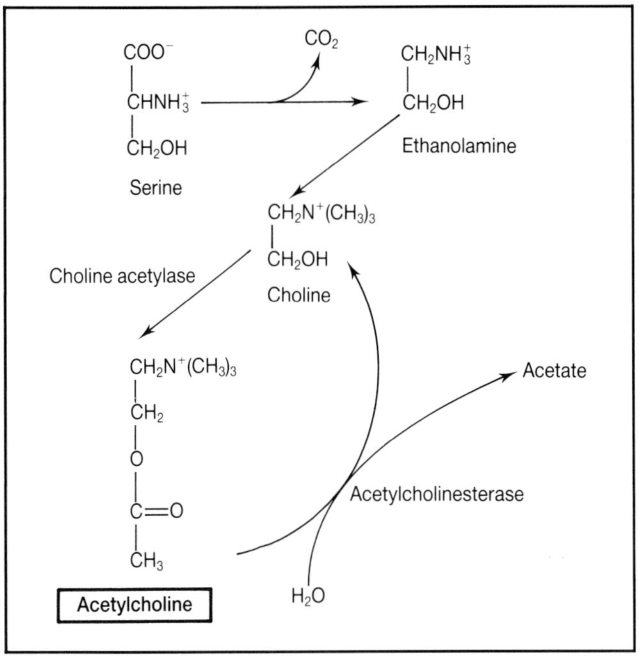

Fig. 3.4. The synthesis and hydrolysis of acetylcholine.

Amino acids as precursors of metabolites

Some of the most important amines derived from amino acids are neurotransmitters. Acetylcholine is formed from choline which in its turn is derived from serine via ethanolamine (Fig. 3.4). Catecholamines are derived from dopamine which in turn is derived from tyrosine via the intermediate L-dopa (used in the treatment of *Parkinson disease*) (Fig. 3.5). Serotonin is a signaling molecule found in the central nervous system and gut mucosa. It is synthesized by the hydroxylation and decarboxylation of tryptophan. The decarboxylation of glutamate produces γ-aminobutyrate (GABA) which is an inhibitor of central nervous system transmission. Histamine is formed by the decarboxylation of histidine.

Glycine and arginine are involved in the synthesis of creatine, an important muscle metabolite. The prime store of muscle energy is phosphocreatine. Hydrolysis of phosphocreatine produces creatinine which is commonly

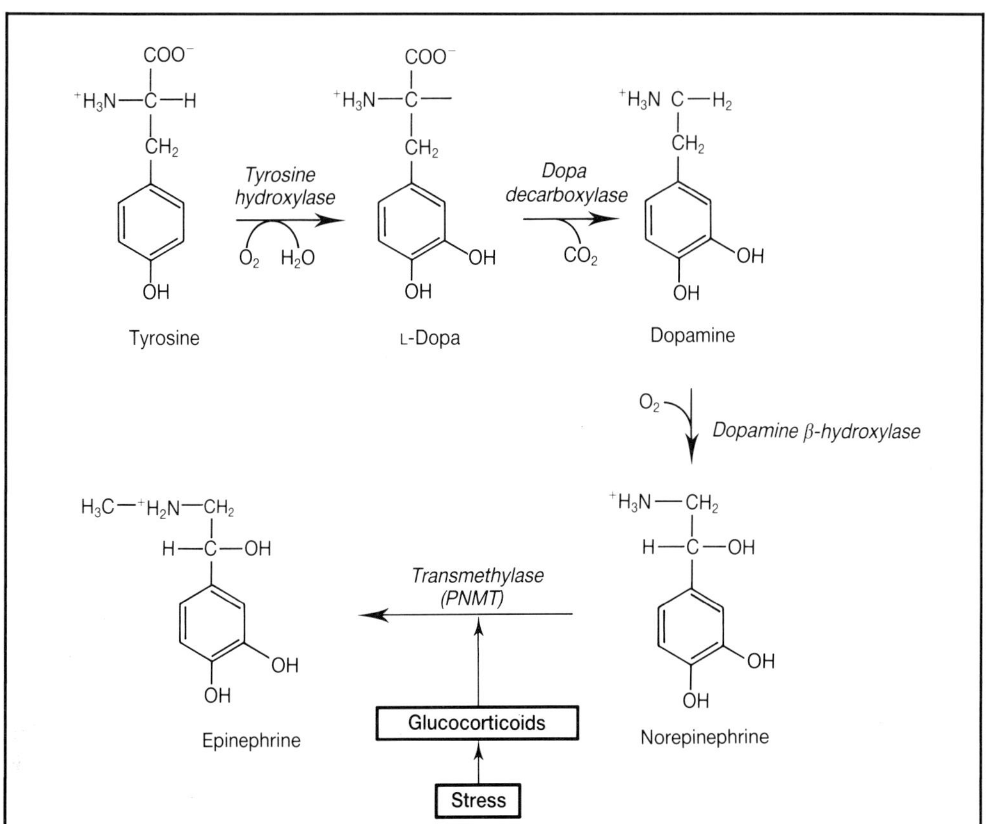

Fig. 3.5. The synthesis of catecholamines.

measured in the blood and urine as an index of both renal function and muscle turnover. Carnitine is a small nitrogen-containing molecule involved in the transport of fatty acids across mitochondrial membranes. It is synthesized from protein-bound lysine. *Inborn metabolic errors of fatty acid β-oxidation* result in a fall in circulating carnitine due to an accumulation of esterified carnitine and dietary carnitine therapy is beneficial.

Protein synthesis and structure

The subject is too complex to be fully tackled here and what follows is an outline to illustrate the principles involved.

Polypeptides are formed by the condensation of amino acids and are linear in form with a free amino group at one end and a free carboxyl at the other. Polypeptides of molecular weight of more than several thousand are called proteins. Each protein or polypeptide has a unique sequence of amino acid residues in its chain which determines both its biological and physicochemical properties. Control of protein synthesis resides in the nucleotide sequences of deoxyribonucleic acid (DNA) and each polypeptide or protein is controlled by an individual gene (see p. 48).

When amino acids link to form polypeptides and proteins the potential for flexible movement is variably restricted by the intrinsic C–N bond, covalent cross-linkages such as –S–S– bonds, hydrogen bonds, ionic interactions and hydrophobic interactions. The gross patterning of polypeptide chains is in a helix or a pleated sheet and both may be found in the same protein. The sequence of amino acids in a polypeptide chain is referred to as the primary structure and the three-dimensional shape assumed by the protein is the tertiary structure. The component of the tertiary structure which is stabilized by hydrogen bonds is known as the secondary structure. Some proteins are composed of subunits and the final aggregated form is referred to as the quaternary structure. The tertiary and quaternary structures of proteins are vital to their roles as binding molecules in which specificity is all important. Examples include the binding of O_2 to hemoglobin, hormones to receptors, and enzymes to substrates.

Proteins have been classified in various ways, e.g. by solubility or by combination with other groups to form conjugated proteins. The characteristics that permit proteins to be separated and quantified are complex and a description of some of the proteins commonly found in blood will serve to illustrate many of their important properties. When blood clots several plasma proteins are consumed in the clot matrix. Serum, the solution associated with a clot, lacks fibrinogen, fibrin and other clotting factors. Plasma is the solution associated with unclotted blood. The normal protein concentration of plasma is 60–80 g/l of which 30–50 g is albumin and 15–30 g a mixture of globulins. Plasma protein concentration is measured densitometrically and individual protein classes are identified by electrophoresis which permits classification into albumin, α_1-globulin, α_2-globulin, β-globulin and γ-globulin. The γ-globulins are primarily synthesized by plasma cells whereas most of the other plasma proteins are synthesized in the liver.

Albumin is the most abundant protein in plasma. It is a globular protein of 66 300 Da consisting of a single polypeptide chain which is strongly negatively charged at physiological pH. The main functions of albumin are to provide osmotic pressure within the capillary and to transport small molecules. Albumin is the prime transporter of poorly soluble molecules such as FFA and bilirubin that need to move from one compartment to another to be metabolized. It also binds poorly soluble drugs such as aspirin, digoxin and barbiturates and all of these may displace natural metabolites. Albumin is the principal transporter of small cations and anions in the blood stream. Half the Ca^{2+} in plasma is bound to albumin.

α_1-Globulins are mainly glycoproteins and high density lipoproteins (HDL). α_2-Globulins include haptoglobin which is the transport protein for free hemoglobin, ceruloplasmin, the copper transport protein, prothrombin (a proenzyme involved in blood clotting), glycoproteins and very low density lipoproteins (VLDL). The major β-globulins are transferrin, the iron transport protein, and low density lipoproteins (LDL). The γ-globulins are immunoglobulins and are grouped into five subclasses each of which is heterogenous, containing thousands of molecules. The synthesis of a particular immunoglobulin (antibody) is provoked by exposure of the plasma cells to a foreign protein or complex carbohydrate (antigen) and the newly made molecule has the characteristic of binding tightly, by specific noncovalent bonds, to produce an antigen–antibody complex which is then eliminated. Five subclasses are recognized—IgG, IgA, IgD, IgE and IgM—and all share a similar general quaternary structure of two light and two heavy polypeptide chains (see p. 667).

Developmental aspects

Before birth

Prenatal growth involves much protein synthesis, especially in the second and third trimesters. The normal human newborn contains about 500 g protein, most of which is accumulated in a linear manner from week 22 to term as the fetus grows from 250 g to 3500 g. The rate of protein synthesis slows as pregnancy advances but it is always greater than in the adult. Increased synthetic rates are accompanied by increased breakdown and the fetal turnover of protein is much faster than occurs postnatally. There is also marked variation between organs in the rate of protein synthesis. Studies in fetal lambs towards term indicate that the half-life of protein synthesized in the liver and heart is approximately 1 day whereas that of muscle is about 1 week. Placental protein turnover is similar to that in the fetal liver and heart. Although protein turnover in all fetal tissues slows with advancing gestation it remains 4–6 fold faster than in the adult. Substrate delivery is the main controlling influence on fetal protein synthesis. Insulin was found to stimulate protein synthesis in muscle only and then only in the presence of hyperaminoacidemia. Insulin-like growth factor I (IGF-I) may also play a role in regulating fetal protein synthesis. In addition to being used for protein synthesis amino acids are important sources of metabolic fuel for the fetus accounting for up to 25 percent of O_2 consumption. This implies an early ontogeny for transamination pathways and nitrogen metabolism.

A consequence of the dynamism of fetal amino acid metabolism is that plasma circulating concentrations are higher than after birth. In contrast maternal circulating amino acid concentrations are low throughout pregnancy and the fetal/maternal ratio is greater than 1, being greatest in the second trimester (approximately 3) and falling towards term (approximately 1.6). The pattern of maternal circulating amino acids differs from that of the nonpregnant woman with glycine, leucine, ornithine, lysine, arginine, serine and α-amino butyrate concentrations all being significantly reduced. In contrast alanine, the amino acid metabolic shuttle between muscle and liver, is elevated. *Toxemia of pregnancy* impairs placental transport of nutrients to the fetus and amino acids in particular. Both maternal and fetal plasma amino acid concentrations rise, but the maternal proportionately more with a consequent fall in the fetal/maternal amino acid ratio. Prolonged pregnancy associated with *intrauterine growth retardation* is also characterized by a drop in the fetal/maternal amino acid ratio due largely to a rise in maternal circulating concentrations. *Overt maternal malnutrition during pregnancy* results in changes in both the mother and newborn infant resembling those seen in *kwashiorkor*. The plasma aminogram of the pregnant woman shows significant increases in ornithine and glycine and a high glycine/valine ratio. In the first hours of life, the aminogram of the infant shows increased concentrations of alanine, proline, glycine and taurine and a slower than normal postnatal fall in branch chain amino acid concentrations. In contrast women from low socioeconomic groups, who subsequently gave birth to light-for-dates babies, had an aminogram that was reduced 20 percent overall but which showed both increases and falls in different groups of amino acids. Ornithine, arginine and aspartic acid were all reduced more than 30 percent, while isoleucine, methionine, valine and cystine were all higher than found in normal pregnancy. The changes again suggest selective alterations in different placental transport groups and/or fetoplacental amino acid metabolism.

Despite fetal amino acid plasma concentrations being higher than maternal, placental cytosolic levels are higher still. The transport of amino acids across the placenta involves both the direct active transfer of essential amino acids from maternal to fetal plasma and placental cytosolic synthesis of nonessential amino acids. The placental concentrations of the metabolically labile straight chain and acidic amino acids are particularly high partly as a consequence of *de novo* synthesis. There are considerable interspecies differences in placental amino acid transport but in humans amino acid transport occurs both by passive diffusion and Na^+-independent and Na^+-dependent carrier-mediated systems (see p. 405).

The concept of an essential amino acid has a new dimension when considering the fetus. Both fetal and placental tissues possess a wide variety of transaminases and deaminases, enabling processing into the mix the fetal tissue needs of those amino acids the placenta can take up. Rapid protein synthesis, coupled with an uneven pattern of enzyme maturation, means that certain amino acids which are nonessential postnatally are essential to the fetus. For example, cystathionase is completely absent from the human fetal liver and the fetus is entirely dependent upon the mother for cystine. The transsulfuration pathway that converts methionine to cystine develops postnatally and it is prudent to regard cystine as remaining essential for some time postnatally. Histidine also appears to be essential for the fetus on the pragmatic evidence that infants fed a low histidine diet show impaired nitrogen retention and poor weight gain. In contrast to the adult the newborn appears unable to make adequate amounts of histidine and by extrapolation so too is the fetus.

Neonatal changes

Big changes in plasma amino acid concentrations occur rapidly after birth. Overall there is a fall in most amino acids which is significant at 4 hours and progresses to become maximal at 24 hours. The fall is greatest in the essential amino acids with the nonessential amino acids and in particular glycine showing a modest rise. The ratio of nonessential amino acids to essential amino acids is 1.3 in the cord blood, rises to a maximum of 2.8 at 24 hours and then remains about 2.0 for several days. Infants born preterm show exaggerated changes and in those suffering *intrauterine growth retardation* the glycine/valine ratio correlates directly with the degree of weight deficit. What the fate of the different amino acids is remains less clear. Protein synthesis continues at a rapid pace immediately after birth and some of the amino acids are consumed in this process. Fat is the principal source of energy in the newborn and it is unlikely that amino acids normally provide a source of calories to milk-fed infants. However, metabolic balance studies on parenterally fed preterm infants show that fat can be replaced as a caloric source by carbohydrate and amino acid.

Selected reading

Felig P. Amino acid metabolism in man. *Annu Rev Biochem* 1975; **44**: 933.

Montgomery R, Conway TW, Spector AA. *Biochemistry, a case oriented approach*. St Louis: CV Mosby, 1990.

B. Ammonia Metabolism: The Urea Cycle

G N Thompson

The fate of dietary protein

The net utilization of dietary protein for protein synthesis varies with age and nutritional state but normally accounts for about 40 percent of intake in infants and 20–30 percent in adults. The majority of the protein ingested is catabolized by oxidative mechanisms and less than 0.5 percent is excreted as urinary free amino acid. The rate of amino acid oxidation increases with feeding and decreases during growth, but there is always a background obligate oxidation of amino acids even during starvation and malnutrition. This obligate oxidation accounts for about 0.3 g protein/kg body weight per day. All amino acids, by definition, contain nitrogen and the common product of amino acid oxidation is ammonia. Ammonia is also generated as a product of purine and pyrimidine metabolism and by metabolism of amines. These reactions take place in a number of tissues but make only a small contribution to total ammonia production. Ammonia is highly toxic and cannot be readily excreted in the urine. A series of enzymes collectively known as the 'urea cycle' converts ammonia to urea which is excreted by the kidneys.

Sources of nitrogen for urea production

Amino acid oxidation takes place in most tissues but the urea cycle is sited exclusively in the liver. The toxicity of ammonia precludes its transport to the liver as a free ion and most nitrogen for catabolic degradation is transported to the liver as alanine or glutamine. Alanine is formed directly as a product of the transamination of glutamate to pyruvate. The reversal of this reaction (Fig. 3.6) forms serine which is in equilibrium with glycine. Glycine also conjugates with benzoate to form hippurate and advantage is taken of this therapeutically in the treatment of *inborn errors of the urea cycle*. Glutamine is formed directly from ammonia via reaction with glutamate through glutamine synthase. While alanine is transported directly to the liver to enter the urea cycle, glutamine is

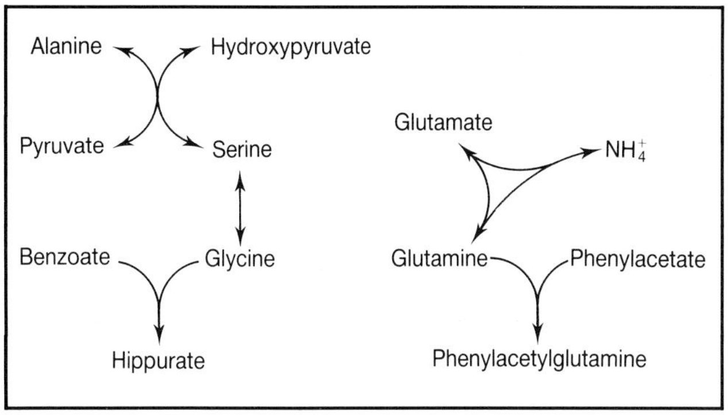

Fig. 3.6. Pathways of waste nitrogen removal by conjugation of amino acids (glycine, glutamine) with therapeutic agents (benzoate, phenylacetate).

mainly metabolized in the gut. Absorptive cells of the small intestine are unusual in that they release ammonia directly into the portal vein for subsequent hepatic metabolism by the urea cycle. The majority of the ammonia produced by intestinal mucosal cells comes from circulating glutamine, but some 30 percent is derived from protein digested in the gut. Glutamine can be conjugated with the drug phenylacetate forming phenylacetylglutamine (Fig. 3.6) which, like hippurate, can be readily excreted in the urine. Since glutamate, the precursor of glutamine, is also in equilibrium with serine, some glutamate nitrogen is removed by benzoate therapy. The combination of benzoate and phenylacetate therapy is very effective in reducing pathological *hyperammonemia*.

There is some support for a role for the kidney in producing nitrogen substrate for the hepatic urea cycle. Citrulline, originating principally from the gut but also from peripheral tissues, may be converted to arginine by the action of arginosuccinic acid synthase and arginosuccinic acid lyase in the kidney. Arginine is then transported to the liver for conversion to urea.

Ammonia toxicity

Hyperammonemia has long been presumed to contribute to the encephalopathy resulting from liver failure, but the multiple accompanying metabolic disturbances make it impossible to distinguish the specific effects of ammonia toxicity on brain function. *Inherited defects of urea cycle enzymes* have given a unique insight into ammonia toxicity as grossly elevated ammonia concentrations are the sole metabolic disturbance common to all these defects. Increased ammonia levels cause vomiting, lethargy and drowsiness, with progression to coma, cerebral edema and death. Histopathological changes include astrocyte swelling and mitochondrial changes without noticeable alterations in neurons. Speculative explanations for these changes include abnormal mitochondrial metabolism, changes in neurotransmitter function, and direct effects on blood flow and astrocytes through osmotic effects of the high concentrations of glutamine that accompany hyperammonemia. Support for the last hypothesis comes from the fact that a rising plasma glutamine is a good predictor of impending coma.

The urea cycle (Fig. 3.7)

The urinary excretion of urea is the main mechanism of waste nitrogen removal in man. The initial steps in the cycle, up to the formation of citrulline, take place in the mitochondria, while the later enzymes are in the cytosol. The mitochondrial enzymes, in particular *N*-acetylglutamate synthase, are susceptible to secondary inhibition by a variety of toxins that may accumulate in inborn errors of metabolism. This explains the hyperammonemia that may occur in disorders such as *methylmalonic acidemia, propionic acidemia* and *fatty acid oxidation defects*. Inherited deficiency of each enzyme in the cycle has been described. Both citrulline and arginosuccinic acid can be excreted in the urine, thereby providing a useful natural route of nitrogen removal if there is a defect in one of the more distal enzymes of ammonia metabolism (e.g. *arginase, arginosuccinate lyase* or *arginosuccinate lyase synthase deficiencies*). This route is unavailable in the more proximal deficiencies, so defects such as *carbamyl phosphate synthase* and *ornithine transcarbamylase deficiencies* tend to cause more severe *hyperammonemia*. Arginine is not normally an essential amino acid in man as it is synthesized in the urea cycle, but it becomes a necessary dietary supplement in the management of urea cycle defects. A deficiency of any urea cycle enzyme, with the exception of arginase, results in a disturbance of arginine production. Arginine is also important as a precursor of ornithine, which is essential to the maintenance of any residual function the urea cycle may have in deficiency states. Arginine also stimulates the activity of *N*-acetylglutamate synthase.

While all enzymes in the cycle are expressed in the liver, expression elsewhere is variable. *N*-acetylglutamate synthase, carbamyl phosphate synthase and ornithine transcarbamylase are present in intestinal mucosal cells, while arginosuccinate lyase and arginosuccinate synthase are expressed in skin fibroblasts and kidney, and arginase is expressed in erythrocytes. These tissue locations are important in reaching a specific enzyme diagnosis of *urea cycle defects*. The concentration of enzymes in the liver means that liver transplantation is an effective therapeutic option particularly in *ornithine transcarbamylase deficiency*.

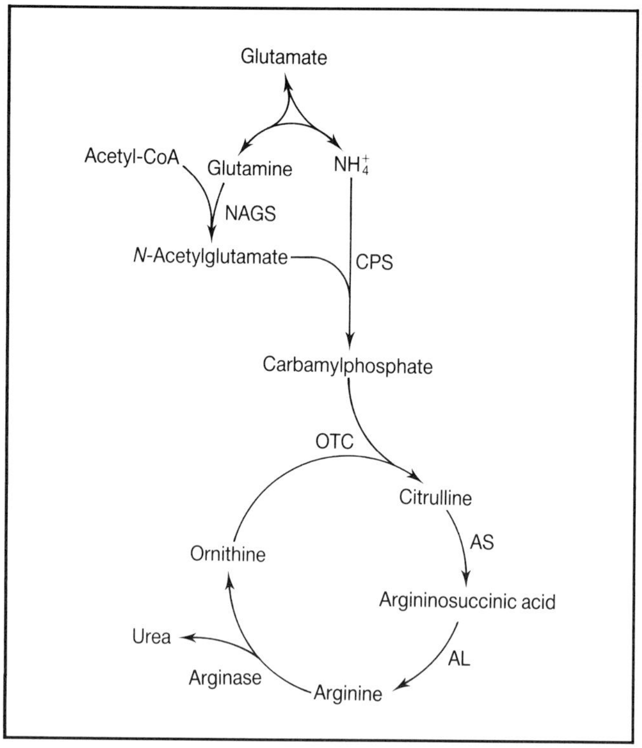

Fig. 3.7. The urea cycle: NAGS, *N*-acetylglutamate synthase; CPS, carbamyl phosphate synthase; OTC, ornithine transcarbamylase; AS, arginosuccinate synthase; AL, arginosuccinate lyase.

Genetics and molecular biology

Ornithine transcarbamylase is located on the X chromosome and defects in this enzyme almost always cause severe *hyperammonemia* in males. Lyonization, the random inactivation of the X chromosome in females, results in the disproportionate representation of either the mutant or the normal allele. When the mutant allele is overrepresented in the liver, female carriers of *ornithine transcarbamylase deficiency* present with severe symptoms, whereas predominance of the normal allele allows a carrier female to remain asymptomatic. Patchy expression of the enzyme in females makes tissue diagnosis of carrier status hazardous as biopsies may be taken from an unrepresentative site. Both deletions and point mutations in the ornithine transcarbamylase gene have been identified and these are helpful in the prenatal diagnosis of *ornithine transcarbamylase deficiency*. Mutations have also been detected in the arginosuccinate synthase gene, although expression of the enzyme product of this gene in fibroblasts means that direct enzyme analysis of accessible tissues such as chorionic villus can be used reliably for prenatal diagnosis.

Developmental aspects

The enzymes of the urea cycle are detectable at 10 weeks' gestation and, by 20 weeks, reach levels similar to those found at birth when the activity is approximately 50 percent of adult values. This is normally sufficient for the unimpaired metabolism of ammonia. Further induction of urea cycle enzyme activity takes place with increased dietary protein intake.

Selected reading

Batshaw ML. Hyperammonemia. *Curr Probl Pediatr* 1984; **14**: 1.

Fernandes J, Saudubray J-M, Tada K, eds. *Inborn metabolic diseases. Diagnosis and treatment*. Berlin: Springer Verlag, 1990.

Newsholme E, Leech AR. *Biochemistry for the medical sciences*. Chichester: John Wiley and Sons, 1983.

Scriver CR, Beadet AL, Sly WS, Valle D, eds. *The metabolic basis of inherited disease*. 6th ed. New York: McGraw-Hill, 1989.

C. Purine and Pyrimidine Metabolism

G N Thompson

Nucleotide synthesis and breakdown

Nucleotides, the structural units of DNA and RNA, have three parts: a nitrogen-containing ring system known as the base, which is either a purine or pyrimidine in nucleic acids; a sugar which is a ribose or deoxyribose sugar in nucleic acids; and one or more phosphate groups. In virtually all living organisms all common nucleotides can be synthesized *de novo* from basic precursors such as ribose phosphate and glutamine. Nucleotides have a wide variety of metabolic roles. They may be polymerized to form the structural backbone of the nucleic acids DNA and RNA. Alternatively, by the action of nucleotidase, nucleosides are formed, the most important of which, adenosine, is phosphorylated to make ATP. Other important biological molecules derived from nucleotides include cyclic AMP, NAD^+, NADH, FAD and coenzyme A.

RNA has a relatively short half-life and is the main contributor to nucleotide catabolism. DNA is not normally broken down except on the death of cells, although dietary DNA may enter the purine and pyrimidine catabolic pathways. The initial step in nucleotide catabolism is conversion to the corresponding bases (adenine, guanine and hypoxanthine in the case of purines, and uracil and thymine for pyrimidines). Further catabolism yields uric acid as the end product of the purine pathway and malonic or methylmalonic acids as the end products of the pyrimidine pathway.

De novo *and salvage pathway synthesis of purines and pyrimidines*

Purines are derived from ribose-5-phosphate by a number of enzymatic steps. Pyrimidines are synthesized from glutamine and bicarbonate which form carbamylphosphate, an early intermediate in the urea cycle (see p. 80). The *de novo* synthesis of nucleotides requires much more energy than recycling the bases to their corresponding nucleotides and 70–90 percent of circulating purines and pyrimidines are derived through the recycling or salvage pathways which are similar for both purines and pyrimidines. The essential steps in the *de novo* and salvage pathways of purine and pyrimidine synthesis and their catabolic pathways are shown in Figs 3.8 and 3.9.

The ubiquitous role of nucleotides is reflected in the diverse symptomatology of inborn errors of purine and pyrimidine metabolism. *Lesch–Nyhan syndrome* is due to a deficiency of hypoxanthine-guanine phosphoribosyltransferase (HGPRT), the enzyme responsible for the salvage of hypoxanthine and guanine, and causes developmental delay, movement disturbance and self-mutilation. Hyperuricemia occurs because of a relative decrease in the recycling of uric acid precursors. By contrast, *adenosine deaminase deficiency* causes *severe combined immunodeficiency*, probably through

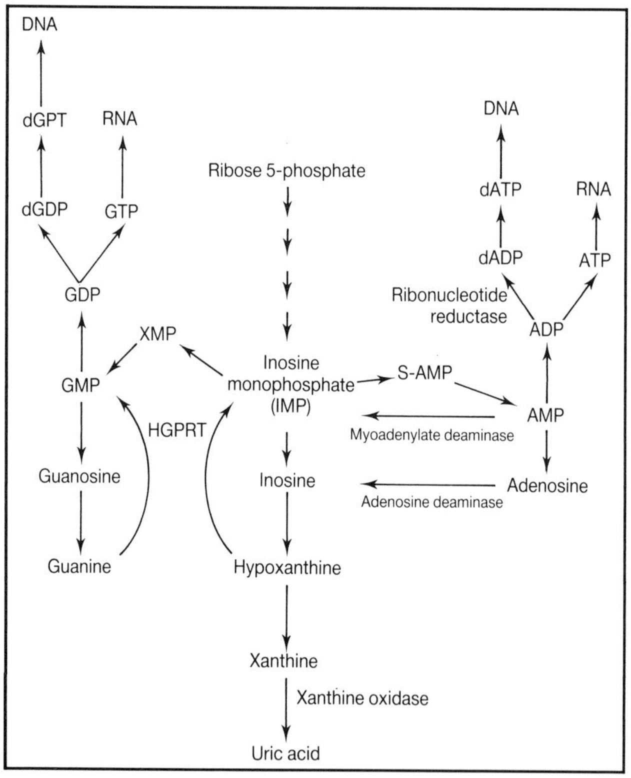

Fig. 3.8. Synthesis and catabolism of purines.

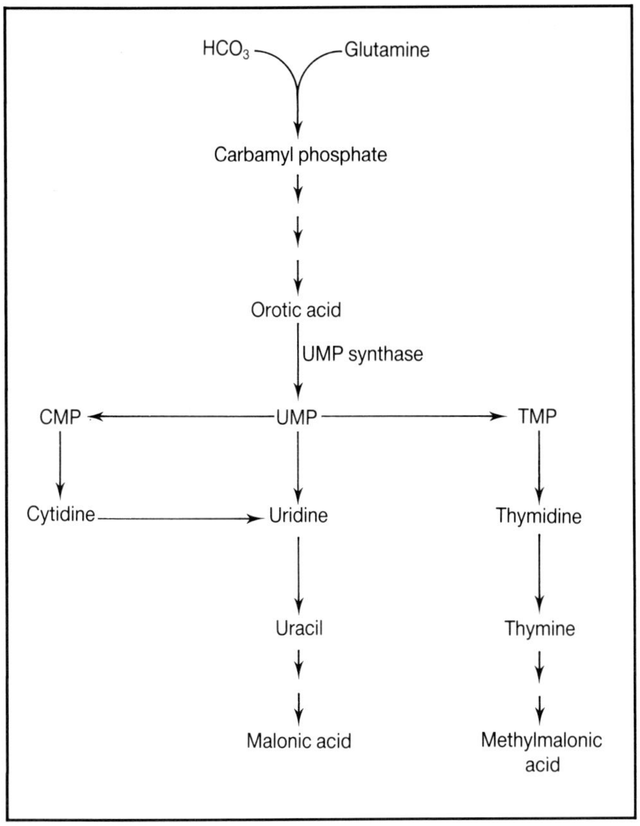

Fig. 3.9. Synthesis and catabolism of pyrimidines.

inhibition of ribonucleotide reductase resulting in less DNA synthesis. Other clinical conditions arising from inborn errors of nucleotide metabolism include *megaloblastic anemia* in *orotic aciduria* due to UMP synthase deficiency, *renal stone formation* in *xanthine oxidase deficiency*, and *muscle cramps* due to *myoadenylate deaminase deficiency* which impairs fumarate production, thereby limiting muscle energy availability.

Hyperuricemia

Uric acid, the end product of purine catabolism, is excreted two-thirds via the kidney and one-third through the gut where it is bacterially degraded. Hyperuricemia causes *gout* by inducing the formation of crystals of monosodium urate which cause inflammation. A number of mechanisms of hyperuricemia have been documented. Inborn errors of carbohydrate metabolism such as *glycogen storage disease type I (glucose-6-phosphatase deficiency), fructosemia (fructose aldolase deficiency)* and *fructose-6-phosphatase deficiency* lead to massive accumulation of phosphorylated carbohydrates, thereby limiting the availability of inorganic phosphate for nucleoside phosphorylation, and to subsequent increased nucleoside catabolism and uric acid production.

Ethanol induces hyperuricemia by increasing uric acid production because of accelerated ATP degradation and inhibition of uric acid excretion due to competition by extra lactic acid production. Decreased production of ATP, as seen in the *metabolic myopathies* such as *glycogen storage diseases III, V and VII* and *myoadenylate deaminase deficiency* also causes hyperuricemia by decreasing the availability of substrates for ATP synthesis. When ATP is degraded during exercise, nucleotides are preferentially degraded to products including uric acid rather than being salvaged. Hyperuricemia may also result from increased nucleic acid turnover seen in the *lymphoproliferative malignancies* and the *tumor lysis syndrome*, from *inborn errors of purine synthesis* and from a primary decrease in uric acid excretion.

The treatment of hyperuricemia depends on increasing uric acid excretion with uricosuric drugs such as probenecid, and decreasing uric acid production with drugs such as allopurinol which inhibits xanthine oxidase.

Selected reading

Fernandes J, Saudubray J-M, Tada K, eds. *Inborn metabolic diseases. Diagnosis and treatment*. Berlin: Springer Verlag, 1990.

Newsholme EA, Leech AR. *Biochemistry for the medical sciences*. Chichester: John Wiley and Sons, 1983.

Scriver CR, Beaudet AL, Sly WS, Valle D, eds. *The metabolic basis of inherited disease*. 6th ed. New York: McGraw-Hill, 1989.

D. Fat and Carbohydrate Metabolism

R D G Milner

The decision to consider carbohydrates and lipids together stems from their great importance as energy sources and the central role of pancreatic hormones in controlling energy delivery. Carbohydrates and lipids also form part of large structural molecules, e.g. myelin and glycoproteins and other molecules of particular pediatric relevance, e.g. surfactant.

The largest fetal energy requirement is for anabolism, but after birth thermogenesis and the skeletal and visceral metabolism associated with homeothermic independence must be added to the total caloric requirement of the infant and child. Glucose plays a special role in energy homeostasis because some tissues, notably the brain, are partially or wholly glucose dependent. Hypoglycemia causes neuronal dysfunction and if sustained, irreversible damage.

Cellular energy balance and the Krebs cycle

The ultimate source of free energy in living organisms comes from oxidative reactions. In biological oxidation, hydrogen is removed from the substrate being oxidized and then reacts with molecular oxygen to form water. Part of the energy released by the oxidation is conserved in the form of compounds with large negative free energies of hydrolysis. These are called high energy compounds. Most high energy compounds are phosphorylated, e.g. adenosine triphosphate (ATP), creatine phosphate and phosphoenol pyruvate, but some are not, e.g. acetyl-CoA. The production of such compounds is termed oxidative phosphorylation in which the oxidative and phosphorylative processes are simultaneous and tightly coupled. This takes place in the respiratory chain located on the inner mitochondrial membrane. Oxidative phosphorylation can be blocked by uncouplers which cause increased oxidation, decreased phosphorylation and the production of extra heat which if excessive may result in *fever*. Synthetic uncouplers include salicylate, dicoumarol and 2,4-dinitrophenol. Natural uncouplers include bilirubin and some bacterial toxins. The physiological uncoupler uniquely present in brown fat mitochondria is a protein, thermogenin (see Chapter 8).

Sugars, fat and amino acids enter a final common energy generating pathway as two to six carbon molecules that are mainly organic acids or acid derivates. This pathway is the tricarboxylic acid cycle, or Krebs cycle (Fig. 3.10), which is the source of most of the CO_2 made in the body, and provides much of the reduced coenzyme pool that enables the respiratory chain to produce ATP. It is also the means whereby excess energy is converted into

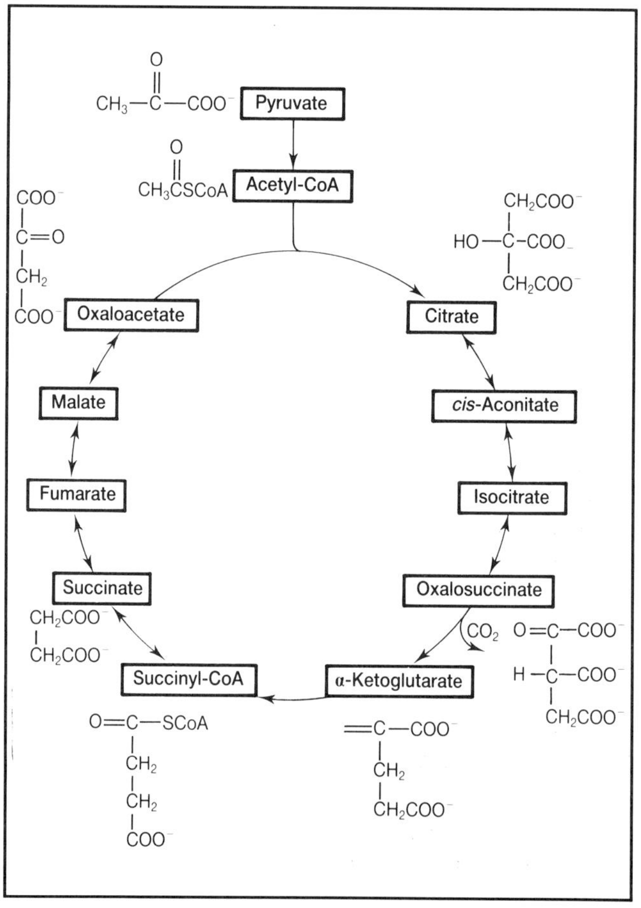

Fig. 3.10. A simplified diagram of the Krebs (citric acid) cycle showing the formulae of only the more clinically important intermediates.

fatty acid, prior to triglyceride formation, and thus to fat deposition. In the Krebs cycle carbohydrates can be converted to fatty acids or amino acids, and amino acids to glucose or fatty acids, but fatty acids cannot be metabolized to glucose. All the enzymes of the Krebs cycle are found on the matrix side of the inner mitochondrial membrane or the matrix space, close by those of the respiratory chain.

A major entry point to the cycle is the two-carbon molecule acetyl-CoA which is formed from pyruvate under the influence of the pyruvate dehydrogenase complex by β-oxidation of fatty acids. Both reactions take place within the mitochondria. The pyruvate dehydrogenase complex is subject to several control mechanisms. It is activated by dephosphorylation (pyruvate dehydrogenase kinase). The kinase is activated by cyclic AMP and ATP. The phosphatase is inhibited by ketosis or a high concentration of fatty acids.

The first step in the Krebs cycle using acetyl-CoA as the starting point is condensation with oxaloacetate to form citrate under the unidirectional control of citrate synthetase which is found only in mitochondria. Citrate is then converted to isocitrate in two steps, both catalyzed by the unidirectional and highly specific aconitase. Isocitrate is next transiently dehydrogenated to oxalosuccinate which remains bound to isocitrate dehydrogenase before being decarboxylated to α-ketoglutarate. This molecule is then decarboxylated by an enzyme complex, α-ketogluturate dehydrogenase, which closely resembles the pyruvate dehydrogenase complex except in its specificity for substrate. The product is succinyl-CoA which is converted to succinate and CoASH by succinate thiokinase with the production of GTP from GDP. This is an example of phosphorylation not involving the respiratory chain and one of the few instances when GDP and not ADP is involved. Succinate passes through the intermediates malate and fumarate *en route* to becoming oxaloacetate in a manner similar to the conversion of citrate to isocitrate. The enzymes involved are succinate dehydrogenase, fumarase and malate dehydrogenase. The net effect of one turn of the wheel is the formation of CO_2 and water from acetic acid yielding the precursors of 12 mol ATP with an efficiency of approximately 40 percent. The Krebs cycle is the largest single source of ATP.

Acetyl-CoA is the principal building block in long-chain fatty acid construction which takes place in the cytoplasm. Under adequate nutrition, it is formed from carbohydrate by glycolysis to yield pyruvate which is converted to acetyl-CoA under the control of pyruvate dehydrogenase, or from protein by the transamination of amino acids which enter the Krebs cycle at various points. Certain amino acids are homologues of Krebs cycle intermediaries, e.g. pyruvate/alanine and α-ketoglutarate/glutamate and these can be converted in either direction as required under the control of transaminases. When amino acid supply exceeds the need for protein biosynthesis the acids are made available to the Krebs cycle in a variety of ways. A homologue is deaminated by an aminotransferase and the carbon skeleton processed through the cycle to yield acetyl-CoA. Direct transamination is possible for only a minority of amino acids such as alanine, aspartate and glutamine. Others, e.g. serine, threonine, glycine and cysteine, are transaminated, converted to pyruvate and processed by that route. A third mechanism is oxidative deamination involving amino acid oxidase to produce ammonium ions or amide groups and carbon skeletons that enter the Krebs cycle.

There is no net synthesis of glucose from fatty acids because each acetyl-CoA entering the cycle generates two molecules of CO_2. Therefore all the fuel entering the cycle is converted into high energy phosphate bonds or heat, leaving no carbon available for glucose synthesis.

While the above pathways provide the major route for the generation of ATP, some high potential electrons must be conserved for biosynthetic purposes. This is done via the synthesis of NADPH as a hydride ion (electron) donor for reductive biosynthesis. The synthesis of NADPH occurs via the pentose phosphate pathway (hexose monophosphate pathway).

$$\text{Glucose 6-PO}_4 + 2\text{NADP}^+ + H_2O \rightarrow \text{ribose 5-PO}_4 + 2\text{NADPH} + 2H^+ + CO_2$$

This pathway is more active in adipose tissue than muscle because large amounts of NADPH are needed for fatty acid synthesis from acetyl-CoA. Because many cells need more NADPH for reductive biosynthesis compared to the requirement for ribose 5-phosphate incorporation into nucleotides, the ribose 5-phosphate can be converted into glyceraldehyde 3-phosphate (and thence to pyruvate), and fructose 6-phosphate by transketotolase and transaldolase, thus creating a reversible link between the pentose phosphate pathway and glycolysis.

Lipid metabolism

Lipids are poorly soluble in water and are found in the body as cell membranes, metabolic fuel, storage forms of energy and emulsifying agents. Lipids can be classified chemically into five groups: **fatty acids** which are a major source of energy and also building blocks for more complicated lipids, **glyceryl esters** which include the triglycerides, the storage form of fatty acids, and phosphoglycerides, the main lipid component of cell membranes, **sphingolipids** which are also membrane components, **sterols** which include cholesterol, bile acids, steroid hormones and vitamin D, and **terpenes** which include the other fat-soluble vitamins (A,E,K). Attention will be focused on fatty acids and the glyceryl esters.

Fatty acids and glycerides

Fatty acids may be represented by the formula R-COOH where R is an alkyl chain composed of carbon and hydrogen atoms. They are commonly classified according to chain length and degree of saturation. Long-chain fatty acids contain 12–26 carbon atoms, medium-chain 6–10, and short-chain 2–4. Almost all naturally derived fatty acids contain an even number of carbon atoms. Fatty acids with one unsaturated bond are monoenoic and polyunsaturated fatty acids are polyenoic. Dietary fat is made up of a mixture of fatty acids mainly present as triglycerides. The fatty acids in animal fat, e.g. butter and lard, are generally more saturated than those in vegetable oils, e.g. olive oil. The unsaturated fatty acid composition of vegetable oils varies, resulting in the need to mix them judiciously in the preparation of commercial infant formulas. Not all polyenoic fatty acids can be synthesized and those that must be obtained from the diet are termed essential fatty acids. In man the linoleic (n-6) and linolenic (n-3) classes are essential. Linoleic acid derivatives are precursors of certain prostaglandins (see p. 103) and linolenic acid metabolites are found in retinal photoreceptor membranes. *Essential fatty acid deficiency* may occur clinically, especially during prolonged *parenteral nutrition*, and is characterized by dermatitis and poor wound healing.

Glycerides are the fatty acid esters of glycerol and may be mono-, di- or tri- depending on the number of glycerol hydroxyl groups esterified. Triglycerides are the most prevalent, being the major storage and transport form of fatty acids. Phosphoglycerides are acylglycerols containing phosphoric acid esterified at the C3-hydroxyl group. They form bilayers when dispersed in an aqueous solution and in this form are the main structural components of cell membranes. Lecithin is the common name for phosphatidylcholine.

Digestion and absorption of fat

(see also Chapter 9)

Most dietary lipid is triglyceride which makes up 20–40 percent of the caloric intake. Fat must be emulsified and hydrolyzed in the intestinal lumen before being absorbed. Emulsification takes place in the aqueous chyme of the duodenum under the influence of bile salts to produce micelles. Micelles are aggregates of molecules made up of both polar (hydrophilic) and nonpolar (hydrophobic) groups. These are known as amphipathic molecules when the molecule is long enough for each end to demonstrate its own solubility characteristics. Phosphatidylcholine is an example of a substance that forms micelles, the nonpolar fatty acid chains being aggregated inwardly while the polar phosphorylcholine groups orient outwards to interact with the surrounding water molecules. Triglyceride and cholesterol esters are not amphipathic, but are able to reside within the nonpolar interior of the micelles where they are digested.

Pancreatic lipase cleaves the fatty acids from positions 1 and 3 of a triglyceride. The resulting fatty acids and 2-monoglyceride are then absorbed by diffusion into the mucosal cells of the upper small intestine. Pancreatic lipase is activated by a cofactor, colipase, also secreted by the pancreas. Colipase binds to the mixed micelle containing triglycerides and facilitates adsorption of lipase to the complex. Once inside the mucosal cell the fatty acids and 2-monoglyceride are resynthesized into triglyceride before passing into the circulation. These reactions consume energy but permit remodeling of the triglyceride entering the circulation. Triglycerides are released into the lymph in the form of a lipoprotein, the chylomicron.

After birth fat quickly replaces glucose as the major energy source, but the mechanisms for lipid digestion and absorption are not fully developed. In the *newborn infant* and especially the *premature* both pancreatic lipase and bile salt concentrations are low. Lipid digestion therefore is mainly intragastric and is under the control of lingual and gastric lipases which have a broad pH optimum (2.5–7.0) and, unlike pancreatic lipase, are not dependent on bile salts. The products of lipolysis, monoglyceride and FFA, compensate for the reduced bile salts by acting as emulsifiers.

Medium chain triglycerides (MCT) do not appear in the food we eat but have an important role in therapeutic diets. They are synthetic triglycerides with fatty acid chains of 8–10 carbon atoms. MCT are absorbed intact by the intestinal mucosal cells where they are hydrolyzed by an intracellular lipase to fatty acid and glycerol. These are not re-esterified but pass directly into the portal vein bound to albumin to be taken up and further metabolized by the liver. MCT are a useful caloric supplement in diseases where one or more of the steps in normal lipid digestion are either not fully developed as in *prematurity* or are defective such as *pancreatic insufficiency* where there is inadequate lipase secreted, or *abetalipoproteinemia* in which chylomicrons cannot be synthesized.

Lipid transport

There are three important routes for lipid movement in the body. Dietary triglyceride is transported from the intestine to the tissues, triglyceride synthesized by the liver is secreted and transported for storage in adipose tissue, and adipose tissue triglyceride is taken to other tissues in the form of free fatty acids (FFA). A small amount of FFA comes from the hydrolysis of triglyceride in chylomicrons and VLDL by lipoprotein lipase at the point of delivery. Cholesterol absorbed from the gut, or synthesized in the liver, must be transported to other tissues as substrate for steroid and membrane synthesis.

Although FFA are only about 3 percent of the total fatty acids in the circulation they are metabolically important. FFA are transported tightly bound to albumin. On average each molecule of albumin binds 1–2 FFA molecules with a dissociation constant in the order of 1 μM. The small amount of unbound FFA is readily taken up by tissue for oxidation or tissue lipid synthesis and the half-life of plasma FFA is only 1–2 minutes.

The remainder of the fatty acids and cholesterol are carried by lipoproteins which have a micellar structure with triglycerides and cholesterol esters in the core surrounded by amphipathic lipids and proteins. There are five main classes of plasma lipoprotein that can be separated by ultracentrifugation (Table 3.2). Chylomicrons are very large molecules, but have the lowest density because they are approximately 98 percent lipid. VLDLs contain about 90 percent lipid of which more than half is triglyceride. They are synthesized in the liver and are primarily responsible for the transport of triglyceride from the liver to other tissues, notably adipose tissue. Triglycerides are transported mainly by chylomicrons and very low density lipoproteins (VLDL), whereas cholesterol esters are carried by low density lipoproteins (LDL) and phospholipids by high density lipoproteins (HDL). Lipoproteins can also be separated by electrophoresis. The band remaining at the origin contains the chylomicrons. The next, called the β-lipoproteins, migrates with the β-globulins and contains the LDL. The band migrating in front of the β region contains the VLDL and is called the pre-β-lipoproteins. The final band, the α-lipoproteins, migrates with the α-globulins and contains the HDL. Lipoproteins contain a wide variety of apoproteins (Apo-) which are synthesized in various organs and have other functions as well as lipid transport. For example, Apo-AI which is the main structural protein of HDL is also an activator of lecithin cholesterol acyltransferase, and Apo-CII which is found in VLDL and HDL activates lipoprotein lipase. *Abetalipoproteinemia* is a rare autosomal recessive condition in which there is deficient synthesis of lipoproteins containing Apo-B. The formation of

Table 3.2. Classes of lipoproteins separable by density and electrophoresis

Lipoprotein	Major lipids	Density range (g/ml)	Electrophoretic mobility
Chylomicron	Triglyceride	<0.94	None
VLDL	Triglyceride	0.94–1.006	Pre-β
IDL	Triglyceride & cholesterol esters	1.006–1.019	β
LDL	Cholesterol esters	1.010–1.063	β
HDL	Phospholipids & cholesterol	1.063–1.21	α

chylomicrons, VLDL and LDL are all deficient with resulting fat malabsorption, ataxic neuropathy, acanthocytosis and ataxic neuropathy.

Lipolysis

The hydrolysis of triglyceride in the circulation is governed by lipoprotein lipase which is present in most tissues including the heart, mammary gland and adipose tissue where its activity is increased by insulin. Lipoprotein lipase is secreted and passes through the capillary endothelium where it binds to the surface membrane of the endothelial cells. The enzyme is activated by apoprotein CII, one of the low molecular weight proteins present in VLDL and HDL. It hydrolyzes triglyceride at positions 1 and 3; the resulting fatty acids are taken up locally and the monoglyceride is transported to the liver where it is metabolized. Intravenous heparin liberates lipoprotein lipase into the circulation from both the capillary endothelium and the liver. The capillary lipase is inactivated by protamine, but the hepatic lipase is not.

Lipoprotein lipase activity can vary between tissues and this may be important in the growth and maturation of individual organs. There is low activity in fetal muscle and heart, but more in the lung possibly related to surfactant biosynthesis. Lipoprotein lipase is present in fetal adipocyte precursors which can hydrolyze exogenous triglyceride and are hormone and heparin sensitive. Lipoprotein lipase activity increases in all tissues immediately after birth irrespective of whether this occurs at term or prematurely. There is impaired clearance of circulating triglyceride in premature infants due to low lipoprotein lipase activity which is directly proportional to the degree of prematurity. When babies are fed parentally using Intralipid, a 10 percent soybean oil emulsion, as a rich caloric source they may develop marked lipemia. Intralipid particles are similar in size to chylomicrons and are also cleared by lipoprotein lipase.

Stored triglyceride, needed as fuel elsewhere in the body, is mobilized from adipocytes by hormone-sensitive lipase which is activated, via the adenylyl cyclase mechanism, by hormones such as glucagon and catecholamines or by sympathetic stimulation. Thyroxine and growth hormone also stimulate lipolysis but do so more slowly, probably by increasing the synthesis of an intracellular regulatory protein rather than by activating adenylyl cyclase.

Triglyceride destined for intracellular catabolism is hydrolyzed by lysosomal acid lipase which has a pH optimum of 5.

Lipid storage

Fat differs from protein and carbohydrate, neither of which has specialized storage arrangements in the body. The only quantitatively important energy reservoir is adipose tissue. There are two kinds of adipose tissue, brown and white.

Brown adipose tissue is important for thermogenesis, white adipose for energy homeostasis. Brown adipose tissue is composed of large multilocular cells packed with mitochondria and has a rich blood supply and sympathetic innervation. Lipolysis is controlled by hormone-sensitive lipase which is stimulated by catecholamines of both sympathetic and adrenal origin. The resulting FFA are oxidized locally in the mitochondria and peroxisomes to produce heat by uncoupled oxidation due to the presence of thermogenin (see Chapter 8). Mitochondria preferentially oxidize saturated medium-chain FFA and peroxisomes long-chain polyunsaturated FFA. Mitochondrial FFA oxidation requires high concentrations of carnitine for transmembrane FFA transport. When endogenous substrate stores are exhausted, brown adipose tissue can take up FFA from the circulation.

White adipose tissue exists as subcutaneous fat and deep body fat. Adipose tissue stores develop late in gestation, the concentration of fetal lipids before 32 weeks being low and constant. In the last 8 weeks of pregnancy subcutaneous fat increases exponentially from 20 to 350 g, and deep body fat from 10 to 80 g. Conditions characterized by fetal hyperinsulinemia, such as *infant of a diabetic mother (IDM)* and *Beckwith syndrome*, are associated with increased adipose tissue development. *Obesity* is associated with an increase in both adipocyte size and number. The extent to which feeding in the first months of life can influence growth of white adipocytes and thereby produce a liability to obesity in later life remains unresolved.

In adipocytes, triglyceride synthesis occurs from FFA, which may be synthesized from glucose metabolism or more likely is delivered to the cell as triglyceride in chylomicrons or VLDL. Insulin stimulates the production of lipoprotein lipase and glucose uptake, thereby enhancing the delivery of both FFA and the glycerol moiety of triglyceride. Lipolysis in adipocytes results in both FFA and glycerol being released into the circulation because adipocytes lack glycerol kinase. Most of the glycerol is metabolized by the liver but the FFA is taken up by nearly all tissues and may be recycled within the adipose tissue.

Fat oxidation

Fatty acids are a major fuel. When catabolized completely to CO_2 and H_2O, 60 percent of the energy is released as heat and 40 percent is conserved to form ATP. Fatty acid catabolism occurs in the mitochondria by β-oxidation in which two carbon fragments are progessively removed in the form of acetyl-CoA which is then catabolized to CO_2 and water in the Krebs cycle. A single β-oxidation yielding 1 mol of acetyl-CoA produces 5 mol ATP and the resulting oxidation of the acetyl-CoA a further 12 mol ATP.

The first step in β-oxidation is formation of the acyl-CoA thioester by combination with CoASH under the control of acyl-CoA synthetase. There are at least three acyl-CoA synthetases for short-, medium- and long-chain fatty acids respectively (Fig. 3.11). The long-chain activating enzyme is located in the outer mitochondrial membrane and endoplasmic reticulum, but the other two are purely mitochondrial. The acyl-CoA formed in the outer mitochondrial membrane must then be transesterified from CoASH to carnitine in order to traverse the inner mitochondrial membrane and arrive at the site of the β-oxidation enzyme system. This is controlled by carnitine acyltransferase located on the inner mitochondrial membrane and is a reversible reaction. Further oxidation takes place within the mitochondrial matrix. Deficiency of an acyl-CoA synthetase results in one of the *inborn errors of fatty acid oxidation, e.g. glutaric aciduria types 1 and 2* which have diverse clinical presentations including hypoglycemia, neurological dysfunction and failure to thrive.

The energy of cardiac contraction comes mainly from fatty acid oxidation and there are important quantitative changes in the perinatal period. Fatty acid oxidation in the fetus is limited by a low concentration of carnitine in the heart and a relative paucity of mitochondria, both of which increase rapidly after birth. Other fetal tissues, such as liver, brain, placenta and lung, also have a limited capacity to oxidize fatty acids, probably due to limited production of palmitoyl carnitine by plamitoyl carnitine transferase A. After birth, fatty acid oxidation increases markedly and remains high until the time of weaning. Carnitine is potentially rate limiting and its inclusion in infant formulae or parenteral nutrients may have an important subsidiary role in the development of fatty acid oxidation. *Carnitine deficiency* may also arise as an inborn metabolic defect in carnitine synthesis, from the trapping and excretion of carnitine esters in *metabolic errors of fatty acid oxidation*, and also from excessive losses in renal conditions such as the *Fanconi syndrome, cystinosis* and *chronic dialysis*.

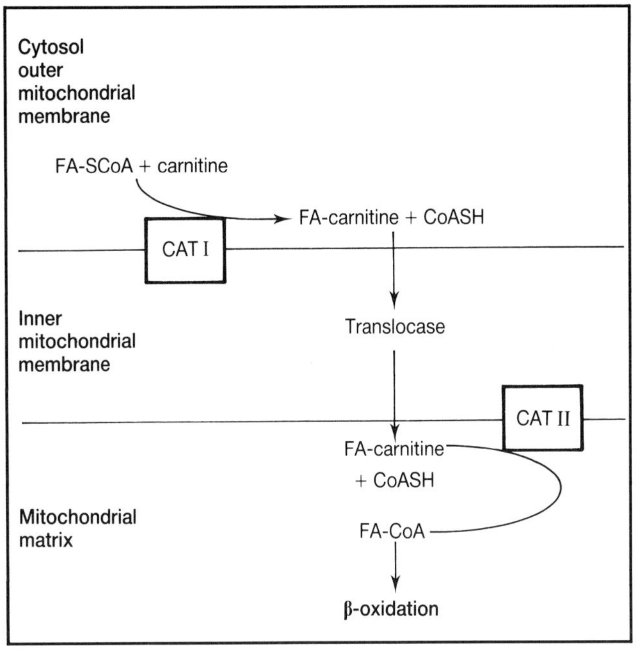

Fig. 3.11. Translocation of long-chain fatty acid acyl groups across the mitochondrial membrane. CAT, carnitine acyltransferase.

Ketones

The efficiency with which two carbon residues can be oxidized in the Krebs cycle depends on glucose availability. If imbalance occurs, as in *starvation* or *diabetes mellitus*, there is an accumulation of acetyl-CoA which is then condensed to form the ketone bodies, acetoacetate, β-hydroxybutyrate and acetone. Ketone body synthesis is blocked by malonyl-CoA, which is the link molecule between glucose and fatty acid metabolism, inhibiting carnitine acyltransferase I. Ketone bodies pass from the liver into the circulation to be used by brain, muscle and heart as an energy source. When the body's capacity to oxidize ketones is saturated they spill into the urine and are exhaled, producing a sickly sweet smell. The ability to smell ketones, which is congenitally absent in some individuals, is almost as important a clinical skill as being able to interpret the underlying pathological biochemistry.

Ketone bodies in the fetal circulation can arise from the partial oxidation of fatty acids, but they may also be of maternal origin, since the placenta is freely permeable. Fasting during pregnancy causes a rapid rise in maternal ketone levels and maternal–fetal ketone body transfer during labor may be appreciable. During the latter part of pregnancy the capacity to oxidize hydroxybutyrate has been demonstrated *in vitro* in fetal liver, brain and placenta. On balance, ketones in the fetal circulation are used more for lipid synthesis than as a source of immediate energy.

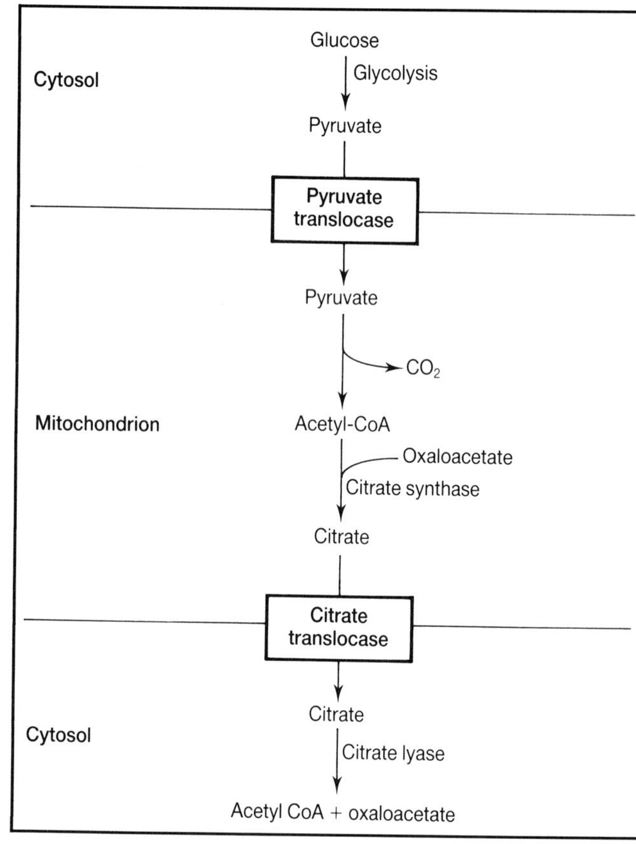

Fig. 3.12. Conversion of glucose to acetyl-CoA.

Lipogenesis

Fatty acids may be synthesized in three ways. The most important quantitatively is *de novo* synthesis from glucose in the cell cystosol. Pyruvate derived from glucose enters the mitochondrion and is converted to acetyl-CoA by the pyruvate dehydrogenase enzyme complex. The acetyl-CoA thus formed cannot traverse the inner mitochondrial membrane and must leave the mitochondrion as citrate to be cleaved by citrate lyase in the cell cytoplasm to produce acetyl-CoA and oxaloacetate (Fig. 3.12). All but one of the acetyl-CoA units that will end up as two carbon blocks in a FFA molecule must first be carboxylated to malonyl-CoA by the enzyme complex acetyl-CoA carboxylase. This is the rate-limiting step in fatty acid synthesis. The assembly of the fatty acid then proceeds under the control of the fatty acid synthetase complex, which consists of six enzymes and a carrier protein. *De novo* fatty acid synthesis always results in an even numbered carbon product because the acetate primer contains two carbons and each malonate unit condensing with it donates two more.

De novo fatty acid synthesis is under short- and long-term control. Short-term control involves modulation of acetyl-CoA carboxylase which is aggregated and activated by citrate and disaggregated by palmitoyl-CoA. Long-term control involves the synthesis of new fatty acid biosynthetic enzymes which have a short half-life. This is stimulated in the liver by glucose and insulin and inhibited during *starvation* or *insulin-deficient diabetes*.

Fatty acid synthesis is active in hepatic cytosol in late fetal life, declines after birth when the diet becomes fat-rich milk, and then increases again at weaning when dietary fat intake falls. Human fetal tissue of 12–20 weeks' gestation is capable of incorporating glucose, fructose, acetate, citrate and amino acids into lipids *in vitro*. The liver also takes up maternal fatty acids which cross the placenta easily. Long-chain unsaturated fatty acids must be provided by the mother. Fetal fatty acid synthesis is stimulated by insulin and inhibited by glucagon or cAMP. Triglyceride synthesis from palmitate has been demonstrated in slices of liver, lung and brain from abortions of 12–16 weeks' gestation.

Phosphoglycerides

Phosphoglycerides are derived from glycerol by two pathways. In the main pathway the phosphoglyceride is produced from glycerol-3-phosphate derived from glucose (Fig. 3.13). This is first converted to a diacylglyerol and then phosphate is removed under the influence of phosphatidic acid phosphatase. This is also the pathway for triglyceride synthesis. The final step is a reaction with a cytidine diphosphate derivative of either ethanol or choline (CDP ethanolamine or CDP choline). Phosphatidylcholine (lecithin) and phosphatidylethanolamine take up about 75 percent of the phosphoglycerides in most tissues and body fluids. All the enzymes involved in phosphoglyceride and triglyceride synthesis are associated with the endoplasmic reticulum. The second pathway bypasses the formation of 1,2-diacylglycerol and involves the reaction between phosphatidic acid and cytidine diphosphate diacylglycerol yielding, in the main, cardiolipin and phosphatidylinositol. Phosphoglycerides are metabolized by phospholipases which remove the acyl residues from the glycerol backbone.

Surfactant is a lipoprotein secreted by pulmonary type II epithelial cells and is essential in lowering the surface tension of the alveoli and permitting normal gas exchange. Surfactant contains a characteristic lecithin, dipalmitoyl phosphatidylcholine, which makes up about half the surfactant lipid. This is an unusual phosphatidylcholine in being saturated; most cell membrane phosphatidylcholine is unsaturated. Another important component of surfactant is phosphatidyl glycerol. The surfactant complex contains two specific proteins, one of 38 kDa and the other 10 kDa. The larger protein molecule is thought to be involved in the secretion of surfactant and the smaller in its recycling. A deficiency of surfactant results in the *respiratory distress syndrome (RDS)* (see Chapter 11).

Sphingolipids

Sphingosine is an 18-carbon dihydric alcohol containing an amino group at C_{17}. It is synthesized from palmitoyl-CoA and serine. Ceramide which is formed by the N-acylation of sphingosine is the key intermediate in sphingolipid synthesis. Ceramide reacts with CDP choline to form choline-P-ceramide (sphingomyelin), UDP galactose to form galactosylceramide and UDP glucose to form glucosylceramide, both examples of cerebrosides. Gangliosides are formed by the addition of hexose residues

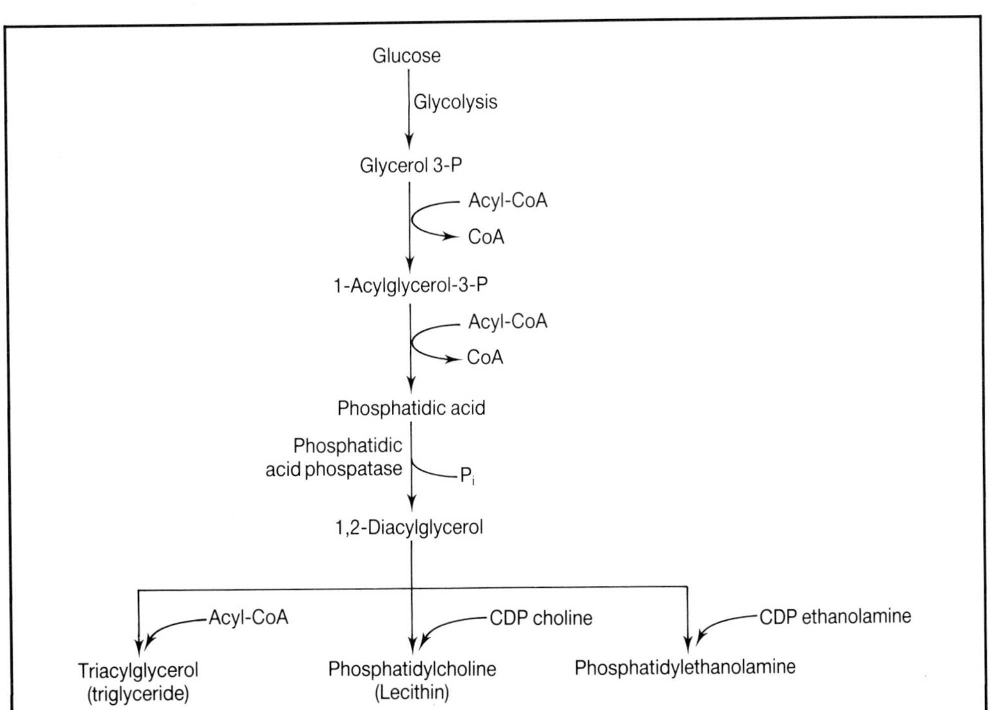

Fig. 3.13. The synthesis of triacylglycerol, phosphatidylethanolamine and phosphatidylcholine from glucose.

to glucosylceramide. Sphingomyelin is degraded by sphingomyelinase which removes the phosphorylcholine residue. Cerebrosides and gangliosides are hydrolyzed by hexosidases which are lysosomal enzymes. Inherited deficiencies of these catabolic enzymes results in the *lipid storage diseases* or *lipidoses* in which there is intracellular accumulation of sphingolipid leading to visceromegaly and neurological degeneration.

Carbohydrate metabolism

The term carbohydrate was used originally to describe naturally occurring compounds such as glucose, sucrose, glycogen, cellulose and starch which can be represented by the formula $C_x(H_2O)_y$ but now also includes more complex molecules which have a sugar in them. Carbohydrates represent about half of the total caloric intake and come mainly from plant sources. The physiologically important monosaccharides are glucose, galactose and fructose. The physiologically important disaccharides are lactose (glucose, galactose), sucrose (glucose, fructose) and to a lesser extent maltose (glucose, glucose). Starch is the most important polysaccharide ingested and glycogen the most important in the body.

Carbohydrate digestion and absorption

(see also Chapter 9)

The glycoside bonds of saccharides are hydrolyzed by glycosidases to give reducing sugars. Mastication stimulates the secretion of salivary amylase which acts on starch in a random manner to produce glucose, maltose and smaller starch fragments called dextrins. Thorough chewing will reduce starch to an average chain length of less than eight glucose units. Amylase action is stopped by the acidity of the stomach, but as the food enters the small intestine and is rendered alkaline by pancreatic juice, digestion of the starch dextrins is continued by pancreatic amylase. The resulting carbohydrate mix from a typical meal is glucose, maltose, isomaltose, lactose and sucrose. Ingested cellulose is nondigestible but contributes to stool bulk.

The important monosaccharides glucose, fructose and galactose can be absorbed across the intestinal mucosa against a concentration gradient, but under normal conditions the intraluminal concentration is greater and the pump functions mainly to prevent sugars leaking back into the intestinal lumen. Disaccharide digestion occurs in the brush border of the upper jejunum where the resulting monosaccharides are absorbed. The postprandial rate of sugar absorption is approximately 1 g/kg body weight per hour. The products of digestion are then delivered to the liver. Apart from a contribution to complex glycoproteins and glycolipids, most galactose and fructose enters the glucose metabolic pool.

Monosaccharide metabolism

There are specific kinases for the initial phosphorylation of the monosaccharides. Cells also contain less specific hexokinases at a relatively constant concentration which convert monosaccharides to the relevant 6-P ester and which are subject to product inhibition. Glucokinase is found only in the liver where its concentration is determined by the circulating insulin level. Skeletal and visceral cellular uptake of glucose occur as a function of the blood glucose and insulin concentrations. Hepatic glucose uptake differs from that in the rest of the body in being dependent on glucokinase which is deficient in insulinopenic conditions such as *diabetes mellitus* or *starvation*. Because glucokinase is not subject to feedback inhibition, glucose uptake is enhanced postprandially when glycogenesis is promoted. In contrast the tissue hexokinase which has a much lower K_m becomes more important during fasting.

Fructose metabolism involves splitting fructose 1-P to two triose fragments by an aldolase (Fig. 3.14). These trioses are glyceraldehyde and dihydroxyacetone phosphate which may then be catabolized by glycolysis or condensed to produce fructose 1,6-diphosphate which is available for glycogenesis via glucose 6-phosphate. Deficiency of the aldolase causes *hereditary fructose intolerance*, a potentially life-threatening condition characterized by vomiting, hypoglycemia, metabolic acidosis and mental retardation. If suspected, a fructose challenge must not be done, it may be lethal.

Galactose is rapidly taken up by the liver, where after phosphorylation by galactokinase, it is converted to glucose 1-phosphate by galactose 1-phosphate uridyl transferase. Deficiency of galactokinase results in *galactosemia*, which is characterized by galactosuria and the development of cataracts. Deficiency of galactose 1-phosphate uridyl transferase results in the accumulation

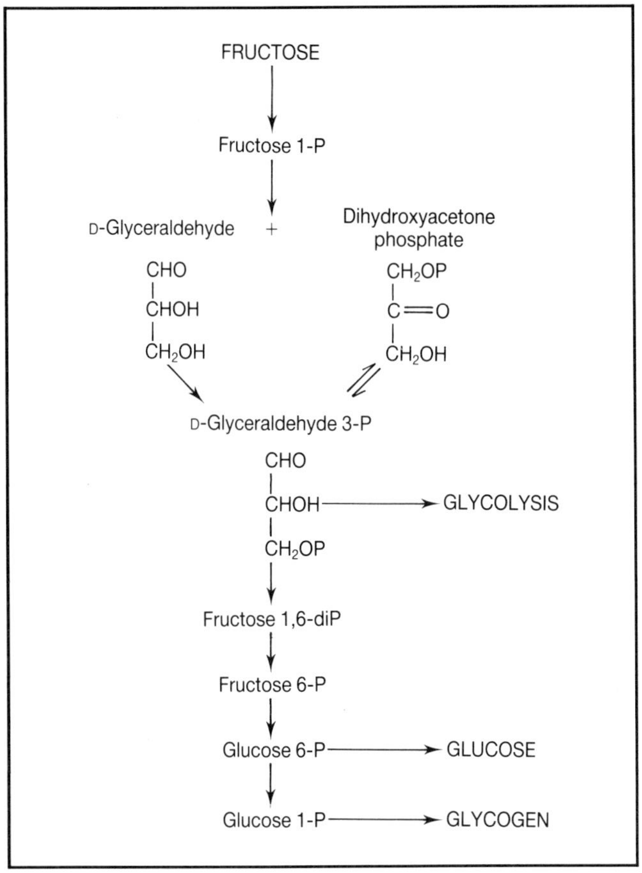

Fig. 3.14. Hepatic metabolism of fructose.

of intracellular galactose 1-phosphate and is the cause of *classical galactosemia*, a serious disease characterized by vomiting, hypoglycemia, cataracts, mental retardation and hepatosplenomegaly.

Glycogen

Glycogen metabolism is at the heart of glucose homeostasis. Glucose 6-phosphatase is the key enzyme in the liver and kidney which permits glucose 6-phosphate, derived from glycogen breakdown, to be converted to glucose and thus access the circulation. Other tissues, such as muscle, may have glycogen synthetic capacity but are obliged to metabolize glucose stores locally by entering glucose 6-phosphate into the glycolytic pathway. Glycogen, mainly hepatic in origin, is the immediate glucose reservoir in times of need. Conversely, when glucose is plentiful there is a finite capacity for glycogen synthesis and any excess glucose is converted to fat.

Glycogenesis is controlled by glycogen synthetase and branching enzyme (D-glucosyl-4,6-transferase) which causes irreversible sequential addition of glucosyl residues to a branched glucose polymer (Fig. 3.15). Glycogenolysis is under the control of phosphorylase and debranching enzymes (oligo-1,4→1,4-glucantransferase and amylo-1,6-glucosidase) which split the terminal glucose residues to yield glucose 1-phosphate (Fig. 3.16). This then must be transferred by phosphoglucomutase to glucose 6-phosphate to allow glucose release. During starvation glycogen stores are rarely completely depleted. A nucleus remains for future glycogen synthesis when refeeding occurs.

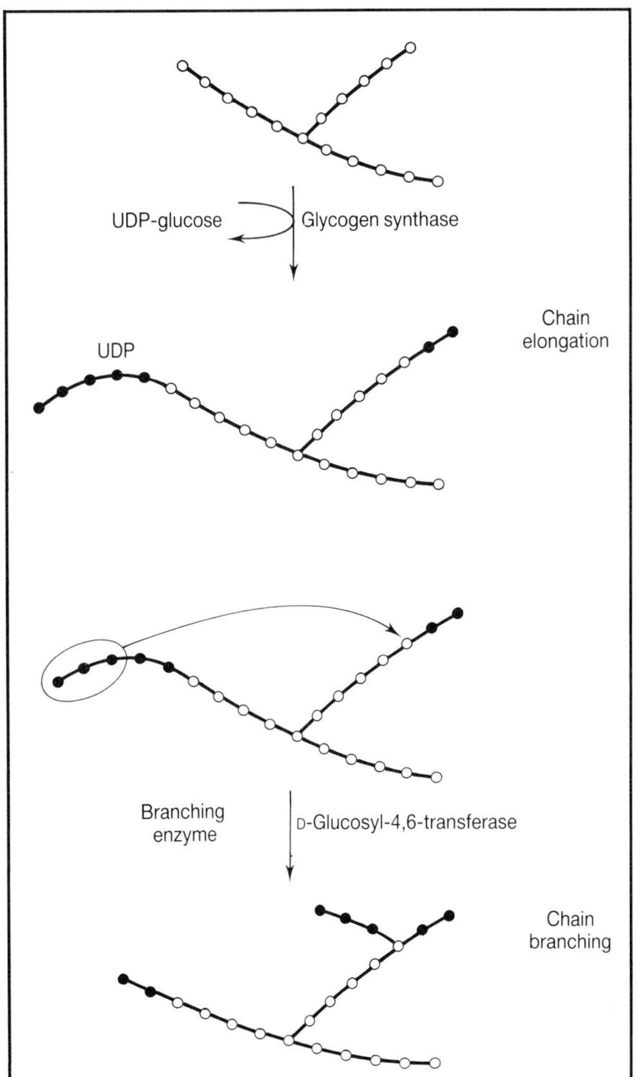

Fig. 3.15. Glycogen synthesis by chain elongation and branching. UDP, uridine diphosphate.

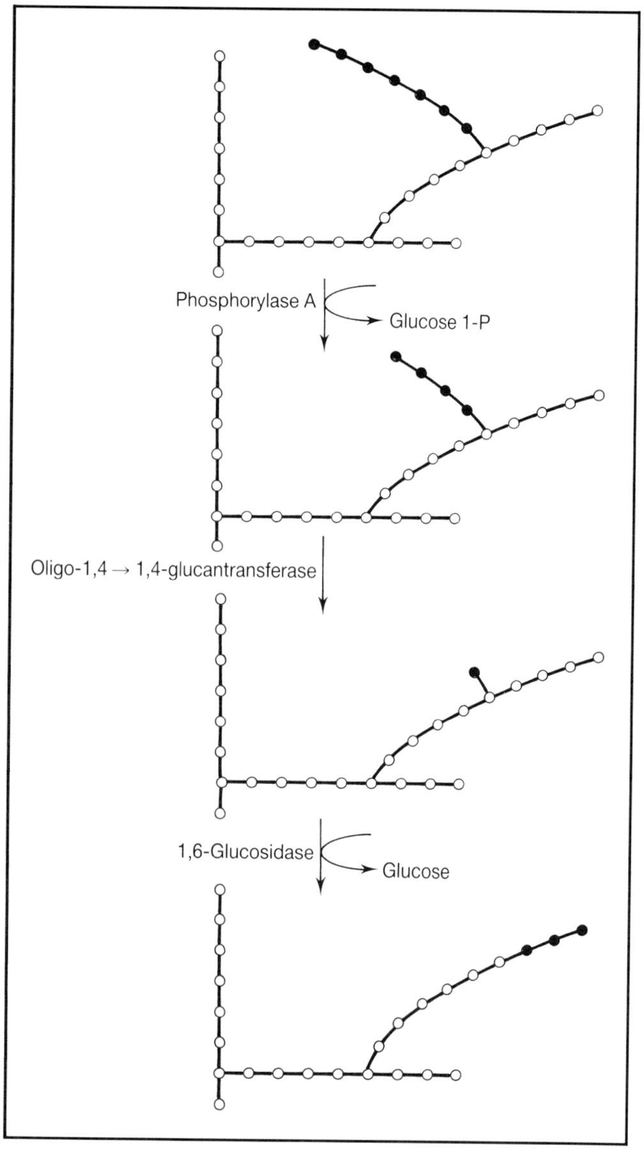

Fig. 3.16. Glycogen breakdown by chain shortening, rearrangement and debranching.

Nearly every cell is capable of glycogen metabolism and the flow of glucosyl units to or from storage is under the hormonal and substrate control of the relevant enzymes. Both glycogen synthetase and phosphorylase exist in two forms, which differ in being phosphorylated or not. The phosphorylation of each pair of enzymes is under the control of ATP and the protein kinase/cAMP/adenylate cyclase cascade. Adenylate cyclase is stimulated by glucagon and catecholamines to result in the production of the active form of phosphorylase (*a*) and the inactive form of glycogen synthetase (I). Glycogen synthetase (I) requires the presence of glucose 6-phosphate to work. Glycogen synthesis is activated by insulin, stimulating glucokinase to produce glucose 6-phosphate and inhibiting phosphorylation of the glycogenolytic enzymes. In adults the balance between glycogen synthesis or breakdown depends largely on the phosphorylation state of the enzymes, but in the fetus the concentration of enzyme, especially that of synthetase, is more important. Towards term there is a rapid accumulation of hepatic glycogen under the control of adrenal glucocorticoids. Both enzymes for glycogenolysis are present in the fetus, but they do not become active until after birth when complete depletion of liver glycogen can occur within 12 hours.

Deficiency of any of the enzymes involved in glycogen metabolism in any tissue results in one of the *glycogen storage diseases* which are variously characterized by hypoglycemia, visceromegaly, muscle weakness and metabolic acidosis.

Glycolysis

Anaerobic glycolysis of one glucose molecule generates lactate and two ATP, whereas aerobic glycolysis to CO_2 and H_2O yields 38 ATP (Fig. 3.17). The three carbon compounds of glycolysis link it to other metabolic pathways, e.g. pyruvate is a precursor of alanine synthesis, glycerol 3-phosphate of triglyceride and phospholipid synthesis and 2,3-diphosphoglycerate is an important erythrocyte metabolite.

In *anoxic* or *hypoxic* conditions, pyruvate acts as a

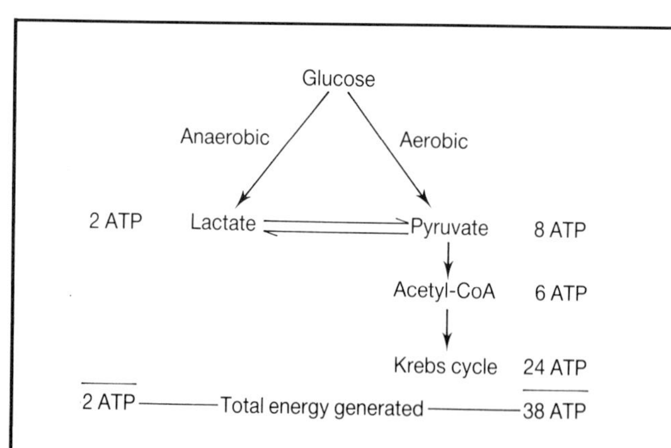

Fig. 3.17. Glycolysis: the energy generated by the anaerobic or aerobic oxidation of glucose.

temporary hydrogen acceptor and lactate is formed, but in normal circumstances hydrogen generated in glycolysis is taken up by NAD^+. This buffering action of pyruvate is an important homeostatic mechanism. Vigorous exercise by a healthy individual produces an O_2 debt and a transient rise of blood lactate, whereas normal exercise by a catabolic, feverish patient may be associated with a sustained rise in blood lactate. *Deficiency of lactic dehydrogenase*, the enzyme converting lactic acid to pyruvate, or of any of the enzymes involved in the synthesis of glucose 6-phosphate from pyruvate or the entry of pyruvate to the citric acid cycle all cause clinically important *lactic acidosis* which may be associated with hypoglycemia, hyperventilation and neurological abnormalities.

Gluconeogenesis

Gluconeogenesis is the synthesis of glucose from noncarbohydrate precursors (see Fig. 3.3, p. 73). The main sites of gluconeogenesis are the liver and kidney which, having glucose 6-phosphatase, are able to release glucose into the circulation. Most other cells have the capacity for gluconeogenesis which is important in the nervous system and erythrocytes but not in muscle. Amino acids are the principal carbon sources for gluconeogenesis. Transamination occurs between amino/keto acid homologues, e.g. pyruvate/alanine and also between nonhomologous pairs such as pyruvate/glutamine and oxaloacetate/glutamine. The blood concentrations of the enzymes controlling these reactions (SGPT and SGOT) are useful clinical markers of disease.

The molecule through which all carbon skeletons must pass in gluconeogenesis is 2-phosphoenol pyruvate (PEP). The enzymes linking PEP and glucose are cytosolic and reversible. In contrast the deaminated keto skeletons, pyruvate, α-ketoglutarate and succinate all traverse part of the Krebs cycle before exiting at oxaloacetate which is converted to PEP under the control of PEP carboxykinase. These reactions are intramitochondrial and irreversible. The key regulatory enzymes in gluconeogenesis are pyruvate carboxylase, PEP carboxykinase, fructose 1,6-diphosphate 1-phosphatase and glucose 6-phosphatase. Pyruvate carboxylase controls the reaction between pyruvate and acetyl-CoA to produce intramitochondrial oxaloacetate and is a crucial meeting point of carbohydrate and lipid metabolism. The 1-phosphatase is inhibited by AMP and ADP whereas the glucose 6-phosphatase is inhibited by glucose and inorganic phosphate. Cortisol stimulates and insulin inhibits the synthesis of all four enzymes.

Pancreatic control of energy homeostasis

Insulin and glucagon are the two islet hormones most intimately concerned with energy homeostasis but they should not be thought of in isolation because they are members of a larger family of peptide signals found in the gut and central nervous system. Attention will be focused on the islet peptides directly involved in fat and carbohydrate metabolism.

Islets of Langerhans

The mature islets of Langerhans are compact round or ovoid groups of polygonal epithelial cells irregularly distributed throughout the exocrine pancreas. Each islet is surrounded by an incomplete pseudocapsule which is continuous with the connective tissue interstitial septa of the exocrine gland. The islet has a rich blood supply of wide, thin-walled, anastomosing sinusoids that form a glomerulus with one afferent arteriole and several efferent capillaries. The islets have both sympathetic and parasympathetic innervation but the physiological importance of this remains unclear.

The islets originate from the primitive ducts of the embryonic pancreas whose cells are pluripotential for development to mature islet cells. There are four undisputed islet cell types: the β cell contains insulin, the α cell glucagon, the δ cell somatostatin, and the PP cell pancreatic polypeptide. The biosynthesis and secretion of each of the four hormones occurs by the same general mechanism. First there is ribosomal synthesis of a preprohormone, from which the leader sequence is removed during passage of the newly formed polypeptide through the endoplasmic reticulum membrane to leave the prohormone in the intracisternal space, from which it passes to the Golgi vesicles where it is stored as granules. The granule contents are secreted by exocytosis in which the granule membrane and cell membrane fuse and break down, allowing release of the granule contents to the circulation.

The proportions of different islet cell types vary depending on the embryological origin of the pancreas which grows as two outpouches of the duodenum that fuse together by the 8th week of gestation to form a ventral and dorsal lobe. The ventral lobe matures to become the uncinate process and posterior part of the head of the pancreas, whereas the dorsal lobe becomes the anterior part of the head, the body and tail of the gland. Islets rich in PP cells are found only in pancreas derived from the ventral lobe. α Cells develop before β cells and islets remain α-cell rich throughout fetal life. β-cell density (the product of cell size and number) increases with development to reach a peak 2 months after birth (11 months gestational age) after which it falls. This phenomenon is clinically important in the histopathological evaluation of pancreas when a diagnosis of *nesidioblastosis* is being considered because comparison with normal pancreas from older infants may give a misleading impression of pathological β-cell overdevelopment.

Abnormal islet development occurs in the *infant of the diabetic mother (IDM)* where there is β-cell and islet hyperplasia together with an increase in the PP cell fraction in the ventral lobe. In *erythroblastosis fetalis* there is hyperplasia of all four islet cell types but only in the islets of the ventral lobe. *Nesidioblastosis* represents a persistent hyperplasia of β cells and the islet may be disorganized with a loss of normal paracrine relationships between different cell types.

Insulin

Structure, storage and secretion

The molecules insulin, relaxin and the insulin-like growth factors (IGF) I and II are structurally related and may be regarded as a family. The insulin gene is on chromosome 11 as a single copy. There is a TATA box 30 base pairs from the starting site for transcription and three exons. Insulin is first synthesized as preproinsulin which contains a leader sequence of 24 amino acids. Proinsulin contains 84 amino acids in a single chain and is cleaved by proteolysis of a 33 amino acid segment to produce insulin which has A and B chains of 21 and 30 amino acids linked by two disulfide bonds. The residue of the cleaved segment is called the connecting or C-peptide and this is retained in the granule and secreted in equimolar amounts with insulin. Insulin, proinsulin and C-peptide can all be measured by competitive protein-binding techniques, most commonly radioimmunoassay. The half-life of circulating insulin is 10 minutes whereas that of C-peptide is appreciably longer, 30 minutes. In some circumstances the measurement of the circulating C-peptide or proinsulin concentration is a more accurate reflection of insulin secretion than the plasma insulin concentration.

Stimulation of secretion

The important nutritional stimuli to insulin secretion are glucose and amino acids. Other monosaccharides also cause insulin release, but glucose is the most important quantitatively. Oral glucose is more potent than intravenous glucose causing the same blood glucose rise. This is due to the enteroinsular axis through which the digestion and absorption of food stimulates the release of messengers from the gut that affect endocrine pancreatic secretion. Messengers with this action have been named incretins. Gastric inhibitory polypeptide (GIP) is a 42 amino acid straight chain arising from the epithelium of the duodenum and upper jejunum. GIP release is stimulated by glucose and galactose transport across the gut. Besides inhibiting gastric activity, GIP is also insulinotropic, but only in the presence of hyperglycemia. It thus fulfils the definition of an incretin. Pancreatic glucagon and the post-translational fragments GLP (1–37) and GLP (7–37) generated by cleavage of proglucagon in the intestine are also insulin secretagogues and potential incretins.

Insulin release is stimulated by amino acids and the mechanism of action of leucine differs from that of other amino acids. Arginine stimulation of insulin secretion is glucose dependent and diazoxide insensitive whereas the opposite is true for leucine. *Leucine-sensitive hypoglycemia* is probably the result of a normal physiological stimulus acting on an increased β-cell mass—this is part of the spectrum of disorders extending to *nesidioblastosis*. The mixture of amino acids resulting from a protein-rich meal is a more powerful insulin secretagogue than any individual amino acid.

Lipids have no consistent effect on insulin secretion. Medium-chain triglycerides (MCT) stimulate insulin release either directly or via a metabolite and their action is synergistic with that of oral glucose. This may be clinically important in patients fed artificial therapeutic diets.

The islets are innervated by the autonomic nervous system and the catecholamines: epinephrine and norepinephrine are powerful inhibitors of insulin secretion. β-Mimetics stimulate insulin release but their use therapeutically, as in asthma therapy, is not thought to be clinically important in glucose homeostasis. The methylxanthines inhibit cyclic 3,5-AMP phosphodiesterase and thereby stimulate insulin secretion. The stimulatory effects of sulfonylureas are pertinent to pediatric practice only in the context of accidental or deliberate poisoning. Diazoxide blocks insulin secretion by interfering with Ca^{2+} uptake and is useful in the management of some *hyperinsulinemic states of infancy and childhood*.

Insulin-dependent diabetes mellitus results from a relative or absolute insulin deficiency in infancy or childhood. *Transient neonatal diabetes* is a self-limiting insulin-dependent diabetes whose pathophysiology is poorly understood. Excessive spontaneous insulin release occurs transiently in the *infant of the diabetic mother* and in the *erythroblastotic newborn*. Sustained or reactive hyperinsulinemia may occur in *nesidioblastosis* and in *Beckwith syndrome*.

Mechanism of action

Insulin binds to specific receptors on the cell surface. The insulin receptor is closely related to the IGF-I receptor and is a glycoprotein of about 350 kDa made up of two pairs of subunits. The α pair of 135 kDa is entirely extracellular and has binding specificity. The β-subunits have a small extracellular domain connecting them to the α-subunits, a transmembrane domain of about 20 amino acids, and a large intracellular domain that is a tyrosine kinase. Insulin binding results in (1) phosphorylation of tyrosine on other proteins, altering their activity, (2) autophosphorylation with increased activity and receptor clustering. The receptor may be deactivated by phosphorylation of serine groups by other kinases, e.g. protein kinase C. Insulin receptors are also found in the cytosol and on the nuclear membrane, possibly as part of a receptor recycling control mechanism. Insulin-sensitive cells such as adipocytes and hepatocytes have higher receptor densities than other cells. Tyrosine kinase may phosphorylate a glucose transporter which is then concentrated at the cell membrane, facilitating glucose entry.

All the actions of insulin are directed towards anabolism and the lowering of blood glucose. Some actions are seen at fasting plasma insulin concentrations, others only in the presence of postprandial raised insulin concentrations. Some actions of insulin are rapid, others slower. Among the slow and longer lasting actions are the induction of enzymes whose gene transcription is under partial insulin control. Transcription may be initiated by the binding of nuclear protein to a *cis*-DNA sequence under the influence of insulin directly or an insulin-derived protein. Enzymes stimulated in this way include glucokinase, pyruvate kinase and glyceraldehyde 3-phosphate dehydrogenase which result in glycogenesis and increased glycolysis. Pancreatic amylase is also stimulated, thereby enhancing starch digestion and saccharide uptake.

Muscle protein is in a state of dynamic flux and its turnover increases with immaturity. Muscle protein turnover of an infant is in the order of 6 g/kg per day whereas that of a middle-aged man is only about 1.5 g/kg per day. Protein synthesis and breakdown in muscle are subject to a number of influences, e.g. muscle activity causes anabolism and excess glucocorticoids induce catabolism. High plasma insulin concentrations that occur postprandially stimulate protein synthesis by increasing the cellular uptake of amino acids and peptide synthesis independently with the consequence that the intracellular concentration of amino acids falls and tissue nitrogen increases. Low plasma insulin concentrations as seen in fasting inhibit but do not abolish proteolysis. Under these conditions muscle produces amino acids, particularly alanine and glutamate which are substrates for hepatic and renal gluconeogenesis. A slight increase of circulating insulin during fasting can depress plasma amino acids and urea nitrogen excretion without influencing circulating lipid metabolites.

Glucose crosses cell membranes by interaction with specific cell membrane proteins, the glucose transporters. These are a superfamily of proteins with 12 transmembrane domains, some of which are primarily located on the cell membrane for constitutive glucose entry. Different members of the family are found specifically in some tissues: e.g. a distinct form is present in neural tissue. Glut 4, the insulin-sensitive transporter found only in fat and muscle, is primarily located in the Golgi apparatus and is translocated to the cell surface in response to insulin. Insulin promotes glucose uptake by increasing the amount of glucose transporter synthesized and by increasing the movement of transporter to the plasma membrane in both muscle cells and adipocytes, but not in hepatocytes which are freely permeable to glucose. Insulin stimulates both glycolysis and glycogenesis. Glycolysis is activated by direct stimulation of phosphofructokinase and unblocking the inhibitory action of fructose 2,6-biphosphate. Glycogen synthesis is promoted by a sequence of events started by the tyrosine kinase of the insulin receptor, leading eventually to the dephosphorylation of both the glycogen phosphorylase and synthetase which are reciprocally inactivated and activated. At low fasting concentrations insulin inhibits hormone-sensitive lipase and thus adipocyte lipolysis. Lipogenesis is promoted by insulin at postprandial concentrations.

Glucagon

The glucagon family

Glucagon is a member of a multigene family which also includes secretin, vasoactive intestinal peptide (VIP), gastric inhibitory peptide (GIP) and glicentin. The glucagon gene is on chromosome 2q36–2q37 and comprises six exons and five introns. Preproglucagon is a 180 residue protein that contains the sequences of glucagon, glicentin and two glucagon-like peptides (GLP), GLP-1 and GLP-2. Glucagon is a 29 amino acid single chain which is synthesized and secreted from the α cells of the islet in a manner analogous to insulin. A fragment of GLP-1: GLP-1(7–37) is 100 times more potent than glucagon as an insulin secretagogue under hyperglycemic conditions and may be physiologically important.

Stimulation of secretion

The stimuli to glucagon secretion and its actions are largely the opposite of those of insulin. Glucagon release is stimulated by hypoglycemia and inhibited by glucose. Fasting increases plasma glucagon concentrations. Both glucagon and insulin release are stimulated by amino acids and arginine is a potent glucagon secretagogue. The simultaneous rise of both hormones after a protein-rich meal ensures the proper conversion of excess glucogenic amino acids to glucose and utilization of the glucose. The α cell is more sensitive to the inhibitory effect of glucose and stimulatory effect of arginine than the β cell. A rise in plasma FFA or ketones inhibits glucagon release and a fall is stimulatory. Other members of the gut peptide family may stimulate glucagon secretion. Catecholamines and sympathetic nervous stimulation result in glucagon release.

Mechanism of action

Glucagon binds to a specific cell-surface receptor which is coupled to adenylyl cyclase by a G_s-protein. Activation of adenylyl cyclase results in the synthesis of cAMP from ATP in the presence of magnesium. This acts on a cAMP-dependent kinase which then adds phosphate groups to the serine and threonine groups of other proteins. cAMP is hydrolyzed by a specific phosphodiesterase that can be inhibited by methylxanthines. Glucagon causes hyperglycemia by promoting glycogenolysis and inhibiting glycogen synthesis via cAMP-induced phosphorylation. At the same time hepatic gluconeogenesis is stimulated by reduction of fructose 2,6-biphosphate concentration, leading to activation of gluconeogenesis and inhibition of glycolysis. Glycolysis raises the blood glucose faster than gluconeogenesis. Adipocyte lipolysis is stimulated via activation of hormone-sensitive lipase. Hepatic lipogenesis is inhibited because acetyl-CoA production from glucose falls with the block of glycolysis. Ketogenesis is stimulated by glucagon induction of carnitine acyltransferase I which is the rate-limiting enzyme for the transfer of fatty acids from the cytosol to the mitochondria.

Intramuscular glucagon injection has a useful clinical role in the treatment of *insulin-induced hypoglycemia* in *diabetes. Glucagon deficiency* is extremely rare but has been reported and results clinically in a presentation characterized by hypoglycemia which is responsive to glucagon therapy, unlike the conditions of insulin excess cited above which are exacerbated by treatment with glucagon.

Other islet hormones

Somatostatin is widely distributed throughout the body in a variety of endocrine cells as well as in the central nervous system. It is a 1.63 kDa peptide containing 14 amino acids synthesized and secreted in a manner analogous to insulin. The stimuli to somatostatin secretion are unknown, but local innervation may be important. The physiological role of somatostatin released from the δ cells of the islets remains unclear; it seems more likely to be a paracrine inhibitor of other islet hormone-secreting cells than a true endocrine messenger.

Synthetic somatostatin analogs have been used experimentally in the treatment of refractory hyperinsulinemic hypoglycemia.

Amylin is a 37 amino acid polypeptide, first isolated from amyloid deposits in pancreatic islet cells from *type II diabetics*. It shows a close structural homology to calcitonin gene-related peptide (CGRP), an alternate splice product of the calcitonin gene. Amylin is a β-cell hormone which colocalizes with and probably is cosecreted with insulin. It appears to inhibit both insulin secretion and the sensitivity of peripheral tissues to insulin and has been implicated as an etiological factor in *type II diabetes*.

Pancreatic polypeptide contains 36 amino acids and is 4.24 kDa. In man both neural and nutritive stimuli are important secretagogues, vagal activity in the anticipatory preprandial phase and protein ingestion both being effective. The actions of pancreatic polypeptide are mainly on the stomach and duodenum where it has a homeostatic action on muscle tone, pancreatic fluid production, bicarbonate and enzyme release, and bile secretion.

Developmental aspects

Before birth

Carbohydrate, predominantly glucose, provides about 60 percent of fetal energy needs. The normal fetus does not produce glucose but receives it by facilitated placental diffusion at a rate of 4–6 mg/kg per minute. In late gestation fetal gluconeogenesis may contribute to fetal and placental glucose utilization if fetal glucose supply is reduced, e.g. maternal fasting or intrauterine growth retardation. A proportion of the glucose taken up by the placenta is metabolized there to produce lactate which then passes to the fetal and maternal circulations. Fetal O_2 consumption is directly related to the sum of the fetal glucose and lactate uptake. Only 50 percent of the glucose taken up by the fetus in late gestation is oxidized, the remainder being converted to glycogen in the liver and muscle, and to fat in the liver and adipose tissue. In the last trimester glucose storage is controlled primarily by insulin but glucocorticoids are also involved in the early ontogeny of glycogen synthetic pathways. Most fetal tissues oxidize glucose preferentially and some, the brain, adrenal medulla, renal cortex and erythrocytes, are obligatory glucose consumers.

The molar transport of lipid molecules may be small in comparison to carbohydrate, but their carbon-rich skeleton may make a significant contribution to fetal metabolism. Net transplacental flux of FFA can occur by (1) direct carrier-mediated transport, (2) placental synthesis and release into the umbilical circulation especially of essential fatty acids produced by chain elongation and desaturation, or (3) lipolysis of complex triglycerides, lipoproteins or phospholipids derived from either the maternal or fetal circulations. Since fetal fatty acid composition varies with maternal diet, placental selectivity in fatty acid transport is probably not of major importance.

Fetal metabolic rate determined by net fetal O_2 consumption is linked directly, but not tightly, to fetal energy supply. The extent to which the placenta determines net glucose and lactate delivery to the fetus influences fetal metabolic rate slightly, but the fact that fetal O_2 consumption remains constant while glucose oxidation varies twofold indicates that a reciprocal relationship exists between glucose oxidation and that of other energy-producing substrates. Amino acids are taken up by the fetus in excess of protein synthetic rates and fetal urea production is high, both indicating a contribution to fetal energy supply. Fetal protein catabolism is regulated by nonprotein energy supply and when necessary the amino acids released are transaminated to glucose or oxidized to maintain fetal and placental metabolic rate, potentially to the detriment of fetal growth.

The placenta is impermeable to both insulin and glucagon, both of which are found in fetal blood from week 10 of gestation. Insulin acts cooperatively with circulating metabolites and paracrine growth factors to maintain an anabolic effect throughout pregnancy. In the first two trimesters the most important insulin secretagogue may be amino acids. Glucose stimulates insulin release in the third trimester only and at this stage of development insulin is both strongly glycogenic and lipogenic. In addition to promoting glucose storage, insulin also stimulates glucose oxidation with a consequent sparing of amino acids. Glucagon secretion is unaffected by acute changes in blood glucose concentration, but increases during chronic fetal hypoglycemia.

During prolonged maternal fasting or subnutrition

there is a fall in both maternal and fetal blood glucose and after several days fetal glucose utilization also declines together with plasma insulin. Fetal glucose delivery is augmented by gluconeogenesis from lactate of placental origin and to a lesser extent from fetal amino acids. This is reflected by fetal glucose utilization remaining higher than umbilical glucose delivery. Hepatic glycogen is not mobilized and is protected for the neonatal transition, even in the face of marked *intrauterine growth retardation*. Fetal and maternal ketones also contribute to fetal energy demands and have a glucose sparing effect. *Fetal hypoxia* is associated with hyperglycemia and a reduced fetal glucose clearance probably due to fetal catecholamine release and inhibition of insulin secretion. There is also increased fetal glucose production possibly arising from catecholamine-stimulated hepatic glycogenolysis.

β-Mimetics are commonly used to suppress uterine contractions in the management of preterm labor and may be administered for periods ranging from hours to weeks. β-Blockers are used less frequently, but women with thyroid or cardiac disease may take them throughout pregnancy. The placenta is permeable to both classes of drug. Treatment with ritodrine, a β-mimetic, has been claimed to improve the growth of small-for-dates fetuses because of increased uterine blood flow and better fetal nutrition, but an alternative possibility, if indeed there is an effect, is the induction of maternal carbohydrate intolerance. The effects of β-mimetics on maternal and fetal lipid metabolism have not been studied. Neonatal hypoglycemia lasting 2–3 days has been reported after maternal propranolol therapy during pregnancy. There are good theoretical reasons to anticipate that transplacentally acquired propranolol could result in disturbed carbohydrate and lipid homeostasis for days after birth.

After birth

Following birth blood glucose is derived from hepatic glycogen for a few hours only, after which gluconeogenesis from lipid is necessary for glucose homeostasis. Tissue fat is mobilized for this purpose until milk intake is adequate. In the normal term infant plasma glycerol concentrations rise sharply in the first minutes of life and FFA in the early hours, while glucose concentrations fall gently. Part of this is associated with the initiation of brown fat thermogenesis. By 12 hours after birth FFA concentrations have stabilized at three to four times the umbilical cord blood concentration, whereas glucose has fallen by approximately one-third. The respiratory quotient of the infant falls over the same interval, from 1.0 to 0.7, signifying a transfer to fat as the principal source of energy. The newborn brain uses both glucose and ketone bodies as fuel. Ketones may provide 10 percent of the energy requirement in normal circumstances and more during starvation.

The rate of FFA mobilization in the newborn depends not only on neuronal and hormonal stimulation and inhibition of lipolysis, but also on changes in the uptake, re-esterification and oxidation of FFA within adipose tissue. Early postnatal lipolysis occurs in a thermoneutral environment due to increased sympathetic activity, but cold exposure can exaggerate the rise in plasma glycerol and FFA. Acidosis has little or no acute effect on lipolysis, but if prolonged is inhibitory. Heparin stimulates lipolysis and when added in low dose to neonatal infusion fluids may have desirable metabolic effects as well as being antithrombogenic.

Fasting is characterized by low but detectable plasma insulin concentrations and modestly raised plasma glucagon concentrations. There is hepatic gluconeogenesis and ketogenesis but no glycolysis or lipogenesis. Similarly there is adipocyte lipolysis and no lipogenesis or glucose uptake. In muscle there is slight proteolysis and no glucose uptake. The hormonal and metabolic responses to feeding vary depending on the nutrient mix. A protein-rich meal causes both insulin and glucagon secretion and stimulates both lipogenesis and gluconeogenesis in the liver, while glycolysis and ketogenesis are suppressed. Glucose uptake is promoted in both muscles and adipose tissue where protein synthesis and lipogenesis, respectively, are stimulated. In contrast, a carbohydrate-rich meal stimulates insulin but not glucagon secretion and causes hepatic lipogenesis and glycolysis but no gluconeogenesis. Glucose uptake is strongly stimulated in both muscle and fat with a consequential promotion of lipogenesis and an equivocal stimulation of protein synthesis. A mixed meal rich in both protein and carboydrate is the strongest stimulus of insulin secretion and causes marginal glucagon release. This is strongly stimulatory to hepatic lipogenesis, glucose uptake by muscle and adipose tissue and the subsequent protein synthesis and lipogenesis.

Hypoglycemia

Hypoglycemia is the commonest clinical manifestation of disordered energy metabolism and is important because the obligatory consumption of glucose by the brain means that sustained hypoglycemia may cause neuronal damage and lead to death. The pathophysiology of hypoglycemia divides neatly into those examples resulting from increased glucose consumption, usually as a consequence of insulin excess, and those due to inadequate glucose production. There are important differences in the etiology of the two mechanisms in the neonate, the toddler and the older child and it is convenient to consider each separately.

The physiological blood glucose range is lower in the newborn, but the absolute glucose concentration is less important than the overall clinical assessment of the baby. *Neonatal hypoglycemia* associated with abnormal physical signs is called 'symptomatic hypoglycemia' and is potentially lethal. Conventional teaching states that 'asymptomatic hypoglycemia' is benign, but recent evidence suggests otherwise and it is prudent to keep a baby's blood glucose above 2.6 mmol/l; there is recent electrophysiological evidence for neurological dysfunction at concentrations lower than this. The *preterm infant*, especially the *very low birthweight infant*, lacks both hepatic carbohydrate and subcutaneous adipose stores, with the result that circulating fuel concentrations are low and may run out, leading to exhaustion of cardiac and respiratory muscle and cerebral damage. *Small-for-dates infants* are also characterized by a tendency to hypoglycemia, the etiology of which is complicated because they are a heterogenous group, some being hyperinsulinemic. *Hypoxia* in the newborn is commonly associated with *respiratory and metabolic acidosis*, so that it may be difficult to disentangle hypoxia from acidosis in clinical problems, but both are associated with an inefficient oxidative metabolism and a tendency to hypoglycemia. *Cold exposure* is detrimental for babies because an increased metabolic rate is necessary to maintain a constant body temperature.

The typical infant of a diabetic mother (*IDM*) has an exaggerated fall in blood glucose and an attenuated rise of FFA because of hyperinsulinemia, but the hypoglycemia is not prolonged past the first few days after birth. Persistent hypoglycemia in an infant clinically resembling but not an IDM should arouse suspicion of abnormal β-cell development as in *nesidioblastosis* or *pancreatic adenoma*. *Beckwith syndrome* is also characterized by hyperinsulinemic hypoglycemia, but the diagnosis is suspected from related clinical abnormalities such as macroglossia, omphalocele and transverse ear creases. *Prenatal exposure to drugs* may have profound clinical effects. Pregnant diabetic women may be treated with *oral sulfonylureas* which cross the placenta. The baby is born hyperinsulinemic and with therapeutic circulating concentrations of an insulinotropic drug that is degraded slowly because of the immaturity of the neonatal liver. These infants suffer profound intractable hypoglycemia and treatment by exchange transfusion may be necessary to remove the drug. Help in recognizing hyperinsulinemic hypoglycemia comes from the absence of urinary ketones and the glucose infusion rate needed to maintain euglycemia. In hyperinsulinemic hypoglycemia this is commonly above 10 mg/kg body weight per minute, whereas substrate shortage is corrected by glucose infusion rates of less than 8 mg/kg per minute.

In addition to the common causes of hypoglycemia such as *malnutrition*, a toddler may have an inborn metabolic error causing inadequate glucose production. In such cases the presence of acidosis and/or hepatomegaly are important clinical clues to which specific biochemical investigations are pertinent (Table 3.3). The *inborn errors of fatty acid metabolism* are unusual because they are the only metabolic defects resulting in nonketotic hypoglycemia. Other uncommon but important conditions that may present as hypoglycemia at this age are *endocrine deficiencies*, in particular *congenital hypopituitarism* and *adrenocortical insufficiency*.

In toddlers and later childhood the principles governing metabolic balance associated with feeding and fasting are no different from those applying to the adult, but the

Table 3.3. Examples of inborn metabolic errors characterized by hypoglycemia associated with acidosis and/or hepatomegaly

Inborn metabolic error	Acidosis	Hepatomegaly
Glucose 6-phosphatase (GSD I)	+	+
Amylo-1,6-glucosidase (GSD III)	−	+
Phosphorylase	+	+
Fructose 1,6-diphosphatase	+	+
Fructose intolerance	+	+
Galactosemia	−	+
Pyruvate carboxylase	+	−

younger the child, the shorter the time during fasting that euglycemia can be sustained. It is important to appreciate that among children of the same age or weight there is a biological spectrum of tolerance of fasting. Some children labeled as having *ketotic hypoglycemia* may have a subtle or partial metabolic defect or they may be examples of one end of the physiological spectrum. The commonest cause of hypoglycemia in childhood is iatrogenic due to insulin overdose in an insulin-dependent diabetic.

Selected reading

Montgomery R, Conway TW, Spector AA. *Biochemistry, a case oriented approach*. 5th ed. St Louis: CV Mosby, 1990.

Senior B, Sadeghi-Nejad A. Hypoglycemia: a pathophysiological approach. *Acta Paediatr Scand Suppl* **352**: 1989.

E. Biochemistry of the Arachidonate Pathway

M S Trautman and M D Mitchell

Pathways of arachidonic acid metabolism

Eicosanoids are derivatives of 20-carbon polyunsaturated fatty acids one of which, arachidonic acid (all *cis*-5,8,11,14-eicosatetraenoic acid), is the precursor of the most important group of eicosanoids, the **prostaglandins**. Formation of these eicosanoids via fatty acid cyclooxygenase requires that arachidonic acid be in the nonesterified form.

Arachidonic acid release

Arachidonic acid is a typical polyunsaturated fatty acid present in cells predominantly in an esterified form, usually in the *sn-2* position of a glycerophospholipid (Fig. 3.18). The liberation of arachidonic acid from glycerophospholipids is a rate-limiting step in the biosynthesis of eicosanoids that is accomplished either directly by the action of phospholipase A_2 or indirectly by action of phospholipase C followed by the action of diacylglycerol and monoacylglycerol lipases (Fig. 3.19).

Arachidonic acid liberated by these reactions is metabolized in **three major pathways** (Fig. 3.19):

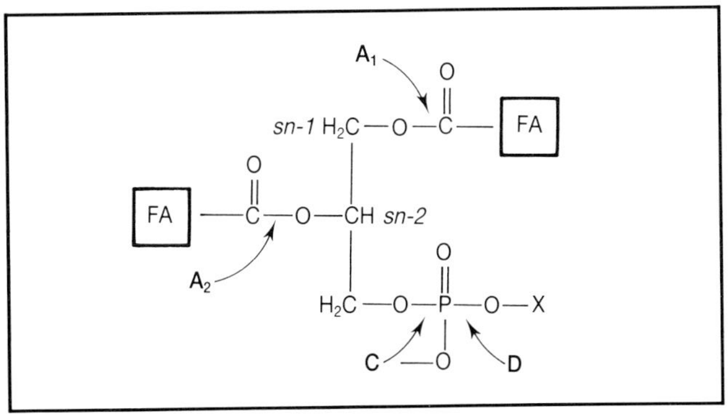

Fig. 3.18. The structure of a generalized glycerophospholipid. Alcohols found in phosphomonoester linkage are depicted as X. Sites of phospholipase hydrolysis are shown by $\mathbf{A_1}$, $\mathbf{A_2}$, **C** and **D**. A saturated fatty acid is typically esterified at the *sn-1* position and a polyunsaturated fatty acid at the *sn-2* position. Fatty acids are represented by FA. (Adapted from Hillier K, ed. *Advances in eicosanoid research*, Dordrecht, Holland: MTP Press, 1978: 109, with permission.)

cyclooxygenase, lipoxygenase and monooxygenase (epoxygenase). Each pathway results in the formation of a variety of biologically active products (Fig. 3.20).

Fatty acid cyclooxygenase

This enzyme is also known as prostaglandin endoperoxide synthase. Arachidonic acid metabolism via this pathway involves the bis-dioxygenation reaction to form the unstable prostaglandin (PG) endoperoxide PGG_2 which is subsequently reduced by a hydroperoxidase to PGH_2. All subsequent PGs are derived from this intermediate.

PGH_2 is converted to thromboxane (Tx) A_2 by thromboxane synthase which is in platelets and a number of cells. TxA_2 is a potent constrictor not only of vascular beds but also of airway smooth muscle.

PGH_2 is converted to prostacyclin PGI_2 by prostacyclin synthase which is in endothelial cells, the uterus and a number of other cells. PGI_2 is a potent vasodilator, particularly of the perinatal pulmonary circulation (see p. 522), and also inhibits platelet adhesion.

PGH_2 is converted to PGD_2 by serum albumin and PGD isomerase. PGD_2 is found in highest concentrations in the central nervous system. When administered systemically it has multiple effects, one of which is pulmonary vasodilatation in the immediate newborn period. PGD_2 is the principal cyclooxygenase product of mast cells.

PGH_2 is converted to PGE_2 by isomerization. PGE_2 is the major arachidonate product of a number of cells and is produced by the placenta. PGs of the E series inhibit gastric secretion and relax bronchial smooth muscle directly by inhibition of acetylcholine release. PGE_2 also dilates the ductus arteriosus (see p. 525 and below). PGE_1, derived from dihomo-γ-linolenic acid, inhibits neutrophil adherence and neutrophil-mediated injury to endothelial cells.

PGH_2 is converted to $PGF_{2\alpha}$ usually by nonspecific reduction. $PGF_{2\alpha}$ acts as a potent bronchoconstrictor and elevated $PGF_{2\alpha}$ concentrations in acute asthma have been reported.

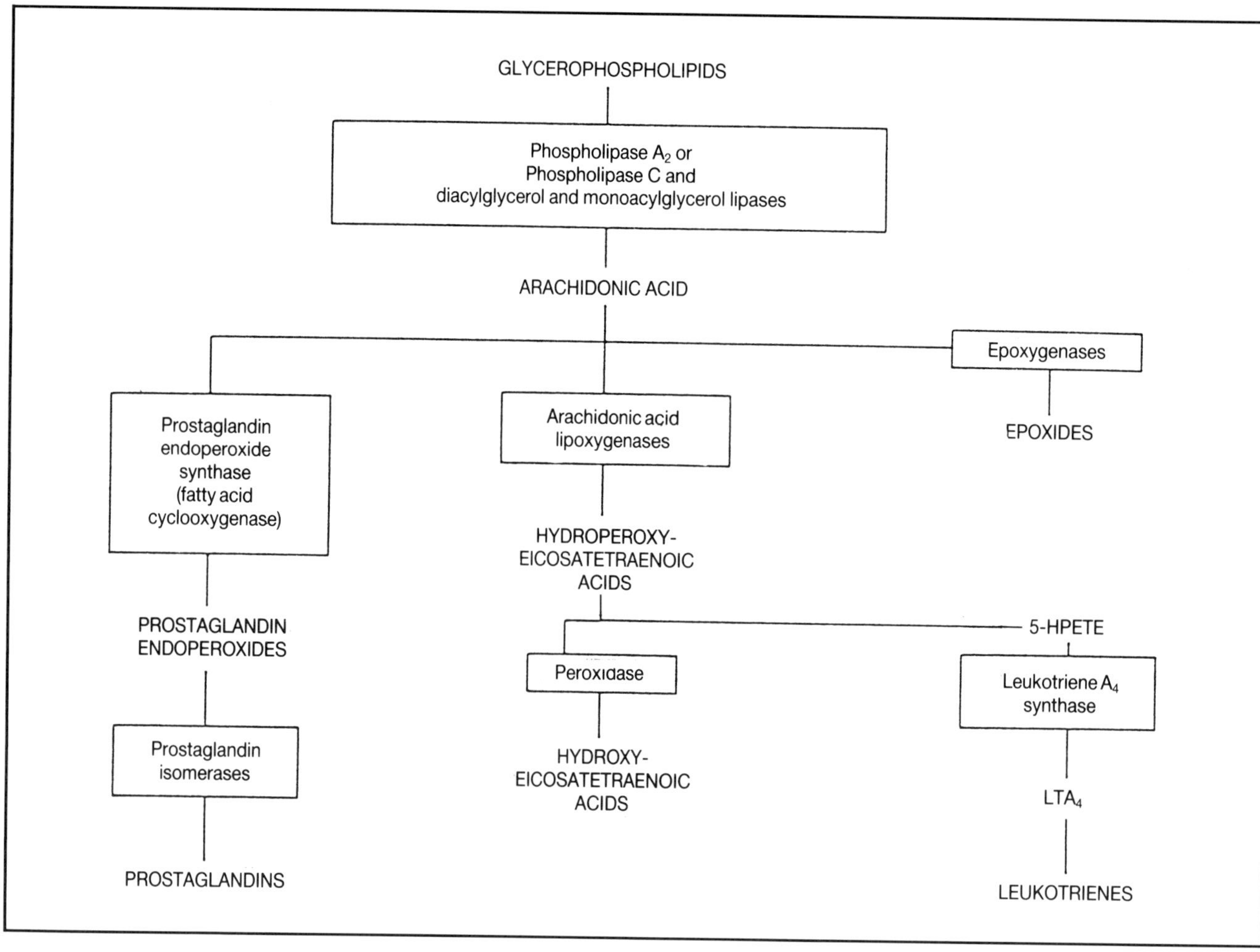

Fig. 3.19. The enzymatic pathways of arachidonic acid metabolism. (From Mitchell MD. *Semin Perinatol* 1986; **10**(4): 243, with permission.)

15-Hydroxyprostaglandin dehydrogenase

The first step in the catabolism of PGs is effected by the cytosolic enzyme 15-hydroxyprostaglandin dehydrogenase (PGDH). The 15-keto derivatives formed are rapidly converted to the 13,14-dihydro-15-keto derivatives which are the major but biologically inactive circulating forms. The lung is a major metabolic venue: almost all biologically active PGs are metabolized during one passage through the lungs. Metabolism occurs by uptake into pulmonary cells and then by the action of PGDH. Biologically active PGs are further eliminated by a series of β- and ϖ-oxidations that result in the formation of products that are excreted in the urine. There are exceptions to this general pattern: PGD_2 is an extremely poor substrate for PGDH and PGI_2 may not be completely metabolized by the lungs since it is a poor substrate for the pulmonary cellular uptake mechanism.

Inhibitors of prostaglandin biosynthesis

The most commonly used inhibitors of PG biosynthesis are the nonsteroidal anti-inflammatory drugs (NSAIDs) such as indomethacin, naproxen, mefenamic acid and ibuprofen. These drugs act at the level of fatty acid cyclooxygenase and block the biosynthesis of all PGs. Glucocorticoids also inhibit PG biosynthesis primarily by an action on the phospholipases via stimulation of antiphospholipase proteins such as macrocortin, lipomodulin, lipocortins and annexins.

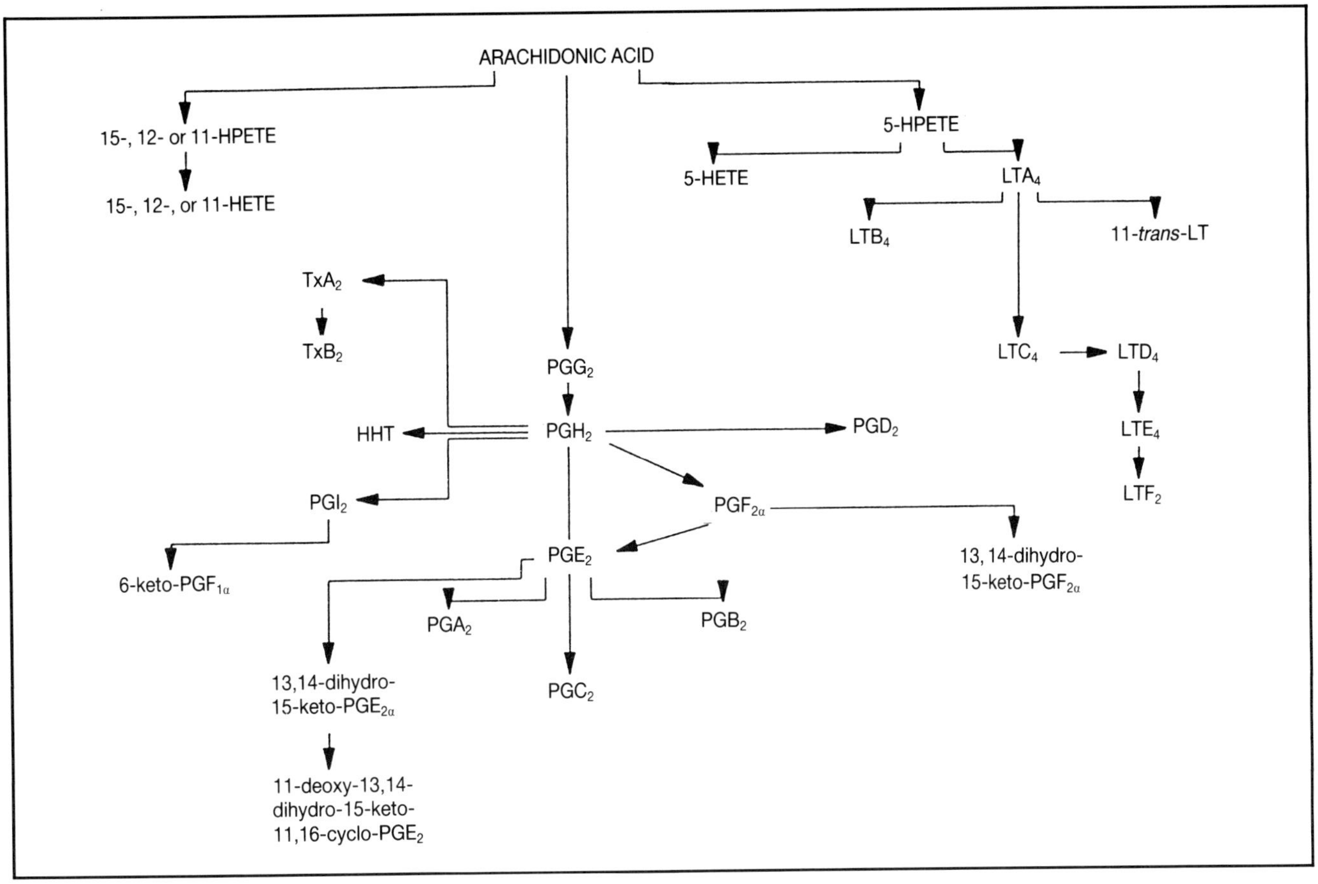

Fig. 3.20. A simplified outline of the pathways of arachidonic acid metabolism. (From Mitchell MD. *Semin Perinatol* 1986; **10**(4): 243, with permission.)

Lipoxygenases

Lipoxygenases are a group of iron-containing dioxygenases which catalyze the insertion of oxygen into polyunsaturated fatty acids including arachidonic acid. Three distinct enzymes insert oxygen at carbons 5, 12, and 15 of arachidonic acid. Additionally, others exist which also insert oxygen at the 8 and 11 positions.

12-Hydroperoxy-eicosatetraenoic acid (12-HPETE) formed by 12-lipoxygenase reduces secretion of neutrophil-specific granules and augments immunoglobulin (Ig)-E-mediated mast cell release. Biological effects of 12-lipoxygenase products are found only at high concentrations.

15-HPETE and its secondary derivatives are the principal products of arachidonic acid metabolism by the 15-lipoxygenases in the lung and eosinophils.

5-HPETE formed by 5-lipoxygenase is the precursor of leukotrienes (LTs) which are important in many inflammatory processes. The key step is the conversion of 5-HPETE to LTA_4 which is then metabolized in a number of ways. Water may be added at C-12 opening the epoxide at C-6 and creating LTB_4, or the epoxide at C-6 may be opened by the sulfhydryl group of glutathione with the formation of LTC_4. LTC_4 may be metabolized further by the sequential elimination of glutamic acid and glycine to form LTD_4 and LTE_4. Conversion of LTE_4 to LTF_4 occurs by addition of a γ-glutamyl residue to the amino group. The further metabolism of LTs is complex.

LTB_4 is a chemoattractant for neutrophils and eosinophils. LTC_4, D_4 and E_4 constrict smooth muscle in airways and vascular and intestinal beds. It should be noted that 15-HPETE can be metabolized by other routes to yield lipoxins that have many important biological properties.

Monooxygenase (epoxygenase)

Metabolism of arachidonic acid by cytochrome P450 leads to various oxygenated products. The epoxy acids exhibit significant biological activity *in vitro*: stimulation of peptide hormone release, mobilization of intracellular Ca^{2+}, and alteration of net K^+ and Na^+ fluxes.

Function of prostaglandins in development

Limited information on the products of the lipoxygenase and monooxygenase enzymes focuses attention on the cyclooxygenase products.

Before birth

Preterm

PGE_2 and $PGF_{2\alpha}$ play a key part in the mechanisms controlling labor (see p. 141) since both contract uterine smooth muscle and soften the cervix at all stages of gestation. They are used as abortifacients. PGE_2 is ten times more potent than $PGF_{2\alpha}$. Inhibitors of PG synthesis such as the nonsteroidal anti-inflammatory drugs have been used to treat *preterm labor*. They should be used with extreme caution or even avoided since results from controlled studies are not available and severe side-effects may occur: e.g. reduction in cerebral blood flow, constriction of the ductus arteriosus. PGI_2 relaxes vascular smooth muscle and inhibits platelet aggregation whereas thromboxane has the opposite actions. Low dose aspirin is used to prevent *pre-eclampsia* and *intrauterine growth retardation* because it alters the PGI_2/thromboxane balance in favor of PGI_2.

Term

Labor at term is initiated in part by increased intrauterine synthesis of PGs. There are substantial increases of both intra-amniotic and plasma PGE_2 and $PGF_{2\alpha}$ concentrations, leading to uterine contractions. Stimuli of fatty acid cyclooxygenase often fail to elicit a release of arachidonate and it is possible that an endogenous activator of phospholipase A_2 or C is likely to be involved to increase PG synthesis during parturition.

After birth

The ductus arteriosus (DA) (see p. 525) is maintained patent by PGE_2 and is relatively unresponsive to other PGs both *in vivo* and *in vitro*. A major source of fetal circulating PGE_2 is the placenta and since only 10 percent of the fetal cardiac output goes to the lungs where PGE_2 is mainly metabolized, the systemic circulating concentration is high. Blocking PG synthesis by cyclooxygenase inhibition causes constriction of the fetal ductus arteriosus and the effect of indomethacin in this respect is greater in immature than mature fetuses. Maturation of ductal PG insensitivity can be triggered by corticosteroids. The fetal ductus arteriosus is open, not because of passive dilatation, but due to a balance between constricting and relaxing stimuli. After birth circulating PGE_2 concentrations fall due to increased pulmonary blood flow and removal of the placenta. This permits the ductus arteriosus to become more sensitive to constricting stimuli such as rising oxygen tension.

Knowledge of the physiological control of the ductal diameter can be applied clinically in *congenital heart defects*. For example: in *aortic arch anomalies* or *left ventricular outflow tract obstruction* the patent ductus supplies most or all of the systemic blood; in *transposition of the great arteries* ductus arteriosus patency allows pulmonary/systemic mixing via bidirectional shunting; and in *right ventricular outflow obstruction* the patent ductus supplies the pulmonary blood flow. PGE_2 has been used to maintain ductus arteriosus patency at infusion rates of 0.02–0.05 μg/kg per minute. PGs influence many systems and their pharmacological use or inhibition of their synthesis will always have multiple effects that must be monitored.

Selected reading

Challis JRD, Patrick JE. The production of prostaglandins and thromboxanes in the feto-placental unit and their effects on the developing fetus. *Semin Perinatol* 1980; **4**: 23–33.

Clyman RI. Eicosanoids and the ductus arteriosus. In

Mitchell MD, ed. *Eicosanoids in reproduction*. Florida: CRC Press, 1990: 273.

Heymann MA. The role of eicosanoids in the fetal and perinatal circulations. In Mitchell MD, ed. *Eicosanoids in reproduction*. Florida: CRC Press, 1990: 285.

Holtzman MJ. Arachidonic acid metabolism. *Am Rev Respir Dis* 1991; **143**: 188.

Mitchell MD. Prostaglandin synthesis, metabolism and function in the fetus. In Jones CT, ed. *Biochemical development of the fetus*. Amsterdam: Elsevier, 1982: 425.

Myatt L. Placental biosynthesis, metabolism and transport of eicosanoids. In Mitchell MD, ed. *Eicosanoids in reproduction*. Florida: CRC Press, 1990: 169.

F. Free Radicals, Oxidants and Antioxidants

C C Winterbourn

The discovery of superoxide dismutase (SOD) in 1968 led to the realization that free radicals must be produced physiologically and opened up the field of free radical biology. It is now clear that not only are free radicals formed during normal metabolism but they are also involved in a number of pathological and toxicological processes. In some cases they are a prime cause of injury. In others they are a consequence, and may either amplify the injury or simply be an epiphenomenon.

Definitions

A free radical is any chemical species containing one or more unpaired electrons. Most free radicals have a lifetime of less than a second and react with a wide range of biological molecules. Some cause oxidation, some reduction, and others, like superoxide, are capable of both. Oxidative reactions are most likely to be injurious.

Molecular oxygen (O_2) is a terminal electron (e^-) acceptor and has a high affinity for electrons. Normally, complete reduction of O_2 via the cytochrome oxidase pathway adds four electrons and produces two molecules of H_2O without releasing any partially reduced intermediates which remain bound to the cytochrome oxidase complex throughout the process. However the partial reduction of O_2 by sequential single electron steps may produce three intermediates, the **superoxide radical** (superoxide anion) ($O_2^{\bullet -}$), **hydrogen peroxide** (H_2O_2) or the **hydroxyl radical** ($OH^\bullet$), each more reactive than O_2 itself.

$$O_2 \xrightarrow{e^-} O_2^{\bullet -} \xrightarrow{e^-/2H^+} H_2O_2 \xrightarrow{e^-/H^+} OH^\bullet + H_2O \xrightarrow{e^-/H^+} H_2O$$

Superoxide is in equilibrium with its protonated form, the hydroperoxyl radical ($HO_2^\bullet$), with a pK_a of 4.8. Superoxide breaks down by spontaneous dismutation to hydrogen peroxide.

$$O_2^{\bullet -} + HO_2^\bullet + H^+ \longrightarrow O_2 + H_2O_2$$

Together these intermediates of O_2 reduction are referred to as either **activated oxygen** or **reactive oxygen species**. Oxidative stress in cells refers to the increased generation of superoxide and hydrogen peroxide. Oxidative damage is the tissue injury caused by free radicals or other strong oxidants.

A **free radical scavenger** is any compound that intercepts radicals without propagating further radical reactions. Some scavengers may be relatively specific, e.g. for hydroxyl or lipid peroxyl radicals; others are more general. Antioxidant defense encompasses both free radical scavengers and enzymatic mechanisms that remove radicals and reactive oxidants.

Sources of free radicals and reactive oxidants

Radiation

Ionizing (nuclear) radiation is harmful because of free radical reactions. Its prime target is tissue water and, in the presence of O_2, the main radical species produced are superoxide and hydroxyl radicals. These water-derived radicals cause damage by reacting with DNA and other macromolecules. Ultraviolet radiation is sufficiently energetic to generate free radicals and also produces electronically excited species that decay by initiating radical reactions. Injury by these mechanisms is seen in *sunburn, porphyria* and *hyperbilirubinemia* treated by phototherapy.

Metabolic generation of radicals

Free radicals are produced during normal metabolism from several sources, the major one being mitochondrial respiration.

Mitochondria

Aerobic life depends on the energy released in the conversion of O_2 to water without forming radical intermediates. This is achieved in the mitochondria by cytochrome oxidase in the respiratory chain. The system is not perfect, however, and there is a continuous flux of superoxide into the cytoplasm.

Xanthine oxidase

Another significant source of free radicals is the oxidation of xanthine and hypoxanthine to uric acid under the control of xanthine oxidase with the concomitant reduction of O_2 to superoxide and hydrogen peroxide (Fig. 3.21). This reaction proceeds normally under the control of xanthine dehydrogenase using NAD as a hydrogen acceptor, but switches to the oxidase in the presence of raised intracellular calcium or ischemia.

Heme proteins

Oxidation of hemoglobin and myoglobin to their met forms is accompanied by the release of heme-bound O_2 as superoxide. Since the met-proteins recycle, there is continuous net generation of superoxide corresponding to the oxidation of about 3 percent of the total hemoglobin per day.

Autoxidations

A number of physiological compounds, e.g. catecholamines, flavins and some sugars, can auto-oxidize to generate radicals.

Drugs and environmental chemicals

Many toxic drugs and environmental chemicals (xenobiotics) such as paraquat are metabolized to free radicals. This may occur either by reduction by NADH or NADPH-dependent reductases that are present in most cells, or by oxidation by cytochrome P450, hemoglobin or peroxidases.

Phagocytes

Free radical production can also be beneficial as in the microbicidal activity of granulocytes and mononuclear phagocytes. Phagocytic stimuli and a wide variety of inflammatory mediators activate an NADPH oxidase located in the cell membrane, causing a burst of O_2 uptake and conversion to superoxide (Fig. 3.22). Superoxide is generated on the external surface of the membrane and released either into the extracellular medium or into the phagocytic vacuole. In *chronic granulomatous disease* superoxide production is absent and recurrent bacterial and fungal infections occur. Superoxide production by phagocytes can be detrimental when host rather than invading cells are the target. This

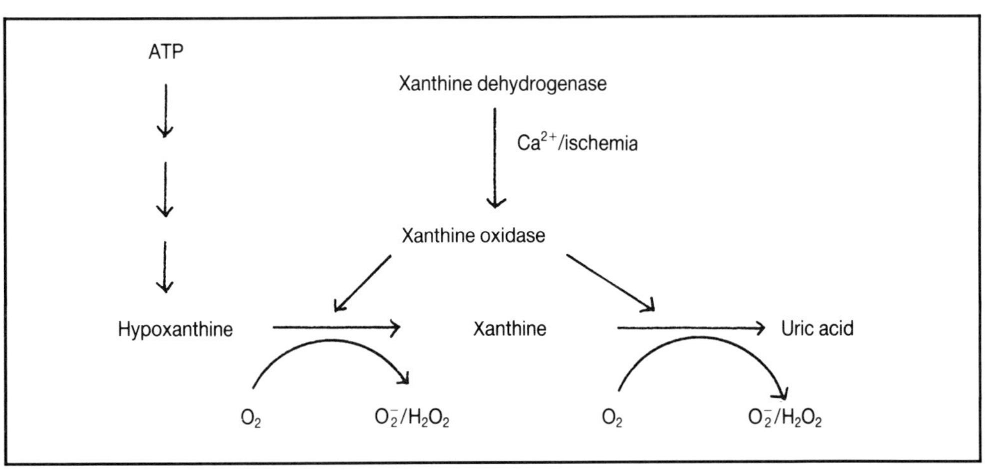

Fig. 3.21. Diagram to illustrate the mechanism of activation of xanthine oxidase and the production of superoxide and hydrogen peroxide from xanthine and hypoxanthine.

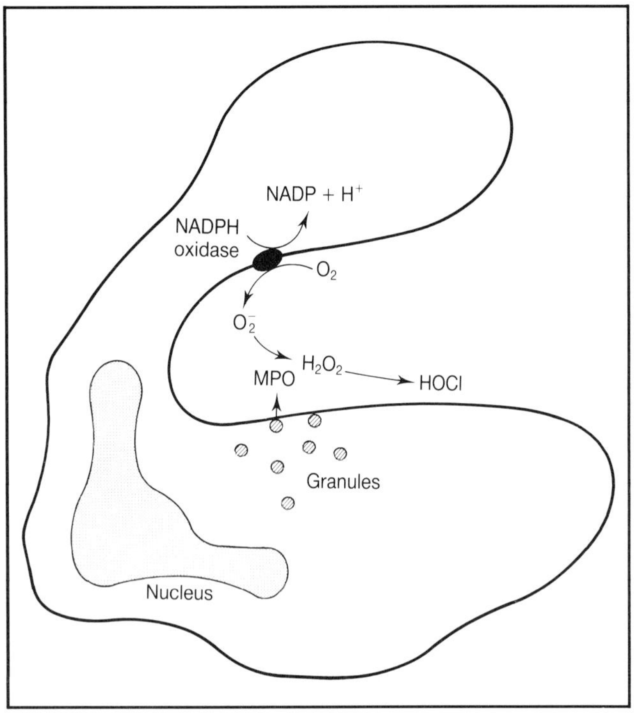

Fig. 3.22. Diagram to illustrate oxidant release by a neutrophil, following phagocytosis of microorganisms or stimulation by inflammatory mediators. Degranulation releases myeloperoxidase (MPO) as well as proteinases, hydrolyases and other antibacterial peptides (see text for abbreviations).

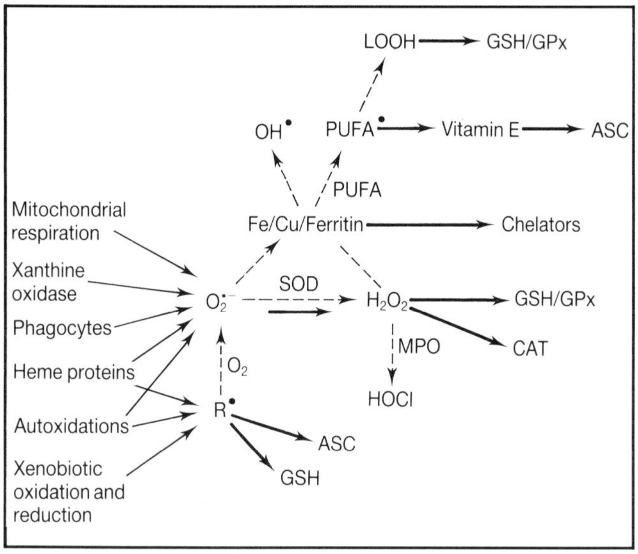

Fig. 3.23. Scheme showing mechanisms of radical production and metabolism. Route of radical production (pro-oxidants) is shown by normal arrows, the interconversion of radicals or reactive oxidants by the broken arrows and radical or oxidant removal by the heavy arrows. R•, unspecified radical; SOD, superoxide dismutase; CAT, catalase; GSH, glutathione; ASC, ascorbate; GPx, glutathione peroxidase; MPO, myeloperoxidase; PUFA, polyunsaturated lipid; PUFA•, lipid radical; LOOH, lipid hydroperoxide (for remainder see text).

is one mechanism by which tissue injury occurs in chronic inflammation.

Although superoxide is the primary product of the oxidative burst, its principal effect in microbicidal activity or host cell killing is via hydrogen peroxide and other reactive oxygen species. Superoxide and hydrogen peroxide have the potential to form hydroxyl radicals and to initiate lipid peroxidation. Although there is little evidence that neutrophils have the iron catalyst required for either reaction, this mechanism may be initiated by catalyst derived from the surrounding medium or target cells.

Hypochlorous acid (HOCl) is a powerful oxidant produced by neutrophils and monocytes from chloride and hydrogen peroxide under the control of myeloperoxidase when the cells are stimulated. HOCl is very reactive with most biological molecules and is a short range oxidant, targeting surface membranes and effectively killing both bacterial and mammalian cells. Myeloperoxidase is not essential for microbial killing, however, as neutrophils have other mechanisms.

Eosinophils contain a related peroxidase that converts bromide to hypobromous acid by an analogous mechanism.

Another free radical produced by phagocytes is nitric oxide (NO), formed from the enzymatic oxidative deamination of L-arginine. Macrophages, when primed by γ-interferon or tumor necrosis factor, produce significant amounts of NO and use it to kill cultured cells. NO is also produced by endothelial cells as the smooth muscle relaxant endothelial derived relaxing factor (see p. 469) and by neuronal dendrites in the brain. The pathophysiological importance of NO is currently being explored.

Antioxidants and free radical scavengers

A complex system of antioxidant defenses preserves the balance between oxidant production and removal. When the balance is upset, by either excess radical production or a defective defense mechanism, oxidative stress and tissue injury can occur. A general scheme for oxidant production and defenses is depicted in Fig. 3.23.

Enzymatic defenses

Antioxidant enzymatic systems are present for removal of superoxide and hydrogen peroxide. Superoxide dismutase (SOD) catalyzes the breakdown of superoxide to O_2 and hydrogen peroxide 1000 times faster than occurs spontaneously.

Superoxide dismutase

$$2O_2^{\bullet -} + 2H^+ \longrightarrow H_2O_2 + O_2$$

SOD is present in all mammalian cells, both as copper/zinc SOD in the cytoplasm and as manganese SOD in the mitochondria. Low concentrations of another copper/zinc SOD are also found extracellularly. The gene for copper/zinc SOD is encoded on chromosome 21 and the concentration of the enzyme is raised in *Down syndrome*.

Hydrogen peroxide is broken down to water and O_2 by catalase.

Catalase

$$2H_2O_2 \longrightarrow 2H_2O + O_2$$

Glutathione peroxidase removes both hydrogen peroxide and lipid hydroperoxides (LOOH) by catalyzing their reaction with reduced glutathione (GSH).

Glutathione peroxidase

$$H_2O_2 \text{ (or LOOH)} + 2GSH \longrightarrow 2H_2O \text{ (or LOH} + H_2O) + GSSG$$

GSH is regenerated by NADPH from the hexose monophosphate pathway and this pathway is therefore necessary for the glutathione cycle. Catalase also requires NADPH for maximal activity. In genetic disorders of the hexose monophosphate pathway, e.g. *glucose 6-phosphate dehydrogenase (G6PD) deficiency*, since both systems for peroxide removal may be compromised, there is a susceptibility to drug-induced hemolytic anemia. Glutathione peroxidase contains the trace element selenium and its activity may be reduced when selenium intake is restricted due to low soil selenium or special diets such as *total parenteral nutrition* or diets for *phenylketonuria* or *cystic fibrosis*. Very low selenium in parts of China causes a *cardiomyopathy (Keshan disease)* but whether low glutathione peroxidase is responsible for this is not known.

Antioxidant enzymes are particularly important in the lung because of the high O_2 environment. They are less important *in utero* and levels remain low until late gestation. Preterm infants may be at risk because of low concentrations at birth.

Low molecular weight scavengers

The most abundant physiological free radical scavengers are vitamin E (α-tocopherol), vitamin C (ascorbic acid) and glutathione. Vitamin E is lipid soluble and found in cell membranes where it intercepts lipid peroxyl radicals and breaks the chain reaction of polyunsaturated fatty acid peroxidation. Ascorbate and glutathione are found in the cytoplasm and other aqueous environments where they intercept primary radicals and repair radical damage to macromolecules. Since the reaction between a radical and a scavenger generates another radical, the scavenger is an effective antioxidant only if its radical breaks down benignly. Ascorbate is particularly good because its radical decays mainly by reacting with itself. α-Tocopherol radicals can do likewise or they may react with ascorbate. The latter reaction permits ascorbate to spare α-tocopherol and provides a link between the aqueous and the lipid phase antioxidants. The glutathione radical probably reacts mainly with O_2 to give superoxide which can be eliminated by SOD. Vitamin A, β-carotene and ubiquinol (coenzyme Q10) can all act as lipid antioxidants in experimental circumstances, but their physiological importance remains to be established.

Vitamin E deficiency in the newborn has several clinical manifestations. One is *hemolysis* due to oxidative injury to the red cell membrane. The *retinopathy of prematurity* may be an oxidative injury which is exacerbated by low vitamin E. Other contributing factors are a high inspired O_2 concentration, light-induced radical generation and immature antioxidant defenses. Vitamin E may also decrease *intraventricular hemorrhage* in the newborn. The etiology of the condition and the role of vitamin E are complex, but it seems probable that oxidative injury due to ischemia and reperfusion plays a part.

Although antioxidants such as vitamins E and C are physiologically important, it does not follow that raising their concentrations therapeutically will be beneficial and in fact they may be harmful. Once a threshold is reached there may be no additional advantage. This is why there is controversy over the use of vitamin E in *retinopathy of prematurity*.

Metal binding

Many free radical reactions require the presence of small amounts of iron or copper. Iron is the more significant physiologically and important facets of antioxidant defense are the storage and transport of iron in an inert form and the maintenance of very low free iron concentrations. The transport proteins transferrin and lactoferrin are inactive as free radical catalysts and ferritin stores iron within a protein shell. However, superoxide and other radicals can release iron from ferritin and this may contribute to their toxicity. Iron overload enhances free radical damage when iron binding capacity is exceeded. The iron chelator, desferrioxamine, has the advantage of a high binding constant and forming an iron chelate that is largely inert.

Radical reactions and oxidative damage

Free radical damage can take various forms, depending on the nature and site of radical formation, and commonly involves the formation of superoxide and hydrogen peroxide. Superoxide is formed directly in a number of biological reactions and also when other radicals react with O_2. Hydrogen peroxide is formed from superoxide either by spontaneous or enzyme-catalyzed dismutation. Both stress the cell by depleting reducing equivalents and energy supplies and also by enzyme inactivation. But their most important toxic action may be as precursors of more reactive species, especially hydroxyl radicals.

Hydroxyl radical production

Hydroxyl radicals are formed when certain ferrous or cuprous complexes react with hydrogen peroxide (Fenton reaction).

$$Fe^{2+} + H_2O_2 \longrightarrow Fe^{3+} + OH^- + OH^\bullet$$

In biological systems, where concentrations of active metal complexes are low, appreciable hydroxyl radical production will occur only if the ferric ions formed in the reaction are recycled to ferrous. Superoxide can do this (via the Haber–Weiss reaction) as can a number of organic radicals. However, iron can also be reduced by compounds such as glutathione and ascorbate that are normally present intracellularly, so the only essential requirements for hydroxyl radical production should be hydrogen peroxide and iron. Radicals such as superoxide might contribute by making this iron available from ferritin.

Hydroxyl radicals react rapidly with most biological molecules. They react close to their site of generation, and this, rather than relative reactivity with different compounds, determines their specificity. Thus hydroxyl radicals generated close to DNA react mainly with DNA, and those generated extracellularly do not penetrate the cell. If the transition metal involved in the Fenton reaction is bound to a target such as a protein molecule, the reactions of the hydroxyl radical can be localized to that molecule. The most abundant compounds, e.g. albumin in extracellular fluid, are likely to be major targets for hydoxyl radicals, although not necessarily critical ones. As hydroxyl radicals are so reactive and nonspecific, any one compound is unlikely to prevent reactions with other tissue constituents. Specific hydroxyl radical scavengers are relatively ineffective *in vivo* because of the high concentrations required.

Lipid peroxidation

Peroxidation of polyunsaturated fatty acids is a classical free radical reaction that occurs in biological membranes and lipoproteins. It is a chain reaction (Fig. 3.24) involving lipid radicals and O_2, that produces unstable and structurally disruptive fatty acyl hydroperoxide groups in the membrane plus a variety of reactive side products. Peroxidation can be initiated by hydroxyl radicals, but mechanisms involving an iron catalyst and a reducing agent such as superoxide or ascorbate, or a heme protein plus peroxide, seem to be more significant.

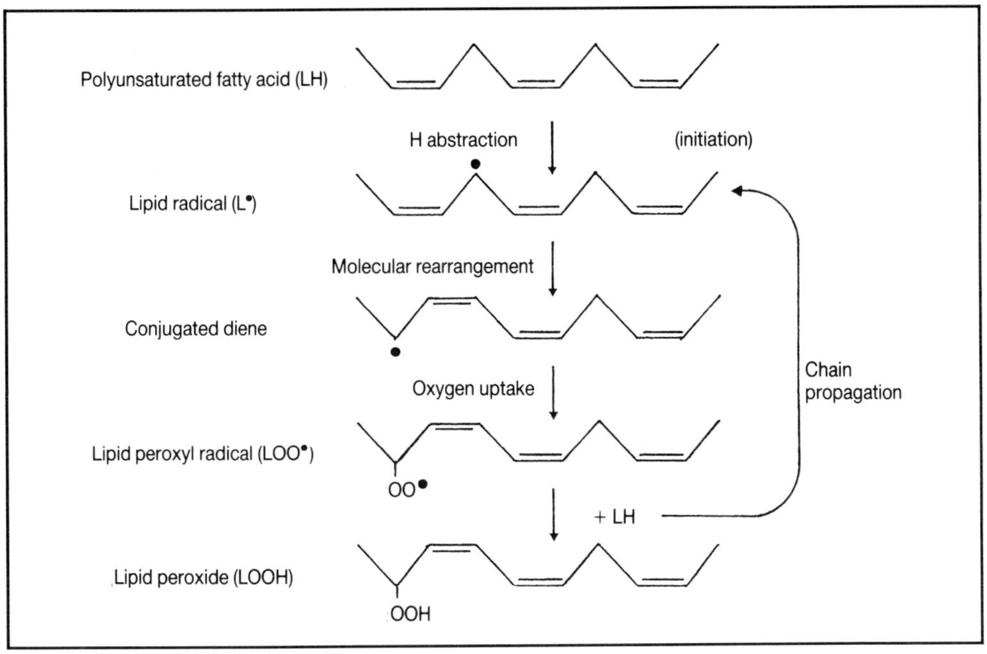

Fig. 3.24. Diagram to illustrate initiation and propagation of lipid peroxidation. Minor breakdown products and relatively unstable lipid hydroperoxides include malondialdehyde, 4-hydroxynonenal and ethane. Various assay methods measure these products.

Lipid peroxidation is a widely measured index of free radical injury. While this can be a definitive and sensitive measure, results with simpler techniques should be interpreted with caution since they are not necessarily specific and have limitations when used for basal tissue concentrations. Furthermore oxidative injury need not cause lipid peroxidation or peroxidation may be secondary to the loss of cellular integrity.

Radical reactions and cytotoxicity

Excessive intracellular free radical production stresses antioxidant defenses, depletes reducing equivalents and energy reserves, and may also inactivate key enzymes involved in energy production. Other enzymes affected include those involved in calcium regulation and alterations of intracellular calcium distribution are a feature of oxidative damage. All of these changes may be cytotoxic.

Proteins, lipids and nucleic acids are susceptible to oxidative damage. Oxidation of DNA results in single or double strand breaks and modification of the bases. Much of the damage is repaired, but persisting modifications at key sites may be mutagenic. Radical reactions can crosslink proteins or oxidize amino acids, resulting in enzyme inactivation or structural alterations to the cytoskeleton or connective tissue. Lipid peroxidation mainly affects cell membrane structure and permeability, and some of the minor peroxidation products react with DNA and proteins. The relative importance of these different effects depends on the tissue type and the nature of the oxidant stress.

Detection of in vivo *oxidative damage*

Although there are strong implications for free radical involvement in a number of diseases, direct evidence has been difficult to obtain. Free radicals are so short lived that they can rarely be detected directly *in vivo* and products of oxidative injury are frequently unstable or metabolized. Radical scavengers and transition metal chelators are useful supportive evidence but not necessarily specific. Recent developments that may be helpful include the measurement of oxidized DNA bases, e.g. 8-hydroxydeoxyguanosine, in blood or urine, detection of oxidatively modified proteins or specific lipid peroxides, and the measurement of the efflux of oxidized glutathione from tissues.

Free radical pathology

Inflammation

Inflammatory cells are a major source of free radicals and oxidative injury is implicated in the pathology of chronic inflammatory diseases including *rheumatoid arthritis* and conditions where there is immune complex deposition. Endotoxemia and complement activation lead to neutrophil accumulation in the lung, providing the potential for oxidative injury in *toxic shock* and the *adult respiratory distress syndrome*. Recent evidence indicates that the products of activated neutrophils and eosinophils are important in the inflammatory component of the pathophysiology of *asthma*.

In experimental systems neutrophil oxidants can kill cultured endothelial and epithelial cells, increase capillary permeability and denature basement membrane and articular cartilage components. α_1-Proteinase inhibitor is inactivated and unable to inhibit neutrophil elastase. This results in neutrophils degrading lung elastin in *emphysema* and is a likely contributor to other inflammatory injury.

O_2 toxicity and chronic lung disease

The toxicity of high O_2 concentrations is best explained by increased oxygen radical generation. Since the lungs have the greatest exposure they are the most susceptible to injury. Preterm infants on ventilators are at risk of developing *bronchopulmonary dysplasia* or *chronic lung disease*. Exposure to elevated O_2 is compounded by barotrauma, the secondary recruitment of neutrophils due to mechanical injury and the low antioxidant defenses due to immaturity. Circumstantial evidence for oxidative damage in such infants is strong and the possibility of antioxidant therapy is being considered.

Ischemia and reperfusion injury

When a tissue is deprived of O_2 due to impaired blood flow, cells are injured and may die. Although restoration of blood flow is essential for recovery, it is now appreciated that providing the ischemia does not do irreversible damage, reperfusion may be responsible for much of the total injury. Despite inhibitors such as SOD and radical scavengers providing dramatic protection in a number of experimental studies, the extent to which oxygen radicals are involved in ischemia/reperfusion injury remains controversial. Results vary depending on the system and index of tissue injury used. Much of the controversy is centered on the heart and *myocardial infarction*. Evidence is stronger for free radicals contributing to *ischemia/reperfusion injury* in the gut, kidney, muscle and particularly brain, arising from trauma, crush or pressure injury and in *perinatal asphyxial encephalopathies*.

Mechanisms by which free radicals can be produced in ischemia/reperfusion include disruption of mitochondrial integrity during ischemia, so that when O_2 is reintroduced there is less control and more superoxide release. A second mechanism involves conversion of xanthine dehydrogenase to xanthine oxidase by ischemia (see Fig. 3.21) thus permitting the accumulation of xanthine and hypoxanthine from the breakdown of adenine nucleotides. This is not a problem during ischemia but reintroduction of O_2 allows the enzyme to act, producing superoxide and hydrogen peroxide. Support for this mechanism comes from studies using the xanthine oxidase inhibitor, allopurinol. Neutrophils are also important since they are recruited in response to the initial injury and amplify the damage by releasing reactive oxygen species.

There is indirect evidence for reperfusion injury in *perinatal asphyxia* and *cerebral trauma* which have many characteristics in common with other brain injuries where oxygen radicals are known to be involved. Observed increases in uric acid concentrations could indicate xanthine oxidase activity, and the rise observed in extracellular glutamate could be due to inactivation of glutamine synthetase which is very susceptible to oxidative inactivation.

Antioxidant therapy

The therapeutic use of oxygen radical scavengers is under active investigation, particularly in relation to inflammatory and ischemic diseases. One approach has been to use the enzymes SOD and catalase. In some cases protective effects have been dramatic, in others not. Both enzymes suffer from short plasma half-lives, inaccessibility to intracellular sites of radical production and inability to cross the blood–brain barrier. Liposomal encapsulation and intratracheal infusion have been used with some success, but overall the initial hopes for enzyme therapy have not been realized. Low molecular weight scavengers have better accessibility and are receiving considerable attention. Scavengers of hydroxyl radicals or HOCl have major limitations because of the high concentrations required. However, inhibitors of lipid peroxidation are effective at achievable concentrations and both natural and synthetic lipid antioxidants are being studied. Thiol compounds such as *N*-acetylcysteine increase antioxidant activity, either directly or via glutathione.

An alternative approach is to prevent oxidant production. Allopurinol is effective when xanthine oxidase is involved and is proving beneficial in some ischemic conditions. Inhibitors of the neutrophil oxidative burst or myeloperoxidase have so far received little attention, but monoclonal antibodies against cell adhesion molecules that prevent neutrophils attaching to the endothelium have shown impressive protection in several animal models of inflammation and ischemia. Since transition metals play an important role in radical reactions, another approach is the administration of chelators such as desferrioxamine. In all these approaches a balance must be preserved between therapeutic effect and preservation of essential physiological functions.

Diet is an important factor, particularly in the neonatal period when intakes of micronutrients may be suboptimal. Low intakes of antioxidant vitamins are reflected in tissue levels and low dietary selenium and sulfur amino acids result in decreased glutathione and glutathione peroxidase activities.

Selected reading

Halliwell B, Gutteridge JMC. *Free radicals in biology and medicine*. 2nd ed. Oxford: Clarendon Press, 1989.

Heffner JE, Repine JE. Pulmonary strategies of antioxidant defense. *Am Rev Respir Dis* 1989; **140**: 531.

Saugstad OD. Oxygen toxicity in the neonatal period. *Acta Paediatr Scand* 1990; **79**: 881.

Vannucci RC. Current and potentially new management strategies for perinatal hypoxic-ischemic encephalopathy. *Pediatrics* 1990; **85**: 961.

Weiss SJ. Tissue destruction by neutrophils. *N Engl J Med* 1989; **320**: 365.

4 • *Phases of development*

Editors: Peter D Gluckman and Michael A Heymann

A. Morphogenesis and Teratogenesis

J A Kuller and M S Golbus

Embryogenesis

Human embryogenesis can be divided into several stages: fertilization and implantation, the embryonic period, and finally, the fetal period.

Mitosis and cleavage of the zygote (formed by fusion of the egg and sperm) result in a ball of cells, the morula. As the morula grows, an inner and outer cell mass and a cell-lined fluid space develop. This structure, called the blastocyst, enters the uterus and implants in the endometrium toward the end of the first post-conceptual week. At the conclusion of the second week, the blastocyst is completely embedded in the endometrium. The outer cell mass or trophoblast then differentiates into an external layer, the syncytiotrophoblast, and an internal layer, the cytotrophoblast. The inner cell mass or embryoblast develops into a two-layered structure composed of the ectodermal and endodermal germ layers.

During the third week the primitive streak becomes evident with a primitive knot at the cephalic end. The primitive streak is a midline thickening of rapidly multiplying ectodermal cells. The embryo becomes polarized with discernible cranial and caudal, and right and left orientations. The invaginating cells of the primitive streak develop a third germ layer, the mesoderm, which forms between the ectodermal and endodermal layers. The chorionic villi also proliferate during this third post-conceptual week, invade maternal vessels, and acquire adequate nutrition and oxygen from the maternal circulation.

The fourth through the eighth post-conceptual weeks comprise the **embryonic period**. This is the time of early embryogenesis and therefore represents the peak vulnerability to the occurrence of major congenital anomalies. As each germ layer differentiates, specific organ systems develop. The **ectoderm** is the source of the nervous system, the sensory organs (eye, ear, nose), as well as the integument. **Mesoderm** develops into the musculoskeletal system, connective tissue, the cardiovascular system, most of the urogenital system, and the adrenal glands. **Endoderm** provides the epithelium of the respiratory and gastrointestinal tracts and the urinary bladder. Endoderm also develops into a variety of glandular organs including the thyroid and parathyroid glands, the pancreas, thymus, tonsils, and liver.

Week 9 begins the **fetal period**, which continues to term. Embryonic growth and early fetal growth occur by cell hyperplasia (increase in cell number). Later, both the size and number of cells increase. The combined cellular hyperplasia and hypertrophy continue throughout the fetal period into the postnatal period. The gross malformations that may result from an insult in the embryonic period rarely occur in the fetal period.

Each organ system develops at slightly different times. The first evidence of **cardiac** development occurs on day 18 or 19 when mesenchymal cells begin to differentiate into angiogenic clusters. These cells proliferate and form a primitive vascular plexus called the cardiogenic area. The cardiogenic area canalizes to become the first cardiac structures. These are called the endocardial heart tubes, which fuse to form the single primary heart tube. As the primary heart tube grows, it begins to undergo looping and segmentation. The four cardiac chambers develop between weeks 4 and 7. Peristaltic contractions of the heart begin on day 22.

Lung development occurs in four progressive phases: the embryonic, pseudoglandular, canalicular, and alveolar periods. Days 22–26 are the embryonic period, during which a ventral endodermal diverticulum evaginates from the embryonic foregut. The epithelial lining of the respiratory tract results from this anlage. The pseudoglandular period begins at 4 weeks, and branching and division of airways and blood vessels occur during this time. At 16 weeks, the canalicular period begins, during which time there is vascular proliferation as well as further development of the bronchial tree. The terminal sac or alveolar period commences with the twenty-fifth gestational week. During this interval, the respiratory tree develops an increased number of respiratory bronchioles and saccules. The surface area for gas exchange becomes sufficient to accommodate extrauterine breathing. Although the fetal lung has no ventilatory function, it is metabolically active.

The **gastrointestinal tract** develops from the primitive

gut, which is an elongated tube extending nearly the entire length of the embryo. It is composed of the foregut, midgut, and hindgut. The foregut develops into the pharynx, lower respiratory tract, esophagus, stomach, proximal duodenum, liver, biliary system, and the pancreas. The midgut evolves into the small intestine, cecum, appendix, ascending colon, and proximal transverse colon. The midgut rapidly elongates and soon outgrows available space in the abdominal cavity. After counterclockwise rotation, the herniated intestine returns to the abdominal space at 10 weeks' gestation. The hindgut derivatives are the distal transverse colon, descending colon, sigmoid, rectum, and superior portion of the anus.

The **urinary system** is complex, and 'three generations' of kidneys evolve. The first generation is called the pronephros; this rudimentary structure disappears by the fourth week. Most of the pronephric ducts are incorporated into the next renal generation, termed the mesonephros. The mesonephric ducts persist in the male to function as genital ducts. In the female they degenerate, becoming only vestigial organs. The third generation, or metanephros, becomes the permanent kidney. Appearing in the fifth post-conceptual week, it begins to function in the eleventh or twelfth week, and the fetus excretes urine into the amniotic fluid. True renal function does not begin until birth because the placenta eliminates metabolic end products from the fetus. The urinary bladder and urethra are derived from the urogenital sinus. The fetal uterus is formed by 18 weeks, at which time vaginal canalization commences. The testes begin to descend at 20 weeks; this is completed at term.

Hematopoiesis progresses through a mesoblastic period, a hepatic period, and a myeloid period. These three maturational stages overlap in time. The mesoblastic period is characterized by the release of cells from blood islands in the yolk sac into the blood stream. This stage begins at 16–19 days and ends at approximately 12 weeks. The second phase of hematopoiesis, the hepatic period, begins at approximately 5 weeks. During this time hematopoiesis occurs primarily in the liver. During the third and fourth month, the spleen also contributes to hematopoiesis. The hepatic period is almost exclusively erythropoietic in nature and ends in the sixth month. Finally, the myeloid period begins between the fourth and fifth months. Hematopoiesis moves to the bone marrow, where it continues throughout postnatal life. During the third trimester of pregnancy the bone marrow becomes the main hematopoietic organ. Erythropoiesis begins when the hemocytoblasts are committed to an erythrocytic line of maturation. This is indicated by the appearance of hemoglobin in the cytoplasm. Erythropoietin probably controls erythropoiesis beginning in the third trimester. Until 36 weeks of gestation, approximately 90 percent of hemoglobin in the fetus is hemoglobin F. Hemoglobin A (adult hemoglobin) is increasingly produced after 36 weeks. Lymphopoiesis is initiated in the third month in lymph nodes and thymus. Mature lymphocytes are first identified in the fetal circulation at this time.

The **central nervous system** develops from ectoderm. The neural tube is formed from the folding and fusion of the neural plate. The cranial neuropore closes on day 25 and the caudal neuropore on day 27. Three primary brain vesicles develop at the expanded cephalic end of the neural tube. These are the forebrain, the midbrain, and the hindbrain. The forebrain eventually forms the cerebral hemispheres and the third ventricle. The midbrain develops into the cerebral aqueduct, the red nuclei, nuclei of the third and fourth cranial nerves, and the substantia nigra. The hindbrain differentiates into the pons, cerebellum and the fourth ventricle. The spinal cord develops from the caudal portion of the neural tube. After the embryonic period, the fetal brain undergoes significant growth of the cerebral hemispheres. The vascular bed of the germinal matrix is the most critical locus of the blood supply to the fetal brain. The vast majority of intraventricular hemorrhages in premature neonates occur in this area.

External fetal characteristics change throughout gestation. At the onset of the fetal period, the head constitutes one half of the total fetal length. The relative size of the fetal head then begins to diminish, and at term occupies only one-fourth of the length of the body. The face becomes more infantile during gestation, and the eyes migrate from the lateral aspect of the face medially. At 26 weeks, the eyes are partly open and eyelashes are visible. The ears are low set at an early age, then later occupy their ultimate position. The limbs lengthen and the external genitalia begin to be discernible at 12 weeks. Intestinal loops, forced from the peritoneal cavity by the enlarging liver, migrate back into the abdomen at 10–11 weeks' gestation.

Teratogenesis

Principles

Teratology, the study of abnormal development, is directed at understanding the causes and mechanisms of maldevelopment. A teratogen is a substance, organism, or physical agent that produces abnormal embryonic structural or functional development. To be considered a teratogen, the agent must act during the embryonic period (Fig. 4.1). An exposure occurring during the fetal period that causes a structural or functional abnormality is called fetotoxic. Fetotoxic effects may mimic defects caused by teratogens, and some teratogens are also fetotoxic (e.g. alcohol).

Approximately 1 in 400 live-born infants has a malformation due to a teratogenic exposure. Teratogens are implicated in approximately 10 percent of all birth defects. Most human teratogens have been discovered by astute clinicians (e.g. *thalidomide syndrome*). Basic science and epidemiological studies have primarily played a confirmatory role in teratogen identification, usually verifying clinical findings after numbers of children with anomalies have been reported. There is approximately a 55 percent correlation between teratogenicity in animals and teratogenicity in humans.

Wilson's principles of teratology

Wilson's six principles of teratology provide a framework of how structural or functional teratogens may act. The first principle is that susceptibility to a teratogen depends on the genotype of the conception and the interaction between the genotype and environmental factors. Teratogenic differences based on genetic susceptibility could be the result of either polygenic inheritance or monogenic inheritance. An example of genetic variability to potential teratogenic agents is that

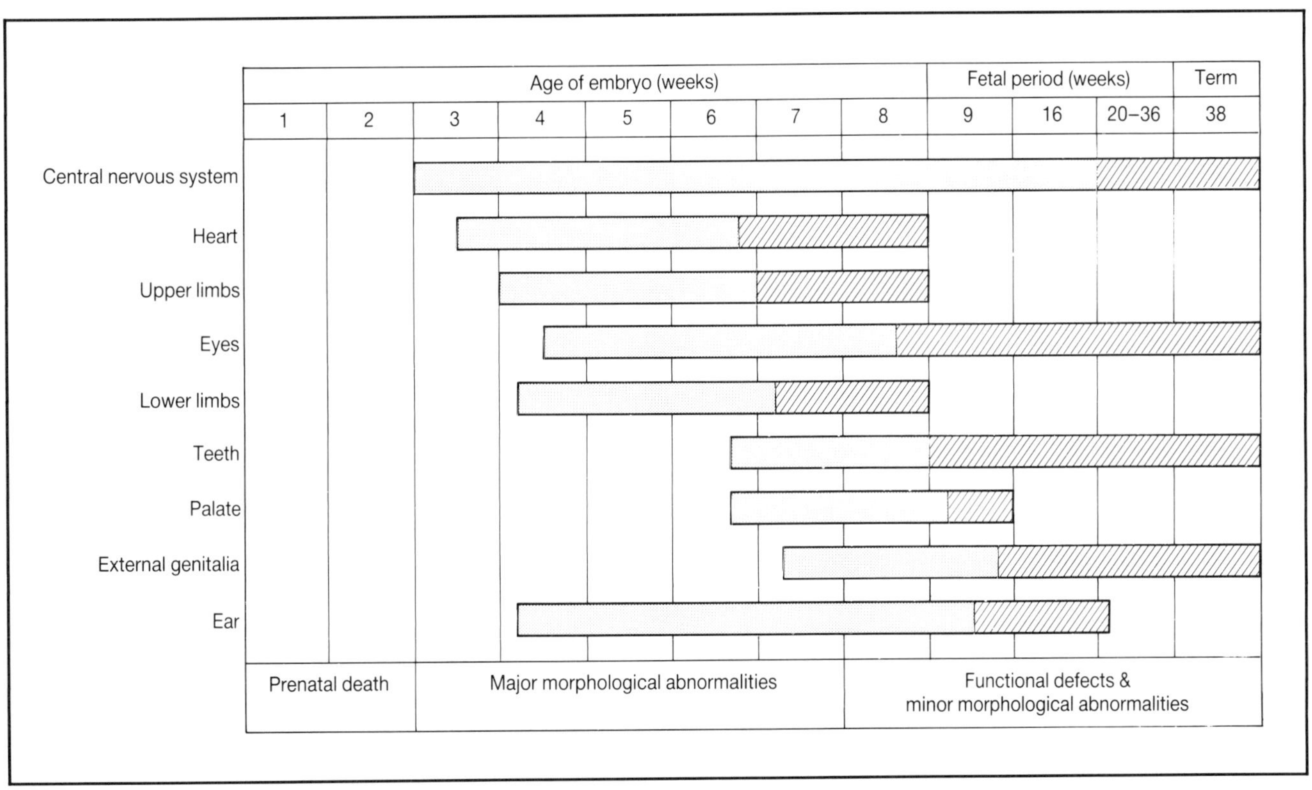

Fig. 4.1. Vulnerable periods in embryonic and fetal development. During the first 2 weeks (predifferentiation stages) of development, the embryo is generally not susceptible to teratogens and a substance either damages all or most of the cells, resulting in death, or damages only a few cells, allowing the embryo to develop without defects. Periods of greatest sensitivity to teratogens are indicated by the stippled portion of the bar; later stages (hatched bar) are less sensitive. (Modified from Moore KL. *The developing human: clinically oriented embryology*. Philadelphia: WB Saunders Company, 1988: p. 143, with permission.)

exposed fetuses with low levels of the enzyme epoxide hydrolase are much more likely to manifest the *fetal hydantoin syndrome* than those with higher levels.

The second of Wilson's principles is that susceptibility of the conceptus to teratogen varies with the developmental state at the time of exposure. During the first 2 weeks of life, the embryo is relatively resistant to teratogenic insults. A large insult may kill the embryo; surviving embryos usually manifest no organ-specific anomalies. During the second to eighth week of development, while organogenesis is occurring, susceptibility to teratogens is maximal. After organogenesis, a teratogen generally only affects the overall growth of the embryo or the size of a specific organ.

Wilson's third principle is that teratogenic agents act by specific mechanisms on developing cells and tissues. A teratogen may act by causing a gene mutation, by chromosome breakage or nondisjunction, by depletion or inhibition of precursors, energy sources, or enzymes, or by causing changes in membrane integrity. These events may result in cell death, decreased cell division, abnormal intracellular interactivity, disruption of cell migration, or mechanical disruption.

Wilson's fourth principle is that the final manifestations of abnormal development are death, malformation, growth retardation, and functional disorders. The teratogenic manifestation may depend on the developmental stage at which exposure occurs.

Wilson's fifth principle is that access of adverse environmental influences to developing tissues depends on the nature of the agent. Some agents are more teratogenic than others. Moreover, an agent may be teratogenic only in a certain species. A perfect example is thalidomide, which produces phocomelia in primates but not in rodents.

Wilson's sixth and final principle is that the degree of abnormal development increases as dosage increases. An embryo may respond to a teratogen in one of three ways. At a low dose, there may be negligible effects or none. At intermediate dosages, organ-specific malformations can result. Finally, at high doses, the effect may be lethal. Route of administration and chronicity of exposure certainly may influence the dosage effect.

Proof of teratogenicity is difficult, but a number of observations may at least implicate a particular agent. First, subjects exposed to the agent should have a particular malformation more often than nonexposed controls. A specific anomaly or pattern of anomalies is consistently associated with the suspected agent. The agent must have been present during the stage of organogenesis when the anomaly should have occurred. The anomaly should be less common prior to the presence of the potential teratogen. Finally, the anomaly can be reproduced in experimental animals.

Human teratogens can be divided into several categories: radiation, illicit drugs, medications, infectious diseases, chemicals, and maternal disease. Each of these will be described in brief.

Radiation as a teratogen

Ionizing radiation is a wave or particle with energy sufficient to break bonds and create ions (see p. 108) capable of causing tissue damage (and therefore teratogenesis). Microwaves, because of their lower energy, cannot produce ionization. Neither can magnetic resonance imaging (MRI) because it utilizes radiofrequency waves. Ultrasound, a mechanical wave, is also incapable of producing ionization. Likewise, video display terminals have not been shown to cause increased risk of congenital anomalies.

Ionizing radiation, the first known environmental human teratogen, was identified around 1920. Both the radiation dose and the gestational age at exposure are critical in determining fetal risk. Moreover, there is virtually no fetal risk associated with a diagnostic study that does not include the maternal pelvis (e.g. chest X-ray, head CT). For larger maternal exposures, the embryonic exposure may need to be calculated in conjunction with a radiation physicist.

An exposure of 5 rad or less (rad is an acronym for radiation absorbed dose) causes no measurable risk to the embryo. The threshold for most radiation effects is in the range of 15–20 rad (0.15–0.20 Gy). Exposures to diagnostic radiation of even 20–50 rad represent an extremely low risk to the embryo. However, more than 50 rad of exposure poses a significant fetal risk regardless of the gestational age at exposure.

It is generally felt that significant radiation exposure earlier than 2 weeks after conception causes an 'all or none' effect, i.e. abortion or a normal fetus. Exposure from 2 to 18 weeks can cause intrauterine growth retardation and mental retardation. In addition, exposure during the embryonic period may result in microcephaly, microphthalmia, and cataracts. Beyond 18 weeks of gestation, the fetus may have effects similar to adult radiation sickness, i.e. hair loss, bone marrow hypoplasia, and skin lesions.

In counseling a pregnant patient after radiation exposure, there is considered to be no medical justification for terminating pregnancy in women exposed to 5 rad or less of ionizing radiation.

Illicit drugs as teratogens

Pregnant women unfortunately have joined the ranks of social and recreation drug users. The prototypic agent is alcohol; it has been estimated that 1–2 percent of women of childbearing age in North America are alcoholics. The *fetal alcohol syndrome (FAS)* is the most common known nongenetic cause of mental retardation. It affects 1/300 to 1/2000 live births and is present in 30–40 percent of children of alcoholic mothers. The threshold amount of alcohol necessary to cause FAS is unknown, but amounts less than two drinks per day carry less risk. The effects on the human fetus from episodic or 'binge' drinking are still unclear.

FAS is characterized by pre- and postnatal growth retardation and cardiovascular, limb, and craniofacial defects. The notable craniofacial features are microcephaly, short palpebral fissures, short upturned nose, midface hypoplasia, thin vermillion border, and smooth philtrum. Children have impaired fine and gross motor functions, impaired speech, and significant developmental delay.

Cocaine use leads to an increased incidence of major and minor congenital anomalies. These are probably secondary to vascular disruption related to the vasoconstrictive and hypertensive action of the drug. Reported malformations include genitourinary tract anomalies, limb reduction defects, disruptive brain anomalies, and segmental intestinal atresia. In addition, there is an increased risk of placental vascular anomalies, particularly *abruptio placentae.*

While tobacco use is associated with an increase in low birth weight infants, no good data indicate an association between congenital anomalies and maternal tobacco use. There is no evidence for marijuana causing teratogenicity. Moreover, congenital abnormalities do not appear to be incurred by infants of mothers who use methamphetamines during pregnancy. Heroin has been shown to cause an increased incidence of intrauterine growth retardation, neonatal withdrawal, and prenatal death. However, the frequency of anatomical malformations has not been found to be significantly increased in several cohort series. Likewise, methadone does not appear to lead to an increase in congenital malformation. Benzodiazepine, barbiturates, and LSD have not been implicated as obvious teratogens. However, making definitive statements regarding teratogenicity is often difficult, as multiple agents may be used simultaneously, especially with alcohol.

Medications as teratogens

To detail the fetal risks of widely prescribed medications is beyond the scope of this chapter. Selected agents will be briefly described. The Food and Drug Administration classifies medications into several categories (Table 4.1). This system has some limitations because pharmaceutical manufacturers rate the drugs, not the FDA.

Thalidomide was a sedative/hypnotic used in the early 1960s. The fetal thalidomide syndrome was characterized by phocomelia, facial hemangioma, esophageal or duodenal atresia, external ear anomalies, and cardiac and renal anomalies.

Diethylstilbestrol (DES) is an estrogenic hormone that was used in approximately six million mothers between 1940 and 1971 to prevent reproductive problems such as miscarriage and premature delivery. The drug later was found to be unsuccessful in preventing these outcomes.

Table 4.1. Food and Drug Administration drug classifications

Category A:	Controlled studies in humans have demonstrated no fetal risk
Category B:	Either animal studies indicate there are no fetal risks and there are no human studies OR Adverse effects have been demonstrated in animals, but not in well controlled human studies
Category C:	No adequate studies are available
Category D:	Evidence of fetal risk, but benefits outweigh risk
Category X:	Proven fetal risk and contraindicated during pregnancy

Females exposed *in utero* before the twelfth week of gestation were first noted to have an increased incidence of a rare malignancy, adenocarcinoma of the vagina. Other female genital tract anomalies were also increased, including uterine anomalies, hypoplastic cervix, vaginal septum, and vaginal adenosis. Males exposed to DES *in utero* are also thought to have an increased incidence of genital abnormalities including epididymal cysts, hypotrophic testis, varicocele, microphallus, and abnormal semen.

Isotretinoin, a vitamin A isomer, has proved very useful in the treatment of severe, recalcitrant cystic acne. It has been estimated that 38 percent of isotretinoin users are women of reproductive age. The teratogenicity of this agent in animals was well documented before its approval for human use. The recently described retinoic acid embryopathy consists of multiple craniofacial anomalies including microtia/anotia, cleft palate, micrognathia, and ocular abnormalities. In addition, heart and central nervous system defects are increased. The critical time of exposure appears to be 2–5 weeks post-conception. By taking the usual daily dose of isotretinoin, a woman is consuming the equivalent of thousands of times the recommended daily allowance of vitamin A. The presumed teratogenic mechanism of isotretinoin and its main metabolite, 4-oxo-isotretinoin, is thought to be from an adverse effect on the initial differentiation and migration of cephalic neural crest cells.

Seizure medications are associated with a two-to-threefold increased risk of fetal malformations. Notably, however, pregnant women with epilepsy who are not receiving anticonvulsant agents are at increased risk for giving birth to infants with congenital anomalies. The prototypic agent is phenytoin, a hydantoin anticonvulsant. The teratogenic effects of phenytoin were recognized in 1964. The *fetal hydantoin syndrome* comprises craniofacial abnormalities, including cleft lip and palate, limb defects, including hypoplasia of distal phalanges and nails, and growth and mental deficiency. Recently, carbamazepine has been found to cause a similar spectrum of anomalies. Decreased amniocyte epoxide hydrolase enzyme activity, which can be measured following amniocentesis, is associated with the highest risk for the fetal anticonvulsant embryopathy.

Valproic acid and its salt form, sodium valproate, are associated with a 1–2 percent incidence of neural tube defects if used between 17 and 30 days after fertilization. No cases of anencephaly, however, have been associated with its use. Various other anomalies have been reported, including craniofacial, urogenital, cardiac, and skeletal abnormalities.

Coumarin derivatives are oral anticoagulants used for treatment and prophylaxis of thromboembolism. First-trimester use of coumarin derivatives may result in an embryopathy (*fetal warfarin syndrome*) in 15–25 percent of exposed fetuses. The common characteristics are nasal hypoplasia and stippled vertebral and femoral epiphyses. Other features that may be present include ocular defects, limb hypoplasia, and mental retardation. The critical period of exposure seems to be 6–9 weeks of gestation. Interestingly, coumarin agents are both teratogenic and fetotoxic.

After years of debate, it is generally felt that first-trimester oral contraceptive exposure does not cause an increased incidence of cardiovascular, central nervous system, or limb defects. In contrast, some synthetic progestogens may cause masculinization of the female infant.

Infections as teratogens

Intrauterine infection may have devastating effects on the developing fetus. The effects of fetal infection, which usually occurs by hematogenous transplacental spread, are diverse and may result in a spectrum of problems including resorption and death of the embryo, intrauterine growth retardation, and congenital anomalies.

Rubella virus is transmitted *in utero* during the course of primary maternal infection. About 10 percent of women of childbearing age do not have antibody to rubella and are at risk for infection. Significant permanent damage is found in approximately 50 percent of children with maternal rubella in the first month of pregnancy, 22 percent in the second month, 10 percent in the third month, and 6 percent in the fourth and fifth months. Classic *congenital rubella* is diagnosed by the presence of cataracts, congenital glaucoma, congenital heart disease, radiolucent bone lesions, hepatosplenomegaly, petechiae, and thrombocytopenia. The most frequent abnormalities are deafness and heart disease.

Cytomegalovirus (*CMV*), a herpes virus, occurs as a primary infection in approximately 1–2 percent of pregnant women. Higher CMV infection rates are reported among child day-care workers. The risk of fetal infection is approximately equal for primary and recurrent maternal infections. However, almost all fetal damage is related to a primary maternal infection. Approximately 40 percent of women who have documented primary infection transmit the infection to their fetuses. However, only 10–15 percent of these infected infants have clinically apparent disease. The most frequently seen permanent damage includes deafness and mental retardation. More severe disease is quite rare and includes microphthalmia, microcephaly, hydrocephaly, chorioretinitis, and hepatosplenomegaly.

Varicella, or *chicken pox,* an acute, highly contagious disease, most commonly occurs in childhood. Approximately 95 percent of adult women are immune to varicella because of infection in childhood. The child with congenital damage due to maternal infection during the first 5 months of pregnancy may have a variety of abnormalities, including low birth weight, skin lesions, eye abnormalities, limb hypoplasia, cortical atrophy, mental retardation, and early childhood death. The mechanism of these anomalies appears to be the development of *in utero* herpes zoster with an associated encephalitis.

The incidence of *syphilis* has been increasing in the USA in the last few years. Damage to the fetus depends on the gestational age at which infection by the spirochete occurs and the time elapsed before maternal treatment. Early congenital syphilis is characterized by prematurity, hydrops, and an enlarged placenta. The newborn may have hepatosplenomegaly, lymphadenopathy, hematological abnormalities, mucocutaneous manifestations, bony lesions, and chorioretinitis. In patients older than 2 years, late congenital syphilis may present with craniofacial anomalies including Hutchinson teeth, mulberry molars, saddle nose, eighth nerve deafness, skin lesions called rhagades, and central nervous system abnormalities including mental retardation, hydrocephalus, convulsions, and paresis.

Toxoplasmosis is caused by a protozoan parasite. Maternal toxoplasmosis may be asymptomatic or present as a mild mononucleosis-like illness. If the pregnant woman acquires the infection in the first trimester, the infection is transmitted to the fetus approximately 15 percent of the time. This rate increases to 25 percent in the second trimester, and 60 percent in the third trimester. Manifestations of congenital toxoplasmosis are likely to be more severe when maternal infection is acquired early. The clinical spectrum of toxoplasmosis in the newborn is characteristic but not specific, and may include chorioretinitis, convulsions, jaundice, hydrocephaly or microcephaly, fever, hepatomegaly, lymphadenopathy, optic abnormalities, rash and pneumonia. Chorioretinitis is the most common single manifestation.

Herpes simplex virus (HSV) infection in the neonate is usually devastating. Most newborn infections are acquired intrapartum by contact of the fetus with the infected maternal genital secretions. Although extremely rare, more than a dozen cases have been reported in which maternal herpes infections early in pregnancy resulted in severe fetal consequences. These included skin lesions, chorioretinitis, microcephaly, hydrocephaly, and microphthalmia. Data suggesting a higher rate of spontaneous abortions in women with genital HSV provide indirect evidence that intrauterine infection from HSV may occur. Because the risk of *in utero* transmission is so small, therapeutic abortion or maternal treatment is not recommended or indicated at present.

Chemicals as teratogens

Exposure to organic mercury compounds is uncommon but is still possible, primarily through the consumption of contaminated fish. Methylmercury easily crosses the placenta and accumulates in embryonic and fetal tissues, particularly the brain. While obvious structural anomalies are not caused by antenatal exposure to mercury, significant neurological abnormalities may result.

The relationship between antenatal exposure to anesthetic gases and reproductive risk has been debated. Chronic first-trimester exposure may increase the risk of spontaneous abortion. Although no recognizable pattern of malformation has been found following maternal exposure to anesthetic gases, some investigations have found an increased rate of all birth defects in infants born to exposed parents. General anesthesia during early pregnancy does not appear to be teratogenic. A number of large studies found no increased risk of congenital malformation.

Maternal disease as a teratogen

Infants of insulin-dependent diabetic mothers (IDM) have a two-to-fourfold increased incidence of major malformations. A derangement in maternal metabolism, primarily maternal hyperglycemia, is the proposed teratogenic mechanism. The congenital defect thought to be most characteristic of diabetic embryopathy is sacral agenesis or caudal dysplasia. This anomaly is found 200–400 times more often in offspring of women with diabetes than in offspring of women without diabetes. Central nervous system abnormalities including neural tube defects and holoprosencephaly are increased tenfold. In addition, cardiac anomalies, especially ventricular septal defects and complex lesions such as transposition of the great vessels, are increased fivefold. Moreover, women whose diabetes is less well controlled are at higher risk for spontaneous abortion and infants with malformations.

Pregnancy in an untreated mother with *phenylketonuria* (*PKU*) exposes the fetus to a very high level of phenylalanine and its derivatives. A high percentage of offspring from women with high phenylalanine levels have mental retardation, growth retardation, and congenital anomalies including microcephaly, congenital heart defects, vertebral anomalies, and craniofacial features resembling the fetal alcohol syndrome. Importantly, infants whose mothers follow a strict low phenylaline diet beginning before conception and whose mothers maintain blood phenylaline levels less than 10 mg/dl appear to exhibit no increased incidence of congenital malformations.

Selected reading

Beckman DA, Brent RL. Mechanisms of teratogenesis. *Annu Rev Pharmacol Toxicol* 1984; **24**: 483.

Briggs GG, Freeman RK, Yaffe SJ. *Drugs in pregnancy and lactation*. 3rd ed. Baltimore: William and Wilkins, 1990.

Grose C, Itani O, Weiner CP. Prenatal diagnosis of fetal infection: advances from amniocentesis to cordocentesis—congenital toxoplasmosis, rubella, cytomegalovirus, varicella virus, parvovirus and human immunodeficiency virus. *Pediatr Infect Dis J* 1989; **8**: 459.

Jones KL. *Smith's recognizable patterns of human malformation*. 4th ed. Philadelphia: WB Saunders Company, 1988.

Moore KL. *The developing human*. 4th ed. Philadelphia: WB Saunders Company, 1988.

Remington JS, Klein JO. *Infectious diseases of the fetus and newborn infant*. 3rd ed. Philadelphia: WB Saunders Company, 1990.

B. The Physiology and Pathophysiology of Fetal Sexual Differentiation

N Josso

Sex differentiation can be defined as the series of events which leads to the development of male or female characteristics in various organs. The gonads, internal genital tract and external genital organs successively become sex oriented during fetal life; gender identity, brain sex and secondary sex attributes differentiate after birth.

Sex differentiation is a complex physiological process, governed by coordinated genetic and hormonal factors operating in an asymmetrical manner. In mammals, the testis imposes masculinity on structures which are programmed to become female. In the absence of testicular hormones, Müllerian ducts persist and develop into uterus and tubes, Wolffian derivatives degenerate and external genitalia do not masculinize. Thus, the binary switch that determines the subsequent steps is the commitment of the primitive gonads to develop either as testes or ovaries, the development of the full sexual phenotype being merely a consequence of that initial decision.

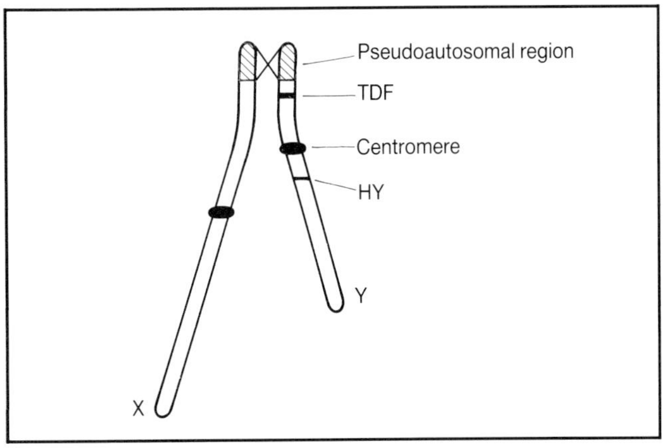

Fig. 4.2. Diagram of sex chromosomes, showing the pseudoautosomal pairing region, and the location of the testis-determining (TDF) and HY genes.

The human testis-determining gene (TDF)

In most vertebrate species, sex differentiation is determined by genetic material present in the heterogametic sex. Sex determination in humans is governed by gene(s) lying on the Y chromosome; the number of accompanying X chromosomes is irrelevant, as shown by the male phenotype of XXY individuals with *Klinefelter syndrome*. Embryos lacking a Y chromosome, whether 46,XX or 45,X, develop ovaries at least initially, unless DNA endowed with testis-determining activity has been transferred to another chromosome, thus giving rise to XX *male* progeny, as discussed below.

The Y chromosome contains a pseudoautosomal region of approximately 2600 kb, which participates in homologous recombination with the X chromosome at meiosis (Fig. 4.2), ensuring that correct segregation of sex chromosomes will occur. Loci proximal to the pseudoautosomal boundary normally abstain from exchange with the X chromosome and exhibit patrilineal inheritance. The location of the testis-determining gene (TDF) in the nonrecombining, Y-specific, region is essential for the chromosomal basis of sex determination. Claims of several Y-located genes to the TDF title have been examined by analyzing the DNA of sex-reversed patients. By definition, the TDF gene can be located only in those Y-specific sequences which are invariably present in XX males and invariably absent in XY women. Recently, the probable TDF gene has been mapped to the most distal part of the Y chromosome short arm, only 10 kb from the pseudoautosomal boundary, and has been named SRY for sex-determining region Y. Earlier, a more proximally located gene, ZFY (Fig. 4.3), was excluded as the candidate TDF because it was shown to be absent in several XX males whose DNA did contain material originating from the Y pseudoautosomal boundary. A former TDF contender, the minor transplantation antigen HY gene, has been tentatively mapped to the Y chromosome long arm, close to the centromere.

The SRY gene is conserved and Y-specific among a wide

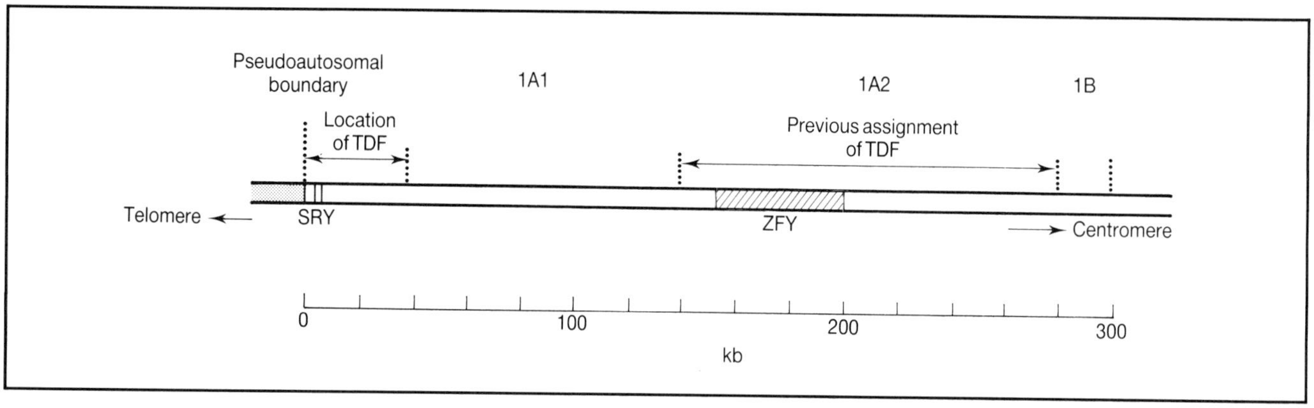

Fig. 4.3. Mapping of TDF: respective localization of SRY and ZFY on the short arm of the Y chromosome. 1A1, 1A2 and 1B represent sections of the Y chromosome identified by probe hybridization. (From Hawkins JR, Sinclair AH. *Semin Dev Biol* 1991; **2**: 251–258, with permission.)

range of mammals and encodes a testis-specific transcript. The gene product contains a DNA-binding domain sharing homology with yeast proteins involved in mating and in chromosomal structure and activity. The related gene in the mouse, SRY, is expressed in the genital ridge just prior to testicular differentiation and in the adult testis.

Gonadal sex differentiation

Testis differentiation

In the mammalian fetus, the gonadal primordium is represented by the gonadal ridge, a thickening of the celomic epithelium covering the anterior surface of the mesonephros, which is progressively colonized by primordial germ cells traveling from the stalk of the allantois through the mesentery and the wall of the fetal gut. The first recognizable event of testicular differentiation, which occurs at 6 weeks in the human fetus, is the development of a new cell type, the primordial Sertoli cell. Sertoli cells soon aggregate to form seminiferous tubules in which germ cells become enclosed. Germ cells in extragonadal locations, such as the adrenal, may survive and differentiate into oocytes. XY oocytes have also been observed in XX/XY female mice, suggesting that the differentiation potential of the mammalian germ cells is predominantly female, and is lost only in a testicular environment, for reasons which remain to be identified. In contrast, sexual differentiation of the gonad is not dependent upon the presence or karyotype of germ cells.

Fetal Sertoli cells are large, clear cells, with abundant cytoplasm containing vesicles of rough endoplasmic reticulum. In these is stored, prior to secretion, a glycoprotein, anti-Müllerian hormone (AMH), which, as shown by the classical experiments of Alfred Jost, is responsible for inhibition of the development of the Müllerian ducts in male fetuses. AMH is the first cognate protein produced by the fetal testis and is expressed immediately after testicular differentiation. Leydig cells differentiate somewhat later, at 8 weeks of gestation in the human fetus. Their number increases dramatically until 12–14 weeks, at which time they begin to degenerate. At birth, very few remain in the interstitial tissue. Fetal Leydig cells produce testosterone, the hormone responsible for the virilization of Wolffian derivatives, urogenital sinus and external genital organs. Initiation of testosterone secretion is constitutive but stimulation by luteinizing gonadotropin (either chorionic gonadotropin or fetal pituitary LH) is necessary for sustained production.

Ovarian differentiation

Slower than the testis to differentiate initially, the fetal ovary eventually reaches a more advanced stage of maturation. Up to the second month of gestation, ovogonia mix freely with somatic cells in the gonadal blastema. Later, growth of connective tissue sheets from the medulla outwards delineates ovigerous cords, containing actively dividing ovogonia, which tend to accumulate near the ovarian surface. At 12–13 weeks, some oogonia, located in the deepest layer of the cortex, have entered meiotic prophase. Maturation progresses from the center of the gonad towards the periphery, until, at approximately 7 months of gestation, all germ cells have entered or completed the meiotic prophase, and mitotic divisions are no longer seen. In parallel, the germ cell pool is severely depleted by waves of degeneration, which preferentially affect cells undergoing mitotic divisions or in the meiotic prophase. Germ cells enclosed in follicles are relatively protected from degeneration.

Primordial follicles can be recognized by 17 weeks, and Graafian follicles by 26 weeks. Fetal granulosa cells produce estrogen at the same developmental stage at which fetal testes produce testosterone, suggesting that the acquisition of the enzymatic activities that allow specific endocrine function by these two tissues may be regulated by similar factors during embryonic development. In contrast, ovarian production of AMH can be demonstrated only after birth.

Normal ovarian development requires the presence of two X chromosomes. Thus, in both classical 45,X and in variant forms of *Turner syndrome* such as XXpi or XXqi, germ cells degenerate, leading to fibrous degeneration of the ovaries. The somatic abnormalities of Turner syndrome are thought to be the result of monosomy for a gene(s) common to the X and Y chromosome, residing on Yp and perhaps on Xq, with the reservation that efforts to map the Turner phenotype on the X chromosome have failed to yield a consistent localization.

Somatic masculinization

In contrast to the recent controversies concerning gonadal sex determination, the concepts regarding sex differentiation of the genital tract have undergone no major change since the now classic contribution of Alfred Jost, who showed that masculinization must be actively imposed upon the genital tract by the hormonal secretions of the fetal testis (Fig. 4.4). Genital primordia can be masculinized only during a short, discrete developmental period, the 'critical stage', which differs for each element of the genital tract.

Müllerian regression: anti-Müllerian hormone

Shortly after gonadal differentiation, the genital tract of male or female fetuses consists of unipotential Wolffian and Müllerian ducts, and bipotential urogenital sinus and external genital primordia. Müllerian regression is the first sign of male differentiation of the genital tract. In the human fetus, the first signs of regression appear in embryos at 8 weeks and regression is more or less complete at 10–12 weeks. Female Müllerian ducts cease to respond to AMH by 8 weeks.

Müllerian regression is mediated by AMH, a 145 000 kDa glycoprotein dimer synthesized by immature Sertoli cells, very soon after testicular differentiation. Serum

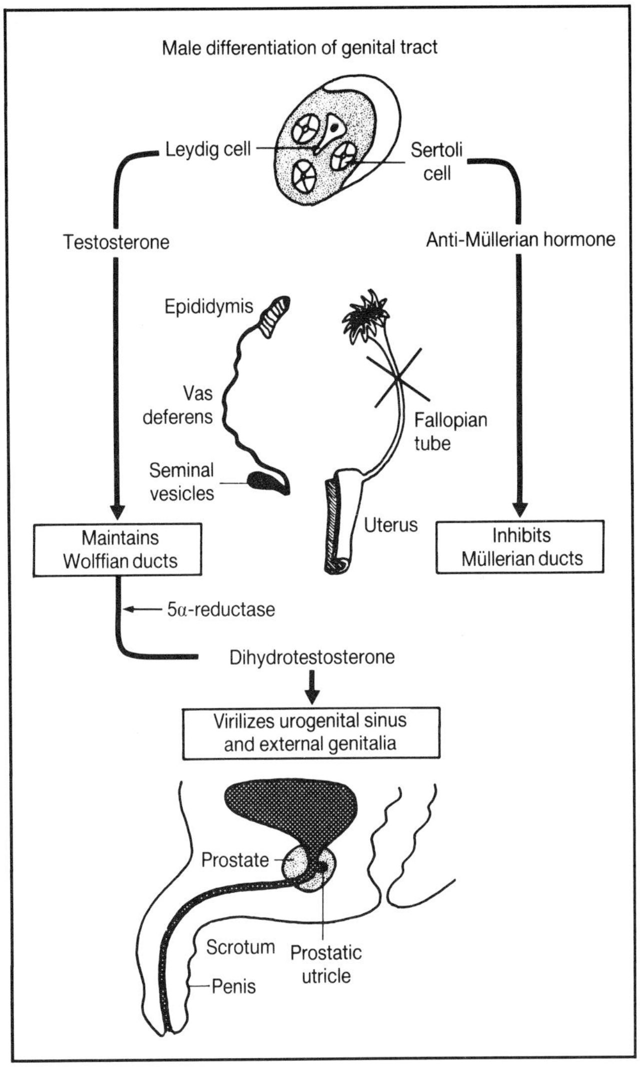

Fig. 4.4. Cartoon of male sex differentiation. Testosterone, produced by fetal Leydig cells, maintains Wolffian ducts and, after reduction to dihydrotestosterone, virilizes the urogenital sinus and the external genital organs. Anti-Müllerian hormone inhibits the development of Müllerian ducts. (From Josso N, ed. In *The intersex child*. Basel: Karger, 1981, p. 6, with permission.)

concentrations remain high until approximately 2 years of age, and then progressively decrease, to become more or less undetectable after puberty. AMH, also called Müllerian-inhibiting substance (MIS) or factor (MIF), is also produced by postnatal granulosa cells, although the function of ovarian AMH has not yet been identified. The 2.8 kb gene has been cloned and mapped to chromosome 19. It consists of five exons, the last one exhibiting a 30 percent homology with members of a superfamily of dimeric proteins involved in growth and differentiation, the TGFβ family. Proteolytic processing of AMH by plasmin yields a TGFβ-like fragment, which carries biological activity.

AMH can now be measured in human serum and has clinical usefulness as a marker of testicular function, particularly as it is produced exclusively by testicular tissue and since prior stimulation by gonadotropins is not necessary for its production. In XY babies in whom the gonads cannot be palpated, AMH measurement can discriminate between *anorchia* and *bilateral cryptorchidism*. In sexually ambiguous XX children, detection of circulating AMH rules out the diagnosis of *female pseudohermaphroditism* in favor of *true hermaphroditism*. The reverse, however, is not true, because dysgenetic testicular tissue may produce little or no AMH. Serum AMH concentrations usually correlate relatively well with Müllerian anatomical status but exceptions are possible, since presence or absence of Müllerian derivatives reflect the biological activity of AMH at 8 weeks of gestation, while serum AMH is a marker of Sertoli cell function at the time of investigation. AMH is detectable in male serum up to puberty, although it has not been shown to play any physiological role in males after Müllerian regression.

Development of Wolffian derivatives, masculinization of external genitalia and testicular descent

Wolffian ducts, originally the excretory canals of the primitive kidney, become incorporated into the genital tract, developing into the vasa deferentia, epididymes and seminal vesicles. Prostatic buds develop around the opening of the ducts at approximately 10–11 weeks of age while fusion of outgrowths of the urogenital sinus forms the prostatic utricle, the male equivalent of the vagina. Testosterone, not AMH, prevents the downgrowth of the vaginal rudiment and the acquisition of a separate perineal opening. In severely masculinized *female pseudohermaphrodites*, a short vaginal canal communicating with the uterus and tubes contacts the wall of the urethra just beneath the bladder neck and may be difficult to opacify radiologically. In contrast, the blind vaginal pouch of *androgen-insensitive male pseudohermaphrodites* has a separate perineal opening (Fig. 4.5). Only the upper part of the vagina is of Müllerian origin and responds to AMH and not testosterone.

At approximately 10 weeks, the genital tubercle elongates and urethral folds fuse over the urethral groove, leading to formation of the scrotum and penile urethra. Male anatomical development is completed at approximately 90 days of gestation, but at that time no appreciable size difference exists between the penis and clitoris. Penile growth occurs between 20 weeks and term, at a time when paradoxically, serum testosterone concentration is declining.

Testicular descent takes place in two phases, transabdominal, which brings the testis to the internal inguinal ring by 12 weeks, and passage through the inguinal canal, which occurs between 7 months and term. The hormonal control of testicular descent is not well

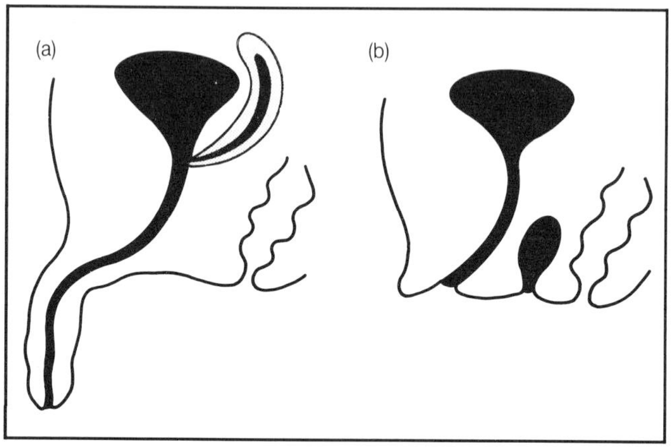

Fig. 4.5. Dissociation between uterine (Müllerian) and vaginal development in intersexuality. (a) Female pseudohermaphroditism with complete virilization of the external genitalia and urogenital sinus for example in severe 21-hydroxylase deficiency: vaginal development has been repressed and the uterus contacts the posterior urethra just beneath the bladder neck. (b) Male pseudohermaphroditism due to complete androgen insensitivity: Müllerian ducts have regressed, but the vagina has developed normally and acquired a perineal opening. It may be short, due to the fact that the upper part of the vagina is of Müllerian origin.

understood; androgens and gonadotropins are apparently implicated only in the transinguinal phase. Testicular insufficiency is often associated with *cryptorchidism*, particularly in cases where Müllerian regression has not occurred. This could be partly due to mechanical causes, since Müllerian derivatives are tightly attached to the testis and may prevent it from reaching the scrotum.

Testosterone: biosynthesis, 5α-reduction and binding to the androgen receptor

Except for Müllerian regression, male sex differentiation is mediated by androgens produced by fetal Leydig cells from 8 weeks onwards. Serum testosterone peaks at approximately 12–14 weeks, and then progressively falls, so that in late pregnancy, testosterone concentration is not significantly different in males and females (Fig. 4.6). Androgen production by the fetal Leydig cell is controlled initially by placental hCG (see p. 312), but fetal pituitary gonadotropins take over during late fetal life, explaining why micropenis and cryptorchidism are frequently observed in *congenital hypopituitarism*. At least five steroidogenetic enzymes are needed for the biosynthesis of testosterone from cholesterol (Fig. 4.7). Because the same enzymes operate also in the adrenal, male

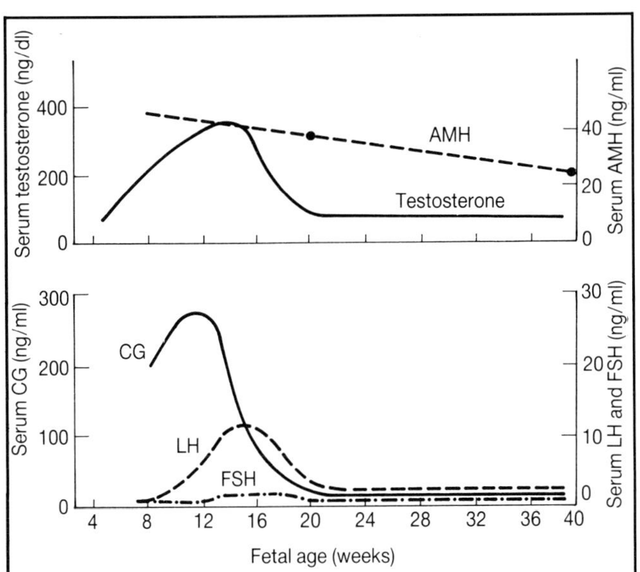

Fig. 4.6. Ontogeny of AMH, testosterone and gonadotropins in human fetal serum. Data for AMH before 20 weeks are extrapolated from measurements performed in fetal bovine serum, which have shown high values. Values at 20 and 40 weeks were measured in human fetal serum in collaboration with Dr Norman Davis, London, UK (Josso *et al. Recent Progress in Hormone Research* 1993, in press). Values for other hormones are taken from Reyes FI, Winter JSD, Faiman C. In *Diabetes and other endocrine disorders during pregnancy and in the newborn*. New York: Alan Liss, 1976: 83–106.

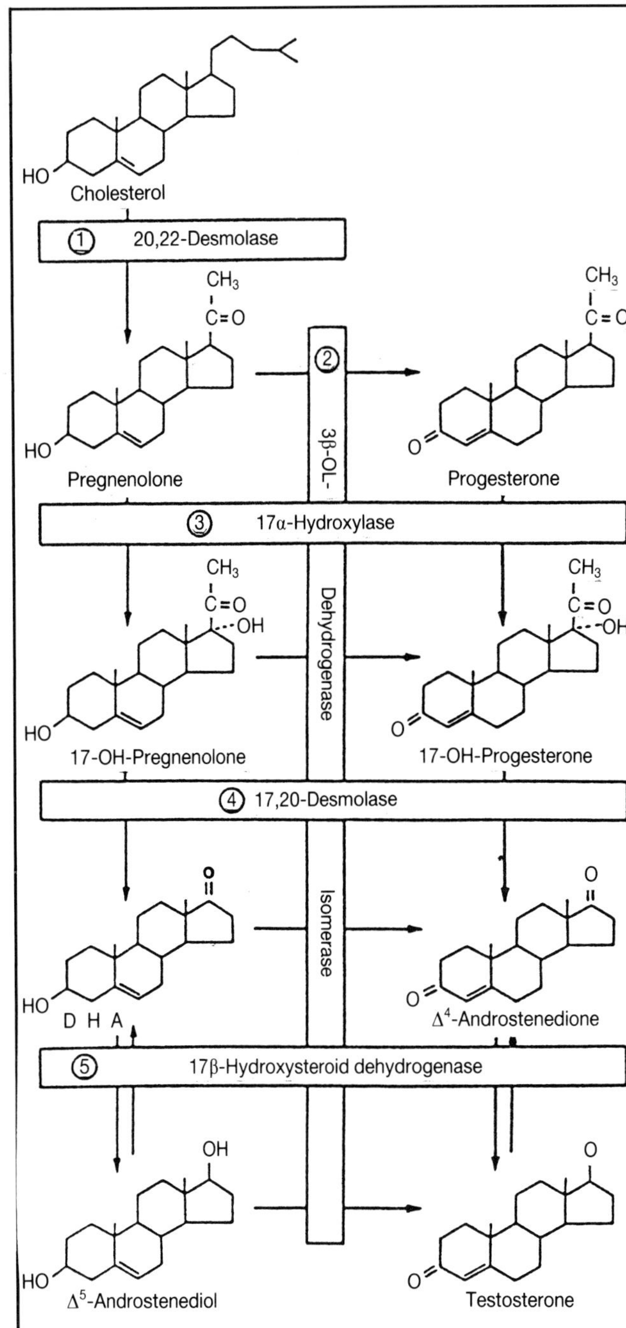

Fig. 4.7. Enzymes necessary to testosterone biosynthesis. (From Forest MG. In Josso N, ed. *The intersex child*. Basel: Karger, 1981: 133–55, with permission.)

pseudohermaphroditism due to steroidogenesis defects is associated with rare forms of *congenital adrenal hyperplasia* (see p. 326).

Testosterone exerts its biological activity by binding to an X-linked receptor molecule. The receptor has much greater affinity for the reduced derivative of testosterone, dihydrotestosterone, than for testosterone itself. Therefore, in tissues such as the urogenital sinus and external genitalia, containing 5α-reductase activity which enables them to generate dihydrotestosterone, the latter is the active androgen. Wolffian ducts, at the time of sex differentiation, do not yet express 5α-reductase activity, and consequently are the only fetal organs controlled by testosterone itself. This is perhaps the reason why they respond only to the high testosterone concentrations achieved by local uptake in the vicinity of the testis, but cannot be maintained by circulating androgen.

The gene coding for the androgen receptor, which has been cloned recently, is located on the X chromosome between the centromere and q13; it belongs to the superfamily of steroid receptors (Fig. 4.8). The human androgen receptor gene, which spans a minimum of 54 kb, is divided into eight exons. Exons 2 and 3 code for the DNA binding domain which consists of two zinc finger domains which are important for recognition and binding of promoter elements of androgen-responsive genes. Mutations in this region have been found in patients with the so-called 'receptor-positive' form of *androgen insensitivity syndrome*, because binding of dihydrotestosterone is not affected. Most mutations, however, have been described in exons 4–8, which code for the steroid hormone binding domain. Deletions and point mutations in this region have been recognized in patients suffering from 'receptor-negative' *androgen insensitivity syndrome*. The N-terminal part of the androgen receptor, encoded by the first exon, is important for transcriptional activation. In contrast to estrogen and progesterone receptors, which reside in the nucleus even in the absence of ligand binding, nuclear localization of the androgen receptor is promoted by androgen. The nuclear targeting signal is located within the hinge region between the DNA and steroid binding domains.

Female development

Female sex differentiation appears to lag behind male organogenesis, although sex determination—defined by the 'critical period' of sensitivity of genital primordia to testicular hormones—occurs at the same time in males and females. In the female, Müllerian ducts persist to form Fallopian tubes, uterus and upper part of the vagina, Wolffian ducts degenerate, and the vagina differentiates at the level of the Müllerian tubercle, between the openings of the Wolffian ducts where the prostatic utricle forms in males. The main difference between male and female organogenesis of the urogenital sinus lies in the downgrowth of the vagina. Whereas in males, the prostatic utricle opens just beneath the neck of the bladder, in females, the lower end of the vagina slides down the posterior wall of the urethra to acquire a separate opening on the body surface.

Feminization of the external genitalia begins by the formation of the dorsal commissure, between the labioscrotal swellings, which give rise to the labia majora. The urethral folds do not fuse and become the labia minora; the stunted phallus develops into the clitoris.

All these steps are constitutive and occur in the absence of hormonal stimulation of any kind. Although the fetal ovary does produce estrogens, female hormones do not

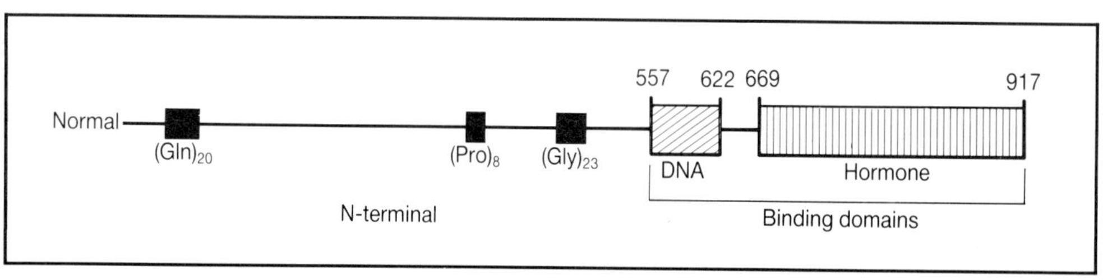

Fig. 4.8. Structure of the androgen receptor protein. Note the stretches of repeated glutamines, prolines and glycines in the first exon and the separate hormone and DNA binding domains. (Modified from Marcelli M, Tilley WD, Wilson CM, Griffin JE, Wilson JD, McPhaul MJ. Definition of the human androgen receptor gene structure permits the identification of mutations that cause androgen resistance: premature termination of the receptor protein of amino acid residue 588 causes complete androgen resistance. *Mol Endocrinol* 1990; **4**: 1105–16. © The Endocrine Society.)

promote female development. A female karyotype does not protect against masculinization by testicular hormones. Female fetuses with *congenital adrenal hyperplasia* may undergo total masculinization of the external genital organs, including formation of a penile urethra. However, in the absence of locally secreted testosterone, no Wolffian ducts differentiate, for reasons discussed above. Under normal conditions, human females are never exposed to AMH during fetal life. However AMH-induced Müllerian regression has been described in bovine freemartins united by placental anastomoses to a male co-twin.

Neurological sex differentiation: brain sex and gender identity

Brain sex

The brain controls the endocrine system through the hypothalamus and pituitary gland. Anatomical differences between male and female brains have been detected in the anterior hypothalamus, thought to control sexual orientation, the anterior commissure and the corpus callosum which could be involved in cognition and patterns of lateralization. From an endocrine perspective, sexual dimorphism lies essentially in the control of gonadotropin secretion. Already in the perinatal period, gonadotropin levels differ between males and females, FSH levels being higher in the latter. At puberty, a cyclic LH preovulatory surge characterizes female reproductive function. In rodents, the ability of the female hypothalamus to release LHRH cyclically can be definitively destroyed by exposure to androgens during a critical period, which ends 5 days after birth; conversely, males castrated during the critical period, but not later, do exhibit a cyclic pattern of LH release at puberty. In humans and subhuman primates, androgen sex imprinting of the hypothalamus is not demonstrated: females exposed to androgens during fetal life, e.g. because of *congenital adrenal hyperplasia*, can ovulate at puberty if treated properly.

Gender identity

Establishment of sexual identity occurs in several stages. The awareness of being either male or female may be evident as early as 13 months of age. Sex-typed behavior is clearly present at 3 years of age or earlier while the orientation of erotic interest emerges with pubertal maturation. The question of the relative influence of hormonal and environmental factors in the determination of gender identity has been heavily debated. It was initially proposed that gender identity was ruled by the sex of rearing and irreversibly established after 3 years of age; however, recent evidence supports the conclusion that in *male pseudohermaphrodites*, unambiguously raised as girls, pubertal masculinization may override social pressure and induce the individual to adopt a male gender role. Examples of successful 'sex-reversal' are rare, however, and every effort should be made to ensure that, in sexually ambiguous children, the sex of rearing chosen in the neonatal period will fit anatomical and endocrine status in adulthood.

Pathophysiology of sex differentiation

The unraveling, albeit incomplete, of the genetic and hormonal mechanisms of normal sex differentiation allows considerable insight into the nature of clinical disorders of sex differentiation. The demonstration that the fetal testis produces two discrete hormones, testosterone and AMH, is central to our understanding sexual ambiguity and gonadal dysgenesis. Normally, genetic, gonadal and somatic sex are coherent, either all male or all female. Inadequate sex differentiation at any level, or discrepancy between its various elements, results in sex ambiguity.

Testes without a Y chromosome: XX males and true hermaphrodites

As discussed above, SRY, the candidate testis-determining gene, not the Y chromosome *per se*, is responsible for testicular differentiation. Transfer of SRY to an X chromosome during paternal meiosis is facilitated by the closeness of SRY to the pseudoautosomal boundary (Fig. 4.9) and results in testicular development in XX individuals. Moreover, *XX maleness* cannot always be explained by transfer of Y-related DNA. Approximately 30 percent of XX males type Y-negative when their DNA is probed with Y-specific probes. These patients are often incompletely masculinized and other *XX males* or *true hermaphrodites* can be traced in the family. Testicular

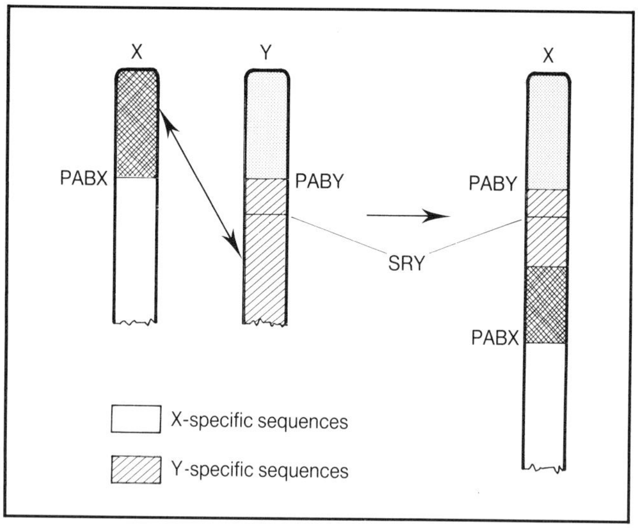

Fig. 4.9. Abnormal X/Y interchange, leading to the generation of XX maleness. Y-specific sequences close to the pseudoautosomal boundary and containing SRY have been involved in crossing over between the X and Y chromosomes during paternal meiosis. The resulting X chromosome carries the SRY gene and will yield male offspring. PABX and PABY, pseudoautosomal boundary from X and Y chromosomes respectively. (Modified from Weissenbach J, Petit C. *Médecine-Sciences* 1990; **6**: 785–90.)

differentiation in *'XX males'* in the absence of Y-related DNA could arise from a mutation in 'downstream' autosomal genes, which mediate the testis-determining activity of SRY; these have not yet been identified in humans.

Masculinization without testes: anorchia and female pseudohermaphroditism

Masculinization of XY individuals with no testicular tissue is due to testicular degeneration during fetal life. The clinical picture in *anorchia* depends upon the timing of gonadal demise. If testes degenerate before 8 fetal weeks, the phenotype is usually female except for the absence of Müllerian derivatives. XY individuals with a female phenotype including an uterus and tubes are classified under the term *pure gonadal dysgenesis* because there is no evidence that testicular tissue developed at any time. If testicular degeneration occurs between 9 and 14 weeks, the clinical picture is that of *male pseudohermaphroditism*, with variable degrees of scrotal fusion and vaginal development. After 14 weeks, the masculine phenotype is complete, but micropenis is usually present.

Female XX pseudohermaphrodites, with sex ambiguity in the presence of normal ovaries, always possess a normal uterus and tubes, since in the fetus, AMH is made exclusively by testicular tissue, which they lack by definition. Masculinization is due to aggression by exogenous androgens, usually of adrenal origin. *Deficiency of 21-hydroxylase* or other steroidogenetic enzymes leads to enhanced androgen secretion, which can produce complete masculinization of the external genitalia. Bilateral cryptorchidism, even without hypospadias, should always be considered with suspicion. Testosterone-dependent masculinization is also reflected in the inhibition of lower vaginal development: the deeper the masculinization, the higher the opening of the vagina in the urogenital sinus. However, not all cases of *female pseudohermaphroditism* are due to testosterone overproduction: malformations, which usually also involve neighboring organs such as the kidney, uterus and terminal gut, may lead to clitoral hypertrophy and labial fusion which mimics the effect of androgens.

Incompetent testes: male pseudohermaphroditism

Failure of testicular tissue to achieve complete masculinization—*male pseudohermaphroditism*—results from many different causes, most associated with an XY karyotype or mosaic cell line. When both AMH and testosterone-dependent steps of sex differentiation are impaired, in other words when persistence of Müllerian derivatives is associated with incomplete masculinization of the external genitalia and urogenital sinus, *testicular dysgenesis* is necessarily involved, since no biochemical cause can explain combined defects in the production or action of a steroid such as testosterone and a glycoprotein such as AMH. The frequent occurrence of testicular degeneration in so-called *'dysgenetic male pseudohermaphroditism'*, characterized by the presence of Müllerian ducts, is therefore not surprising. *True hermaphrodites* have a similar phenotype; their lack of masculinization is due to an insufficient amount of testicular tissue, and also to severe testicular dysgenesis.

When Müllerian regression has occurred normally, biochemical defects affecting testosterone synthesis or peripheral effect should be sought for. Mutations of enzymes necessary for testosterone production (Fig. 4.7) are rare, also affect adrenal steroidogenesis and can be recognized through measurement of hormone precursors. Decreased testosterone production, even in the absence of Müllerian derivatives, can also be due to the late occurrence of testicular dysgenesis; in this case, circulating AMH concentrations are also low. Since testosterone action requires transformation into dihydrotestosterone and its binding to an androgen receptor, biochemical defects of androgen target organs can also lead to sex ambiguity limited to testosterone-dependent steps. In *5α-reductase deficiency*, target organs are unable to produce dihydrotestosterone, and only testosterone is available for binding to the androgen receptor. Paradoxically, although the external genitalia are very poorly masculinized at birth, virilization occurs at puberty with the marked rise in sex steroid production that ensues. 5α-Reductase deficiency is seldom encountered outside highly inbred isolates, such as have been described in the Dominican Republic. *Androgen insensitivity*, an X-linked disorder due to lesions of the androgen receptor gene, is a much more common disorder, and displays a variety of phenotypes. From a clinical standpoint, androgen insensitivity may be complete or partial, with either female or ambiguous genitalia. Biologically, the capacity of the androgen receptor to bind dihydrotestosterone is either impaired ('receptor negative form') or normal ('receptor positive form'), suggesting abnormalities in distinct domains of the androgen receptor gene (see above).

Finally, in rare instances, the external genitalia and urogenital sinus are normally masculinized, but Müllerian ducts do not regress. This condition, *the persistent Müllerian duct syndrome*, is heterogeneous. In some cases, no testicular or circulating AMH can be detected; an abnormality of the AMH gene is the most likely possibility. Elsewhere, AMH levels are normal for age, and study of AMH bioactivity is required to distinguish between the secretion of an abnormal, immunoreactive but biologically inactive, AMH and a target organ defect.

Selected reading

Goodfellow P, Lovell-Badge R, eds, *Seminars in developmental biology, sex determination and the Y chromosome* **2**(4): August 1991.

Josso N, Cate RL, Picard JY, *et al*. Anti-Müllerian hormone, the Jost factor. *Recent Prog Horm Res* 1993; **48** (in press).

Jost A. Genetic and hormonal factors in sex differentiation of the brain. *Psychoneuroendocrinology* 1983; **8:** 183–93.

Wilson JD. Syndromes of androgen resistance. *Biol Reprod* 1992; **46**: 168–73.

C. Placental Physiology

J E Harding

Transport and metabolism

The placenta is the interface between the maternal and fetal circulations. As such it has a primary role in ensuring the fetus is supplied with all metabolic requirements for growth and survival and in the removal of waste products. This role does not involve only transport of materials between the two circulations. In many cases important metabolism of substrates occurs within the placenta, providing both modified substrates essential to the fetus and ensuring the continued survival of placental tissues which have a very high metabolic rate. Thus the dual placental functions of transport and metabolism need always be considered together in any discussion of placental function.

Mechanisms of placental transport

Substances may cross the placenta in a number of different ways (Table 4.2). Small lipid-soluble molecules cross the placenta readily by simple diffusion across cell membranes. The rate of diffusion provides no significant barrier to placental transfer for these substances, and transfer is largely dependent upon placental blood flow.

Small water-soluble molecules cross the placenta by diffusion down their concentration, osmotic and electrochemical gradients. This diffusion possibly occurs through notional pores in the placental membrane, although the physical existence of such channels has not been demonstrated on electron microscopy. Transfer of these substances depends upon placental permeability, which may change with gestational age, possibly by changes in surface area or barrier thickness.

Transport of some molecules across the placenta is faster than can be accounted for by simple diffusion. Such transport, which is carrier mediated but does not require energy, occurs by facilitated diffusion. Specific larger molecules may also cross the placenta by active transport; an energy-requiring, carrier-mediated process, often against a concentration gradient. Finally, large molecules may cross the placenta by endocytotic processes, which are probably also carrier mediated.

Table 4.2. Mechanisms of placental transport for different substances

Mechanisms	Example
Diffusion, flow-limited	O_2, CO_2, unconjugated bilirubin
Diffusion, membrane-limited	Na^+, K^+, urea, water
Facilitated diffusion	Glucose
Active transport	Amino acids, Ca^{2+}
Endocytosis	IgG, iron, vitamin B_{12}

Glucose

Transport

Glucose crosses the placenta by facilitated diffusion down a concentration gradient from mother to fetus. Carriers have a high K_m with a saturation well above the physiological range for maternal blood glucose. Carriers are found on both the maternal and fetal sides of the placenta, consistent with bidirectional fluxes across the placenta, and capacity is higher on the fetal side.

Metabolism

Placental glucose consumption is very high, amounting to up to two-thirds of the total glucose taken up from the uterine circulation. This contributes to the maternal/fetal glucose gradient and a low fetal glucose concentration. Most placental glucose utilization is from glucose in the fetal rather than the maternal circulation, so that placental glucose consumption largely depends on fetal glucose concentrations. Pathways of glucose metabolism in the placenta are poorly understood. Glucose may be used for glycolysis and glycogen synthesis although both processes decrease as gestation proceeds. Some glucose is also used for lactate production, with return of lactate to both the fetal and maternal circulations. Gluconeogenesis, i.e. *de novo* glucose synthesis, does not occur in the placenta.

Regulation

Glucose transfer is largely determined by the maternal/fetal concentration gradient. Glucose carriers are insulin independent, similar to those found in the brain. Insulin may affect glucose transfer only indirectly by altering arterial glucose concentrations in either the fetal or maternal circulations.

Amino acids

Transport

Total plasma amino acid concentrations are approximately twice as high in the fetal as in the maternal circulations. For most, although not all, amino acids, placental concentrations are even higher than the fetal levels. Amino acids are thus transported up a concentration gradient into the placenta by active, carrier-mediated, energy-requiring transport mechanisms. The mechanism of their release to the fetal circulation may be by diffusion down the concentration gradient, or may be carrier mediated. For at least some amino acids there are large bidirectional fluxes across the placenta, suggesting the likelihood of carriers on the fetal side of the membrane. Of the six well described amino acid carrier systems, three (A type and ASC type [Na^+ dependent] and L type [Na^+ independent]) have definitely been identified in the human placenta. However, many more carrier systems have also been reported, several of which may be placenta specific and even exist in specific fetal isoforms. There is much overlap of amino acids between the different carriers and competition between different amino acids for the same carrier. Thus the transport of any one amino acid may affect the transfer of several others. For example, high phenylalanine concentrations inhibit placental tyrosine and tryptophan uptake *in vitro*. Since these amino acids are required for neurotransmitter synthesis, this mechanism may contribute to mental retardation in infants of mothers with uncontrolled *phenylketonuria*.

Metabolism

Net placental amino acid uptake is normally small, although the placenta requires some amino acids for oxidation, tissue synthesis and synthesis of protein hormones such as hCG and placental lactogen. The placenta also contributes to important metabolic cycling of amino acids to the fetus. Glutamate, aspartate and serine produced by the fetal liver are taken up by the placenta with the production of the metabolically related glutamine, asparagine and glycine which are returned to the fetus. The placenta also produces ammonia, some of which is taken up by the fetal liver, possibly as a mechanism for conserving nitrogen in the fetal circulation. The placenta has a large capacity for transamination of amino acids, and for deamination with release of the corresponding keto acids, although the significance of these pathways is as yet unknown. In *intrauterine growth retardation*, as total uterine substrate supply decreases, amino acids account for an increasingly large proportion of placental oxidative fuel requirements. In late gestation this high demand may be met by placental uptake of amino acids, particularly branched-chain amino acids, from the fetal circulation, resulting in net fetal amino acid loss and thus fetal wasting.

Regulation

A prolonged decrease in maternal amino acid concentrations causes an increase in placental amino acid transport, apparently by inducing synthesis of new carriers. Similarly, a long-term increase in maternal concentrations causes a decrease in transport, possibly by transinhibition of carriers. Hormonal regulation of amino acid transport such as occurs in many other tissues has not been described for the placenta. Insulin does not appear to have an effect, and a postulated role for acetylcholine remains to be confirmed. Both *alcohol* and *nicotine* inhibit placental amino acid transfer and this effect may contribute to *fetal growth retardation* seen in fetuses of mothers who use these drugs.

Oxygen

Transport

Oxygen diffuses across the placenta down a concentration gradient from mother to fetus. In the human placenta, membrane permeability imposes no significant barrier to diffusion, and O_2 transport is therefore determined by uterine and umbilical blood flows, i.e. is flow limited under normal circumstances. The regulation of uterine and umbilical blood flows are discussed in Chapter 10 (see p. 540).

Metabolism

Placental O_2 consumption is high, accounting for as much as 50 percent of O_2 taken up from the uterine circulation. On a weight-specific basis placental tissues at term have an O_2 requirement four to five times that of the fetus which in turn is twice that of the adult. It is not known what proportion of this O_2 consumption is required for different placental functions such as transport or protein synthesis.

Regulation

Placental O_2 transfer depends on maternal and fetal placental blood flows, and the O_2 carrying capacities of the maternal and fetal blood. According to the Fick principle, uterine O_2 delivery is equal to uterine blood flow times the arteriovenous difference of O_2 content across the uterine circulation. When uterine blood flow is decreased, e.g. with uterine contractions, maternal exercise or smoking, the continued rapid diffusion of O_2 out of the maternal blood results in a fall in uterine venous O_2 content and thus an increase in arteriovenous difference, resulting in increased O_2 extraction. This increase in extraction maintains uterine O_2 delivery until uterine blood flow falls by more than 50 percent (Fig. 4.10). Thus increased uterine extraction results in a wide margin of safety for O_2 delivery to the uterus under normal circumstances. Under some circumstances, there may be further adaptation to maintain uterine O_2 delivery. For example, maternal exercise results in hemoconcentration, thus increasing O_2 delivery to the uterus despite a decrease in uterine blood flow. The shift in the maternal hemoglobin O_2 dissociation curve caused by increased temperature and acidosis also improves O_2 delivery (see p. 547) and may contribute to this adaptation.

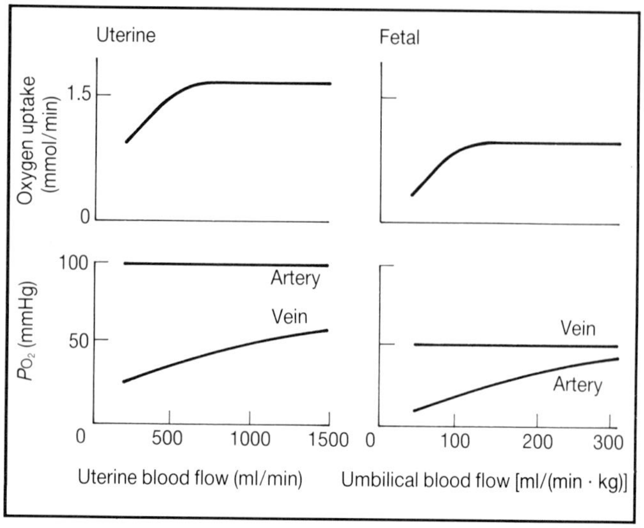

Fig. 4.10. The effect of decreases in placental blood flow on O_2 uptake and Po_2. As blood flow decreases, the increasing arteriovenous difference results in increasing O_2 extraction, so that O_2 uptake is not reduced until blood flow is reduced by more than 50 percent. The figure is a diagrammatic representation derived from experimental data in the sheep.

Fetal O_2 uptake is similarly a product of the umbilical blood flow and the arteriovenous differences for O_2 content across the umbilical circulation. Once again, reduced umbilical blood flow such as may be seen in cord compression results in no change in umbilical venous O_2 content because of rapid O_2 diffusion across the placenta. If fetal O_2 demand is unchanged, this results in a fall in fetal $Pa{O_2}$ as the reduced amount of oxygenated fetal blood mixes with the deoxygenated blood reaching the heart. This in turn results in decreased umbilical arterial $Pa{O_2}$, increasing the arteriovenous difference for O_2 across the placenta and thus increasing fetal O_2 extraction. Once again, there is a relatively wide margin of safety, and acute falls in umbilical blood flow result in no change in fetal O_2 uptake until the flow is reduced by more than 50 percent (Fig. 4.10).

Essential to this remarkable capacity to increase O_2 extraction in the face of decreased blood flow to either side of the placenta is the capacity of the placenta to allow rapid gas transfer. Since O_2 transfer across the placenta is by diffusion down a concentration gradient, persisting rapid transfer requires no decrease in the concentration gradient. To achieve this, O_2 must be unloaded from maternal hemoglobin efficiently, and removed on the fetal side of the placenta by rapid binding to fetal hemoglobin. In this way, the high affinity of fetal hemoglobin for O_2 helps maintain transfer and allows increased extraction as the supply decreases if either uterine or umbilical placental blood flows decrease. If the affinity of hemoglobin on the fetal side of the placenta is decreased, e.g. by *exchange transfusion* with adult hemoglobin, or has reduced carrying capacity, e.g. *fetal anemia*, this capacity to increase extraction in the face of reduced supply is decreased and thus the margin of safety is decreased. Likewise, increased maternal hemoglobin O_2 affinity, e.g. maternal *hemoglobinopathies*, or reduced maternal hemoglobin O_2 carrying capacity, e.g. carbon monoxide from maternal cigarette smoking displacing O_2 from maternal hemoglobin, will result in no acute decrease in fetal oxygenation, but a reduced margin of safety in the face of any changes in blood flow.

It is possible that other adaptive mechanisms contribute to the capacity of the fetus to increase O_2 extraction from the maternal circulation when required. For example, fetal hypoxemia may result in a rise in umbilical venous tone and pressure, thus potentially opening previously underperfused fetal/placental vessels and increasing the available exchange area in the placenta for O_2 extraction. When O_2 supply or umbilical blood flow is reduced chronically, it is also likely that placental O_2 demand is reduced in order to improve fetal O_2 supply. If decreased O_2 supply is maintained, there appears to be a gradual reduction in fetal O_2 uptake, with a resultant reduction in the O_2 gradient across the placenta and reduced placental O_2 transfer, e.g. *intrauterine growth retardation*.

Lipids

Transport

Transport of lipids into the placenta may occur by at least three different mechanisms, and the mechanism of release from placenta to fetus is unclear. First, fatty acids may be taken up from the maternal plasma by specific carriers. This probably accounts for the majority of lipid transfer across the placenta, although carrier details are unknown. Secondly, triacylglycerol in maternal very low-density lipoproteins (VLDL) is hydrolyzed by lipoprotein lipases on the maternal placental surface and the released fatty acids are transported across the placenta, possibly by carriers as already described. Thirdly, maternal low-density lipoproteins (LDL) bind to receptors on the maternal side of the placenta, are taken up by endocytosis and are degraded in placental lysosomes with release of cholesterol. Other lipoproteins probably also bind to the placental surface but their roles are unclear. Mechanisms of transport for related substances such as fat-soluble vitamins, choline and carnitine are poorly understood.

Metabolism

Lipids are extensively metabolized in the placenta. Fatty acids which have been taken up from the maternal circulation, hydrolyzed in the placenta or synthesized *de novo* may be modified by desaturation, elongation or partial oxidation before release to the fetus. In particular, chain modification in the placenta may result in increased transfer of medium-chain fatty acids to the fetus. This may be important because of the limited fetal capacity to oxidize long-chain fatty acids due to low fetal carnitine levels. Placental fatty acids may also be esterified to complex lipids and then be released directly to the fetus or further hydrolyzed before release. Cholesterol from maternal LDL is an important placental precursor for steroid hormone synthesis. Thus maternal *hypobetalipoproteinemia*, resulting in low circulating LDL and VLDL cholesterol, results in *low maternal progesterone, estradiol and estriol levels*.

Regulation

Fatty acid transport across the placenta increases with gestation. The rate of transfer is largely determined by the transplacental gradient, i.e. by maternal levels and fetal utilization. Transfer may also be affected by placental blood flows and by circulating albumin concentrations since albumin binds to free fatty acids. Increased maternal plasma lipoprotein and free fatty acid concentrations and increased placental fatty acid binding capacity are seen in *maternal diabetes* and result in increased lipid transfer to the fetus.

Proteins

Many plasma proteins cross the human placenta in very small amounts by diffusion under the physiological restraints of the membrane. However, most are broken down in the placenta so that maternal protein acquired by the fetus is negligible relative to fetal protein synthesis. FSH, LH, insulin, glucagon and growth hormone apparently have negligible transfer across the placenta. In contrast, IgG crosses the placenta in significant amounts by pinocytosis, probably after binding to a specific receptor such as the Fc receptor.

Water and electrolytes

The human placenta appears to be very permeable to small electrolytes such as Na^+ and Cl^-, which cross the placenta by rapid diffusion along concentration and electrochemical gradients. Placental transport of these and many other ions such as K^+, sulphate, H^+, iodide and bicarbonate are all determined not only by diffusion but also by electrochemical gradients established by the numerous co- and counter-transport mechanisms, many linked to Na^+ pumps. Water crosses the placenta by diffusion and by filtration, following the balance of osmotic and hydrostatic pressures. The mechanism of disturbance in this balance such as occurs in *hydrops fetalis* is not well understood.

Minerals

Calcium

Fetal Ca^{2+} concentrations are higher than maternal in late gestation, and Ca^{2+} is transported actively across the placenta by an ATP-dependent, saturable, magnesium-dependent transporter on the fetal surface of the placenta. Ca^{2+} transport is probably regulated by fetal $1,25(OH)_2D_3$ concentrations via a specific vitamin D-dependent calcium binding protein in the placenta. Fetal parathormone probably affects placental Ca^{2+} transport largely via its effects on vitamin D synthetic rates. It is unknown if fetal parathormone or calcitonin also directly affect placental Ca^{2+} transport. Newborns with *vitamin D-dependent rickets* ($1,25(OH)_2D_3$-1α-hydroxylase deficiency) are normal at birth, implying that adequate placental Ca^{2+} transport can occur with very low hormone concentrations. It is unclear if maternal hormones also regulate placental Ca^{2+} transport. However, placental Ca^{2+} transport does appear to reflect chronic changes in maternal calcemia, since transient *neonatal hypoparathyroidism* occurs in newborns of hypercalcemic mothers, and *neonatal hyperparathyroidism* in newborns of hypocalcemic mothers.

Phosphate

Phosphate is actively transported across the placenta by sodium-dependent saturable carriers on the maternal surface. Regulation is poorly understood.

Iron

Fetal iron concentrations are higher than maternal in late gestation. Iron appears to cross the placenta by receptor-mediated endocytosis. Maternal transferrin binds to specific receptors on the placental surface and is taken up by endocytosis. The iron is then detached from transferrin and incorporated into ferritin in the placenta. The mechanism of transfer from placental ferritin to the fetal circulation is unknown. Placental receptors increase late in gestation and transfer is possibly regulated by placental ferritin levels, but it is still controversial whether any significant increase in placental iron transfer occurs during maternal *iron deficiency anemia*.

Selected reading

Carter AM. Factors affecting gas transfer across the placenta and the oxygen supply to the fetus. *J Dev Physiol* 1989; **12**: 305.
Carter BS, Moores RR, Battaglia FC. Placental transport and fetal and placental metabolism of amino acids. *J Nutr Biochem* 1991; **2**: 4.
Coleman RA. The role of the placenta in lipid metabolism and transport. *Semin Perinatol* 1989; **13**: 180.
Faber JJ, Thornburg KL. *Placental physiology*. New York: Raven Press, 1983.
Hay WW. Energy and substrate requirements of the placenta and fetus. *Proc Nutr Soc* 1991; **50**: 321.
Shennan DB, Boyd CAR. Ion transport by the placenta: a review of membrane transport systems. *Biochim Biophys Acta* 1987; **906**: 437.
Sibley CP, Boyd RDH. Control of transfer across the mature placenta. *Oxf Rev Reprod Biol* 1988; **10**: 382.

D. Parturition

G C Liggins

The mechanism initiating parturition in a number of animal species is known to result from the release of prostaglandin $F_{2\alpha}$ ($PGF_{2\alpha}$) from the uterine epithelium, stimulated at term by a rapid fall in progesterone levels and a sharp rise in estrogen. The changes in steroid synthesis result from rising concentrations of cortisol in the fetal circulation which induce the activity of 17α-hydroxylase, a placental enzyme necessary for the conversion of progesterone to estrogen (Fig. 4.11). The placenta of primates, including man, lacks the enzyme and parturition is not preceded by an alteration in the ratio of progesterone:estrogen. Nevertheless, $PGF_{2\alpha}$ and prostaglandin E_2 (PGE_2) are released in substantial quantities in human labor and are almost certainly responsible for the various changes in the uterine smooth muscle and connective tissue that lead to labor and delivery. The factors responsible for the control of uterine prostaglandin synthesis in human pregnancy remain uncertain. However, most investigators agree that human parturition is the outcome of paracrine rather than endocrine events. The most favored hypothesis proposes that the paracrine interaction involves a maternal tissue (decidua) and fetal tissues (amnion and chorion).

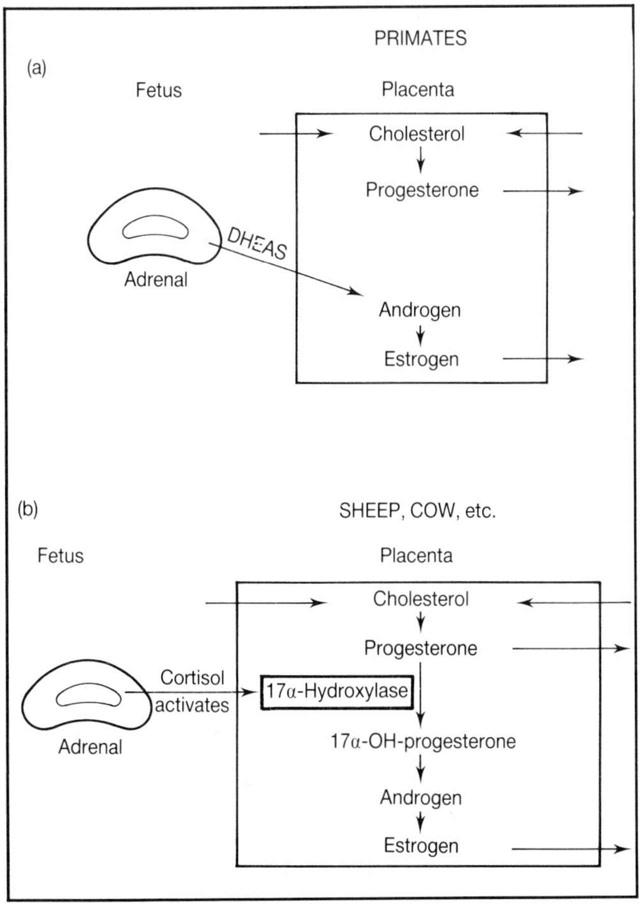

Fig. 4.11. Pathways of steroid synthesis in the placenta in various species demonstrating the fundamental difference depending on the presence or absence of 17α-hydroxylase. The primate (including human) placenta lacks the enzyme and depends on the fetal adrenal for substrate for estrogen synthesis. DHEAS, dehydroepiandrosterone.

Evidence implicating PGs

1. The concentrations of $PGF_{2\alpha}$ and PGE_2 in amniotic fluid and of their stable metabolites in plasma rise sharply after the onset of labor.
2. Treatment with small amounts of $PGF_{2\alpha}$ or PGE_2 induces labor which reproduces exactly the events of spontaneous labor.
3. Inhibitors of PG synthesis such as aspirin or indomethacin can prolong pregnancy or arrest labor.

Actions of PGs on the uterus

The administration of PGs to women at any stage of pregnancy leads to abortion or delivery provided that sufficient time (8–12 hours) is allowed for uterine responses involving protein synthesis to evolve. The changes involve both the smooth muscle and the connective tissue of the cervix and fetal membranes. The smooth muscle cells exposed to $PGF_{2\alpha}$ or PGE_2 develop gap junctions that transmit spike potentials, thereby propagating an electrical wave from a single pacemaker site. The resulting coordinated contraction of the whole uterus is effective in expelling the fetus whereas the local, uncoordinated contractions that occur throughout pregnancy are ineffective. $PGF_{2\alpha}$ and PGE_2 are oxytocic (i.e. stimulate contractions) and, in addition, enhance the sensitivity of smooth muscle cells to oxytocin. Prostacyclin (PGI_2) relaxes smooth muscle and may contribute to uterine quiescence during pregnancy. Both $PGF_{2\alpha}$ and PGE_2, particularly the latter, cause changes in the uterine and amniotic connective tissues akin to those occurring in inflammation or tissue remodeling. Specifically, enhanced activity of collagenolytic enzymes causes mature, 'tough' collagen to be degraded and partly replaced by young, more fragile collagen with fewer crosslinks. The concentration of strongly charged, sulfated glycosaminoglycans in the proteoglycan matrix is halved, leading to loosening of the tight packing of the collagen bundles. The overall effect of these biochemical changes is a 12-fold decrease in the mechanical strength of the intrapartum cervix compared with the nonpregnant cervix. Similar biochemical events in the amnion weaken this tough membrane sufficiently to allow labor contractions to burst it. Relaxin as well as PGE_2 and $PGF_{2\alpha}$ increase the compliance of the pregnant human cervix when applied topically but whether relaxin has a physiological role in cervical ripening in women as it has in many animals is uncertain.

Synthesis of uterine PGs

(see also p. 103)

The various uterine tissues have different spectra of PG synthesis. The predominant PG released by the myometrium is PGI_2 whereas the decidua forms mainly $PGF_{2\alpha}$ and the amnion and cervix release PGE_2. It is likely that $PGF_{2\alpha}$ of decidual origin is the major PG initiating labor. As in other tissues, uterine PGs require arachidonic acid as the mandatory substrate. Arachidonic acid is present in abundance in the phospholipids of uterine tissues which are specifically enriched with this fatty acid, probably as a response to high levels of progesterone. Free arachidonic acid is converted by cyclooxygenase to unstable endoperoxides (PGG_2 and PGH_2) which are rapidly transformed by specific synthases to the various prostanoids including the primary PGs, prostacyclin and thromboxane. Thus the availability of free arachidonic acid determines the rate of synthesis, cyclooxygenase imposes a maximal production rate and the relative activities of the synthases determine the spectrum of end products (Fig. 4.12).

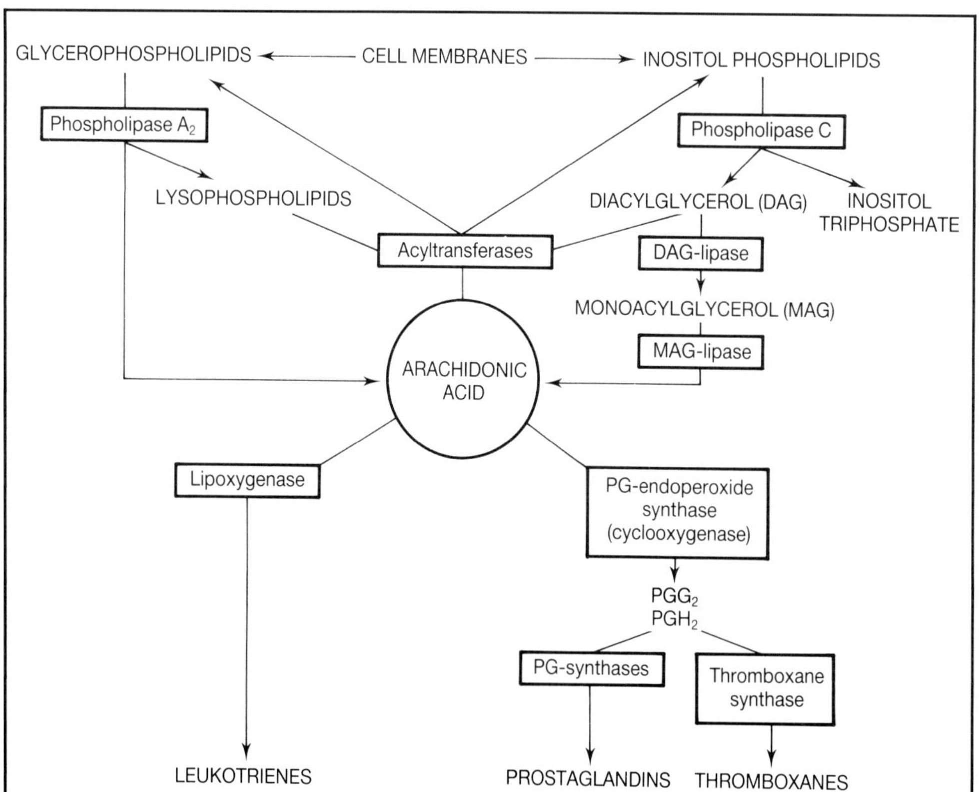

Fig. 4.12. Simplified diagram of pathways of prostanoid synthesis in uterine tissues. Free arachidonic acid is either metabolized to end products or reincorporated into phospholipids.

Control of PG synthesis

Arachidonic acid is liberated by hydrolysis at the *sn-2* position of glycerophospholipids such as phosphatidylcholine and phosphatidylethanolamine through the action of phospholipase A_2 (PLA_2) which is present intracellularly in an inactive, membrane-bound form capable of almost instantaneous activation. An alternative source of arachidonic acid is phosphatidylinositol which is hydrolyzed successively by phospholipase C and di- and monoacylglycerol lipases. This pathway also liberates inositol triphosphosphate (IP_3) which mobilizes free Ca^{2+} and enhances the activity of the Ca-dependent PLA_2. A wide variety of physical, chemical, and bacteriological factors stimulate activity and many of them, such as stripping placental membranes, or intrauterine placement of hypertonic solutions, irritant solutions or foreign bodies, have been used clinically to induce labor or abortion. However, the physiological stimulus of PLA_2 in the human uterus remains uncertain.

Progesterone

Progesterone has multiple actions on the uterus including stimulation of hypertrophy of smooth muscle cells, inhibition of gap junction formation, inhibition of oxytocin receptor synthesis and other effects that promote uterine quiescence. In addition, progesterone inhibits the activity of PLA_2 and the synthesis of PGs. A fall in the concentration of progesterone, by reversing these inhibitory effects, leads to increased uterine action and labor in some species. The weakness of the 'progesterone withdrawal' hypothesis in human pregnancy is the absence of a prepartum fall in progesterone concentrations in plasma, myometrium or myometrial nuclear receptors. Some researchers have proposed that progesterone concentrations fall locally in target tissues despite maintained levels elsewhere. However, this is not supported by direct measurements of the concentrations of progesterone.

The progesterone receptor antagonist, mifepristone (RU486), causes abortion when administered before 8 weeks of pregnancy but thereafter requires additional treatment with $PGF_{2\alpha}$ to be reliably effective.

Estrogen

Estradiol-17β is a potent stimulus of myometrial hyperplasia, gap junction formation, oxytocin receptor synthesis, PLA_2 activity and PG synthesis. However, like progesterone, estrogen shows no prepartum trends in concentration. Furthermore, administration of large amounts of estrogen to women at term is ineffective in inducing labor. Local concentrations of estrogen could be raised by conversion of the high concentration of estrogen sulfates in amniotic fluid to unconjugated estrogen. However, steroid sulfatase present in fetal membranes is no more active in tissues obtained at delivery than in tissues obtained before labor.

Oxytocin

Oxytocin is the most powerful oxytocic agent known, yet its administration is ineffective in inducing labor, despite producing powerful contractions, unless the pregnancy is near term. The reason for this failure is that the various changes in the muscle and connective tissue induced by PGs are absent; the contractions are incompletely propagated and the cervix remains non-compliant. Recently, oxytocin has been found to stimulate decidual synthesis of $PGF_{2\alpha}$. The concentration of oxytocin in plasma remains low throughout pregnancy and rises only in the second stage of labor; the concentration of receptors increases with the onset of labor. Thus it is possible that oxytocin plays a part in initiating parturition by stimulating both contractions and decidual synthesis of $PGF_{2\alpha}$. The stimulus to oxytocin receptor synthesis is unknown, although estrogen stimulates receptors in experimental animals: the absence of an increase in estrogen concentrations before parturition in women excludes this as a cause. Uterine sensitivity to oxytocin increases during treatment with $PGF_{2\alpha}$ or PGE_2, suggesting an increase in oxytocin receptors but a postreceptor change cannot be excluded.

Secretory component (gravidin)

Amniotic fluid contains secretory component of IgA, a 78 kDa protein that binds tightly to IgA and facilitates passage of IgA through epithelial membranes. The protein is a potent inhibitor of PG synthesis by blocking the activity of PLA_2. Cultures of chorionic cells generate this secretory component in greater quantities when the cells are harvested before than when harvested during or after labor. These observations suggest that secretory component contributes to the maintenance of uterine quiesence to term and that a fall in the rate of synthesis may be one of the factors responsible for the liberation of $PGF_{2\alpha}$ associated with the onset of labour.

Platelet activating factor

Platelet activating factor (PAF) is a potent stimulus of smooth muscle contractility by raising the intracellular concentrations of Ca^{2+} as in its action on platelets. It is absent from amniotic fluid of women before labor starts but is usually present during labor. A PAF antagonist administered to rats prolongs labor but not the duration of pregnancy, suggesting that PAF is not an important component of the mechanism initiating labor. The production of PAF, a phospholipid-derived factor, may be a byproduct of PLA_2 activity during PG synthesis.

The role of PGs in preterm labor

Preterm labor is of two types involving primarily the connective tissue. In the first type, the connective tissue of the cervix undergoes the biochemical changes normally seen at term and dilates prematurely, painlessly and without uterine contractions; the membranes bulge through the cervix and rupture and the fetus is delivered after a brief second stage of labor. This so-called *incompetent cervix syndrome* presumably reflects the premature release of PGE_2 in cervical tissue but the stimulus is unknown. The second type of preterm labor results from premature activation of myometrial contractions; it mimics term labor and is probably dependent on release of $PGF_{2\alpha}$. In some instances, the cause is clearly related to an obstetric complication such as hemorrhage, uterine malformation, trauma or infection. In most instances, no cause is apparent and there is a tendency to recurrence in successive pregnancies. The extent to which infection contributes to preterm labor is controversial. Some investigators claim that subclinical *amnionitis* is the cause of most cases of idiopathic preterm labor. Others consider that the common occurrence of low-grade amnionitis in preterm labor is a result rather than a cause. However, there is agreement that a variety of organisms have the ability to stimulate PG synthesis. The endotoxin lipopolysaccharide, which is usually present in amniotic fluid in association with Gram-negative amnionitis, is a potent stimulus of PLA_2 activity and PG synthesis. Cytokines such as interleukin-1α, interleukin-1β and tumor necrosis factor that mediate the inflammatory response stimulate PG synthesis.

Controlled clinical trials of antibiotic in women at high risk of preterm labor have so far been unsuccessful in consistently reducing the incidence.

Selected reading

Bleasdale JE, Johnston JM. Prostaglandins and human parturition: regulation of arachidonic acid mobilization. *Perinat Med* 1985; **5**: 151.

Casey ML, MacDonald PC. The role of prostaglandins in labor. In McNellis D, Challis J, MacDonald P, Nathanielsz P, Roberts J, eds. *The onset of labor: cellular and integrative mechanisms*. Ithaca: Perinatology Press, 1988: 141.

Challis JRG, Lye SJ. Parturition. In Clarke JR, ed. *Oxford reviews of reproductive biology*. Vol. 8. Oxford: Clarendon Press, 1986: 61.

Liggins GC. The paracrine system controlling human parturition. In Jaffe RD, Dell'Acqua S, eds. *The endocrine physiology of parturition and the peripartal period*. New York: Raven Press, 1985: 205.

E. Puberty

E O Reiter and P M Martha Jr

Puberty is that period of transition between childhood and adulthood, during which individuals undergo a striking growth spurt, realize the appearance of secondary sexual characteristics, achieve fertility and experience substantive psychological changes. The endocrine events of pubertal maturation are but a part of a developmental continuum extending from initial sexual differentiation through senescence.

Reproductive endocrine system

(see p. 311)

Suprahypothalamic sites

Higher cortical centers and the limbic system influence synthesis and secretion of the decapeptide gonadotropin releasing hormone (GnRH) by the arcuate nucleus of the hypothalamus. In addition, it is quite clear that many neurotransmitters, as well as sex steroids and varied gonadal peptides, affect the production of GnRH.

Hypothalamus

The arcuate nucleus of the medial basal hypothalamus and its transducer neurosecretory neurons release GnRH in a periodic oscillatory fashion. This decapeptide is then transported from the median eminence to the anterior pituitary gland via the primary plexus of the hypothalamic pituitary portal circulation.

Anterior pituitary gland

Upon reaching the anterior pituitary gland, molecules of GnRH bind to surface receptors on specialized cells, called pituitary gonadotropes, which synthesize and store the glycoprotein hormones luteinizing hormone (LH) and follicle stimulating hormone (FSH). In response to this intermittent GnRH stimulation, LH and FSH are secreted in a pulsatile fashion, to enhance gonadal steroidogenesis and maturation of the germinal epithelium. The concept that the LH secretory bursts are temporally related to a central episodic process such as GnRH release is supported by the finding that volleys of electrical activity have been recorded from the medial basal hypothalamus coincident with LH pulses.

Gonads

In the female, ovaries are the site of sex steroid production in follicles and thecal tissue; ova are the germinal products. In the male, sex steroid production occurs in testicular Leydig cells, while spermatogenesis occurs in the germinal epithelium of the seminiferous tubules. Multiple peptides, including the insulin-like growth factors, the inhibin family, and diverse cytokines are also produced by the gonads.

Patterns of gonadotropin release

The availability of sensitive and specific immunoassays and bioassays for the gonadotropins has permitted their quantitation, both at the extremely low levels present through mid-childhood years and then at the rising levels which characterize pubertal change. Most likely due to the molecular heterogeneity of circulating LH and FSH, qualitative as well as quantitative changes in concentrations of circulating gonadotropins affect gonadal steroidogenesis and maturation of germinal tissues. The highly sensitive immunofluorometric assays (IFMA) appear to measure the circulating molecular forms responsible for the bioactive gonadotropin levels traditionally quantified by *in vitro* bioassays.

Changes in levels of gonadotropins

Production of gonadotropins by the human fetal pituitary is demonstrable by 10 weeks of gestation, with hormonal secretion occurring by 11–12 weeks. In pituitary glands and serum of fetuses, gonadotropin concentrations reach adult castrate levels by mid-gestation, with a decline thereafter to reach typical childhood values by term. Following the decrease in sex steroids during the first several days after birth, concentrations of FSH and LH increase again and exhibit wide fluctuations during the first months of life. These intermittent high gonadotropin concentrations are associated with pubertal levels of testosterone in male infants and, to a less striking extent, increased estradiol concentrations in females. By 6 months of age in the male and 1–2 years in the female, concentrations of LH and FSH decrease to low levels, which then persist throughout childhood until the onset of puberty (Fig. 4.13).

In the immediate peripubertal period basal gonadotropin concentrations again begin to increase. In girls, FSH levels rise during the early stages of puberty and then plateau, whereas LH levels tend to rise during later stages. In boys, FSH concentrations rise progressively throughout puberty, and LH levels increase sharply during early pubertal development and then gradually rise throughout the remainder of the pubertal years.

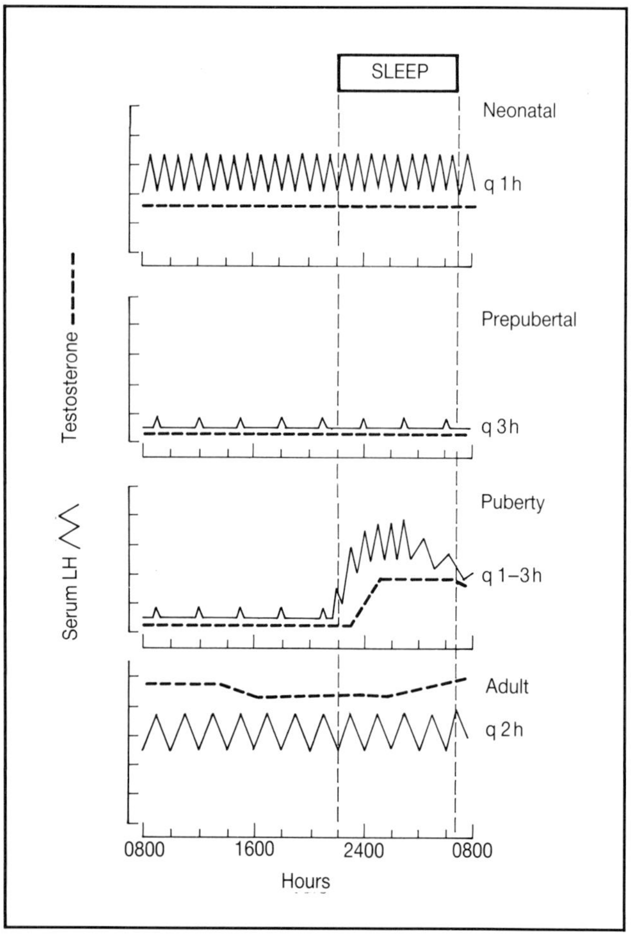

Fig. 4.13. LH and testosterone secretory patterns throughout sexual maturation in males.

In addition to these changes in immunoreactive gonadotropins, changes in the levels of biologically active LH (measured by sensitive, *in vitro* rodent interstitial cell testosterone generation assays) have been quantitated throughout fetal life and in all stages of extrauterine life. In human studies, bioactive LH concentrations are generally undetectable during prepubertal years, then rise dramatically during pubertal maturation. The increment in mean LH levels from prepuberty to puberty is substantially greater when determined by bioassay than with standard immunoassay techniques. The utilization of IFMA measurements of LH confirm the striking increase of LH from prepuberty to adulthood, ranging to as high as 100-fold. This strong correlation between LH levels determined by bioassay and IFMA, in contrast to immunoassay, techniques stresses the importance of using highly specific and sensitive measuring systems when assessing the very low gonadotropin levels of early prepubertal children.

Episodic circadian secretion

LH is secreted in a pulsatile (episodic) manner even in prepubertal children, but with a frequency and an amplitude lower than that in pubertal children or adults. The increment of mean LH levels during puberty corresponds to a rise in both the magnitude of LH pulses and the frequency of its secretory episodes. A generally similar pattern occurs in FSH pulsatile release. In addition to these episodic bursts of LH and FSH secretion, a circadian rhythm exists which is augmented in late childhood and adolescent years. In prepubertal children, a small but detectable nocturnal enhancement of LH release is present.

During puberty, sleep-enhanced LH secretion increases progressively until the late pubertal years when the pattern of LH secretion appears to stabilize throughout the 24-hour period and is comparable to that seen in the adult. It appears, thus, that the increased levels of LH during pubertal years are amplifications of pre-existing patterns of episodic and circadian gonadotropin release that have been demonstrable even during the period of mid-childhood gonadotropin secretory quiescence.

Regulation of gonadotropin secretion

The generous secretion of LH and FSH by the fetal and neonatal pituitary diminishes by the third year, after which the entire reproductive endocrine system becomes relatively quiescent until the onset of puberty. Two different processes (i.e. a 'dual mechanism of restraint') have been postulated to explain these developmental changes in gonadotropin secretion: one is a sex steroid-dependent mechanism, i.e. a highly sensitive hypothalamic–pituitary–gonadal negative feedback system; the other is an apparently sex steroid-independent mechanism by which the central nervous system modulates gonadotropin secretion, presumably by altering GnRH synthesis and release.

Sex steroid-dependent control

To explain the sex steroid-dependent negative feedback system, it has been postulated that the hypothalamic–pituitary–gonadotrope system is highly sensitive and rapidly responsive to suppressive effects of tiny quantities of circulating sex steroids during the middle childhood years. With the onset of puberty, the hypothalamic arcuate nucleus and the pituitary gonadotropes appear to become progressively less sensitive to inhibitory effects of sex steroids on GnRH release, resulting in increased pulsatile GnRH release (altered frequency and heightened amplitude) with consequent increased secretion of gonadotropins. The site of steroid action may involve both hypothalamic and pituitary cells with appropriate steroid receptor systems. The sensing mechanism for this set point regulation of negative feedback control has been referred to as the 'gonadostat'. Though the concept of the gonadostat has proved useful in explaining many aspects of the normal physiological changes in gonadotropin levels, it seems unlikely that a gonadostat change is the sole initiator of the fall of gonadotropin levels during the midpubertal quiescent period. Nonetheless, in adult females, acquisition of an appropriate set point for negative feedback may be a prerequisite for appropriate gonadotropin fluctuations during the early follicular phase of the menstrual cycle to allow appropriate ripening of a mature ovum.

Sex steroid-independent control

The diphasic pattern of gonadotropin secretion from infancy through adulthood (i.e. higher in the first 1–3 years of life than in the next 8–10 years with a subsequent secondary rise in adolescence into adulthood) is qualitatively similar in normal individuals and in patients with functional agonadism. The fall in gonadotropin synthesis and secretion in children with agonadism (best studied in children with gonadal dysgenesis) has suggested the presence of intrinsic inhibitory CNS influences, largely independent of gonadal sex steroid production, that may also act to diminish gonadotropin production and release during middle childhood years and thus restrain the onset of puberty. The mechanism of this central nervous system inhibitory action remains unknown; endogenous opiates and the pineal gland, though well studied, seem not to be involved.

Suprahypothalamic control

Recent studies in both primates and rodents demonstrate that GnRH or at least GnRH mRNA is present in abundant quantities in the hypothalami of immature monkeys and in rodents, suggesting adequate synthetic capacity for GnRH. Further, GnRH and consequent gonadotropin release are quickly evoked by administration of excitatory neuroamines, such as *N*-methyl-D-aspartate, to juvenile animals. Direct measurements of portal GnRH levels after electrical stimulation of the basal hypothalamus indicates that the capacity for GnRH release is similar to that for prepubertal and pubertal monkeys. Such data confirm an early potential for GnRH synthesis and secretion, supporting the notion that suprahypothalamic neuroregulatory factors may have major importance in the timing of puberty and in the regulation of function of the hypothalamic arcuate nucleus. A 'desynchronization' of neurosecretory activity within the family of GnRH neurons may be associated with uncoordinated continuous low-grade GnRH release that must be 're-synchronized' to escape the prepubertal quiescent period.

LH and FSH appear always to be secreted in a pulsatile

or episodic fashion with discrete bursts of hormone release from the gonadotropes, separated by intervals of quiescence. Modulation of frequency and amplitude of such secretory bursts occurs through an interaction of GnRH in its oscillatory rhythm, with sex steroids and gonadal inhibins/activins at the pituitary gonadotrope. This generates a pulsatile ultradian gonadotropin concentration profile in the peripheral circulation. The frequency of GnRH pulses and the intermittent nature of its activating signal upon the gonadotropes appear critical in maintaining the responsiveness of the gonadotropes and also normal LH and FSH secretion. In the absence of exposure to pulsatile GnRH, the gonadotrope is unresponsive. Paradoxically, continuous infusion of GnRH will also inhibit gonadotropin secretion through a process of 'desensitization', or 'down-regulation' of the GnRH receptors on the gonadotrope cell membranes.

Interaction of synthetic gonadotropin releasing hormone with pituitary gonadotropin secretion

Since the augmented secretion of LH and FSH at the onset of puberty apparently results from decreased neurohormonal restraints on synthesis and pulsatile secretion of GnRH, the disinhibition of the arcuate GnRH oscillator should lead to increased GnRH pulses (frequency and amplitude) initially, followed by increased gonadotropin secretion by the pituitary gonadotropes and, finally, enhanced sex steroidogenesis by the gonads. GnRH secretion cannot be readily measured in humans; nonetheless, endogenous GnRH release may be assessed indirectly and qualitatively by the gonadotropin response to exogenous synthetic GnRH. With the availability of this synthetic decapeptide, pituitary sensitivity to GnRH and the dynamic reserve or readily releasable pool of pituitary LH and FSH have been carefully examined throughout the life cycle, as well as in many disorders of the hypothalamic–pituitary–gonadal system.

Results of such studies support the concept that the prepubertal stage is characterized by functional GnRH insufficiency. It must be noted that such studies do not clarify the issue of the primary or secondary nature of this functional GnRH insufficiency, but merely reflect a state of low exposure of pituitary gonadotropes to endogenous GnRH. The release of LH following administration of GnRH is minimal in prepubertal children beyond infancy, increases strikingly at the peripubertal period and throughout puberty, and further in adult males and females. The change in the maturity-related patterns of FSH release after administration of GnRH is quite different from that of LH and results in a striking reversal of the FSH:LH ratio of gonadotropin release. It appears that differing pulse frequency of endogenous GnRH accounts for the discordance of FSH and LH that evolves during sexual maturation. Prepubertal and pubertal females release much more FSH than males at all stages of sexual maturation. Prepubertal girls, indeed, appear to have a larger releasable pool of pituitary FSH than either pubertal girls or prepubertal or pubertal males. Circulating levels of serum FSH and LH (a summation of basal secretion) are similar in prepubertal children, a dramatic qualitative contrast to the amount of gonadotropin release evoked by GnRH administration (the immediately available stores). The heightened LH release by pituitary gonadotropes in response to exogenous GnRH in peripubertal children, who do not yet exhibit physical signs of sexual maturation, provides evidence of slowly increasing levels of endogenous GnRH which augment pituitary responsiveness to exogenous GnRH. It should be noted that an enhanced nocturnal release of LH also is seen in this peripubertal period. The degree of previous exposure of gonadotropes to endogenous GnRH appears to affect both the magnitude and quality of LH responses to a single dose of GnRH.

Before puberty, the low set point of the hypothalamic–gonadostat to inhibitory feedback effects of low concentrations of plasma sex steroids and intrinsic CNS factors suppress secretion of GnRH. As a result, the prepubertal pituitary gonadotropes have small pools of releasable LH and, thus, diminished responsivity to an exogenous bolus of synthetic GnRH. With the onset of puberty, increased release of endogenous GnRH increases the number of LH receptors on the gonadotrope, enhances pituitary sensitivity to exogenous GnRH, and enlarges the reserve of LH within the gonadotrope. The above-noted phenomenon of gonadotrope desensitization by chronic GnRH exposure was discovered during a series of experiments in which exogenous GnRH was administered both by intermittent and also by continuous intravenous infusion. When GnRH was given intermittently, gonadotropin secretion was fully re-established in animals with lesions of the medial basal hypothalamus in which the arcuate nucleus (and its GnRH neurons) had been obliterated. It was also observed that GnRH, administered to prepubertal monkeys in a pulsatile manner, led to the establishment of spontaneous menstrual cycles. When GnRH was administered by a continuous infusion, pituitary gonadotropin secretion was almost eliminated and required pulsatile GnRH dosing to re-establish normal patterns of LH and FSH release.

Such data dramatically emphasized the importance of the pattern of GnRH administration (or endogenous production) and showed that puberty could be induced in prepubertal monkeys through discontinuous administration of GnRH pulses and eliminated by continuous infusion. These studies in monkeys led to extensive investigation of the efficacy of exogenous GnRH administration to patients with varying degrees of hypogonadotropic hypogonadism. In such clinical trials, the administration of GnRH in a pulsatile manner results in the appearance of a pubertal pattern of gonadotropin secretion and a maturation of pituitary-gonadal function.

Positive feedback and ovulation

In normal adult women, the midcycle gonadotropin secretory surge is attributed to a **positive feedback** effect of an increased, critical concentration of estradiol for a sufficient length of time during the latter part of the follicular phase. This stimulatory effect of estradiol is a late maturational event, not occurring before midpuberty, and absent in prepubertal and early pubertal girls. The development of positive feedback of estradiol requires: (1) ovarian follicles primed by FSH to secrete adequate estradiol and maintain critical levels in the circulation; (2) pituitary gonadotropes sensitized by estradiol to amplify and augment the GnRH effect and containing enough readily releasable LH to provide an LH surge; (3) adequate GnRH stores for the hypothalamic GnRH neurosecretory neurons to increase GnRH acutely in response to estradiol stimulation; and (4) a sufficiently insensitive negative feedback system to allow estradiol levels to rise sufficiently to elicit an LH surge without blunting GnRH and gonadotropin release. Estrogen-induced positive feedback occurs directly upon pituitary gonadotropes which are simultaneously exposed to GnRH. It does not appear that frequency or amplitude modulation of the GnRH pulse is a prerequisite of the midcycle LH surge; nonetheless, changes in GnRH release at this period probably also occur.

Estrogen presumably exerts a positive feedback effect at both the pituitary gonadotropes and the hypothalamic GnRH neurons.

Control of the time of onset of puberty

The complexity of the specific mechanisms involved in the timing of pubertal onset have defied elucidation. The average age at menarche has followed a secular trend toward earlier occurrence over the past century. This decrease in the age of puberty has been explained by improvements in socioeconomic conditions, nutrition, and general health. That trend appears to have slowed or ceased during the past several decades in developed nations. Nonetheless, influences other than socioeconomic ones affect the age of puberty. An important role for nutritional factors and body composition upon the time of pubertal onset has been suggested by the earlier age of menarche in moderately obese girls, by delayed sexual maturation in the presence of malnourishment and chronic illness, and by the relationship of amenorrhea to states of diminished body fat such as anorexia nervosa and voluntary weight loss. Conditions of excessive energy expenditure, such as vigorous physical conditioning, may independently affect the onset and progression of the pubertal process. Metabolic signals potentially may affect pubertal maturation.

Differences in utilization of energy stores by younger than older primates, perhaps relating to rates of energy consumption or availability of energy substrate, have suggested some association between metabolic alterations during growth and the timing of pubertal onset. The pineal gland-melatonin system and the opioidergic network do not appear important in the pubertal process, but the activity of the noradrenergic system parallels GnRH release. Excitatory neuroamines, additionally, may fully activate the hypothalamic–pituitary–gonadal axis in primates, demonstrating their role as potential suprahypothalamic regulators of GnRH release. The temporal regulation of these processes remains undefined.

Abnormalities of pubertal maturation

Delayed sexual maturation

The first sign of pubertal development in boys is testicular enlargement, largely based upon increased volume of the seminiferous tubules; this should occur by age 14. Breast budding is the initial physical manifestation of puberty in girls and should occur by 13 years of age. A higher incidence of *delayed sexual maturation* appears to be present in boys than in girls. The causes of delayed pubertal maturation are shown in Table 4.3 and demonstrate that there may be disorders of general health, of the central nervous system, as well as of gonadal function. The most common cause, however, is the syndrome of so-called *'constitutional delay of adolescence'* (or the 'syndrome of slow growth and delayed maturation'). This syndrome is characterized by: (1) familial late maturation; (2) delayed skeletal maturation; (3) an attenuated progression through the pubertal process; (4) an ultimate height that is generally within normal range for family. Differentiation between constitutionally delayed pubertal maturation and the syndrome of *hypogonadotropic hypogonadism,* especially in early adolescence, is quite difficult. The diagnosis will surely become apparent by late adolescent years, but simply waiting until then is not generally an acceptable clinical option. Administration of exogenous GnRH has been used in an attempt to separate these two syndromes, but remarkable degrees of overlap occur in the readily releasable pools of LH and FSH, so that a definitive diagnosis is not possible based on the GnRH test results.

When considered in the light of the dual mechanism of restraint of puberty during normal mid-childhood, the syndrome of delayed adolescence is characterized by a more prolonged and intense degree of inhibition of hypothalamic GnRH synthesis and secretion. This results in a more profound and exaggerated period of GnRH insufficiency. In true hypogonadotropic hypogonadism, either the central nervous inhibition does not disappear or there is an intrinsic abnormality of the synthesis in secretion of GnRH.

Isosexual precocious puberty

A child is considered to have *precocious puberty* in North America when there is an appearance of testicular enlargement or pubic hair growth in the male prior to age 9 or breast budding or pubic hair growth in the female prior to age 8. This is based upon ages of mean pubertal onset 2.5 SD below the mean. Those children in whom evidence of sexual development occurs between ages 6 and 8 may have a syndrome variant that should be referred to as 'constitutional precocious puberty'; this is simply an earlier onset of puberty without the accelerated pubertal maturation seen in those children with an even earlier onset of precocity. The differential diagnosis of true isosexual precocious puberty is shown in Table 4.4. 'Complete' or 'true' precocious puberty is dependent upon early initiation of gonadotropin secretion consequent to premature attainment of a pubertal pattern of GnRH production by the arcuate nucleus of the hypothalamus. In this condition, the above noted dual mechanism of restraint of puberty becomes attenuated at an early age so that the inhibitory controls of hypothalamic arcuate nucleus pulsatile GnRH secretion are diminished and gonadotropin secretion increases. Activation of the

Table 4.3. Causes of delayed pubertal maturation

Generalized disease	Central nervous system	Gonadal
Malnutrition	Constitutional delay	Gonadal dysgenesis
Gastrointestinal	Congenital anomalies, e.g. craniopharyngioma	Noonan syndrome
Endocrine	Neoplasms	Orchitis
Renal	Post-inflammation states	Testicular regression syndrome
Cardiorespiratory	Trauma	Trauma
Hematology/Oncology	Hypogonadotropic states (Kallmann, Prader–Willi)	Neoplasms
Collagen–vascular		Errors of testosterone biosynthesis

Table 4.4. Causes of isosexual precocious puberty

Gonadotropin (and GnRH)-dependent	
	Idiopathic
	Structural CNS abnormalities
	Neoplasms
	Congenital anomalies (e.g. septo-optic dysplasia, midline defects)
	Post-infection, trauma, irradiation
Gonadotropin (and GnRH)-independent	
	hCG-producing neoplasm
	Sex steroid-producing neoplasms of the gonads or adrenal
	Extragonadal androgen (males)—congenital adrenal hyperplasia
	Abnormalities of 'intragonadal regulators', e.g. McCune–Albright syndrome, ovarian cysts, Leydig cell hyperfunction (testotoxicosis)
Normal variants of development	
	Precocious thelarche
	Precocious adrenarche

hypothalamic–pituitary–gonadal axis is similar, then, to that seen in normal children but occurs at an earlier age. There are pubertal levels of sex steroid production, gonadotropin concentrations in the pubertal range with the expected frequency of episodic secretion and circadian variability, and a mature level of GnRH-induced LH release. The fact that continuous administration of GnRH leads to diminished release of pituitary gonadotropins through a process of down-regulation of pituitary GnRH receptors has led to a major therapeutic advance in this area. Potent long-acting GnRH agonists, behaving like a continuous infusion, are now the standard of care for children with gonadotropin-dependent sexual precocity. The hypothalamic–pituitary–gonadal axis is suppressed with concomitant slowing of sexual maturation and growth and an increase in final adult height outcome.

Variants of pubertal maturation

Precocious thelarche

Premature breast development without any other evidence of progressive sexual maturation is referred to as premature thelarche. This syndrome does not appear to be dependent upon prolonged activation of the hypothalamic–pituitary unit, but rather is due either to transient secretory burst of GnRH and the gonadotropins or to a period of primary ovarian dysregulation of estrogen synthesis and secretion. The differential diagnosis of premature thelarche includes true sexual precocity and ovarian cysts or tumors. There do not appear to be any long-term developmental consequences of this variant of normal development.

Precocious adrenarche (pubarche)

The appearance of sex hair prior to age 8 in girls or 9 in boys without any other evidence of progression of sexual development defines the syndrome of precocious adrenarche (pubarche). It is more common in girls, especially those who are taller, heavier and having slightly advanced skeletal maturation. The regulation of adrenal androgenesis remains poorly understood. There is a significant increase in adrenal androgen secretion by age 8 in both boys and girls, antedating the pubertal increases of gonadotropin and gonadal steroid production. The increasing levels of adrenal androgens correlate with development of the zona reticularis of the adrenal cortex. In general, maturation of this process of adrenal androgenesis and of the hypothalamic–pituitary–gonadal axis appear independent. The enhanced adrenal androgenesis seems to be, in part, an ACTH-dependent process, though other portions of the pro-opiomelanocortin (POMC) molecule have been implicated in the activation; changes of intra-adrenal enzyme action favoring synthesis and secretion of androgens have also been demonstrated. The differential diagnosis of precocious pubarche includes unusual cases of late-onset *congenital adrenal hyperplasia* and adrenal or gonadal *androgen-producing neoplasms*. Most commonly, however, this syndrome of early adrenal androgenesis is a variant of the normal. Onset of other pubertal events, the age of menarche and final adult height appear to be normal. The long-term risk of development of polycystic ovarian disease in association with this syndrome remains to be characterized.

Selected reading

Drop SLS, deMuinck Keizer-Schrama S. Pubertal development and gonadal function. *Curr Opin Pediatr* 1991; **3**: 701.

Grumbach MM, Styne DM. Puberty: ontogeny, neuroendocrinology, physiology, and disorders. In

Wilson JD, Foster DW, eds. *Williams textbook of endocrinology*. 8th Ed. Philadelphia: WB Saunders Co, 1992: 1139.

Marshall JC, Kelch RP. Gonadotropin releasing hormone: role of pulsatile secretion in the regulation of reproduction. *N Engl J Med* 1986; **315**: 1459.

Plant TM. Puberty in primates. In Knobil E, Neill JD, eds. *The physiology of reproduction*. New York: Raven Press, 1988: 1763.

Reiter EO, Grumbach MM. Neuroendocrine control mechanism and the onset of puberty. *Annu Rev Physiol* 1982; **44**: 595.

Rosenfield RL. The diagnosis and management of delayed puberty. *J Clin Endocrinol Metab* 1990; **70**: 559.

5 ◆ *Growth*

Editor: Peter D Gluckman

A. Cell and Tissue Growth

D J Hill and V K M Han

The regulation of cell growth and differentiation

Growth of the embryo, fetus and child is a multifaceted process involving not only cell replication, hypertrophy and differentiation, but also the ordered migration of cells to defined anatomical sites, their condensation into organs, profound morphological events such as the formation of three germ layers, and programmed cell death. The integrated process of growth and development requires precise intercellular communication. The communication routes used are often not centrally controlled by the nervous system or circulating endocrine hormones, but depend on local cell–cell interactions via peptide growth factors and membrane-associated recognition molecules. Knowledge of how growth factors interrelate with each other and in the context of extracellular matrix and intercellular recognition molecules is central to understanding tissue development.

Growth factors and oncogenes

Peptide growth factors are peptide or glycoprotein hormones which are widely expressed in body tissues, and regulate aspects of tissue hyperplasia, differentiation, morphogenesis and cell migration. As a class of messengers, they typically act close to their sites of synthesis as paracrine or autocrine hormones, rather than as endocrine hormones transmitted via the circulation. This distinction is not mutually exclusive. For instance, the insulin-like growth factors (IGFs), also known as somatomedins, are widely expressed during development, yet are also present in blood. In addition to IGFs, the other major types of growth factors that are involved in cellular growth and differentiation are epidermal growth factor (EGF), and its analog transforming growth factor α (TGFα), platelet derived growth factor (PDGF), fibroblast growth factors (FGFs), transforming growth factor β (TGFβ) and nerve growth factor (NGF). Several of these terms are generic and cover a family of related molecules.

Growth factor structure

There are two types of IGF, IGF-I and IGF-II, and two classes of receptor, type I and type II. The IGFs are mitogenic for isolated cell types derived from all three primitive germ layers. IGF-I typically has an ED_{50} of 1–3 nM while IGF-II is an order of magnitude less active. IGFs are almost never found in free form but are complexed in tissues and biological fluids to a family of specific binding proteins (BPs). At least six IGFBPs exist, designated IGFBP-1 to 6. In addition to extending the biological half-life of IGFs, IGFBPs are capable of modulating IGF bioactivity in either an augmentative or an antagonistic manner. For further discussion of the IGF system see p. 180.

EGF is a single-chain polypeptide with molecular weight 6 kDa. Mouse EGF was first isolated from the submaxillary glands of male mice and the equivalent human peptide from urine. A structural analog of EGF is TGFα which shows a 30–40 percent amino acid homology. TGFα is more abundantly expressed than EGF prior to birth. Both peptides share a high affinity cell receptor. Platelet derived growth factor (PDGF) was first identified in the α storage granules of platelets. It exists as either homodimers or heterodimers of two separate peptide units, A and B, which are products of separate human chromosomes. In platelets, PDGF is always found as A-B heterodimers. The PDGF B chain is analogous to the product of the v-*sis* oncogene. The high affinity PDGF receptor also has two subunit components, α and β, and can exist in homo- or heterodimer forms. Both EGF and PDGF act as mitogens for isolated mesenchymal cells with ED_{50} values of 0.5–2.0 nM. EGF additionally has proliferative effects on epithelia.

The FGF family contains at least eight members, the best characterized of which are basic and acidic FGF. Various molecular sizes of FGF exist between 18 kDa and 26 kDa. Both acidic and basic FGF bind avidly to acidic sulfated glycosaminoglycans such as heparan sulfate and syndecans. Neither FGF has a signal peptide and they cannot be exteriorized by cells via the endoplasmic reticulum. However, abundant basic FGF is found in association with cell membranes and extracellular matrix, suggesting that it may be released complexed to glycosaminoglycans. Although basic FGF is an extremely potent mitogen for isolated connective tissue cell types with an ED_{50} of 10–100 pM, its most dramatic effects are as an angiogenic agent. Proliferating endothelial cells express abundant basic FGF mRNA.

Transforming growth factor β also exists as multiple isomers of which $TGF\beta_1$, β_2 and β_3 are expressed in mammalian development. TGFβ is a homodimer of 25 kDa originally identified in platelets and as a tumor cell product. It is a potent inhibitor of epithelial cell proliferation and a bifunctional regulator of mesenchymal cell growth. Its growth inhibitory effects have been linked to an altered phosphorylation state of the retinoblastoma gene product, while its limited ability to promote cell growth may be mediated by an up-regulation of PDGF B-chain expression. TGFβ binds avidly to extracellular matrix molecules such as decorin and is stored in large amounts in bone matrix. When released by cells it exists as a precursor form which is biologically inactive. The active TGFβ molecule can be released from the 'latent' form experimentally by heat or acidic pH, while this may result from proteolytic activation by target tissues *in vivo*. An ability of TGFβ to greatly increase fibronectin and type I collagen production by fibroblasts underlies its ability to induce a fibrotic response and hasten wound healing *in vivo*.

Nerve growth factor (NGF) is a basic peptide of 13 kDa and shares 25 percent homology with the A and B chains of insulin. The storage form of NGF comprises three subunits, α, β and λ, existing in a dimeric structure (so-called 7SNGF). The β-subunit is the biologically active component (NGF). At least two other neurotropins with structural analogy to NGF are present in the mammalian brain; brain derived neurotropic factor (BDNF) and neurotropin 3 (NT-3). NGF interacts with two types of receptors in neural tissues: the high affinity, low capacity receptor and the low affinity, high capacity receptor. The high affinity receptor is a heterodimer comprising the trk peptide and the low affinity NGF receptor. BDNF and NT-3 interact with related receptors involving trk-B and trk-C peptides in heterodimers with the low affinity NGF receptor. Each of the neurotropins has a different ontogeny and spatial distribution in the brain and different tropic activities on various neuronal phenotypes. The predominant effect of NGF is to promote the survival, differentiation and axonal outgrowth of sensory and sympathetic ganglia. It also has a weak mitogenic action for lymphoid tissues, which have the low affinity, high capacity receptors. NGF is selectively produced by peripheral tissues to which the neurites of the developing sensory and sympathetic neurons are attracted by chemotaxis. NGF is then transported retrogradely to the neuronal cell bodies, where it provides the crucial function of survival. For further discussion of NGF see p. 215.

Expression and distribution of growth factors in early development

Messenger RNA encoding basic FGF is present at low levels in the oocyte but is absent following fertilization, to reappear as a product of the embryonic genome at the time of neurulation. Messenger RNAs for two other members of the FGF family, kFGF and *int*-2, are present in as early as the four-cell stage in mouse embryo and predominate prior to organogenesis. TGFβ mRNA and peptide is found in the four-cell mouse embryo and blastula respectively, as is mRNA for the related peptide, activin.

During later embryonic development, basic FGF mRNA steadily increases in abundance until day 16 of gestation in mouse. Expression is greatest in the tail, face and developing limbs. Conversely, the FGF-related oncogene *int*-2 is expressed in parietal endoderm, primitive mesoderm, the pharyngeal pouches and neuroepithelium of the hindbrain between 7.5 and 9.5 days of gestation. Different members of the FGF family appear to have distinct anatomical and ontological patterns of expression, which together cover almost every embryonic and fetal tissue. Similarly, $TGF\beta_1$, β_2 and β_3 have distinct patterns of expression in the rat fetus but are collectively expressed in every tissue. TGFβ mRNA is predominantly found in epithelial cells, but the peptides are predominantly found on mesenchyme following immunocytochemistry. This is likely to reflect the ability of TGFβ to bind to matrix elements in mesenchyme such as decorin.

From studies with isolated embryonal carcinoma cells, it would appear that IGFs appear later in development than FGF or TGFβ. Undifferentiated cell lines do not express IGFs, but will produce IGF-II consequent to differentiation into either mesoderm or endoderm following exposure to retinoic acid. Similarly, IGF-II mRNA could not be detected in human embryos fertilized and cultured *in vitro* to the formation of blastocysts, but was detected in differentiated trophoblast from abortus tissue as early as 35 days post-conception. IGF-I mRNA does not appear in the rat embryo until around day 11 of gestation. In the late embryonic and fetal rat, abundant IGF-II mRNA was localized by *in situ* hybridization to the yolk sac, liver, skeletal muscle, precartilaginous mesenchymal condensations, chondrocytes, periosteum and centres of intramembraneous ossification. The importance of IGF-II to fetal growth was demonstrated by studies in which one allele of the IGFBP gene was disrupted in the mouse embryo by homologous recombination. Animals which failed to express one IGF-II gene were smaller than wild type mice at birth, but postnatally grew at the same rate. Postnatally, IGF-II mRNA levels decline to negligible levels by weaning in most tissues except for brain, which continues to express IGF-II mRNA in the choroid plexus and leptomeninges. Conversely, IGF-I mRNA levels increase during neonatal life and achieve adult levels in rat liver, and other tissues, by 50 days of life. One rat tissue which expresses abundant IGF-I mRNA postnatally is the epiphyseal cartilage of the growth plates within long bones. It therefore seems likely that the ability of IGF-I to potentiate longitudinal skeletal growth depends at least partly on a local synthesis within the growth plate.

In the human fetus of late first or early second trimester, IGF-II mRNA is present in every body tissue, but is most abundant in stromal tissues around and within organs. Conversely, immunocytochemistry has shown that IGF peptides are concentrated on epithelia in the gut, kidney and lung and in differentiated muscle. Since several IGFBPs show a similar immunocytochemical distribution it seems likely that the IGFBPs may direct the cellular distribution of IGFs.

Both IGF-I and II are detectable in human fetal plasma from at least 15 weeks of gestation. From 32 weeks until term, concentrations of both peptides increase twofold, but still remain lower than in the adult. Conversely, in the rat fetus, circulating IGF-II levels are 20- to 100-fold greater than in maternal serum. Despite an abundance of IGF-II in blood, correlations between circulating levels and weight or length of the fetus or newborn are poor. A positive correlation exists between these parameters and circulating IGF-I in the fetus. Cord blood levels of IGF-I are depressed in infants who are small for gestational age. For further discussion see p. 165.

Control of growth factor expression and release

Most information on the control of growth factor release has been obtained with IGFs and is reviewed on p. 180. Before birth, the presence of IGF-I does not primarily depend on the availability of pituitary growth hormone (GH). Although fetal tissues show little specific binding of radiolabeled GH, recent *in vitro* studies have detected both mRNA and immunoreactive peptide for the GH receptor in several tissues. This suggests that the GH receptor may be expressed *in utero* but may be functionally immature. Another potential anabolic hormone in the human fetal circulation is human placental lactogen (hPL). While hPL was shown to stimulate amino acid transport, glycogen synthesis and IGF-I release by fetal liver *in vitro*, there is no direct evidence that hPL modulates IGF expression *in vivo*.

The importance of insulin to prenatal growth is acutely obvious. Insulin availability is closely associated with circulating levels of IGFs in the fetus, especially IGF-I (see p. 164).

Two variables dominate IGF-I gene transcription in the growing child; pituitary sufficiency and nutritional adequacy (see p. 181). Other hormones also influence IGF-I expression in a tissue-specific manner. Estradiol increases IGF-I mRNA expression in uterus and ovary while parathyroid hormone has a similar effect on isolated osteoblasts. Prior to puberty there is a positive correlation between serum IGF-I levels and growth velocity, and abnormally low IGF-I may be indicative of an endocrine-based growth disorder.

Biological actions of growth factors during development

An early embryonic expression of several peptide growth factors is logical with regard to the known synergistic interactions of growth factors during the cycle of cell replication. Studies with mouse Balb/c-3T3 fibroblasts showed that PDGF and basic FGF predominantly acted at the G_o/G_1 boundary and rendered cells 'competent' to enter the cell cycle. In the same model, EGF acted in early G_1, and IGFs in late G_1, to allow the cells to progress to S phase and initiate DNA synthesis; they have therefore been termed 'progression factors'. Thus the controlled expression of a variety of growth factors may provide a fine control of cell proliferation rate in discrete tissues. During tissue remodeling, the release of proteolytic enzymes such as plasminogen activator will lead to local extracellular matrix degradation, which will in turn liberate additional stored growth factors such as TGFβ. This may serve to limit the proliferative events.

Such interactions between growth factors are well demonstrated in *in vitro* models of cell differentiation. The differentiation of the L6 rat myoblast cell line into postmitotic myotubes is prevented by basic FGF and EGF, but potentiated by IGF-I or II. $TGF\beta_1$ has little effect on myoblast proliferation rate but has an inhibitory effect on cell differentiation. Thus, altered local expression of particular growth factors can trigger specific events of cellular differentiation.

Both basic FGF and $TGF\beta_2$ are able to mimic the actions of an endogenous morphogen and induce the development of mesoderm from primitive animal pole ectoderm removed from the *Xenopus* embryo. Messenger RNA encoding basic FGF is present in the *Xenopus* embryo at this time, and mesoderm-inducing activity can be partly neutralized with anti-basic FGF antiserum. Proof that the endogenous members of the FGF family were responsible for mesoderm formation was provided by expression of a dominant negative mutant of the FGF receptor in *Xenopus* embryo. Serious defects in gastrulation and in ventral mesoderm formation resulted, with no development of the somites of the tail. The β form of activin mRNA appears in *Xenopus* embryo coincident with mesoderm formation, and activin may be responsible for the development of dorsal mesoderm. A *Xenopus* ectodermal cell line releases a mesoderm-inducing activity which can be mimicked with activin or $TGF\beta_2$, and blocked by antiserum against $TGF\beta_2$. Thus, basic FGF and activin may jointly regulate the formation of the trilaminar embryo.

Transforming growth factor α and FGF are angiogenic and may contribute to the high density of uterine capillary formation around the site of embryonic uterine implantation. TGFα is expressed by the embryo in negligible amounts at this time compared to a massive expression in the maternal decidua adjacent to the embryo. TGFα mRNA levels were greatest at the time of implantation of the rodent embryo and subsequently showed a slow decline in parallel with decidual resorption. A surge of estrogen at the time of implantation may greatly increase the uterine expression of EGF/TGFα receptors. *In situ* hybridization of mRNA for PDGF B chain showed localization in trophoblasts as early as 21 days postconception in man, suggesting that PDGF may contribute to the invasive growth of placental implantation.

$TGF\beta_1$ and β_2 are analogous to bone-derived factors previously known as cartilage-inducing factors A and B with the ability to induce chondrocyte formation from embryonic mesenchymal explants. Exposure of undifferentiated mesenchyme from primitive limb buds to $TGF\beta_1$ or β_2 induced the appearance of chondrocytes. It is likely that TGFβ is responsible for specific events of differentiation in developing connective tissues, since $TGF\beta_1$–β_3 mRNAs have been localized to chondrogenic areas in both the rat and human embryo.

Oncogenes

Oncogenes are normal components of the genome, which through an inappropriate degree of expression, translocation, or point mutation, are no longer under precise developmental control. This can lead to the expression of structurally or quantitatively aberrant oncogene-encoded proteins which can either be markers of neoplasia, or may contribute to the growth and metastasis of tumors. A pivotal finding was that viral oncogenes introduced into cells by retroviruses were homologous to normal cellular genes involved in the control of growth and differentiation. The virally inserted RNA is converted to DNA by host cells which express the aberrant oncogenic protein. The first published example of this was the finding that the v-*sis* oncogene encoded a peptide related to the B-chain form of PDGF. Other oncogenes encode proteins which represent normal or altered growth factor receptors (v-*erb* is related to the EGF receptor, c-*met* is the hepatocyte growth factor receptor); intracellular second messenger components (c-*src* and c-*ros* encode tyrosine-specific protein kinases, c-*ras* encodes a GTP binding protein); or DNA-binding proteins (c-*fos* and c-*myc*). The normal cellular equivalents of these oncogenes are expressed as part of the controlled pattern of embryogenesis and fetal development, often under the control of peptide growth factors. During the replicative cycle of fibroblasts, basic FGF will induce a transient elevation of c-*myc* and c-*fos* expression at the beginning of G_1. Later in G_1 a transient elevation of c-*ras* will occur in response to EGF. Within whole tissues a high expression of c-*myc* was found in the trophoblast during uterine invasion which declined as placental invasive growth ceased. The *src* gene appears to be preferentially active in embryonic neural tissues such as eye and brain of the embryo, while c-*ras* is expressed at high levels, compared with adult, in the human fetal brain and lung.

Matrix development and cell–cell interaction

Extracellular matrix consists of two major classes of molecules: proteins such as collagens, fibronectin and laminin; and mucopolysaccharides such as hyaluronic acid, heparan sulfate, and chondroitin and keratin sulfate. Most epithelia are tightly attached to a basal lamina, or basement membrane, which is rich in type IV collagen and forms a connection with the fibrillar forms of collagen within the connective tissue stroma. The formation of the basal membrane and type IV collagen is stimulated by TGFβ, which is expressed by many developing epithelia. Basement membranes are also rich in laminin, a structure of three polypeptides with total molecular weight 820 kDa which forms a connecting bridge between matrix components and the cell membranes. Laminin has high affinity binding sites for type IV collagen, heparan sulfate, and the integrin class of receptors on cells. Extracellular matrix pathways rich in laminin are thought necessary for the migration of dendritic and axonal projections of neurites during the development of the central nervous system.

In the extracellular matrix of connective tissues, the role of laminin is served by fibronectin. Fibronectins also form a bridge between cells such as fibroblasts and other matrix components such as type I collagen. Cellular attachment is via a family of integrin receptors with an Arg-Gly-Asp amino acid recognition sequence in the binding domain. Integrins are linked to actin within the intracellular cytoskeleton by the connecting peptides vinculin and talin. By their attachments fibronectin molecules are able to regulate cell shape during development, which is important during cell migration and differentiation. An example of this is the migration of neural crest cells during embryogenesis. Cells leave the area of the neural tube to become the peripheral nervous system, the adrenal medulla, and the melanocytes of skin. Migration routes are defined by tracts of fibronectin-rich mesenchymal matrix. These tracts are also rich in hyaluronic acid, an hydrophilic molecule which creates a loose gel through which migrating cells can pass easily. Hyaluronic acid is bound to the membrane of migrating cells, and appears to inhibit intercellular adhesion. When undifferentiated muscle cell precursors migrate into the embryonic limb buds from the somites they have pericellular hyaluronic acid coats. This phenotype is maintained by the presence of FGF molecules derived from the surrounding mesenchyme. When migration ceases, a reduction in hyaluronic acid presence allows muscle cell adhesion, and fusion following terminal differentiation. An important feature of tissue remodeling and cell migration is the ability of the tissue to produce neutral proteases such as plasminogen activator. The subsequent activation of plasminogen to plasmin results in the destruction of extracellular matrix at the site of remodeling. The ability of cells to release plasminogen activator is potentiated by basic FGF, and inhibited by TGFβ.

During organogenesis it is important for cell condensation that specific cell–cell adhesion be encouraged. This can be achieved by cell membrane-bound recognition molecules of which there are two types. Cadherins are calcium-dependent adhesion molecules divided into E-, P- and N-cadherin subgroups. Each is a glycoprotein of 720–750 amino acids. E-cadherin is responsible for the close association of epithelial cells within epithelial layers as in the kidney tubule, gastrointestinal tract, or parenchyma of liver. P-cadherin is found on the trophoblast cells of placenta and heart, while N-cadherin is rich in the central nervous system and embryonic mesoderm. The calcium-independent class of intercellular recognition molecules is called 'cell adhesion molecules' (CAMs). N-CAMs are a family of sialic acid-rich proteins, particularly abundant in the developing central nervous system, which promote neuron–neuron adhesion. N-CAMs are also expressed by differentiating muscle and glial cells.

Programmed cell death

In addition to cellular proliferation, differentiation and migration, selective death of a population of cells plays a crucial role in the final morphology of the tissues and structures of the developing embryo. This process, called the programmed cell death, or apoptosis, is important in the development of the brain, limbs and palate. In the limbs, areas of cell death known as the necrotic zones are essential for the separation of the digits and development of their shape. Programmed cell death also plays an important role in the development of the central nervous system, e.g. cell death is necessary for the separation of the developing neural tube from the contiguous epidermis.

Factors that regulate programmed cell death are not well understood, although it appears that this process may be programmed into the genome of the cells that are destined for death. Some of the genes responsible for this process have been cloned in invertebrates. Soluble factors produced by interacting cells may also regulate cell death. In the nervous system, cell death occurs in neurons that fail to make contact with appropriate targets. This results from the lack of uptake of neurotropic factors, such as NGF, BDNF or NT-3 produced by the targets, which may be another neuronal body, gland or muscle.

The regulation of organ growth

The growth and functional maturation of several organs has been linked to the local expression of peptide growth factors and their interactions with endocrine hormones. Three examples will be given: the adrenal gland, placenta and brain. The adrenal gland is an extremely active steroidogenic organ *in utero* producing cortisol and $\triangle^5$ steroids such as dehydroepiandrosterone (DHA) and its sulfated derivative, DHAS. The latter are further metabolized by placenta to estrogens. The human fetal adrenal expresses large amounts of mRNA for IGF-II in early second trimester, and this was increased *in vitro* by exposure of adrenal tissue to adrenocorticotropic hormone (ACTH) or dibutyryl cAMP, the second messenger activated by ACTH. Human fetal adrenal also contains mRNA for basic FGF, which is also up-regulated by ACTH. Proliferation of fetal adrenal cells is enhanced by IGFs, suggesting that they may partly mediate the tropic actions of ACTH on fetal adrenal hyperplasia, which is largely limited to the cortex. Extrapolation from studies with postnatal adrenal tissue suggests that growth factors may also contribute to adrenal function. When bovine fasciculata cells were maintained *in vitro* in the presence of IGF-I, receptors for angiotensin II were increased and ACTH-induced corticosterone and pregnenolone output elevated three- to sixfold. IGF-I most likely increased the availability of cholesterol and/or its transport to the mitochondria.

The finding of abundant IGF-II mRNA expression in the human cytotrophoblast and a high density of both type I and II IGF receptors on placental tissues suggests a role for IGFs in placental growth and perhaps function. IGFs promote the replication of isolated placental fibroblasts. Both IGF-I and insulin stimulate 3β-hydroxysteroid dehydrogenase activity, the rate-limiting enzyme in the conversion of pregnenolone to progesterone in isolated trophoblasts. In the same model IGF-I inhibited the activity of trophoblast aromatase necessary for estrogen production. While IGFs may regulate trophoblast function, this may be aided by a local expression of EGF or TGFα which will increase the differentiation of cytotrophoblastic cells into a functional syncytium *in vitro*. A high expression of basic FGF in placenta may contribute to endothelial cell proliferation, angiogenesis being a major feature of placental growth.

Multiple transcripts of IGF-I and II mRNA are found in the fetal and neonatal rat brain, as are IGF type I and II receptors. Cultured fetal rat neuronal and astroglial cells also release both IGF-I and II. Glial cells proliferate in response to exogenous IGF-I, and other growth factors such as EGF and basic FGF. The mitogenic actions of EGF are mediated in part by increased endogenous synthesis of IGFs. IGF-II will also promote the embryonic neurons and neurite formation in isolated rat sensory and sympathetic ganglia, and in human neuroblastoma cells. In these models IGF-II was synergistic with nerve growth factor. IGF-I was shown to increase the commitment of mixed glial cell cultures from the newborn rat cerebrum to form oligodendrocytes. The IGFs may also serve as neurotransmitters within brain since IGF-I was shown to stimulate acetylcholine release from rat cortical brain slices, and to cause the differentiation of catecholaminergic precursors in cultures of dorsal rat ganglia.

Selected reading

Han VKM, Hill DJ. The involvement of insulin-like growth factors in embryonic and fetal development. In Schofield P, ed. *The insulin-like growth factors, structures and biologic functions*. Oxford: Oxford University Press, 1990: 178–220.

Hill DJ, Strain AJ, Milner RDG. Growth factors in embryogenesis. In Clarke JR, ed. *Oxford reviews of reproductive biology*. Vol. 9. Oxford: Clarendon Press, 1987: 398.

Lee DC, Han VKM. Expression of growth factors and their receptors in development. In Sporn MB, Roberts AB, eds. *Peptide growth factors and their receptors II*. New York: Springer-Verlag, 1990: 611.

Sharpe PM, Ferguson MWJ. Mesenchymal influences on epithelial differentiation in developing systems. *J Cell Sci* 1988; **Suppl 10**: 195.

Sporn MB, Roberts AB, eds. *Peptide growth factors and their receptors*. Berlin: Springer-Verlag, 1990.

B. Prenatal Growth Control

R D G Milner

An overview

The control of prenatal growth resides in the mother, the placenta and the fetus. Growth control can be considered in terms of immutable effects such as the genetic contribution and variable effects through which the genetic mechanisms are modulated. It is helpful to first review fetal growth control when there is no environmental or nutritional constraint. Under such circumstances control resides in the fetal genome which coordinates cellular multiplication, migration, differentiation and death to achieve normal organ growth and development. Then, separately, the contribution of the placenta and the maternal environment are considered to illustrate how optimal fetal growth can be modulated and pathological influences are mediated.

The human fetus undergoes the equivalent of some 42 successive mitotic divisions in progressing from a fertilized ovum to a term infant, with only five more divisions being necessary to achieve adult size. Growth velocity expressed as fractional change per unit time is greatest for length at approximately 20 weeks and for weight at 34 weeks (Fig. 5.1). The slowing of the rate of weight gain that occurs thereafter is due to uterine constraint. Growth occurs by changes in cell number and size: in the first trimester growth is by increase in cell number, in the second there is a stable rate of cellular division accompanied by an increase in cell size, while in the third trimester the rate of mitosis slows while growth by cellular hypertrophy continues. Any disturbance of growth in the first trimester is likely to result in abortion. In the second or third trimesters intrauterine growth retardation (IUGR) can be caused by slowing of the mitotic rate or prevention of cellular hypertrophy. The earlier IUGR occurs, the more likely it is to be irreversible. Chronic growth retardation produces a short, underweight infant but acute growth arrest at the end of pregnancy results in a long, skinny baby. These are also referred to as proportionate and disproportionate IUGR.

Multiple gene loci contribute to the birth weight of the normal fetus. Models have been developed that partition

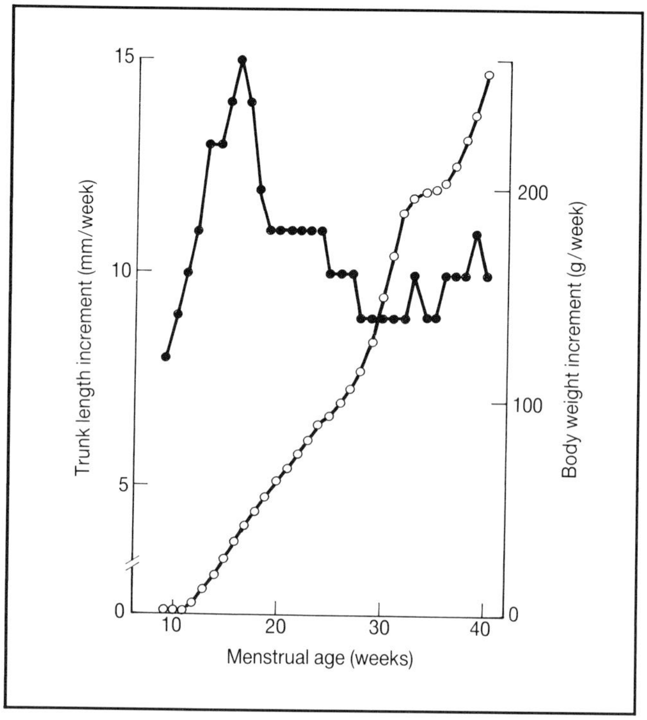

Fig. 5.1. Increase in sitting height (closed circles) and body weight (open circles) shown as a function of menstrual age. (Data taken from Streeter GL. *Contrib Embryol* 1921; **55**: 143.)

the contribution of genetic and environmental factors in determining birth weight (Table 5.1). Variation in birth weight can be roughly partitioned: one-third to genetic factors, one-third to recognizable environmental factors, and one-third unknown. Of the 38 percent that is genetic, the maternal genotype (20 percent) is more important than the fetal genotype (15 percent), and the paternal contribution is solely via the fetal genotype. Chromosomal abnormalities that give rise to recognizable syndromes such as *Turner syndrome* (45,XO) or *Down syndrome* (trisomy 21) characteristically produce small babies. This is thought to be the result of a reduced rate of cell division.

In the last trimester the fetus doubles its body weight, from approximately 1.5 to 3.0 kg, due mainly to the rapid

Table 5.1. Partitioning of birth weight variation

Genetic		
Maternal genotype	20%	
Fetal genotype	16%	
Fetal sex	2%	
		38%
Environmental		
General maternal environment	18%	
Immediate maternal environment	6%	
Maternal age and parity	8%	
Unknown	30%	
		62%

acquisition of protein and fat. In the first 1.5 kg body weight acquired over 28 weeks there is about 50 g fat, whereas in the second 1.5 kg there is 500 g fat. At term the male fetus is heavier and has a greater lean body mass and less body fat than the female, possibly due to the effect of fetal testosterone production. Lipid accumulation by the fetus in the third trimester is the most important determinant of a newborn baby being overweight or underweight and is determined by nutrient availability and fetal insulin secretion.

Fetal determinants

Optimal expression of the fetal genome in controlling prenatal growth depends on adequate delivery of nutrient to the fetus. Nutrient supply depends on the maternal environment producing the right mix of substrate and maternoplacental cooperation in delivering the goods to the fetal compartment. The fetus is commonly perceived as being both the gross and net recipient of metabolic fuels but under some circumstances the fetus contributes to placental metabolic needs when these are not fulfilled from the maternal side. When this happens fetal growth is compromised to ensure fetal survival. If the fetus becomes catabolic in the last trimester, the losses of fetal protein exceed those of lipid and fetal wasting may occur, which is detectable by ultrasound. For the purpose of clarity the fetus will be considered here as receiving optimal nutrition, thus enabling attention to be focused on endocrine and growth factor control mechanisms. Disturbances to fetal nutrition are considered further on p. 165.

Hormones

Fetal peptide hormones and growth factors do not cross the placenta with the possible exception of limited permeability to thyroxine. In contrast, steroid hormones are secreted and metabolized by the materno–placento–fetal unit in its entirety. Both peptides and steroids play a part in fetal growth and organ maturation.

The role of growth hormone (GH) in postnatal growth makes the pituitary a plausible focus of attention in prenatal growth. Pituitary GH is present in the fetal circulation from week 12 of gestation and by midpregnancy plasma concentrations are in the 100 ng/ml range and greater than at any other time before or after birth. The fall in GH which occurs in late gestation is thought to be related to maturation of, and institution of, tonic inhibitory tone in the hypothalamo–hypophyseal axis (see p. 295). Despite the abundance of GH in the circulation the hormone is not thought to be the major endocrine determinant of fetal growth because *anencephalic fetuses* are characterized by a relatively normal body weight. *Laron syndrome* is a heterogenous group of autosomal recessive conditions due to a lack or dysfunction of GH receptors. The normal birth weight of such infants and those with congenital GH deficiency has been used as an argument for the unimportance of GH in prenatal life, but recent studies have shown a reduced birth length and relative obesity. Furthermore, GH receptors have been demonstrated on a variety of fetal cells in the second trimester and experimental studies have shown that the pituitary axis is important in producing the correct number and size of cells in different organs. GH receptors develop on fetal hepatocytes at about week 30 and may be responsible for the initiation of insulin-like growth factor binding protein 3 (IGFBP-3) synthesis and have some influence on fetal IGF-I secretion late in gestation. GH itself has little role in regulating fetal growth; however, IGF-I, as will be discussed later, appears to have a central role.

The pituitary–thyroid axis operates from week 10 of gestation and fetal thyroid function is characterized by reverse triiodothyronine (RT3) being secreted in excess of triiodothyronine (T3), but RT3 is not thought to have significance for fetal development. Late in gestation T3 production rises due to an effect of cortisol on hepatic deiodinase. This is important for fetal lung maturation and explains the increased incidence of *respiratory distress syndrome* in *congenital hypothyroidism*. Fetal hypothyroidism which may arise from a structural anomaly or inborn error of metabolism results in delayed osseous and neuronal maturation but has no significant effect on body size overall. For further discussion of the fetal thyroidal axis see p. 308.

The fetal pituitary–adrenal axis secretes more high molecular weight precursors and low molecular weight fragments of adrenocorticotropin (ACTH) than occur after birth. They may play a part in the development and function of the fetal zone of the adrenal cortex which secretes large quantities of dehydroepiandrosterone (DHA) and DHA sulfate. Glucocorticoids in the fetal circulation originate in the mother and placenta as much as from the fetal adrenal. They have a general permissive role in fetal growth and a specific stimulatory action on the development of certain enzyme systems, such as those involved in surfactant and glycogen biosynthesis.

The importance of insulin for fetal growth is acutely obvious. When insulin is grossly deficient in the human fetus, as in *pancreatic agenesis*, term birth weight is in the range of 1200–1500 g, muscle mass is deficient and adiposity absent. Fetal hyperinsulinemia is associated with excessive birth weight, primarily due to increased adiposity, in the infants of poorly controlled diabetic mothers.

Fetal insulin secretion is stimulated by amino acids up to 28 weeks of gestation and by glucose and amino acids thereafter. Cellular anabolism progresses to replication under the influence of growth factors. Growth factor synthesis and release are promoted not only by intracellular events such as the delivery of fuel, which is augmented by insulin, but possibly also by placental lactogen (PL) and placental GH which may be acting on many tissues in a manner analogous to that of GH on the hepatocyte postnatally. Finally, there is a long loop in which insulin reinforces the anabolic process by stimulating PL secretion.

There are a number of interactions between insulin, circulating IGF-I levels and nutritional availability in the fetus. For example, fetal pancreatectomy in the sheep results in a much-reduced circulating IGF-I as does experimental fetal growth retardation induced by maternal fasting or uterine vessel occlusion. Experimental fetal hyperinsulinemia elevates circulating levels of IGF-I and IGF-II. Similarly, infants with *transient neonatal diabetes mellitus* have a reduced plasma IGF-I. Conversely, *infants of diabetic mothers* have normal cord blood IGF-I levels, but if the analysis is restricted to those heavy for dates, circulating IGF-I is elevated. Fetal nutrient availability also affects the IGFBPs (see p. 181). IGFBP-1 in cord blood is inversely related to birth weight and may restrict the availability of IGFs to tissues. The interaction between these three factors is critical in the regulation of the growth of the late gestation fetus.

Migration, adhesion and growth factors

Cellular and tissue interactions in the embryo and fetus are subject to at least three types of control: the deposition and subsequent modification of extracellular matrix molecules, the expression of cellular recognition molecules and the appropriate expression of intercellular messengers such as peptide growth factors.

Neural crest cells migrate to form the peripheral nervous system, dermal pigment cells and connective tissues of the head. Migration is preceded by the expression of tenascin along the pathway and its removal immediately afterwards. Tenascin is structurally related to fibronectin and is also thought to play a role in the epithelial–mesenchymal interactions that initiate the formation of certain tissues and the differentiation of mesenchymal cells.

Cells recognize their anatomical position within developing structures by the expression of intercellular recognition molecules. These are categorized into the cell adhesion molecules (CAMs) that do not require calcium and the cadherins which are calcium dependent (see p. 159). Identical recognition molecules are expressed on the membranes of homotypic cells during tissue condensation and between heterotypic cells during mesenchymal–epithelial interaction. For example, when uterine decidual cells become associated with the extraembryonic cells of the embryo to form the primordial placenta, both layers express placental cadherin.

The peptide growth factors are typically synthesized in, or adjacent to, the cells on which they will act. They are thus primarily autocrine or paracrine rather than endocrine messengers. They are synthesized *de novo* on demand and when released act on cell-surface receptors which are glycoproteins. Following stimulation there is a spectrum of intracellular metabolic signals which have a uniform final common path. This involves increased amino acid and glucose uptake, RNA and protein synthesis. DNA synthesis and cell replication may follow but not all growth factors are stimulatory; some, such as transforming growth factor β and tumor necrosis factor, inhibit cellular multiplication.

Insulin-like growth factors

There is considerable evidence that the insulin-like growth factors (IGFs) play a major role in the regulation of fetal growth. The biochemistry and general physiology of the IGFs are reviewed on p. 180. The IGFs stimulate cellular multiplication and differentiation, but they have also an insulin-like pharmacological action which results in hypoglycemia. The main site of IGF synthesis in the fetus is mesenchyme and connective tissue, but IGFs act on all types of cell regardless of embryological origin. Some IGF-I has been recovered immunochemically from all human fetal tissues tested. Lung and intestine have the highest concentration and liver the lowest. The multiple sources of IGF-I which may all contribute to circulatory levels, although the liver is the primary source, make the biological interpretation of blood IGF concentrations difficult. The difficulty is compounded by the fact that nearly all circulating IGF is bound to carrier proteins which extend the half-lives of IGF-I and IGF-II and alter their bioavailability (see p. 180).

IGFs can be detected in fetal blood from week 13 and a direct correlation has been found between umbilical cord IGF-I and birth weight, but not in IGF-II which is similar in concentration in the fetal and adult circulation. A correlation has been made experimentally between bioassayable serum IGF and fetal undergrowth and a number of reports of reduced IGF-I levels in spontaneous intrauterine growth retardation have been published. The interaction between insulin, nutritional status and fetal IGF-I secretion was reviewed earlier.

The action of IGF and other growth factors depends as much on the ontogeny of receptors as on the messenger peptide. Most fetal tissues possess receptors for both IGF-I and IGF-II. The type I IGF receptor is similar but not identical to the insulin receptor and quite unlike the type II IGF receptor (see Fig. 5.1). Each receptor recognizes its own signal preferentially. The insulin receptor is sensitive to insulin and less so to IGF-I. The type I IGF receptor is sensitive to IGF-I and less so to both IGF-II and insulin. The type II IGF receptor recognizes IGF-II primarily and insulin not at all. Fetal tissues have greater concentrations of both types of IGF receptor than adult tissues.

Circulating IGF is complexed to a family of binding proteins (see p. 180). The largest (IGFBP-3) is an acid-stable molecule of 53 kDa which reacts with IGF and an acid-labile nonbinding protein to produce a complex of approximately 150 kDa. It is synthesized mainly in the liver under pituitary GH control and is the most important IGF transporter in the last trimester. Its ontogeny may be related to the development of GH receptors on fetal hepatocytes.

IGFBP-1 is a 28 kDa peptide which binds to IGF to produce a complex of approximately 34 kDa (see p. 184). In the first trimester fetal IGFBP-1 can be detected immunohistochemically in the adrenal cortex, Leydig cells and small mononuclear cells in the liver. In the second trimester it is the major circulating binding protein for IGFs and is found in a wide range of fetal tissues. At birth umbilical cord and maternal IGFBP-1 levels are similar and inversely related to birth weight.

IGFBP-2 is intermediate in size with a weight of 29.6 kDa. Less is known of its function; its concentration is higher in the fetal circulation than postnatally and is influenced by metabolic factors. It is the primary form of binding protein found in the cerebrospinal fluid and human breast milk.

Other growth factors of importance to fetal growth, including epidermal growth factor (EGF), the fibroblast growth factor (FGF), platelet derived growth factor (PDGF), and the transforming growth factor β (TGFβ) are reviewed on p. 155. These paracrine or autocrine growth factors interact with insulin and nutrients such as glucose and amino acids in a mutually reinforcing manner to provide a permissive stimulating environment for cellular anabolism.

Metabolism

The fetal metabolic rate as reflected by net fetal oxygen consumption is only slightly associated with energy delivery to the fetus. The relative constancy of fetal metabolic rate at widely differing glucose concentrations indicates that there are important alternative substrates. In view of the limited availability and/or oxidation of other nonprotein energy sources, it is likely that there is a reciprocal relationship between glucose and amino acids in fulfilling fetal energy requirements. The net uptake of amino acids is more than is needed for fetal protein synthesis and what is left over is oxidized or transaminated and stored as lipid. When a shortfall of metabolic delivery to the fetus occurs, fetal protein catabolism permits the release of amino acids for gluconeogenesis or direct oxidation and preservation of metabolic rate even at the cost of fetal growth. Under these circumstances the fetus may even be a net energy provider to the placenta, its lifeline.

Placental determinants

The placenta grows faster than the fetus and reaches maximum weight at about 33 weeks of gestation, though surface area and vascularity continue to develop thereafter. The placenta affects fetal growth mechanically by being the transport system via which nutrients and oxygen are brought to the fetus and waste products removed. Equally important are the metabolic and endocrine aspects of placental function which include steroid hormone metabolism and peptide hormone production.

Mechanics

Morphological abnormalities such as a bilobate or reniform placenta or a placenta with an accessory lobe do not appear to influence fetal development, but abnormalities of the umbilical cord do. Reduced birth weight is commonly associated with velamentous insertion of the umbilical cord or battledore placenta and also with a single umbilical artery, which is, however, often a marker of other abnormal fetal morphology. Microscopic changes in the placenta, such as intervillous thromboses, placental infarction, or degeneration of the syncytiotrophoblast in *pre-eclamptic toxemia*, are all associated with fetal growth retardation.

The principal determinants of fetal placental perfusion are cardiac output and the distribution of blood in the fetal circulation. The fetal placenta has a low vascular resistance and receives about half the cardiac output. The umbilical arterial wall is muscular and is not thought to be innervated outside the abdomen, but is sensitive to vasoactive peptides. Important umbilical artery vasoconstrictors include angiotensin, vasopressin, bradykinins, serotonin, adrenergic agonists and the prostaglandins (see p. 544). Increased renin–angiotensin secretion in *maternal hypertension* might cause reduced umbilical flow and thereby fetal growth retardation.

Umbilical blood flow is highly dependent on fetal heart rate since there is little variation in umbilical resistance (see p. 540). Flow increases with body size but not proportionately, since in late gestation a greater fraction perfuses fetal organs. Hypoxemia causes a redistribution of blood flow between fetal organs but little alteration in umbilical vascular resistance. In early gestation hypoxemia causes fetal tachycardia and increased umbilical blood flow, whereas later on there is bradycardia coupled with increased arterial pressure which helps to preserve umbilical blood flow. Morphine and other central nervous system depressants cause fetal bradycardia. The resulting fall in umbilical blood flow may partly explain the intrauterine growth retardation seen in the offspring of *drug abusers*.

Placental gaseous exchange is by passive diffusion (see p. 138). The major physiological determinants of oxygen delivery to the fetus are maternal and fetal blood flow and the relative affinities of fetal and maternal hemoglobin for oxygen. If placental surface area is reduced or the diffusion distance increased by thickening of the placental membrane, reduction in the overall oxygen diffusion capacity may restrict fetal growth. This can occur as a result of placental infarction or intervillous fibrin deposition.

Hormones

The placenta synthesizes and secretes into the maternal circulation a growth hormone variant, hGH-V, which is also known as placental GH. It differs from pituitary GH in only 13 amino acid residues. First detected in midpregnancy, placental GH levels increase to term but the actions and biological significance of this peptide remain to be defined. What, if any, role it plays in the fetus is not known. Placental GH does not appear to be essential for successful pregnancy because normal fetal development has occurred in a woman who had a deletion of both the hGH-V and placental lactogen (PL) genes.

The placenta makes large amounts of PL (also known as chorionic somatomammotropin), a molecule with close biological and chemical similarities to pituitary GH. More than 99 percent of PL is secreted into the maternal circulation where it is lipolytic and diabetogenic. PL secretion is responsible for the exaggerated oscillations of fuel metabolites that occur during fasting and postprandially in pregnancy. Despite plasma concentrations in the fetus being 100-fold less, the hormone may play a part in fetal anabolism. Many fetal cells have PL receptors and PL stimulates protein synthesis and cell division both directly and via an action on insulin release. PL may thus have an important role in normal fetal growth, but this action is permissive or superfluous, as are the actions of other lactogenic hormones such as hGH-V, since there are case records of successful pregnancies in which the mother has a congenital inability to synthesize PL.

Since the placenta links fetus and mother in the complicated pools and pathways of steroid metabolism, it is appropriate to consider the effects of steroids, principally glucocorticoids, on fetal growth under a placental heading. The fetoplacental contribution to steroid production becomes quantitatively important from week 8 of gestation. The placenta then becomes the most important source of C_{18} and C_{21} steroids in both fetal and maternal circulations. The fetal adrenal cortex, in particular the fetal zone which makes up 80 percent of the gland, is the chief source of fetal steroid precursors, in particular C_{19} steroids (see p. 319).

Cortisol enhances the maturation of a number of important enzymes involved in tissue and organ preparation for extrauterine life. From 32 weeks the choline phosphotransferase pathway becomes increasingly important in the manufacture of pulmonary surfactant and this is under the control of cortisol in association with thyroxine, prolactin and estrogens. Cortisol is involved in the maturation of glycogen synthetase upon which the accumulation of hepatic glycogen stores depends in the last trimester. Norepinephrine is converted to epinephrine in the adrenal medulla by phenylethanolamine-*N*-methyltransferase which is induced by cortisol (see p. 341).

Metabolism

The placenta influences fetal metabolism principally by regulating the transport of metabolites to the fetus. There are transporters or carriers for most substrates, some of which, e.g. glucose and fatty acids, diffuse passively whereas others, e.g. amino acids, are moved actively and largely uphill (see p. 136). The amount of selected nutrients that passes to the fetus is affected by local placental metabolism. Developmental changes in placental transport capacity result in a changing fetal diet throughout gestation. In the sheep, halfway through gestation, placental weight is greater than at term but glucose transport capacity is low. In the second half of gestation placental weight decreases by 20 percent but glucose transport capacity increases eightfold.

The near-term placenta contains a large variety of enzymes capable of metabolizing amino acids through pathways such as amino acid oxidation, protein synthesis, gluconeogenesis and glycogen synthesis. Experimental studies have shown that the net umbilical uptake of amino acids provides more than half the fetal carbon and more than one and a half times the nitrogen required for normal growth and development. This is reflected in a high fetal urea production rate. Not all amino acids contribute equally to the nitrogen excess; glycine, lysine, histidine, asparagine/aspartate and glutamine/glutamate are all taken up in amounts similar to net carcass accretion and any deficiency in maternal supply would be harmful to fetal growth. The capacity of the fetus to oxidize excess fetal amino acids appears to develop early in gestation.

The placenta and fetus cycle amino acids. Both the placenta and the fetus produce ammonia and that from the placenta passes into both the maternal and umbilical circulations. Glutamine and glycine are taken up by the fetus from the placenta and by the fetal liver from the umbilical circulation, whereas the metabolically related products glutamate and serine are produced by the liver and taken up by the placenta. The importance of these interactions to fetal and placental wellbeing is not apparent yet, but their existence implies a more sophisticated fetoplacental relationship than had hitherto been imagined.

Lipid transport from mother to fetus is quantitatively slight, but the high carbon content of lipid molecules makes their contribution to fetal metabolism disproportionately great. Since fetal fatty acid composition varies with the maternal diet, it seems unlikely that the placenta exerts a significant selectivity in lipid delivery.

Maternal determinants

Nutrition

Fetal caloric requirements are 95 kcal/kg per day, of which 40 are committed to growth and 55 are oxidized. To this minimum caloric cost of pregnancy must be added the maternal metabolic burden of carrying the conceptus and preparing for lactation. Direct measurement has shown the extra caloric requirement for pregnancy to be in the order of 20 000 kcal or less than 100 kcal/day, but there are marked individual and ethnic differences between women in this respect. The basal metabolic rate (BMR) of pregnant women in Europe rises slightly in the first trimester and then progressively thereafter. In contrast, Gambian women show a fall in BMR in the first trimester and a gradual rise to a level at term that is just above prepregnancy reference values.

Despite the relatively high optimal plane of maternal nutrition, underfeeding has a relatively small effect on fetal growth. Starvation, as experienced in Holland in 1944–45, led to a small fall in birth weight only when maternal intake fell below 1500 kcal/day in the third trimester. Conversely, food supplementation during pregnancy of marginally undernourished women causes an increase in birth weight. Adequate cellular delivery of nutrient is an overriding condition for normal intrauterine growth. Nutrient oversupply is not known to influence growth before 28 weeks of gestation, but can influence weight gain in the third trimester by stimulating pancreatic β-cell ontogeny and fetal insulin secretion.

Hormones

The changes in maternal circulating GH and GH-like peptides which occur during pregnancy all combine to have a diabetogenic or anti-insulin effect on the mother so that metabolites such as glucose and free fatty acids oscillate more wildly during feeding and fasting than in the nonpregnant state. This has important implications for fetal substrate delivery. Inadequate compensation by the maternal β-islet cell may result in fetal overgrowth.

Disease

Maternal disease influences fetal development by altering placental perfusion or by producing placental transfer of abnormal molecules. Impaired delivery of oxygen to the placenta occurs in *maternal cyanotic heart disease* or *chronic debilitating lung disease*. Maternal *pregnancy-associated hypertension* is often associated with poor intrauterine growth. This may be related to thromboses in the placental microvasculature or to associated renal involvement. A corollary is that factors increasing uterine blood flow, such as bed rest, stimulate fetal growth.

Maternal drug abuse may retard fetal growth directly as in the toxic effects of acetaldehyde on placental hormone synthesis and fetal cellular mitosis, or indirectly via reducing maternal food intake. *Smoking* has a dose-related effect on fetal growth; 20 cigarettes a day brings the birth weight down by 200 g. The toxic agents are both nicotine and carbon dioxide. Nicotine increases uterine vascular resistance and decreases blood flow, leading to fetal hypoxia and hypercapnia. Carbon monoxide leads to tissue hypoxia in both mother and fetus by the formation of carboxyhemoglobin. It may also bind to cytochrome and impair placental nutrient transport.

Maternal metabolic disorders characterized by excess circulating concentrations of one or more metabolites might be expected to affect fetal growth, the most commonly cited being *phenylketonuria* which can cause microcephaly and congenital heart disease. Conditions having in common immunoglobulin overproduction may influence fetal development in a variety of ways; in *systemic lupus erythematosus* transplacental passage of IgG causes fetal tissue damage. In *maternal thyrotoxicosis* the passage of long-acting thyroid stimulating immunoglobulins may cause fetal thyrotoxicosis.

Maternal infections have a spectrum of harmful effects on the fetus. *Malaria* inhibits fetal growth by impairing placental blood flow. Serious systemic bacterial infection, particularly *Gram-negative septicemia*, at any stage of pregnancy may kill the fetus whereas *viral or protozoal infections* such as *rubella, cytomegalovirus*, or *toxoplasmosis* all cause fetal tissue damage and growth retardation along with specific pathology characteristic of the infection.

The only environmental factor with an unequivocal effect on human fetal development is altitude. Infants born at 15 000 ft have a mean birth weight 16 percent less than those born at 500 ft. Fetal growth retardation in these circumstances results from decreased oxygen delivery.

Selected reading

Clemmons DR, Underwood LE. Nutritional regulation of IGF-I and IGF binding proteins. *Annu Rev Nutr* 1991; **11**: 393.

De Pablo F, Scott LA, Roth J. Insulin and insulin-like growth factor I in early development: peptides, receptors and biological events. *Endocr Rev* 1990; **11**: 558.

Hill DJ, Hogg J. Growth factors and the regulation of pre- and postnatal growth. *Baillière's Clin Endocrinol Metab* 1989; **3**: 579.

C. Postnatal Growth

C1. Postnatal Growth–an Overview

G R Ambler and P D Gluckman

Postnatal growth is determined by a complex interaction between genetic, environmental and hormonal influences. At birth these influences replace the dominant maternal and placental influences of the fetal growth period (see p. 162).

Normal growth patterns

Mean birth weight at term is approximately 3.5 ± 0.4 kg and length 48 ± 2 cm. Postnatal linear growth is most rapid immediately after birth, being up to 45 cm/year during the first 3 months, falling rapidly to around 15 cm/year from 9 to 12 months of age. Similarly weight velocity falls from approximately 10 kg/year in the first 3 months to around 3 kg/year from 9 to 12 months of age. From the age of 1 year there is a gradual fall in linear growth rate, reaching a nadir just before the onset of puberty. If puberty is delayed, then late prepubertal growth velocity may be very low. Throughout childhood there is a fairly consistent growth rate of 5.0–7.5 cm/year and weight gain of 2–3 kg/year. At puberty, a rapid increase in growth rate occurs with a peak height velocity averaging 9.5 cm/year in boys and 8.2 cm/year in girls. For descriptive purposes Karlberg considered the human growth curve in three components: the rapid but rapidly decelerating growth of infancy, the more steady growth rate of the childhood period and the growth spurt associated with puberty (see Fig. 5.2). The legs grow faster than the body in childhood, with an exponential fall in the upper to lower body segment ratio from approximately 1.7 at birth to 1.0 in the female and 0.9 in the male adult.

Organ and tissue growth in general parallels skeletal growth, with some notable exceptions. The eyes and brain are highly developed at birth and attain most of their adult size within the first few years of life. Lymphoid tissue mass increases throughout childhood, reaching a

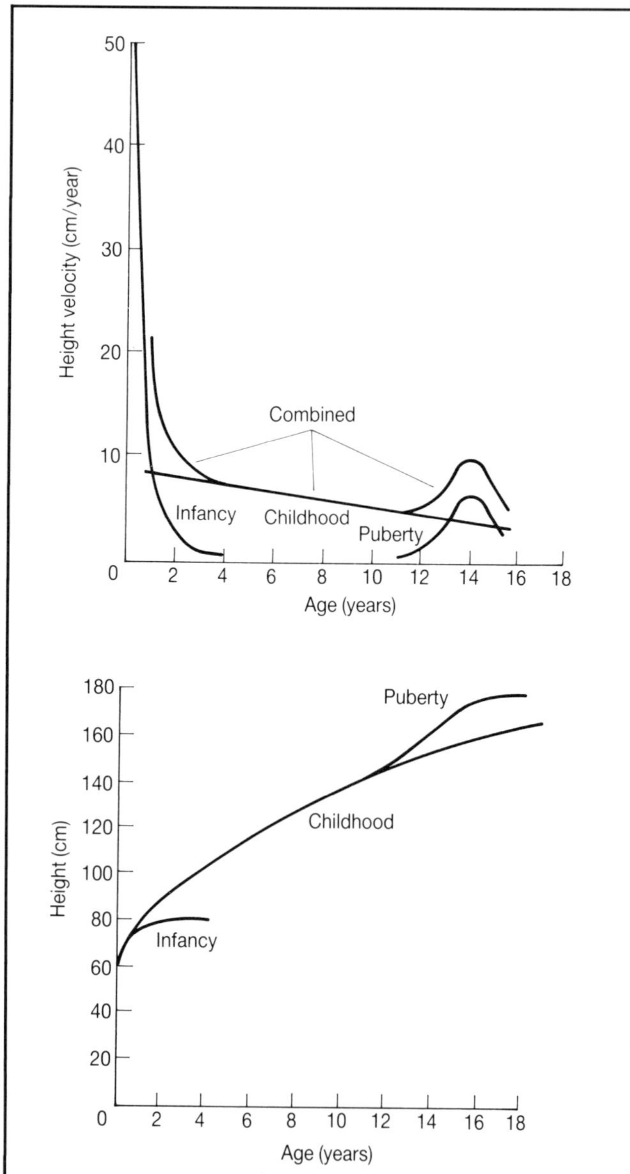

Fig. 5.2. The Infancy–Childhood–Pubertal Growth model of Karlberg, shown here for boys. Upper: the mean values for height velocity for each component (infancy, childhood, puberty) and their sum (combined velocity). Lower: the model for attained height (50th centile shown). (From Karlberg J. *Acta Paediatr Scand Suppl* 1989; **356**: 29. Published with permission. Copyright © 1987, Karlberg J, ISBN 91–7900–265–X; copyright © US, Karlberg J, TX 2 560 182.)

maximum just before puberty, and then declines throughout adult life. Reproductive tissues are relatively undeveloped until the onset of puberty when they grow rapidly and attain mature size within a few years.

Factors influencing growth

Genetic and ethnic influences

The effects of racial and genetic differences on birth size and growth are difficult to assess because of associated environmental differences such as nutrition, maternal health and disease prevalence. Fetal genotype makes a minor contribution only to size at birth (see p. 163); however, postnatal growth and stature are strongly genetically determined. Correlation of length with final adult height is low at birth ($r=0.3$), increasing by 1 year ($r=0.7$) and reaching a stable prepubertal level ($r=0.8$) by 2 years of age. By 2 years of age, a significant correlation of stature to parental height is evident, and this strengthens with age. Monozygotic (MZ) twins become progressively more concordant for height with age ($r=0.93$ by 8 years), while dizygotic (DZ) twins become less concordant ($r=0.49$ at 8 years).

There is a also a significant genetic contribution to the timing of pubertal maturation. MZ twins have a much higher correlation of age at menarche ($r=0.93$) than DZ twins ($r=0.62$). In individual families, children experiencing late puberty often have a family history of delay in one or both parents.

Racial groups vary significantly in size, body proportions and the timing of maturational events. The Dinkas and the Watutsi tribes of Africa are amongst the tallest races with males often reaching 196 cm, while the pygmies of the Congo are one of the smallest with mean adult male height around 128 cm. In most instances this is assumed to be a polygenic trait. It has been suggested that there is a specific defect in the tissue growth hormone receptor in the pygmy; however, this is not proven. Amongst different racial groups, social conditions are the predominant influence on age at menarche; however, this is overridden by racial differences in some instances. In similar social circumstances, African children mature more quickly than European children in all respects. Ideally growth standards used should be appropriate for racial group. Differences in body proportions also occur; for example, Africans have longer legs than Caucasians, and Europeans have broader shoulders in relation to their hips.

Sex differences in growth are also seen. Male fetuses have a slightly higher average birth weight than female fetuses. Growth rate during childhood is not significantly different between the sexes although boys are on average slightly taller than girls. The pubertal growth spurt occurs on average 2 years later in boys than girls, giving boys an average of 2 years more prepubertal growth (approximately 10 cm) before the onset of puberty. This, coupled with the greater magnitude of the male pubertal growth spurt, accounts for the mean adult height difference of 13 cm between the sexes.

Abnormalities in sex chromosomes have significant effects on growth and stature. For example in *Turner syndrome* (45,XO or mosaic forms) mean birth weight and length are reduced by approximately 500 g and 3 cm respectively, childhood growth rate is low and there is absence of a spontaneous pubertal growth spurt. In *Klinefelter syndrome* (46,XXY) tall stature is often a feature and hypogonadism is present. Abnormalities in autosomes may also have profound effects on growth such as in *Down syndrome (trisomy 21)* where mean adult height is reduced by approximately 20 cm in males and 14 cm in females. A large number of genetically determined disorders affect skeletal growth and stature (e.g. *achondroplasia*). Other metabolic and organ system diseases such as *cystic fibrosis* and inborn errors of metabolism may affect growth indirectly via nutritional and other secondary effects.

Specific genetic defects affecting endocrine function may also occur. It has been recently recognized that deletion of part of the hGH gene on chromosome 17 results in absence of circulating GH and severe growth failure (*isolated GH deficiency type 1A*). Genetic defects in the growth hormone receptor and serum growth hormone binding protein have also been recognized in disorders of growth hormone resistance such as *Laron syndrome*.

Environment

Nutrition influences growth profoundly, and protein-energy malnutrition is a major worldwide cause of poor growth and failure to reach genetic height potential. Among populations not characterized by either undernutrition or overnutrition, however, the relationship of diet to growth is less clear. The secular trend of increasing population height and weight and decreasing age of puberty in developed nations is most attributable to nutritional effects, but also to other health and environmental influences. For optimal growth to occur the diet must be sufficient in calories, essential amino and fatty acids, vitamins and trace elements. Children who have been severely malnourished *in utero* or infancy may subsequently show catch-up growth with adequate nutrition; however, in up to 40 percent of cases this catch-up growth is incomplete or nonexistent. This may relate to the duration, severity and earlier onset of nutritional deficiency. This phenomenon is as yet incompletely understood. Decreased growth rate during periods of malnutrition can be considered an adaptive response to allow nutrients to be channelled into essential metabolic and homeostatic functions.

Nutritional status interacts with the endocrine regulation of growth. Indeed, the somatotropic axis can be viewed as the mediator of the interaction between the genetic drive to grow and environmental factors such as nutrition. Severe undernutrition is associated with increased mean serum GH levels and increased GH pulse amplitude. Serum IGF-I levels are, however, decreased by undernutrition, and experimentally this has been demonstrated to be associated with a down-regulation of the number of tissue growth hormone receptors. Since IGF-I has been implicated as an anticatabolic hormone, this may be an adaptive response allowing preferential utilization of mobilized substrates to maintain homeostasis rather than for cell growth or proliferation. The onset of puberty (as studied by age at menarche in girls) is significantly influenced by social and environmental influences. The secular trend to an earlier age of menarche (menarche occurring earlier at an average rate of 3–4 months per decade over the last 100 years) is believed to be related to nutritional and environmental influences.

In addition to inadequate food availability, a number of disease processes may lead to malnutrition and consequent effects on growth. These include a wide range of malabsorptive conditions such as *celiac disease* and *cystic fibrosis*, chronic disease processes outside the gastrointestinal system and disorders of increased energy utilization such as *diabetes mellitus*.

Other environmental factors interact in a complicated manner with nutrition and the endocrine system to influence growth. These include disease prevalence, hygiene standards, socioeconomic class, physical activity and emotional wellbeing. Thus, growth is often used by public health officials as a retrospective parameter of population health status. *Emotionally deprived or abused* children have been shown to have decreased growth hormone secretion, low serum IGF-I levels and abnormalities of ACTH secretion and thyroid function. In general these return to normal, along with growth rate, on removal from the harmful environment. Growth in children may also be seasonal, often with more rapid linear growth in the spring and summer than autumn and winter. In domestic animals marked seasonality of GH secretion has been noted with lesser secretion during declining day lengths. Girls who are blind or deaf experience significantly earlier menarche then controls, and menarche may be delayed in girls who exercise excessively, presumably because of altered gonadotropin release.

Hormonal regulation

Major hormones influencing somatic growth are growth hormone, IGF-I, thyroxine, corticosteroids, sex steroids and insulin. It is now recognized that additional peptide growth factors have important local tissue effects through autocrine and paracrine mechanisms, such as epidermal growth factor, transforming growth factors, fibroblast growth factors, etc. (see p. 155).

Growth hormone and IGFs

Growth hormone and IGF secretion and action are discussed in detail subsequently (see pp. 174 and 180).

Thyroid hormone

Athyrotic infants are normal size at birth, suggesting that thyroid hormone does not play a major role in fetal growth. Such infants, however, may exhibit delayed osseous and neurological development. Postnatally, thyroid hormone is critical to neurological and somatic growth and untreated hypothyroid infants manifest severe growth failure and mental retardation. The role of thyroid hormones in growth is permissive rather than primary, and growth retardation in *hypothyroidism* is believed to be mediated in part by deficient pituitary GH secretion and also by deficient action of thyroid hormone on cartilage growth and ossification. Appropriate thyroid hormone replacement normalizes growth in hypothyroid infants and children, and there is often a period of catch-up growth followed by resumption of a normal growth rate. *Hyperthyroidism* results in a mild acceleration of linear growth with moderate acceleration of osseous maturation, and usually with weight loss because of increased metabolic rate.

Insulin

Insulin also has an important permissive role in growth by its role in regulating substrate availability to cells. It may also function as a stimulator of growth. In fetal life, hyperinsulinism is well known to be associated with fetal overgrowth in conditions such as *infants of diabetic mothers* and *Beckwith–Wiedemann syndrome*, whereas insulin deficiency as occurs in *pancreatic agenesis* or in insulin resistance (e.g. *leprechaunism*) is associated with small infants. Postnatally, insulin deficiency inhibits growth as occurs in inadequately treated *diabetes mellitus*. Some of the growth promoting effects of insulin may be mediated through the type I IGF receptor, or through influences on levels of IGF binding proteins.

Glucocorticoids

Normal glucocorticoid secretion and stress response is required for normal homeostasis; however, the importance of glucocorticoids in growth relates to the inhibition of growth in states of glucocorticoid excess. Normal daily glucocorticoid production is approximately 6–12 mg/m^2 per day of cortisol, and linear growth may be affected by endogenous or exogenous provision of only two to three times this secretion rate. Growth effects are most likely by direct inhibition at target tissues, especially skeletal tissues, rather than through effects on the somatotropic axis. Glucocorticoids promote protein catabolism and insulin resistance in tissues. The most common clinical situation encountered is exogenous glucocorticoid administration for control of chronic inflammatory disease.

Sex steroids: gonadal steroids and adrenal androgens

The gonadal steroids, predominantly testosterone and dihydrotestosterone in males and estrogens in females, are of importance in normal growth only from the onset of puberty. In early infancy gonadotropin levels are relatively high and in the male, testosterone levels may be as high as midpubertal levels in the first month of life, falling rapidly over the first 6 months or so to very low levels which are maintained until the onset of puberty (see p. 145). In female infants there may be mild elevation of estradiol levels. At puberty, circulating concentrations of gonadal steroids increase under control of pulsatile gonadotropin secretion. Both androgens and estrogens have a major influence on GH secretion and have been shown to increase the amplitude of GH secretory episodes without affecting frequency. Sex steroids also up-regulate the tissue GH receptor; this may in part be indirect through effects on GH secretion. Associated with this up-regulation are increases in serum IGF-I levels. There is also evidence to suggest that sex steroids may have direct effects on skeletal growth, independent of the somatotropic axis.

Excess endogenous androgen production in the prepubertal child such as in *precocious puberty*, *androgen producing tumors* or *congenital adrenal hyperplasia* is associated with accelerated linear growth rate and weight gain and accelerated osseous maturation. Exogenous androgen administration has similar effects. Estrogens have similar effects; however, they tend to stimulate linear growth at low doses, with attenuation at higher doses.

Adrenal androgens (such as DHEA, DHEAS and androstenedione) show a progressive increase in serum levels in both males and females from about age 7 years until about 13–15 years. The adrenal component of pubertal maturation is termed adrenarche (see p. 326), but the interactions between adrenal and gonadal steroids in the process of puberty are poorly understood. The bulk of evidence suggests the adrenal and gonadal steroid axes are independently regulated. The increase in adrenal androgens in late childhood may contribute to growth of pubic hair before significant increases of gonadal steroids occur. A normal pubertal growth spurt can occur in the absence of adrenal androgens. Some have attributed a small mid-childhood growth spurt to adrenal androgen production, but this is not proven. Early onset of adrenal androgen effects is termed *premature adrenarche*, and may be associated with normal or mildly advanced height and bone age.

Parathyroid hormone and calcium homeostasis

Normal growth requires normal calcium and phosphate homeostasis and is adversely affected in *hypoparathyroidism* or parathormone resistance (*pseudohypoparathyroidism*) and a wide range of related disorders affecting bony mineralization.

Selected reading

Falkner F, Tanner JM, eds. *Human growth. A comprehensive treatise.* Vol. 2, 2nd ed. New York: Plenum Press, 1986: Chapters 1–12.

Hindmarsh PC, Brook CGD. Normal growth and its endocrine control. In Brook CFD, ed. *Clinical paediatric endocrinology*. 2nd ed. Oxford: Blackwell Scientific, 1989: 57.

Sinclair D. *Human growth after birth*. 4th ed. New York: Oxford University Press, 1985.

C2. The Role of Growth Hormone in Postnatal Growth and Metabolism

A Nilsson, J Isgaard and O G P Isaksson

Biochemistry

Growth hormone (GH) was isolated from the human pituitary in 1956 and the complete amino acid sequence was established in 1971 as a single polypeptide chain consisting of 191 amino acids with two disulfide bridges. The molecular weight is 22 kDa, often referred to as 22K GH, and contributes to 70–75 percent of circulating GH. Other forms of GH found in the pituitary and circulation are 20K GH, $22K_{Asp\ 152}$ GH and $22K_{Glu\ 137}$ GH. 20K GH is formed by alternate splicing of the pituitary GH gene. Humans have a total of five GH-related genes present on chromosome 17 coding for pituitary GH, placental variant GH (hGH-V) and three placental lactogen-related genes. The physiological significance of the different molecular forms of GH is unclear but experimental results indicate that the various forms have different affinity to the GH receptors.

Recently, the receptor epitopes of the human GH have been shown. There are three discontinuous polypeptide determinations in human GH which modulate the binding to the liver GH receptor: the loop between residues 54 and 74, the central portion of helix 4 to the carboxyl terminus and, to a lesser extent, the amino terminal region of helix 1.

The patterns of GH secretion

The hypothalamus controls and regulates the GH secretion through two peptides with opposite effects which are secreted into the portal vessel and affect the GH-producing somatotropes of the pituitary. Growth hormone releasing factor (GRF), which stimulates GH production and secretion, is produced both in the ventromedial and arcuate nucleus of hypothalamus. Somatostatin (SRIF), which originates from the anterior periventricular region and arcuate nucleus, is released in an episodic manner and blocks spontaneous and GRF-induced GH release. The control of GH secretion is discussed in detail on p. 295. However, certain aspects are specifically relevant to understanding the actions of GH. The interaction between the two hypothalamic peptides generates a pulsatile release of GH with regular GH peaks at 3–4-hour intervals separated by periods of low or undetectable GH plasma levels (Fig. 5.3).

The pattern of GH release is different in male and female rats and this sexual dimorphism has functional consequences. The male pattern consists of regular large

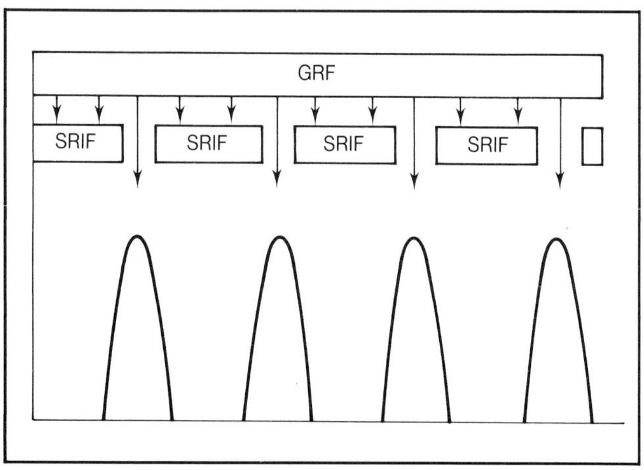

Fig. 5.3. Schematic presentation of GH secretion through actions of growth hormone releasing factor (GRF) and somatostatin (SRIF).

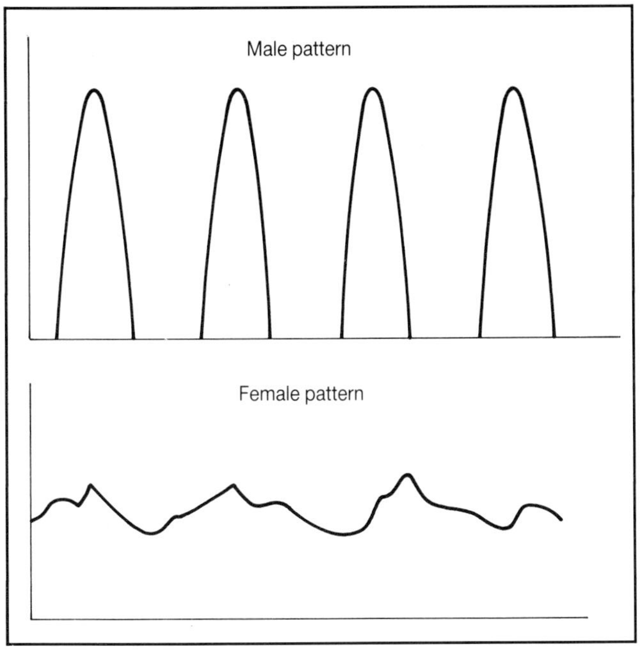

Fig. 5.4. Illustration of the male and female GH secretory pattern.

multicomponent GH peaks separated by intervals of very low or undetectable levels of GH. In females, the plasma pattern is more irregular with more frequent pulses of lower amplitude and a constant elevated baseline secretion (Fig. 5.4). The intermittent responses to GRF in male rats could be explained by cyclic variations in SRIF tone whereas the uniform GH responses to GRF in the female rat may reflect a more continuous release of SRIF. In humans the differences between the sexes in the GH secretory pattern are less pronounced than in the rat.

The sex differences in GH secretion are due to differential exposure to sex steroids. There are indications that testicular androgen secretion during a critical period of neural development (e.g. neonatal rat) influences the mature GH secretory pattern. This process appears analogous to the critical period in neural development when androgens determine other sexually dimorphic characteristics (see p. 133).

Pulsatile GH secretion is more favorable for body growth than continuous GH release; this explains why male rats grow faster than females. A pulsatile infusion of GH stimulates increased weight gain and longitudinal bone growth more effectively than continuous infusion of GH. The GH secretory pattern also influences carbohydrate, lipid and protein metabolism. The effect on carbohydrate metabolism is mainly diabetogenic (anti-insulin-like) but GH also exerts a transient insulin-like effect under certain experimental conditions. The diabetogenic effect of GH is exemplified by the fact that 40–60 percent of the *acromegalic* patients have impaired glucose tolerance with elevated serum levels of insulin. GH administration to experimental animals or man results in increased protein accretion, decreased lipid deposition, improved food efficiency and increased galactopoiesis.

The importance of the pattern of GH secretion for the metabolic effects of the hormone is not fully understood. It has been shown that the total plasma phospholipid concentration, which is higher in females than in males, appears to be regulated by the GH secretory pattern since continuous, but not intermittent, GH treatment increases the phospholipid levels in hypophysectomized rats. Finally, the pattern of GH release explains the difference in serum levels of apolipoprotein E and cholesterol between the sexes in the rat.

The activity of several metabolic enzymes in the liver, including 5α-reductase, 5β-hydrolase, 16α-hydroxylase, carbonic anhydrase and serum cholinesterase, is also regulated by the pattern of GH secretion. The most dramatic effect is on the 16α-hydroxylase activity which is markedly elevated by the pattern of GH secretion. By intermittent GH administration the activity is increased and during continuous exposure the levels in hypophysectomized rats are decreased.

GH secretion also influences the concentration of other peptide hormone receptors. The prolactin receptor concentration in the liver is higher in female rats than in male rats: this has been shown to be due to the continuous GH release in the female rat. In contrast, the episodic secretion of GH in male rats increases the number of hepatic epidermal growth factor receptors. The ontogeny of GH secretion is discussed on p. 297.

The physiological significance of GH in adults has only recently been studied. Adults with *hypopituitarism* have so far received replacement therapy with thyroid hormones, adrenal and sex steroids, but not GH. However, the recent availability of recombinant GH has made it possible to study the effect of GH replacement therapy. Deficient adults are overweight, exhibit reduced bone mineral content and in social life show lower rates of employment and marriage. Replacement therapy with GH decreases body fat mass on average by 20 percent and adipose tissue was redistributed from abdominal to peripheral locations. Recent studies also show an increase of extracellular fluid volume, total body nitrogen, muscle volume and physical strength as well as vigor, ambition, sense of wellbeing and quality of life. By conventional replacement therapy with thyroid hormones, adrenal and sex steroids to hypopituitary patients, changes like decreased basal metabolic rate, cardiac output, glomerular filtration rate, and blood volume have not been restored. This may indicate yet other important physiological functions of GH extending into adult life.

The GH receptor and the GH binding protein

The biological actions of GH are initiated when GH binds to specific GH receptors on the plasma membrane of the target tissue. GH receptors have been detected in several tissues including the liver, kidney, heart, muscle, ovary and the epiphyseal growth plate. The human GH receptor was recently cloned and shown to be a protein consisting of 620 amino acids (aa) with a single transmembrane domain. The extracellular domain contains 246 aa, the transmembrane and the intracellular domain 24 and 350 aa respectively. The extracellular domain has five potential N-linked glycosylation sites and seven cysteine residues forming three disulfide bonds. The function of the unpaired cysteine, located close to the plasma membrane, is not yet fully understood but it could be involved in the receptor dimerization which may be essential to activation of the receptor or interaction with membrane-associated proteins.

The human GH receptor gene contains at least 10 exons, spanning more than 85 kb. The extracellular domain of the receptor is encoded by exons 3–7, the transmembrane domain by exon 8, and exons 9 and 10 encode the intracellular domain. The GH receptor is closely related to a superfamily of hormone peptide receptors including the prolactin receptor, receptors of interleukins 2, 3, 4, 5, 6, 7 and the granulocyte-macrophage colony stimulatory factor receptor as well as the erythropoietin receptor. Some experimental results suggest that subpopulations of slightly modified GH receptors may exist with different structures, binding characteristics or functions. These receptors are generated by alternative splicing of the GH receptor mRNA.

Studies in several species support the concept that the GH receptor is expressed at low levels at the time of birth with increased expression with age. GH receptors are present in some areas of the fetal brain, although their function remains suppositional.

In serum, a specific binding protein (BP) for GH has been found in several species, including man, rabbit, rat and mice. In the rabbit the binding protein has an amino acid sequence identical to the extracellular portion of the GH receptor and consequently could originate from proteolytic cleavage from the GH receptor. On the other hand, in rodents specific mRNA encoding the BP has been cloned. This transcript is homologous to the extracellular domain of the GH receptor but the transmembrane and the intracellular domains have been substituted by a short hydrophilic sequence. It was recently shown that circulating GHBP in rat is derived from an alternative spliced transcript of the GH receptor gene. It remains to be established by which mechanism the GHBP is generated *in vivo* in humans.

The function of the BP is not fully understood. In the rat the GHBP transcripts are coexpressed with the GH receptor in all analyzed tissues. Circulating GHBPs have been shown to attenuate GH plasma peaks, diminish the troughs of the GH secretion, and inhibit GH elimination from the blood. This implies that the physiological function of the BP may be to modulate the half-life of GH in serum or modulate the amount of free GH at the receptor of the target cell.

Laron syndrome or *GH resistance syndrome* is an autosomally recessive inherited disease which is characterized by growth failure, low serum IGF-I and increased GH secretion and resistance to GH therapy. Recently, it was shown that these patients lack serum GHBP and preparations of hepatic membranes have low GH binding activity. Such patients have mutations or deletions in the extracellular domain of the GH receptor. Theoretically, a mutation or deletion on the internal part of the GH receptor, which is thought to be of importance to the signaling mechanism, should also result in symptoms similar to the *Laron syndrome* and this may explain the recent observation that some children with this syndrome have normal levels of GHBP in their plasma.

The GH receptor is regulated by a number of factors. GH itself increases the number of GH receptors in liver, muscle, adipose tissue and in chondrocytes. Sex steroids enhance hepatic GH receptor number and thus may be one mechanism operative in the pubertal growth spurt. Thyroid hormone may also affect the GH receptor. Undernutrition is associated with a reduction in GH receptor number at least in the liver and this effect may be mediated by insulin.

The signaling mechanism of the GH receptor

The GH receptor sequence provided no evidence for earlier described signaling mechanisms (see p. 26) such as ATP/GTP binding sites or the presence of tyrosine kinase in the intracellular domain of the receptor, although GH has been demonstrated to stimulate tyrosine phosphorylation of the receptor.

Recently, the crystal structure of the extracellular domain of the human GH receptor with bound GH was identified and has been used to infer the mechanism of GH–GH receptor interaction. The complex consists of one GH molecule and two molecules of the GH receptor. Moreover, there was also a substantial contact surface between the carboxyl-terminal domains of the receptors, providing a mechanism for receptor dimerization. The current hypothesis is that the receptor dimerization is the first step in GH action. Thus it may be that GHBP could be involved in the signaling mechanism by complexing with GH bound to the membrane-anchored GH receptor. Cytosolic GHBP has also been shown present in many cells and is identical in structure to the circulating GHBP. Immunoreactive GH receptor or GHBP have been found in the nuclei of several cell types, suggesting that GHBP could be involved in GH regulation of nuclear events.

Another possible mechanism is that the GH–GH receptor/BP complex interacts with a transmembrane protein which then transmits the signal to the nucleus through a mechanism such as tyrosine phosphorylation. Such heterodimeric receptor protein interaction is used by IL-2.

GH regulation of tissue growth

The absence of *in vitro* effects of GH resulted in the hypothesis that GH acts primarily on the liver and that the liver, in response to GH action, produces somatomedins (later renamed the insulin-like growth factors or IGFs) which are released into the blood stream. Although many of the *in vivo* effects of GH can be mimicked by IGF-I, there are several points of discrepancy between their actions.

By studying the growth, differentiation and proliferation of preadipose cells, Green and co-workers (1985) made the important observation that GH has a specific stimulatory effect on preadipocyte cell conversion to adipocytes, which forms the basis of the 'dual effector theory'. According to this theory GH stimulates the differentiation of progenitor cells which subsequently become responsive to growth factors like insulin-like growth factor I (Fig. 5.5). The role of the IGFs is discussed in detail on p. 180.

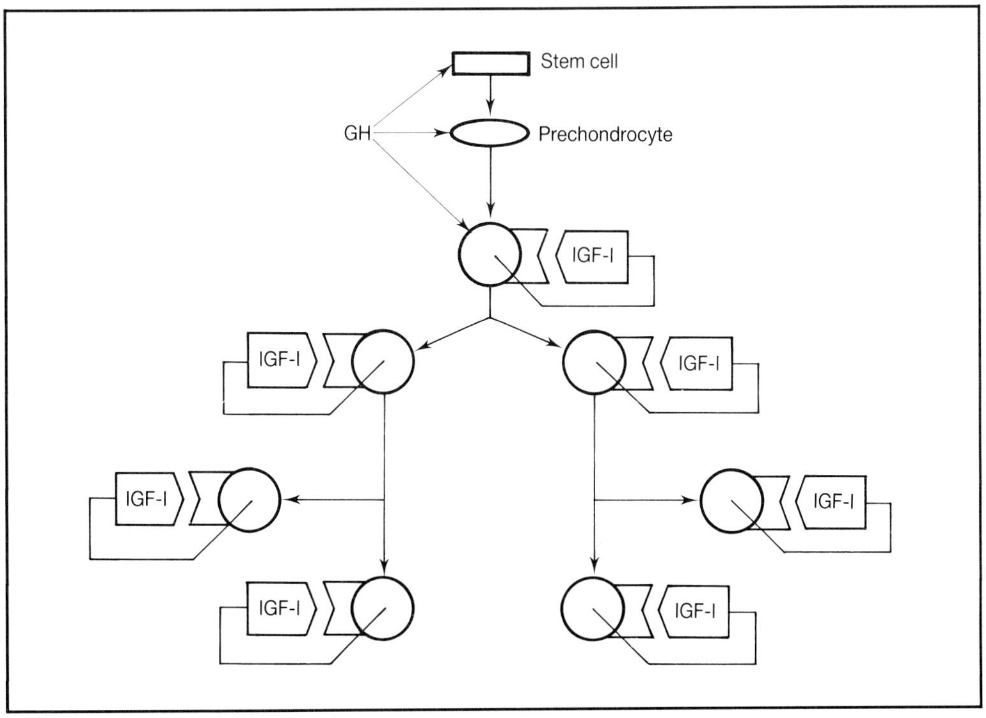

Fig. 5.5. A hypothetical model of GH action on the longitudinal bone growth, based on the dual effector theory.

The epiphyseal growth plate and longitudinal bone growth

A large number of hormones and nutritional factors affect mammalian growth but only GH has been shown to stimulate postnatal longitudinal bone growth in a specific and dose-dependent manner. In humans complete lack of GH, such as in *GH deficiency type Ia* due to a gene deletion, results in a final height of 120–130 cm while overproduction of GH leads to *gigantism* before puberty or *acromegaly* in adults.

Longitudinal bone growth is the result of cell proliferation in the epiphyseal growth plates which are located in the proximal and distal part of the long bones (Fig. 5.6). The growth plate has a strict cellular organization with the germinative, proliferative, hypertrophic and degenerative cell layers. The germinative cell layer consists of rarely dividing cells, i.e. stem cells or progenitor cells. During the process of growth, stem cells initiate their program of differentiation and enter the proliferative cell layer, where frequent cellular divisions occur, forming continual cell columns. Subsequently, these cells stop dividing, mature and hypertrophy in the hypertrophic cell layer. Finally the chondrocytes degenerate and the matrix becomes a site for calcium deposition. As new progenitor cells continuously start their program of differentiation, the growth plate could be regarded as a constantly renewing tissue pushing the bony epiphysis further away from the center of the long bone.

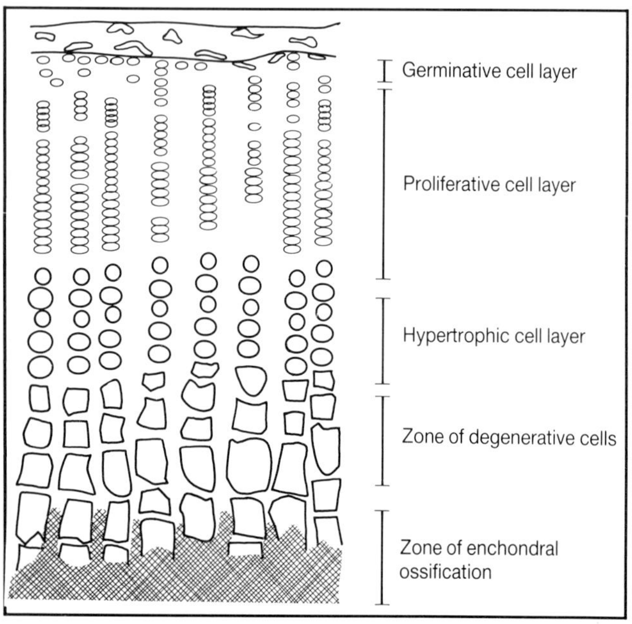

Fig. 5.6. A schematic presentation of the proximal tibial growth plate and its cellular organization.

Bone growth is the result of the recruitment of new cells from the stem cell layer and the number of cell divisions in the proliferative cell layer together with increasing size of cells within the hypertrophic cell layer. Under normal conditions the rate of stem cell recruitment, the cell proliferation and the mineralization are in balance, retaining the same thickness of the growth plate.

GH action on longitudinal bone has mostly been studied in hypophysectomized rats. In this animal model it has been shown that locally injected, or locally infused, GH results in unilateral bone growth without a concomitant rise in serum IGF-I. Local GH treatment resulted also in local expression of IGF-I mRNA as well as increased presence of IGF-I protein. By co-infusing IGF-I antibodies with GH locally, the growth stimulation of GH was abolished. *In vitro*, culture of epiphyseal growth plate chondrocytes derived from GH-treated hypophysectomized rats showed increased response to IGF-I in subsequent culture. The application of the dual effector theory to these findings forms the basis for the proposed mechanism of action for GH on the epiphyseal growth plate. GH preferentially acts on the prechondrocytes, or young differentiating chondrocytes, in the germinative cell layer that have a high potential to divide. During the process of differentiation the cells become responsive to IGF-I and the gene encoding IGF-I is expressed, resulting in local IGF-I production. As a result IGF-I stimulates the differentiating cells by an autocrine or paracrine mechanism.

Skeletal muscle

In skeletal muscle, it has been demonstrated that GH stimulates growth by increasing the number of cells rather than the cell size. Thus, GH stimulates DNA replication in skeletal muscle. In analogy with GH effects on prechondrocytes, according to the dual effector theory it is possible that GH interacts with skeletal muscle progenitor cells. The proposed progenitor cells for myoblasts are the satellite cells. However, it remains to be determined whether GH can interact directly with these cells. *In vitro*, it has been demonstrated that the differentiation of a cell line of myoblasts and the expression of myotubes were GH dependent.

The role of IGF-I in muscle growth is not yet clarified. Several *in vitro* studies have demonstrated effects of IGF-I on a number of anabolic processes related to increased muscle mass or function, including stimulatory effects on proliferation and promotion of differentiation of myoblasts to myotubes following cell division. *In vivo* IGF-I has been shown to stimulate skeletal muscle protein synthesis and inhibit breakdown.

Studies regarding muscle regeneration in rats following ischemic injury have revealed increased expression of GH receptor mRNA and also increased expression of IGF-I, both on messenger and protein level, indicating a role for both GH and IGF-I during muscle regeneration. However, in regenerating muscle of hypophysectomized rats, IGF-I expression was also seen, suggesting that production of IGF-I may in part be independent of GH during certain conditions.

Adipose tissue

Apart from its effects on somatic growth, GH is also an important regulator of intermediary metabolism. *GH deficiency* results in an increase of body fat, whereas excessive levels of GH, as in *acromegaly*, result in a decrease in body fat. When *GH-deficient* patients are treated with GH, there is a decrease in total adipose tissue. Moreover, the distribution of adipose tissue was affected since subcutaneous adipose tissue was decreased less than visceral adipose tissue.

A number of studies have demonstrated that GH regulates the number of fat cells. This is illustrated in patients with short stature secondary to *GH deficiency* who, despite large total fat cell mass, exhibit a low number of fat cells. The same relation has been found in hypophysectomized rats where GH administration results in a reduced total fat cell mass and an increased fat cell number. Mature adipocytes are regarded as terminally differentiated cells unable to proliferate. Thus, increased fat cell number is the result of recruitment of cells from a preadipocyte population. During the process of adipose conversion a marked change in the cellular phenotype occurs. Synthesis of structural and membrane proteins is reduced, enzymes responsible for triglyceride synthesis are induced and hormonal sensitivity is modified. This process of fat cell differentiation has been extensively studied during experimental conditions and the velocity of the process has been found to be GH dependent. Pretreatment of preadipose cells with GH increases the responsiveness of the cells to subsequently added IGF-I in terms of thymidine incorporation and the rate of adipose conversion, thus demonstrating that IGF-I was more effective at a later stage of differentiation.

Concluding remarks

It is thus clear that both GH and IGF-I have important biological functions for the promotion of somatic growth. However, it remains to be established that the dual effector theory is applicable to all GH-dependent tissues. Assuming that this mechanism of action of GH is a generalized phenomenon, IGF-I, either locally produced or circulating, may not substitute for the effect of GH on progenitor cells and consequently may have a more limited ability to stimulate growth. On the other hand, IGF-I expression has been demonstrated in regenerating tissues in hypophysectomized animals indicating that some IGF-I is produced locally independent of GH.

Selected reading

Daughaday WH, Rotwein P. Insulin-like growth factors I and II. Peptide, messenger ribonucleic acid and gene structures, serum and tissue concentrations. *Endocr Rev* 1989; **10**: 68.

Green H, Morikawa M, Nixon T. A dual effector theory of growth hormone action. *Differentiation* 1985; **29**: 195.

Isaksson OGP, Lindahl A, Nilsson A, Isgaard J. Mechanism of the stimulatory effect of growth hormone on longitudinal bone growth. *Endocr Rev* 1987; **8**: 426.

Laron Z, Pertzelan A, Karp M, Kowadlo-Silbergeld A, Daughaday WH. Administration of growth hormone to patients with familial dwarfism with high plasma immunoreactive growth hormone: measurement of sulfation factor, metabolic and linear growth responses. *J Clin Endocrinol Metab* 1971; **33**: 332.

C3. Insulin-like Growth Factors

W F Blum

The discovery of insulin-like growth factors (IGF) is based on an observation in 1957 that the stimulatory effect of growth hormone (GH) on sulfate incorporation into cartilage matrix is mediated by a soluble substance termed 'sulfation factor'. During the following years multiple GH-dependent factors were identified which were designated 'somatomedins' and subsequently were renamed insulin-like growth factors in view of their evolutionary relationship to insulin. The isolation of pure peptides revealed the existence of two major peptides, IGF-I and IGF-II. Somatomedins A and C were shown to be identical with IGF-I and multiplication stimulating activity (MSA) was recognized as the rat homolog of IGF-II. IGFs have pivotal roles in the regulation of proliferation, differentiation and specific functions of many cell types and in regulating body growth and metabolism.

In contrast to many other peptide hormones, especially those with short-term metabolic effects, IGFs are noncovalently bound to specific binding proteins (IGFBP). Only about 1 percent of circulating IGFs exist in their free form.

Biochemistry

IGF-I and IGF-II

IGF-I and IGF-II are single-chain polypeptides with 62 percent sequence homology. IGF-I is a basic peptide of 70 amino acids (mol. wt=7649). IGF-II is a slightly acidic peptide of 67 amino acids (mol. wt=7471). Both are about 30 percent homologous to proinsulin. By analogy to proinsulin their amino acid sequences can be divided into domains B, C, A and a short extension D at the C-terminus. The major sequence differences are in the C-peptide region. Several variant forms are described which may arise from alternative splicing of the primary gene transcript, incomplete processing of the prohormone, or proteolytic cleavage of the mature peptide. A truncated IGF-I form, lacking the first three amino acids, is a potent stimulator of IGF-I specific effects and has been identified in neural extracts and in colostrum. However, it does only weakly bind to some IGFBPs.

Different regions of the molecules are involved in the binding to the IGF type I and type II receptors and also to IGFBPs. Both IGFs are synthesized as prepropeptides with a molecular size of approximately 20–22 kDa. Processing of the propeptide includes cleavage of the so-called E-domain which extends the length of the mature IGF peptides at the C-terminus. Pro-IGF forms are present in the circulation in certain clinical situations, e.g. *chronic renal failure* or in *non-islet cell tumor induced hypoglycemia* (NICTH) which is caused by large tumors that produce excessive amounts of IGF-II.

IGF binding proteins

Six classes of IGFBPs (IGFBP-1 to 6) have been identified. They show a high degree of sequence homology (about 40 percent) especially within the N- and C-terminal regions where a relatively large number of cysteines is conserved. Biochemical characteristics of the various IGFBPs are listed in Table 5.2. IGFBP-1 and IGFBP-2 contain an Arg-Gly-Asp (single letter code: RGD) sequence near the C-terminal which is thought to facilitate binding

Table 5.2. Biochemical characteristics of the human IGF binding proteins

IGFBP	Amino acids	Mol. wt (kDa)	Cysteine	Glycosylation	RGD sequence
IGFBP-1	259	28.1	18	–	+
IGFBP-2	289	31.3	18	–	+
IGFBP-3	264	28.7[1]	18	+	–
IGFBP-4	237	26.3	20	+	–
IGFBP-5	252	28.6	18	+	–
IGFBP-6	216	22.8	16	+	–

[1] Glycosylated molecular weight 42–45 kDa.

to integrin receptors on the cell surface. Cell-surface adherent IGFBPs may modulate IGF-receptor interactions. IGFBP-4, IGFBP-5 and IGFBP-6 contain glycosylation sites. The carbohydrate moieties do not affect IGF binding to IGFBP-3, although they may influence interactions with the cell surface or the metabolic clearance. A further mechanism of post-translational modification of IGFBPs is phosphorylation which may modulate the affinity of the IGFBPs for IGFs.

IGFBP-2 and IGFBP-6 preferentially bind IGF-II whilst the other IGFBPs have a similar affinity for either IGF peptide. The affinity constants compare with the affinity constants of the IGF-I and IGF-II receptor. The association of IGFBP-3, the major circulating IGFBP, with either IGF is rapid. In contrast, the dissociation reaction is extremely slow with a half-time in the range of 17 hours. Despite this very slow dissociation rate physiological concentrations of free IGF would be restored within 10–30 minutes due to the high levels of the IGF/IGFBP-3 complex in the circulation. Although the mass action law could explain the release of IGF from the complex, it may be facilitated by specific proteases or by binding of glycosaminoglycans.

IGFBP-3 is unique among the IGF binding proteins in that after association with either IGF-I or IGF-II it is then able to bind a so-called acid-labile subunit (ALS) thus constituting a large molecular weight ternary complex of 125–150 kDa. ALS is a single-chain protein with a molecular size of 70 kDa and is glycosylated, resulting in a total molecular weight of 84–86 kDa. Although its affinity for the IGF/IGFBP-3 complex is clearly lower than the affinity of IGF for IGFBP-3, most of the IGF in the circulation is found in the large molecular weight range. This is caused by an excess of ALS which promotes the rapid formation of the ternary complex as soon as IGFs have bound to IGFBP-3.

In addition the extramembranous portion of the type II receptor is found in the circulation. This binds only IGF-II and is particularly high in fetal blood. Whether it acts as a further form of binding protein is unclear.

Molecular biology

The IGF-I gene is located on the long arm of chromosome 12 and the gene for IGF-II at the end of the short arm of chromosome 11 contiguous to the insulin gene. Both genes are remarkably long and complex as compared to other peptide hormones. The IGF-I gene spans about 95 kb and contains six exons. Multiple mRNAs are found due to the alternative use of different exons, alternative splicing of the primary transcript and to variable polyadenylation at the 3′ end of the mRNAs. The mature IGF-I peptide is encoded by exons 3 and 4: exons 1 and 2 are used alternatively leading to class 1 or class 2 mRNAs. Most of the E-domain is encoded by exons 5 and 6. By alternative splicing of the primary transcript either of these two exons is used resulting in two propeptides with different E-domains, Eb and Ea respectively. The human IGF-II gene spans 35 kb and contains nine exons and four promotors adjacent to exons 1, 4, 5 and 6 at their 5′ ends. The mature IGF-II peptide is encoded by exons 7 and 8 and part of exon 9. Various mRNAs differing in length are found due to the alternative use of the various promotors and their adjacent exons.

The physiological meaning of the heterogeneity of IGF mRNAs is not fully understood but it may be relevant for the post-transcriptional regulation of IGFs. Large IGF-I mRNAs have a shorter half-life than smaller variants and the use of alternative 5′ sequences leads to different leader peptides which may be important for alternative targeting of the translation products. The concept that the heterogeneity of IGF mRNAs is physiologically relevant is supported by findings which show that the mRNA patterns are tissue and development specific.

Regulation

The regulation of IGFs is very complex owing to (1) the involvement of multiple regulatory factors, (2) their endocrine and paracrine modes of action and (3) the importance of IGFBPs for maintenance of physiological concentrations. While the regulation of circulating IGFs and IGFBPs may differ from local regulation, the major regulators of IGF-I (GH and nutrition) elicit a similar influence at both levels.

The regulation of circulating IGF-I and IGF-II cannot be regarded independently from IGFBPs. The most abundant IGFBP in blood is IGFBP-3, which represents 90 percent of total circulating IGFBP in children and adults. A molar 1:1 ratio between total IGF (IGF-I plus IGF-II) and IGFBP-3 is found in the circulation in all situations except *chronic renal failure*. The reason why this 1:1 ratio is observed is that the metabolic half-life of free IGF-I and IGF-II is very short (4–15 minutes). Therefore only

IGFBP-bound IGFs remain in the circulation. Consequently, total IGF-I and IGF-II serum levels are primarily determined by the IGFBP-3 levels. As IGF-I and IGF-II may displace each other from IGFBP-3, the ratio of IGF-I and IGF-II may be quite variable.

While the kidneys are not a primary site of IGF clearance, renal function plays a major role in the removal of IGFBPs from the circulation. In *chronic renal failure* IGF-I and IGF-II levels are normal and IGFBPs are markedly elevated due to the accumulation of small molecular weight forms.

The plasma levels of both IGFs and the IGFBPs show age dependence but the patterns are quite different for each peptide (see Fig. 5.7).

IGF-I

Growth hormone

The major hormonal regulator of IGF-I, both in the circulation and in peripheral tissues, is GH. IGF-I serum levels are decreased in *GH deficiency* (GHD) and are increased in *acromegaly*. Administration of GH in patients with GHD, or in GH-deficient animals, produces a marked increase of IGF-I in the blood maximal after 12–24 hours due to induction of hepatic IGF-I synthesis. In addition, IGF-I expression is stimulated in multiple tissues including epiphyseal cartilage, which may be of particular importance for longitudinal growth (see p. 178). As in many other hormonal regulatory systems there is a negative feedback loop mediated by IGFs on GH secretion at both the hypophyseal and hypothalamic levels. Thus in *undernutrition* or in *Laron syndrome* where there is GH resistance, IGF-I levels are low and circulating GH is high.

In patients with *hyperprolactinemia* normal IGF-I levels may be found despite obvious insufficient GH secretion. This can be explained by the weak affinity of PRL to the GH receptor.

Other adenohypophyseal hormones

Other pituitary hormones besides GH or PRL have no direct influence on IGF-I serum levels. They are, however, involved in the regulation of paracrine IGF-I synthesis in their specific target cells. TSH stimulates IGF-I production by thyroid follicular cells; LH (or hCG) stimulates IGF-I expression in granulosa and Leydig cells; FSH stimulates IGF-I in granulosa and Sertoli cells. This effect is mediated by cAMP and is modulated by the presence of other peptide growth factors.

Patients with *hypothyroidism* have impaired IGF-I serum levels that increase upon thyroxine substitution. The thyroxine effect is thought to act via the stimulation of GH secretion. In *hyperthyroidism* IGF-I levels are unchanged.

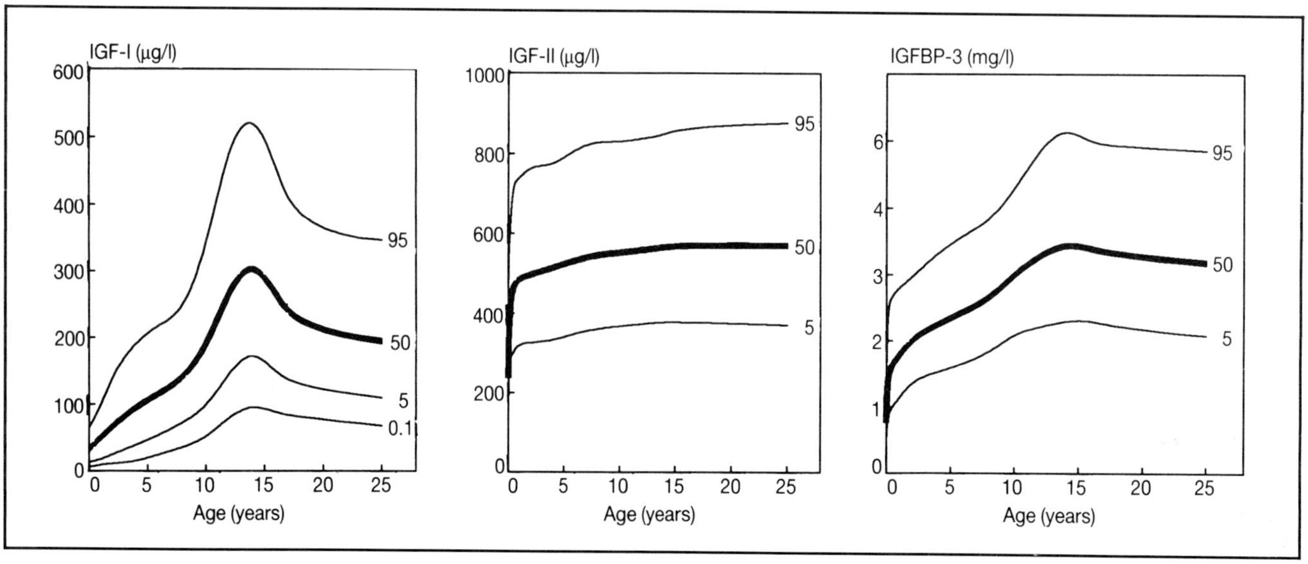

Fig. 5.7. Age-dependent normal ranges of IGF-I, IGF-II and IGFBP-3 serum levels.

Steroidal influences

Low dose estrogen replacement therapy in *hypogonadal* patients increases serum IGF-I, possibly through the stimulation of the GH secretion. On the other hand, pharmacological doses of estrogens suppress IGF-I levels in normal individuals or in patients with *acromegaly*. This effect may be due to a direct inhibition of IGF-I expression in the liver as shown experimentally. From a clinical point of view it may also be relevant with respect to treatment of girls with *tall stature* with high doses of estrogens in order to reduce final height. In contrast to the liver, IGF-I expression is stimulated by estrogens in the uterus underlining the divergent regulation of circulating IGF-I and local IGF-I production. In humans no direct effect of androgens upon IGF-I serum levels has been demonstrated. The increase observed in hypogonadal patients after androgen treatment is thought to be secondary to an increase of GH secretion. Also, the stimulatory effect of oxandrolone, an anabolic drug which is widely used in patients with *constitutional delay of growth and adolescence* to improve height velocity, may be explained by its weak androgenic activity.

In patients with *Cushing syndrome* or during chronic high dose corticosteroid therapy, IGF-I levels are normal or slightly elevated, contrasting with impaired growth, and suggesting glucocorticoids inhibit the effects of IGF-I. In addition there may be local effects as suggested by suppression of IGF-I production in osteoblast cell cultures.

Other hormonal influences

PTH induces IGF-I synthesis in osteoblasts or bone tissue culture. However, it does not influence IGF-I serum levels.

IGF-I serum levels are decreased in untreated *diabetes mellitus* and normalize upon insulin treatment. It appears that insulin has a permissive effect on GH-stimulated IGF-I production in the liver and other tissues perhaps by affecting the GH receptor.

There are a variety of paracrine peptide growth factors that stimulate local IGF-I production alone or in combination with tropic hormones (see p. 155). These include platelet derived growth factor (PDGF), epidermal growth factor (EGF), transforming growth factor α (TGFα), and basic fibroblast growth factor (bFGF). TGFβ has inhibitory and stimulatory effects.

Nutritional factors

The second most potent regulator of IGF-I serum levels besides GH is the nutritional status. IGF-I declines exponentially during fasting within a few days and is restored upon refeeding. This decrease is caused by a reduction of hepatic IGF-I gene expression which is also seen in nonhepatic tissues. Both protein and calorie intake play a role. If in human adults the daily caloric intake falls below a threshold of 12 kcal/kg, insensitivity to GH develops secondary to a decrease of GH receptor density and impairment of post-GH receptor events. IGF-I measurements can therefore be used to monitor nutritional status.

Other influences on IGF-I secretion

In patients with *sepsis* IGF-I serum levels and IGF-I production in the liver decline and cannot be restored by GH administration. This may be due to a decrease in hepatic GH receptor density in the liver due to tumor necrosis factor (TNF). In patients with large *solid tumors* or with *leukemia*, IGF-I levels are significantly decreased and normalize during chemotherapy despite severe nutritional problems and cytotoxicity due to the treatment. This finding again indicates possible regulation of IGF-I by so far unknown immunological factors.

From experimental studies it is known that lesions of various tissues including muscles, tendons, nerves, blood vessel endothelium, kidney, and subcutaneous or epidermal cells cause a local transient increase of IGF-I production lasting about 3–5 weeks. Moreover, IGF-I may be released at the site of the lesion by platelets or macrophages. These findings suggest an important role of IGF-I in wound healing. Despite the local stimulation of IGF-I synthesis at the site of tissue lesions, IGF-I serum levels decline in severely traumatized patients, or after severe abdominal surgery, within a few days and are slowly restored within 2–3 weeks. This decline occurs even under calorically adequate parenteral nutrition. The mechanisms that are involved in this down-regulation are unclear.

As the liver is the main source of circulating IGFs and also IGFBPs it is therefore not surprising that IGF-I serum levels decline in liver disease. A significant correlation is found with conventional indicators of liver function.

IGF-II

Little is known about the regulation of IGF-II. This may in part be due to the divergent developmental patterns of IGF-II in different species. Whereas in the rat, for example, IGF-II serum levels decline postpartum to almost unmeasurable concentrations, they rapidly increase in humans during the first few weeks of life (Fig. 5.7). This makes the extrapolation of experimental findings in animal studies to the human situation difficult. A second problem arises from the fact that IGF concentrations in blood are largely determined by the IGFBP-3 levels. This is especially true for IGF-II which follows closely the IGFBP-3 concentration in many situations. It is therefore difficult to recognize whether IGF-II levels are directly controlled by a certain factor or whether any changes are secondary to variations of the binding proteins.

While GH is a firmly established regulator of IGF-I and IGFBP-3, it is doubtful that it also directly regulates IGF-II serum levels. In *growth hormone deficiency* IGF-II serum concentrations are decreased and they increase during GH treatment following the increase of IGFBP-3. In contrast, in normal individuals a transient decrease of IGF-II levels is observed upon high dose GH treatment, probably due to the displacement from IGFBP-3 by IGF-I. Moreover, in patients with *acromegaly* IGF-II levels are normal. In various other conditions IGF-II serum levels are diminished, closely paralleling the pattern of the decrease of IGFBP-3 rather than IGF-I: fasting or *malnutrition*, *malignancies*, trauma, severe surgical trauma, and *hepatic insufficiency*.

An increase of IGF-II mRNA following GH administration was found in rat brain, skeletal and cardiac muscle, whereas hepatic mRNA remained unchanged. Cortisol suppressed IGF-II mRNA in the liver. In human fetal adrenals and human granulosa cells, ACTH and FSH respectively stimulated IGF-II expression. These findings and others suggest that at least locally produced IGF-II may indeed be subject to the regulation of various hormonal factors.

IGF binding proteins

A most striking feature of IGFBP-1, IGFBP-2 and IGFBP-3 is that their control is quite independent, suggesting different biological functions of these peptides. Knowledge on the regulation of IGFBP-4, IGFBP-5, IGFBP-6 is still sparse.

IGFBP-1

Basal circulating IGFBP-1 levels are high at birth (in humans mean 0.070 mg/l), decline until adolescence (mean 0.016 mg/l) and increase again with aging. In contrast to IGFBP-2 and IGFBP-3, IGFBP-1 levels exhibit a marked circadian fluctuation with high levels at night which depend on food intake. Fasting causes a rapid rise of IGFBP-1 whilst refeeding suppresses IGFBP-1 levels. An increase of IGFBP-1 can also be induced by extreme physical exercise. These changes are related to the secretion of insulin which strongly impairs IGFBP-1 gene expression. Experimental evidence suggests that the insulin effect is mediated by the availability of intracellular glucose. As a consequence, IGFBP-1 levels are significantly increased in *diabetes mellitus* and decline upon successful treatment.

IGF-I has a similar suppressive effect to insulin. There is an inverse relationship between IGFBP-1 and GH secretion. Local production of IGFBP-1 may be controlled by other factors such as progesterone and relaxin, e.g. in the decidualized cells of the endometrium.

IGFBP-2

The age-dependent pattern of IGFBP-2 serum levels resembles that of IGFBP-1, although absolute levels are higher by an order of magnitude. There is, however, no circadian variation and insulin does not appear to have a major effect on IGFBP-2 levels. However, like IGFBP-1, IGFBP-2 shows an inverse relationship with the GH status. Interestingly, IGF-I administration to humans has an opposite effect, resulting in a moderate increase. A major regulator appears to be IGF-II which strongly binds to IGFBP-2. In patients with *non-islet cell tumor induced hypoglycemia* secreting large amounts of IGF-II or its prohormone forms, IGFBP-2 levels are excessively elevated and can be used as a diagnostic marker.

IGFBP-3

In contrast to IGFBP-1 and IGFBP-2, IGFBP-3 serum levels are low at birth. They rise rapidly during the first few weeks of life and show a peak at the time of puberty (see Fig. 5.7). There is no circadian rhythm. The regulation of IGFBP-3 serum levels resembles in many aspects the regulation of IGF-I. The major regulator is GH. Levels are decreased in GHD and normalize upon treatment with GH within several days. On the other hand, IGFBP-3 levels are markedly elevated in *acromegaly* and normalize after successful therapy. Although *in vitro* studies suggest that IGF-I may directly stimulate IGFBP-3 production, IGF-I administration to normal humans, patients with GHD or patients with *GH receptor deficiency (Laron syndrome)* does not affect IGFBP-3 serum levels, indicating that the GH effect on circulating IGFBP-3 is not mediated by IGF-I.

Minor influences upon IGFBP-3 levels are exerted by thyroid hormones which may act via GH. The absence of sex steroids has no influence whereas in *precocious puberty* IGFBP-3 levels are markedly increased. Whether this effect is due to increased GH secretion remains unclear. In *Cushing syndrome* IGFBP-3 levels are slightly increased, suggesting some regulatory influence of corticosteroids. IGFBP-3 concentrations are decreased by a number of nonhormonal factors, although the kinetics of the changes are slower and not as pronounced as with IGF-I: the conditions include fasting, polytrauma, severe surgical trauma, large tumors, *leukemia*, and impaired hepatic function.

Actions of the IGFs

IGF receptors

Both IGF-I and IGF-II act through membrane-bound receptors on the cell surface. Two classes of IGF receptors can be distinguished. The type I IGF receptor (or IGF-I receptor) consists of a heterotetramer and is highly homologous to the insulin receptor. The type II IGF receptor (or IGF-II receptor) consists of a single chain peptide which is identical to the cation-independent mannose-6-phosphate receptor. Both receptors are substantially glycosylated in the extracellular domains. Both IGF-I and IGF-II cross-react with the insulin receptor. Their affinities, however, are about 100-fold lower than the affinity of insulin which makes possible interactions unlikely under physiological conditions.

IGF-I receptor

The gene is located on chromosome 15. The receptor is synthesized as a precursor protein consisting of 1337 amino acids with the α-domain at the amino terminus. Processing of the proreceptor involves proteolytic cleavage leaving two subunits, α and β (mol. wt 100–135 kDa and 90–95 kDa, respectively), that are linked by disulfide bridges. While the α-subunit is localized extracellularly, the β-subunit spans the cell membrane carrying a tyrosine kinase domain at the cytoplasmic portion. For full receptor activity the dimerization of two αβ-hemireceptor molecules is required. The affinity for IGFs and insulin decreases in the order IGF-I > IGF-II >> insulin. There is some receptor heterogeneity in various tissues, possibly due to different post-translational processing, which causes variability in the binding affinities for IGF-I and IGF-II.

The understanding of the events that take place after receptor activation by IGF is still vague. By analogy to the insulin receptor, tyrosine kinase seems to play a pivotal role. On binding of the ligand the β-subunit is autophosphorylated by an intramolecular reaction activating tyrosine kinase. There is evidence that further signal transmission involves stimulation of phospholipase C generating 1,2-diacylglycerol and inositol 1,4,5-triphosphate as second messengers. Also, interactions with the adenylate cyclase system may occur. After binding of IGFs to the type I receptor, phosphorylation of various intracellular proteins is observed.

IGF-II receptor

The gene is located on chromosome 19 and the receptor protein is expressed in virtually every cell type. The single-chain polypeptide has a calculated molecular mass of 270 kDa. There is a short hydrophobic membrane-spanning domain and an unusually short cytoplasmic portion. Ninety-two percent of the receptor is extracellular, consisting of 15 conserved repeats. Confusingly, the receptor bears two binding sites for two totally unrelated ligands: one for mannose 6-phosphate (Man 6-P), which serves as a recognition marker for lysosomal enzymes, and one for IGF-II. Its affinity for IGF-I is lower by two orders of magnitude and is virtually absent for insulin. The role of this receptor in targeting acidic hydrolases from the *trans*-Golgi network, or from the cell surface to lysosomes, is well established. Less clear is the significance of IGF-II binding to the same protein. Since IGF-II impaired binding of Man-6-P labeled peptides, it has been speculated that IGF-II may be involved in the control of lysosomal enzymes that are secreted into the extracellular compartment during tissue remodeling. The type II receptor is also found in the circulation particularly in the fetus where it may act as an IGF-II specific binding protein.

Most IGF-II effects appear to be mediated via the IGF-I receptor. Scattered evidence, however, suggests that at least in some cell types activation of the IGF-II receptor is involved in IGF-II stimulated DNA synthesis or specific cellular functions. These observations are supported by the finding that the short cytoplasmic portion of the receptor contains a binding domain for G_i-proteins, in particular for the G_i-2α-subunit. G_i-2 directly induces calcium influx through a voltage-independent cation channel. Activation of G_i-2 is inhibited by Man-6-P binding to the receptor which may provide a basis for the modulating effects of Man-6-P containing growth factors (e.g. TGFβ). It was further shown that IGF-II activates phospholipase C via the IGF-II receptor inducing an increase of inositol triphosphate and 1,2-diacylglycerol generation.

Physiological role of IGFs

IGF-I and IGF-II influence a multitude of cell types of ectodermal, mesodermal and entodermal origin by stimulating (1) proliferation, (2) differentiation, (3) specific cell functions and (4) insulin-like metabolic effects. Examples where IGFs promote differentiation are myoblasts, chondroblasts, osteoblasts, neuroblasts, preadipocytes, lens cells and hematopoietic cells. Examples where IGFs stimulate specific functions of differentiated cells include the synthesis of proteoglycans and collagens by chondrocytes, steroidogenesis in gonadal cells, synthesis of thyroid hormones in thyroidal cells, or seemingly remote actions such as potentiation of natural killer cell activity. Many of these effects are of utmost importance in the growing organism. *In vivo* administration of IGF-I in animal models or in patients with *Laron syndrome* resulted in a clear promotion of linear growth.

The diversity of cells that respond to IGFs and of the responses that are promoted by these peptides raises the question of the physiological significance of such apparently unspecific signals. In particular, what is the information transmitted to the cells by IGFs? An answer cannot be given without considering the bimodal nature of IGF action: 'autocrine/paracrine' versus 'endocrine'. An autocrine/paracrine mode of action means that IGFs elicit their effects at or in the near vicinity of their site of production. This view is supported by a number of findings:

1. IGF-I and IGF-II are synthesized in many tissues and by many cell types, especially in cells of mesodermal origin.
2. Their local expression is developmentally regulated.
3. The regulation of local IGF synthesis is subject to tissue-specific hormonal or to nonhormonal factors.
4. Local application of IGF-I promotes tissue repair or hypertrophy.

An endocrine mode of action means that IGFs are transported by the blood stream to a distant site of action. Evidence in favor of this view includes:

1. While the main source of circulating IGFs is the hepatocyte, these cells are poor in IGF-I receptors, suggesting that they are not a target for locally produced IGF-I.
2. Blood has the highest concentrations of IGF-I and, in humans, of IGF-II.
3. Systemic application of IGF-I has metabolic effects, e.g. nitrogen retention, and promotes growth in the absence of GH, e.g. in *Laron syndrome*.
4. Blood-borne IGF-I is rapidly transferred to peripheral tissues, where it is unevenly distributed mainly to functionally active cells.

Obviously, both modes of IGF action, autocrine/paracrine and endocrine, are of importance and the question is, how both perspectives can be reconciled to obtain a comprehensive understanding.

A general feature of IGFs is that they primarily act on cells which are ready to proliferate or to perform a specific function. This particular status of a cell may be triggered by specific signals such as other peptide growth factors or tissue-specific tropic hormones. This view may be exemplified by the proliferation of fibroblasts. Quiescent fibroblasts are rather unresponsive to IGF-I. If these quiescent fibroblasts are exposed to so-called 'competence factors' like platelet derived growth factor (PDGF) or basic fibroblast growth factor (bFGF), they become competent for proliferation. That is, the cells enter into the phase G_1 of the cell cycle. To further traverse through G_1 into the S-phase, where DNA replication takes place, requires the presence of so-called 'progression factors', particularly IGF-I. The overall observable effect of IGF-I on the proliferation of quiescent fibroblasts would then be a synergistic potentiation of the mitogenic effect of PDGF or bFGF.

Similarly, IGF-I is synergistic with FSH, LH and hCG to promote steroidogenesis in granulosa cells, ovarian theca-interstitial cells, Leydig cells and Sertoli cells; with TSH to stimulate thyroid hormone synthesis in thyroid derived cells; with erythropoietin to stimulate erythropoiesis; with granulocyte-monocyte colony stimulating factor to stimulate granulopoiesis; with interleukin-2 to stimulate natural killer cells and also with several other systems. It is thus evident that the IGFs are part of a complex interplay of diverse regulatory factors. A number of tropic hormones stimulate IGF expression in their target tissues (see above), thereby generating an auxiliary mechanism to potentiate their local effects (Fig. 5.8).

How do circulating IGFs fit into this scenario? Blood-borne IGFs may further increase local concentrations in the interstitial compartments. The major regulators of IGF-I in the blood are food intake and GH. IGF-I therefore provides information on the nutritional status of the organism at the cellular level. For cells which have become competent for proliferation it would be inappropriate to proliferate at a maximal rate if nutrient supply is insufficient due to chronic malnutrition. Decreases in IGF-I may thus decelerate mitosis or other cellular functions and adapt cellular activity to the nutritional situation. GH, on the other hand, integrates signals from the central nervous system (CNS) and the GH-IGF axis may therefore serve as a line of communication from the CNS down to the peripheral tissues. This may be exemplified by *psychosocial growth retardation*. If a child is raised in an unfavorable social environment, GH secretion becomes insufficient and consequently, IGF-I serum levels decline, resulting in poor growth. In summary, circulating IGFs and in particular IGF-I may provide information at the cellular level about the nutritional and environmental status of the organism and coordinate the whole body metabolic state (see Fig. 5.8).

Physiological role of IGFBPs

Direct evidence for one or the other physiological role of the IGFBPs is still scarce but it appears that the various proteins have distinct functions. This is suggested by (1) their largely divergent patterns in different compartments, (2) their different developmental patterns and (3) their different regulation by hormonal or nonhormonal factors. While IGFBP-3 is by far the most abundant IGFBP in the circulation after the first few

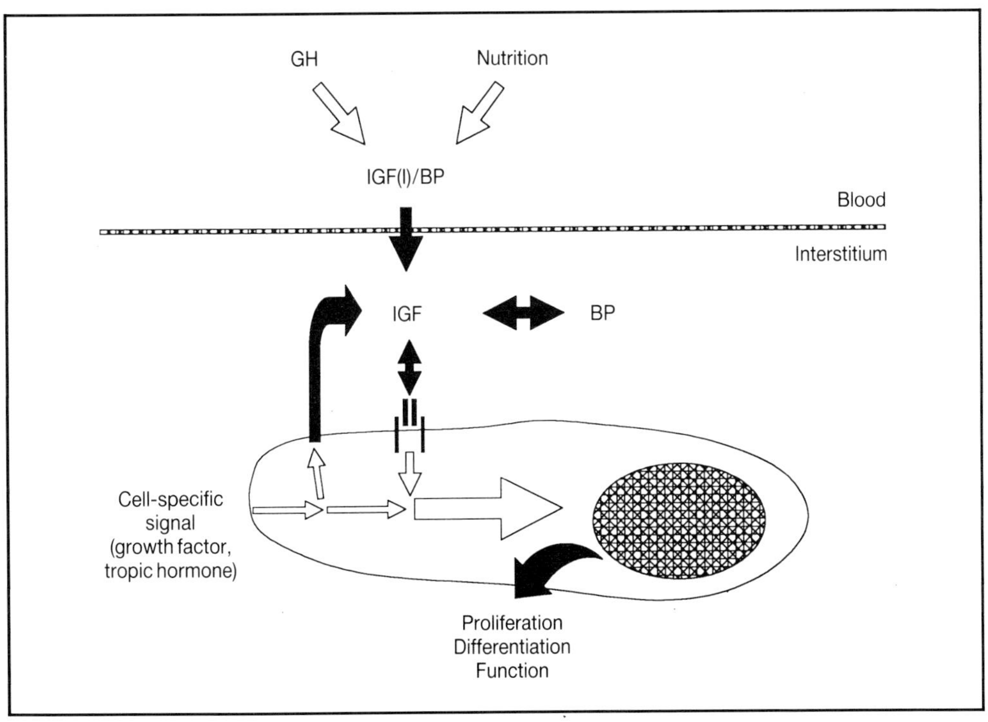

Fig. 5.8. Schematic representation of the biological action of IGF. IGF synthesis is stimulated by cell-specific signals such as other peptide growth factors or tropic hormones. In addition IGFs are transferred from the circulation to the interstitium. They reversibly interact with their binding proteins (BP) and receptors on the cell surface. Activation of the receptor will then potentiate the response triggered by the cell-specific signal.

weeks of life, it is very low in cerebrospinal fluid, where IGFBP-2 and IGFBP-6 predominate. Similarly in human milk and in seminal plasma IGFBP-2 is present at very high levels. The pattern in the lymph varies considerably between different tissues.

The role of circulating IGFBP-3 as a reservoir for IGFs is widely accepted: it serves as a buffer preventing large fluctuations of free IGF. Formation of the ternary complex by binding of the ALS subunit may be of particular importance as the large complex is no longer subject to glomerular filtration. It may also prevent the transfer of IGFBP-3 to other extravascular compartments. Why is such a reservoir and buffer for IGFs necessary? First, there is no intracellular storage pool of IGFs. These peptides are secreted as they are synthesized. Secondly, large fluctuations would be unfavorable with respect to the physiological role of IGF-I in transmitting information on the nutritional and GH secretory status of the organism to the cells. Teleologically, acute food intake or a single GH pulse would be irrelevant for a competent cell to decide whether or not proliferation should take place at a maximal rate. Rather, the long-term nutritional or GH secretory status is important. The presence of a large pool of circulating IGFs releasing the peptides slowly provides a mechanism for integration of these factors over days.

Because of the very slow dissociation rate of the IGF/IGFBP-3 complex, the metabolic half-life of complexed IGF is markedly prolonged as compared to free IGF. Due to the very high affinity of IGFBP-3 for IGFs, free IGF is kept in a concentration range that would allow binding to the IGF receptors, but not to the insulin receptor, preventing acute insulin-like effects despite the very high total concentrations of IGFs.

IGFBP-1 and IGFBP-2 may be involved in the fine tuning of free IGF-I and IGF-II. IGFBP-1 is acutely suppressed by glucose ingestion. This suppression could make free IGFs available, thereby complementing the effect of insulin. IGFBP-2 is consistently found to increase in situations where free IGF-II must be expected to be elevated. IGFBP-2 may therefore function as a buffer for free IGF-II, preventing acute insulin-like effects. In addition to these possible roles of IGFBP-1 and IGFBP-2 in the regulation of free IGFs, there is some evidence that they may also be involved in the transfer of IGFs to the extravascular space and in their specific targeting.

The influence of IGFBPs on IGF activity at a cellular level is controversial. Both inhibitory and stimulatory effects were found which are, however, not necessarily mutually exclusive and may depend on the experimental set-up or the particular IGFBP preparations used. An excess of IGFBP inhibits IGF activity by competing for IGFs with their receptors. With IGFBP-1 and IGFBP-3 stimulatory effects on IGF-I activity can also be observed, especially when IGF-I and IGFBP are applied at an equimolar ratio. Although the exact molecular mechanisms are yet unclear, a constant supply of IGFs by release from the IGF/IGFBP complex may be causative. Modifications of the IGFBP molecules such as phosphorylation may be involved in determining an inhibitory or stimulatory function.

Specific developmental aspects

Embryogenesis and fetal life

IGF-I and especially IGF-II have been assumed to play a role in fetal development. The evidence was, however, vague and circumstantial until recently, when direct evidence for the importance of IGF-II for embryonic growth was demonstrated. In mice, who bear a disrupted IGF-II allele, IGF-II expression is markedly reduced and embryonic growth is impaired.

In mouse embryos IGF-II is expressed along with the IGF-II receptor by the two-cell stage. In preimplantation 64-cell blastocytes IGF-II expression is found in every cell. During organogenesis, and later in mid-gestation fetuses of various species including man, there is abundant IGF-II mRNA in every organ mainly in cells of mesodermal origin. The IGF-II receptor is abundant and ubiquitous until late gestation when it significantly declines. IGF-I expression commences later but not before embryo implantation, although type I IGF receptor mRNA could be demonstrated in mouse embryos as early as in the eight-cell stage. IGF-I and type I IGF receptor expression are widespread in every organ. Many cells express both IGF peptides, but this is not uniform.

With the appearance of IGF receptors cells become responsive to IGF-I or IGF-II. Exogenous administration of either peptide stimulates embryogenesis. In early gestation, when no functional circulation has yet developed, their mode of action must necessarily be autocrine/paracrine. Later, circulating IGFs may also become important. From animal experiments it appears that GH has indeed some influence on fetal IGF-I levels.

This is supported by the clinical observation that newborns with *Laron syndrome* or *congenital GH deficiency* have a somewhat reduced birth length. Nutritional deprivation has also a suppressive effect on fetal serum IGF-I.

IGFBP-1 and IGFBP-2 are expressed in a variety of fetal tissues with the highest abundance in liver. Their serum levels in human fetuses are several-fold increased as compared to young children, whereas the levels of IGFBP-3 are several-fold decreased. Although the expression and the concentrations of the various IGFBPs are different in the fetus, their control is qualitatively similar to that described postnatally.

Pregnancy

During pregnancy maternal IGF-I and IGF-II serum levels rise until late gestation and decline rapidly after delivery. IGF-I, but not IGF-II, was shown to positively correlate with birth weight and length, suggesting that maternal IGF-I may be important for fetoplacental development. The rise of IGFs may in part be due to a rise in IGFBP-3 which is high normal or slightly augmented in the second and even more in the third trimester. However, the IGFBP-3 circulates mainly in pregnancy as a 30 kDa fragment which is generated from the complete protein by a specific protease. Although this protease is also present in other situations, e.g. severely ill patients, its activity is particularly high after the seventh week of gestation in humans. The 30 kDa form still binds IGFs and is able to constitute the ternary complex but its affinity for IGFs is somewhat reduced. The protease may therefore provide a mechanism to facilitate IGF release from the complex. IGFBP-1 levels clearly increase by mid-gestation whereas IGFBP-2 levels decline during pregnancy and both normalize after delivery.

Interestingly, IGF-I, IGF-II and IGFBP-3 levels normalize in pregnant women with *GH deficiency*. This strongly suggests that placental factors such as placental lactogen (hPL) or placental GH (variant GH) regulate IGF-I and IGFBP-3 during pregnancy and substitute for GH of hypophyseal origin.

Postnatal life

Circulating IGFs and IGFBPs exhibit characteristic age-dependent patterns (see Fig. 5.7) which differ within various species. While IGF-II and IGFBP-3 rise rapidly after birth in humans, IGF-I increases slowly in early childhood with a most prominent peak at the time of puberty. IGF-I levels fall continuously in adult life whereas IGF-II and IGFBP-3 decrease only slowly between the third and sixth decade and decline more rapidly thereafter. In contrast, the IGFBP-1 and IGFBP-2 serum levels are high at birth, decline until adolescence and increase again with aging. The physiological significance of these patterns remains unclear. There is good evidence that the pubertal peak of IGF-I and IGFBP-3 is caused by an increase of GH secretion at that time and it may be involved in the control of the pubertal growth spurt.

Clinical applications

Diagnostic use

The importance of IGFs for growth and development makes them interesting parameters for evaluation of growth disorders. Special care must, however, be taken to avoid interference of the IGFBPs in the IGF measurements which can cause grossly erroneous results.

IGF-I and IGFBP-3 and, with limitations, also IGF-II are shown to be of great interest in the evaluation of *growth retardation*. Subnormal levels indicate insufficient production due to one of the causes listed in Table 5.3. The combination of IGF-I and IGFBP-3 levels is particularly useful in identifying GH-responsive children with borderline GH secretion.

In tall young patients, or adult patients with clinical signs of *acromegaly*, elevated serum levels of IGF-I and IGFBP-3, but normal levels of IGF-II, are suggestive of pathologically increased GH secretion and further GH testing is required.

Therapeutic use

The availability of recombinant IGFs and IGFBPs makes their use as therapeutic agents conceivable. Although this wide field is still at a very preliminary stage, first results of experimental studies and of clinical trials are promising. IGF-I may be beneficial for such diverse indications as: growth in patients with *Laron syndrome*, changing the catabolic to an anabolic state post-surgery, improving wound healing in polytraumatized or severely

Table 5.3. Clinical situations with abnormal serum levels of IGF-I, IGF-II and IGFBP-3

Diagnosis	IGF-I	IGF-II	IGFBP-3
GH deficiency	−(−−)	−(−−)	−(−−)
Laron syndrome	−−−	−−−	−−−
Diabetes mellitus	−	−	−
Hypothyroidism	−	−	−
Malnutrition/malabsorption	−−	−	−
Liver insufficiency	−(−−)	−(−−)	−(−−)
Malignancy	−(−−)	−(−−)	−(−−)
Acromegaly	+(++)	n	+(++)
Precocious puberty	+	n	+
Chronic renal failure	n	n(+)	+(++)

n, normal levels; −, low levels; +, increased levels.

burned patients. With respect to wound healing experimental results suggest that the administration of IGF-I complexed to IGFBP-3 is particularly effective.

Selected reading

Blum WF. Insulin-like growth factors and their binding proteins. In Rank MB, ed. *Functional endocrinologic diagnostics in children and adolescents*. Mannheim: J & J Verlag, 1992: 102.

Daughaday WH, Rotwein P. Insulin-like growth factors I and II. Peptide, messenger ribonucleic acid and gene structures, serum, and tissue concentrations. *Endocr Rev* 1989; **10**: 68.

Rechler MM, Nissley P. Insulin-like growth factors. In Sporn MB, Roberts AB, eds. *Handbook of experimental pharmacology*. Vol. 95/I. *Peptide growth factors and their receptors I*. Berlin: Springer-Verlag, 1990: 263.

Spencer EM, ed. *Modern concepts of insulin-like growth factors*. New York: Elsevier, 1991.

6 ◆ *The nervous and muscle systems*

Editor: Hugo Lagercrantz

A. Overview

H Lagercrantz

The human brain has a weight of 300–400 g at birth, which is about one-tenth of the body weight. The brain continues to grow rapidly after birth. By 1 year it has a mean weight of 900 g and by 3 years it has achieved 80 percent of adult brain weight (1350 g). The human infant is probably relatively immature at birth as compared with other primates.

There has been a philosophical question whether the brain of the newborn infant is a 'tabula rasa', as suggested by Aristotle and Locke, or whether the infant is born with some conceptions about the extrauterine world as believed by Descartes and Kant. However, a number of studies have now demonstrated that the infant is born with an innate conception of the world. He recognizes the human face, voice and smell (see p. 256).

The infant is born with a central pattern generator of locomotion and can make walking movements even if he is born prematurely (see p. 241). The infant rapidly develops oral communication (see p. 260). The infant soon starts to sort sound categories simply on the basis of the distribution of sounds in the parent's voice.

Thus the innate visual and auditory conceptions, the oral and locomotion patterns must be genetically determined. However, it is intriguing to understand how the blueprint for the wiring of the 10^{12} neurons and connectivity of the 10^{14} synapses can be contained in the human genome. There are probably only 30 000 genes within the human genome which affect the development of the CNS.

There are probably basic genetic programs for proliferation, migration and localization of neurons in the cortex. The basic framework of columns of six layers is very similar over the whole cortex. Furthermore the development occurs in cascades (see p. 203). For example, in the cerebellum the Purkinje cells develop first and then determine the formation of the granule cells.

There are also cascades of expression of various neurotransmitters, which probably have important tropic functions during development (see p. 217). For example, at a certain stage nearly one out of four synapses contain norepinephrine in one cortical layer of the rat brain, as compared with less than 1 percent in the adult brain. It is possible that these noradrenergic neurons function as pioneering structures. A second wave of increased expression of tyrosine hydroxylase and turnover of norepinephrine occurs around birth, which might be of importance for neonatal adaptation (see p. 264).

To some extent the brain of the newborn infant is more complicated than the adult brain. There is a redundancy of neurons, synapses and dendrites and a number of redundant neuronal connections. During development there is a reorganization of the neuronal wiring which includes programmed cell death, pruning of axonal arborization, phagocytosis of redundant synapses, etc. These processes are probably dependent on interactions between neurons and their targets and to what extent the neurons and their dendrites and synapses are used. The classical example is the degeneration of neurons in the visual cortex which will occur if the eyelids are kept closed during a critical period in infancy (see p. 209).

On the other hand there is probably a great plasticity in the newborn brain. If there is a lesion of certain areas, other areas compensate (often with increased axonal arborization) or develop more. One example is *dyslexia*, where the left Wernicke's language area is underdeveloped, but there is compensatory overdevelopment of other areas.

We are born with genetically determined innate behavioral and motor functions. The limited number of genes have to diversify their actions by combining their effects in time and space, which explains the importance of critical periods and environmental factors for development of the brain.

Selected reading

Changeux JP. Neuronal man. In *The biology of mind*. Oxford: Oxford University Press, 1985.

Mehler J, Dupoux E. *Naitre humaine*. Paris: Editions Odile Jacob, 1990.

Patterson PP, Purves D. *Readings in developmental neurobiology*. Cold Spring Harbor: Cold Spring Harbor Laboratory, 1982.

Purves D, Lichtman JW. *Principles of neural development*. Sunderland, MA: Sinauer Associates, 1985.

von Euler C, Forssberg H, Lagercrantz H, eds. *Neurobiology of early infant behavior*. London: Macmillan, 1989.

B. Development of the CNS

B1. Development and Differentiation of the Neural Tube

R S Nowakowski

There are four major reasons for studying the development of the CNS. First, it is easier to understand the basic organizational plan because the organization of the immature CNS is less complex than that in the adult. Second, a substantial portion of the nomenclature used to describe the adult brain is derived from embryological principles. Third, because the CNS is not completely mature at birth, either at term or even less so in premature infants, knowledge of the state of development and maturity at various stages is essential in order to design rational therapies for pediatric neurology. Finally, there are numerous abnormalities that affect the developing CNS.

The problem and the basic questions

The adult nervous system contains approximately 10^{12} neurons, each of which makes hundreds or, perhaps, thousands of synapses with other neurons. Each of the variety of divisions and subdivisions of the neuraxis has its own characteristic structure and function, and accordingly each is organized into a different pattern of nuclei and/or laminae. The problem faced by the neuroembryologist is to understand: (1) how this tremendous diversity is generated, and (2) how these diverse portions of the CNS are integrated to produce a functional entity. Modern biology requires that these issues be addressed not only in terms of relatively gross changes in the architecture of the developing CNS but also and, perhaps more importantly, in terms of characteristics of its constituent cells: their behavior, their interactions with other cells and with respect to changes in gene expression within them. For this reason, the 'life history' of the neurons of the CNS is of primary importance in understanding CNS development. In particular, it is important to define the common features, influences, and capabilities of the differentiating neurons of the CNS. As is true in any developmental analysis, the elucidation of such similarities provides a set of concepts or 'rules' that make understanding a complex system easier.

Conceptualization of the complicated events and processes that contribute to the development of the CNS involves answering a series of simple questions such as 'When?', 'Where?', 'What?', and 'How?'. Answering these is not a simple task, because many different issues and simultaneously occurring processes must be taken into account (e.g. Which cells and cellular interactions affect the fate of other cells? Which genes are expressed in which cell type, and when are they expressed? Does the maturation of one region of the CNS affect the maturation of other regions of the CNS? etc). Nevertheless, the use of these simple questions provides a useful framework for the discussion, in this and the following section, of the major issues confronted by contemporary neuroembryologists in the analysis of CNS development.

'When?': a question of time and timing

'When?' addresses the time that an event (a 'what?') occurs. For example: When do neurons first appear? When do axons grow into a certain region? When is a particular behavioral competency first achieved? Questions of 'when?' can be answered in two ways: (1) in terms of an absolute time frame (i.e. 'time'), and (2) in terms of the time relative to the occurrence of other events (i.e. 'timing').

For most species used in experimental studies, an absolute developmental time frame is usually measured simply as days after conception and days after birth. In Table 6.1 the gestation periods of some common laboratory animals are listed. Sometimes, for greater precision, staging systems based on readily observable features of the embryo (e.g. eye opening, fusion or separation of fingers and toes, etc.) are used to reduce problems resulting from genetic heterogeneity, differences in diet or environment, or simply because some species (e.g. chick) develop rapidly—and to allow valid comparisons between individual specimens. For defining the absolute age of human embryos and fetuses,

Table 6.1. Gestation periods of various species

Species	Length of gestation period
Chick	21 days
Chinese hamster	13 days
Mouse	19 days
Rat	21–22 days
Cat	65 days
Rhesus monkey	165 ± 5 days
Human	40 ± 1 weeks after last menstrual period; 38 weeks after conception

gestation is generally measured from the time of occurrence of the last menstrual period rather than from the day of conception. Human gestation is considered to be 40 weeks long, even though the conceptus is present for only 38 weeks. The staging system for human embryos and fetuses relies upon easily measurable features such as greatest length (GL) or crown-to-rump length (CRL).

With respect to issues of the time of occurrence of particular developmental events, it is critical to consider the species being examined before any general conclusions are made. A major reason for this is simply that the relative maturity at the time of birth varies from species to species and birth is not correlated with most measures of the maturity of the CNS. This means that events which occur prenatally in some species may occur postnatally in other species. One example of this variation is the maturation of the cerebral cortex. In rats and mice most of the cells destined to comprise the cerebral cortex are generated during the second half of gestation, during a period that ends only a few days before birth. In contrast, in monkeys and humans these same events are completed about the time of the end of the second trimester, well before birth. It is also of great significance that the development of the CNS is not confined to the gestational period. For example, in humans during the intrauterine period the brain grows from nothing to about 350 g. Most of the neurons of the CNS are produced during the first half of this period (see below). After birth the brain continues to grow, mostly by modifications of the numbers, sizes and connections of the neurons generated before birth, reaching a size of about 1350 g at 20 years of age. Most of the postnatal growth occurs within the first 3 or 4 years after birth, but changes in myelination and in other measures of maturation (e.g. cortical surface area, numbers of glial cells, etc.) continue to be apparent even at 70–80 years after birth.

The sequence of occurrence and the relative timing of events is a second critical component of 'when'. The general principle is that development occurs as a cascade of events and that any one event may influence those that follow it but not those that precede it. Knowledge of the order of occurrence of developmental events can provide information about the presence or absence of a causal relationship between the two events. Relative timing can be thought of as a simple cascade of events, such as A → B → C (Fig. 6.1a). If event A occurs before event B, then it is possible for A to influence B but not for B to influence A (Fig. 6.1b). In addition, events that occur

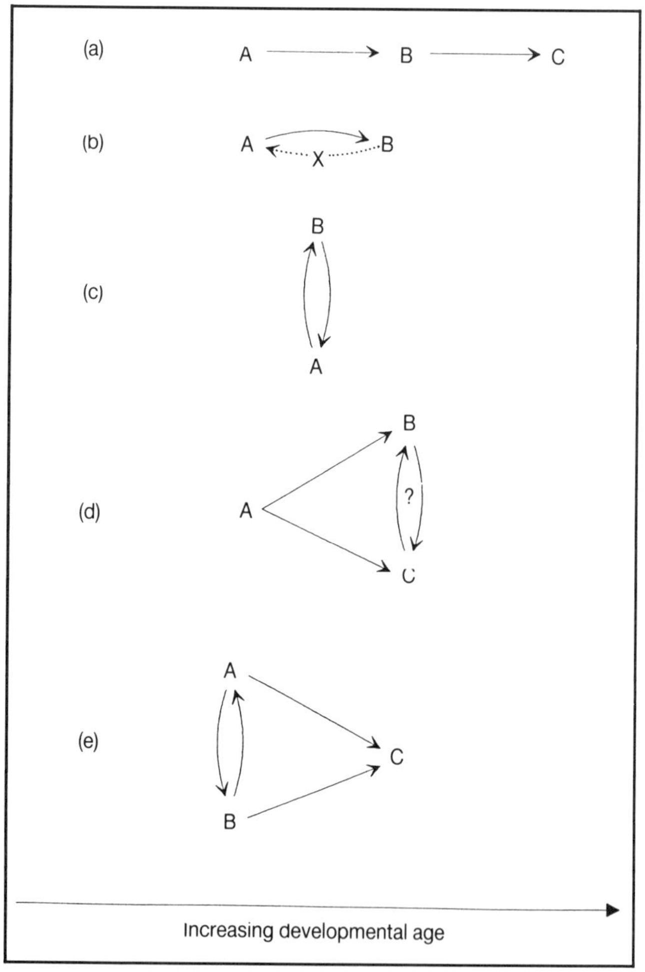

Fig. 6.1. Examples of how events during development influence each other in different ways. (a) Events which follow each other in a sequence can be causally related. (b) A late occurring event cannot influence an earlier occurring event. (c) Two events occurring at the same time can influence each other. (d) One early occurring event can influence two (or more) later occurring events which may or may not influence each other. (e) One event may be dependent on the interaction of two (or more) earlier occurring events.

simultaneously can influence each other (Fig. 6.1c). It does not, however, necessarily follow that just because A precedes B and C that A influences either B or C; it is also possible that B proceeds independent of A, or that both A and B are influenced by some common event which occurs prior to (or concurrent with) both of them. In many cases a more detailed analysis of relative thinking can provide some insight into the issue of causality. A corollary to the cascade concept is that the earlier during development that a particular event occurs, the greater is its potential influence on subsequently occurring events. This also means that the disruption of an early event is likely to have a greater effect on the adult structure than the disruption of a later occurring event. The reason for this is not just because of the existence of simple cascades (Fig. 6.1a) but also because of the interaction of developmental events. For example, one early occurring event can influence more than one later occurring event which may or may not interact (Fig. 6.1d), or two early occurring events might need to interact in order for some later event (Fig. 6.1e) to occur.

Knowledge of when something occurs can be used to corroborate and/or eliminate possible biological bases for issues such as behavioral critical periods or to identify the etiology of a developmental malformation. For example, a behavioral-enriched environment during the postnatal period can lead to an increased cell number in the adult neocortex. Since it is known that the events associated with the proliferation and production of cells comprising the adult cortex occur before this critical period, the enriched environment cannot affect adult cell number by influencing cell proliferation. However, it is also known that in many areas of the CNS, a large fraction of the neurons generated die as part of the normal developmental process; therefore, the most likely mechanism involved is a reduction in cell death. Another striking example of inferences that can be made from this sort of temporal analysis comes from work examining the relationship between mental retardation in children who were exposed *in utero* to the high radiation levels associated with the atomic bombs dropped on Hiroshima and Nagasaki and the gestational age of the fetuses at the time of the exposure. For fetuses exposed during a critical period lasting from the eighth to the fifteenth week of gestation, the risk of presenting with mental retardation at some time after birth was directly proportional to the dose of radiation received. However, if the exposure occurred before the eighth week the risk of mental retardation was no greater than in the general population, and if it occurred after the fifteenth week the risk of mental retardation was less than one-fifth of the risk associated with exposure during the critical period. The time of occurrence of this critical period implicates a radiation-induced compromise in the proliferation and migration of neurons destined for the cerebral cortex (see p. 202 for a description of these processes).

'Where?': the three dimensions of the neural tube

Early during the development of a vertebrate embryo, the structures that will give rise to the CNS are formed from the primitive ectoderm by a process known as neurulation (Fig. 6.2), which begins near the end of the third week after conception. During neurulation, the neural tube and neural crest are formed by the folding in upon itself of the ectoderm, which is the outer surface of the embryo. At the beginning of neurulation the shallow neural groove just above the notochord marks the position of the neural plate (Fig. 6.2a). As the neural groove deepens (Fig. 6.2b), the lateral edges of the neural plate fuse to form the neural tube (Fig. 6.2c). The lumen of the neural tube eventually becomes the ventricular system of the mature CNS. The wall of the tube produces and becomes the cells and tissue of the mature brain. The cells just lateral to the edge of the neural plate and some of the cells from the dorsal portion of the neural tube become the neural crest which produces a variety of structures in the periphery, including most of the peripheral nervous system.

The fact that the early nervous system is a tube defines a coordinate system that can be used for the recognition and localization of the various subdivisions of the adult CNS. Like any other tube, the neural tube can be considered to have three dimensions—longitudinal, circumferential, and radial (Fig. 6.3). This coordinate system with reference to a developmental configuration is useful because developmental subdivisions precede and presage functional subdivisions and also because the complex organization of the adult CNS is somewhat easier to understand when the less complex precursor organization of the developing CNS is understood. Differential differentiation (i.e. differences in cell proliferation, neuronal migration, etc.) of the wall of the

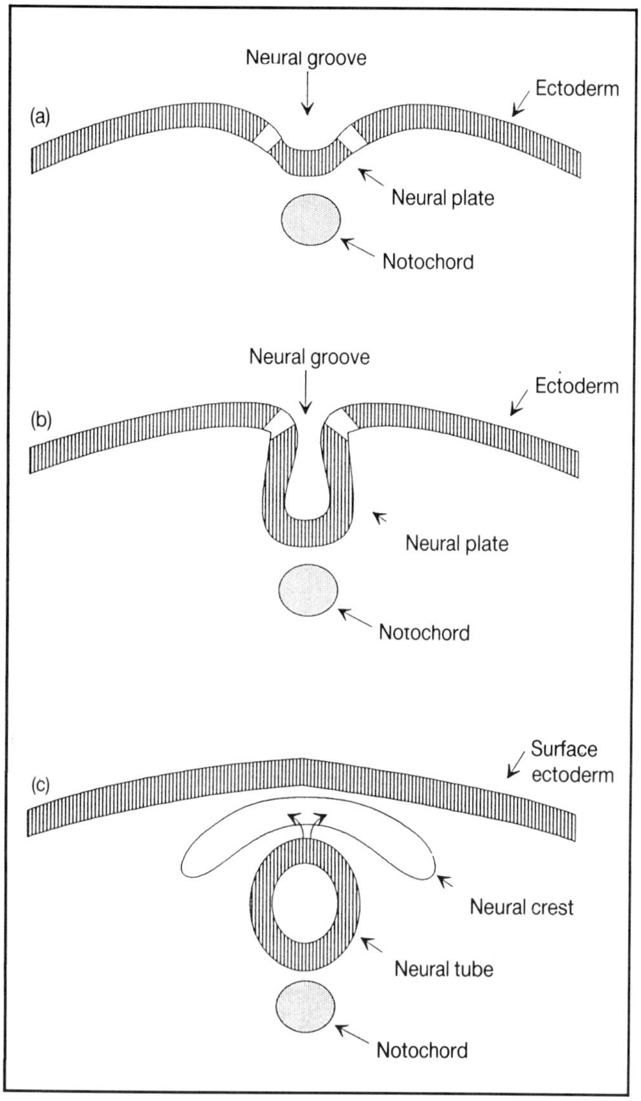

Fig. 6.2. Neurulation. Neurulation, which in humans begins near the end of the third week after conception, is the process in which the ectoderm (the outer surface of the embryo) is induced to fold in upon itself to form the neural tube. (a) At the beginning of neurulation there is a shallow groove just above the notochord; this neural groove marks the position of the neural plate. (b) and (c) As the neural groove deepens, the lateral edges of the neural plate fuse to form the neural tube. The cells just lateral to the edge of the neural plate and some of the cells (arrows) from the dorsal portion of the neural tube become the neural crest. The CNS is derived from the neural tube. The neural crest cells produce a variety of structures in the periphery including most of the peripheral nervous system.

neural tube along each of these three dimensions during subsequent development is, to a substantial degree, responsible for the complex and diverse anatomy of the mature brain. (1) Differential differentiation along the longitudinal dimension produces the major subdivisions

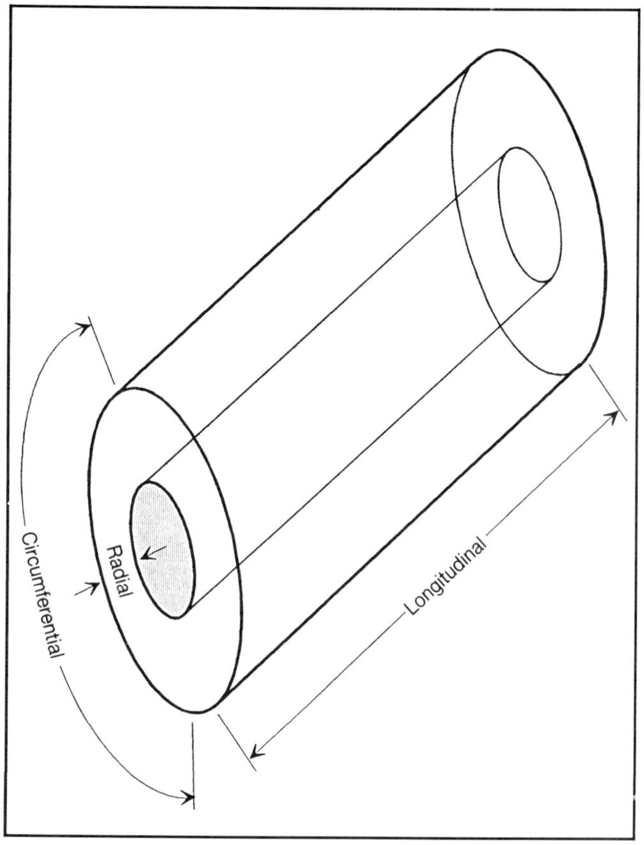

Fig. 6.3. A schematic diagram of the neural tube. The neural tube has three dimensions: longitudinal, circumferential, and radial. Differentiation along each of these three dimensions proceeds in a different way. (See the text for further details.)

of the CNS. (2) Within each of these major subdivisions, differential differentiation in the circumferential dimension gives rise to the development of structurally and functionally distinct areas. (3) Finally, within each area along the radial dimension the wall of the neural tube develops laminae or nuclei that are distinct for each subdivision.

Differentiation along the longitudinal dimension

The head and tail ends of the embryo have already been determined before the beginning of neurulation, and neurulation proceeds at a different rate in the different parts of the neural tube. Eventually, about 50 percent of the tail or caudal end of the neural tube becomes the spinal cord which acquires a segmental organization, i.e. it becomes organized in repeating units called segments, each of which is associated with the sensory and motor innervation of a part of the body. The head or cephalic portion of the neural tube acquires, for the most part a 'suprasegmental' organization, which means that: (1) its organization is not based on a repeating unit, and (2) a substantial portion of its input and output is not devoted to or derived from a single body region but rather provides connections to (and from) the segmentally organized portions of the nervous system. It is this suprasegmentally organized part of the neural tube that becomes the brain. The brainstem, which develops from intermediate portions of the neural tube, acquires a pattern of organization which is in part segmental (i.e. the motor and sensory components of the cranial nerves) and in part suprasegmental.

The cephalic portions of the neural tube (i.e. the head portions, see Table 6.2) exhibit tremendous growth relative to the remainder of the neural tube; this disproportionate growth of the suprasegmental portions of the neural tube is referred to as 'encephalization'. Even before the closure of the neural tube is complete, the cephalic end of the neural tube differentiates into three primary vesicles (i.e. 'bulges') that form from its wall (see Fig. 6.4). From rostral-to-caudal (i.e. from front-to-back, literally 'beak-to-tail') these vesicles are: (1) the prosencephalon or forebrain, (2) the mesencephalon or midbrain, and (3) the rhombencephalon or hindbrain. Subsequently, the prosencephalon becomes subdivided into the telencephalon rostrally and the diencephalon caudally, and the rhombencephalon becomes subdivided

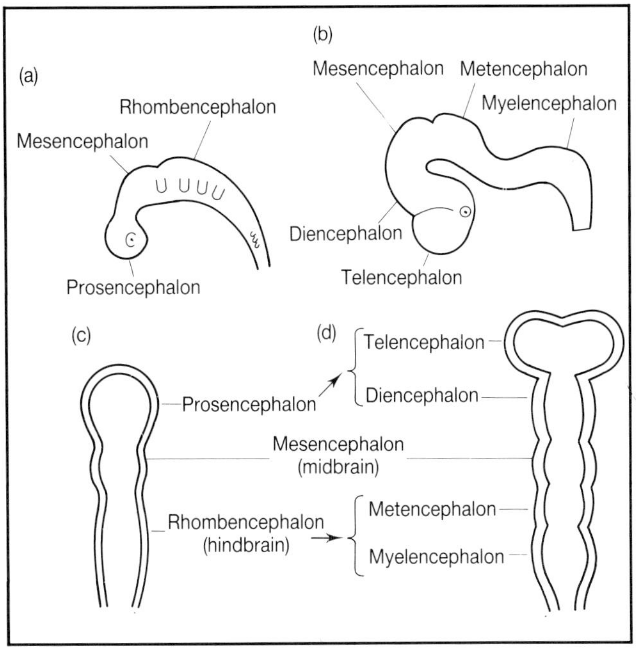

Fig. 6.4. Longitudinal differentiation of the neural tube. Differential differentiation along the longitudinal axis produces the major subdivisions of the CNS. In a 4-week-old human embryo there are three primary brain vesicles: the prosencephalon, mesencephalon, and rhombencephalon (a, b). During the following 2 weeks the primary vesicles become subdivided. The prosencephalon becomes the telencephalon and diencephalon, and the rhombencephalon becomes the metencephalon and myelencephalon (c, d).

Table 6.2. The encephalons

Primary vesicle	Secondary vesicle
Prosencephalon (*proso*, forward + *enkephalos*) forebrain	Telencephalon (*telos*, end + *enkephalos*) endbrain
	Diencephalon (*dia*, through or across + *enkephalos*) 'throughbrain' (many ascending and descending pathways cross or pass through the diencephalon on their way to or from the telencephalon)
Mesencephalon (*mesos*, middle + *enkephalos*)	Mesencephalon midbrain
Rhombencephalon (*rhombos*, rhombic + *enkephalos*) 'rhombic brain' (at this level of the brain, the ventricle is shaped like a rhombus)	Metencephalon (*meta*, after or post + *enkephalos*) 'afterbrain'
	Myelencephalon (*myelos*, marrow + *enkephalos*) medulla (the spinal cord is the 'marrow' of the vertebral column and the medulla is the spinalmost portion of the brain)

At first, the names of the subdivisions of the embryonic brain seem formidable, but an examination of their root meanings facilitates their usage. In all cases, the second part of the name is derived from the Greek word *enkephalos* (*en*, in + *kephalos*, head). Each prefix has a similarly descriptive root that is derived either from its relative position in the neural tube or some other salient feature. See Fig. 6.4.

into the metencephalon rostrally and myelecephalon caudally, thus forming five secondary vesicles. In the human embryo, these five secondary vesicles are already recognizable at the fifth week of gestation, thereby defining at a very early developmental stage the major structural subdivisions of the adult brain. In fact, the names of these vesicles are frequently used to refer to parts of the adult brain. Major adult structures are derived from each of these secondary vesicles; for example: (1) the cortex is derived from the telencephalon; (2) the thalamus and hypothalamus are derived from the diencephalon; (3) the midbrain is derived from the mesencephalon; (4) the pons and cerebellum are derived from the metencephalon; and (5) the medulla is derived from the myelencephalon.

Developmental errors in neural tube closure and in the subsequent longitudinal parcelation of the nervous system lead to profound malformations of the nervous system, presumably because these are two of the earliest events of CNS development. The two most common places for the failure of the neural tube to close are at its two ends, i.e. in the spinal cord and prosencephalon. Failure of the neural tube to close at its caudal end results in a severe form of *spina bifida* known as *rachischisis*. In rachischisis, the spinal cord, the vertebrae and the overlying skin are malformed such that the central canal of the spinal cord (i.e. the cavity of the neural tube) remains open to the surface. As a result this malformation is detectable by ultrasonography and/or by measurement of serum α-fetoprotein. Rachischisis is the result of a very early failure of neural tube closure; failures at later stages of closure result in less deleterious forms of *spina bifida*. Similar features of neural tube closure at the rostral end of the neural tube result in *anencephaly*, a malformation in which the derivatives of the prosencephalon do not form. The precise etiologies of neural tube closure defects are in many cases unknown. In some cases viral infections have been implicated, and in addition neural tube closure defects may be genetic. For example, in the mouse, mutations (at the splotch locus and the T-locus) produce neural tube defects which resemble those seen in humans. Also, recently a family of genes containing the homeobox element (so named because it is found in the homeotic mutations of the fruit fly, *Drosophila melanogaster*) has been localized to specific longitudinal subdivisions of the neural tube. It can be expected that the molecular genetic bases of the processes associated with the formation of the longitudinal subdivisions of the CNS will soon become amenable to analysis.

Differentiation in the circumferential or tangential dimension

Once the basic longitudinal subdivisions have appeared each of them is subsequently modified by further differentiation in the other two dimensions of the neural tube. The specializations that develop circumferentially around the neural tube (i.e. tangential to its surface; see Fig. 6.3) are most easily described in the region destined to become the spinal cord. Here the neural tube can be divided into four circumferentially defined zones or 'plates': the floor plate, paired lateral plates, and the roof plate (Fig. 6.5); each of the two lateral plates is divided into a basal plate and an alar plate on either side of the sulcus limitans. The structures of the adult spinal cord develop predominantly from the alar and basal plates, which become the dorsal (sensory) and ventral (motor) horns of the spinal gray matter, respectively (Fig. 6.5a,c). These same four circumferential subdivisions exist in the brainstem, where the relationship of sensory and motor derivatives of the alar and basal plates to the sulcus limitans is retained (Fig. 6.5b,d) despite the fact that

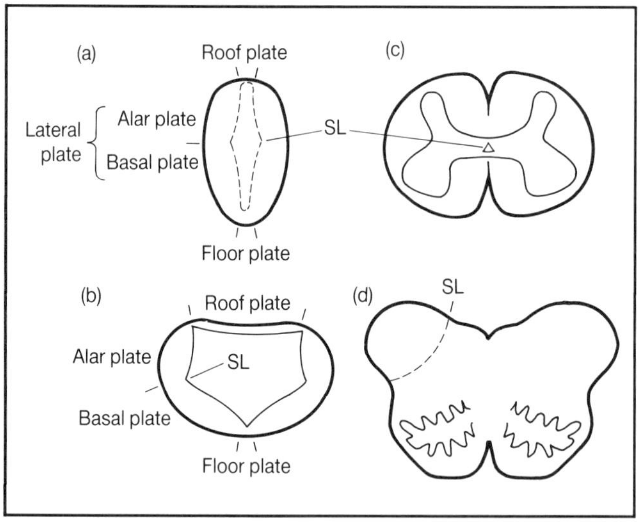

Fig. 6.5. Circumferential differentiation of the neural tube. In the spinal cord there are four circumferential zones or plates: a roof plate, an alar plate, a basal plate, and a floor plate. The names of these plates are derived from their position around the tube (the Latin word *ala* means wing.) In the medulla, the alar and basal plates are displaced laterally by the expansion and attenuation of the roof plate. In both the spinal cord and medulla the sulcus limitans marks the border between the basal and alar plates; in the adult the morphological relationship between the sensory and motor derivatives of the alar and basal plates is similar although their orientation around the sulcus limitans shifts from dorsoventral in the spinal cord to mediolateral in the medulla.

growth and expansion of the roof and floor plates distort the shape of the neural tube. The extension of the alar, basal, roof and floor plates is difficult to define in the prosencephalic derivatives. However, differentiation in the tangential dimension is still obvious. For example, in the diencephalon three sulci divide the wall of the diencephalon into four zones that become, from dorsal to ventral, the epithalamus, dorsal thalamus, ventral thalamus and hypothalamus. Similarly, in the telecephalon cortical subtypes are derived from different regions of the wall of the hemisphere: the archicortex is derived from the medial wall of the lateral hemisphere, the neocortex from the dorsolateral wall and the paleocortex from the lateral wall of the hemisphere.

An important feature common to differentiation in both the longitudinal and circumferential dimensions is that the underlying developmental processes produce subdivisions of the neural tube that are discernible very early during the development of the CNS and that, to a significant degree, the early appearance of these subdivisions precedes the functional differentiation of the CNS. From this observation it can be inferred that the wall of the neural tube, even at very early stages, is a mosaic, i.e. each portion has different potential and developmental capabilities. The existence and nature of these differences continues to be the subject of a wide variety of investigations. For example, molecules (e.g. LAMP or limbic system-associated membrane protein) that are associated with differences between the various subdivisions are beginning to be identified. At later stages of development the degree of mosaicism within each subdivision is uncertain. For example, within the neocortex if one area of developing neocortex is transplanted into the position of a different kind of neocortex at an early enough stage the transplant will develop the functional and molecular characteristics of the host cortex. More recently, it has been shown that single cells which are part of the same clone (i.e. descended from a single progenitor cell) can ultimately reside in different cortical regions and thus subserve different functions. In contrast, the laminar position of the cells within the cortex (and hence some of their functional characteristics) is determined before the cells leave the proliferative zones (see p. 204) during the last cell cycle (specifically during the G_2-phase) occurring prior to the cells becoming permanently postmitotic. Thus it appears that to some extent the functional characteristics of cells within a single subdivision are imposed on the cells both by the position in the neural tube in which they ultimately reside and by the position in the neural tube from which they arise.

Differentiation in the radial or laminar dimension

From the description outlined above it should be clear that differentiation of the neural tube along its length and circumference defines its basic organizational plan and that the different areas of the CNS are discernible early during development. However, the structure of the CNS undergoes tremendous further differentiation and refinement before it can be considered to be mature. For the most part this additional refinement, which builds on the internal organization established by longitudinal and circumferential differentiation, is brought about by differentiation in the radial dimension that produces a variety of laminar and nuclear schemes in various parts of the neural tube. What is happening to produce this variety of lamination patterns in the various parts of the CNS is discussed in the following section.

Selected reading

Barbe MF, Levitt P. The early commitment of fetal neurons to the limbic cortex. *J Neurosci* 1991; **11**: 519.

Keynes R, Lumsden A. Segmentation and the origin of regional diversity in the vertebrate central nervous system. *Neuron* 1990; **2**: 1.

Nowakowski RS. Basic concepts of CNS development. *Child Dev* 1987; **58**: 568.

O'Leary DDM. Do cortical areas emerge from a protocortex? *Trends Neurosci* 1989; **12**: 400.

Otake M, Schull WJ. In utero exposure to A-bomb radiation and mental retardation; a reassessment. *Br J Radiol* 1984; **57**: 409.

Rakic P. Specification of cerebral cortical areas. *Science* 1988; **241**: 170.

Sidman RL, Rakic P. Development of the human central nervous system. In Haymaker W, Adams RD, eds. *Histology and histopathology of the nervous system*. Springfield, Illinois: CC Thomas, 1982: 3.

Walsh C, Cepko C. Widespread dispersion of neuronal clones across functional regions of the cerebral cortex. *Science* 1992; **255**: 434.

B2. Cell Proliferation and Neuronal Migration in the Developing CNS

R S Nowakowski

The basic organizational plan of the central nervous system (CNS) is defined early during development by differentiation along the length and around the circumference of the neural tube (see p. 195). Additional structural refinements and differentiation in the internal organization of each CNS subdivision are, to a considerable extent, the result of a series of changes in the radial dimension which produces a variety of laminar schemes in different parts of the neural tube. To understand the variety of laminar organizational schemes which exist in the different parts of the adult CNS it is necessary to understand three distinctly different cellular processes: cell proliferation, cell migration, and cell differentiation. Together these three steps can be considered to comprise 'the life history' of a single neuron or glial cell; each cell must pass successively through all three of these steps in order to become a mature component of the CNS. Within each division and subdivision of the developing CNS, cell proliferation, cell migration, and cell differentiation occur simultaneously, but for a single cell these steps represent a cascade of developmental events. Cells which pass through the cascade early can influence the fate of those cells which pass through the cascade at subsequent times. In any part of the nervous system cells in the same or even in different states of maturation can interact and affect each other's fate.

Cell proliferation

Cell proliferation in the developing CNS occurs, for the most part, in two specialized zones which line the lumen of the neural tube, i.e. the future ventricular system. These two zones are the ventricular zone, which is immediately adjacent to the ventricular surface, and the subventricular zone (Fig. 6.6). The first of these two zones to appear is the ventricular zone. The ventricular zone is present in all portions of the developing CNS, and in some places it is the only proliferative zone to appear. The cells of the ventricular zone form a pseudostratified columnar epithelium; they are attached to the ventricular surface and have a long, pially directed process which ends either on the pial surface or on a blood vessel. Mitosis occurs at the ventricular surface, after which the nucleus of a newly divided ventricular zone cell moves out to the border of the ventricular zone, where it re-enters the DNA-synthetic phase (or S-phase) of the cell cycle, and begins to move back towards the ventricular surface (Fig. 6.6a); this 'to-and-fro' movement is known as interkinetic nuclear migration. The subventricular zone appears in some, but not all, parts of the developing CNS (Fig. 6.6e and 6.6g vs 6.6d and 6.6f). It differs in two key ways from the ventricular zone. First, the subventricular zone cells are not attached to either surface. Second, the nuclei of the subventricular zone cells do not undergo a 'to-and-fro' movement with different phases of the cell cycle. The subventricular zone is a phylogenetically 'newer' feature, which is present only in the 'newer' portions of the CNS. For example, all of the neurons of the major subdivisions (areas CA1, CA2, and CA3) of the hippocampus, an archicortical or 'old' cortical structure, are derived from the ventricular zone. In contrast, a substantial subventricular zone is present in the developing neocortex and probably contributes large numbers of neurons to that phylogenetically newer structure. The differences in the distribution of the two proliferative zones along the ventricular surface appear early, just as the first neurons are being produced; this indicates that the ventricular surface of the developing nervous system is a mosaic, and that the differentiation of major subdivisions of the CNS follows distinctly different patterns even at early stages.

The proliferative zones of the CNS are present transiently during the developmental period during which time they produce the neurons and glia that will eventually comprise the adult nervous system. The neurons are produced over a period of several days to weeks, and the time of production of a neuron is referred to as its 'birthday'. Both the length of the period of production and the time of its occurrence during development are characteristic of the specific region of the CNS. For example, in the human all of the neurons of the neocortex are produced between the tenth and eighteenth weeks of gestation, but the neurons of the cerebellar cortex are produced over a much longer period that begins about the same time (for the Purkinje cells) but does not end until about the third postnatal month (for the cerebellar granule cells). The length and time of occurrence of these periods of production also vary

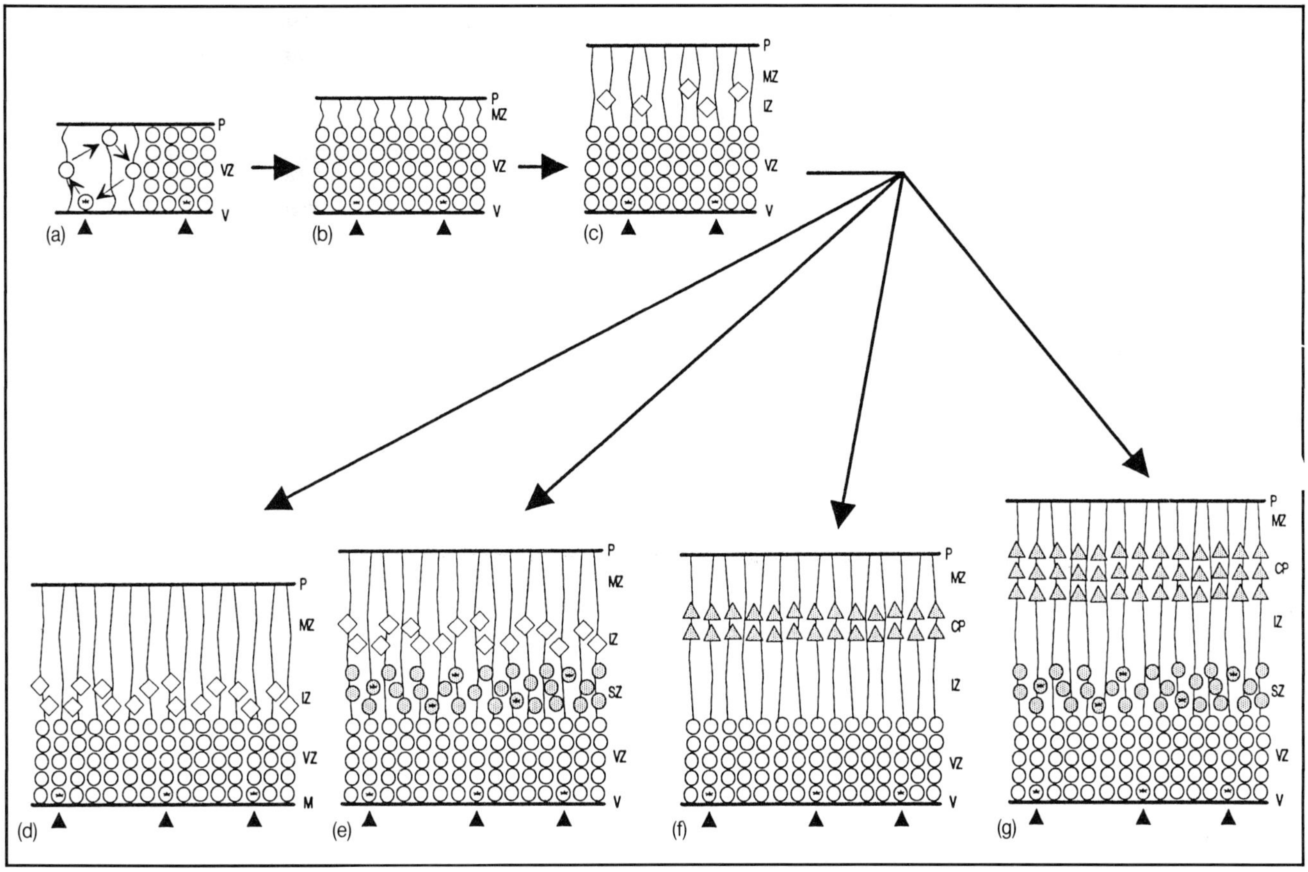

Fig. 6.6. Differentiation in the radial dimension. (a, b and c) The early stages of the differentiation of the neural tube. All parts of the early developing CNS have a ventricular zone (VZ) and eventually develop a marginal zone (MZ) just subjacent to the pial surface (P). The VZ is a pseudostratified columnar epithelium, which means that the nuclei of the cells are stratified, but each cell has contacts that reach the ventricular (V) and pial surfaces of the neural tube. (a) The left side of the drawing illustrates the movement of the nucleus of a single cell as it passes through the various phases of the cell cycle; DNA synthesis occurs in the outer half of the VZ and mitosis (i.e. cell division) occurs adjacent to the ventricular surface. This movement of the cell's nucleus is known as interkinetic nuclear migration. Shortly after neurulation the neural tube consists of only the VZ. (b) The next zone to appear is the MZ, which is an almost cell-free zone just subjacent to the pial surface. (c) Shortly after the formation of the MZ an intermediate zone (IZ) forms; this zone contains the first postmitotic cells of the nervous system. The IZ is located between the VZ and MZ. (d, e, f and g) After achieving the stage represented in (c), the development of different regions of the CNS varies. Four possible alternatives for the subsequent radial development of the CNS can be defined by whether movement of postmitotic neurons is by passive displacement (d and e) or active migration (f and g) and by the presence of one (d and f) or two (e and g) proliferative zones. (d) and (e) show areas in which passive displacement occurs. (f) and (g) show areas in which active migration occurs. (d) In some parts of the neural tube the only proliferative zone present is the VZ. The postmitotic cells derived from the VZ aggregate and mature in the IZ, immediately adjacent to the VZ. One portion of the nervous system which has this pattern of radial differentiation is the spinal cord. (e) In other portions of the nervous system postmitotic cells also aggregate in the IZ and differentiate there, but some of these cells are derived from the subventricular zone, SZ. The dorsal thalamus is an example of a portion of the nervous system which follows this pattern of development. (f) In the hippocampus (an archicortical region) all of the postmitotic cells are derived from the VZ. They migrate across the sparsely populated IZ and form a cortical plate (CP). (g) In the neocortex both a VZ and a SZ are present. Again the derivatives of these two proliferative zones migrate across the IZ and form a CP. Abbreviations: V, ventricular surface; VZ, ventricular zone; SZ, subventricular zone; IZ, intermediate zone; CP, cortical plate; MZ, marginal zone; P, pial surface.

considerably in different species. In each region, the neurons are produced in a characteristic sequence, such that there is a correlation between neuronal birthdays and cell class and distribution. In general, the first neurons to be produced in each region are the large projection neurons and, for the most part, the glial cells are produced after most of the neurons have been produced. However, among the first cells to be produced are a population of astrocyte-like cells called radial glial cells that play an important role in neuronal migration, as described below. Recently, experiments using single cell markers to locate the position of cells of a single clone have revealed that in some regions of the CNS a single proliferating cell can produce both neurons and glia, but in other regions the neuronal and glial lineages separate at a relatively early period of time.

Neuronal migration (passive displacement vs active migration)

The final position of most of the neurons in the adult nervous system is usually distant from the ventricular surface. Therefore, a mechanism for the movement of cells from their site of proliferation to their final position is necessary. The patterns of movement of the postmitotic neurons vary in different portions of the nervous system. In some regions, neurons leaving the proliferative population remain in an 'intermediate zone' immediately adjacent to the proliferative zones (Fig. 6.6c, 6.6d, 6.6e). In contrast, in other regions, the neurons leaving the proliferative population move some distance away from the proliferative zones and eventually coalesce to form an incipient cortex referred to as a 'cortical plate' (Fig. 6.6f, 6.6g).

There are two basic and quite different ways that neurons move from the sites of cell proliferation to their final position. While both of these ways are generally referred to as 'neuronal migration', only one seems to involve the active participation of the young neuron itself. Therefore, they will be distinguished here as passive cell displacement and active neuronal migration. Both passive cell displacement and active neuronal migration produce a correlation between a neuron's final position and its time of origin or 'birthday'. As its name implies, passive cell displacement does not seem to require active locomotory movement by the postmitotic neuron. In this case a postmitotic neuron leaves the proliferative population (influenced to do so by some unknown signal or signals) and is displaced only a very short distance from the border of the proliferative zone (Fig. 6.7a). Thereafter, as the new postmitotic neurons are similarly displaced outward from the proliferative zone, the original cells are passively displaced even further from the proliferative

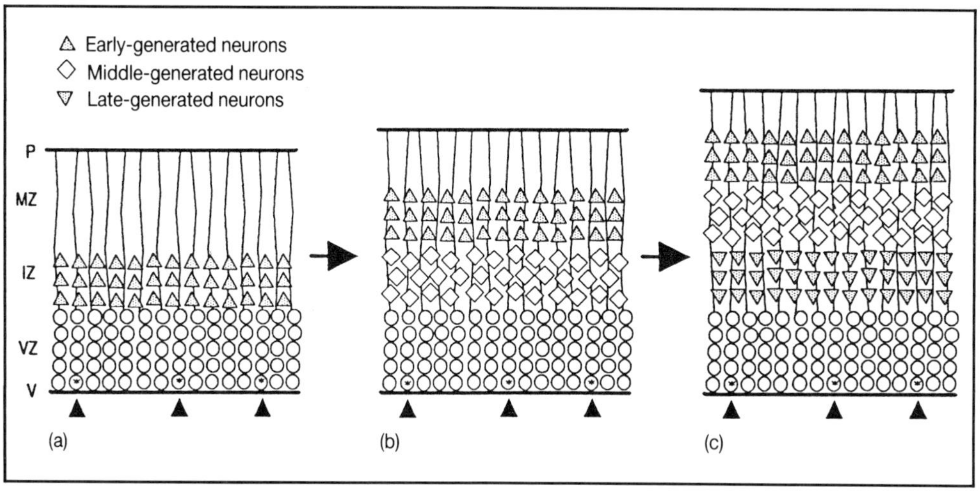

Fig. 6.7. The sequence of events associated with passive displacement. In some areas of the developing nervous system movement of postmitotic neurons is by passive displacement. The early generated neurons leave the ventricular zone (VZ) and take up a position only a short distance from it. Later, as additional cells are produced by and leave the VZ, the earlier produced cells are displaced outward. (a) through (c) illustrate the progressive passive displacement of the previously generated neurons away from the ventricular surface by subsequently generated neurons. (a) The earliest generated neurons which leave the VZ are shown as triangles. (b) The next group of neurons to be generated are represented by diamonds. Their movement out of the VZ displaces the earlier generated neurons toward the pial surface. (c) The last neurons generated, represented by inverted triangles, displace both of the earlier generated populations of neurons. This sequence of events produces a specific distribution of neurons known as an outside-to-inside spatiotemporal gradient. Abbreviations: V, ventricular surface; VZ, ventricular zone; IZ, intermediate zone; CP, cortical plate; MZ, marginal zone; P, pial surface.

zone by the interposition of the subsequently generated neurons (Fig. 6.7b). In those parts of the CNS in which passive cell displacement occurs, the first neurons that leave the proliferative population are, in general, ultimately located farthest from the proliferative zone; the subsequently generated neurons are found at levels progressively closer to the proliferative zone (Fig. 6.7c). Thus, passive cell displacement produces a correlation between time of origin and final position that is referred to as an 'outside-to-inside' spatiotemporal gradient. Note that outside and inside are both defined with respect to the position of the cells relative to the proliferative zone; therefore, outside is usually towards the pial surface, and inside is towards the ventricular surface, although this is reversed in the cerebellum where granule cell proliferation occurs adjacent to the pia. Areas of the nervous system in which the outside-to-inside spatiotemporal gradient is manifest include the thalamus, the hypothalamus, the spinal cord, many regions of the brainstem, the retina, and the dentate gyrus of the hippocampal formation.

The second way by which young neurons move from the proliferative zone to their final positions requires the active participation of the postmitotic neurons in producing: (1) a displacement away from the proliferative zones, and (2) a bypassing of earlier generated neurons. In this case, neurons leave the proliferative zone and move through the intermediate zone (Fig. 6.8a); the progressively later generated neurons bypass neurons produced earlier and occupy positions sequentially closer

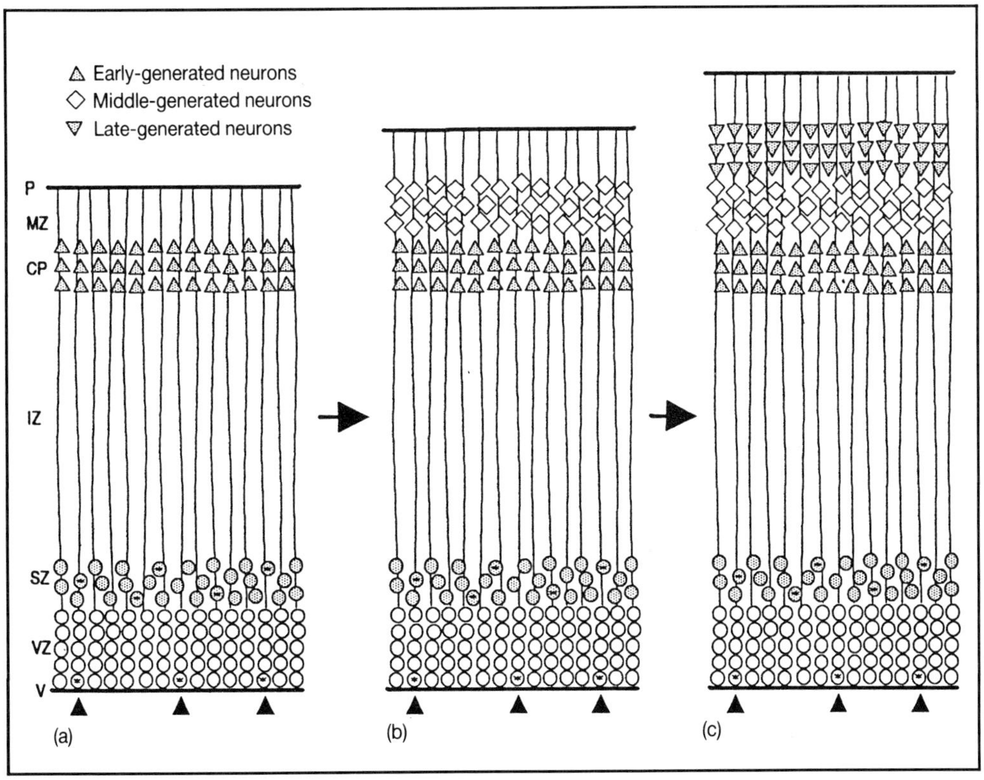

Fig. 6.8. The sequence of events associated with active neuronal migration. In some parts of the developing CNS, neurons leaving the proliferative zone move a great distance before reaching their final position. (a) The early-generated neurons (triangles) leave the proliferative zone and assemble in a formation known as the cortical plate (CP), which is situated between the intermediate (IZ) and marginal zones (MZ). (b) Later generated groups of neurons (diamonds) leave the proliferative population and move across the IZ and past the earlier generated cells to take up a position on the top of the CP. (c) The last generated neurons (inverted triangles) migrate across the IZ and past both groups of earlier generated cells to take up residence at the top of the CP. This type of distribution of neurons is known as an inside-to-outside spatiotemporal gradient. Abbreviations: V, ventricular surface; VZ, ventricular zone; IZ, intermediate zone; CP, cortical plate; MZ, marginal zone; P, pial surface.

to the pial surface (Fig. 6.8b and 6.8c). Thus, in regions of the developing CNS in which the migrating young neurons actively contribute to their own displacement away from the proliferative zones the result is an 'inside-to-outside' spatiotemporal gradient. In this pattern the earliest generated cells remain closest to the proliferative zone and comprise the deepest layers, while the last generated cells move past the earlier generated neurons to the farthest position from the proliferative zone and occupy the most superficial layers. Inside-to-outside spatiotemporal gradients are found in most portions of the cerebral cortex and in several subcortical areas. Areas in which spatiotemporal gradients of the inside-to-outside type occur are, in general, well laminated structures with layers oriented tangential to the radial dimension of the CNS, i.e. that run parallel with the surface of the proliferative zones.

Some neurons, notably the granule cells of the cerebellar cortex and the granule cells of the dentate gyrus, migrate part of the way to their final destination using some features from each of these two 'migratory' methods. In both the cerebellum and the dentate gyrus the young neurons actively participate in the initial part of their migration as they move away from the site of their production but, upon reaching the vicinity of their final destination, they do not bypass the earlier generated cells but push the earlier generated cells further away from the proliferative zone.

Neuronal migration and radial glial fibers

During their migration many neurons are guided to their final position by radial glial fibers, which provide the 'scaffolding' for the future adult neocortex as well as for other cortical and noncortical structures. The radial glial fibers are the long, pially directed processes of an astrocyte-like cell whose soma is usually found in the ventricular or subventricular zone (Fig. 6.9). During early development the radial glial cells have an attachment to both the ventricular surface and the pial surface; they are

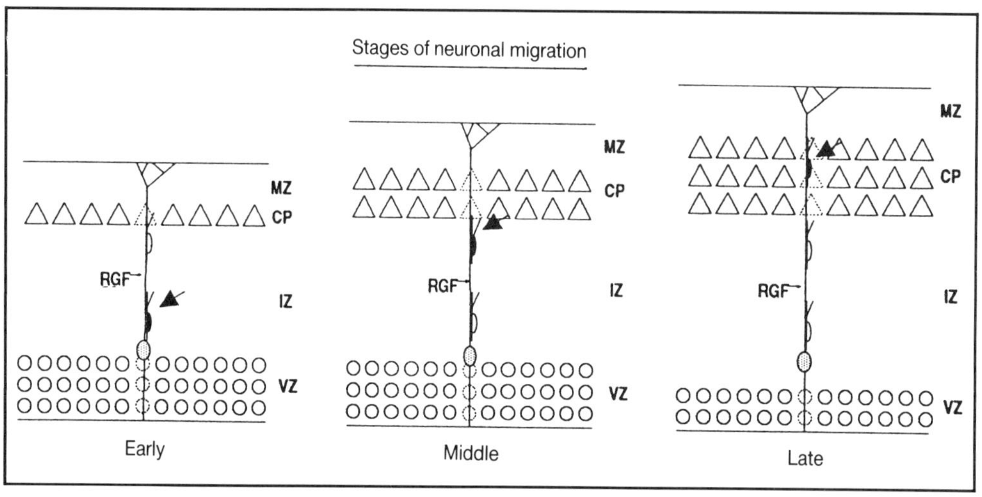

Fig. 6.9. A schematic illustration of the interaction between migrating neurons and radial glial fibers. After leaving the proliferative zone (VZ), a young neuron moves toward its final position in the cortical plate (CP) along a radially aligned glial cell (shaded ellipse) which has attachments to both ventricular and pial surfaces. The progression of one such young neuron from the VZ through the intermediate zone (IZ) to the CP is illustrated by a single black cell marked by an arrow in each of the three drawings (a), (b) and (c). The migratory process can be divided into three stages. (a) As a young neuron leaves the proliferative zone it becomes apposed to a radial glial fiber (RGF) and acquires a polarity directed toward the pial surface. (b) Next, the young neuron enters the locomotory phase and traverses the IZ, maintaining its apposition to the radial glial fiber and its polarity. Subsequently generated young neurons (shown with a white cell body) leave the proliferative zone and become apposed to the same radial glial fiber. (c) When the young neuron reaches the top of the CP, it loses its apposition to the radial glial fiber and reorganizes its polarity in order to differentiate into a mature neuron. Disruption of any of the three steps of the migratory process can result in ectopic neurons. Abbreviations: VZ, ventricular zone, IZ, intermediate zone; CP, cortical plate; MZ, marginal zone.

aligned radially, and more-or-less uniformly, in an arrangement similar to the hub-to-rim organization of the spokes of a bicycle wheel. However, as development proceeds differential growth in some parts of the CNS, such as the cerebral cortex, produces distortions in the radial glial fiber system such that the once relatively straight path delineated by each radial glial fiber becomes a curved or even tortuous path. Thus, the radial glial fibers map the proliferative zones onto the wall of the neural tube; in principle the neurons that are produced by the proliferating cells from a small area of the ventricular zone will migrate along the surface of the same (or adjacent) radial glial fibers and will end up in close proximity to each other in the mature CNS.

The process of neuronal migration (Fig. 6.9) is a complicated one and consists of at least three phases. The three phases are: initiation of migration, a locomotory phase, and a termination phase. During the initiation phase a newly divided cell makes the transition from neuroblast (i.e. a proliferating cell) to young neuron (i.e. a non-proliferating, permanently postmitotic cell) and leaves the proliferative population. The young neuron then becomes apposed along its length to a radial glial fiber, thus establishing an axis of polarity away from the ventricular surface. The second, or locomotory, phase of migration begins once the young neuron is aligned with the radial glial fiber. During this phase a young neuron moves actively along the surface of a radial glial cell, retaining its apposition to the radial glial fiber and its axis of polarity. Upon reaching the vicinity of its final position at the border of the cortical plate and the marginal zone, a young neuron stops its migration and becomes detached from the radial glial fiber, thus freeing up space on the radial glial fiber for subsequently generated neurons. Its migration completed, the young neuron continues its differentiation process by growing dendrites and sending out an axon that eventually makes contact with other neurons. The locomotory phase can be very long as, for example, in the cerebral cortex where a migrating neuron can move along a radial glial fiber which may be tens of millimeters long.

Disruptions of migration

Disruption of any of the three phases which comprise the process of neuronal migration results in an abnormality in cell position. Neurons which fail to reach their appropriate final positions are said to be ectopic (or heterotopic). In humans, the best studied examples of defects in neuronal positioning are in the cerebral cortex where abnormalities in neuronal migration have been associated with a variety of disorders and syndromes ranging from severe mental retardation to 'rather minor' behavioral disorders. The presence of ectopic neurons and disruptions of the migratory process has been associated with the sequelae of *hydrocephalus*, *lissencephaly*, *methylmercury poisoning*, *methanol exposure*, some *craniofacial anomalies*, and a variety of other conditions. In addition, ectopic neurons have been found in some patients with mental retardation and seizures and in area CA1 of the hippocampus of patients with *schizophrenia* and in the language areas of patients with *dyslexia*. It is difficult to assess in such human pathological material the developmental fate of neurons that fail to migrate to their proper positions. It is not known, for example, whether the connections made by these abnormally positioned neurons are with their normal targets or with some other targets. Most importantly it is not known how such abnormalities in connectivity (if they exist) might affect the function of the area of the brain in which the ectopic cells were normally destined to reside. Some insight into these issues is beginning to emerge from studies in mutant mice that have defects in neuronal migration and from experimental disruptions of the migratory process.

Neuronal differentiation

The final phase in the life history of a neuron is its differentiation. This is an extraordinarily complex process which is responsible for a large proportion of the diversity, in all its many aspects, of the adult CNS. During differentiation a neuron acquires its mature morphological and functional characteristics. Thus, the process includes the elaboration of an axon and dendritic processes and the expression of neurotransmitter phenotype. Also, some neurons will elaborate a signal which causes their axon to become myelinated; others will not. All of these aspects of the differentiation process have a specific manifestation which differs for different cell classes. For example, the dendrites grow out and form an arborization pattern characteristic for each particular cell class. Similarly, the specific neurotransmitter enzymes which are characteristic of that cell class are also produced; in addition, at each of its postsynaptic sites the neuron must produce the specific receptors it needs to receive input from its various presynaptic partners. Just as neurons acquire their mature properties, glial cells also differentiate. During their differentiation, glial cells become separated into distinct lineages committed to produce particular cell types (i.e. oligodendrocytes or astrocytes); these 'glioblasts' continue to proliferate even after this commitment. The processes of differentiation can continue for many years after the basic plan of the CNS is laid down and neurons have been formed. For example, in humans it is known that the myelination of most pathways in the CNS continues long after birth, and that changes can be detected even into the eighth decade of life. In fact, the sequence of myelination of major pathways during the perinatal period was the original basis for the traditional classification of neocortical areas into primary, secondary and association cortices. A thorough treatment of the complex processes of cell differentiation in the CNS is beyond the scope of this review; therefore, the discussion below will be confined to the limited aspect of axon–target interactions.

Axon–target interactions

(see also p. 210)

During differentiation a neuron extends its axonal process from the cell soma to a postsynaptic cell or target. As it grows the axon must find its way through a complicated terrain populated by other cells and their processes to the area of its potential target. Once there it must locate and 'select' not only the appropriate target cell but also the appropriate part of that cell's dendritic tree in order to make its synapses. Clearly this process depends on a variety of mechanisms in order to be successful, and it is likely that different mechanisms, or sets of mechanisms, are used by different populations of growing axons. For example, one mechanism might be needed to guide an axon over long distances to reach its target, and once the appropriate target has been reached a second, different mechanism, might be needed to direct the terminal arbors of the growing axon to the specific cell and site upon which it will form synapses. There is considerable evidence that the mechanism of axonal guidance involves interactions among laminin, fibronectin, N-CAM (see p. 60) and other molecules in (or on) the axons themselves and in their environment.

During the formation of connections in the developing CNS, axons do not simply grow directly and only to their final target. Quite the contrary, a feature common to many axons in the developing CNS is that they grow exuberantly, which means that they form transient connections with specific cells and areas of the nervous system that they do not normally innervate in the adult. Two types of transient connections are made: divergent and convergent. Divergence (Fig. 6.10a) means that during development one axon, one neuron, or one population of neurons innervates a greater number of cells and/or a greater area of the CNS than it normally does in the adult (Fig. 6.10a′). Convergence (Fig. 6.10b) is the converse of divergence; this means that during

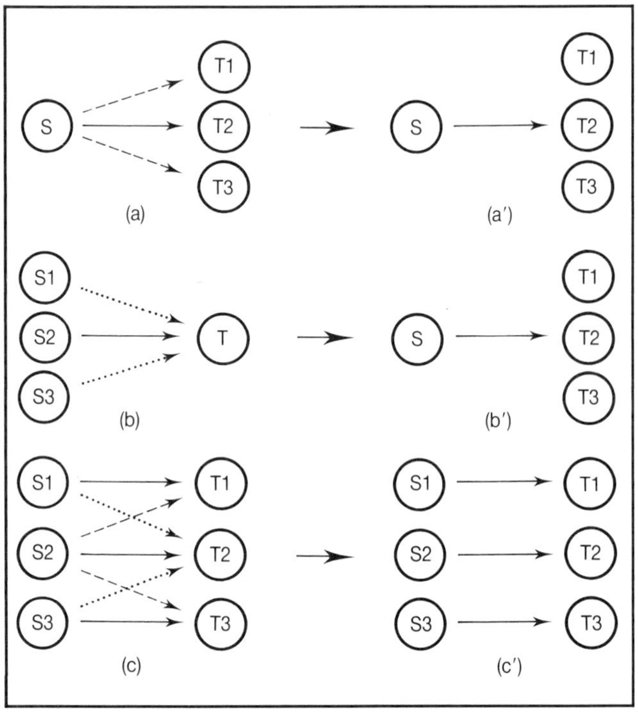

Fig. 6.10. During development of the CNS two types of exuberant connections occur. (a) Transient divergence: a single source (S) of axons (either a single cell or a single population of neurons) projects to several targets (T1, T2, T3) in an area broader than its eventual adult distribution. A subsequent withdrawal of a portion of the projection produces the adult pattern (a′). (b) Transient convergence: Axonal projections from more than one source (i.e. from more than one cell or population of neurons, S1, S2, S3) terminate on a single target (T). Subsequent withdrawal of the projection from some of the sources produces the adult pattern (b′). (c) Transient divergence and convergence in combination: In this situation some exuberant projections of both types must be withdrawn to produce the adult pattern of connections (c′). Note that in some cases the elimination of projections that diverge from one source involves the same connections that are convergent to some particular target.

development one target neuron, or population of neurons, can be innervated by several axons, or axons from several sources, even though in the adult that target might be innervated by only one of these afferent sources (Fig. 6.10b′). Divergent and convergent transient axonal projections are not mutually exclusive, and it is probable that both occur within single populations of neurons (Fig. 6.10c). At a later stage of development the normal adult pattern of connectivity (and perhaps an ordered map of connections) is established by the elimination of the extra (or exuberant) divergent and convergent axon collaterals (Fig. 6.10c′).

Elimination of transient features

Three distinctly different phenomena appear to be responsible for the elimination of exuberant axonal connections: the retraction of axon collaterals, naturally occurring neuronal death, and the reorganization of axonal and dendritic trees. These three mechanisms involve the elimination of transiently present features and are, therefore, regressive events. (1) In the case of neurons which have exuberant projections to a target that they do not normally innervate in the adult, the transient connections seem to be removed by retraction of one of the axon collaterals. For example, during development pyramidal neurons in the visual cortex send transient collaterals to the spinal cord, which they do not normally innervate in the adult. Later in development this transient innervation is eliminated by retraction of the spinal projecting collaterals of these axons while their cells of origin and their normal projections to other subcortical targets persist. (2) When a population of neurons projects to a wider target area during development than in the adult, the transient connections can be eliminated by a process of selective cell death; those neurons which project beyond the normal adult innervation territory die. It has been hypothesized that such selective cell death is, in part, a mechanism of 'error correction'. (3) During development the terminal arbors of axons may project to an area that is broader than normal. Such transient connections can be eliminated by a shrinking or retraction of the terminal arbor of the axons. All three of these phenomena seem to contribute to the elimination of both divergent and convergent connections, and the attainment of the adult pattern of connections usually involves more than one of these mechanisms. This can be illustrated by the development of the connections between the retina and the lateral geniculate nucleus. During development approximately 50 percent more retinal ganglion cells are produced than are normally found in the adult; moreover, the ganglion cells of one retina project to the entire volume of the lateral geniculate instead of to restricted layers as in the adult. As development proceeds, the 'extra' ganglion cells die, and the 'exuberant' axonal arbors are retracted until the adult laminar pattern emerges.

The significance of regressive events

The development of a complex organ, such as the nervous system, is generally considered to consist of a series of progressive events which build upon each other to produce the final adult structure. It is clear, however, that axonal elimination and neuronal cell death eliminate transient structures and are, therefore, regressive events which occur normally during the development of the CNS. There are numerous other types of regressive events during normal development. For example, concomitant with the loss of axons and axon collaterals in most systems there is also a net decrease in numbers of synapses and synaptic densities, as well as spatial reorganization of synapses (not necessarily accompanied by a change in their numbers). Presumably at the functional level there are also changes in synaptic efficiency. Biological control of these regressive events is generally believed to involve a number of factors alone and/or in combination; these factors include competition either for limited postsynaptic space or for usage of growth factors available in limited quantities, the interaction of different neurons by means of electrical activity, and the effects of systemic factors such as hormones. It seems likely that all of these mechanisms will be found to contribute to the elimination of transient exuberant connections. During normal development the interaction between progressive and regressive events eventually reaches a stable (or semi-stable) equilibrium that characterizes the normal state of the mature brain.

Exacerbation or interruption of either a progressive or regressive event will disrupt the establishment of a stable equilibrium and produce a pathological condition. The nature and severity of the functional disturbance produced will depend on the influences of the new 'balance' of progressive and regressive processes on the establishment and maintenance of connections. The general presumption is that normal functional competence is not achieved, at least in part because the neurons involved either die or do not make normal connections. However, an additional (and often overlooked) consideration is that because development proceeds as a cascade (see p. 196) any disruption can have a variety of sequelae, which can ultimately influence neurons that were not directly affected by the initial disruptive event. In addition, it is crucial to emphasize that the control and disruption of both progressive and regressive processes is likely to be regionally specific, reflecting underlying regional differences in gene expression. Specific genetic disruptions, therefore, could affect specific regions or areas of the developing CNS, and the nature of the pathological conditions which would result depends both on the process that was disrupted directly and on the subsequent consequences to other processes active in the specific region involved. In addition, these underlying regional differences in gene expression (reflected in variations in development in different regions of the CNS) mean that even a systemically mediated disturbance of development could produce an abnormality in a relatively confined area of the CNS. Similarly, differences in timing of developmental events in different regions means that the same disruption occurring at different times could produce markedly different pathological changes in the mature CNS. For example, syndromes in which the processes of neuronal migration, cell proliferation, or cell death have been stimulated or disrupted in some way could produce either ectopic neurons, a deficiency of neurons, or 'extra' neurons. The functional disturbance produced in each of these cases would depend on what part of the CNS is affected and on how well the cells that were directly, and indirectly, affected are able to make and maintain normal connections.

Selected reading

Jacobson M. *Developmental neurobiology*. 3rd ed. New York: Plenum, 1991.

LeDouarin N. *The neural crest*. Cambridge: Cambridge University Press, 1982.

Nowakowski RS. Basic concepts of CNS development. *Child Dev* 1987; **58**: 568.

Nowakowski RS. Development of the hippocampal formation in mutant mice. *Drug Dev Res* 1988; **15**: 315.

Rakic P. Cell migration and neuronal ectopias in the brain. *Birth Defects* 1975; **11**(7): 95.

B3. Development of Neuronal and Neuromuscular Connectivity

S Cullheim and B Ulfhake

Precise connections between nerve cells are achieved by two different sorts of mechanisms. First, outgrowing axons are led by various molecular guidance cues from specific areas to particular target regions which are rather broadly defined (see p. 204). The second stage includes an exact point-to-point matching between each axon and the specific target neurons. This is achieved by intricate interactions between the nerve cells involved. In the following, the attention will primarily regard the second type of events. A large part of the description will focus on the neuromuscular junction as it has been extensively used as a model for the study of synapse development.

Axonal development

Polarization of neurons

Neurons are highly polarized cells with two types of extensions from the cell body. In general, the axon mediates electrical signals from the neuron to other nerve cells, while the dendrites receive the electrically mediated information from other neurons. There are clear structural differences between axons and dendrites, particularly in the organization of the cell membrane and the cytoskeleton. The development of axons and dendrites seems to be preceded by a nonpolarized period when all processes extending from the cell body have the same undifferentiated characteristics. It then seems as if the initial outgrowth of the axon is predetermined in the neuron, but the direction of further elongation is determined by factors in the tissue through which the axon grows.

Axon growth

Once formed, the axon will grow along a specific pathway in order to contact specific target cells. The axon extends at its growing tip by means of a specialized enlargement of the axon shaft called the growth cone, and the directed growth of the axon is accomplished by interactions between the growth cone and its environment. Such interactive mechanisms may include (1) mechanical routing by oriental structures in the pathways; (2) a differential adhesiveness between the growing axon and molecules of surrounding tissue elements; (3) influence from electrical fields in the tissue; and (4) release of factors promoting or inhibiting axon growth by cells in the axonal pathways and by axonal targets. Although each of these factors probably has some merit, none of them can by itself explain all features of axon growth. Instead, it is plausible to believe that a number of mechanisms act together with a proper timing to lead axons to their targets. Following this initial crude adjustment, a second set of events takes over to match each axon to a specific target neuron.

Synapse formation

The second type of events leads to the formation of synapses between neurons. A synaptic contact has a number of ultrastructural features, including opposed plasma membranes of the pre- and postsynaptic elements, a synaptic cleft between the membranes, and synaptic vesicles containing transmitter substances, close to or in contact with the presynaptic membrane. Receptors for the transmitters are located in the postsynaptic membrane. By release of transmitters the presynaptic neuron may induce electrical and/or chemical short- and/or long-term changes in the postsynaptic cell.

The development of the synapse involves an interaction between the pre- and postsynaptic elements and a number of factors may act in combination to achieve a functional development of a synapse. One obvious such factor is that the two elements involved are in close proximity at the appropriate time for establishment of the connection. It seems likely that, in addition, there must exist a biochemical compatibility or affinity between pre- and postsynaptic elements. However, much remains to be revealed about the molecular nature of such an affinity.

The interplay between developing pre- and postsynaptic structures *in vivo* has been most extensively studied at the neuromuscular junction. Such studies have shown that the presynaptic motor nerve terminal, using acetylcholine (ACh) as transmitter substance, has a major role in the formation of synaptic contacts. Thus, before the arrival of the motor nerve, nicotinic ACh receptors are distributed rather uniformly over the surface of muscle fibers (Fig. 6.11). After innervation of the muscle fiber, the density of receptors is increased at the site of innervation, and decreased at extrasynaptic sites. This effect seems to be mediated by electrical activity and diffusible factors other than ACh, e.g. calcitonin gene-related peptide (CGRP), released by the presynaptic nerve terminal. Initially, the newly formed synapse is rather labile, as exemplified by the short half-life of ACh receptors in the postsynaptic membrane. With increasing time, a stabilization of the synapse occurs, with a decreasing lateral mobility and a longer half-life of the receptors. Also the functional channel properties of the receptors show a progressive change after the initial innervation.

Neuron death (see also p. 209)

The studies of the development of the neuromuscular junction have given strong indications that substances released from the presynaptic motoneuron nerve terminal may have an influence on the production of postsynaptic receptors. Other evidence provided from this type of study suggests that there is an influence also in the reverse, retrograde direction. An obvious example of such a retrograde influence is seen in the mechanisms involved in motoneuron death during the time period for muscle innervation. Thus, during this period about half the population of spinal motoneurons die. This death is completed before birth in mammals. Ample evidence has been provided that the number of surviving motoneurons depends on the number of muscle fibers available for innervation. Thus, early limb amputation results in a much larger loss of motoneurons, while grafting an additional limb increases the number of surviving neurons. This implies that the cell death does not occur because the motoneurons are intrinsically defective. Rather, it appears as if the motoneurons, after the initial axon outgrowth, compete for trophic factors which are essential for the survival of developing motoneurons.

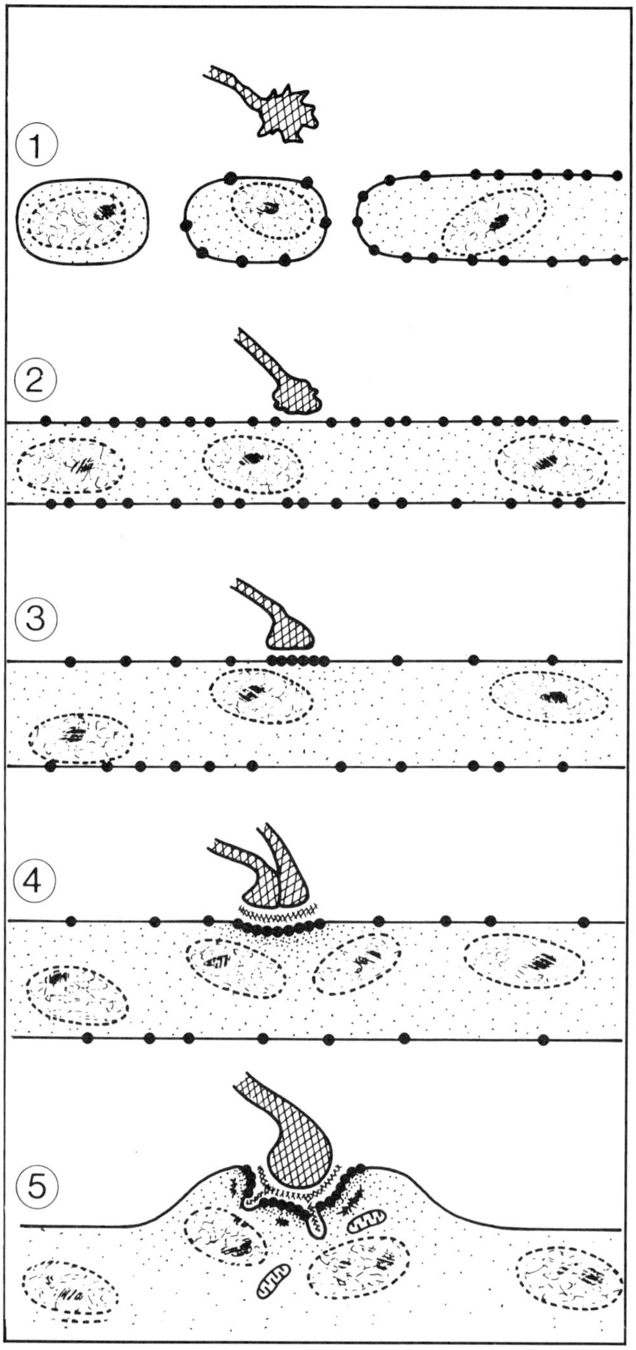

Fig. 6.11. Schematic illustration of the formation of a synapse between a nerve and a skeletal muscle during development in the rat. (1) The growth cone arrives at the surface of mononucleated myoblasts, which have started to express acetylcholine receptor (AChR) molecules (filled circles) all over the surface of their cytoplasmic membranes. (2) Fusion of myoblasts into myotubes is accompanied by an increase of AChR biosynthesis. (3) The growth cone is immobilized and receptor molecules are accumulated beneath the nerve terminal. The expression of the genes encoding the AChR subunits becomes restricted to fundamental nuclei under the end plate. (4) A multiple innervation is transiently seen and receptors outside the synapse are gradually disappearing. (5) The maturation of the motor end plate includes stabilization of the receptor and change in the mean opening time of ion channels. (By courtesy of Professor Jean-Pierre Changeux, Institut Pasteur, Paris.)

Trophic effects on the presynaptic element

It has been assumed that the trophic effects of the postsynaptic muscle fiber on the presynaptic motoneuron are exerted by at least two mechanisms. First, the muscle probably releases a factor which makes the terminal motor axon arborize or sprout. Secondly, in order to survive, the motoneuron must innervate muscle fibers with a number of terminals which is sufficient to obtain an adequate amount of muscle-derived neurotrophic factor. Such a trophic factor is, with all probability, locally released at the synaptic site and then transported retrogradely to the motoneuron cell body. Furthermore, it has been shown that neural activity may be important for the production of trophic factors. Thus, a pharmacological blockade of neuromuscular transmission during the sensitive period may result in rescue of motoneurons that otherwise would have died. This may be explained by a larger production of neurotrophic substances by inactive muscle fibers.

Synapse elimination

In mammals, motoneuron death appears completed before birth. At birth each muscle fiber may be innervated by several different motoneurons, but this polyneuronal innervation is eliminated during the first few weeks of postnatal life to give the adult innervation pattern, i.e. a muscle fiber is innervated by one motoneuron only (Fig. 6.12a). The mechanism for this elimination seems to be a withdrawal of the presynaptic branch into the parent motor axon. Although the number of inputs to a muscle fiber in this way decreases during development the complexity of the remaining ones increases, forming more synaptic boutons and release sites. The same development has been described for a number of regions of the adult and peripheral nervous systems. Thus, synapse overproduction followed by synapse elimination has been shown in peripheral ganglia (Fig. 6.12b), as well as in the cerebellar and cerebral cortices.

Regulation of synapse elimination through trophism

The elimination of neuromuscular synapses requires muscle contraction and is delayed after transection of muscle tendons or after blocking the synaptic

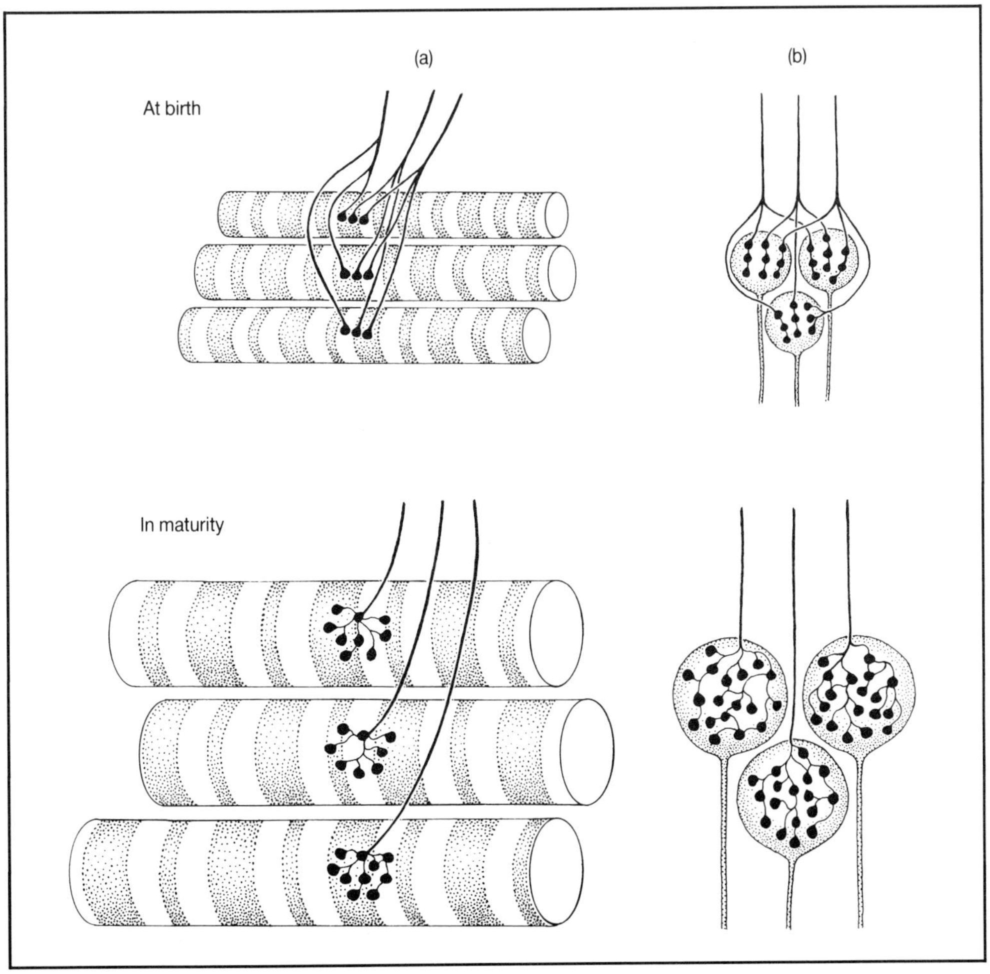

Fig. 6.12. Schematic illustrations of postnatal synaptic rearrangements in mammalian muscle (a) and ganglia (b). At birth, each axon innervates more target cells than in maturity, but the terminal arborizations display a larger complexity in the adult animal. (Reprinted by permission of the publishers and author from *Body and Brain: a trophic theory of neural connections* by Dale Purves, Cambridge, Mass: Harvard University Press, Copyright © 1988 by the President and Fellows of Harvard College.)

transmission. The mechanism of this activity-dependent synapse elimination is not known, but also in this case it has been speculated that a competition between nerve terminals for trophic factors released by the muscle forms the basis for the elimination. It has been speculated that the release of trophic factors only occurs during depolarization of the muscle fibers and that these factors can only be taken up by simultaneously active terminals. Thus, asynchronous activation of the nerve terminal and the muscle fiber would lead to a lack of trophic support to the terminal, thereby triggering a withdrawal of the presynaptic branch. The overall purpose of these events would be to match an appropriate number of innervating axons to each target cell and vice versa.

Synaptic rearrangements in neurons with a complex connectivity

At this stage, it should be noticed that the experiments which form the basis for the mentioned hypothesis were made in studies of rather simple systems. Since most central neurons are geometrically complex, it may be very difficult to verify a synaptic rearrangement in these cases. Attempts to study the development of the synaptic connectivity of a richly innervated neuron, the spinal motoneuron, have revealed a much more intricate rearrangement of the synaptic input.

Synaptic boutons are present on the initial axon segment of the spinal motoneuron at birth, but they disappear during the first few weeks of life. There is also a postnatal loss of boutons from the cell body and the motor axon collaterals with projections in the cord lose terminal branches. In all these regions, there is an elimination of synapses in line with what is found in the periphery. When including the dendrites in the study, however, another pattern emerges. Thus, the total number of synapses on the dendrites appears the same, about 50 000, irrespective of postnatal age. This constant number seems to be the result of an elimination of some inputs and a formation of others (Fig. 6.13). This process may still be explained by the trophism hypothesis, but it certainly requires a much more complex set of events, probably involving a number of different trophic substances. It has been proposed that the mentioned changes reflect a shift in the control of the spinal motoneuron from local to supraspinal levels. It has also been suggested that the central parts of the motoneuron

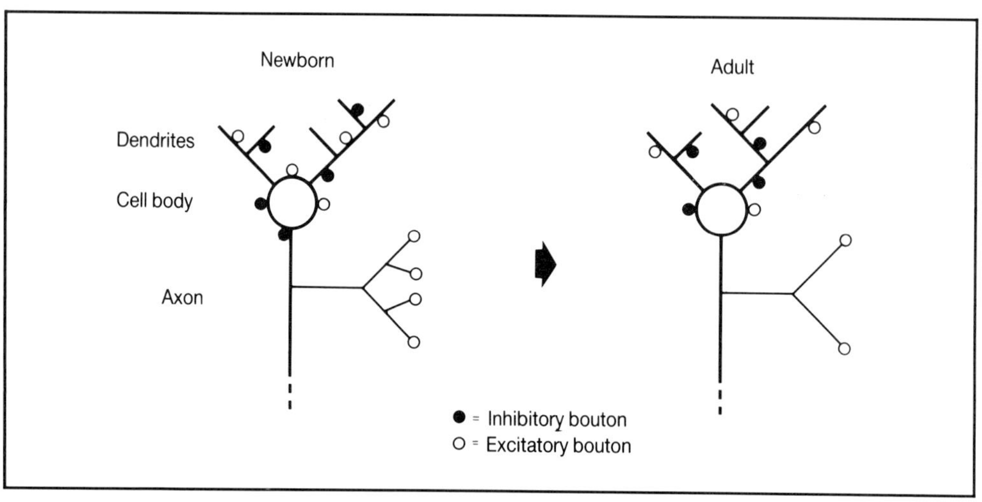

Fig. 6.13. Scheme for intramedullary synaptic rearrangements in cat α-motoneurons postnatally. The number of synaptic terminals of the axon collateral system is reduced by half within a constant terminal field. Half the number of synapses on the cell body and all synapses (predominantly inhibitory) on the initial axon segment are removed. The dendrites are apposed by a constant number of synaptic boutons reflecting a balance between the establishment and removal of synaptic connections. The dendrites are to some degree remodeled during their invasion of new territories, but the total number of dendritic end branches remains constant. (From Cullheim S, Ulfhake B. Postnatal synaptic reorganization of cat motoneurons. In *Neurobiology of early infant behaviour*. London: The Macmillan Press, 1988. Reproduced with permission of The Macmillan Press.)

may be under an inhibitory influence during the rearrangement period. This may be important to suppress any inadequate electrical activity elicited during the rebuilding process. Be that as it may, studies of the development of a complex synaptic input system have, not surprisingly, given a more complicated picture than what has been provided from studies of a simple synaptic organization.

Concluding remarks

There is accumulating evidence that some of the mechanisms controlling the development of connectivity in the nervous system involve an intricate competition for substances which are necessary at an early stage for survival of neurons, or later for survival of nerve terminals. Such a 'trophic' interaction may indicate the importance of establishing a particular type of nerve connection at a critical period of time, after which the connection can no longer be made. Critical periods have been demonstrated for instance in the formation of the synaptic connectivity in the visual cortex, but it is highly plausible that this is a general phenomenon involving also higher functions, such as language. On the other hand, trophic mechanisms may also open the possibility to compensate for the loss of some synaptic inputs by expanding others by a larger degree of nerve cell survival, less retraction of nerve end branches and even formation of new axon terminals.

Selected reading

Jacobson M. *Developmental neurobiology*. 3rd ed. New York: Plenum Press, 1991.

Jessell TM. Neuronal survival and synapse formation. In Kandel ER, Schwartz JH, Jessell TM, eds. *Principles of neural science*. 3rd ed. Amsterdam: Elsevier, 1991.

Kandel ER, Jessell TM. Early experience and the fine tuning of synaptic connections. In Kandel ER, Schwartz JH, Jessell TM, eds. *Principles of neural science*. 3rd ed. Amsterdam: Elsevier, 1991: 945.

Purves D. *Body and brain. A trophic theory of neural connections.* Boston, MA: Harvard University Press, 1988.

B4. Nerve Growth Factors

T Ebendal

Specific neurotrophic factors (neurotrophins) are produced in limited amounts in the target tissues and mediate the cell interactions regulating neuron survival during development. The release of these proteins is also believed to regulate the extent of innervation of the target tissues. In addition to their role in neuronal development, neurotrophic factors are important in the functioning of the adult nervous system. Besides nerve growth factor (NGF), the neurotrophins include brain derived neurotrophic factor (BDNF) and neurotrophin-3 (NT-3). Recently, neurotrophin-5 (NT-5), a possible mammalian homolog to NT-4 described in the frog *Xenopus*, has been cloned in man and rat.

Nerve growth factor is synthesized as a 305 amino acid long prepro-NGF from which the mature basic 118 amino acid NGF protein is generated by proteolytic cleavage at dibasic amino acid residues to act as a trophic factor for many sensory and sympathetic neurons in the peripheral nervous system.

Functional properties

Nerve growth factor is also present in the brain, where it serves to function in the development and maintenance of cholinergic neurons of the basal forebrain. An increased activity of cholineacetyltransferase (ChAT) in the basal forebrain of neonatal rats has been seen after the injection of NGF. BDNF and NT-3 are trophic to a broader range of neurons.

A remarkable property of the neurotrophic factors is their ability to stimulate a pronounced neurite outgrowth response in immature peripheral ganglionic neurons. This has been much studied in tissue culture and it is obvious from such studies that the different neurotrophins each stimulate different, but partially overlapping, populations of peripheral sensory and autonomic ganglionic neurons. Such stimulation evoked by locally produced neurotrophins forms the basis for the stimulated ingrowth of peripheral, and also possibly central, ingrowth of nerve fibers to different target areas (see p. 211). The administration of antibodies to NGF to the newborn rat or mouse causes a severe reduction in the development of the sympathetic chain ganglia (immunosympathectomy).

Anatomical distribution

The distribution of neurotrophin mRNAs in the adult rat brain studied by *in situ* hybridization, histochemistry, and RNA blotting, has shown remarkable regional specificity with high levels in the hippocampus where expression is confined to subsets of pyramidal and granule neurons. Of the neurotrophins, BDNF mRNA is the more widely distributed in the brain, although the highest levels are found in the hippocampus followed by the cerebral cortex, pons and cerebellum. In the periphery, NGF has been found to be produced in densely innervated tissues such as the iris, heart and vas deferens. After lesions of peripheral nerves, NGF is also produced locally by cells in the nerve including Schwann cells and fibroblasts.

Structure

The structure of NGF has very recently been clarified from crystallographic data. The form of the mature NGF protein is markedly flat with two subunits held together along the flat surfaces mainly by hydrophobic residues coming in contact at the interface. The amino acid sequences of the neurotrophins have been ascertained by analysis of DNA clones isolated from the human genome. The similarities between the different neurotrophins are substantial; however, variable regions give specificity to the different family members. From studies of the recombinant neurotrophins it is evident that NGF, BDNF and NT-3 each have unique biological activities and may cooperate to support the development and maintenance of the nervous system.The final number of neurotrophins involved in such a network of cell interactions functioning in brain development remains to be determined.

Receptors

The neurotrophins stimulate survival and differentiation of a range of neurons by binding to cell-surface receptors. Low affinity binding of all tested neurotrophins is mediated via a 75 kDa glycoprotein (LNGFR) that has been cloned and characterized. The function of LNGFR is not well understood at present.

Recently, a 140 kDa tyrosine protein kinase encoded by the proto-oncogene *trk* has been found to bind NGF with high affinity and to evoke the cellular neurotrophic responses. In addition, a protein encoded by the *trk*-related gene *trkB* has been shown to bind BDNF and NT-3 with high affinity. Very recently, a third member of the *trk* family, *trkC*, has been cloned and demonstrated to function as a high affinity receptor for NT-3. Even though there are obvious preferences for binding of a particular neurotrophin to only one of the *trk* family of receptors, there is some promiscuity, especially if the concentration of neurotrophins is raised.

The expression of *trk* and LNGFR mRNA are colocalized in the rat brain to the medial septum nucleus and the nucleus of Broca's diagonal band housing the NGF-responsive magnocellular cholinergic neurons projecting to hippocampus and cerebral cortex. High affinity binding of NGF has been demonstrated for scattered neurons in the striatum, but immunohistological detection of the LNGFR protein has been difficult in this area. It is now clear that the lateral parts of the striatum of the rat, known to bind NGF at high affinity, expresses *trk* mRNA in scattered neurons, without a concomitant expression of the LNGFR.

In sharp contrast, the pattern of expression of *trkB* is widespread in many areas of the cortex (piriform, frontal, cingulate) as well as lateral septum and the ependymal lining of the lateral ventricles. The neocortex showed labeling with *trkB* in several of the layers, most notable in areas likely to correspond to layers II, III and V. A similar layered pattern is also observed for BDNF, a ligand for the *trkB* protein. This suggests possible auto- or paracrine functions for BDNF and *trkB* in the development and maintenance of the cerebral cortex.

Development

The pattern of expression of neurotrophins and their receptors are changing with development in brain and in other organs including testis and ovary. Several studies have described the developmental appearance of NGF in the brain and spinal cord. NGF mRNA is present only in trace concentrations in the fetal rat brain and increases postnatally, approximately 20-fold, until 3 weeks after birth, when adult levels have been reached. Binding of radiolabeled NGF to sections of the chick embryo suggested the early expression of NGF receptors, not only in the classical target neurons for the NGF protein, but also in a variety of other cells, in particular skeletal muscle cells and neurons in the lateral motor column of the spinal cord. In contrast mRNA coding for BDNF is present in the immature brain in relatively high concentrations.

Brain damage

Lesion-induced alterations in the level of neurotrophins have been reported in a number of experimental systems. Thus denervation of the rat iris increases the levels of detectable NGF. Surgical or excitotoxic lesioning of the brain also rapidly increases the levels of BDNF and to some extent also NGF. The functional significance at a detailed level is still not clarified but it is likely that the neurotrophins participate in a cascade of protective mechanisms activated by brain damage.

Clinical applications

The rapid progress made in the study of neurotrophic factors has led to an understanding of how these proteins may be of clinical use in situations of *neurodegenerative disease*. NGF may be of clinical use in *Alzheimer disease* since the trophic action of NGF is directed towards the severely affected cholinergic neurons of the forebrain. Another neurodegenerative disease where NGF might find a clinical application is *Huntington disease*, where NGF may support the degenerating cholinergic interneurons expressing the *trk*-encoded high affinity NGF receptor. Studies of the regulation of NGF in the brain of patients with *Down syndrome*, sharing some neurodegenerative traits with Alzheimer disease, would be worthwhile. Also some other growth factors have been found to stimulate neurons in the brain. Such factors include insulin-like growth factor I, basic fibroblast growth factor and ciliary neuronotrophic factor. It is likely that brain development and maturation and the response to neural injury is regulated by the interaction of several of these factors with the neurotrophins.

The first clinical trials with NGF infused into the human brain have been carried out: one case concerns the use of NGF to support grafted adrenal medullary tissue transplanted to the putamen of a patient with *Parkinson disease*; a second case concerns a patient with *Alzheimer disease* receiving a 3-month period of intraventricular NGF infusion. In both cases, representing models for possible future application of NGF therapy, beneficial effects but no ill-effects were documented, encouraging further limited studies.

Selected reading

Ebendal T. NGF in CNS: Experimental data and clinical implications. *Progr Growth Factor Res* 1989; **1**: 143.

Ebendal T, Söderström S, Hallböök F, *et al*. Human nerve growth factor: biological and immunological activities, and clinical possibilities in neurodegenerative disease. In Timiras PS, Privat A, Giacobini E, *et al.*, eds. *Plasticity and regeneration of the nervous system*. *Adv Exp Med Biol* 1991; **296**: 207.

B5. Expression and Regulation of Chemical Neuroregulators

D M Katz

Intercellular communication in the nervous system is mediated by chemical neuroregulators that are released by neurons and act on postsynaptic target cells. A hallmark of the mature nervous system is the enormous diversity of chemical neuroregulators (neurotransmitters, neuromodulators) and of the receptor molecules to which they bind. Therefore, normal development of the nervous system requires a precise orchestration of transmitter and receptor expression so that neurons and their targets achieve an appropriate neurochemical match. Recent studies in animal model systems indicate that neurochemical ontogeny is not simply 'hard-wired' and immutable; rather, development of transmitter properties is a dynamic process that can be influenced by multiple epigenetic influences. A challenge for clinicians and basic scientists, therefore, is to understand how perturbations of development may derange maturation of neurochemical function.

Transmitter diversity in the mature nervous system

Multiple classes of neuroactive molecules are synthesized and released by neurons in the central and peripheral nervous systems. The most ubiquitous transmitters are probably the excitatory and inhibitory amino acids, including glutamate and γ-aminobutyric acid, respectively. Other important molecules include the neuropeptides, such as substance P, somatostatin and enkephalin, as well as the 'classical' monoamine transmitters serotonin, dopamine, norepinephrine, epinephrine and acetylcholine. It is important to recognize that one neuron may release multiple neuroactive molecules that can interact both pre- and postsynaptically. Moreover, patterns of nerve cell activity can differentially regulate release of each colocalized molecule.

Transmitter ontogeny

De novo expression, as well as quantitative maturation of transmitter properties, are temporally and spatially regulated in the developing nervous system. Thus, neurochemical development spans embryonic, fetal and postnatal life, with different transmitter systems appearing and maturing with diverse time courses. Some transmitter properties that appear early during embryogenesis may disappear at later stages. The functional significance of such transient expression is unknown; however, it is possible that some neuroactive molecules play trophic roles during early development independent of their functions as mediators of synaptic transmission at later stages. Animal studies have demonstrated, for example, that embryonic neuronal survival, proliferation and differentiation can be influenced by vasoactive intestinal polypeptide, a molecule believed to act as a synaptic modulator in the mature nervous system. It is important to note that patterns of transmitter expression during ontogeny are often accompanied by parallel changes in transmitter receptors. Therefore, transmitter systems in the developing embryo and fetus must be considered potential targets of maternally administered receptor agonists and antagonists.

Regulation of transmitter development by environmental influences

As noted above, transmitter development can be influenced by multiple factors in the neuronal microenvironment. These include nerve impulse activity, factors synthesized by non-neuronal cells (i.e. glia and Schwann cells) and neuronal target tissues, trophic peptides, including NGF and circulating hormones, such as adrenal corticosteroids. Studies in animal models demonstrated, for example, that the normal postnatal development of noradrenergic transmitter properties in peripheral sympathetic neurons requires presynaptic impulse activity. Administration of exogenous glucocorticoids, on the other hand, has been shown to alter the normal time course of transmitter expression in neurons of the developing enteric nervous system in rats. Recent studies indicate that transmitter development may also be regulated by the very tissues that receive neural innervation. The postnatal development of cholinergic properties in the sympathetic innervation of sweat glands, for example, is mediated by a factor or factors secreted by the gland tissue. Prior to innervation of the glands, these sympathetic neurons are noradrenergic; they switch to the cholinergic phenotype under the influence of their target. Thus, transmitter expression in at least some neural systems exhibits considerable plasticity and can be altered by perturbations of normal cell–cell interactions.

Molecular mechanisms of transmitter regulation during development

Environmental influences can alter neurotransmitter development and function by acting through multiple mechanisms, including regulation of gene transcription, translation of messenger RNA, and post-translational modification of gene products. Regulation of gene transcription and translation are important not only for *de novo* synthesis of transmitter-related molecules but also for quantitative regulation of transmitter levels. Any single transmitter-related molecule may be regulated by multiple pathways. For example, nerve impulse activity raises levels of tyrosine hydroxylase activity, the rate-limiting enzyme in catecholamine synthesis, by increasing synthesis of new enzyme molecules and by phosphorylation-activation of existing enzyme molecules; the net effect of both mechanisms can be an increase in transmitter synthesis.

Perinatal changes in chemical neuroregulators

The perinatal period is accompanied by particularly marked changes in the neurochemical milieu of the fetus and newborn. A well known example is the surge in circulating catecholamines associated with normal parturition; increased norepinephrine levels play an important role in the transition from intra- to extrauterine life: for example, by initiating thermogenesis (see p. 357). Perinatal changes in transmitter systems have also recently been described in the central nervous system. For example, animal studies indicate that in specific regions of the brain, such as cerebellum, fetal levels of somatostatin and substance P are several fold higher than in the adult, decreasing dramatically in the perinatal period. Similarly, in human infants, brainstem levels of somatostatin and met-enkephalin decrease significantly during the first months of postnatal life. On the other hand, levels of substance P mRNA in the nucleus tractus solitarius, a region involved in autonomic regulation, appear to increase markedly during the first day of extrauterine life. At present, we speculate that changes in CNS transmitter expression associated with birth may in part reflect alterations in neuronal function that are critical for adaptation to the extrauterine environment.

Selected reading

Black IB. Regulation of autonomic development. *Annu Rev Neurosci* 1978; **1**: 183.

Black IB, Adler AE, Dreyfus CF, *et al.* Neurotransmitter plasticity at the molecular level. *Science* 1984; **225**: 1266.

Lagercrantz H, Slotkin TA. The 'stress' of being born. *Sci Am* 1985; **254**: 100.

Landis SC. Target regulation of neurotransmitter phenotype. *Trends Neurosci* 1990; **13**: 344.

C. SENSORY PHYSIOLOGY

C1. Somatosensory Function during Development

M Fitzgerald

The somatosensory system begins to develop extremely early in fetal life, before either the auditory or the visual systems. At 7–8 weeks of gestation in the human and 15 embryonic days in the rat (E15; where birth is at E21.5) the first connections are made between the peripheral processes of primary sensory neurons in the trigeminal ganglion and their targets in skin and muscle, and also between their central processes in the Vth nerve and neurons in the brainstem. Since motoneurons make contact with muscles at about the same time, the components of a reflex arc are established and stroking the upper or lower lip with a light hair causes a reflex response at 8 weeks. These first sensory connections develop in an approximate rostrocaudal sequence so that at 10.5 weeks the hands are sensitive and by 13.5–14 weeks almost the entire body surface can evoke reflex responses on skin stimulation. A similar sequence is observed in the fetal rat over embryonic days 14–17 (E14–17) and much of the information discussed below is derived from laboratory studies in this species. Other than a basic difference in developmental timetable (the rat is born very immature at approximately the equivalent of the beginning of the third trimester in the human) the events taking place in the developing somatosensory system are very similar in the two species.

The early onset of somatosensory reflexes indicates the formation of sensory connections at the segmental or local level but tell us nothing about the stage at which sensory information is transmitted to higher levels in the thalamus or cortex. In the rat, projection fibers from the spinal cord and brainstem begin to grow into the thalamus in the late fetal period and continue to do so over the early postnatal period. Somewhat later, perhaps triggered by the sensory input, descending cortical fibers arrive in the thalamus, arranging themselves in a lattice around the spinothalamic and trigeminothalamic terminals. Thalamic projection fibers arrive at the cortical plate at birth making an organized pattern of terminals by postnatal day 4 (P4) in the rat and approximately 29 weeks in the human fetus, coinciding with the appearance of somatosensory evoked potentials. The maturation of thalamic and cortical connections takes place over a considerable postnatal period.

Establishing a functionally organized somatosensory system

The task of the somatosensory system is to signal events on the body surface to the central nervous system and to do so effectively it needs to be able to provide the following information: (1) the nature or modality of the signal, i.e. is it touch, pressure, temperature etc.?; (2) the intensity of the signal; and (3) the location of the signal on the body surface. In order to understand somatosensory function during development, it is not enough therefore to establish when appropriate sensory connections are made. We need to study how the signals are transmitted from the periphery and how they are processed centrally at each developmental stage.

The development of peripheral sensory receptors

Information about the nature or modality of a peripheral stimulus is provided by specific sensory afferents, each responding to a particular type of stimulus. Experiments in rats have established that this specificity is present from very early in fetal life, i.e. from the time sensory nerves first reach the skin. At this stage, when as yet no specific end organs (such as hair follicles, Pacinian corpuscles, etc.) have developed and all the sensory nerve endings are apparently homogeneously distributed in a plexus of free nerve endings, it is already possible to distinguish low threshold, rapidly adapting 'touch' receptors from high threshold, slowly adapting 'pressure' receptors and polymodal nociceptors and so on. In other words, these properties are intrinsic to the sensory afferents themselves and are not imposed on them by any anatomical receptors in the target skin. Clearly then, in fetal life information provided by the peripheral afferents to the central nervous system is specific with respect to stimulus modality. The extent to which this specificity is transmitted centrally is not so clear. Again, studies in rats demonstrate that the processing of information within the spinal cord takes much longer to mature.

Maturation of peripheral receptor properties

The ability of peripheral sensory afferents to accurately reflect stimulus intensity in terms of frequency of firing shows great changes through fetal and neonatal life. So although the ability to produce a specific signal to, say, light touch of the skin, is present from the outset, that signal will initially be of a very low amplitude and the frequency response will be very poor. In an adult, very fine alterations in stimulus intensity can be accurately monitored by alterations in firing frequencies of low threshold receptors. Such receptors may fire at 500 Hz or more. Such fine tuning is not present in the fetus and develops gradually, partly with myelination of the axons (which allows more rapid conduction) but especially with the growth and innervation of peripheral end organs. End organs, such as hair follicles and Meissner's corpuscles appear to act as amplifiers and improve the frequency response of primary afferents. Those primary afferents that do not ever innervate such end organs and remain unmyelinated do not change their firing properties from fetal life. C-fiber nociceptors, discussed in more detail on p. 223, have the same properties in fetal life as they do in the adult.

Maturation of central sensory processing in the spinal cord and brainstem

Recordings in the newborn rat and kitten spinal cord and brainstem show that the slow maturation of central synapses greatly restricts the transfer of information into the central nervous system. Central cells are able to fire action potentials only infrequently and easily become fatigued. Their ability to code information about the temporal nature of the stimulus is severely restricted. In the rat, the cells in the spinal cord show reasonably mature responses by P14, but those in the cortex will take considerably longer.

The development of somatotopic maps

Information on the location of a signal on the body surface is, of course, initially provided by the primary afferents whose receptive fields lie within the stimulus site. However, in order to preserve that information centrally, primary sensory afferents are arranged in such a way that they terminate in a highly ordered pattern within the spinal cord or brainstem. Particular peripheral nerves have exclusive non-overlapping terminal fields within the spinal cord and these border with adjacent peripheral nerves to provide an ordered map of the body surface. The result is that neighboring cells in the central nervous system have receptive fields on adjacent areas of skin and the map of the body surface or somatotopic map is preserved at each level of the somatosensory system. This map gives us an accurate image of our body surface and allows us to locate stimuli anywhere on it. When primary sensory afferents first grow into the spinal cord early in fetal life, they do so in the same highly ordered pattern later observed in the adult. The growth is specific and organized and so from an anatomical perspective there is every reason for information concerning stimulus location to be as accurately signaled to the CNS in the fetus as in the adult. However, when recordings are made from neonatal spinal cord cells in the rat it is clear that receptive fields are relatively much larger than in the adult. In other words, the central somatotopic map is smeared and stimulus location will be less accurate. The reason for this appears again to arise from lack of central inhibition in neonatal spinal cord. In the adult, inhibitory processes act to 'focus' or fine tune the somatotopic map, reducing the size of central cells' receptive fields and therefore reducing their overlap with those of their neighbors. This inhibition is lacking in the fetus and neonate, leaving receptive fields larger and the map less focused. Larger receptive fields will act to increase the chance of a given signal actually exciting a central cell, which may be important in the fetus and neonate. However the increased chance of activation is at the expense of accurate information on stimulus location.

Events at higher levels of the nervous system

Much less is known about the functional development of somatosensory processing above spinal cord and brainstem level. Recent results show thalamic afferents reaching the cortical plate at P0 in rats, earlier than was previously thought. These terminals rapidly organize themselves into adult form by P4. There is good evidence that the pattern of thalamocortical afferent projections and organization of cortical sensory cells is determined by the periphery. Experiments using the development of the highly organized sensory pathways for the vibrissae show that a 'blueprint' for constructing an organized 'barrel' of cortical cells related to a single vibrissa is initiated in the periphery. This is transferred to the cortex via a sequentially developing chain of afferent connections, through trigeminal axons, brainstem projections and thalamocortical axons through to the cortical cells. The physiological maturation of cortical cells' receptive fields takes some time. At P7 cells have a clear columnar organization but receptive fields are larger than in the adult, latencies very long and frequency following poor. The same processes almost certainly take place in human infants following the arrival of thalamic afferents in the cortex at 29 weeks and taking place over the following weeks and months.

Injury in the developing somatosensory system

Peripheral sensory nerves are highly sensitive to injury up to the first postnatal 10 days in the rat. Damage to peripheral axons will result in irreversible cell death in the dorsal root ganglion and therefore permanent denervation to that body region. Central cells are dependent on their primary afferent input to develop normally and deafferentation of neonatal rat spinal cord results in permanent growth retardation of spinal cord cells. Central adjustments are made, however, to this peripheral loss. Dorsal roots from nearby intact sensory afferents sprout into the deafferented region, resulting in a permanent distortion of the somatotopic map such that cells in the region will therefore represent fields of inappropriate areas of skin. This phenomenon is seen right up to the cortical level and reorganization of connections within the cortex results in a disproportionately large amount of CNS devoted to surrounding innervated skin at the expense of the denervated region.

Conclusion and comments

While peripheral sensory afferents are capable of signaling stimulus location, modality, and to some extent intensity from early in fetal life, much of this is not processed accurately by the CNS for some time. Synaptic transmission is weak and it appears that one of the primary functions of the immature CNS is amplification of the signal in order to send it centrally. This amplification is at the expense of signal accuracy. Temporal and spatial aspects of sensory stimuli are traded for increasing the chance of evoking activity in central cells. Activity evoked by sensory input is likely to be important for the overall normal development of the nervous system. Peripheral nerve damage in fetal and neonatal life results in permanent alteration in the formation of connections within the somatosensory system.

Selected reading

Coleman JR, ed. *Development of sensory systems in mammals*. Chichester: John Wiley & Sons Inc., 1990.

Fitzgerald M, Shaw A, MacIntosh N. Postnatal development of the cutaneous flexor reflex: comparative study of preterm infants and newborn rat pups. *Dev Med Child Neurol* 1988; **30**: 520.

Hanson MA, ed. *The fetal and neonatal brain-stem—developmental and clinical issues*. Cambridge: Cambridge University Press, 1991.

Rowe M, Willis WD, eds. *Development and plasticity of somatosensory brain maps*. New York: Alan Liss, 1985.

Willis WD, Coggeshall RE, eds. *Sensory mechanisms of the spinal cord*. 2nd ed. New York: Plenum Press, 1991.

C2. Development of Pain Pathways

M Fitzgerald

A useful definition of pain is 'an unpleasant sensory and emotional experience associated with actual or potential tissue damage, or described in terms of such damage'. This chapter concentrates on the sensory rather than the emotional aspects of pain and the first part of this section is a discussion of the basic anatomy (see Fig. 6.14), physiology and pharmacology of developing pain pathways and the associated descending control pathways as understood from laboratory studies. Next, pain behavior in human infants and the methods by which their pain can be assessed is described and interpreted in the light of the underlying neurobiology. Finally, the possible consequences of injury and pain to the developing infant nervous system are considered.

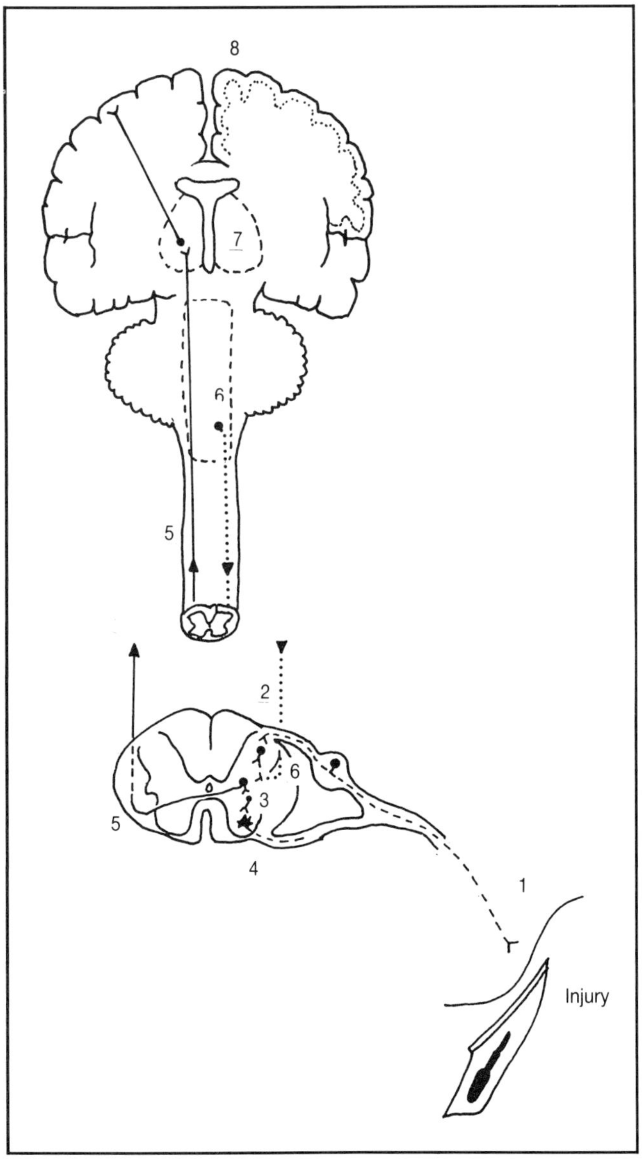

Fig. 6.14. A summary diagram of the key aspects of pain pathway development discussed in this chapter. 1. Peripheral nociceptors in injured tissue. 2. Primary sensory afferent central terminals. 3. Central spinal cord circuits. 4. Nociceptive reflexes. 5. Ascending pathways. 6. Descending inhibitory pathways from the brainstem. 7. Thalamic connections. 8. Cortical mechanisms.

The anatomy and physiology of developing pain pathways

The development of pain pathways has been largely studied in the rat pup and, where possible, complemented with investigation in human infants. The first 3–4 postnatal weeks in a rat spans the late gestational and early neonatal period in the human and the sequence of events appears very similar in the two species.

While all the peripheral sensory receptors appear to develop early in fetal life, the major group of afferents responsible for signaling tissue damage, C-fiber nociceptors, are notable in that their receptor properties in the fetus are exactly the same as in the adult. They are polymodal receptors, responding to mechanical, thermal and chemical noxious stimuli with a characteristic low frequency of firing and fairly slow onset and long after-discharge. As such, these properties appear to be fairly 'primitive' and are established in the fetus with no further need for maturation. Aδ-nociceptors, which are mechanical and heat nociceptors with thinly myelinated axons, do change over the postnatal period, but only in their frequency of firing rather than in a fundamental change in sensitivity.

Despite the early development of their receptor properties, C-fibers are slow to establish mature central synaptic connections. In the rat, they grow into the spinal cord at birth, but do not make connections for at least a week after this. This is quite different from the myelinated sensory afferents which grow into the cord well before birth and rapidly make effective synaptic connections. For the first postnatal week, C-fiber terminals are present in the spinal cord, and are capable of releasing neuro-transmitter when stimulated, but cannot evoke action potentials in central spinal cord cells to allow information to be transmitted to higher centers. In this immature state, the release of neurotransmitters by C-fibers in response to noxious stimulation, is in a rather general 'nonspecific' way, raising the overall excitability of the spinal cord and increasing the responses of subsequent stimuli, rather than activating specific groups of spinal cord cells in the central nociceptive pathway. It is not clear yet whether the same slow development of C-fiber processing takes place in human infants but if so it would suggest that responses to noxious stimuli, particularly those involving tissue damage and inflammation that activate C-fibers, may be present but more diffuse and less specific than in the adult.

Developmental neurochemistry of pain

Substance P and other neuropeptides appear in small diameter C-fiber afferents before birth in the rat and can be released into the spinal cord on electrical stimulation. Levels do not reach those in the adult, however, until postnatal day 15 (P15). Substance P binding sites take a long time to mature. In the neonate, they are diffusely distributed in high density all over the spinal gray matter and only by P21 become organized into discrete areas, confined to superficial dorsal horn and ventral nuclei. In the human spinal cord, substance P appears at about 9 weeks but levels remain low until birth. Enkephalin is one of the last peptides to appear at 14 weeks in the human cord and in the rat at P0. Opiate receptors also undergo considerable postnatal maturation. The appearance of functionally active kappa receptors precedes mu receptors, and this coincides with the onset of κ- and μ-mediated analgesia in rat spinal cord.

The development of ascending and descending pathways

In the rat, the postnatal period sees an enormous increase in the development of central spinal cord circuitry, the growth of ascending and descending pathways and the maturation of the higher centers in thalamus and cortex. In the human infant this takes place over the whole period of infancy. We know remarkably little about pain pathways in these higher centers but since mature somatosensory evoked potentials are not recorded from the rat until P12 and the human until 29 weeks of gestation, it seems that pain processing before then is subcortical. That does not make it any the less important, however, in terms of potential physiological damage.

A particularly important pathway in pain processing is the descending axons that travel down from brainstem control centers onto sensory cells of the spinal cord and trigeminal system. Such descending fibers form an important part of the endogenous pain control system in adults, whereby a noxious input is inhibited at spinal cord level and the resultant pain transmission to higher levels greatly reduced. These descending fibers are present from before birth in the rat but do not become effective until the second postnatal week. In fact, stimulus produced analgesia from the periaqueductal gray cannot be elicited until P21 in the rat. As a result, there is no endogenous dampening down of noxious inputs to the CNS in the immature infant. This may be partly due to the low levels of the transmitters 5-hydroxytryptamine (5-HT) and norepinephrine in these descending inhibitory axons at this time, but also due to immature interneurons (some enkephalinergic) in the spinal cord.

Pain responses in infants

From the above discussion it is not surprising that even the most premature human infants display responses to painful or noxious stimuli. Such responses are difficult to assess due to lack of verbal cues but nevertheless reliable measures have been obtained using facial expression, body movement and cry. Of these, facial expression is the most reliable, characterized by a 'cluster' of facial actions comprising brow bulging, eyes squeezed shut, deepening of the nasolateral furrow and open mouth. Physiological measures such as heart rate, blood pressure and palmar sweating have also been shown to be useful although the immaturity of the autonomic nervous system may confound assessment. Considering the wealth of evidence for such reactions to infant pain and the clear physiological evidence for functional pain pathways, it is interesting that infant pain was ignored and denied for so long. Even now, many pediatric health care workers remain unconvinced that infants 'feel' pain. The reason for this may well lie in the emphasis on 'short, sharp' pain, such as that evoked by a heel lance or needle as an example of pain reactions. Many reports demonstrate the inherent inter- and intrasubject variability in response to such brief noxious stimuli. Physiological studies provide evidence for it. Sensory C-fibers have not formed mature synaptic contacts in the spinal cord and responses must be evoked by weak synaptic transmission from Aδ-fibers. But such 'short, sharp' pain may have little relation to pain in a clinical setting such as postoperatively or during intensive care procedures. When such longer term pain in infants is studied, there is no doubt about their response.

Hormonal and metabolic responses provide very clear indication of pain in infants following surgery for ligation of a *patent ductus arteriosus* and support the use of fentanyl in both pain relief and reducing postoperative complications. Studies using sensory reflex thresholds after repeated (rather than single) heel lances to show that a clear hyperalgesia or tenderness develops in the site of a local skin injury in the youngest premature infant. Therefore, while individual infants may give somewhat unreliable responses to a single painful stimulus, there is no doubt that the infant nervous system is capable of mounting a very clear response to a more established, clinically relevant pain.

Potential long-term consequences of pain in infancy

Tissue damage produces pain by activating nociceptive sensory afferents which then trigger central changes in the CNS. While these central changes are incompletely understood, it is clear that the balance of central excitation is altered such that previously ineffective 'subthreshold' sensory inputs become capable of exciting central cells. The developing central nervous system is especially vulnerable to alterations in its sensory inputs. The effects of peripheral nerve damage on the subsequent development of the somatosensory system is discussed on p. 222. Excessive or noxious inputs may be equally powerful in altering the pattern of connections in the developing CNS. The infant spinal cord lacks descending inhibition from the brainstem. This may be advantageous to the normal developing CNS by maximizing all sensory inputs but it means that abnormal noxious stimuli are not dampened down at all at spinal cord level as in the adult. Effective pain relief has now been shown to reduce postoperative morbidity in premature infants. It may also ensure normal sensory development in infants exposed to trauma during a critical stage of development.

Selected reading

Anand KJS, Sippell WG, Aynsley-Green A. Randomized trial of fentanyl anaesthesia in preterm babies undergoing surgery: effects on the stress response. *Lancet* 1987; **i**: 243.

Fitzgerald M. Development of pain mechanisms. *Br Med Bull* 1991; **47**: 667.

Fitzgerald M. The developmental neurobiology of pain. In Bond MR, Charlton JE, Woolf CJ, eds. *Pain research and clinical management*. Amsterdam: Elsevier, 1991: 253.

Lloyd-Thomas A. *Practical pain control in children*. Oxford: Oxford University Press, in press.

McGrath P. *Pain in children*. New York: The Guildford Press, 1990.

McGrath PJ, Unruh AM. Pain in children and adolescents. In Bond MR, Charlton JE, Woolf CJ, eds. *Pain research and clinical management*. Vol. 1. Amsterdam: Elsevier, 1987.

Schechter N, Berde C, Yaster M. *Pain management in children and adolescents*. Baltimore: Williams & Wilkins, in press.

C3. Development of the Auditory System

A G Pettigrew and D J Henderson-Smart

The development of speech and intellectual processes of language depend on adequate auditory function from a very early age. The development of mental and psycho-motor function also appears to depend on binaural processing for sound localization during the early postnatal period. The auditory system is, however, vulnerable to adverse prenatal and postnatal influences and these factors can have long-term consequences on the behavior and function of the individual.

Development of the peripheral auditory system

The human pinna achieves an adult-like structure by about 20 weeks of gestation and continues to grow until about the age of 10 years. The ear canal in newborn infants is only slightly shorter than that of adults, but it is narrower, more oval in shape, and because it is surrounded by only a thin layer of cartilage it is very soft. This feature has important implications for auditory assessment in neonates because false negative diagnosis of auditory deficit can arise from compression of the outer canal. During infancy, the canal wall and the cartilage thicken to produce a more rigid meatus and the position of the tympanic membrane changes relative to the wall of the canal.

The ossicles of the middle ear cavity and the tympanic ring (which supports the tympanic membrane) grow to adult size during the period of 10–22 weeks of gestation. At this age the ossicles are cartilaginous, but ossification is completed by about 32 weeks of gestation. The maturation of the tympanic ring is protracted and includes completion of the ring structure and growth of lateral processes which contribute to the outer canal. Maturation of the middle ear muscles occurs during the fourth month of gestation. The maturation of the tympanic membrane is completed by about 6.5 months of gestation although slight changes in its orientation occur postnatally. Clearance of the middle ear cavity occurs during the last month of gestation but the cavity becomes enlarged postnatally. All of these changes contribute to the development of middle ear function and an increase in middle ear compliance in the neonatal period. The functional development of the middle ear is probably the determining factor in the development of auditory sensitivity.

Development of the cochlea

The cochlea in the human begins to develop at about 3 weeks after conception. The organ of Corti differentiates between 10 and 25 weeks of gestation, by which time it has reached its adult form. The inner hair cells differentiate prior to the outer hair cells and this occurs first in the middle of the basal turn of the cochlea and then proceeds to the remaining part of the basal turn and towards the apex. The axons of cochlear ganglion cells enter the developing cochlea very early and innervate the hair cells in a basal to apical sequence soon after they differentiate. Synaptogenesis between the axons and the hair cells occurs prior to formation of the stereocilia (week 15 versus week 22). The growth and myelination of the cochlear axons occurs in the same basal to apical sequence, myelination having begun at about 6 months of gestation.

Development of the auditory pathway

The central axons of the ganglion cells penetrate the medulla at about 8 weeks of gestation, just after the differentiation of the brainstem auditory nuclei. The differentiation of the higher nuclei of the central auditory pathway occurs over the next few weeks and myelination of the central pathway begins in the brainstem at about 6 months of gestation and slightly later at higher levels of the pathway.

Onset of function

It has been estimated that the human cochlea has sufficient structural development at 18 weeks to provide auditory input. However, the onset of hearing in the human probably occurs at about 26–27 weeks of gestation. It is at or soon after this age that acceleration of the heart rate, movements of the body and eye-blinks of the fetus *in utero* can be detected in response to loud sounds delivered to the maternal abdomen. These responses are best evoked using tones below 2 kHz; responses to tones of higher frequency appear to develop slightly later. It is also at 27–28 weeks post-conception that neurophysiological evidence of central neuronal activity in response to brief sounds (see below) can be recorded in premature infants.

Development of auditory sensitivity

Several methods have been developed to assess the auditory sensitivity of newborn infants. Some of these methods rely on the behavioral response of the infant to a sound. Whilst these techniques are relatively simple, the interpretation of data can be complicated by changes in the state of arousal of the infant.

The most popular objective method for determining the auditory sensitivity of a neonate is to record auditory evoked responses. These responses are recorded by averaging samples of the electroencephalogram detected from electrode pairs at conventional locations on the scalp following each of a train of brief auditory stimuli of known intensity (either broad-band clicks or tone pips). With appropriate amplifier filters and time samples it is possible to record submicrovolt waveforms that are generated in the brainstem (brainstem auditory evoked response, BAER, Fig. 6.15), or larger and longer waveforms that are generated in the midbrain and cortex (middle latency evoked and cortical evoked responses). Unlike the latter two evoked responses, the BAER is unaffected by the state of arousal of the infant, is a highly reproducible potential and is ideal for determining the auditory sensitivity of an infant.

It is generally accepted that the thresholds for sounds of various types are higher in preterm neonates than in young infants and adults. Relatively few studies, however, have examined the development of auditory sensitivity in neonates in detail. This is an important question because steps to facilitate the earliest possible detection of hearing deficit in infants must be considered relative to the time course of normal auditory development. Recent reports in the literature indicate that whilst some preterm neonates can have BAER thresholds to click stimuli of 40 dB hearing level (HL) at 28–34 weeks of gestational age, other preterm infants, who subsequently have normal hearing, have BAER thresholds at considerably higher levels (70–80 dB HL) at this early age (Fig. 6.16). On the other hand, a small percentage of preterm infants who have thresholds at this level at this age can exhibit long-lasting moderate to profound hearing deficits. On the basis of longitudinal and cross-sectional studies of preterm and term infants using BAERs, it appears that those infants who achieve thresholds of 30 dB HL or better by term equivalent age can be expected to have normal auditory sensitivity. Furthermore, it has been recommended that any screening procedure for early detection of auditory deficits is best performed at or as close as possible to term equivalent age. Tests prior to this age can reveal thresholds that are elevated but which subsequently resolve over as little as 2 days and the infants subsequently have normal hearing. It has also been recommended that any evidence of elevated auditory thresholds at term age be confirmed by follow-up testing using BAERs and behavioral methods.

Functional capacity of the auditory system in the newborn

Sound localization

Provided certain procedural and stimulus conditions are observed, it is possible to demonstrate that infants of only a few days of age are capable of orientating their head towards an off-center sound such as that of a rattle. This ability is lost after about the first month postnatal, and re-emerges at 4–5 months postnatal. It has been proposed that the first period of orientation ability is associated with reflex mechanisms in the brainstem and that the subsequent decrease and re-emergence of orientation ability reflects changes in cortical control of the behavior. This possibility has received support from studies in

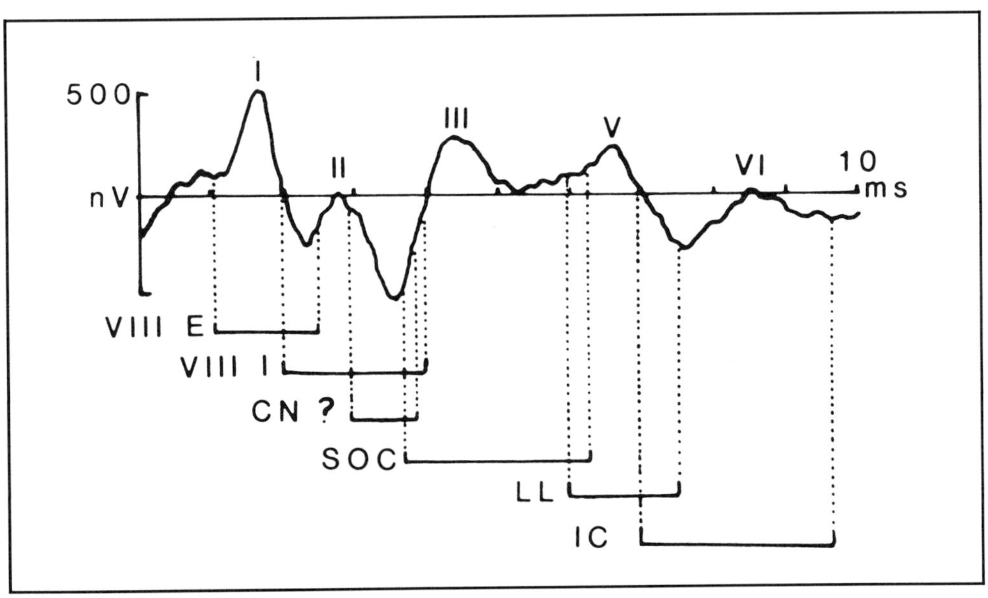

Fig. 6.15. BAER recorded from an infant and possible sites of neural activity generating the response. VIII E, extracranial auditory nerve; VIII I, intracranial auditory nerve; CN, cochlear nuclei; SOC, superior olivary complex; LL, lateral lemniscus; IC, inferior colliculus. (Taken in part with permission from Henderson-Smart *et al.* In Hanson MA, ed. *The fetal and neonatal brainstem*. Cambridge: Cambridge University Press, 1991.)

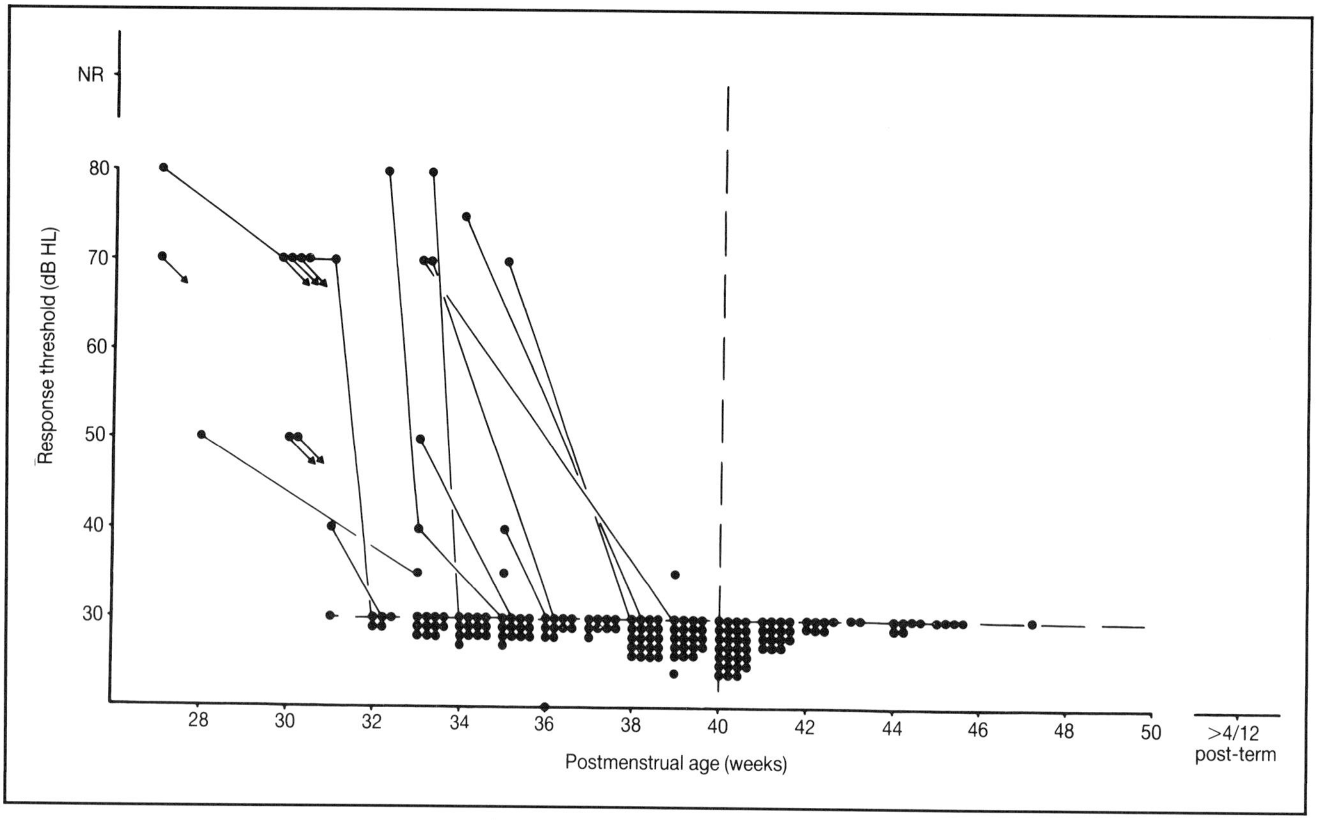

Fig. 6.16. BAER thresholds (dB hearing level, HL) in a group of preterm and term infants. Arrows indicate that the thresholds in those infants were 30 dB HL or lower at or after term equivalent age. Lines connect data points for other individual preterm infants and indicate that auditory thresholds can fall quickly in the postnatal period. (Data in part from Pettigrew *et al. Early Hum Dev* 1986; **14**: 109.)

which the precedence effect was used to examine the role of cortical processing in auditory localization in infants. Infants were only able to localize sounds under these conditions during the second phase of orientation responses to simpler sounds. Even though other explanations of this age-related change in behavior can be proposed, the data indicate that the use of orientation responses for testing auditory sensitivity in young infants must be made with care.

Speech discrimination

It has been established for some time that infants can discriminate between speech sounds which differ in vowel content, voicing and initial or final consonants. Indeed, behavioral studies suggest that the processing of auditory signals by infants at 1 month of age may be adequate for speech perception and language comprehension. Recent research has also shown that infants as young as 2 days of age and at 1 month exhibit a preference for so-called child-directed speech ('motherese') which is characterized in comparison to adult-directed speech by higher overall pitch, wider excursions in pitch, and slower tempo. Newborn infants also prefer their mother's voice to that of another female saying the same words and they can discriminate two languages when one of the languages is native to their culture. These abilities have been attributed to the capacity of the auditory system in the newborn to respond to psychophysical properties of speech sounds. Infants at this age also show left–right preferences for tones and syllables. These and other behavioral observations indicate that auditory function during the last stages of gestation and in the newborn period is well developed and exerts an important influence on behavior. The recording of averaged cortical potentials evoked by different speech sounds during development of newborn infants has also been undertaken and variations in the responses with electrode location, stimulus content, arousal and maturation have been reported.

Tests for auditory dysfunction in neonates

The series of deflections in the normal BAER waveform have a fixed pattern and the latencies of these deflections vary with sound intensity and postnatal age. The latencies of all peaks in the response are affected equally by sound intensity and hence the interpeak intervals in the response remain constant with changes in stimulus intensity (or peripheral sensitivity). On the other hand, delays or absence of peaks in the response have been associated with abnormal function of the central auditory pathway. Because the waveform of the BAER is generated from a series of sites in the brainstem, the identification of peaks and the measurement of interpeak intervals obtained in this non-invasive test can be used to provide information about neural function at different levels in this sensory pathway. The advantage that this technique offers in providing objective evidence of auditory and brainstem neural function underlies its current popularity.

Methods such as the auditory cradle or 'crib-o-gram' and habituation techniques, which rely on infant movement following a sound, have been used and provide a relatively inexpensive first level screen for auditory dysfunction. Follow-up assessment of infants who have failed to reach criteria with these and other behavioral methods are essential.

A newer method for the assessment of peripheral auditory function is the recording of evoked otoacoustic emissions. When a normal hearing ear is exposed to a brief sound such as a click, there follows after a few milliseconds delay a low level sound in the external meatus which can be detected by a sensitive microphone. This otoacoustic emission is generated within the cochlea and is unaffected by the state of arousal of the patient. Furthermore, the emission is not measurable when the ear under test has a hearing loss of more than 15–30 dB HL. The technique has been recommended for auditory screening but when a negative result is detected, hearing should also be assessed using BAERs.

Factors that influence auditory development

Certain perinatal factors place an infant at risk of auditory dysfunction. The list of these factors most often includes (1) family history of deafness, (2) maternal infection during pregnancy (*toxoplasmosis*, *rubella*, *cytomegalovirus*, or *herpes simplex*), (3) neonatal infection (especially *meningitis*), (4) *congenital malformations* and (5) complications commonly associated with preterm delivery. The possibility that auditory deficits in older infants may have followed exposure to loud sounds for extended periods should also not be overlooked.

The highest incidence of auditory deficit is consistently reported to be amongst infants who have survived very early preterm delivery, and in particular those preterm infants who have suffered severe *hyperbilirubinemia* and relatively long-term exposure to ototoxic antibiotics. However, just as one factor might be prominent for one infant, another infant with the same insult can have normal hearing. Thus the general view has been put that auditory deficits in preterm infants are associated with a complex interaction of factors which occurs during a less-than-optimal perinatal course.

Changes in the auditory pathway with abnormal development

The development of neuronal populations and the interconnection between neurons within the auditory system can be severely disrupted by abnormal development of the peripheral auditory system. For example, lesions of the cochlea at a very young age are associated with substantial loss of neurons in the cochlear nucleus and rearrangement of connections between neurons in these and other brainstem auditory nuclei. On the other hand, unilateral conductive hearing loss does not appear to affect the number of neurons in the cochlear nucleus on the affected side, but it does interfere with the organization of connections between the cochlear nuclei and the inferior colliculus. Several studies also indicate that activity within the auditory axons has an important influence on the transneuronal regulation of cell size in the auditory nuclei. These experimental data should be borne in mind when the development of the auditory system in neonates is under threat. It cannot be assumed that strategies for the alleviation of auditory deficits in newborn infants and young children will be operating through a normal auditory pathway.

Selected reading

Edelman GM, Gall WE, Cowan WM, eds. *Auditory function. Neurobiological bases of hearing*. New York: John Wiley and Sons, 1988.

Moore DR. Anatomy and physiology of binaural hearing. *Audiology* 1991; **30**: 125.

Muir DW, Clifton RK, Clarkson MG. The development of a human auditory localization response: a U-shaped function. *Can J Psychol* 1989; **43**: 199.

Pettigrew AG, Edwards DA, Henderson-Smart DJ. Screening for auditory dysfunction in high risk neonates. *Early Hum Dev* 1986; **14**: 109.

Pettigrew AG, Edwards DA, Henderson-Smart DJ. Perinatal risk factors in preterm infants with moderate-to-profound hearing deficits. *Med J Aust* 1988; **148**: 174.

Romand R, ed. *Development of auditory and vestibular systems*. New York: Academic Press, 1983.

Stevens JC, Webb HD, Hutchinson J, *et al*. Evaluation of click-evoked oto-acoustic emissions in the newborn. *Br J Audiol* 1991; **25**: 11.

C4. Development of the Visual System

J Atkinson

Development of the visual system can be thought of as consisting of three overlapping and interacting parts:

1. Increased sensitivity during development to different visual attributes such as contrast, detail, velocity of motion, orientation or slant. Here development is in both the peripheral system (e.g. the photoreceptors in the retina) and in central pathways of the cortex. Many different segregated pathways develop differentially, carrying information from the eye to the brain, with analysis and reanalysis en route.
2. Improvements in the eye movement control systems, linked in many instances to mechanisms responsible for selective attention.
3. Development of interpretive mechanisms to understand incoming information and initiate appropriate motor actions.

It is not always possible to separate these three processes in any observable overt visual behavior. For example, if a 9-month-old child learning to crawl falls down a step, is this because the child cannot detect and perceive depth changes, or because he can analyze disparity cues but cannot interpret them, or merely because he has poor integration between perceptual and motor actions? The deficit in development could be in any one of these systems or in all of them.

Assessment of the developing visual system

To attempt to dissociate different sensory, perceptual, cognitive and motor operations, a number of different techniques and methodologies have been developed. These can be broadly specified as behavioral, electrophysiological or photorefractive.

Behavioral assessment

Here overt visual behavior is observed and measured. Two such methods are preferential looking and habituation. In preferential looking the ability to detect differences between two simultaneously presented displays is gauged from the child's preference for looking at one display rather than the other. Preferential looking has been used extensively to measure acuity (see below). More complex visual and cognitive discriminations (e.g. between different textures) have been tested in infants using habituation/dishabituation paradigms. When the same pattern is presented repeatedly an infant's responsiveness (assessed either by looking time or measures of arousal) declines; the infant is said to be habituated to the pattern when a certain criterion or decrement in responsiveness is reached. Following this a novel pattern is presented. If responsiveness now increases then the infant must have been able to detect a difference between the old and the new patterns—this is called dishabituation or recovery.

Electrophysiological assessment

The visual evoked potential response (VEP) is a small electrical potential recorded from scalp electrodes. The

VEP is obtained by synchronizing recording with the stimulus (which may be a pattern either appearing or reversing in contrast). To increase the signal-to-noise ratio the stimulus is presented repeatedly and the electrophysiological response is averaged. Cortical and subcortical activity specific to the stimulus are thus magnified relative to other electroencephalographic activity. The significance of the response depends on sophisticated statistical analysis comparing the phase, amplitude and latency of the electrical response with changes in the eliciting visual pattern. In clinical testing phase reversing checkerboard patterns are often used. 'Designer stimuli' which specifically elicit responses from particular types of neurons for dissociating cortical from subcortical responses are described below.

Photo/videorefraction

Recently a family of techniques has been devised for measuring the optics of the eyes in infants and young children; these are called photorefraction or videorefraction. The technique depends on measurement of a light reflex on the retina from a small flash source.

Theories of visual development

Data obtained over the last 20 years using these techniques has led to several theoretical models of visual development. These are briefly discussed below, together with some of the evidence pertaining to them.

The idea of 'two visual systems' arose out of comparative studies of vision across different species. It was suggested that subcortical systems control orienting responses which define crudely 'where' an object is located and trigger foveation to this location, while cortical mechanisms are used to define 'what' is actually in the foveated area. Using this idea, Bronson (1974) put forward a model of human visual development, suggesting that newborn vision was totally subcortically controlled—the cortex matured at around 2 months postnatally. Atkinson (1984) put forward a modified 'two visual systems' model suggesting that the newborn visual system was 'largely' subcortically controlled, with different cortical mechanisms starting to function at different times postnatally.

In adult vision a 'where' and a 'what' system have been defined solely within the cortical pathways—a largely parietal module is concerned with localizing objects within a spatial array, while those involving the temporal lobe contain mechanisms tuned to 'what' aspects such as form and color. A second model of adult visual processing, arising out of the first, is based on two types of anatomically and morphologically distinct ganglion cells of the retina (parvocellular and magnocellular). The two streams are separate at the subcortical levels with parvocellular and magnocellular neurons projecting to different regions of primary visual cortex, V1. A parvocellular based system subserves detailed form vision and color, while the magnocellular system subserves movement perception and some aspects of stereoscopic vision. Anatomical and physiological findings have allowed identification of populations of neurons specific for detection of separate visual attributes within these cortical streams. Information for different attributes within these cortical streams appears to be segregated at many different levels of the cortex. Using these adult and primate models, it is possible to consider infant development in terms of onset of function in specific cortical streams. Below we consider the development of selectively tuned pools of neurons for visual processing of a number of different attributes.

The development of visual function

Visual acuity and contrast sensitivity

The commonest measure, clinically, is that of visual acuity (VA). Three different measures can be defined: (1) Detection acuity—the smallest object or line that can be detected. (2) Resolution acuity—the finest detail that can be resolved. Resolution acuity is often measured in infants, young children and pediatric patients with very limited communication skills by means of preferential looking. (3) Recognition acuity—the smallest letter stroke width to allow correct letter identification. Snellen measures of this type are universally used to measure adult visual acuity (expressed as a fraction or decimal compared to a standard adult norm of stroke width equal to 1 minute arc). Modifications using letter matching in preschool children have been devised. Recognition acuity in adults is slightly lower for letters in a crowded array than for isolated single letters. This 'crowding effect' is more marked in preschool children, amblyopes and some dyslexics.

VA specifies only how well the system handles fine detail. The quality of functional vision depends also on how well more coarse, but possibly fainter, patterns of light and dark can be detected, measured in the contrast sensitivity function (CSF). Grating patterns with sinusoidal luminance profiles are used, varying both spatial frequency (broadness of the stripes) and contrast (the intensity difference between the brightest and darkest points of the grating). In adults the CSF is approximately U shaped, with lower sensitivity at both low and very high spatial frequencies. Resolution acuity represents the special point on this function where even a grating of 100 percent contrast can only just be detected.

There is very rapid development of both acuity and contrast sensitivity over the first 6 postnatal months (simulated in Fig. 6.17). This is followed by gradual increases up to adult levels for resolution acuity by 3–5 years and for recognition acuity of single letters by 5–6 years. Newborn acuity, measured at near distances, has been estimated at around the 30 minute arc. If this is approximately converted to an adult distance acuity it would place the individual on the legally blind register! However the newborn's vision is adequate for distinguishing between many large objects and is better than that needed for independent mobility in partially sighted adults.

Information on detail and contrast is carried by both subcortical and cortical visual pathways. Three steady changes in underlying processes over the first postnatal year of life, each likely to be limiting factors, are: the differentiation of the fovea, myelination of the visual pathways, and increases in the number of synapses. In addition, optical refractive errors (in particular marked astigmatism) may be a major limiting factor in infants over 6 months of age. Several models have shown that both retinal and neural limitations underlie acuity changes in infants, and it is not easy to separate subcortical from cortical contributions to these limitations.

Orientation or slant

There is now general agreement that infants can discriminate between static grating patterns, differing in orientation or slant of the lines. A statistically reliable steady state VEP (OR-VEP) can be elicited by a 90 degree change in orientation. This can be taken as evidence for orientation-selective mechanisms which are only found in cortical visual pathways and not subcortically. At a rapid reversal rate between the two orientations (e.g. 8 reversals per second) a significant response is found only in the second postnatal month. With slower alternations (3 reversals per second), the median age for the response is 3 weeks. Interestingly, this rapid improvement in temporal sensitivity appears to be specific to the orientation response and not to nonorientational mechanisms.

Directional motion

It is well established that young infants prefer moving to static visual displays. However, this in itself cannot be taken as evidence of the operation of true motion mechanisms. Any moving stimulus also produces a temporal modulation and it is well known that infants show a preference for full field flicker, i.e. temporal modulation without coherent motion. In general, true motion detectors are in evidence if a differential response to different directions of motion can be demonstrated. To measure such mechanisms designer stimuli can be used, consisting of two-dimensional random dot displays, which can have a particular direction of motion without the confounding presence of any dominant orientation component. In a similar way to the OR-VEP, a VEP can thus be generated to a change in the direction of motion of a set of random dots. The first significant motion VEP for a velocity of 5 degrees per second appears at around 2 months of age, with onset for higher velocities occurring later. Parallel behavioral studies show once again that the velocity is a critical determinant in obtaining discrimination of relative motion at different ages.

The magnocellular stream running from ganglion cells to the cortical regions V1, V2, V3 and MT is related to information about direction. In the previous section we saw that some discrimination of orientations was possible at birth and it seems strange that information about direction of movement should not also be a built-in capability of the newborn, to provide fundamental information about 'where'? Indeed the newborn does have a crude directional system already operating as is evidenced by the optokinetic system giving optokinetic nystagmus (OKN)—a largely subcortical stabilizing mechanism which is present in the visual system of virtually every species. Thus it seems that the infant has at least two potential 'where' systems—the

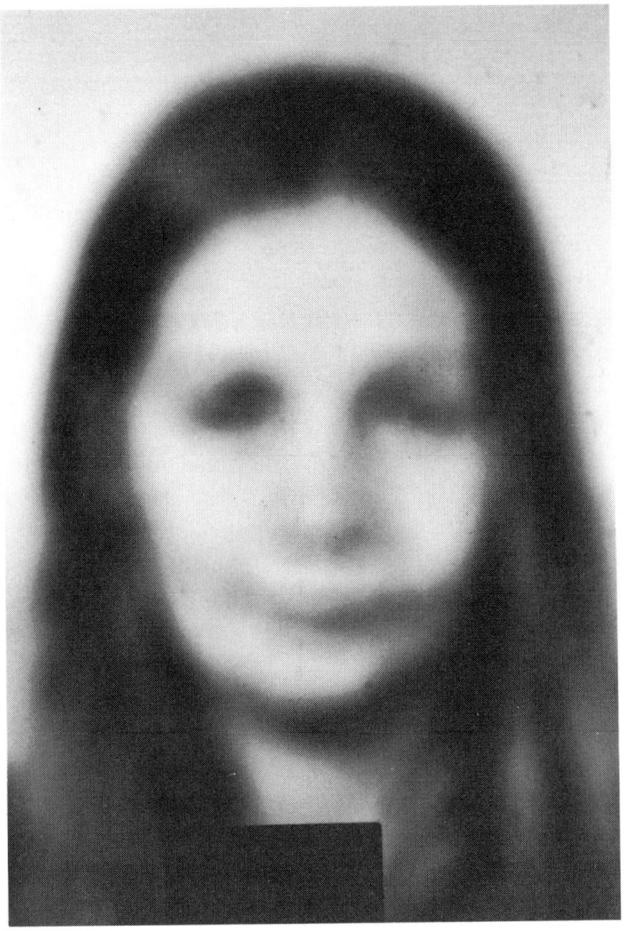
(a)

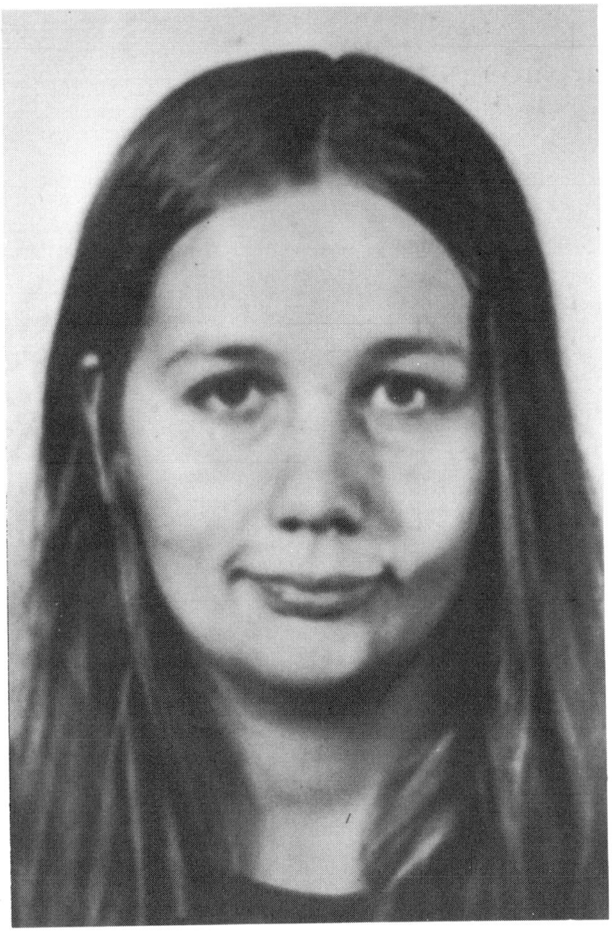
(b)

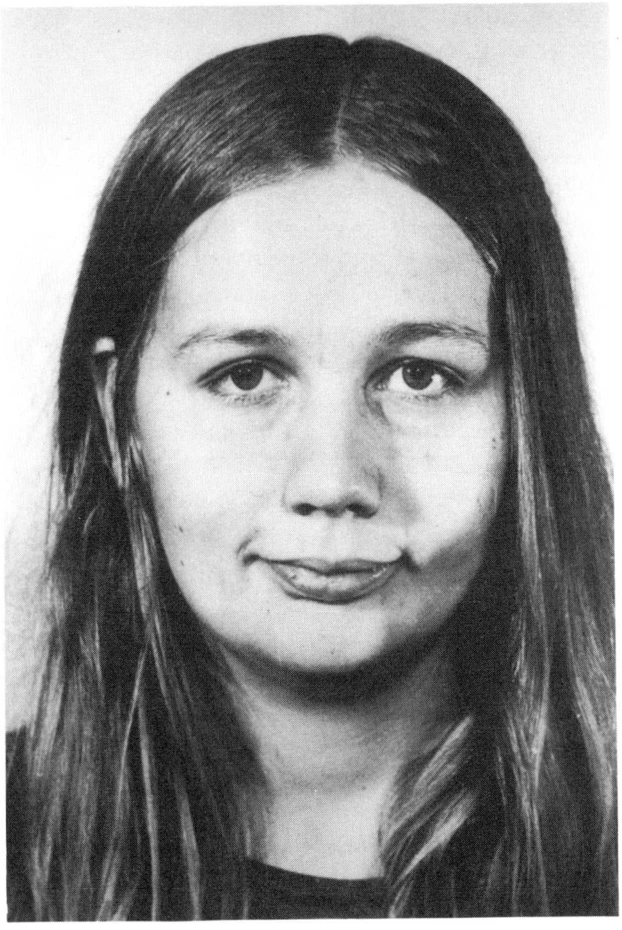
(c)

Fig. 6.17. (a) Simulation, using experimental acuity values and an optical blur function, of the image a newborn would have of a face, viewed at 25 cm distance; (b) similar simulation for 3-month infant; (c) fully focused image seen by an adult.

OKN mechanism (operating maximally when the whole visual field is moving in a uniform direction) and a cortically controlled system (to fixate and smoothly track a single object in the field of view). This later cortical system presumably operates within the magnocellularly based system and in developmental terms becomes functional later than the subcortical system (i.e. a few months postnatally).

Binocularity

As signals from the two eyes first interact at the cortex, any response dependent on detection of binocular correlation or disparity must be dependent on the operation of cortical rather than subcortical mechanisms. Such responses are first seen on average around 3–4 months post-term with adult values in stereoacuity being reached by 4–5 years or possibly a little earlier. These studies and models indicate that the onset of functioning of cortical binocular mechanisms is postnatal and such mechanisms cannot be used in any depth or distance judgements involved in spatial localization made prior to 3 months of age. The magnocellular system is thought to be the predominant location of disparity-selective neurons.

Differential onset in parvocellular and magnocellular streams

The findings on development of three types of cortical detectors have been considered above. Each type is specific for coding information concerning a particular spatial attribute: orientation (necessary for shape analysis), directional movement (for analyzing an object's trajectory), and correlation/disparity detection (for judging the object's relative depth or distance from other objects). Development of sensitivity to these attributes takes place postnatally and must depend on cortical, rather than subcortical, analysis.

Infants show sensitivity to changes of orientation before they show differential responses to the direction of movement and before they detect disparity change. Although not discussed here, infants in the first few weeks after birth show relatively sophisticated ability to detect differences based on color alone, using isoluminant displays. The above data suggest that certain parts of the parvocellular system become functional slightly before parts of the magnocellular system.

Development of eye movement systems and attentional control mechanisms

Many eye movement control systems are subcortical. However, effective oculomotor behavior requires not only selection of a fixation target but also disengagement of attention from one object to switch to another. These abilities, involving cortical control of subcortical circuitry, show striking improvements in the first few postnatal months. The newborn has difficulty disengaging fixation from a continuously present central target to a second one in the peripheral field. This 'sticky' fixation can be likened to *Balint syndrome* patients (with bilateral parietal damage). Difficulties in shifting attention, monitored using photorefraction, show that the newborn only change their focus for targets over a fairly narrow near range (2–3 feet). However, by 6 months this ability is almost adult-like.

Changes in refraction with age, abnormal refractions and links to strabismus

Statements about refraction and refractive errors usually refer to the focusing power of the eye when accommodation is completely relaxed, for instance by a cycloplegic drug. Where the eyes are focused in normal vision depends on whether the eyes are myopic, emmetropic or hyperopic when relaxed, and on the degree of active accommodation at that instance. Two different refractive states are seen in the newborn depending on whether cycloplegia is used or not; the average cyclopegic refraction is slightly hyperopic while the newborn tends to accommodate freely myopically. Very few marked spherical myopic cycloplegic refractions are seen in the first few years of life, although there is a high incidence of both myopic and hyperopic astigmatisms and spherical hyperopia. These errors tend to reduce in most infants by 2 years of age. Any marked error persisting beyond 2 years may lead to *amblyopia*.

Marked hyperopia in the first year of life is predictive for *strabismus* and *amblyopia* in the preschool years.

Successful prevention of *strabismus* and *amblyopia* may be achieved by spectacle correction for refractive errors in infancy.

Disruption of normal vision in one eye early in life can seriously disrupt development of binocular vision. The resulting *amblyopia* means that this eye cannot perceive forms and shapes normally.

Misalignment of the two eyes (*strabismus*) usually results in the visual cortex not encoding the information from the deviating eye (suppression). If a squint is present early in life and left untreated for years, late surgery will be largely cosmetic with little vision recovered. Very few squints are manifest at birth, although the newborn can be intermittently strabismic for several months. It is possible that some infants develop *strabismus* because of a congenital lack of potential binocularity; e.g. albinos lack the uncrossed visual pathways so information from the two eyes is not combined in the cortex. Others develop normal disparity detection at 4 months postnatally, but lose it as the result of a developing *strabismus*. Early surgery is thought more likely to restore normal binocular development, although even with early treatment good stereoacuity is rarely achieved.

Here, visual development has been considered largely in isolation from other developing systems. However sensory, perceptual, cognitive, and social development is heavily linked. It may be that delays in the development of one visual mechanism affect not only other visual circuitry, but also other integrative systems crossmodally. It may be that there are often delays common to all brain mechanisms in a single individual. As yet there is debate about whether these relationships are correlations or causations.

Selected reading

Atkinson J. Human visual development over the first six months of life: a review and a hypothesis. *Hum Neurobiol* 1984; **3**: 61.

Atkinson J. Assessment of vision in infants and young children. In Harel S, Anastasiow NJ, eds. *The at-risk infant: psycho/socio/medical aspects*. Baltimore: Paul H Brookes Publishing Co. Inc., 1985.

Atkinson J. Infant vision screening: prediction and prevention of strabismus and amblyopia from refractive screening in the Cambridge photorefraction program. In Simons K, ed. *Infant vision: basic and clinical research committee on vision*. Commission on Behavioral and Social Sciences and Education, National Research Council. New York: Oxford University Press, in press.

C5. Ocular Motor Control

G Lennerstrand and J Ygge

The eyes are part of a moving head that in turn is part of a moving body, and the visual search of the space around us involves a smooth coordination of all these movement systems.

Eye movement types

The need for eye movements is twofold: first the visual system performs best when images are steady on the retina. Since the head and body are in motion most of the time, eye movements must compensate for this to maintain an appropriate vision. The vestibulo-ocular reflex and optokinetic system serve this function. Secondly, with the evolution of a fovea, the central part of the retina where the highest visual acuity resides, eye movements are needed to bring the object of interest onto that part of the retina. The saccadic system serves this function. When at the fovea, the smooth pursuit system holds moving targets there.

Studies on eye movements in adults are extensive, but only recently have attempts been made to record eye movements of infants. The technique of electro-oculography (EOG) has been used almost exclusively, since other more sensitive and accurate methods are either too intrusive or require too much cooperation on the part of the child.

Development of ocular motor function

Eye muscles and motor nerves are formed in the sixth week of fetal life, and fetal eye movements have been demonstrated by ultrasonic investigations already in the sixteenth week of gestation. These eye movements are at first slow changes in eye position but tend to be more related to fetal behavior by the end of the third trimester.

The eye muscles are probably functioning by birth in a manner similar to that of the adult, with the exception of speed of contraction which is probably slower due to thinner muscle and nerve fibers. Very little is known about the development of the brainstem mechanisms controlling eye movements.

Congenital defects of eye muscles, motor nuclei and nerves are uncommon. Aplasia of the abducens nucleus can occur and leads to misdirected innervation of the lateral rectus muscle by the oculomotor nerve in the *eye retraction syndrome of Stilling–Türk–Duane*. Eye motor defects may be due to more common congenital brainstem and cerebellar anomalies: *myelomeningocele* with the *Chiari malformation*. The defects include horizontal gaze palsy, strabismus and nystagmus.

The vestibulo-ocular reflex (VOR)

Existing data indicate that the VOR time constants increase during the first 3–5 months of life to reach nearly adult values. The gain of the VOR is larger in infancy and declines during childhood and perhaps adolescence to adult rates.

Ophthalmological nystagmus of the fixation type such as *congenital nystagmus* is probably not connected with VOR dysfunction but is more likely with other abnormalities of the brainstem or cerebellar control of eye movements.

Saccades

Saccades (sudden jerky movements), the fastest of all eye movements, serve to redirect the line of sight to a new target of interest. During the first postnatal months the tendency to change fixation increases and older infants become more attentive to peripherally located visual stimuli. The saccadic latencies are longer in infants than in adults and increase with target eccentricity. Large saccades are usually hypometric in infants and seem to be programmed in smaller, stepwise movements due to some motor or sensory constraint. However, the saccadic system can function without hypometria if appropriate targets are supplied and free scanning of the visual scene is allowed. The saccadic system thus appears to be the first well coordinated motor system of human development. However, the age at which the size, the latency and the sequencing of saccades reaches adult levels is not known.

Saccades are among the few eye movements that can be executed voluntarily. *Oculomotor apraxia* is a congenital defect of horizontal, but not vertical saccadic movements. Refixations are instead elicited with head thrusts, which are very characteristic of the condition.

Pursuit

The smooth pursuit system serves to track an object of interest and to keep that target on the fovea. Pursuit is generally believed to reflect foveal function, and infants are known to have immature foveas.

Smooth pursuit in young infants is dependent on the size and the speed of the moving target. Stimulation with large targets at low speed may activate not only the fovea but also parafoveal retinal areas and therefore elicit optokinetic responses and not actual pursuit movements. Saccadic pursuit or 'cog-wheeling' is easily evoked in infants, as well as combinations of the eye and head movements. At 2 months of age smooth pursuit movements were seen but they were lagging the stimulus. An adult-like smooth pursuit had not evolved even at 8 months of age, but the exact age of maturation is not known. However, horizontal pursuit movements seem to develop earlier than vertical movements.

Optokinetic nystagmus (OKN)

Within a few hours of birth OKN can be evoked, although with subnormal slow phase velocity which progressively reaches adult levels. With monocular testing there is a clear directional preponderance in the infant below some 4–5 months of age, and the nasally directed stimuli elicit stronger OKN than temporally directed ones. The asymmetry disappears with the development of binocular vision, but it is retained in individuals with early onset *convergent strabismus* (see below) who do not develop proper binocularity. The OKN abnormality is also believed to be an important factor for the development of *latent nystagmus* in children with this type of strabismus.

Vergence movements

Proper vergence movements are the requirements for normal development of binocular functions. The system is functional in the newborn although with limitations in range and accuracy. Sensory constraints in the form of low accommodation accuracy and poor disparity detection limit vergence functions in the first months of life. However, there is a gradual improvement and at 6 months consistent responses to changes in binocular parallax and retinal disparity are obtained. Dysfunction of the vergence system is a hallmark of *strabismus*, but it is unclear if the initial defect in this group of diseases is in the vergence system or in the binocular functions that supply the command signals for vergence movements.

There is a strong coupling between the vergence system and accommodation (increase in refractive power of the lens in order to allow proper near vision). Abnormalities of vergence movements without strabismus are usually of psychogenic origin, but can also be due to accommodation deficits.

Strabismus

Strabismus is defined as a pathological deviation of one eye with respect to the other. It is generally a childhood disease with a strong familial trait. Binocular functions always suffer in childhood strabismus, but it is mainly in its effects on monocular vision, i.e. as a creator of *amblyopia* that strabismus causes ophthalmological concern.

The cause or causes of manifest childhood *strabismus* are known to a very limited extent. Interference with the mechanisms to fuse the images of the two eyes into one is an established factor, but how this inadequacy comes about in childhood strabismus is a matter of controversy, particularly whether the fusion defect is congenital or acquired, or if it is sensory or motor (vergence disturbance). In children with neurological abnormalities, for instance those with *Down syndrome*, *cerebral palsy*, *hydrocephalus* and other more generalized brain disease, strabismus is common (40–60 percent) in addition to other abnormalities of ocular motility. Sometimes specific brainstem lesions can be connected with strabismus: e.g. the *Duane* and *Möbius syndromes*.

Refractive errors play an important part in the etiology of squint. For example, uncorrected hyperopia may cause a disproportionately large convergence impulse and convergent strabismus. However, it does not account for more than 20–30 percent of strabismus cases.

Selected reading

Aslin RN. Motor aspects of visual development in infants. In Salapatek P, Cohen LIS, eds. *Handbook of infant perception*. Vol. I. Orlando: Academic Press, Florida, 1987; 43.

Aslin RN. Normative oculomotor development in human infants. In Lennerstrand G, von Noorden GK, Campos E, eds. *Strabismus and amblyopia*. London: Macmillan, 1988: 133.

Leigh RJ, Zee DS. *The neurology of eye movements*. 2nd ed. Contemporary Neurology Series. Philadelphia: FA Davis Co, 1991.

Shupert C, Fuchs AF. Minireview: Development of conjugate eye movements. *Vision Res* 1988; **28**: 585.

Taylor D with Avetisov E, Baraitser M, Brazier J, *et al.* *Pediatric ophthalmology*. Boston: Blackwell Scientific Publications, 1990: 595.

von Noorden GK. *Burian and von Noorden's binocular vision and ocular motility*. St Louis: CV Mosby, 1990.

D. Motor Functions

D1. Development of Motor Function

H Forssberg

Innate motor patterns

Innate motor patterns develop endogenously during ontogeny. They are crucial for survival of the species and provide vital functions such as respiration (e.g. breathing), nutrition (e.g. sucking, mastication, swallowing, defecation, micturition), reproduction (e.g. sexual behavior, labor, nursing) as well as movements of the body (e.g. locomotion and posture). Innate movements are present in all vertebrates, although the form varies depending on the anatomy of the species and the surrounding environment (e.g. different forms of locomotion in water, air and on ground). In mammals, and particularly in primates, more sophisticated movements are innate (e.g. facial expression of emotions). There is no sharp border between innate and learned movement, and most innate movements depend on practice to develop properly.

Neural substrate

Innate motor patterns are produced and controlled by neural networks in the brainstem and spinal cord, i.e. at a low level in the motor control system. In invertebrates and lower vertebrates, these networks have been explored in detail concerning types of neurons, connections between neurons, transmitter substances and membrane properties. The significant feature of these networks is the capability to generate a pattern of signals to appropriate motoneurons producing the intended movement. For several movements the pattern is cyclically repeated, e.g. in breathing, mastication and locomotion. The neural networks are then organized to generate an oscillatory activity. Such networks are called central pattern generators, since they are capable of generating motor patterns without sensory information. However, the sensory information, evoked during the movement, is critical in determining the final motor pattern. The same networks may be used to produce different motor patterns when influenced by different sensory input, or by various neurotransmitters and neuromodulators. Sensory information is also important in the adaptation of the motor activity to the environment, e.g. after a perturbation of an ongoing movement.

The neural networks can be triggered from sensory afferents and are then usually called reflexes although the motor pattern is very complex, e.g. swallowing reflex and grasp reflex. Similar movements can also be voluntarily initiated, e.g. swallowing and grasping. The same neural networks are then initiated by signals from higher levels in the motor control system, i.e. neural circuits in the brainstem, basal ganglia, or motor cortex (Fig. 6.18).

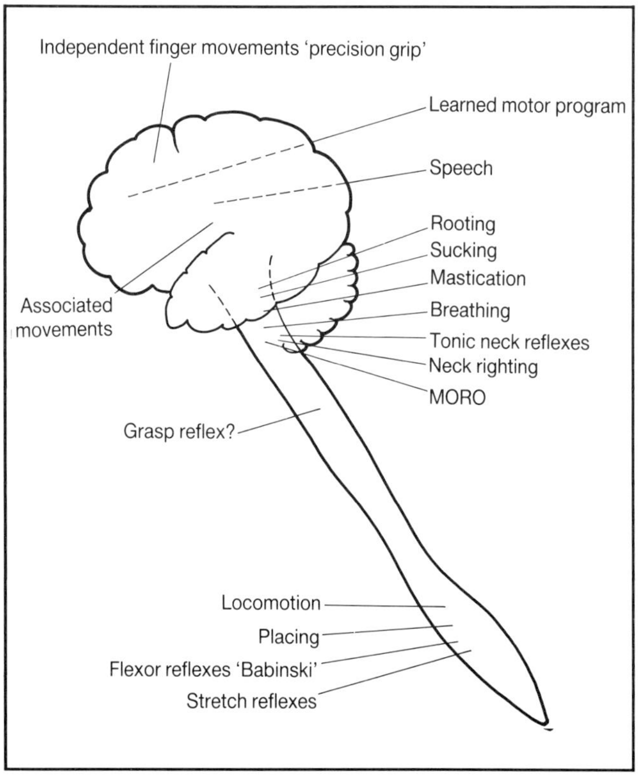

Fig. 6.18. The anatomical location of neural networks primarily involved in the control of various movements emerging during the fetal period and the first postnatal years.

Development

Innate movements develop early, usually during the fetal period. They are endogenously initiated without any external stimulus. Sensory neurons do not establish connections with the motoneurons until after the first movements have occurred. This indicates that the organization of the neural networks are genetically determined and that they can produce the motor pattern without sensory feedback from peripheral afferents. However, sensory information obtained during movements influences the motor pattern and may also contribute to the final shaping of the neural networks. Several innate movements retain the same pattern through all phases of the development, e.g. swallowing, while some change dramatically, e.g. locomotion, and others are only present during a short period of development.

Movements in the newborn

The immediately newborn infant has a repertoire of innate motor patterns, required for survival, e.g. respiration, swallowing. These have been organized and practised during a major part of the fetal life. Several of the movements have a reflexive character, i.e. they are triggered by external stimuli. Various reflexes, such as the swallowing reflex or the blink reflex, are present in their adult form and will remain the same throughout development. Other reflexes can only be elicited during some phase of the infant period, i.e. developmental reflexes. The infant also has frequent episodes of 'general movements' when body, head and extremities are spontaneously moved.

Protective reflexes

Protective reflexes, important to defend the infant from destructive agents, are present directly after birth and remain through life. The blink reflex, the cough and sneeze reflexes, are examples of such reflexes. The flexor reflex, responding with a flexion of the limb after a noxious stimulus, is also present after birth. However, during infancy all physiological flexor muscles of the leg, including the dorsal flexors of the toes, are activated. This gives a 'toe up' response or a 'Babinski sign' when the plantar response is tested. This response probably disappears during the second year in favor of an extensor response, which plantar-flexes the toes, at the same time as the gait is transformed into a plantigrade pattern.

Muscle tone and stretch reflexes

The muscle tone, i.e. the tension of the muscles at rest, is modified during the last trimester of fetal life and during the first months of postnatal life. The muscles are flaccid before the twenty-eighth week of gestational age. Tone first increases in distal segments and in a caudo-cephalic direction. It develops faster in flexor muscles than in extensor muscles, resulting in flexion of most joints. Flexor tone peaks at term. Muscle tone is dependent on the gestational age and has been used to estimate the gestational age of preterm infants. Premature infants have less flexor dominated tone. Muscle tone is due both to current neural activity of the motoneuron and to passive mechanical components, i.e. muscle fibers, tendons and ligaments, etc. The early dominating 'active' flexor tone depends on spinal mechanisms with enhanced cutaneous (flexor) reflexes and reduced tonic (extensor) stretch reflexes. Postnatally the extensor tone develops gradually in a craniocaudal direction due to development of tonic γ-motoneuron control and supraspinal inhibition of the interneurons mediating the inhibition of extensor motoneurons in cutaneous reflexes.

Early damage to the central nervous system often results in decreased muscle tone during the first postnatal months. This is usually followed by increased muscle tone, which is one of the first predictors of a later disturbed motor development with spasticity, paresis and dyscoordination.

The stretch reflex is known to be a simple monosynaptic reflex, with an afferent fiber (type Ia) from the muscle spindle projecting directly to the motoneuron of the same muscle (see Fig. 6.19). Its function is to regulate the activity in the motoneuron depending on length changes of the muscle. In infants the projection is much wider and a tendon tap does not only activate the agonist, but also antagonist muscles and more distant muscles, e.g. tap on the Achilles tendon elicits reflex responses in the calf muscle, pretibial muscles and hamstrings muscles. A tap on the patellar tendon also evokes responses in the contralateral leg, i.e. crossed adductor response.

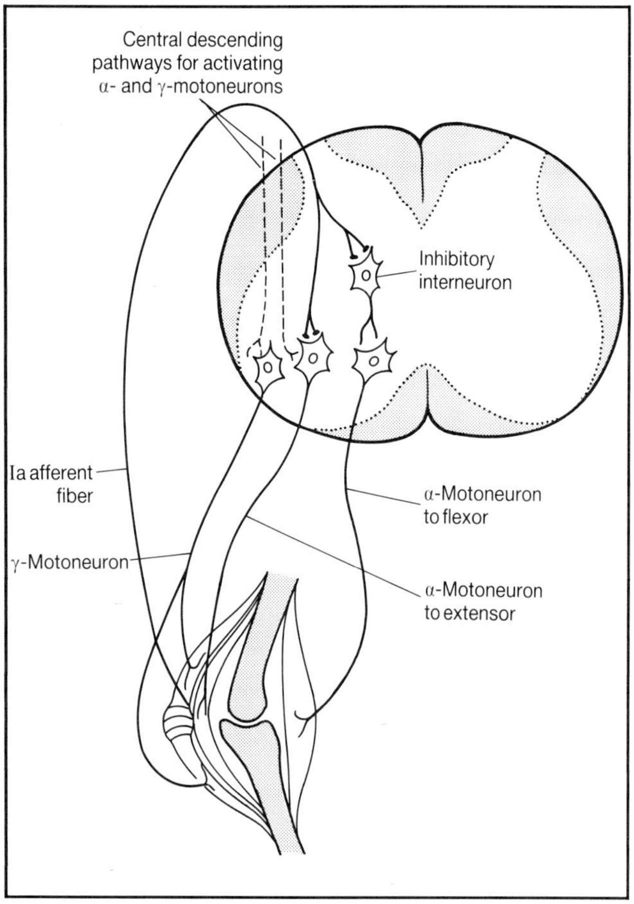

Fig. 6.19. Connections for stretch reflex. Sketch of two antagonistic muscles, an extensor and a flexor, together with some of their connections in the spinal cord that are activated through sensory discharges from a spindle. When the extensor muscle is briefly stretched, the α-motoneuron is excited monosynaptically (the stretch reflex) while the flexor is inhibited via interneurons (reciprocal innervation). Thereby antagonistic muscles cooperate. Central descending pathways activate α-motoneurons to initiate voluntary movements and excite γ-motoneurons to maintain sensory discharges during contraction. (From Kuffler SW, Nicholls JG, Martin AR, eds. *From neuron to brain*. 2nd ed. Sunderland, MA: Sinauer Associates Inc. Publishers, 1984: 399. Reproduced by permission of Sinauer Associates Inc.)

Table 6.3. Developmental reflexes and voluntary movements during the first postnatal year

Movement	Appears	Disappears
Moro	Birth	4–5 months
Infant stepping	Birth	1–4 months
Placing reactions	Birth	1–4 months
Protecting reflexes	Birth	Persist
Babinski	Birth	1–2 years
Rooting	Birth	?
Sucking, swallowing	Birth	Persist
Pre-reaching	Birth	Voluntary reaching
Grasp reflex	Birth	Voluntary grasping
ATNR	2–3 weeks	4–6 months
Crossed adductor response	2–3 months	7–8 months
Voluntary reaching and grasping	3–4 months	Persist
Neck righting reflexes	4–6 months	?
Side-fall reflexes	5–7 months	Persist
Parachute reaction	6–8 months	?
Unsupported sitting	6–8 months	Persists
Supported locomotion	7–12 months	Independent walking
Precision grip	9–11 months	Persists
Independent walking	9–18 months	Persists

Developmental reflexes

Several responses and reflexes during the neonatal period are transient and represent ontogenic adaptations (see Table 6.3). They are triggered by a sensory stimulation. In several cases, a similar movement can later be voluntarily induced. Often the motor pattern is complex (e.g. infant stepping). Most developmental reflexes are present at birth, but some mature late during gestation and are absent in preterm infants. The purpose of these movements is often obscure. Some may be evolutionary remnants while others may be important for organization of neural networks later used for other movements. The threshold to elicit a developmental reflex varies considerably depending on the behavioral state of the infant. Some examples of the best known developmental reflexes are presented. The Moro reflex consists of an abduction–extension of the arms followed by an adduction and flexion. It is elicited by vestibular afferents, e.g. following a sudden extension of the neck. If the threshold is low or vestibulum absent, it may also be induced by dynamic stretch receptors in the neck muscles as well as by other afferents. The reaction is modified if the child is grasping an object, i.e. a mild passive stretching of the arms changes the pattern into flexion–adduction. In human infants the Moro reflex has no obvious function, while a similar movement is efficient for the monkey infant to attach to the mother during her movements. The Moro reflex is present at birth in all children.

The asymmetric tonic neck reflex (ATNR) is elicited by a

tonic activation of stretch receptors in the neck muscle following a rotation of the head. The response is controlled by neural networks in the brainstem since it can be elicited after decerebration. The appearance of ATNR is not consistent. It is usually not present in the newborn but appears after 2–4 weeks. It is most prominent during the second postnatal month and disappears before 5 months. A too strong and easily elicitable ATNR is pathological. There are several other neck, labyrinthine and righting reflexes, initiated by muscle receptors in the neck, or by vestibular mechanisms which influence the position of head and body.

The grasp reflex can be elicited in hands and feet. It may be elicited by tactile stimulation of the palms but also by proprioceptive stimulation achieved while stretching the arm. The grasp reflex involves distal finger muscles as well as proximal arm muscles which are initially activated in 'flexor synergy', i.e. all flexor muscles at all joints are activated *en bloc*. The grasp reflex becomes more difficult to elicit when the child starts to grip voluntarily. The network controlling the grasp reflex and the voluntary grasp are probably the same. Initially all joints are coupled, but later, the networks become divided into smaller fragments controlling individual joints and fingers. A short latency grasp reflex may also be used during manipulation when an object slips.

Rooting and sucking are part of an autonomous feeding behavior initiating undulatory searching movements of the head and sucking. Rooting develops gradually under afferent control from tactile stimuli around the mouth and becomes totally directed. Sucking is elicited from lip afferents and afferents inside the mouth. Both patterns may also occur spontaneously. The threshold and the intensity of these responses are highly dependent on hunger and satiation.

Infant stepping is a locomotor-like behavior with alternating leg movements. It can be induced by holding the infant erect with the feet placed on an horizontal surface, letting the infant support some of the body weight and slowly pulling the infant forward. The stepping movements are usually present the first month after birth and then fade away. Several children, however, maintain the stepping until they start walking with support. Daily exercise may improve the locomotor movements and prevent the disappearance. Infant supine kicking with alternating leg movements resembles stepping movements. Tactile placing reactions are elicited when the dorsal aspect of a foot contacts, for example, the edge of a table. It consists of a flexion and forward movement of the leg followed by a placing of the foot. Both tactile and proprioceptive stimuli may elicit the response.

These developmental reflexes are innate motor patterns produced by neural networks in the spinal cord and brainstem. They are initiated by external stimuli but the neural networks reflexly stimulated may be complex, producing complicated movement patterns. During the early infant period the networks can operate autonomously, without influence from higher levels of the motor control system. The excitability of the network, i.e. the threshold of the reflex, is, however, influenced by other factors such as the behavioral state of the infant. Later, during development, higher subcortical and cortical structures develop and begin to influence the performance of the movement, usually by inhibiting the neural networks. In other cases, e.g. grasping, the reflex initiation of the grasp is inhibited by prefrontal centers, while other centers in the motor cortex may use the same 'grasp networks' during voluntary grasping. The networks are maintained although they are inhibited and not used. Responses resembling the infantile reflexes, e.g. rooting, sucking, grasp reflex, may often reappear after *dementia* and brain damage in adults when the inhibiting centers have been affected. However, these responses are caricatures reflecting a damaged, and not a developing, central nervous system.

There have been several studies on the significance of various infantile responses and reflexes in the newborn infant, but they do not predict the outcome. In contrast, persisting reflexes indicate brain damage which will interfere with the motor development. This is because, while the reflex arcs are situated in the spinal cord and brainstem, networks at a higher level controlling and inhibiting the reflexes may be damaged during the perinatal period.

General movements

In addition to externally triggered reflex movements infants frequently move spontaneously the head, body and all extremities during minute long sequences several times every hour. These movements start slowly, build up to a crescendo and then cease gradually. They are variable in speed and amplitude. General movements in preterm infants are considerably affected in *encephalopathies*. They become stereotyped and 'cramped', involving only parts of the body with abrupt onset and termination. Such abnormal movements can predict an adverse developmental outcome.

Postural control

Postural control implies: (1) supporting the body against gravity, (2) maintaining proper position of the body segments, and (3) keeping the equilibrium. The newborn has several transient tonic neck and righting reactions that control the position of the body segments in relation to each other but does not require muscle activity for antigravity support or equilibrium. Muscle control for support and equilibrium develops in a craniocaudal direction with most infants gaining head control already within the first weeks. Successively the body can be lifted and supported on the under arm, on the hands and on all four limbs, respectively. Independent sitting and standing require elaborate equilibrium control due to the reduction of the support surface. The extensor muscles of the legs are usually strong enough to carry the body at 4–6 months of age.

Equilibrium control

The equilibrium control system strives to project the center of mass within the support surface. The vestibular, visual and somatosensory systems provide continuous information about the body position. A deviation of the body is immediately monitored and initiates postural adjustments which resist the deviating movement and brings the body back to equilibrium. The somatosensory system is the first to respond and initiates sharp bursts of muscle activity 90–100 ms after the perturbation during standing. This is followed by responses evoked by the vestibular system with (latency about 180–200 ms). Motor activity evoked by the visual system is slower and important for achieving the final position. The responses have invariant muscle activation patterns for certain disturbances and contain a whole set of muscle contractions, e.g. a forward sway of the standing body is counteracted by a wave of muscle contractions on the dorsal side of the body beginning in the calf muscles and continuing up to the neck muscles. The responses can, however, be adapted and modified depending on the nature of the disturbance, e.g. if the support phase is rotated or translated or during weightlessness. The adaptation is a function of an integration between the three sensory systems and requires an intact cerebellum.

The vestibular, visual, and somatosensory system are functioning in the fullterm newborn, but it is only after several weeks that postural adjustments can be elicited by external perturbations. Side-fall reflexes and parachute reactions first develop after 6 months. The development of neural networks responding to sensory stimuli and producing the adequate motor pattern is the factor limiting their appearance. The postural adjustment and their muscle activation patterns resemble those in adults, e.g. children just able to sit without support activate the same muscles as adults and in the correct order. The muscle responses only have more variable amplitudes and longer latencies. Because of lack of integration between the sensory systems, young children lack the capability to adapt the responses to the environment. This develops around 5–7 years, whereafter the responses also become less variable and the latencies shorter.

Delayed and disturbed postural development is common in several neurological disorders and may be caused by defect sensory function or more likely by defective processing of sensory information to activate appropriate neural networks. In children with *cerebral palsy* the muscle activation patterns deviate from the normal sequential order, leading to inefficient compensatory forces.

Integration between posture and movement

The equilibrium is disturbed during voluntary movements due to reaction forces of the moving limb and transition of the center of mass. In adults, the neural control of voluntary movements includes activation of postural muscles, counteracting the perturbance evoked by the movement. This activity is initiated prior to the movement and is called anticipatory postural activity. This implies a process calculating the effect the programmed voluntary movement will have on the equilibrium as well as the programming and release of compensatory postural muscle activity. This process depends on frontal motor areas and on the basal ganglia. It is not known when anticipatory postural control emerges but it is present during the second year. In children with mental retardation and delayed motor development the emergence of anticipatory postural control is delayed.

Locomotion

Locomotor stages

The development of locomotion can be divided into several consecutive phases (see Table 6.4). Locomotor-like movements are performed endogenously *in utero* and also in a reflexive manner after birth, i.e. infant stepping. In the majority of infants the stepping movements can only be elicited during the first postnatal months. This is followed by an inhibitory period until supported locomotion occurs at 6–9 months. During this stage the infants can voluntarily induce the locomotion and direct their gait in a certain direction. They can also support their body weight on one leg but need support to maintain the equilibrium. During this time they are also usually able to crawl and creep on all four limbs. At 9–18 months they can release the external support and are capable of maintaining balance while walking. Finally the gait pattern is transformed into the adult plantigrade form (Table 6.4).

Table 6.4. Stages of human locomotor development

1. Fetal locomotor like movements
2. Infant stepping
3. Inactive period
4. Supported locomotion
5. Independent walking
6. Transformation to plantigrade gait

Transformation to plantigrade gait

The principles of human locomotion are similar to those of quadrupedal mammals, i.e. cyclical alternating leg movements support the body and propel it forward. In certain aspects the human gait pattern is unique, being adapted to the bipedal posture about 3–4 million years ago. This is not the case in other bipedal primates. There are several specific determinants for the bipedal, plantigrade gait, which contributes to reduce the vertical oscillation of the body and to increase the step length resulting in lower energy expenditure (see Table 6.5). The development of a prominent heel strike is of special interest. This is due to an active dorsiflexion of the foot, provided by contractions of the pretibial muscles and inhibition of the calf muscle activity during the end of the swing phase. This is achieved by a specific individualized pattern of muscle activity and rotates the ankle joint out of phase with the knee and hip. None of the plantigrade determinants is present in the early stages of locomotion. In contrast, all muscles are activated in conjunction. Ankle, knee and hip joints are flexed and extended together. The foot is placed on its toe or forefoot. A large proportion of all infants are still walking on their toes (never contacting the floor with the heel) when they start to walk independently. In addition short latency reflexes are induced after foot contact in both flexor and extensor muscles. Not until independent walking has been established is there a slow transformation of the gait pattern; the plantigrade determinants then successively develop. During the same period muscle strength and postural control develop, allowing the child to make longer steps, increase the speed, narrow the base and later, around 2 years, allowing running.

Table 6.5. Plantigrade determinants

1. Foot movement—heel strike
2. Knee movement—stance leg flexion
3. Intralimb coordination—joint rotations out of phase
4. Pelvic movement—rotation, tilt, translation
5. Muscle activity—individual temporal pattern for each muscle

Neural models

From studies in other vertebrates it is evident that the basic locomotor rhythm is produced by neural networks in the spinal cord. Sensory afferents from the moving limbs provide a powerful influence on the central network and can modify the pattern. This modulation is of great importance to adapt the locomotion to the external environment. Several neural networks generate the locomotor pattern—at least one network for each limb. The interaction between these networks determines the interlimb coordination, e.g. walk, trot and gallop. Supraspinal mechanisms are required to achieve a purposeful locomotion; to induce activity in the spinal networks; to set the speed of the locomotion; to maintain equilibrium; to steer the direction of the locomotion; to avoid obstacles; and to guide the placement of the paws, etc. Centers in the brainstem control the spinal networks via reticulospinal pathways. These centers can initiate and halt the locomotor activity as well as determine the rate of activity. These reticular centers are influenced by circuits in both motor cortex and basal ganglia. Other centers of the reticular system influence the muscle tone in the limbs and the power of the contractions. Cortical circuits are involved in fast corrections of the ongoing locomotor movements in order to avoid visible obstacles. The cerebellum is provided with information from the moving limb by sensory afferents and from the activity in the spinal locomotor generating circuits. This information is used to activate proper adjustments to comply with the environment.

It is likely that a similar organization is present also in humans. Stimulation of the locomotor centers in the brainstem induces locomotion in monkeys. The fetal locomotor-like movements and the infant stepping are thought to be produced by autonomous neural networks in the spinal cord, either initiated spontaneously or under afferent influences. Stepping movements cannot be induced beyond the newborn period probably due to supraspinal inhibition while proper supraspinal connectivity is developing. The emergence of voluntary, goal-directed locomotion may reflect the maturation of locomotor centers in the brainstem and their proper contact with the spinal locomotor networks via the reticulospinal system. The onset of independent walking is probably the result of the maturing postural control in cerebellar and vestibular structures. The brain has to mature to a certain degree before it is ready to execute a certain motor skill. On the other hand, instructions and practice seem to be involved in the achievement of independent walking, since children deprived from normal human contact may not develop bipedal gait.

The emergence of plantigrade gait is unique to the human species. The slow and gradual transformation of the locomotor pattern after the onset of independent walking suggests, however, that the original neural networks are used and that they are gradually influenced by other neural mechanisms.

Development after early brain lesions

Prior to independent locomotion children with *cerebral palsy* (diplegia or hemiplegia) exhibit an immature locomotor pattern similar to that of nonimpaired children. At the time when children normally transform their locomotor pattern into a plantigrade gait, children with *cerebral palsy* retain the immature nonplantigrade pattern. All muscles are activated together in a uniform pattern with a high degree of antagonistic coactivation. The sharp short-latency reflexes after foot contact remain. The foot is placed on the toes or forepart of the foot and several children walk on their toes as a result of the premature activation of the calf muscles during the swing phase. In addition to the disturbed coordination of the locomotor movements, the gait of these children is also disturbed by muscle weakness (paresis) and spasticity, which may altogether prevent the children from walking. A similar retained immature gait pattern may also be seen in other neurological diseases such as *mental retardation* and *autism*. In *habitual toe walkers* the immature gait pattern is retained up till school age, without other neurological symptoms.

The retained immature gait pattern after early brain lesions suggest that supraspinal mechanisms are responsible for the transformation to plantigrade gait, and that these are disturbed in *cerebral palsy* and some other diseases, and that they mature slowly in *habitual toe walkers*. This rigid system, depending on maturing neural circuits, also explains the meager effect of locomotor training during physical therapy.

Eye–hand coordination and reaching

Movements in extrapersonal space require information from several sensory modalities. When a hand movement to a visible target is generated the position of the target is defined in a visual coordinate system while the hand position is derived from somatosensory information into a body-oriented coordinate system. The sensory information and motor commands must be coordinated. This type of integration and transformation is present in an immature form in the newborn infant, who may perform pre-reaching movements, e.g. moving the hand towards an object without grasping. This implies that parts of the mechanisms are innate. A similar capacity is innate in other vertebrates, e.g. a frog catching a fly with its tongue. After about 3–4 months the infant can reach out and grasp an object. At this time the movement consists of several segments, i.e. accelerations and decelerations. The segments decrease in number with age, and after the first year there is usually only one large initial segment followed by a few small segments.

This development of the movement trajectory reflects a

transition from several small motor commands, each moving the hand a bit closer to the target, to a single motor program bringing the hand the entire distance. There is thus a change in the strategy from a feedback controlled movement in which the trajectory is continuously monitored and new small motor commands consecutively initiated, to a feedforward controlled program, in which the entire movement is programmed in advance of the movement being initiated. The small segments at the end of the movement are correcting movements based on visual information during the movement and required to guide the last part of the movement.

When an infant starts reaching for objects the movement trajectory of the hand may vary from straight to circumferential. The body is moved forward and rotated to get closer to the object. Initially the hand is open until the object is contacted. Around 9 months of age it begins to be shaped according to the form of the object and during the second year the hand starts to close before contact of the object. When mature, the reaching movements thus involve two motor programs activated in parallel. Hand shaping is controlled by the motor cortex while the movement of the hand is governed by brainstem mechanisms.

'Clumsy children' often have a reduced capability to process and utilize the sensory information required to program movements to targets in the extrapersonal space. Similar deficits may be seen in children with *cerebral palsy* and *spina bifida*. The deficit affects the capability to program movements in advance, and these children rely mainly on a feedback strategy, i.e. they perform several smaller movement segments while monitoring the outcome of the movement with sensory information. Children with *congenital blindness* have large problems performing movements in extrapersonal space. However, they initially do not use their hands as perceptual organs to obtain information about external objects. Instead the hands are used for eating, pulling objects etc., so-called 'blind hands'. Motor development in blind children is generally delayed. This delay includes tasks that do not directly rely on visual information.

Manipulation and grasping

During the first postnatal months a power grasp can be reflexively elicited. Probably the grasp reflex is determined by neural networks in the cervical spinal cord. When voluntary grasping emerges between 3 and 4 months, it is still in the form of a power grasp, i.e. including all fingers and other joints of the arm. Subsequent development is characterized by a fractionation of the power grasp and an increased degree of freedom, i.e. the thumb and fingers can be individually controlled. At 9–11 years the precision grip develops, i.e. a small object can be picked up between the tips of the thumb and index finger. The emergence of independent finger movements and precision grip reflects a change in the control from one neural network controlling all fingers in conjunction, to several networks controlling one finger each. This development is achieved by the maturation of the motor cortex and corticospinal tracts.

Manipulation of objects requires an adequate control of the forces grasping and lifting the object. The grip force is adapted to the friction between the object and the skin by cutaneous mechanoreceptors in the finger tips recording small microslips of the object when the grip force is getting too small. If the object starts to slip, grip reflexes instantly (60 ms) increase the grip force. Similarly, short loading reflexes increase the vertical lift force when required. When infants start to use the precision grip, their grip force is considerably higher than required. They also initiate the grip by squeezing the object before lifting, i.e. initiating the grip force well before the lift force. (By this strategy they manage to lift objects without dropping, although the capability to adapt the grip force to the friction is not yet developed and they have slow and small grip and loading reflexes.) When the child is about 2 years old he can adapt the grip force to the friction of the object. The reflex latencies continue to shorten during the subsequent 4–5 years.

When small children lift objects with the precision grip, they increase the isometric force in segments, i.e. the force rate is increased and decreased several times. This stepwise force increases until the lift force overcomes the gravitational force of the object, i.e. the object lifts off. The force increase is terminated by sensory information from the lift-off, i.e. feedback control. During the second year, children gradually change to feedforward strategy. The grip force and load force are initiated together in one force pulse targeting the weight of the object. This means that the motor command is programmed in advance and is based on an internal neural representation of the object, e.g. the weight. This is formed during earlier manipulation of the object and stored until next time the object is lifted. The capability to program the force pulses adequately continues to develop until 8–10 years of age. Proprioceptive information of an object's weight can be used from 2 years of age, while visual size information (transformed into weight) can be used first after 3 years.

Inability to perform task-related individual finger movements are common in children with *cerebral palsy*, due to the early damage of the motor cortex or corticospinal tract. In addition these children retain a sequential initiation of the forces, which are increased in successive steps, i.e. they do not program the entire force output in advance. They use an excessive grip force, although they have some capability to adjust the grip force to the friction of the object. Hence, they continue to use a feedback strategy and have an inefficient sensorimotor integration correcting the force output.

Learned motor skills

Complex motor skills such as writing, playing instruments and performance of various athletic skills, require instruction and practice before they can be skilfully performed. The movement is practised during intense mental concentration. They gradually become automatized and finally perform, without special attention. Sensory information is significant for the progress during the learning period. The afferent inflow from the movement is compared to the 'ideal' movement and corrections are made until the next time the movement is executed, i.e. the sensory information is not used for feedback control but for programming of the next movement. As the training procedure advances, a central motor program is gradually shaped. After a proper program has been established, sensory information is no longer crucial. Hence, learned movements may continue to be performed following deafferentation. The afferent information is, however, normally used to parameterize the movement, i.e. to scale the strength and duration of the motor program. Afferents compensate for perturbations of the movement. Often learning implies a change from segmented movement trajectories into faster one-segment movements. This is usually accompanied by a transformation from coactivation of antagonistic muscles to reciprocal muscle activity, often in a triphasic pattern. A complex program contains several parts, or subprograms, which are activated together or in sequence. These subprograms may be innate or learned movements, integrated into the learned movement complex. In certain motor patterns, several complex motor programs are successively initiated, e.g. picking up an object from the floor, walking a couple of steps and putting the object on a shelf. To achieve such a smooth movement the motor programs are coordinated into a motor plan.

The neural substrate for learned motor programs and motor plans are not known, but the control is likely distributed between several systems. Learned sequences of finger movements are controlled from the premotor area via the motor cortex. The cerebellum is crucial for other learned movements, while motor planning and procedural memories are disturbed after dysfunction of the basal ganglia.

Development of motor skills during childhood is a result of neural maturation as well as of learning processes. Often it is not possible to separate the two mechanisms. Generally the motor patterns during early development depend mainly on maturation, i.e. innate movements, while movements developing later are achieved with learning and practice. However, the maturation of the brain continues over a long time and may be the limiting factor for the learning process. Complex motor skills are the most vulnerable and dys-coordination or clumsiness is a common motor problem in children without other neurological impairments.

Selected reading

Euler C, Forssberg H, Lagercrantz H. In *Neurobiology of early infant behavior*. Wenner-Gren International Series. London: Macmillan, 1989.

Forssberg H, Hirschfeld H. In *Children with movement disorders: motor control theories and therapeutic concepts*. Basel: Karger, 1992.

Forssberg H, Stokes VP, Hirschfeld H. Basic mechanisms of human locomotion development. In Gunnar M, Nelson C, eds. *The Minnesota Symposia on Child Psychology*. Vol. 24. New Jersey: Erlbaum and Associates, 1992: 37.

Prechtl HFR, ed. *Continuity of neural functions from prenatal to postnatal life. Clinics in Developmental Medicine*. Oxford: Blackwell, 1984.

Prechtl HFR, ed. *The neurological examination of the fullterm newborn infant*. 2nd ed. *Clinics in Developmental Medicine* **63**. London: Heinemann, 1977.

D2. Fetal Movements

J G Nijhuis

That a fetus moves *in utero* has been known for centuries. However, only after the introduction of ultrasonographic techniques, has it been possible to observe the movements of the fetus in its natural environment. Not until 1976 was it shown that the fetus indeed moved spontaneously *in utero* under normal circumstances. Movements occurred in the first trimester of pregnancy. It was emphasized that absence of fetal movements may indicate impending fetal death. Therefore, the first aim of observing fetal motility is to assess fetal status. The second aim is to get more insight in the development of the nervous system. In longitudinal studies the first appearance of several movements was analyzed (see Table 6.6). A categorization of movement patterns was introduced with a description of how the individual movements were performed in terms of speed, force and amplitude.

In the second and third trimester, much attention has been paid to the observation of breathing movements and gross body movements. It was supposed that breathing movements would provide a useful indicator for fetal wellbeing. However, their measurement has been of limited value because they are not continuously present (see p. 605). Furthermore, it has been shown that breathing movements disappear just before and during labor. In cases of threatening premature labor, the presence of breathing movements can therefore be very reassuring.

Body movements have been recorded using several techniques, but the variation of the number of movements that can be recorded under standardized conditions is such that there is as yet no uniformly accepted criterion for the number of movements that would indicate *fetal distress*. A trend in an individual pregnancy appears to be of greater importance. It has been shown that under hypoxic conditions the fetus stops moving. Fetal breathing is one of the first movements to stop. For example, if a mother starts smoking, breathing movements will immediately cease. When hypoxia is sustained, general movements will also diminish. Finally the quality changes and the fetal tone disappears. These observations have led to the development of a biophysical profile of the fetus, a score which is used to predict the fetal condition. Items that have been included in this profile are the heart rate, pattern, fetal breathing movements, fetal body movements, fetal tone and the amount of amniotic fluid. It will be clear that not only hypoxia, but also narcotic drugs may influence fetal motility dramatically.

As gestational age progresses the length of epochs in which breathing and body movements may be absent increases dramatically. While in the first trimester periods without movements will not be longer than 10 minutes, in the term period it is not unusual for breathing movements to be absent for 120 minutes.

Table 6.6. Overview of a number of fetal movements which can be observed ultrasonographically and their first appearance

Movement observed	Gestational age (menstrual weeks)
Just discernible movements	7–8
General body movements	8–9
Isolated movements of arm or leg	9–11
Breathing movements	10–12
Yawning	12–15
Sucking movements / swallowing	13–15
Eye movements	16–17

Selected reading

Drogtrop AP, Ubels R, Nijhuis JG. The association between fetal body movements, eye movements, and heart rate patterns between 25 and 30 weeks of gestation. *Early Hum Dev* 1990; **23**: 67.

Manning FA, Platt LD, Sipos L. Antepartum fetal evaluation: development of a fetal biophysical profile. *Am J Obstet Gynecol* 1980; **136**: 787.

Nijhuis JG, ed. *Fetal behaviour. Developmental and perinatal aspects*. Oxford: Oxford University Press, 1992.

de Vries JIP, Visser GHA, Prechtl HFR. The emergence of fetal behaviour. II. Quantitative aspects. *Early Hum Dev* 1985; **12**: 99.

de Vries JIP, Visser GHA, Prechtl HFR. The emergence of fetal behaviour. III. Individual differences and consistencies. *Early Hum Dev* 1988; **16**: 85.

E. Behavior, Sleep and Rhythms

E1. Fetal Behavior

J G Nijhuis

If a child is quiet asleep nobody would expect him/her to walk or talk. If a child wakes up one would be very surprised if he made no sound at all. This shows that what one expects from a child depends on its 'behavioral state'. For the neonate, this concept consists of five states, 1–5: quiet sleep, active sleep, quiet awake, active awake and crying, respectively. It is increasingly recognized that fetal motility and fetal heart rates are not independent variables and provide the basis of our concepts of fetal behavior.

Fetal behavior and behavioral states

The study of fetal motility and fetal heart rate is of interest not only from a developmental physiological point of view, but specially in terms of fetal surveillance. However, one of the crucial differences between the observation of fetal motility and the recording of fetal behavior is that several variables are assessed at the same time to provide better insights into the fetal condition. While fetal motility (fetal body and limb movements, breathing and eye movements) is observed using ultrasound techniques, the fetal heart rate pattern (FHRP) is simultaneously recorded by cardiotocography. It must be emphasized that the observation of fetal behavior is very time-consuming; the optimal recording time is 1–2 hours!

Four fetal behavioral states have been defined in the last weeks of pregnancy which are similar to the neonatal states. These states have been called 1F through 4F, 1F being similar to state 1, non-REM sleep; state 2F is similar to state 2, REM-sleep; state 3F is similar to state 3, quiet awake, and state 4F is similar to state 4, active awake. Each state has its own fetal FHRP, A through D (Table 6.7): FHRP A is stable with a small oscillation bandwidth and only isolated accelerations; FHRP B has a wider bandwidth and frequent accelerations; FHRP C has wide oscillations and no accelerations; FHRP D has long-lasting accelerations. Although the states are similar to the neonatal states it is not proven that the fetus is really awake *in utero*. Immediately prior to term the fetus spends 30–40 percent in state 1F, and 40–50 percent in state 2F. Only 10 percent of the recording time can be recorded as states 3F and 4F.

Table 6.7. Schematic representation of state criteria

	Body movements	Eye movements	FHRP
State 1F	Incidental	Absent	A
State 2F	Present	Present	B
State 3F	Absent	Present	C
State 4F	Continuous	Present	D

For explanation of fetal heart rate patterns (FHRP) A, B, C and D, see text.

Behavioral states are certainly present during the last 4 weeks of pregnancy. Before that time the fetal behavior seems to be less 'organized', although a certain linkage between movements and FHRP, or between eye movements and body movements can often be observed.

Fetal breathing movements are not continuously present and were therefore not included in the state definitions. Their incidence and regularity is state dependent: if a fetus is in state 1F, fetal breathing is much more likely to be absent than present. However, if breathing movements are present they are much more regular during 1F. Other behaviors appear to be state dependent (e.g. fetal voiding).

Consequences for clinical practice

Cardiotocography (CTG) is certainly the most widely used technique for fetal surveillance and in that respect the 'silent CTG' is probably the most frequently occurring 'suspect' tracing. The CTG may be silent or nonreactive during 45 minutes (FHRP A) before a transition to a more reactive pattern (FHRP B) may occur. Other 'suspect' patterns are the sinusoidal-like FHRP which can be seen during fetal sucking, and the 'tachycardia with decelerations' which can be recorded during 'fetal jogging' (state 4F).

Because of a lack of understanding of fetal behavior

many obstetricians have adopted techniques to arouse the fetus. Vibroacoustic stimuli are applied for this reason via the maternal abdominal wall. Although it is certain that the fetus can respond to such powerful stimuli, it is a nonphysiological approach, thus limiting its interpretation. Using these stimuli, transitions can be seen from a silent pattern A (state 1F) into a very reactive pattern D (state 4F), a transition which is never observed under normal circumstances. Although fetal behavior reflects the quality of the fetal CNS it is very difficult to interpret behavior as 'normal' or 'abnormal' in an individual fetus because of the large variability of behavioral variables that can be observed in a group of fetuses.

Selected reading

Arduini D, Rizzo G, Caforio L, *et al*. Behavioral state transitions in healthy and growth retarded fetuses. *Early Hum Dev* 1989; **19**: 155.

Bekedam DJ, Visser GHA, de Vries JJ, Prechtl HFR. Motor behavior in the growth retarded fetus. *Early Hum Dev* 1985; **12**: 155.

Nijhuis JG, ed. *Fetal behavior. Developmental and perinatal aspects*. Oxford: Oxford University Press, 1992.

Prechtl HFR. The behavioral states of the newborn infant (a review). *Brain Res* 1974; **76**: 185.

E2. Sleep

S L Davis

The physiology of sleep

In the human adult the waking state is defined by the purposeful quality of responses to the environment and by the presence of intact memory. However, any behavioral definition of the transition between waking and sleep is difficult to apply in practice and for clinical purposes this transition is defined by the electroencephalogram (EEG). The waking EEG is characterized by rhythmic activity in the alpha frequency range (8–12 Hz). Drowsiness (stage 1 'sleep'), with loss of visual fixation and appearance of slow eye movements, is accompanied by the reduction in amplitude of alpha activity and the intrusion of theta frequency activity (4–7 Hz). Specific EEG transients, spindles and K-complexes, define the onset of true sleep and are characteristic of stage 2 sleep. If sleep is maintained, high voltage delta activity (0.5–3 Hz) becomes increasingly prominent. Stage 3 sleep is defined by the presence of high voltage delta activity during 30–70 percent of the record; stage 4 sleep by the presence of high voltage delta activity during greater than 70 percent of the record. The quality and duration of delta sleep is dependent to some degree on the time of day but is mostly influenced by the sleep history, i.e. the amount of delta activity is determined by the duration of waking prior to sleep onset and tends to decline as sleep continues. Behaviorally, sleep stages 2, 3 and 4 are characterized as nonrapid eye movement sleep (nonREM). In nonREM sleep postural (tonic) muscle tone is high, especially in antigravity muscles of the jaw and neck including muscles that maintain the patency of the upper airway. In contrast, phasic muscle activity including eye and limb movement, is absent.

When sleep is maintained for more than 90 minutes, a transition to rapid eye movement sleep (REM) may occur, especially during the night. This transition is often heralded by isolated rapid eye movements. At REM sleep onset, a body movement is followed by a sudden fall in postural muscle tone. Bursts of rapid eye movements then become prominent. The EEG reverts to a low voltage pattern resembling that seen in the drowsy state. REM sleep persists for up to 30 minutes before tonic muscle activity is reinstated following a body movement and stage 2 sleep transients reappear; a second sleep 'cycle' begins. Both the propensity for REM sleep and the duration of REM sleep episodes are determined by an endogenous circadian rhythm and are linked to the nadir of the body temperature cycle.

An individual entrained to the day–night environment and sleeping 7–9 hours per night experiences most delta sleep in the first 2–4 hours of the sleep period and most REM sleep in the early morning hours just prior to waking. This is in accordance with the association of delta sleep with prior waking and the linkage between REM sleep and the nadir of the body temperature rhythm. There is a circadian rhythm of sleep propensity evident in the latency to sleep onset of individuals studied in a constant environment and in the proportion of sleep achieved by individuals studied using an ultradian (e.g. 30 minute) sleep–wake schedule. There is a peak of sleep propensity in the mid-afternoon followed by a period of wake maintenance in the early evening when sleep initiation is impossible. The wake maintenance zone is followed by a 'gate' after which the nocturnal increase in sleep propensity is expressed.

Development of sleep and waking states

Preterm infant

The developmental aspects of sleep physiology are highly related to brain maturity and to a lesser degree are affected by experience. Therefore, it may be appropriate to extrapolate information gained from the study of infants born prematurely to the fetus *in utero*.

The behavioral and EEG characteristics of sleep states in infancy are summarized in Table 6.8. Prior to 28 weeks conceptual age the preterm infant displays little temporal organization of behaviors although there may be some clustering of eye and limb movements after 22 weeks. The EEG shows an invariate discontinuous pattern of low amplitude activity intermittently interrupted by bursts of high voltage sharp and slow activity (trace discontinu). At 28–32 weeks conceptual age periods of activity alternating with periods of relative quiescence become synchronized with fluctuations in the variability of heart rate and respiratory efforts. The state of relative inactivity with regular heart rate and breathing is clearly a precursor of the nonREM sleep state. Between 28 and 36 weeks conceptual age the behavioral differences between active and quiet sleep states become increasingly clearcut and the association between the specific EEG patterns and behavior increasingly distinct. At 36 weeks conceptual age the discontinuous EEG pattern has matured manifesting an increase in voltage of activity between bursts and decreased interburst interval compared to the more immature pattern, and is uniquely linked to the quiet sleep state. Active sleep, characterized by bursts of rapid eye movements superimposed on rolling slow eye movements, frequent fine face and limb movements and occasional body movements, is a precursor of the REM sleep state. By 36 weeks this behavioral state is closely associated with a continuous EEG pattern similar to that seen in drowsy waking. However, a significant proportion of sleep time in the preterm remains unclassified, with incomplete coordination between behavior, cardio-respiratory patterns and EEG.

There is little information yet available regarding a diurnal variation in behavioral states in the human fetus or preterm; however, a diurnal rhythm in heart rate variability, not apparently determined by maternal food intake or sleep state, has been reported.

Term infant

In the term infant, waking is recognized by eye opening to stimulation and visual fixation (state 3 of Prechtl). However, states of high activity (state 4) and crying (state 5) are also classified as waking. The transition from

Table 6.8. Summary of human infant sleep states

	Active sleep	Quiet sleep
28–36 weeks gestation	Coalescence of body, limb and eye movements High heart rate variability Irregular breathing	No movements Low heart rate variability Regular breathing
36–40 weeks gestation	Continuous EEG	Discontinuous EEG
40–44 weeks gestation	Absent tonic activity in postural muscles **REM sleep**	Sustained tonic muscle activity Discontinuous EEG (*trace alternans*) or continuous low voltage slow EEG
1–6 months		Continuous low voltage slow EEG with sleep spindles after 6 weeks
6 months–adult		Stage 2 **nonREM sleep** (spindles, K-complexes) Stage 3 & 4 **nonREM sleep** (high voltage delta)

waking to sleep cannot be clearly defined in the newborn; slow eye movements appear with the onset of drowsiness; superimposed rapid eye movements that appear at the transition to a sleep-onset active sleep state are not always readily distinguished from saccadic movements seen in waking. The EEG pattern during the transition from quiet waking, to drowsiness, to active sleep demonstrates an increasing amount of low voltage slow activity without a clear distinction between states. After an interval of active sleep usually lasting up to 10 minutes, eye movements cease and the EEG progresses to an alternating pattern of high and low amplitude activity with a periodicity of 3–8 seconds (trace alternans) characteristic of quiet sleep (state 1 of Prechtl). After 10–20 minutes of quiet sleep there may be a transition to waking marked by movement, eye opening or crying, or if sleep is maintained, to active sleep (state 2). At term, active sleep has all of the characteristics of REM sleep as described above; there are phasic movements of eyes and limbs on a background of reduced tone in postural muscles; the EEG shows a low voltage continuous pattern.

The cycle of alternating quiet and active states has a periodicity of approximately 60 minutes in the newborn. The infant sleeps from 16 to 17 hours out of 24 hours. There is usually no diurnal clustering of waking and sleep at birth, although some infants may already demonstrate some prolongation of sleep periods at night and of waking periods during the day in the first week of life.

Birth to 6 months

The character and timing of sleep changes dramatically during the first 6 months of infancy. A mature nonREM sleep state evolves and a diurnal rhythm of sleep and waking is established. Despite these changes the infant continues to sleep for 16–17 hours out of 24 hours throughout the first year of life.

In quiet sleep a continuous EEG pattern characterized by low to moderate voltage 2–4 Hz delta activity emerges after birth and gradually replaces the alternating EEG pattern over the next 4 weeks. From 6 weeks sleep spindle-like activity appears and becomes increasingly prominent during quiet sleep. The EEG pattern of stages 3 and 4 sleep, characterized by high voltage slowing, emerges between 3 and 6 months. At 6 months, with the appearance of K-complexes in association with sleep spindles during stage 2 sleep, nonREM can be adequately described in terms of the adult EEG stages. The mature pattern of sleep onset, via quiet sleep, is increasingly frequent, especially in the laboratory setting, between 3 and 6 months. However, in a familiar environment the transition from drowsy to an active sleep state at sleep onset is frequently seen throughout the first year of life.

There is a high degree of interindividual variation in the age of appearance of a diurnal rhythm. Term-born infants living in the home environment typical of westernized countries will achieve a higher propensity for sleep during the hours of darkness by 6 weeks. The prolongation of periods of waking during the daylight hours and shortening of waking duration at night play a major role in the evolution of a diurnal rhythm. Night-time consolidation of 2–4 hour sleep periods characteristic of the newborn to form sleep periods of 6–8 hours' duration occurs subsequently as an infant learns to re-enter sleep after brief waking without intervention of the caretaker. It must be noted that the timing of sleep and waking in infancy is highly dependent on culturally determined environmental factors and on the timing of the behavior of infant caretakers. The influences of an endogenous rhythm of sleep propensity and of behavioral conditioning are probably both additive and interdependent.

Infancy and childhood

Sleep stages 3 and 4 become increasingly prominent after 6 months and reach a lifetime peak at 2–4 years in both duration per sleep cycle and in a tendency to recur in successive cycles. The duration of the nonREM–REM sleep cycle lengthens from 60 minutes to 90 minutes during childhood with prolongation of nonREM sleep duration. After 6 months sleep is usually maintained for at least 6 hours at night but a high propensity for sleep continues during the daytime. Multiple daytime naps consisting of one to two sleep cycles gradually consolidate into a single afternoon nap which persists at least to the age of school entry. This increase in sleep propensity in the mid-afternoon is analogous to that experienced by the adult especially under conditions of sleep deprivation or fragmentation.

State-related phenomena

Breathing

From about 28 weeks conceptual age in the human infant the regulation of breathing is strongly influenced by state. In the human fetus, breathing movements detected by ultrasound are linked to the behavioral state characterized by the presence of activity, eye movements and high heart rate variability and are otherwise infrequent. Studies of breathing in the ovine fetus indicate that breathing movements are inhibited in association with the high voltage EEG state and that this inhibition is released by a lesion of the pons (see p. 604). This inhibition is also released at birth when breathing becomes continuous throughout waking and sleep. However, there remain fundamental differences in the regulation of breathing between waking and REM sleep, and nonREM sleep. In nonREM sleep respiratory drive is dependent on metabolic factors, e.g. oxygen and carbon dioxide tensions and pH, and stretch reflexes. In waking and REM sleep there is an additional 'waking' drive arising from supramedullary centers. Hence, in the *congenital hypoventilation syndrome (Ondine curse)* ventilatory failure characteristically occurs in nonREM. On the other hand, the atonia of postural muscles which include intercostal and upper airway maintaining muscles, may have profound effects on breathing during REM sleep in infancy. Upper airway dysfunction may be exacerbated in REM sleep and paradoxical movements of the chest wall are commonly seen in this state in young infants.

Thermal regulation

The regulation of body temperature is influenced by an endogenous circadian rhythm (see p. 254) and by sleep state. Conversely, both diurnal variations in body temperature and sleep state organization are influenced by environmental temperature and by the history of thermal exposure.

In mammalian species basal metabolism and consequently heat production falls and the hypothalamic temperature set point is adjusted downwards at the onset of nonREM sleep (see p. 361). In a thermoneutral environment there is an overall decrease in body thermal conductance associated with vasoconstriction of superficial blood vessels. In a high thermal environment an increase in body conductance may be necessary to adjust body temperature downwards during nonREM sleep. In many mammalian species REM sleep is associated with a loss of hypothalamic temperature regulation, so that body temperature changes passively with environmental temperature during brief REM sleep episodes. The situation is not clear in the human infant, but there is some evidence that active thermoregulation is maintained during REM sleep. A circadian rhythm of body thermal conductance causes a fall in body temperature and in trunk skin temperature, and a rise in peripheral skin temperature, during the night in an entrained individual in a thermoneutral environment. The changes in body and skin temperature associated with sleep are superimposed onto these diurnal rhythms. The night-time fall in body temperature is minimal in the first weeks of infancy and becomes clearly present and independent of environmental temperatures after 6–12 weeks.

Sleep disorders

Insomnia

When sleep is delayed or interrupted by pain, illness or environmental stimuli the effects are twofold. First, there is a cumulative loss of sleep and secondly, there is a disruption of circadian regulation. Sustained sleep loss can have profound effects on behavior, cardiovascular function, thermoregulation and breathing. Irritability, hyperactivity and deficits in attention are prominent in the infant and young child who is sleep deprived. The direct relationship between waking duration and delta sleep propensity means that stages 3 and 4 sleep occur earlier and persist for longer when sleep has been disturbed. Breathing disorders related to reduced respiratory drive during sleep which include *congenital hypoventilation syndrome* and *obstructive sleep apnea syndrome* are exacerbated by sleep loss and by sleep fragmentation. The loss of the diurnal rhythm that facilitates sustained sleep at night places great stress on the families and caretakers of infants and young children. The desynchronization of endogenous circadian rhythms has possibly more wide ranging effects, e.g. disrupting the response to thermal stress or infection.

Some infants who have demonstrated age appropriate sleep behavior in the first 6 months of life subsequently experience difficulty initiating sleep and in maintaining sleep beyond 2–4 hours. Parents of such infants have often determined that sleep can only be initiated or reinstated if the infant is held, rocked, walked or driven in the car. These requirements may dominate the family's activities. It has been postulated that in these circumstances the infants have been conditioned to initiate sleep only with the specific assistance of the caretakers and that the infants need to relearn how to relax and enter sleep using their own resources. Various regimens have been advocated which require the parents to gradually withdraw their interventions.

Parasomnias

Several sleep disorders that are common to the preschool child are associated with defective arousal from extreme delta sleep. Stage 4 sleep is most prominent in the child at 2–4 years of age and many sleep problems resolve spontaneously with advancing age. These disorders include *night terrors*, *sleep walking* and *enuresis*. They are all exacerbated by factors which increase the amount and depth of delta sleep and include sleep loss, excitement and physical activity on the preceding day. They are ameliorated by the avoidance of these precipitating factors.

Sleep-related upper airway dysfunction

During quiet breathing, pressures generated in the upper airway are of the order of -2.0 to -0.5 cmH_2O in infants as in adults. Collapse of the airway is prevented by its structural integrity and by the dilating actions of various muscles acting to pull the base of the tongue forwards and pull the lateral walls of the oropharyngeal airway apart (see p. 617). Some upper airway dilating muscles are phasically active with inspiration; some show sustained tonic activity throughout the respiratory cycle; some show both tonic and phasic inspiratory activity, e.g. the genioglossus muscle. Drive to the upper airway muscles comes from the respiratory center which in turn receives input from volume and flow mediated reflexes arising in the lungs and upper airway itself. When the upper airway is anatomically altered in the presence of *craniofacial anomalies*, hypertrophy of lymphatic tissue, presence of mucosal swelling or airway secretions to produce luminal narrowing, the pressures generated in order to maintain tidal volume increase disproportionately. In this situation upper airway maintaining muscles may be acting maximally to maintain airway patency during quiet breathing. Any decrease in respiratory drive, as occurs at sleep onset, may then result in a tendency for the airway to narrow on inspiration, causing flow limitation and hypopnea, or in complete airway collapse on inspiration, causing *obstructive apnea*. Flow limitation is frequently associated with vibration of the airway structures and snoring. *Obstructive apnea* may be silent but is usually interrupted by snorting as the airway reopens in association with arousal.

Both *hypopnea* and *apnea* disrupt sleep and may become more prolonged as sleep loss accumulates; they are both accompanied by marked increases in negative inspiratory intrathoracic pressures and pulsus paradoxus; they may be associated with significant hypoxemia. Many children snore when they suffer from *upper respiratory tract infections*. A child who snores consistently over months or years warrants otolaryngologic examination for *enlarged tonsils and adenoids*. Children with *craniofacial anomalies*, large tongues (e.g. in *mucopolysaccharidoses*), *obesity* (e.g. *Prader–Willi syndrome*) may be prone to sleep-related upper airway dysfunction. The question of a role for upper airway dysfunction in the causation of some cases of *sudden infant death syndrome* (SIDS) has not yet been fully resolved. Prolonged *obstructive apnea* has been associated with subsequent *SIDS*. Some cases of recurrent *SIDS* in families may relate to a familial craniofacial appearance characterized by a small lower jaw accompanied by an anatomically narrowed upper airway.

Selected reading

Guilleminault C, ed. *Sleep and its disorders in children*. New York: Raven Press, 1987.

Reppert SM, Rivkees SA. Development of human circadian rhythms: implications for health and disease. In Reppert SM, ed. *Research in perinatal medicine. Vol. IX. Development of circadian rhythmicity and photoperiodism in mammals*. Ithaca, New York: Perinatology Press, 1989: 245.

Thorpy M, ed. *Handbook of sleep disorders*. New York: Marcel Dekker Inc., 1990.

E3. Biological Rhythms

I C McMillen

Definitions

In biology there are a wide range of processes which repeat in a predictable manner. There are circannual rhythms such as the reproductive rhythms in seasonally breeding animals which have a period of about a year. Infradian rhythms are biological rhythms with a periodicity of more than 28 hours, whereas circadian rhythms are approximately 24 hours in length. Finally ultradian rhythms are rhythms which recur with a periodicity of less than 20 hours. This section will focus on the development of circadian rhythms, review the evidence that the circadian rhythm generating system is functional before birth and examine the changes which occur in the circadian system in the 3–6 months immediately after birth.

Circadian rhythms

The pattern of activity of many normal physiological functions (such as sleep and wakefulness, body temperature, urinary electrolyte excretion, melatonin and cortisol secretion, etc.) follow a circadian rhythm. Circadian rhythms are endogenously generated by a 'body clock' or circadian 'pacemaker' which oscillates with an inherent periodicity within the central nervous system. In the absence of any information about the external environment, circadian pacemakers oscillate with a periodicity of around, but not exactly, 24 hours, i.e. their activity and the activity of the rhythms they generate are said to 'free run'. In the presence of external time cues, e.g. light and dark cycles, the activity of the pacemakers is entrained to an exact 24 hour cycle. Whilst the main external time cue (or zeitgeber) is considered to be the light/dark cycle, other cues, including external temperature variations and social cues, are also thought to be important in the entrainment of circadian pacemaker activity. It has been found that in human subjects kept isolated from the range of daily time cues two main groups of endogenous circadian rhythms maintain different periodicities over several months. The rhythms of REM sleep, urinary K^+ excretion, plasma cortisol concentrations and core body temperatures are linked, but the periodicity of these rhythms under conditions of temporal isolation is different from that of the rhythms in skin temperature, urinary Ca^{2+} excretion and slow wave sleep. This phenomenon of internal descynchronization of rhythmic functions suggests that there are at least two circadian oscillators which control circadian rhythm generation in the human. In the presence of external time cues the pattern of activity of these oscillators must be coordinated to maintain an exact 24 hour periodicity of all physiological functions which show circadian rhythmicity.

The circadian pacemaker and entrainment

Evidence from experimental studies in the rat and other rodents suggests that major circadian pacemaker activity is present in the bilateral suprachiasmatic nuclei (SCN) which are located in the anterior hypothalamus. *Anterior hypothalamic tumors* disrupt the normal periodicity of the human sleep and wakefulness cycle and the SCN may therefore be an important pacemaker in the human. Entrainment of the activity of neurons in the SCN to an exact 24 hour periodicity by light is mediated by the retinohypothalamic tract which forms part of the optic tract and extends from the retina and terminates in the SCN.

Development of the circadian pacemakers

In the rat, there is a circadian variation in the metabolic activity of neurons in the SCN from as early as day 19 of gestation (term = 21 days) and it has been shown that the metabolic activity rhythm in the fetal SCN is entrained to the activity rhythm in the maternal SCN. Whilst it is clear that activity of the fetal SCN has an endogenous circadian rhythm, this rhythm is present at a time when the SCN are morphologically immature and have few synaptic connections. Further, hormonal and behavioral rhythms are only present in the newborn rat from the end of the first postnatal week. Therefore it is unclear whether the activity rhythm in the fetal rat SCN has any role in prenatal life. In longer gestation species, including man, there is limited information on the structure and function of the developing circadian pacemakers. In the human, however, there are 24 hour rhythms in a range of fetal physiological parameters which are present during late gestation. A key question is whether these fetal rhythms are endogenously generated by the fetal circadian pacemakers which are entrained by the influence of external times cues. Such time cues could be maternal in origin, e.g. hormonal signals generated by the maternal circadian pacemaker which is itself entrained to the external day/night cycle. The presence of some fetal rhythms may, however, simply reflect the fetal behavioral or hormonal responses to certain stimuli (e.g. the metabolic consequences of maternal feeding) which tend to occur at the same time each day. In order to understand the origin and source of fetal rhythms it is necessary to compare data from studies in the human with those in the experimental animal, the sheep.

Source of daily fetal rhythms

Daily rhythms are found in the human fetus from around 20 weeks of gestation. The fetal heart rate shows a clear 24 hour rhythm from as early as 22 weeks of gestation and the incidence of human fetal body movements peak in the early hours of the morning (02:00–04:00) during the last 10 weeks of pregnancy. In the experimental animal, the fetal sheep, there is a daily variation in the incidence and amplitude of breathing movements which is present from around 125 days of gestation (gestational length of 147 days). It appears that this fetal rhythm is not a consequence of the maternal feeding regimen or of diurnal changes in fetal plasma glucose or prostaglandin concentrations. It is interesting, however, that an 8 hour phase advance in the time onset of external darkness (i.e. from 19:00 to 11:00) produces a shift in the phase of the rhythm in breathing movements in the fetal sheep. This change in the time of darkness is associated with a change in the phase of the maternal and fetal plasma melatonin rhythms and it has been suggested that the maternal melatonin rhythm may act as a transplacental signal to entrain fetal behavioral activity to the external day/night cycle as the fetal melatonin rhythm is derived entirely by transplacental passage of maternal melatonin which is of pineal origin. It is unknown whether melatonin acts to entrain the activity of the fetal SCN to the external day/night cycle or whether it acts directly at the respiratory centers in the fetal brainstem.

Whilst there is some evidence therefore that fetal behavioral rhythms may be endogenously generated, there is no evidence that the rhythm in human fetal adrenal function is endogenously generated by the human fetal circadian pacemaker. In late pregnancy there is an inverse relationship between the 24 hour profiles of maternal plasma concentrations of cortisol and estriol. Measurements of maternal estriol provide a useful measure of fetal adrenoplacenta function. The presence of an inverse relationship between the 24 hour rhythms of cortisol and estriol in late pregnancy is consistent with the hypothesis that maternally derived glucocorticoids act via negative feedback in the fetal hypothalamic–pituitary axis. This is supported by the observation that exogenous glucocorticoids suppress the maternal cortisol rhythm and also abolish the diurnal rhythm in maternal estriol. These observations are interesting because they indicate that whilst there are a range of 24 hour rhythms in fetal behavioral and hormonal patterns, each rhythm may be generated by a different fetal or maternal mechanism and the presence of such rhythms is not necessarily evidence that the human fetal circadian pacemakers are active before birth.

Postnatal circadian rhythms

There is a delay after birth in the emergence of entrained circadian behavioral and hormonal rhythms. The earliest age at which entrained rhythms in sleep and wakefulness and in plasma cortisol and melatonin concentrations emerge is at around 8–12 weeks after birth. It is unknown if the postnatal delay in the emergence of entrained circadian rhythms is a consequence of the time required for the maturation of central pathways which carry information about the light/dark cycle to the circadian pacemaker or the time required for maturation of the synaptic connections of the circadian pacemaker. A further possibility also exists which is that it is consistent exposure to external time cues such as the daily light/dark cycle which determines the rate at which circadian entrainment develops. It has been widely accepted that the emergence of an entrained sleep–wake profile in the human infant is predominantly the result of maturation of the CNS. This is supported by the demonstration using spectral analysis that sleep–wake activity has a more prominent 24 hour component in term infants when compared with preterm infants at the same postnatal age. However, it may be misleading to compare the development of sleep–wake rhythms in pre-

and full-term infants without taking into account that after birth the preterm infant will spend some time in a hospital neonatal nursery where there is often constant illumination through the day and night and where there are several different care givers in any 24 hour period. In one study it has been shown that the circadian sleep–wake rhythm in a group of preterm infants entrained after a similar time of exposure to an environment with daily time cues (i.e. light/dark cycles and a single care giver) but at an earlier post-conceptional age when compared with the term group. Therefore the length of exposure to environmental time cues may be as important as neurological maturity in determining the development of entrainment of circadian rhythms in the human infant.

Summary

It is clear that there are 24 hour rhythms present in behavioral and hormonal profiles before birth. The source of these rhythms remains to be identified and it is not yet clear that the circadian pacemaker is endogenously active in the human before birth. There is evidence, however, that maternal melatonin may provide the fetus with circadian information and may act to entrain some patterns of fetal behavior to the external day/night cycle. After birth there is a 2–3 months delay in the emergence of entrained circadian rhythms and this delay may be related to maturation of the circadian pacemaker and its afferent and efferent connections. It is also the case that consistent exposure to external time cues is important in determining the rate of synchronization of an infant's circadian state with the external day/night cycle. A better understanding of the ontogenesis and development of coordination of circadian rhythmicity will ultimately lead to an improved definition of the optimal environment for neonatal intensive care.

Selected reading

Reppert SM, ed. *Development of circadian rhythmicity and photoperiodism in mammals*. Ithaca, NY: Perinatology Press, 1989.

E4. Psychological Development During the First Years of Life

M Heimann

The early competence of the human infant

The newborn child has several capacities that prepare him to participate in early social interactions. These capacities might be considered as early social 'building blocks' that are used within the emerging relationship with the mother or father. Some basic biological assumptions concerning the early development are:

1. The cortex is immature but not nonfunctional at birth and some processing within cortical areas can take place very early in life.
2. Subcortical areas can govern complex behavioral responses since animal studies have clearly demonstrated that a complex response can be controlled by subcortical areas during infancy, while at later stages cortical areas 'take over' control of the behavior.
3. There is a relationship between psychological and biological growth, for example, a change in visual attention during the second and third month of life parallels a rapid increase in myelination within the central nervous system.
4. All senses are functional to some degree at birth and the infant is able to respond to sensory information received, for example, the newborn child has reduced visual acuity compared to the adult but is able to focus on an image at a distance of 15–25 cm. The visual system develops rapidly over the first year and visual acuity reaches adult levels before the child's first birthday.

The following presentation focuses on some of the more important 'building blocks' for early social development: the development of cognitive and communication skills during the first years of life.

Early social development

Voice recognition

The neonate is capable of differentiating the mother's voice from another woman's voice at 2–3 days and prefers the mother's voice. Also, a female voice is preferred to a male voice. The infant most probably has learned to recognize the mother's voice while still *in utero*. When the voice of the mother is filtered so that it sounds as it would to the infant in the womb the infant less than 1 day old prefers the filtered to the unfiltered voice of the mother.

Face recognition

Newborn infants, as early as 37 minutes after birth, display an increasing selectivity for face-like forms. Neonates show a preference for following a slowly moving face as compared with a scrambled face pattern or blank stimulus. This preferential tracking is most evident during the first month of life. The capacity declines between 4 and 6 weeks of age. It is not clear why this is so, but one suggestion is that the capacity demonstrated by the newborn infant is governed by noncortical systems. Thus, the decline is explained by the maturation of cortical systems aimed at more sophisticated face recognition processes. As the child grows older moving stimuli as well as real faces become more salient and more motivating. However, the newborn infant can also discriminate between real persons. Some observations of infants aged 1–2 days show that the neonate can detect the difference between the mother's face and that of another woman.

Neonatal imitation

One of the more fascinating capacities of the newborn infant is an early imitative ability. The newborn will imitate mouth opening and tongue protrusion, head turning, finger movements, lip protrusion and sounds. Since infants have been observed to imitate within the first hours after birth, this capacity is most likely innate. The imitative capacity seen at birth, however, is not the same as the more mature imitative capacity that emerges around 9 months of age. There have been no longitudinal studies of imitation starting from birth so that it is unknown if the imitative capacity observed in the neonate is a precursor of later imitation or if it has a significance of its own.

There are some cues as to how to interpret neonatal imitation:

1. Imitation has been observed for a wide range of gestures so reflex mechanisms do not explain the phenomena.
2. There is some decline in imitation around 3 months of age.
3. There are large variations in imitation between individual neonates.
4. The imitative capacity observed during the first months of life has been linked to the mother–child interaction. Infants displaying a strong tendency to imitate, avert their gaze to a lesser degree while interacting with the mother than do infants with a weak tendency to imitate.

In conclusion, neonatal imitation is a robust phenomenon, but there is insufficient information to date to allow inclusion of neonatal imitation in any assessment of the psychological wellbeing of a young infant. It is possible to speculate on a possible social function for neonatal imitation. This early imitative capacity can be viewed as a factor that facilitates each participating individual's sensitivity to social cues within an ongoing interaction.

Eye-to-eye contact

An increased level of alertness at birth in many infants, thought to relate to high levels of catecholamines, enables the parents to interact with a visually active and attentive newborn. This early visual contact between the parents and their child is often a strong emotional experience. Studies investigating the effect of extended contact between mother and child directly after delivery tend to find some short-term effects (the physical contact and the time spent in eye-to-eye contact increases) but no clear and consistent effects beyond the first 3 months of life. The importance of eye-to-eye contact increases dramatically as the child grows older. Observations of mothers interacting face to face with their infants have found that visual contact dominates during the first 2–3 months of life. The interaction is primarily regulated by the mother during this early phase since the infant is incapable of sustaining contact for a long period of time. However at 2 months infants interacting with their mother spend 80–90 percent of their time looking at the mother's face. This intensive eye-to-eye contact is easily interrupted. It decreases dramatically if another adult enters the room or if the mother is asked to display a 'passive face'. The child will try to keep eye-to-eye contact using movements and vocalizations, but will grow more passive and uninterested if not successful. Thus, the child knows already at 2 months what to expect from an interaction with an adult.

Visual contact continues to be important throughout the child's psychological development, but the amount of time spent in actual eye-to-eye contact diminishes rapidly between 3 and 6 months of life. The infant becomes more and more interested in exploring both objects and the broader environment, and the focus of the dyadic interaction between mother and child slowly expands to include an increasing number of objects.

Smiling

Smiling can be observed as early as the first days or weeks of life. This early smile ('endogenous smile') is incomplete, includes only parts of the infant's face (e.g. the mouth region) and it is not elicited by external stimulation. It is frequently observed during sleep especially during REM sleep phases. In the second and third weeks of life a smile ('exogenous smile') can be easily elicited by external stimulation, by a touch while awake or by a soft high-pitched voice.

The human face becomes the most salient stimulus early in the second month making the smile a more obvious 'social' response. This later emerging smile resembles the adult smile in that it includes the whole face, both the mouth region and the eyes. The early social smile is elicited by a person interacting with the infant. A clear change can be observed between 3 and 6 months as the child gradually limits the response to familiar persons.

Additional competencies

The newborn infant has several other areas of competence that can be used in a social context, e.g. the neonate's capacity to recognize the mother's odor, to display prereaching behavior, to show differential crying and to use early vocalization ('cooing') within a face-to-face interaction.

Some milestones in early cognitive development

Cognitive development during the first 6 years of life is divided into two main periods. First, there is the sensorimotor period which covers the first 24 months of life. During this period the basic assumption is that the child's response to the surrounding world is primarily sensory and motor. The child responds to the stimuli that are present. There is no planning of behavior and there are no internal representations (no words or mental pictures representing the world). Secondly, the preoperational period starts at 2 years of age and continues until 6–7 years. Two of the early milestones within this period are the fast emerging capacity for symbolic activity, for example role-playing and make-believe plays, and the rapidly increasing language skills. The child's way of thinking is, however, primarily egocentric in that the child has difficulties in taking the perspective of someone else. The child also cannot solve tasks requiring the use of general principles or rules.

Object permanence

In order to understand and interpret the world as adults or older children do, the very young child must develop a set of rules that are called 'perceptual constancies'. These rules enable the child to understand that a certain image reflects the same object even when the object moves away from the child. Size constancy develops early so that a child can interpret and act upon depth cues when 6 months old; some size constancy is already evident at 2 months of age. Shape constancy exists in some rudimentary form at 2–3 months. Color constancy is mastered at a basic level when the child is 4 months old.

These constancies form the basis for the development of an 'object concept'. An important milestone in the development of the object concept is the understanding that an object continues to exist when not visible. This 'object permanence' develops over the first year. The first sign of object permanence can be observed at 2 months; the infant displays a surprise reaction when a toy suddenly disappears. However, the child does not try to search for the toy before 6–8 months and it is not until 9–12 months that the child actively and successfully searches for a toy that has been completely hidden.

Multimodal perception

An infant is able to combine information from different senses very early in life. Four to five month old infants are able to connect sound rhythms with movements and to look at a person mouthing a sound that corresponds to the sound they are actually hearing. Furthermore, the neonate's ability to imitate mouth opening and tongue protrusion indicates a multimodal capacity is already present at birth.

Deferred imitation

It was previously thought that the infant's capacity to imitate after a delay of several hours or days (deferred imitation) did not emerge until 18–24 months. However, recent reports have indicated that 9-month-old infants can imitate actions after a 24 hour delay. Thus, we must assume that both the memory and representational capacities necessary for deferred imitation are within the child's ability by this age.

Internal representation

The capacity to form internal representations means that the child can form inner mental pictures about the world and is able to manipulate those images or words mentally. It was previously thought that this ability evolved at 18–24 months, but new findings indicate that some capacity for forming internal representations occurs much earlier. The data on deferred imitation is but one of these new pieces of evidence. There are also reports indicating that 3-month-old infants can visually recognize an object they have previously only felt. This comparison requires at least some rudimentary representational ability.

Pretend play

The first signs of pretend play are seen around the child's first birthday. A common example is the child that takes a toy spoon and pretends to feed himself. The capacity to play develops rapidly over the second year and a change can be observed at around 15–21 months of life when the child begins to incorporate other actions or toys, e.g. when the 18-month-old child takes a cup and gives her doll something 'to drink'.

The child starts to manipulate objects in a more complex manner, e.g. using a baby bottle to comb the doll's hair, between the second and third birthday. This ability is called 'substitute pretend play' and continues to develop throughout the preschool years.

Another type of play emerges between 4 and 5 years of age. The child is now able to role-play and this is a period when many parents become astonished by the vivid imagination they observe in the play of their child. By 6–7 years this 'sociodramatic play' is gradually decreasing, although it does not disappear. At this age games with specific rules become more popular.

Communicative development

Prelinguistic development

The infant is equipped with several behaviors that communicate to the parents. The neonate can discriminate between different human voices and by 3–4 months can discriminate between different language sounds, e.g. letters, syllables, intonation patterns, to a higher degree than most adults. In contrast, the child's own sounds are limited; crying is the most common sound during the first weeks of life, cooing sounds, i.e. sounds made up of single vowels like 'uuuu' are heard by 1 month. New vowels are added and the child becomes more and more competent in changing the intonation pattern during the next couple of months.

Between 6 and 10 months the infant starts to combine vowels and consonants to produce new and different syllables, e.g. 'dah dah'. This babbling becomes frequent and as the child reaches 9–10 months the intonation pattern becomes more like the pattern of the language that child hears. It is also at this age that the child starts to use gestures in trying to communicate. The child might stretch the arm and hand towards a toy he wants and make whining sounds. Pointing is also a gesture that is first observed between 9 and 12 months.

Verbal language

The child speaks his or her first word towards the end of the first year. There are large variations in normal children so that the first word occurs between 8 and 18 months. The first word is quite often an idiosyncratic utterance that the child has made up. It is important that it is used consistently to mean something, e.g. naming a toy or a person or indicating a specific request.

Language progresses relatively slowly in the beginning. It takes the child approximately 3 months to add the next 10 words to the vocabulary. Language development proceeds very quickly after the 50-word point at 16–20 months old. On average, the 2-year-old child knows 300 words; the 3-year-old has a vocabulary of some 1000 words; and the 6-year-old has a vocabulary of about 14 000 words!

The first sentence is uttered before the child's second birthday. Early sentences are short and usually consist of two words like 'I do' or 'eat cookie'. However, the child has conveyed complex requests before this happens. A child of 17 months might grab the hand of his mother and say 'cookie' meaning 'give me a cookie'. This communicative strategy to combine a word and a gesture in order to communicate is often called a 'holophrase'.

The child's first sentences are grammatically short and simple. Since only words critical to the message are included it is called 'telegraphic speech'. More complex structures like plurals, auxiliary verbs and prepositions are added as the child grows older. The first signs of complexity come as early as 24 months. The child's language continues to be immature for a long period and not before 4 years is it similar to adult language.

Concluding remarks

This chapter has emphasized development taking place within the social, cognitive and language domains during a child's first year. It has been shown that the neonate is already equipped with important competencies that help the child and parents build a mutual relationship. However, compared with his later achievements the newborn is immature and in many ways helpless.

The first relationship starts to develop right after birth, but it is not until the child is 6–12 months old that we can observe formation of a strong affectional bond. Functionally, the early attachment between mother and child serves to give the child security and protection. Thus it is most often in situations of distress or separation we observe that the child has developed a strong attachment. Increased separation anxiety and a fear of strangers is seen between 6 and 8 months. A secure relationship succeeds in comforting the infant after a short separation period. An increase in behaviors in which the child checks out where the mother or father is can be seen around 10 months. One example of this social referencing is when a child looks in the mother's face to try to understand emotional expressions. Thus, by interpreting the mother's cues, the child can judge if a new object or an unfamiliar situation is fearful or not.

Selected reading

Berk LE. *Child development*. Boston: Allyn and Bacon, 1989.

Heimann M. Neonatal imitation: a social and biological phenomenon. In Archer T, Hansen S, eds. *Behavioral biology: neuroendocrine axis*. Hillsdale NJ: Lawrence Erlbaum Associates, 1991: 173.

Johnson MH, Morton J. *Biology and cognitive development: the case of face recognition*. Oxford: Blackwell, 1991.

Kolb B, Fante B. Development of the child's brain and behavior. In Reynolds CR, Fletcher-Jantzen E, eds. *Handbook of clinical child neuropsychology*. New York: Plenum Press, 1989: 17.

Meehler J, Fox R, eds. *Neonate cognition: beyond the blooming buzzing confusion*. Hillsdale, NJ: Erlbaum, 1985.

F. Vegetative Functions

F1. Thirst and Hunger

M Rundgren

Thirst (see also p. 331)

A dynamic balance between intake and output of water normally keeps the body fluid content and tonicity within narrow limits. The maintenance of water balance depends on the ability to alter renal water excretion via adequate changes in antidiuretic hormone (vasopressin, AVP) release and an efficient thirst mechanism which ensures that inevitable water loss is replenished. Water intake, induced by absolute or relative lack of water in one of the fluid compartments, is called 'primary drinking', while water and/or fluid intake not associated with any water deficit is called 'secondary drinking'. The latter is the usual manner in which water is supplied, i.e. we drink in advance of apparent need. This terminology is not to be confused with *primary* and *secondary polydipsia* which means respectively, augmented water intake without or with preceding increased fluid loss. The regulation of AVP secretion is discussed on p. 330.

Thirst is a general sensation and in its genuine form (i.e. caused by water deficit) one of our strongest motivational drives. The feeling of thirst is usually associated with dryness of the mouth and throat, but local moistening of these parts gives only partial and transient relief of the sensation. Damage to the hypothalamic region of the brain (e.g. trauma, tumor, infarction, hemorrhage) may cause various degrees of thirst deficits (*hypodipsia* and *adipsia*) resulting in chronic dehydration and hypernatremia. Selective injuries to the hypothalamo–neurohypophyseal vasopressin system (*central diabetes insipidus*) lead to excessive renal water loss with compensatory *secondary polydipsia*. Sometimes pathological processes in the anterior hypothalamic region (e.g. tumors, *third ventricle cysts*) are associated with *primary polydipsia*, apparently due to nonspecific irritative stimulation of neuronal circuits involved in thirst control.

Regulation

Primary drinking and increased AVP release are elicited by absolute and relative dehydration. Hyperosmolality is the most important stimulus in both conditions and about 1–2 percent change in plasma tonicity is sufficient to activate these water conserving mechanisms. The threshold for thirst is at a somewhat higher plasma osmolality than for AVP secretion, i.e. water loss is reduced before the urge to drink is aroused, which seems a suitable arrangement for terrestrial life. The hyperosmolality is detected by sensors in or close to the anterior wall of the third cerebral ventricle. The sensors have not been identified histologically and controversies exist whether they are osmoreceptors in a general sense (i.e. activated by cell dehydration) or in some manner specifically sensitive to the extracellular sodium concentration. Osmotic changes on either side of the blood–brain barrier (BBB) (i.e. in the vascular and cerebroventricular compartments) influence the apparent activity of the sensors. Recent evidence indicates that they may be located in some of the circumventricular organs, i.e. structures lacking an effective BBB (see Fig. 6.20). The extracellular fluid (ECF) volume is another major determinant of primary drinking. The hypovolemia accompanying absolute dehydration (water deficit) may account for up to 30 percent of the dipsogenic stimulus in this situation depending on species and degree of dehydration. Intense thirst is also commonly experienced during isotonic hypovolemia (e.g. *hemorrhage*). Hypovolemia and/or hypotension may stimulate thirst via both reflex and humoral mechanisms. In the former instance, release of reflex inhibition from arterial baroreceptors and cardiopulmonary distension receptors is thought to increase water intake. However, this kind of influence on thirst is less apparent than for the AVP release. Reduced ECF volume may also stimulate thirst via the elevated plasma levels of angiotensin II (AII) which, at least in experimental conditions, is a potent dipsogen. Circulating AII is thought to stimulate water intake via the so-called circumventricular organs mentioned above. The central AII system may also be involved (see p. 331). The physiological and pathophysiological roles of AII in thirst control still remain to be defined, however.

The neuronal circuits involved in relaying different relevant stimuli for thirst are only partially resolved and the cerebral site(s) where these signals are integrated into an urge to drink water is unknown. Current ideas about the cerebral organization of control of primary drinking are summarized in Fig. 6.20.

Secondary drinking is commonly associated with meals and after hot spiced food. This intake of various beverages is evoked by oropharyngeal factors or specific appetite drives and not by any particular urge for water. Thus, secondary drinking may be influenced by a multitude of factors characteristic to ingestive behavior in general and it is largely unknown whether it is under any regulatory control. However, in certain conditions a specific urge for water is apparent, like the thirst felt by the mother just before or at the onset of breast feeding and that often experienced during *hemodialysis*. This may well be caused by hitherto unknown factors or known hormonal or volumetric influences unappreciated in these particular situations.

Satiation of thirst

Afferent information of poorly defined modalities (osmolality? distension? temperature?) from several orogastrointestinal levels contributes to an early preabsorptive termination of drinking. However, ingested water has effects on plasma osmolality within minutes, and diminished osmotic stimulation of thirst may be of importance to satisfy the urge to drink in humans who restore a water deficit rather slowly. Although the preabsorptive inhibitory signals in dehydrative thirst are exact and potent they appear insufficient to affect the fluid intake in most instances of secondary drinking when a surplus of water is commonly ingested.

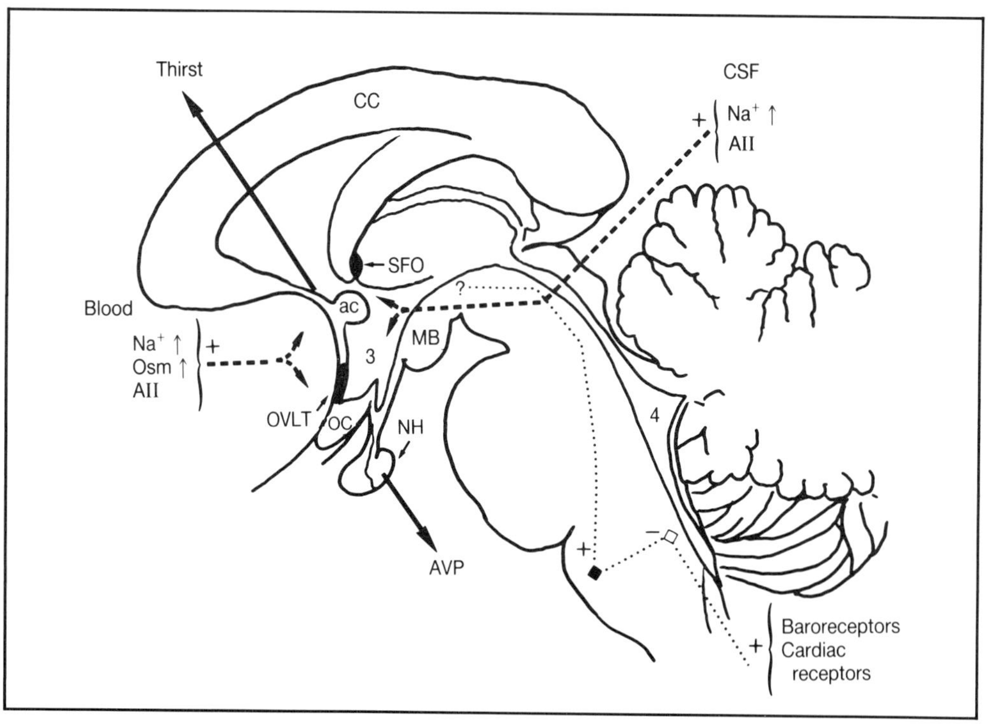

Fig. 6.20. Cerebral control of water balance. The indicated changes in blood and CSF composition are thought to act on sensors close to the anterior wall of the third ventricle. The two circumventricular organs (OVLT and SFO) in this region may play a key role in this respect. Baroreceptor afferents are relayed in the medulla, from where second or third order neurons influence both water intake and AVP release, the latter via projections to the AVP-secreting neurons in the hypothalamus. + = stimulatory influence; − = inhibitory influence. Abbreviations: ac, anterior commissure; AII, angiotensin II; AVP, vasopressin; CC, corpus callosum; CSF, cerebrospinal fluid; NH, neurohypophysis; oc, optic chiasm; Osm, osmolality; OVLT, organum vasculosum of the lamina terminalis; SFO, subfornical organ; 3, third ventricle; 4, fourth ventricle.

Specific developmental aspects

Water drinking appears to be an innate behavioral capacity although initial control of thirst mechanisms is not critical for survival in mammals since the mother's milk is sufficient for maintenance of water balance. At the time of weaning, however, it is essential that a regulatory control of water intake is functional. Rat pups respond to thirst challenges such as hypertonic saline, hypovolemia and AII during the first week of life, i.e. 2 weeks before weaning. Still, the suckling of milk is not influenced by dehydration in this species, but rather governed by feeding control. Little is known about the maturation of thirst control in humans. Water is usually aversive to newborn babies, but may be readily taken by a few weeks of age. Severe forms of congenital *diabetes insipidus* (central or nephrogenic) may cause extreme dehydration leading to neonatal death or mental retardation, but the inability to match water intake with the fluid losses in these situations is usually not a manifestation of immature thirst control. It is important to understand more about the development of thirst control in infants, not only because dehydration is common but also since hypertonicity in itself, by causing vomiting and diarrhea, may contribute to further fluid loss, possibly leading to brain damage.

Several disorders during fetal life, infancy and adolescence (e.g. *congenital cerebral malformations, hydrocephalus, intraventricular cysts, craniopharyngioma*) may cause severe damage to the hypothalamic region with consequent effects on many autonomic functions, causing a plethora of clinical symptoms. Both *polydipsia* and *hypodipsia/adipsia* may appear. In the former instance it is essential to judge whether the increased water intake is secondary to augmented renal fluid loss or not. Reduced or absent thirst is a prerequisite for the occurrence of chronic hypernatremia if water is available and there are no motor deficits to disable fluid ingestion. The plasma Na^+ concentration is commonly higher than expected from the estimated water deficit in these patients who may fail to increase sodium excretion during dehydration.

Hunger

Hunger provides the motivational drive for the complex act of feeding which involves seeking and ingestion (and preparation) of food. Feeding is part of the homeostatic control of energy balance by providing the metabolic fuel (calories). Like water drinking, food intake is also influenced by psychological and sociocultural factors. Quite often we experience a more or less strong desire (i.e. appetite) for food and/or drink of certain flavor, which sometimes may reflect an actual need for specific substances (e.g. salt appetite in sodium deficiency).

Regulation

The classical concept of the cerebral control of food intake with dual feeding (or hunger) and satiety centers in the lateral and ventromedial hypothalamus respectively, has been revised. It has become apparent that relevant visceral information (mainly gastrointestinal and hepatic afferents) and visual, gustatory and olfactory stimuli project to several cortical and subcortical areas, including most parts of the limbic system. Additionally, the strong influence of associative factors, learned behavior, stress, etc., on food intake implicates a rather widespread cerebral involvement in hunger and satiety control. However, without doubt the hypothalamus is crucially involved in the cerebral regulation of feeding. Damage to its ventromedial parts, without apparent effects on pituitary function, causes hyperphagia and obesity (*hypothalamic obesity*) and large lesions in the lateral hypothalamus induce *aphagia*, and other behavioral deficits. Further analysis of hypothalamic lesions has revealed that these effects to a large extent are caused by destruction of fibers of passage rather than of 'integrating centers'. Damage to other parts of the limbic system may cause similar disturbances in feeding control (particularly *aphagia*) but the effects are usually less dramatic.

Plasma glucose levels, or rather the cellular glucose metabolism, are normally inversely correlated with hunger feelings. However, the strong reinforcement of hunger by the sight, smell, taste and initial intake of palatable food hints at the complex constellation of nonmetabolic factors which makes it difficult to identify the relative importance of possible metabolically related 'signals' for initiation of feeding. Peripheral, as well as central, administration of a number of endogenous substances such as transmitters and neuropeptides causes satiated animals to eat, but this probably reflects pharmacological activation or inhibition of neuronal systems involved in feeding behavior rather than indicating roles as messengers from deprived energy depots for the arousal of hunger.

Eating is terminated before any significant uptake of nutrients has occurred. Both stomach fullness and the composition of ingested food are of importance for the degree of satiety. Additionally, gustatory and olfactory influences and the act of swallowing seem to contribute since direct intragastric administration of food is less satiating than an orally ingested meal. Several gastrointestinal peptides appear to be involved in mediating 'satiety signals' between the gut and brain. Recent evidence suggests that cholecystokinin (CCK) activates vagal afferents peripherally, which in turn via unknown mechanisms, lead to release of the CCK in the brain where it acts as a satiety agent.

Specific developmental aspects

Initial feeding behavior is probably mainly governed by the sucking reflex since this capacity is present in *anencephalic babies* and in decerebrate animal pups. However, it is generally believed that crying babies who eagerly take the breast and suck intensely express hunger. Little is known about whether the caloric intake is under any regulatory control during the early stages of life when large amounts of nutrients are needed for the rapid rate of growth. Apparently, insufficient feeding in newborn full-term or preterm babies is commonly due to a poorly developed sucking reflex, general weakness or respiratory problems. During development the control mechanisms of feeding go through several stages of encephalization with a gradual change to food which, at least initially, appears to be less palatable.

Feeding disorders (e.g. *anorexia*, *obesity*, *bulimia nervosa*) appear during childhood and adolescence. The neural and 'humoral' basis for hunger and satiety control briefly summarized above has offered relatively little to the understanding of etiological factors for these disturbances. Hypothalamic damage of various causes (see above under thirst) may, depending on its extent and location, induce *hyperphagia* and *obesity* as well as *anorexia*. However, in most instances of these conditions the possible involvement of hypothalamic or other neural malfunction is unknown.

Selected reading

Fitzsimons JT. Thirst and sodium appetite. In Lightman SL, Everitt BJ, eds. *Neuroendocrinology*. Oxford: Blackwell Scientific, 1986: 207.

Le Magnen J. *Neurobiology of feeding and nutrition*. New York: Academic Press, 1992.

Robbins TW. Hunger. In Lightman SL, Everitt BJ, eds. *Neuroendocrinology*. Oxford: Blackwell Scientific, 1986: 252.

F2. The Autonomic Nervous System

H Lagercrantz and D Walker

The autonomic nervous system was defined by Langley (1921) as 'all the nerve cells and nerve fibers by means of which efferent impulses pass to the tissues other than multinucleate striated muscle'. We now know that there is also a sensory component with afferent fibers intermixed with motor fibers in nearly all visceral nerves. Visceral sensation and pain are an undeniable reality.

Traditionally, the autonomic nervous system has been divided into sympathetic and parasympathetic components. The enteric system in the gut is now also considered as a separate entity since it is neither adrenergic nor cholinergic in nature. The autonomic motor neurons consist of a two-neuron chain in contrast to somatic motor neurons which innervate their target organs directly. All autonomic preganglionic neurons use acetylcholine as the transmitter. Almost all sympathetic postganglionic neurons use noradrenaline as transmitter, while parasympathetic neurons use acetylcholine. Many of these neurons also contain neuropeptides and ATP which are released as cotransmitters or neuromodulators. In the enteric nervous system there are probably also purinergic (i.e. ATP-releasing) nerves besides cholinergic and adrenergic neurons.

The sympathetic nervous system is often regarded as a part of a larger sympathoadrenal system. The other part is the chromaffin tissue in the medulla of the adrenals and the paraganglia which might be of particular functional importance around birth (see p. 341). The adrenal glands are innervated by cholinergic preganglionic nerves, although this innervation matures after birth in some mammals.

Development

The preganglionic fibers originate from the neural tube, while the postganglionic neurons develop from the neural crest. A regionalization of the nervous system can be recognized at an early stage; the sympathetic chain including the adrenal medulla, is developed from the entire length of the neural crest. Enteric neurons migrate from the cranial part of the neural crest to the foregut where they give rise to the Meissner's and Auerbach's plexa. The vagal innervation of organs in the thorax and abdomen is derived from cells originating from both the hindbrain and the vagal ganglia within the cranium. These cells extend in a tract to innervate the heart, lungs, stomach and upper intestines.

The sympathetic nerve trunk takes form by about the seventh week after conception in the human. The adrenal medulla and the paraganglia start to become differentiated from the tenth to twelfth weeks (see p. 341). The sympathetic innervation of visceral organs matures much later, after birth in the immature rat, but it is started around mid-gestation in the fetal sheep. We can assume by extrapolation that in the human, innervation of the viscera is not fully developed at birth (see below).

Differentiation and plasticity

An important question is whether the ultimate fate of the cells is already determined by the position they initially occupy along the axis of the neural crest, or whether their differentiation is determined by their route of migration and the position they finally occupy in the body. Experiments using transplantation of neuroblasts between chick and quail embryos has given invaluable insight into this complicated question. When cells from the vagal neural crest of the quail were introduced into the adrenomedullary region of the chick neural crest, these cells became adrenomedullary in phenotype. Conversely, when quail cells from the adrenomedullary region were placed in the vagal region of the chick embryo's neural crest, these cells colonized the gut and were transformed into cholinergic ganglia and peptidergic neurons. These experiments show that neural crest cells are 'pluripotent' and that the phenotype expressed is determined by signals received during migration and/or by the target tissue in which the cell is ultimately embedded.

The microenvironment therefore seems to be very important for the differentiation and choice of transmitters that a neuron will develop (see p. 217). For example, it has been shown that immature sympathetic ganglion cells in tissue culture first contain nor-epinephrine, but change their transmitter production to acetylcholine in the presence of a cytoplasmic factor in the culture medium. In the absence of this crucial substance the ganglia cells retain norepinephrine as their principal transmitter. The expression of neurotransmitter can also be modified by corticosteroids.

As in other parts of the nervous system (see p. 209), the precursor cells of the autonomic nervous system are overproduced and there is a period of time when some cells are selected to survive and others die. It is now generally accepted that immature neurons compete with each other to make contacts with the target tissue, and that survival and trophic factors are then produced which are taken up by nerve cells and promote further growth and development. One such factor is NGF (see p. 215), which has been shown to be very important in the development of catecholamine-containing nerves in the sympathetic nervous system, and of central cholinergic neurons in the brain.

Expression of receptors

There appears to be no direct correlation between the adrenergic and cholinergic innervation of an organ and the expression of the respective transmitter receptors by the tissue. α-Bungarotoxin binds to nicotinic receptors on cultured sympathicoblasts and skeletal muscle. Chick hearts bind the specific muscarinic antagonist 3-quinyclidinyl benzylate (3-QNB) from at least 70 hours of incubation age. The binding of 3-QNB increases with age, but there is no alteration in the rate of increase around the time that the vagal fibers invade the myocardium, or at the time when vagal transmission can first be demonstrated.

There seem to be significant differences in the expression of adrenergic receptors in various organs (see Fig. 6.21). In the heart the number of β-adrenergic receptors is fairly constant from birth until adult life.

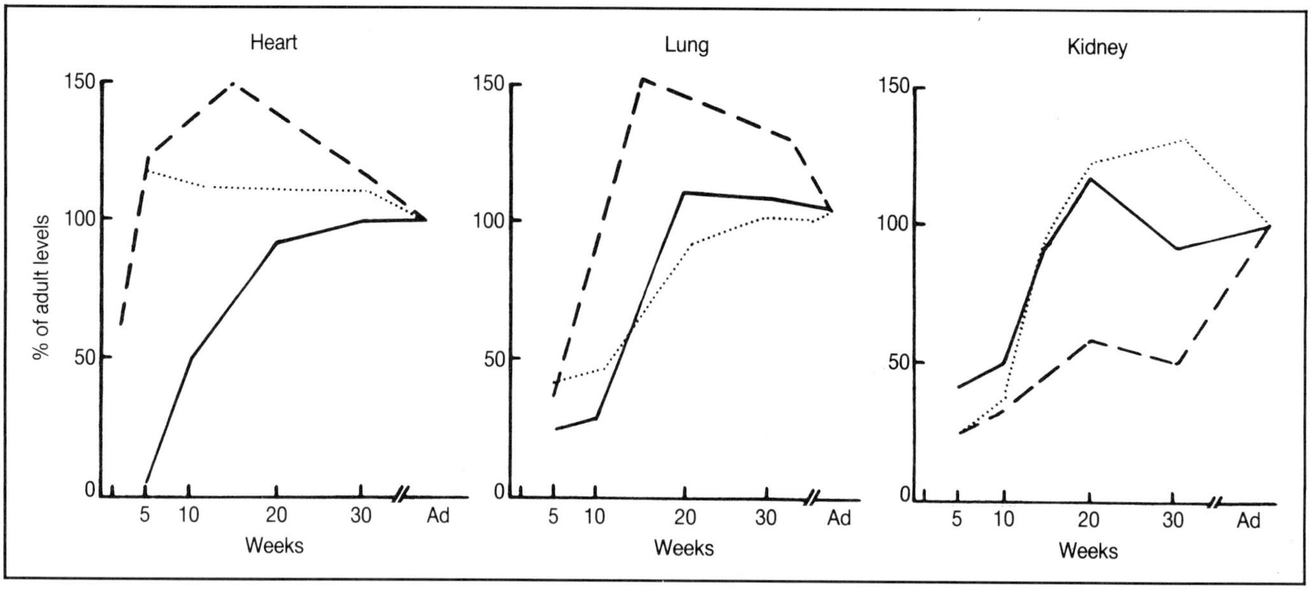

Fig. 6.21. Development of sympathetic innervation and adrenoreceptors in rat. —— Sympathetic synapse concentration (norepinephrine concentrations in the tissues); ----- α-adrenoreceptor density; ..... β-adrenoreceptor density; Ad, adult. (From Lagercrantz H, Marcus C. Sympathoadrenal mechanisms during development. In Polin RA, Fox WW, eds. *Fetal and neonatal physiology*. Philadelphia: WB Saunders Co, 1992: 160. Reproduced with permission of WB Saunders Co.)

α_2-Adrenergic receptors seem to dominate in infant fat tissue which leads to inhibition of lipolysis. In the lung a marked increase of β-adrenergic receptors just before birth has been demonstrated in the fetal rabbit and sheep. The development of these receptors seems to be promoted by glucocorticoids and thyroid hormones. Stimulation of the pulmonary β-adrenergic receptor inhibits lung fluid production.

Not only the number of receptors can change during development, but also the coupling between the receptor and its signaling system. Furthermore, only a fraction of the receptors is probably necessary to achieve a maximal effect by the tissue, while the remaining receptors are called 'spare' receptors. Their numbers seem to increase after birth.

Assessment of the function of the autonomic nervous system

Relatively few studies have been done recording sympathetic nerve activity directly in the fetus and the neonate. Spontaneous discharge has been observed in the major visceral nerve trunks in anesthetized newborn piglets. A functioning sympathetic innervation to the adrenal medulla and splanchnic vasculature has been demonstrated shortly after birth in these animals. Renal nerve activity has been recorded in unanesthetized fetal and newborn sheep, and it is now known that the renal and adrenal nerves are important in mediating part of the response to stress in this species. Much of the cardiovascular response to stress in fetal sheep (e.g. hypoxia, asphyxia, hemorrhage) is attributed to reflex alteration of the distribution of cardiac output, so it seems that much of the efferent sympathetic nervous system is functional before birth. Less is known about the human fetus, but heart rate has been studied in detail and some of the changes observed before and during labor have been shown to be blocked by atropine, and the parasympathetic innervation of the heart is therefore functional before birth. Little is known about the development of vasodilator fibers in the fetus and newborn (e.g. to muscle and skin).

Most of our present knowledge about the sympathetic nervous activity in the fetus and the newborn is also based on determination of plasma and to a lesser extent urinary catecholamines. However, plasma catecholamines also reflect the activity of the adrenal medulla and paraganglia. However, after adrenalectomy of fetal sheep the plasma norepinephrine level was essentially sustained at the same level as in sham-operated animals, while epinephrine was not detectable. This indicates that there is a low sympathetic nervous tone in the fetus. During hypoxia the norepinephrine release is substantially lower in adrenalectomized fetal sheep than in the controls, indicating that the adrenals become important during hypoxic stress.

The plasma concentrations of prostaglandin E_2 and adenosine are relatively high in the fetus, and much of this production is probably of placental origin. Because both of these substances are either physiological antagonists of catecholamines or inhibit release of norepinephrine from sympathetic nerve terminals, it has been suggested that the placenta provides an inhibitory influence on the sympathetic nervous system during fetal life. At birth the removal of the umbilical circulation means that this inhibitory influence on sympathetic activity is lost. This would allow a number of catecholamine-dependent phenomena such as non-shivering thermogenesis to be established at birth (see p. 367).

Nervous versus hormonal control

The sympathetic nervous system is poorly developed in the newborn rat, and less arborized in the newborn lamb and probably also in the human infant at birth. On the other hand, there is probably more chromaffin tissue in the adrenal gland and paraganglia of the newborn than of the adult mammal (see p. 341). These well established findings indicate that circulating catecholamines might be of greater importance than the norepinephrine released from sympathetic nerve terminals. This is also corroborated by the finding of a supersensitivity of, for example, the neonatal heart, probably due to lower norepinephrine reuptake of the immature sympathetic nerve terminals.

During hypoxia and asphyxia fetal animals respond by redistributing the cardiac output away from skeletal muscles, kidney and the gut circulations so that more of the cardiac output goes to the heart and brain. This ensures that these organs retain an adequate supply of oxygen even though the amount of oxygen in the blood is reduced. The response is signaled by oxygen-sensitive receptors in the aortic and carotid bodies which increase sympathetic nerve activity to the muscle, renal and mesenteric vascular beds. This response occurs rapidly at the onset of the hypoxic or asphyxic stress. At the same time catecholamines are released into the circulation from the adrenal medulla. There is evidence that the initial reflex vasoconstriction is not maintained for more than a few minutes and the slower increase of plasma norepinephrine concentrations produce a longer lasting constriction of these 'non-essential' vascular beds. For example, denervation of the kidney in fetal sheep blunts the initial fall in renal blood flow, but does not reduce the degree of vasoconstriction which develops more slowly.

Preparation for birth

The maturation of the adrenal cortex, resulting in the induction of the enzyme PNMT and synthesis of epinephrine toward the end of pregnancy means that the adrenal gland releases substantial amounts of this catecholamine only as term approaches. Epinephrine is more potent than norepinephrine in inhibiting production of liquid by the lung epithelium. The rise of epinephrine concentrations in plasma, before and during labor have the effect of decreasing the amount of liquid in the alveolar spaces of the lung and the actual resorption may occur during labor so that the lung is ready for gas exchange from the moment the first breath of air is taken. Endogenous catecholamines also promote the release of surfactant into the alveolar spaces. There is only a sparse innervation of the pulmonary vasculature, and although this is functional, neural activity is not thought to play a significant role in the control of the volume of lung liquid or release of surfactant.

The sympathetic nervous system has a very important role in regulating the activity of brown fat. Brown fat is an important site of heat production in the newborn (see p. 362). Heat is produced because a specialized protein within the mitochondrial membrane (thermogenin) causes the proton electrochemical gradient derived from fatty acid breakdown to be released as heat. The activity of thermogenin is increased after stimulation of the sympathetic nerve fibers, or after injection of norepinephrine into the circulation but it is probable that the nervous system is the most important physiologically. Although brown fat depots are laid down during fetal life, they appear to be refractory to activation by norepinephrine or sympathetic nerve stimulation until after birth. It has been suggested that a placental inhibitory substance is responsible for this inactivity *in utero*. At birth although there is a surge of release of norepinephrine and epinephrine from the adrenal medulla, recent experiments suggest that the increased activity of the sympathetic innervation is more important in inducing a prompt response in brown fat depots.

Transition at birth

The sympathoadrenal system of the fetus is considerably activated during parturition. There is a dramatic increase in activity of the sympathetic nervous system, especially the activity of the baroreceptors and chemoreceptors in the carotid bodies. There is also a great increase in the plasma concentrations of both norepinephrine and epinephrine. There is probably a parallel activation of both the sympathetic and adrenal systems. The parasympathetic nervous system is also activated, particularly if the delivery is complicated as shown by the large decreases of heart rate which often occur during labor. So-called early decelerations of the heart rate are often seen during uterine contractions, which have been assumed to be due to pressure on the fetal head having the effect of activating nuclei in the brainstem. By determining the PQ time interval of the fetal ECG in relation to the RR interval, a considerable level of vagal input to the fetal heart can be demonstrated in the hypoxic fetus.

There also seems to be a parallel central activation of the noradrenergic system in the brainstem immediately after birth. A threefold increase of norepinephrine turnover was found in the brainstem of the 1-hour-old rat as compared with the mature fetus. The change of behavior of the infant from the sleep-like states observed *in utero*, to the wide awake, aroused state present immediately at birth, has been attributed to activation of central catecholamine pathways, especially those arising from the locus ceruleus in the brainstem.

Development after birth

The newborn infant seems to be subject to a high level of sympathetic activity in the first hours after birth. The heart rate is elevated; the peripheral blood flow is low; the pupils are dilated; the intestines probably have little motility. The ability to increase the sympathoadrenal activity substantially during asphyxia is of vital importance for survival and the presence in the circulation of drugs which block adrenergic receptors markedly decreases the chances for survival during severe asphyxia.

After birth there is substantial maturation of the parasympathetic nervous system. The vagus nerve becomes essential for gastrointestinal function very soon after birth. Various methods of assessing autonomic function in the newborn infant have been described, although none is very precise. Sympathetic nervous activity can be assessed by measuring the heart rate, blood pressure and peripheral blood flow changes during head-up tilting. The infant responds with first an increase of the heart rate and then a decrease; this response reflects first the sympathetic and then the vagal input to the heart. Limb blood flow is decreased after tilting, due to increased vascular resistance.

Vagal responses can be tested by bulbar compression (a rather crude method), laryngeal stimulation with water, or by cold stimulus to the face. Various tests of this type have indicated some relationship between high vagal tone and occurrence of apneas and bradycardias. Autonomic instability has also been assumed to be an important factor responsible for the *sudden infant death syndrome* (SIDS), and also in instances of the so-called *'near miss' SIDS*.

Selected reading

CIBA Foundation Symposium. *Development of the autonomic nervous system*. Tunbridge Wells: Pitman, 1981.

Gootman PM. *Developmental neurobiology of the autonomic nervous system*. Clifton, New York: Humana Press, 1986.

Lagercrantz H, Slotkin T. The stress of being born. *Sci Am* 1986; **254**: 100.

Lagercrantz H, Edwards D, Henderson-Smart D, *et al.* Autonomic reflexes in preterm infants. *Acta Paediatr Scand* 1990; **79**: 721.

Loewy AD, Spyer KM. *Central regulation of autonomic functions*. New York: Oxford University Press, 1990.

G. Nutrition of the Brain and Asphyxia

G1. The Blood–Brain Barrier

K Møllgård

The structure of the blood–brain barrier

The concept of a blood–brain barrier arose more than 100 years ago from investigations which demonstrated that certain dyes injected intravenously in experimental animals stained most tissues but not the brain. Later it was shown that these dyes were bound to plasma proteins so that the barrier to the dyes was actually a barrier to dye–protein complexes, i.e. to macromolecules. More recently the concept has been extended to include a series of mechanisms that control the internal environment of the brain. While the term blood–brain barrier (BBB) implies an overall impermeability, the BBB is best considered as selectively permeable.

Essential to the function of the BBB is the occurrence of a diffusion restraint provided by membrane specializations called tight junctions. Electron microscopic studies have shown that protein in the circulating blood is excluded from the brain because the cells at the interfaces between blood and brain tissue, or blood and CSF, are joined by tight junctions. These interfaces are present at three main sites, and constitute the physical–morphological barrier of the blood–brain and blood–CSF barriers: (1) between the nonfenestrated endothelial cells of cerebral blood vessels (the blood–brain barrier), (2) between epithelial cells of the choroid plexus (the blood–CSF barrier), and (3) between the cells of the arachnoid (the blood–arachnoid barrier).

Tight junctions exclude blood-borne macromolecules such as proteins from brain extracellular fluid (ECF) and CSF. They also restrict the penetration into brain and CSF of smaller lipid-insoluble molecules such as inulin or sucrose. Various 'active' mechanisms responsible for the selective permeability (e.g. carrier-mediated transport, receptor-mediated transcytosis) of the brain barrier system reside in luminal and abluminal cell membranes and depend upon intracellular properties of cerebral endothelial cells, choroid plexus epithelial cells and arachnoid cells. These mechanisms are responsible for the transport of essential materials (e.g. glucose, amino acids, electrolytes) into and out of the brain, building up gradients between brain and plasma, and brain and CSF. Thus, apart from keeping macromolecules out of the brain, the BBB has important functions in maintenance of brain electrolyte levels, modulation of substrate entry (saturable transport systems, endothelial cell enzymes), protection from systemic neurotransmitters and hormones and exclusion of blood-borne toxic substances.

Surrounding each capillary is a basement membrane that probably provides some restraint on overdistension of the capillary but that offers no impediment to the diffusion of even large tracer molecules. The basement membrane is the combined product of endothelial cells and perivascular glial cells. Via astrocytic end feet, astrocytes induce and maintain the specific functions of brain endothelial cells including increased development of tight junctions. In the presence of most brain lesions which cause pathological changes, brain capillaries undergo structural changes to resemble systemic generally permeable capillaries. This 'loss' of the BBB probably represents a failure of astrocytes to carry out their role in maintaining the BBB.

The BBB is not complete everywhere in the CNS. In certain regions of the brain, the normal nonfenestrated endothelial cells are replaced by highly permeable fenestrated capillaries that permit brain neurons to monitor substances in the blood and neurosecretory neurons to release secretory material into the systemic circulation. Such regions, devoid of a BBB but sealed towards the CSF by a blood–CSF barrier, include the pineal gland, the subfornical organ, the organum vasculosum of the lamina terminalis, the median eminence, the neurohypophysis, and the area postrema. Due to their relationship to the ventricular system these structures are collectively referred to as circumventricular organs.

Barriers in the developing brain

The general belief appears to be that the blood–brain barrier in the fetus or newborn is immature. The mechanisms that control the internal environment of the human brain appear sequentially during development. Tight junctions that prevent the intercellular passage of protein appear very early, probably as soon as blood vessels invade the brain or the choroid plexuses begin to differentiate. Although these junctions are probably 'tight' to protein as soon as they form, recent tissue culture evidence suggests that they may be more permeable to other molecules early in development. The barrier to protein is present very early indeed; other barrier mechanisms develop at different times, probably not related to the time of birth, which in relation to brain development, occurs at very different times in different species.

Not only are the blood–brain, blood–CSF and (pia-)arachnoid barriers to protein present very early in brain development, but there is a fourth barrier at the CSF–brain interface in the immature brain that is not present in the adult. This CSF–brain barrier is dependent on specialized intercellular junctions (strap junctions) between adjacent neuroepithelial cells which prevent intercellular passage of protein from CSF to the brain ECF. The presence of this barrier correlates with the presence of very high concentrations of plasma protein in CSF of the immature brain. These proteins probably enter the CSF from plasma via epithelial cells of the choroid plexus, not because of immaturity of the blood–CSF barrier, but because of the presence early in brain development, of transcellular protein-specific transfer mechanisms in the choroid plexus. Many different plasma proteins have been demonstrated to be present within choroid plexus epithelial cells, especially in early human brain.

The high concentration of proteins in immature CSF may in some as yet unknown way be involved in the excessive cell proliferation that occurs in the ventricular zone which lines the entire ventricular system. Apart from the neuroepithelial cells at the CSF–brain interface, brain cells develop within an ECF with a very low protein concentration. This relative isolation of the developing brain from extracellular protein may be an important prerequisite for normal neuronal migration and differentiation and for establishing the initial neuronal networks. Furthermore rather confusingly, some proteins that are immunologically indistinguishable from plasma proteins are found intracellularly in both neurons and glial cells in the developing brain; there is now evidence that some of these proteins may be synthesized *in situ*, although some are also taken up at specific sites and by specialized mechanisms.

However, it is true that low molecular weight compounds and many nutritionally important compounds such as amino acids do penetrate to a greater extent in the developing brain than in the adult brain; but this is probably only the case much earlier in brain development than at stages equivalent to the newborn in humans. Whether this greater permeability to certain compounds early in brain development is a reflection of 'immaturity', or is due to developmental specialization is not clear. The fact that it is selective suggests that the latter is more likely.

It should be obvious from the previous paragraphs that the general statement that the blood–brain barrier in the fetus or newborn is immature is misleading. It is important to specify which barrier (virtually nothing is known about the developing human pia-arachnoid) to which material and at which stage of brain development.

Pathophysiology of barriers in the developing brain

Kernicterus occurs in infants exposed to high levels of unconjugated bilirubin. This has often been cited as evidence that the blood–brain barrier is immature because hyperbilirubinemia does not cause encephalopathy in adults. However, this interpretation does not take account of the fact that the bilirubin which may accumulate in the brains of newborn infants is due to an accumulation of unconjugated bilirubin. Accumulation of unconjugated bilirubin beyond the neonatal period is very unusual. However, it is found in the rare congenital deficiency of glucuronyl transferase that occurs in the *Crigler–Najjar syndrome*. Such patients do show clinical signs of bilirubin encephalopathy in the adult.

Unconjugated bilirubin binds to albumin and it seems clearly established both in animal experiments and in clinical practice, that *kernicterus* only occurs when the binding capacity of albumin for bilirubin is exceeded. In premature infants and some very severely ill neonates this can occur at unexpectedly low levels of bilirubin. Additional mechanisms therefore have to be considered. A breakdown of the blood–brain barrier might allow bilirubin bound to albumin to enter the brain under pathological conditions. Another possibility is that hypercapnia (see below) might result in a transfer of bilirubin bound to albumin into brain and CSF. It has been suggested that *kernicterus* follows when the rate of deposition becomes very high as a result of high bilirubin concentrations, low albumin reserve binding sites, low pH, after administration of displacing drugs, or if the bilirubin oxidase system has been affected by asphyxia. Such a complex pathophysiology would appear to account for many clinical findings that have previously appeared contradictory.

It has been known for some time that high levels of carbon dioxide in the blood result in an increase in penetration of various molecules such as albumin and sucrose into both brain and CSF in the adult. The mechanism is not known. As indicated above the blood–brain and blood–CSF barriers to low molecular weight substances are much more permeable in the immature than in the mature brain. The effect of hypercapnia superimposed upon the intrinsically high normal permeability may result in a considerable penetration of smaller molecules into brain and CSF.

There have been extensive studies of the effects of different forms of hypoxia (anoxic, ischemic, and histotoxic) on blood–brain barrier properties in adult animals, but in the fetus and neonate much less is known. A series of permeability studies performed in dead fetuses and newborn showed that the barrier to proteins was remarkably resistant to postmortem changes and remained intact for many hours after death.

It has been stressed above that the blood–brain barrier to protein appears to be formed very early in brain development, probably as blood vessels first invade the nervous tissue of the very immature brain. Nevertheless, these vessels do appear to be more fragile than in the adult.

The advent of non-invasive methods for the examination of brains in neonates has revealed a remarkably high incidence of *subependymal hemorrhages* in premature infants. Many of these hemorrhages are 'silent' and do not give rise to immediate clinical manifestations, although it is less clear whether they result in subsequent brain malfunction. A proportion of the *subependymal hemorrhages* progress to *intraventricular hemorrhage*, some of which have serious effects on the infant. The hemorrhages begin within the ventricular zone or subependymal layer, particularly in the ganglionic eminence which is a site of very active angiogenesis.

Circumvention of developing and mature brain barriers via retrograde axonal transport

The brain barrier system can be circumvented by transport via axons from motor neurons in the spinal cord and cranial nerve nuclei in the brainstem. These motor neurons project to the external environment. Due to both receptor-mediated uptake and endocytosis followed by retrograde axonal transport, substances such as viruses, bacterial toxins, and various plasma protein-bound ligands (heavy metals, dyes) that are present in the external environment can reach the neuronal perikarya within the brain. The brain barrier system is circumvented equally well in the developing and mature brain.

Selected reading

Møllgård K, Saunders NR. The development of the human blood–brain and blood–CSF barriers. *Neuropathol Appl Neurobiol* 1986; **12**: 337.

Møllgård K, Dziegielewska KM, Saunders NR, *et al.* Synthesis and localization of plasma proteins in the developing human brain. Integrity of the fetal blood–brain barrier to endogenous proteins of hepatic origin. *Dev Biol* 1988; **128**: 207.

G2. Nutrition of Neurons

A Schousboe and B Quistorff

Energy metabolism and enzymes

Neurons

Under normal conditions the main substrate for energy metabolism in neurons is glucose. Neurons contain all enzymes necessary for conversion of glucose to either lactate or carbon dioxide (CO_2) and water via the pyruvate dehydrogenase reaction and the tricarboxylic acid (TCA) cycle. While oxidation of glucose to CO_2 yields 36–38 molecules of ATP per glucose, its conversion to lactate via anerobic glycolysis leads to production of only two molecules of ATP per glucose. Under conditions with an adequate oxygen supply the lactate production is small and glucose is oxidized almost entirely through pyruvate dehydrogenase and the TCA cycle. Under conditions where the supply of glucose is inadequate, neuronal energy metabolism can utilize ketone bodies (acetoacetate and β-hydroxybutyrate) when present in high concentrations, or amino acids such as glutamine and branched chain amino acids (valine, leucine and isoleucine). With regard to ketone bodies, it has been shown that the metabolic rate of neurons in culture is similar when glucose is substituted for by acetoacetate. Glutamine also appears to be an excellent substrate to maintain oxidative metabolism in most neurons. It should, however, be emphasized that in glutamatergic neurons, glutamine serves as an energy source only under extreme conditions of glucose deprivation because it is acting as the precursor for neurotransmitter glutamate. The branched chain amino acids, although being metabolized in neurons, are unlikely to play any major role in the maintenance of ATP levels in neurons.

Neurons contain essentially all enzymes pertinent for metabolism of the above mentioned substrates. It should be underlined, however, that two important enzymes are not expressed in neurons. These are glutamine synthetase (GS) and pyruvate carboxylase (PC), both of which are present only in astrocytes and possibly other types of glial cells (see below). The functional consequence of the lack of GS is that neurons are unable to synthesize glutamine from glutamate and therefore are dependent on a supply of this amino acid from astrocytes since supply from blood appears to be negligible. This is particularly serious in case of glutamatergic (see above) and GABAergic neurons (neurons utilizing γ-aminobutyrate (GABA) as the neurotransmitter) since glutamine serves as the precursor for these neurotransmitter amino acids. In other words, it appears that these neurons are dependent on astrocytes with regard to supply of the substrate for biosynthesis of their neurotransmitters. Neurons also lack PC. This enzyme which by fixation of CO_2 converts pyruvate to oxaloacetate, a TCA constituent, is necessary in order for a cell to maintain normal levels of TCA cycle constituents. Since glutamate and GABA could be synthesized not only from glutamine but alternatively also from α-ketoglutarate, a TCA cycle constituent, neurons could have overcome the dependency on the astrocytes concerning glutamine supply if they had the ability to perform a net synthesis of TCA cycle intermediates from glucose. However, due to the lack of PC, the neurons are also totally dependent on astrocytes as far as this alternative pathway for neurotransmitter amino acid biosynthesis is concerned, since again supply from the circulatory blood appears to be negligible. The implication of this functional metabolic compartmentation is not clear, but is the topic of active research.

Astrocytes

Like neurons, astrocytic energy metabolism is normally maintained with glucose as the major substrate and, like the neurons, the astrocytes are capable of utilizing other substrates such as ketone bodies and amino acids when the concentration becomes appropriately high. Compared to neurons, astrocytes in culture have much more active glycolysis, leading to lactate production. However, in the brain *in vivo* this is unlikely to occur since the overall lactate formation of the brain is rather modest and since neurons do not appear to take up lactate. It is interesting that astrocytes synthesize considerable amounts of citrate, a TCA cycle constituent, which subsequently may become available for neurons. This ability of the astrocytes to perform a net synthesis from glucose of TCA cycle constituents is obviously in agreement with the unique presence of PC in these cells.

Glycogen which is exclusively stored in astrocytes can be converted to glucose upon stimulation of astrocytes by neurotransmitters/neuromodulators including vasointestinal polypeptide (VIP) and norepinephrine. Thus neurons can utilize such molecules to signal surrounding astrocytes to mobilize glucose. It is conceivable that this glucose could subsequently be transferred to the neurons. This requires the hydrolysis of glucose 6-phosphate to glucose by glucose 6-phosphatase, an enzyme present in astrocytes. The amount of glycogen stored is, however, modest compared with other glycogen storing tissues like muscle and liver and it is not clear to what extent glycogen plays a functional metabolic role in brain energy metabolism.

Ontogenetic aspects

Regulation of glucose metabolism to either lactate or acetyl-CoA is dependent among other factors upon the subunit composition of lactate dehydrogenase. This enzyme consists of five isoforms known as LDH 1–5 and the relative amount of each one of these five isoenzymes appears to determine whether pyruvate will be converted to lactate or will be oxidized to acetyl-CoA (see p. 94). Other key factors are, of course, the regulation of pyruvate dehydrogenase and the redox state of the cytosol, i.e. the $NAD^+/NADH$ ratio. In adult brain, the LDH isoenzyme composition favors oxidative metabolism but at early ontogenetic stages, the LDH isoenzyme composition allows anerobic glycolysis, i.e. lactate formation to take place. This means that in newborns the brain is better equipped for ATP operation via anerobic glycolysis during hypoxia. However, significant lactate production takes place only to the extent that there is a net NADH production in the cell which is not compensated for by oxidative phosphorylation in the mitochondria. This change in the LDH isoenzyme composition during early ontogenesis appears to take place both in neurons and astrocytes. The lactate production of the newborn is an efficient ATP generating pathway only because here the lactate release from the brain is more efficient than in the adult brain, probably due to a higher permeability of the blood–brain barrier to small molecules (see p. 269).

Glucose utilization by the brain

Normally in the brain there is a distinct regional heterogeneity of blood flow and a tight coupling between blood flow and metabolic activity. This coupling may, however, be disrupted during *ischemia* and reflow after ischemia where low flow regions may exhibit a very high glycolytic activity which appears to be associated with histologically verifiable damage. In fact, a deranged ratio of glucose metabolism to flow on a regional basis has been suggested as one general mechanism of neuronal damage. The basis of this hypothesis was the important observation that food deprived monkeys apparently withstood circulatory arrest much better than animals given intravenous glucose prior to the ischemic insult. The observation of relative protection against ischemia by substrate depletion has been repeatedly confirmed in adults and correlates strongly with the degree of brain lactate concentration. It is not clear, however, whether the enhanced damage after hyperglycemic ischemia is caused by the increased H^+ concentration or by the accumulation of lactate and/or glycolytic intermediates *per se*.

It is well known that upon reflow after even short periods of ischemia the brain will show multiple small foci of impaired reperfusion. A consistent finding has been swelling of perivascular glial cells which may lead to obliterative compression of capillaries. Alternatively, it has been suggested that the no-reflow phenomenon could be caused by increased blood viscosity. Perhaps the glial swelling mechanism may deserve further attention since excessive lactate formation may take place in particular in these cells due to their high glycolysis, thereby giving rise to a possible increase in intracellular osmotic pressure. In this context, it should be noted that release of large amounts of taurine from astroglial cells may play an important role in the maintenance of osmotic equilibrium.

Extracellular glutamate increases during ischemia and plays an important role in regional brain damage (see p. 278). Whether this is related to the increased rate of glycolysis in astrocytes is not clear, but one could speculate that since the mechanism needed for glutamate production from pyruvate is present in the astrocytes, increased glutamate output could result from the accumulated lactate during the reperfusion.

The clinical conditions seen after a hypoxic insult involve an initial phase of hyperperfusion where the normal coupling between blood flow and metabolism is deranged. This situation could be caused by the increased extracellular acidosis leading to arterial vasodilation. The length of this initial phase of vasodilation varies sometimes up to 12 hours followed by a hypoperfusion period.

Selected reading

Benveniste H, Drejer J, Schousboe A, Diemer NH. Elevation of the extracellular concentrations of glutamate and aspartate in rat hippocampus during transient cerebral ischemia monitored by intracerebral microdialysis. *J Neurochem* 1984; **43**: 1369.

Ginsberg MD. Local metabolism responses to cerebral ischemia. *Cerebrovasc Brain Metab Rev* 1990; **2**: 58.

Hertz L, Drejer J, Schousboe A. Energy metabolism in glutamatergic neurons, GABAergic neurons and astrocytes in primary cultures. *Neurochem Res* 1988; **13**: 605.

Lassen NA, Ingvar DH, Raichler ME, *et al.*, eds. *Brain work imaging*. Alfred Benzon Symposium 31, Munksgaard, Copenhagen, 1991.

Passoneau JW, Hawkins RA, Lust WD, Welsh FA, eds.

Cerebral metabolism and neuronal function. Baltimore: Williams & Wilkins, 1980.
Siesjö BK. *Brain energy metabolism*. Chichester, New York: John Wiley & Sons, 1978.

G3. Perinatal Asphyxia and Neonatal Seizures

M I Levene and M Y Anthony

Asphyxia occurring prior to, or during delivery remains an important cause of permanent neurological deficit in surviving infants. Despite considerable research no single intervention has been shown to protect against functional damage occurring as a result of the birth process. Understanding the pathophysiological processes underlying asphyxial insults may open new avenues for effective therapeutic interventions.

Asphyxia results from failure of normal respiratory gas exchange with resulting hypoxia, hypercapnia and metabolic acidosis. *Postasphyxial encephalopathy* in the neonate shows a consistent pattern of neurological features which can be relatively easily divided into mild, moderate and severe (Table 6.9). Infants with mild encephalopathy recover fully by 48 hours after birth and convulsions are not a feature. Infants with moderate encephalopathy have convulsions, but these may be subtle and unrecognized by inexperienced staff. Coma is a feature of severe HIE together with marked flaccidity and severe respiratory depression.

Susceptibility to asphyxia

It is well known that the immature animal withstands asphyxia better than those that are more mature. It has been found that mature fetal rats survived more than 25 times longer in an atmosphere of pure nitrogen than adult rats subjected to the same insult. One-day-old rat pups survived approximately 10 times longer than adult rats. This protective effect is partly due to the immature heart sustaining a cardiac output for significantly longer than in mature animals but, quite independently the immature brain appears to be more resistant to the effects of asphyxia.

For the purposes of this section we will consider asphyxial injury that occurs as the result of compromise in the intrapartum period although there is increasing evidence of asphyxial encephalopathy occurring well

Table 6.9. A clinical grading system for hypoxic-ischemic encephalopathy (HIE)

	Mild	Moderate	Severe
Level of consciousness	Hyperalert	Lethargic	Stuporous
Neuromuscular control			
Muscle tone	Normal	Mild hypotonia	Flaccid
Posture	Mild distal flexion	Strong distal flexion	Intermittent decerebrate
Stretch reflex	Overactive	Overactive	Decreased or absent
Segmental myoclonus	Present	Present	Absent
Complex reflexes			
Suck	Weak	Weak or absent	Absent
Moro	Strong: low threshold	Weak, incomplete, high threshold	Absent
Oculovestibular	Normal	Overactive	Weak or absent
Tonic neck	Slight	Strong	Absent
Autonomic function			
Pupils	Generalized sympathetic mydriasis	Generalized parasympathetic miosis	Both systems depressed Variable, unequal, poor light reflex
Heart rate	Tachycardia	Bradycardia	Variable
Bronchial secretions	Sparse	Profuse	Variable
Gastrointestinal motility	Normal or decreased	Increased diarrhea	Variable
Seizures	None	Common, focal or multifocal	Uncommon (excluding decerebrate)

before birth. The infant's response to asphyxial events depends both on the condition of the fetus and the type of insult. The mature fetus is well adapted to the process of labor and these adaptations are described below. If the infant is already stressed prior to labor then these physiological adaptations may be compromised. Fetal growth impairment is a common and important maladaptation. The growth retarded and metabolically compromised fetus is likely to withstand the rigors of labor less well than a fetus who is well grown with adequate metabolic reserves.

There are two important components of the asphyxial insult: severity and duration. Severity refers to the intensity or completeness of the insult, the most intense being *cardiac arrest*. This only very rarely occurs without prolonged compromise prior to the myocardial collapse. A more common rapid onset lesion without prior compromise is *placental abruption*. If this is massive then placental perfusion will be critically reduced with consequent rapid fetal asphyxiation. The duration of the asphyxial insult will clearly determine the final outcome. Different parts of the brain appear to be preferentially damaged by insults of different duration. Acute and total asphyxia, such as occurs with complete cessation of blood flow (e.g. *umbilical cord prolapse*) causes a lesion affecting spinal cord, brainstem and thalamus. Episodes of partial asphyxia (as may occur during a long and complicated labor) produce a different pattern of cerebral injury affecting mainly cortical and subcortical structures. The reasons for the different distribution of lesions depends on the redistribution of regional cerebral blood flow during asphyxia and the degree of neural maturation.

Systemic injury

The human infant possesses a number of adaptive mechanisms to protect vital body functions during asphyxia. The two most vital organs, the brain and the heart, receive oxygenated blood in preference to the kidneys, lungs, gut and skin. These adaptive mechanisms will spare the brain and myocardium until the severity of the asphyxia surpasses the threshold and once exceeded there will be a failure of energy supply to these vital organs. The resulting compromise to cardiac function may cause ischemic damage to already hypoxic tissues. This may produce arrhythmias or systemic hypotension which causes further impairment to the brain.

The preferential shunting of blood away from the immediately less vital organs results in the systemic complications of asphyxia. *Renal failure* and *necrotizing enterocolitis* are the two most important clinical complications that occur following severe perinatal asphyxia, but recognized clinical complications may affect almost any organ system.

Mechanisms of tissue injury

Lactic acidosis

Glucose and oxygen are the two main substrates of cerebral metabolism in the immature brain (see p. 271). In the absence of oxygen only anerobic glycolysis can occur which generates lactic acid. Although lactic acid can under normal circumstances be a metabolic substrate, excessive production may compromise cerebral function and exacerbate the development of cerebral oedema. Lactic acid may be neurotoxic in high concentrations, and the glia appear to be more vulnerable than neurons. There is some evidence in adults that asphyxia occurring in the presence of elevated levels of plasma glucose fuels the anerobic pathway leading to excessive production of lactic acid and more severe cerebral injury. More recent studies have shown that in immature animals treatment with glucose prior to asphyxia actually prolonged survival and may reduce neuropathological injury. It therefore appears that there is a fundamental difference in the metabolism of glucose between immature and adult animals.

Cerebral edema

Injury to the cerebrum may cause cerebral edema which has been considered to be an important initiator of further cerebral compromise due to a progressive fall in cerebral perfusion with the development of brain swelling. Cerebral edema is thought to be due to both vasogenic and cytotoxic mechanisms. Vasogenic edema occurs as the result of increasing capillary leakiness with fluid extravasation from the capillaries into the extracellular compartment of the brain: this has been shown to occur in immature rat pups. Cytotoxic edema is due to failure of membrane pumps (see below). Although cerebral edema occurs following asphyxia, there is no good evidence in the immature animal that vasogenic edema causes progressive failure of cerebral perfusion. Infants who have suffered severe intrapartum asphyxia develop raised intracranial pressure due to cerebral edema and in some there is progressive reduction in cerebral perfusion. This occurs about 24 hours after birth but it is associated with an increase in cerebral blood flow velocity which may be due to vasoparalysis (see below). The reason for the intracranial hypertension is more likely to be due to increased cerebral blood volume than edema.

Measurement of cerebral blood volume during life is possible in human neonates by means of near infrared spectroscopy (NIRS). This technique measures changes in oxy- and deoxyhemoglobin within the brain and total intracerebral hemoglobin can be calculated. NIRS has shown a progressive increase in cerebral blood volume following severe birth asphyxia.

Failure of membrane pumps

Cellular integrity is maintained at least in part by the control of intracellular ion gradients. During severe asphyxia, neuronal depolarization occurs with rapid ionic fluxes. The main intracellular cation is K^+. The ratio of Ca^{2+} and Na^+ inside and outside the cell is maintained by membrane pumps. These pumps require ATP to restore intracellular ionic equilibrium. It is estimated that under normal circumstances, 50–60 percent of intracellular energy consumption is directed towards ion pumping. Once the energy supply is depleted there follows a progressive accumulation of intracellular Ca^{2+} and Na^+ and an increase in extracellular K^+. Rescue mechanisms of the mitochondria to clear excessive Ca^{2+} accelerates the depletion of the available ATP. The intracellular levels of ATP decrease with a concomitant rise in the concentrations of purine nucleotide catabolic products, such as xanthine and hypoxanthine.

Using magnetic resonance spectroscopy (MRS) it is possible to evaluate ATP generation/depletion directly or indirectly by assessing the ratio of phosphocreatine (PCr) to inorganic orthophosphate (P_i). Cerebral intracellular pH can also be measured from the difference in resonance frequency between PCr and P_i. It has been shown that there is a progressive rundown in the substrate PCr and an increase in P_i after the first 24 hours of life following severe birth asphyxia in human newborn infants (Fig. 6.22).

The combination of energy failure and ion shifts into the cell results in cellular damage and cytotoxic edema, which in turn may impede the delivery of substrates. The infant's relatively low level of brain glucose may also contribute towards the rapid failure of energy. Accumulation of excessive Ca^{2+} within the neuron causes proteolytic activity with further damage and influx of Ca^{2+} (see below).

Free radicals

Oxygen is required for transforming substrates, releasing energy, oxidizing endogenous compounds and detoxifying xenobiotics. For these purposes oxygen acts as a terminal four-electron acceptor and its end state is stable as water. If the reduction of oxygen is incomplete, as occurs during asphyxia, a series of highly reactive chemical intermediates are produced, such as the superoxides and hydroxyl species. These are known as oxygen derived free radicals (see p. 108). Enzymes exist to deactivate the free radicals produced under normal aerobic conditions. Superoxide dismutase, selenium-dependent glutathione peroxidase and catalase are the main biologically active enzymes present in a variety of organs. Free radicals can initiate chain reactions with the proliferation of new free radicals. Tissue injury occurs as the result of lipid peroxidation affecting mitochondria and cell membranes.

Degradation of ATP results in increasing concentration of hypoxanthine which under normal circumstances is converted to uric acid by xanthine oxidase. During asphyxia, increased levels of hypoxanthine are found and very high levels have been reported in the cerebrospinal fluid of asphyxiated newborn infants. Reoxygenation after asphyxia (as occurs with resuscitation) causes hypoxanthine to be oxidized to uric acid with the production of oxygen free radicals. There is a substantially increased production of superoxide radicals in the brains of newborn pigs who have been asphyxiated and then reventilated compared with control animals. Treatment with superoxide dismutase and catalase prior to asphyxia in newborn lambs prevented abnormalities in postasphyxial cerebral blood flow.

Neuronal Ca^{2+} influx activates phospholipid degradation of the cellular membrane leading to high concentrations of free fatty acids. Simultaneously the production of oxygen free radicals is highly destructive, causing widespread indiscriminant oxidation and

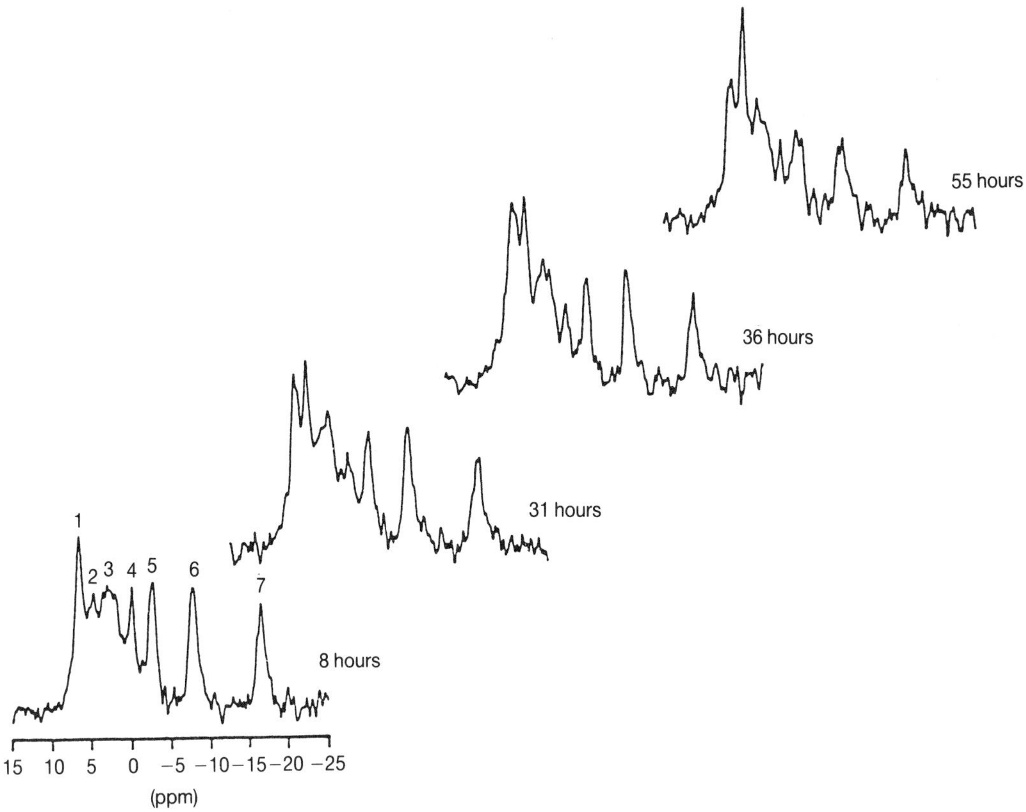

Fig. 6.22. Phosphorus spectra from a baby born at 37 weeks of gestation who has sustained severe birth asphyxia. The peaks (1–7) are attributable to phosphomonoesters, P_i; phosphodiesters, PCr; γ, α and β phosphorus nuclei of ATP, respectively, and the age at the time of each study is indicated. At 8 hours the spectrum was normal, but [PCr]/[P_i] fell to a minimum value of 0.32 at 55 hours, when [ATP]/[total phosphorus] also fell to 0.04. Intracellular pH rose to a maximum of 7.28 at 36 hours. The infant died aged 60 hours. (From Wyatt *et al. Arch Dis Child* 1989; **64**: 953. Reproduced by permission of the editors of *Archives of Disease in Childhood*.)

peroxidation of proteins, DNA and lipids such that a cascade of free fatty acid metabolites is released, producing derivatives of arachidonic acid including thromboxanes, prostaglandins and leukotrienes many of which further disrupt the cellular metabolic pathways. These vasoactive substances may then cause further secondary underperfusion. Indomethacin when given to asphyxiated newborn pigs inhibits the production of superoxide radicals presumably by blocking these pathways. It has been proposed that oxygen free radicals release neurotransmitters, further damaging the brain (see below).

Following asphyxial injury there is both activation of brain resident macrophages (microglia) and invasion of blood-borne macrophages. These may also release cytotoxins including superoxide radicals.

Vasoactive species generation

Immediately following resuscitation of animals subjected to experimental asphyxia, there is a marked increase in cerebral blood flow. This is followed within 10–30 minutes by a period of cerebral hypoperfusion, sometimes called the 'no reflow phenomenon' which is believed to be due to arteriolar vasospasm secondary to endothelial injury. The state of arteriolar tone is dependent on the relative activity of endothelium derived relaxing factors (EDRFs) and constricting factors. Vasoconstrictors such as endothelin-1 oppose the vasodilating effect of EDRFs (primarily nitric oxide). Free radicals are generated by endothelial cells following hypoxia and reoxygenation and these substances have been shown to stimulate the production of EDRFs.

In the human infant, Doppler ultrasound studies of the cerebral circulation have shown a marked increase in cerebral blood flow velocity and a reduction in resistance following severe birth asphyxia. These changes suggest that there is progressive vasodilatation of the cerebral arterioles following birth asphyxia. It is of interest that these changes occur in the second 24 hour period after the asphyxial event and may be related to oxygen free radical damage to the endothelium of the cerebral vasculature.

Endothelin-1 (see p. 468) is produced by the endothelium in low basal concentrations insufficient to cause vasoconstriction. However, following asphyxia or the administration of calcium in animals the levels rise after a lengthy delay. How this peptide fits with the observations of delayed vasodilatation and vasoparalysis is unclear but it would seem possible that the endothelial damage that occurs during hypoxic-ischemic insults may well play an important role in altering the hemodynamics of the cerebrum.

Excitatory amino acid release

Excitatory amino acid neurotransmitters are released in excess as the result of an asphyxial insult. Glutamate is one such neurotransmitter and its ligands *N*-methyl-D-aspartate (NMDA), AMPA (formerly quisqualate) and kainate activate Na^+ and Ca^{2+} channels allowing entry of these ions into the neuron. Glutamate acting via the NMDA receptor has been implicated as the major neurotransmitter in the pathogenesis of delayed neurotoxicity. Excessive release causes the receptor operated channels to open with entry of toxic concentrations of Ca^{2+}. This initiates the cascade of intracellular damage which is evident 24–48 hours after the asphyxial insult described above. The immature animal has a marked preponderance of NMDA receptor sites compared to the adult and this is an important reason for the predisposition of the developing brain to this type of injury. The distribution of receptor sites may well partly explain the regional differences in neuronal damage following hypoxic-ischemic insults, for example, the predilection for the striatal neurons and the hippocampus. Blockage of NMDA receptor sites with specific antagonists appears to prevent this form of injury (see below).

Seizures

Following an asphyxial insult, depending on its duration and severity, an infant may suffer from seizure activity. Many neurons in a damaged area will malfunction transiently before recovering, other disrupted cells will die. The creation of dysfunctional neuronal circuits may well result in seizure activity. The abnormal neurons may act as epileptogenic zones and trigger electrical discharge. The propagation of these discharges will be enhanced by the release of excitatory neurotransmitters (especially glutamate) and by the reduction in the firing threshold caused by the ionic shifts, particularly of Ca^{2+} and K^+. It is also possible that this situation is exacerbated by the disturbance of inhibitory neurons.

Prolonged seizures may cause further cerebral compromise due to excessive metabolic demands on the neuron which may outstrip its substrate delivery. Excessive production of intracerebral lactate may occur, but it is not clear that this is a major cause of neuronal injury. In addition, prolonged convulsions may interfere with the infant's respiration, leading to hypoxia.

In newborn animal models where status epilepticus has been induced, subsequent marked reduction in brain weight and cerebral DNA concentration has been found. The seizures were not severe enough to cause neuronal necrosis but permanent impairment of brain growth did occur and was most severe in those animals who had the longest duration of convulsions. Evidence in the human newborn that seizures cause further cerebral injury is lacking. It is rare for neonates to have prolonged convulsions and data from animal studies may not be relevant in this respect.

Treatment strategies

Haldane described the effects of asphyxia as not only stopping the machine but wrecking the components. This concept is now well accepted and we are beginning to understand the mechanisms by which the wreckage comes about by understanding the intracellular processes involved. To date there are no methods proven to prevent the cascade of events that follows severe intrapartum asphyxia, but application of the mechanisms described above in controlled clinical trials may improve outcome in the future.

Management of birth asphyxia has traditionally been

directed towards treating complications, but new methods will attempt to intervene early in the cascade of intracellular events. Cerebral edema occurs following asphyxia and measurement of raised intracranial pressure may allow directed therapy. Management has included hyperventilation, dehydration and the use of a variety of drugs including osmotic agents, corticosteroids and diuretics, but there is no evidence that either the prevention or clinical management of this condition is of any benefit in improving functional outcome.

In view of the lack of convincing data that neonatal convulsions cause further cerebral injury and the potential adverse effects of these drugs on the developing central nervous system, we feel that the use of anti-convulsants should be reserved for infants with frequent or prolonged clinical convulsions.

Attempts have been made to prevent oxygen free radical disease by two strategies. The first is directed towards the administration of oxygen free radical scavengers and the second involves the use of a xanthine oxidase inhibitor (such as allopurinol) to suppress hypoxic-ischemic injury. To date there are no convincing data on their effectiveness in human neonates.

Calcium channel blockers act in several ways, possibly by altering cerebral blood flow during or after the hypoxic-ischemic insult. Alternatively they may reduce entry into cells following the insult and increase the cellular resistance to ischemic injury. There are few studies assessing the effects of the calcium channel blockers on preventing injury to the immature brain.

Flunarizine, a drug which crosses the blood–brain barrier well, has been shown to protect the brain of immature rat pups if given prior to the asphyxial insult. As flunarizine is a free radical scavenger it may have other actions in apparently limiting hypoxic-ischemic damage. There are few data from the human newborn, but water-soluble nicardipine was administered to four severely asphyxiated and comatose full-term newborn infants. Two of the four developed severe hypotension due probably to its vasodilating and negative inotropic effects. This effect has also been reported in immature animals. The effect of calcium channel blockers on the cardiovascular system must be very carefully evaluated before further human studies are undertaken.

There are a number of studies on the neuroprotective effect of NMDA receptor antagonists in the asphyxiated immature animal's brain. MK-801 has been widely evaluated as a noncompetitive NMDA antagonist and has been shown to have impressive effects on reducing the extent of neuronal infarction when given up to 2 hours following experimental asphyxia. Unfortunately MK-801 is toxic and its dose–response curve has not yet been carefully evaluated.

Experimentally postasphyxial central administration of several growth factors including insulin-like growth factor 1 and basic fibroblast growth factor has been shown to improve neuronal survival. The mechanisms of these trophic effects are not known but the expression of growth factors by both neurons and glial cells is markedly increased after an asphyxial insult.

It has been known for many years that hypothermia protects the brain during periods of underperfusion. It has more recently been shown that cerebral hypothermia occurring immediately after global ischemia also protects the brain from neuronal injury. This raises the intriguing possibility that the immature brain may be protected by a relatively simple physical treatment and this deserves further evaluation.

Selected reading

Choi DW. Cerebral hypoxia: some new approaches and unanswered questions. *J Neurosci* 1990; **10**(8): 2493.

Kjellmer I. Prenatal and intrapartum asphyxia. In Levene MI, Bennett MJ, Punt J, eds. *Fetal and neonatal neurology and neurosurgery*. Edinburgh: Churchill Livingstone, 1988: 357.

Levene MI. The asphyxiated newborn infant. In Levene MI, Bennett MJ, Punt J, eds. *Fetal and neonatal neurology and neurosurgery*. Edinburgh: Churchill Livingstone, 1988: 370.

Levene MI. *Neonatal neurology*. Edinburgh: Churchill Livingstone, 1987.

Saugstad OD. Neonatal oxygen radical disease. In David TJ, ed. *Recent advances in paediatrics*. No. 10. Edinburgh: Churchill Livingstone, 1992: 173.

Vannucci RC. Current and potentially new management strategies for perinatal hypoxic-ischemic encephalopathy. *Pediatrics* 1990; **85**: 961.

Wyatt JS, Edwards AD, Azzopardi D, Reynolds EOR. Magnetic resonance and near infrared spectroscopy for investigation of perinatal hypoxic-ischemic brain injury. *Arch Dis Child* 1989; **64**: 953.

H. Development of Skeletal Muscle

L Edström and L-E Thornell

The muscle fiber

The vertebrate striated muscle fiber is a single, multinucleated (syncytial) cell, typically 10–100 μm in diameter and several centimeters long. Its cell membrane–the sarcolemma–is composed of a plasma membrane to which a basal lamina is attached. Every muscle fiber is innervated by a terminal motor axon which is related to a specialized synapse—the neuromuscular junction. The postsynaptic membrane, the motor end plate, is a specialized area of the sarcolemma containing acetylcholine receptors. In immature muscle fibers acetylcholine receptors are widely distributed over the sarcolemma: this distribution is also reproduced in denervated mature muscle fibers. One single motoneuron and its muscle fibers constitute the motor unit, the smallest functional unit of the motor system.

The main muscle fiber constituents are myofibrils 1–3 μm in diameter, nuclei, sarcoplasmic reticulum, the T-system, mitochondria and cytoskeletal organelles.

The myofibril

The ultrastructure of the myofibril is demonstrated in Fig. 6.23. The striation pattern of dark and light bands of the myofibril repeats with a periodicity of 2–3 μm. Each unit is called a sarcomere—the fundamental contractile element of the striated muscle fiber. The band pattern is determined by a precisely ordered arrangement of contractile filaments within the myofibril (Fig. 6.23). The A-band contains an array of thick (15 nm diameter) myofilaments, in longitudinal register parallel to the fibril axis. The thick filaments are interconnected by the M-line. The I-bands contain the thin (8 nm diameter) filaments which are anchored to the Z-disc. The thin filaments also overlap the thick filaments in the A-band. The H-zone is less dense than the rest of the A-band owing to the absence of overlapping thin filaments. The thick filaments are mainly composed of myosin molecules. The thin filaments are composed of actin, troponin and tropomysin molecules. The myosin molecules (Fig. 6.23) contain six

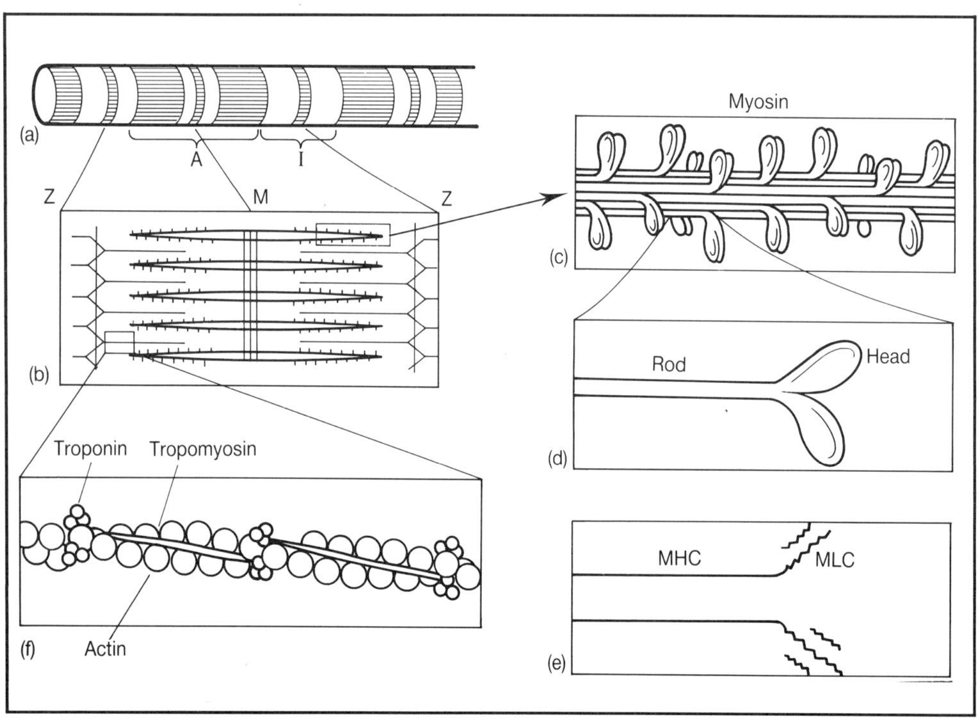

Fig. 6.23. Schematic model of the structure and composition of the thick and thin filaments. (a) Myofibril. (b) A sarcomere interdigitating thick and thin filaments. The thick filaments are anchored in the M-band and the thin filaments in the Z-discs. (c) The thick filaments are composed of myosin molecules which have two heads and a rod portion (d). (e) Two myosin heavy chains (MHC) form the rod and the major portion of the heads, which in addition contain two pairs of myosin light chains (MLC). (f) The thin filaments are composed of a helix of ball shaped actin molecules with thin strands of tropomyosin and troponin molecules located at regular intervals.

polypeptide chains: two heavy chains (MHC, 200 kDa) and two pairs of light chains (MLC, 15–27 kDa). The myosin heavy chains form a rod and a head portion. The head has both a functional and a structural domain, i.e. it contains the actin binding sites and myosin ATPase activity.

T-system and sarcoplasmic reticulum

The T-system of a muscle cell is a network of tubular invaginations of the plasma membrane. Specific functional associations, triads, are formed with the sarcoplasmic reticulum (SR). The SR is equivalent to the endoplasmic reticulum of other cells and thus represents an intracellular tubular system. It captures, stores and releases Ca^{2+}.

Cytoskeletal organelles

Eukaryotic cells contain cytoplasmic fibrillar elements which play a central role in establishment and maintenance of cell shape, cell movement, cytoplasmic flow, etc. They are important for cellular and subcellular morphogenesis. The cytoskeletal organelles are of special significance in the muscle cell where resistance to mechanical stress is crucial. The intermediate filaments (IF) are a heterogenous class of insoluble cytoplasmic filaments containing desmin which are intermediate in size between thin (actin) and thick (myosin) filaments. They have been observed in practically all eukaryotic cells.

Titin (connectin) and nebulin are two families of proteins, the subunits of which are among the largest so far described in biology. Titin with a molecular weight of 1.2–1.4 mega-Dalton (MDa) and nebulin 600 kDa are a part of the intrasarcomeric cytoskeleton. α- and β-actinin are actin-related proteins which are important constituents of the Z-disc. One congenital myopathy is characterized by an inherited abnormality of the Z-disc, i.e. *nemaline body myopathy*, and it is suggested that a basis for the disorder is an abnormal development of Z-disc due to actinin abnormalities. A peripheral cytoskeletal system is proposed containing actin, vinculin, ankyrin, spectrin and dystrophin. These membrane associated components may be linked to the integral proteins and to the IF connecting the Z-disc to the cell surface.

Summary of events resulting in muscle contraction

The T-system has the function of carrying electrical depolarization into the cell to activate contraction by causing Ca^{2+} release from the SR. The myofibrillar proteins actin and myosin are responsible for the transduction of chemical energy into mechanical work when muscle contracts. The actin–myosin complex hydrolyzes ATP. Troponin is a Ca^{2+}-binding protein. In combination with tropomyosin it is a regulator of the contractile activity of muscle. At low levels of Ca^{2+} the actin–myosin interaction is inhibited by troponin–tropomyosin resulting in low ATPase activity and a relaxed muscle. When the muscle is stimulated to contract, Ca^{2+} is released from SR, increasing the concentration of Ca^{2+} in the sarcoplasm. Troponin then binds Ca^{2+}, the inhibitory effect of troponin–tropomyosin is removed, actin and myosin are able to interact, ATPase activity increases and the muscle contracts.

Muscle fiber development

Nomenclature and definition of myogenic cells

The skeletal muscle cells originate from mesodermal cell populations. The early sign of myogenesis is the appearance of bipolar spindle shaped myoblasts with a distinct morphological appearance. The spindle shape is characteristic for myoblasts in culture as well as *in vivo* and may reflect specific cytoskeletal equipment. Myoblasts are defined as postmitotic, mononucleated cells capable of fusion and of synthesizing contractile proteins. They are immediate descendants of presumptive myoblasts which can neither fuse nor synthesize muscle-specific gene products.

As a result of myoblast fusion, long cylinder-shaped, multinucleated cells are formed called myotubes. These syncytial cells exhibit central nucleation and peripherally located myofibrils. In parallel to these primary myotubes (first generation myotubes) are longitudinally oriented myoblasts which subsequently fuse to form secondary myotubes (second generation myotubes). Initially the primary myotubes and their associated myoblasts as well as secondary myotubes are coupled by gap junctions and share a common basal lamina. During maturation the secondary myotubes transform into independent myofibers with separate basal laminae. In the myofiber the nuclei shift to a subsarcolemmal position typical of the mature cell.

Central nuclei are commonly found in mature muscle fibers in association with pathological processes. They may be an important marker for an ongoing myopathic process. For example muscle fibers with multiple central nuclei are typically observed in *myotonic dystrophy*. *Centronuclear myopathy* (*myotubular myopathy*) is a rare hereditary muscle disorder with a characteristic muscle biopsy appearance. Single centrally located nuclei are observed surrounded by a myofibrillar-free zone which is reminiscent of a myotube; this condition has been suggested to be partly the result of an arrest in normal muscle fiber maturation.

Development of the sarcoplasmic reticulum and T-system

During cell differentiation the SR is formed from the rough-surfaced endoplasmic reticulum and develops simultaneously with the formation of the myofibrils and the T-system. In embryonic muscle cells the early SR is seen as tubular extrusions from the endoplasmic reticulum, which forms reticular networks around the developing myofibrils. An early association between the Z-disc of the myofibril and the SR has been observed. At first early SR form irregular associations with the developing T-tubules. Later on there is formation of triads which are then composed of SR and T-system components.

Myofibrillogenesis and cytoskeleton

The first recognizable step in myogenesis is the expression of desmin in replicating presumptive myoblasts. Other muscle-specific proteins appear in the following order: α-actinin, titin, the muscle-specific actin, myosin heavy chains and finally nebulin. Myofibrillogenesis starts with the formation of Z-brushes composed of α-actinin and actin to which titin becomes linked. The primitive A-bands are formed independently and at a later developmental stage the interaction of the Z-brushes and the A-bands occur to form the sarcomeres in the myofibrils. Desmin is not essential for early stages of myofibrillogenesis.

Desmin may, during some part of the muscle development, coexist with another IF subunit, vimentin, which is found in most mesenchymal cells and is commonly observed also in presumptive myoblasts at stages of development when desmin is not yet detectable. As myogenic cells start to express muscle-specific gene products, there is a marked accumulation of desmin. Desmin filaments may be important for the alignment of the sarcomere.

Actin exists in a number of polymeric forms and its role in muscle contraction is supplemented by its cytoskeletal functions when it interacts with a number of actin, associated proteins. Our knowledge of such proteins increases rapidly. As the state of actin polymerization is related to its viscosity the cytoplasmic viscosity could be regulated by actin.The amount of actin exceeds that of myosin in myogenic cells early during development.

Dystrophin is a spectrin homolog recently identified as the product of the mutant gene in Xp21 locus; abnormalities of this gene lead to X-linked *muscle dystrophies* of *Duchenne* and *Becker* varieties. In *Duchenne muscular dystrophy* there is an almost total lack of dystrophin. In *Becker muscular dystrophy* there are changes in the amount of protein expressed and/or expression of an abnormal protein. The mechanism of muscle fiber degeneration is not fully understood and there are reasons to believe that genetically encoded abnormalities of other cytoskeletal components are of importance for abnormal muscle development and muscle fiber degeneration. The susceptibility for muscle fiber degeneration in dystrophin deficiency is related to muscle fiber type. Fast twitch muscle fibers with large cross-sectional area seem to be more vulnerable. It is possible that the increase in the size of the muscle fibers during maturation and growth is an important factor in the progressive muscle degeneration in *Duchenne/Becker muscular dystrophy*.

Origin and diversification of muscle fiber types

Most skeletal muscles can be described as slow or fast twitch types based on physiological, morphological, histochemical and biochemical characteristics. The speed of contraction is related to the myosin ATPase content of the fiber. Fast twitch and slow twitch fibres are organized into separate motor units where the muscle fiber type is matched to the motoneuron discharge properties. Thus typical slow twitch motor units are responsible for postural muscular function and typical fast twitch motor units are responsible for rapid movements. There are structural differences between typical slow twitch and fast twitch muscle fibers. The Z-disc is broader in slow twitch than fast twitch fibers and the M-line morphology is specific to fiber type. ATPase activity is linked to the heavy chains (MHC) of the myosin molecule and separate myosin isoforms (slow or type 1, type IIA, IIB, IIX) are related to slow twitch and fast twitch fiber types. Embryonic and fetal isoforms are related to immature muscle fibres.

The traditional view is that fiber type is the result of innervation by a motoneuron with a specific activity pattern during development. More recent findings suggest, however, that innervation is not necessary for the primary formation of fast and slow muscle fibers from myoblasts. A family of proteins (MyoD1, myogenin, myf5, MRF4, etc.) convert nonmyogenic cells into cells capable of myotube formation and muscle-specific gene expression by interacting with specific DNA sequences. This multiplicity of regulatory proteins suggests that each might regulate a different subset of muscle-specific genes and contributes to the formation of different types of fast and slow twitch muscle fibers.

Development of muscle fiber innervation

Individual motoneurons preferentially innervate specific types of muscle fibers. Thus intrinsic properties of muscle cells are partly responsible for the formation of motor units. Early interaction with neural tissue is important in the formation of some myoblasts from nonmyogenic precursor cells. Later there seems, however, to be two phases in myogenesis; first, where myogenesis and fiber type formation is independent of innervation, and later a phase where further development of fiber types is motoneuron dependent.

The initial stages of motoneuron formation are largely independent of interactions with muscle cells. The local interaction between nerve and muscle cell seems to be important for innervation of different types of muscle fibers by the appropriate motoneuron. Thus fast and slow twitch muscle fibers differ in surface components including proteins that mediate cell adhesion such as laminin and NCam. Fibers are initially innervated by multiple neurons and inappropriate synapses are successively eliminated (see p. 210). Nerve and muscle fibers which match each other perfectly might then form the most successful synaptic contact in a competitive situation. In a less competitive situation a less appropriate motoneuron may be able to innervate a certain muscle fiber and modify it. Such a situation is observed in muscle reinnervation after nerve lesions in the mature neuromuscular system.

Intrafusal muscle fibers

Muscle spindles are stretch-tension receptor organs in muscles. They are composed of long fibers of small diameter—intrafusal muscle fibers—innervated by both afferent and efferent nerves and surrounded by a capsule (see p. 239). Nuclear bag fibers contain a bag of nuclei at the central part of the fiber whereas nuclear chain fibers have their nuclei in a chain. Three types of intrafusal fibers can be distinguished on the basis of their expression of myosin heavy chains. Bag fibers are of two types expressing predominantly slow types of myosin heavy chains (MHC) whereas chain fibers express fast isoforms. A special MHC isoform, slow tonic myosin, is regionally expressed in the bag fibers and is never expressed in extrafusal fibers in mammalian limb muscle. By 10 weeks of gestation a subpopulation of the primary generation of myotubes express the slow tonic MHC and seem destined to become intrafusal muscle spindle fibres. Second generation fibers found in close relation to each spindle precursor initially express only fetal and embyronic MHC. Later one or more of these secondary myotubes express slow tonic and slow twitch MHC and give rise to nuclear bag fibers. The rest become nuclear chain fibers.

The afferent innervation seems to be of ultimate importance for the initiation of muscle spindle differentiation. Defective spindle function during development might be one causative factor in *arthrogryposis*.

Selected reading

Barbet JP, Thornell LE, Butler-Browne GS. Immunocytochemical characterization of two generations of fibers during the development of the human quadriceps muscle. *Mech Dev* 1991; **35**: 3.

Fischman DA. Myofibrillogenesis and morphogenesis of skeletal muscle. In Engel AG, Banker BQ, eds. *Myology*. New York: McGraw-Hill, 1986: 5.

Konigsberg IR. The embryonic origin of muscle. In Engel AG, Banker BQ, eds. *Myology*. New York: McGraw-Hill, 1986: 39.

Miller JB. Myoblasts, myosins, myoDs, and the diversification of muscle fibers. *Neuromusc Dis* 1991; **1**: 7.

Pette D, Staron RS. Cellular and molecular diversities of mammalian skeletal muscle fibers. *Rev Physiol Biochem Pharmacol* 1990; **116**: 2.

7 ◆ *The endocrine system*

Editor: Peter D Gluckman

A. General Principles of Endocrinology

P D Gluckman

An overview

As one of the two systems of extracellular communication, the endocrine has been defined in terms of hormones secreted into the blood stream acting at sites distal to their production. Increasingly it is recognized that this is an inadequate definition. Chemical messengers may act either on their own cell of production in an 'autocrine' manner or on neighboring cells in a 'paracrine' manner (Fig. 7.1). The possibility of some hormones acting on their own cell of production without extra-cellular secretion in an 'intracrine' manner has also been raised. The endocrine system is critically involved in the processes of growth, reproduction, cellular nutrition and energy homeostasis as well as in other physiological mechanisms such as thermal, cardiovascular and fluid homeostasis. Thus it is not surprising that there are marked ontogenic changes in all endocrine axes and that many disorders of the endocrine system in childhood manifest with altered growth.

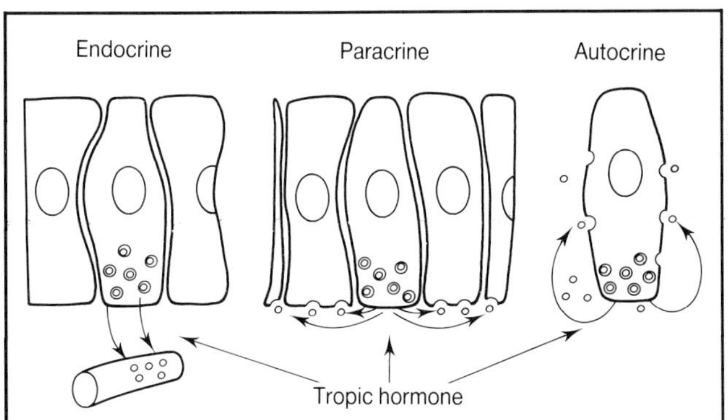

Fig. 7.1. Schematic representation of modalities by which hormones and growth factors reach target tissues. Whereas traditional hormones are formed in glands of internal secretion and are transported to distant sites of action through the blood stream (endocrine modality), peptide growth factors are more often produced locally by the target cells themselves (autocrine modality) or by neighboring cells (paracrine modality). Regardless of where they are formed, production is regulated in a similar fashion by tropic hormones and other regulatory influences. (From Underwood LE, Van Wyk JJ. Peptide growth factors other than somatomedins. The relationship to traditional hormones: paracrine and autocrine versus endocrine modes of action. In Wilson JD, Foster DW, eds. *Williams textbook of endocrinology*. 8th ed. Philadelphia: WB Saunders Co., 1992: 1087. Reproduced by permission of WB Saunders Co.)

The endocrine system is full of many interactions. It is characterized by feedback loops which may be inhibitory or stimulatory (see p. 292). In addition hormones may regulate the number or affinity of their own or heterologous receptors: e.g. pituitary growth hormone (GH) up-regulates the concentration of high affinity GH receptors (see p. 176), insulin up-regulates the type II insulin-like growth factor (IGF) receptor but down-regulates its own receptor. Hormones may also compete with heterologous receptors; e.g. most actions of testosterone in the brain are due to binding to the estradiol receptor. Several hormones are obviously tropic to the release of others in well defined axes (e.g. the thyrotropin releasing factor (TRF)–thyroid stimulating hormone (TSH)–thyroid axis) but other hormones can have indirect effects on other components of the endocrine system. For example, the action of follicle stimulating hormone (FSH) on granulosa cell proliferation may involve stimulation of autocrine production of IGF-I (see p. 112).

Hormone action depends on the interaction of the hormone with a receptor which may be either membrane bound, cytosolic or nuclear. A number of distinct signaling systems (see p. 26) are then utilized which then manifest in hormone action. There are two major groups of hormones: those that are peptides or amino acids, and those that are steroids or sterol derived (e.g. vitamin D). Polypeptide/amino acid hormones, with the exception of thyroid hormones, bind to membrane-bound receptors. As with the hormones there can be close evolutionary relationships between hormone receptors which can be classified in receptor superfamilies. However, as many peptide hormones (e.g. insulin) are internalized in association with their membrane receptor after binding, the possibility that such internalization may be part of signal transduction as well as for degradation cannot be ignored. Steroid/sterol hormones diffuse into cells and act on intracellular receptors.

Hormone action is targeted. In large part this is

achieved by tissue-specific expression of hormone receptors. However, other mechanisms exist. Circulating and tissue binding proteins may prevent high levels of free hormone acting at inappropriate sites. Thus many steroid hormones and some peptide hormones (e.g. IGF-I, GH, thyroid hormones) have specific binding proteins. There is evidence that the IGF binding proteins may target IGFs to specific cell types. Some hormones are localized by virtue of secretion into the hypophyseal or gastrointestinal portal vessels. The paracrine route of secretion is increasingly recognized as a major means of hormone targeting and specificity of action. Under some circumstances the 'hormone' is metabolized to its active derivative within the target tissue (e.g. brown fat converts thyroxine to triiodothyronine).

Pathophysiological disturbance of the endocrine system may be due to hormone excess or deficiency, or to abnormalities of the receptor/postreceptor mechanisms leading to hormone resistance. Abnormalities of hormone secretion may also be due to the secretion of an abnormal hormone; e.g. single point mutations in insulin may lead to rare forms of *diabetes mellitus*. In malignancy incompletely or incorrectly processed hormones may be secreted. Tumors may inappropriately express hormones ectopically. Another form of inappropriate hormone receptor stimulation can occur when an immunoglobulin capable of binding to the receptor and activating signal transduction is circulating (e.g. thyroid stimulating antibodies in *thyrotoxicosis*).

Thus the interpretation of a hormone level in blood is not always straightforward. Many hormones are sensitive to stress (e.g. prolactin (PRL), catecholamines) or to changes in posture (e.g. renin) or to acute (e.g. insulin) or chronic (e.g. IGF-I) changes in nutrition. A high plasma level of a hormone may reflect inappropriate and pathological hypersecretion (e.g. high lutenizing hormone (LH) and FSH levels in *central precocious puberty*); they may appropriate because they are secondary to abnormalities of binding protein (e.g. the high thyroxine levels associated with *hereditary excess of thyroid binding globulin* (TBG). A high level of hormone may also be secondary to a defect in feedback—either as a consequence of receptor or postreceptor defects (e.g. high levels of GH in *Laron syndrome*) or because of end-organ failure (e.g. high gonadotropin levels in *Turner syndrome*).

Many hormones are secreted in characteristic temporal patterns. Some are markedly pulsatile (e.g. GH), making single time point measurement uninterpretable. Some show diurnal rhythms (e.g. melatonin, cortisol, GH, PRL) and others show longer cycles (e.g. menstrually related changes in LH, FSH, estradiol, progesterone, PRL).

Given these complexities and the problems of interpretation of isolated hormone measurements, the assessment of the endocrine system generally involves carefully standardized tests of the dynamic interplay between different components of the axis.

Peptide hormone secretion and action

The synthesis of peptide hormones, as for other proteins, involves first transcription of DNA to pre-mRNA followed by post-transcriptional processing by way of excision of introns, polyadenylation of the 3′ end and capping of the 5′ end. At this step diversity may occur. Several hormones arise as a result of alternate splicing during post-transcriptional processing (e.g. 20 kDa variant GH arises from the pituitary GH gene, calcitonin gene related peptide (CGRP) is formed by alternate splicing of the calcitonin gene). Some hormone genes show remarkable complexity with long sequences of uncoded 5′ or 3′ nucleotides, complex intron/exon structures with multiple splicing alternatives, multiple promotor and polyadenylation sites. Such complexity is particularly notable for IGF-I and IGF-II genes presumably reflecting their diverse paracrine, autocrine and endocrine roles and the consequent need for multiple sites of regulation (see p. 180). The 5′ region of the gene contains the regulatory sequences including tissue-specific and metabolic/hormone response elements which are specific binding sites for regulatory proteins. In the case of the metabolic/hormone response promotor these may be the intracellular hormone receptors themselves (e.g. steroid hormone receptors) or *trans*-acting factors whose production is under hormonal regulation: e.g. the cAMP response element (CRE) is activated by the CRE-binding protein (CREB). Introns may also contain regulatory elements.

The translation of the genetic information from mRNA into a peptide occurs on the endoplasmic reticulum and the peptide formed is not the mature peptide but is a prepeptide with an amino terminal signal sequence. This prepeptide then undergoes post-translational processing before secretion. The presence of a signal peptide is an essential characteristic of a peptide that is to be secreted as it enables its sequestration in the cisterna of the endoplasmic reticulum which is the first step in the export from the cell of a secreted protein. The signal peptide is 15–30 amino acids in length, is hydrophobic and recognizes specific sequences on the endoplasmic reticulum to allow translocation into the cisterna. Most post-translational processing then occurs in the Golgi region. If, after removal of the signal peptide by proteolytic cleavage, the remaining peptide is active the prepeptide is known as a prehormone; however, most hormones are synthesized as preprohormones, i.e. after cleavage of the signal peptide the remaining peptide will require further post-translational cleavage to release the mature hormone. This may lead to the release of other peptides from the prohormone of unknown biological significance (e.g. neurophysin is coreleased with AVP). A single preprohormone may be the precursor to one (e.g. preproinsulin) or several hormones (e.g. preproopiomelanocortin is the precursor of β endorphin and ACTH; preproenkephalin contains multiple copies of both met- and leu-enkephalin). Other forms of post-translational modifications include glycosylation, phosphorylation, sulfation, acetylation and finally folding into tertiary structure. In rare cases the post-translational steps may vary for a single prohormone (e.g. in the anterior lobe of the pituitary proopiomelanocortin is cleaved to adrenocorticotropic hormone (ACTH) and β endorphin whereas in the intermediate lobe ACTH is processed further to α melanocyte stimulating hormone (αMSH) and corticotropin-like intermediate peptide (CLIP)).

Within the Golgi apparatus the prohormones are processed and packaged into secretory vesicles which bud off from the Golgi stack of smooth endoplasmic reticulum. Generally these mature by condensation of the protein into a more tightly packed granule and the application of a second membrane to the vesicle. Under the appropriate stimuli the granules migrate to the cell surface and by fusing to the cell membrane exocytose their contents from the cell.

The regulation of hormone secretion can take place at each level in this complex process. However, in practice the major sites of regulation are either translational or at the secretory step. Most hormone-secreting cells maintain significant prepacked hormone for release and the primary event is to stimulate secretion but, in some cases, hormones are not prepackaged ready for release (e.g. IGF-I) and enhanced synthesis is the primary event.

Membrane-bound receptors can be classed in several superfamilies. Members of these superfamilies have evolutionary relationships and are presumed to have formed by gene duplication. The major classes are reviewed on p. 18 and include the G-protein-linked receptors, tyrosine kinase receptor family and the GH/PRL/cytokine receptor superfamily.

The binding of a hormone to the membrane-bound receptor is rapid and determined by the number of, and affinity of, unoccupied receptors on the cell surface. As hormones generally circulate in low concentration, hormone receptors must have high affinities to have physiological significance. Further, they must have relatively low capacity to be saturable and have specificity. This specificity is not always absolute (e.g. at high levels insulin has some affinity for the type I IGF receptor and this may explain somatic overgrowth in fetal hyperinsulinemia). For most larger peptides the binding structure relies on the three-dimensional structure of the hormone and thus a single point mutation may affect affinity. The signal transduction system which amplifies the signal is dependent on the class of receptor. As discussed on p. 19, activation of G-protein-linked receptors affects intracellular cyclic AMP, the phosphoinositol cycle, cytosolic calcium and indirectly ion channels. The tyrosine kinase receptors contain intrinsic enzyme activity and when activated by ligand binding initiate a cascade of intracellular phosphorylation. The signal transduction system for other hormone receptors, including the GH/PRL receptor family, is not known. The relationship between receptor occupancy and hormone action is not linear. Complex mechanisms exist to allow the appropriate response under conditions which would not be favorable for simple linear coupling. These mechanisms involve both changes in binding properties and postreceptor events. In addition, most hormones either up-regulate or more often down-regulate their own receptor, thus offering a greater degree of complexity of regulation.

Membrane receptors are in a dynamic state. Like other proteins they are synthesized on the endoplasmic reticulum but lacking the signal peptide they are not processed for exocytosis but following post-translational modification are inserted into the cell membrane by membrane fusion. A characteristic of many membrane-associated receptors is that after ligand binding they aggregate on the cell surface. This appears important for signal transduction. After aggregation the receptor is internalized through special regions known as coated pits. These are clathrin rich and eventually pinch off into the cytoplasm and form endosomes. These carry the receptor–hormone couplet into the cell. These endosomes then fuse with lysosomes, the hormone is degraded and the receptor is either degraded or recycled. This cycle may itself be under endocrine regulation (e.g. insulin enhances cycling of the type II IGF receptor to the cell surface). Not all hormone is degraded in this manner and in many cases membrane-bound or circulating proteases are more important than receptor-mediated degradation.

The secretion and action of steroid hormones

The regulation of steroid synthesis and secretion is dependent on the provision of cholesterol as the substrate. Most is provided from circulating low-density lipoproteins (LDL). These contain a protein moiety, apolipoprotein B, which binds to a cell-surface receptor and is internalized via a coated pit/endosomal pathway in an identical process to that for other protein hormones and thus liberates cholesterol into the cell. Small amounts of cholesterol may be synthesized *de novo* in the cell from acetate or mobilized from intracellular cholesterol ester pools. Cytosolic free cholesterol is actively regulated; for example LDL uptake inhibits *de novo* cholesterol biosynthesis.

The tropic hormones that stimulate steroid synthesis do so primarily by stimulating side-chain cleavage and the formation of pregnenolone, the rate-limiting step in steroid biosynthesis. However, all the relevant enzymes are subject to a degree of endocrine control as are some steps in cholesterol supply (e.g. LDL receptor number is enhanced by ACTH).

Steroids, vitamin D, thyroid hormones and retanoids have similar modes of action. They enter the cell by diffusion and bind either to cytosolic or nuclear receptors of a single superfamily. Estrogen and progesterone receptors are nuclear irrespective of whether steroid occupied or not; the intracellular location of glucocorticoid receptors is still unresolved. The vitamin D and thyroid receptors are always nuclear associated. It is thought that in the absence of a ligand, some steroid receptors are inactivated by binding in the cytoplasm to heat shock protein 90 (HSP). This appears most likely for the glucocorticoid receptor (see p. 24) but it may be a more general mechanism. In the presence of the steroid ligand, the receptor undergoes a conformational change which allows its transduction into the nucleus (if initial binding was cytosolic) where binding domains on the receptor can bind to steroid response units at the 5′ untranslated region of the target gene which is then activated and transcription is initiated. The receptor contains thus two binding sites—one for the hormone and the other a zinc finger motif for DNA binding. The steroid receptors are 80–100 kDa proteins. They tend to dimerize when occupied by hormone and this appears to facilitate binding to DNA. The synthesis of steroid receptors is also subject to endocrine influences.

Recent evidence suggests other forms of steroid mediated action may occur. In the brain some actions are rapid and may occur via steroid–membrane interactions.

Selected reading

Habener JF. Genetic control of hormone formation. In Wilson JD, Foster DW, eds. *Williams textbook of endocrinology*. 8th ed. Philadelphia: WB Saunders, 1992: 9.

B. Neuroendocrine Mechanisms

G E Richards

Neuroendocrinology encompasses the processes by which various homeostatic systems are regulated by the central nervous system. Although exceptions exist, the majority of this communication is mediated by the hypothalamus.

Functional hypothalamic–pituitary relationships

Hormonal homeostasis is maintained by multiple interacting regulatory loops which act by determining the secretory activity of several discrete hypothalamic–pituitary regulatory systems. A group of well developed hypothalamic nuclei at the base of the third ventricle, whose neurons project to the medial eminence and the posterior lobe of the pituitary, are responsible for integration of signals from the brain and body and translation of those signals into an appropriate level of hormone secretion.

Neurons in these areas regulate the hormonal secretions of the pituitary in several ways. Some neurons, such as those of the supraoptic and paraventricular nuclei which secrete vasopressin and oxytocin, project directly to the posterior pituitary. Their cell terminals form the posterior lobe of the pituitary. Thus when a stimulus to oxytocin or vasopressin release occurs in the brain or the periphery, the signal is received in the supraoptic or paraventricular nucleus and hormone is released from the same neuron's terminals within the posterior pituitary (see p. 330).

A second type of neuron, found more commonly in the arcuate nucleus, has cell bodies in one of the hypothalamic nuclei and nerve endings abutting on the hypothalamic–pituitary–portal capillaries (primary capillary plexus) in the median eminence. These neurons release their peptide hormone message into the hypophyseal–portal circulation, which ends as a secondary capillary plexus among the pituicytes of the anterior lobe of the pituitary. The unique anatomical features of this portal system are the small distance traversed and the complexity of the multihormonal milieu of the anterior pituitary.

A third type of hypothalamic neuron which plays an important role in hormonal regulation has its cell body in one nucleus and its terminal on another neuropeptide secretory neuron in the same or another nucleus. These neurons probably have modulatory and integrational roles in hormone secretion.

These three kinds of neuronal connections describe the functional relationship of the hypothalamus and pituitary. The pituitary itself consists of the anterior lobe, whose cells produce and secrete growth hormone (GH), luteinizing hormone (LH), follicle stimulating hormone (FSH), prolactin (PRL), thyroid stimulating hormone (TSH), and adrenocorticotropic hormone (ACTH). The posterior pituitary secretes vasopressin (AVP) and oxytocin (OT).

In the fetus a distinct intermediate lobe forms from the posterior limb of Rathke's pouch. This is corticotrope rich but, in contrast to the adenohypophysis, it appears to be regulated by direct innervation by dopaminergic neurons arising in the arcuate nucleus. The post-translational processing of the proopiomelanocortin (see p. 322) also differs in the intermediate lobe. The intermediate lobe is less apparent postnatally and its biological significance is unknown.

Patterns of hormonal regulation (Fig. 7.2)

Input from both the internal and external environment affects hypothalamic–pituitary functioning through combinations of open loop and feedback loop systems to integrate the effects of nutrition, temperature, day/night light cycles, pain, affective factors and different schedules of intrinsic rhythms. The regulation of individual pituitary hormones are discussed in more depth in subsequent chapters.

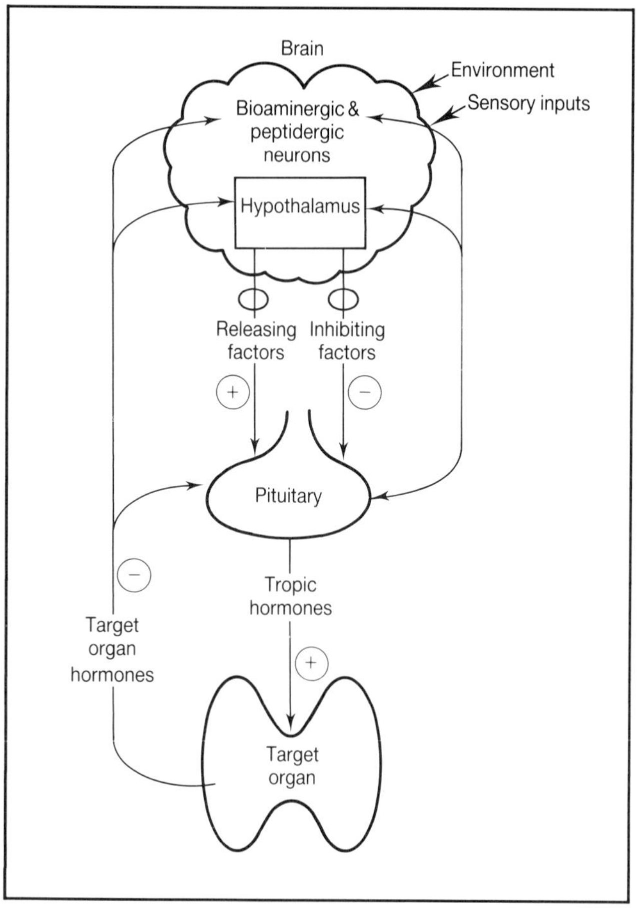

Fig. 7.2. Regulatory feedback loops of the hypothalamic–pituitary–target organ axis. Being a combination of both stimulatory and inhibitory factors, hormones often act in concert to maintain homeostatic balance in the face of physiological or pathophysiological perturbations. (From Habener JF. Genetic control of hormone formation. In Wilson JD, Foster DW, eds. *Williams textbook of endocrinology*. Philadelphia: WB Saunders Co., 1992: 16. Reprinted with permission of WB Saunders Co.)

Feedback loops

To maintain homeostasis, hormone release must be closely regulated by a series of feedback systems. For such a system to work there must be discrete outputs to be regulated, receptors and processors to receive signals and recognize discrepancies between a set point and current amount of activity. Three examples of feedback mechanisms can be used to illustrate these general principles.

Long loop feedback mechanisms typically involve a three-step signaling sequence, such as hypothalamus–pituitary–target organ. In this type of system, the output of the target organ signals the hypothalamus to decrease (negative feedback) or increase (positive feedback) its specific output to the pituitary. Most anterior pituitary hormones have a long loop feedback system. For example, thyrotropin releasing hormone (TRH) from the hypothalamus stimulates the pituitary to secrete thyroid stimulating hormone (TSH) which in turn stimulates the thyroid gland to secrete thyroxine. When circulating thyroxine decreases, the secretion of TRH and subsequently TSH increases, encouraging more secretion of thyroxine from the thyroid gland.

Short loop feedback is a direct signal from a target organ to the source of that organ's regulation. An example of this mechanism is the ability of growth hormone to influence the output of growth hormone releasing hormone and somatostatin (SRIF).

Ultrashort (paracrine) feedback is the ability of a cell to influence the output of cells of a similar cell type: for example, prolactin can decrease further the secretion of prolactin by lactotropes in the pituitary.

Many hormonal feedback systems involve two or all three of these mechanisms. In addition, there are distinct inputs from many parts of the central nervous system which are not known to be regulated in any manner by the hormones which are affected (for example the effect of cold on TSH release). This situation is known as **open loop** input.

Neuroendocrine rhythms

Most pituitary hormones are released by periodic bursts of active secretion with, or without, a background amount of constant (or tonic) secretion. Onto this short-term rhythm of secretion may be imposed ultradian or circadian (e.g. ACTH) patterns of medium-term increases and decreases in activity of the loop. In some instances an even longer term pattern of seasonal activity (e.g. prolactin) or developmentally regulated activity of the loop (e.g. gonadotropins) exists. Further regulatory influences such as nutrition, exercise and affective factors can modulate the activity of a feedback system.

Development of the hypothalamic–pituitary unit

Anatomy

The human pituitary takes shape by 5 weeks of gestation with the formation of Rathke's pouch from the primitive pharyngeal stomodeum. The hypothalamus, pituitary stalk and posterior pituitary have formed from the primitive ventral neural ridges by 7 weeks. By 9 weeks of gestation capillaries have begun to develop around the portion of the diencephalon adjacent to Rathke's pouch. These capillaries differentiate into the hypothalamic–hypophyseal–portal system by about 11 weeks of gestation. Rathke's pouch will form the anterior and intermediate lobes of the pituitary gland. The area known as the hypothalamus at maturity is recognizable as discrete nuclei by about 15 weeks. The functional integrity of both the portal system and hypothalamic nuclei continues to mature until late in gestation. The general scheme by which these nuclei are formed is by migration of neurons from the outside of the primitive brain anlage inward to the place of nuclear organization. Further organization and interconnection of nuclei occurs until about 18 weeks. By this time, the fetus is able to regulate its internal environment in a sophisticated and autonomous manner. The details of regulation of specific hormones will be discussed in subsequent sections.

Several clinical syndromes can result from incomplete development of the hypothalamic–pituitary unit. For example, *anencephaly* deprives the fetus of any hypothalamic function, although the pituitary gland itself forms normally. More subtle functional abnormalities of the hypothalamus are observed in children with the syndrome of *septo-optic dysplasia* and other midline anatomical abnormalities. Failure of Rathke's pouch migration can result in a pituitary gland which is not connected to its regulatory input. This *isolated pituitary syndrome* is probably the most common cause of *congenital hypopituitarism*. The differentiation of specific cell types within the anterior pituitary is dependent on extrinsic and intrinsic factors. Abnormalities of a specific pituitary differentiation and transcription factor (pit-1) may result in abnormal formation not only of GH producing cells, but of TSH and PRL producing cells for which pit-1 is also a necessary transcription factor. This results in a rare autosomal recessive form of *congenital hypopituitarism*. Tumors of the cells of Rathke's pouch (*craniopharyngioma*), can disrupt the normal hypothalamic–pituitary anatomical relationship and cause pituitary dysfunction.

The development of neuroendocrine sexual dimorphism

The human, as many other species, has a sexually dimorphic brain. Differences between males and females include the preoptic hypothalamic area, in which females undergo loss of cells between the ages of 4 and 10 years; the functional significance of this region is not known. The factors responsible for the multiple dimorphic features of the brain are not well understood. It is possible that the pattern of sex steroid secretion in the perinatal period and the selective presence of receptors for steroids on specific neurons combine to orchestrate different patterns of cell development and cell death in males and females. The observation that male and female fetuses regulate gonadotropins differently suggests that these sex differences may be programmed very early in development. There are numerous examples in animals of anatomical and behavioral changes induced by manipulation of the sex steroid milieu during a critical period of development.

Functional maturation of neuroendocrine regulation

Hypothalamic–hypophyseal function requires the completion of a large number of developmental processes, which are only beginning to be understood. The ability to communicate by neurosecretion presupposes that the neuron has the ability to synthesize a specific neurotransmitter and/or neuropeptide. The message emitted by one cell must be received by another cell or cells, which is dependent upon the development of specific receptors. Furthermore, the appropriate intracellular second messenger systems must be sufficiently mature to effect the appropriate cellular response. These receptors and intracellular elements must be functional at all levels of the feedback loops described above. Thus the development of one receptor (or any one particular element) in a feedback regulatory system can be the developmental regulator of the function of the entire system. It is more likely that the components of a feedback system are individually developmentally regulated in such a way that the system functions differently at different times to suit the needs of the organism as a whole. Understanding of this complex developmental orchestration is primitive.

Although there are significant differences in the signals for neuroendocrine regulation among the pituitary hormone systems, which will be discussed in later sections, there are common developmental patterns which suggest an overall scheme by which regulatory systems are built. The first of these patterns is the increasing pituitary content of hormone as development progresses. The second is a tendency for plasma hormone concentrations to increase during gestation, sometimes with a subsequent decrease toward term. These two patterns together imply gradual acquisition by the fetus of the ability to restrain pituitary secretion. The time during the second half of gestation when these phenomena can occur corresponds in the human with the progressive development of the hypothalamic nuclei and neuronal tracts which have been demonstrated to modulate neuroendocrine function in the mature animal. The third pattern is the asynchronous development of specific hypothalamic inputs which either stimulate or suppress pituitary hormonal secretion. For example, the responses of both PRL and GH to various pharmacological stimulants and suppressants do not develop all at once, but follow a program specific to both the stimulus and responding hormone. The result is a gradual accumulation of an increasing number of modulating inputs to hormone secretion. A fourth consideration is the asynchronous development of the ability to manufacture and secrete a hormone and the receptors for that hormone. For example, the role of GH in regulating growth is relatively less in the neonate because of receptor immaturity; thus in *congenital growth hormone deficiency*, birth length is only slightly reduced (see p. 163).

Role of the maternal–placental unit

A final influence on the development of neuroendocrine regulatory systems to consider is the effect of the fetal hormonal milieu resulting from maternal and placental hormone production. This influence includes placental production of a wide variety of both steroid and protein hormones, some of which (chorionic gonadotropin, estrogen, etc.) are integral parts of developing feedback systems.

The placenta may perform other functions which modulate fetal neuroendocrinology, such as metabolizing hormones to inactive compounds, selectively regulating fetal exposure to maternal hormones, and production of growth factors.

Neuroimmunoendocrinology

There are three major ways in which the neuroendocrine and immunological systems interact. It is well recognized that many hormones have dramatic effects on immune function. The effects of glucocorticoids on all aspects of lymphokine synthesis and action (see p. 325) are the most obvious example. Secondly, the lymphokines produced by the immune system have significant effects on neuroendocrine function. The multiple actions of interleukin-1 on the adrenocorticotropic and gonadotropic axes are examples. Thirdly, cells of the immune system produce hormones and peptides which have been associated with classic neuroendocrinology, such as ACTH, GH, TSH and enkephalins. The developmental aspects and teleology of these findings are not well understood.

Selected reading

Fisher DA. Endocrinology of fetal development. In Wilson JD, Foster DW, eds. *Williams textbook of endocrinology*. Philadelphia: WB Saunders Co., 1992: 1049.

Gluckman PD, Grumbach MM, Kaplan SL. The neuroendocrine regulation and function of growth hormone and prolactin in the mammalian fetus. *Endocr Rev* 1981; **2**: 363.

Hokfelt T, Meister B, Villar MJ, *et al*. Hypothalamic neurosecretory systems and their messenger molecules. *Acta Physiol Scand Suppl* 1989; **583**: 105.

Jacobson M. *Developmental neurobiology*. 3rd ed. New York: Plenum Press, 1991: Chapters 7 and 8.

Mulchahey JJ, Di Blasio AM, Martin MC, *et al*. Hormone production and peptide regulation of the human fetal pituitary gland. *Endocr Rev* 1987; **8**: 406.

C. Growth Hormone

F de Zegher

Growth hormone (GH) is the principal hormone regulating longitudinal growth during childhood (see Fig. 7.3). The assessment of GH secretion is important in the evaluation of children with growth disorders. Recombinant human GH is therapeutically used in an increasing range of disorders. This section will focus on the regulation of GH secretion; GH action is discussed more extensively on p. 174.

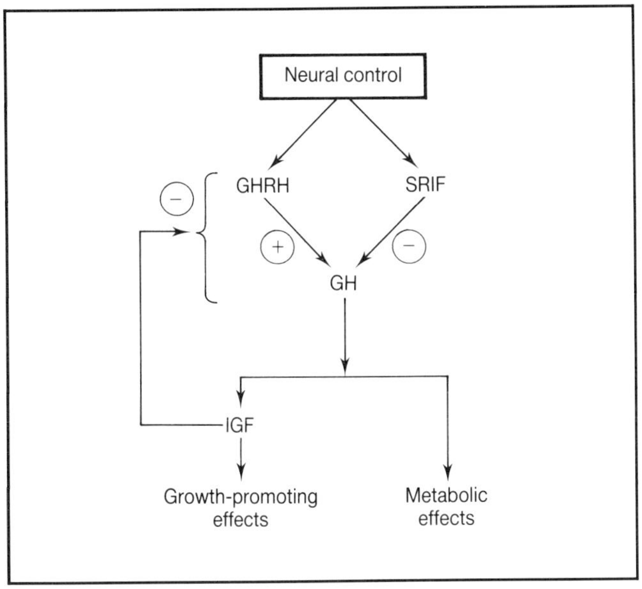

Fig. 7.3. Simplified concept of the mature somatotropic axis.

Origin and biochemistry

The GH and prolactin gene evolved from a common precursor gene. The GH gene, located on chromosome 17, is part of the GH gene family also encoding for placental lactogen and placental GH. Deletions of the gene are responsible for type Ia form of *familial growth hormone deficiency*. GH is a single chain 22 kDa peptide of 191 amino acids synthesized and secreted from storage granules by the somatotropes of the anterior pituitary. Somatotropes and lactotropes are derived from a common ontogenic precursor cell: they depend in part on the activity of the pit-1 gene for their differentiation. Defects in pit-1 expression result in *congenital hypopituitarism* associated with GH, PRL and TSH deficiency. Variant forms of the GH may also be secreted by the adenohypophysis. The most important is 20 kDa GH which represents about 10 percent of secreted GH and is a consequence of alternate splicing of the GH gene such that a second mRNA species coding for a GH missing 15 residues is formed. Its biological significance is unclear.

GH circulates in the blood partly complexed with a binding protein that is structurally similar to the extracellular domain of the GH receptor. It is unclear whether GH binding protein is formed by alternate splicing of the GH-receptor gene or by proteolytic cleavage of the extramembranous portion of the GH receptor. This GH binding protein appears to modulate the half-life of circulating GH which normally approximates 20 minutes in children. In those cases of *Laron syndrome* where the mutation affects the binding domain of the GH receptor, the GH binding protein is also absent from the circulation; this can be useful diagnostically.

Regulation of GH secretion

GH secretion is under the regulatory control of the central nervous system. Complex networks of neurotransmitter neurons modulate the release of two hypothalamic hormones, the stimulatory GH releasing hormone (GHRH) and the inhibitory somatostatin (somatotropin release inhibiting factor, SRIF); these are the principal final mediators of metabolic, endocrine and neural influences on GH secretion. The net effect of these hypothalamic influences is stimulatory and in structural or functional disorders of the hypothalamic–pituitary connection such as in *congenital hypopituitarism*, GH secretion is deficient.

A host of neuropeptides and neurotransmitters are capable of modulating GH secretion. Many of them, including enkephalins, neurotensin, GABA, dopamine and neuropeptide Y, have been localized in the hypothalamic arcuate nucleus–median eminence complex. They may act at the level of the GHRH and/or SRIF producing neurons; some may also directly influence GH secretion at the pituitary level.

GHRH is a 44 amino acid amide. The GHRH gene is located on chromosome 20. *In vivo*, GHRH is rapidly degraded to a biologically inactive product through cleavage at the N-terminus. In the brain, GHRH is found only in cell bodies of the ventromedial and arcuate nuclei from where fibers project to the median eminence and make contact with portal vessels. Serum immunoreactive GHRH appears to be mainly from extrahypothalamic origin, probably from the gut and pancreas. Hypothalamic GHRH synthesis and/or release is stimulated by α_2-receptor agonists, opioids, thyroid hormones and GABA, and is inhibited by SRIF, GH, and IGF-I. The actions of GHRH on the somatotrope are mediated by G-protein-linked membrane receptors, that are up-regulated by glucocorticoids and down-regulated by GHRH itself. GHRH elicits an immediate release of preformed GH through the intramembranous adenylyl cyclase system of the somatotropes. GHRH activates the adenylyl cyclase, while SRIF exerts an inhibitory effect. The activated adenylyl cyclase converts ATP to cAMP, that stimulates GH release. Calcium mobilization also participates in GHRH-mediated GH release, either at the adenylyl cyclase level or at a step distal to cAMP. GHRH stimulates GH gene transcription and GH synthesis in the somatotropes; these actions appear to be independent of calcium mobilization and GH release. GHRH is also able to induce somatotrope proliferation.

SRIF-14, a cyclic tetradecapeptide, is the most important product processed from preproSRIF in SRIF-containing cells. A larger molecular weight form, SRIF-28 was initially thought to be a mere prohormone but may also play some physiological role as it has a distinct subclass of receptor. SRIF is an important inhibitory neurotransmitter widely distributed in the brain, but also in the gastrointestinal tract. The highest density of SRIF-containing cells is found in the anterior periventricular region of the hypothalamus. Axons of a major part of the periventricular SRIF cells sweep laterally, then caudally and again towards the midline, thus forming an SRIF pathway ending in the median eminence at the level of the ventromedial nucleus. Hypothalamic SRIF release is calcium dependent with the neurotransmitters dopamine, acetylcholine and norepinephrine enhancing SRIF release, and β-adrenergic blockers, GABA and serotonin inhibiting SRIF release. Similarly, the peptides glucagon, insulin, neurotensin, GHRH and bombesin stimulate, whereas opiates and galanin inhibit SRIF secretion. GHRH, GH and IGF-I all stimulate hypothalamic SRIF release and SRIF inhibits its own release. Binding of SRIF to the G-protein-linked membrane SRIF receptors of the somatotropes inhibits the catalytic subunit of the adenyl cyclase system, which results in an inhibition of basal and GHRH-stimulated GH release. However, SRIF does not inhibit GH gene transcription and GH synthesis. SRIF can partly inhibit GHRH-stimulated somatotrope proliferation. SRIF is also able to down-regulate its own pituitary binding sites.

The complex interaction of GHRH and SRIF on the somatotropes results in an intermittent release of GH into the circulation, thus eliciting a pulsatile plasma GH profile. The regulation of GH secretion is completed by a variety of feedback loops at both the hypothalamic and the pituitary level, in which at least GHRH, SRIF, GH itself, IGFs and intrapituitary paracrine modulators (e.g. acetylcholine) are involved. Finally, some metabolic substrates and circulating cytokines are also known to participate in the regulation of GH secretion: free fatty acids decrease GH release, whereas hypoglycemia and interleukin-1 induce GH secretion.

The normal pulsatile profile of plasma GH in children consists of long trough episodes with low or undetectable GH levels, alternating with shorter bursts during which GH concentrations are elevated (see p. 174). Throughout childhood, these GH pulses of variable amplitude occur approximately over every 3 hours. Augmented GH peaks are associated with slow wave sleep (stages 3 and 4) possibly through a serotoninergic mechanism. GH pulses provoked by vigorous exercise and by physical or emotional stress are probably of adrenergic origin. Sex steroids, thyroid hormone and low amounts of glucocorticoids increase the amplitude of GH peaks. Spontaneous GH secretion is decreased in alimentary *obesity* and increased in conditions of *starvation, kwashiorkor* and *marasmus,* in part through modulation of the feedback actions by IGFs and their binding proteins.

Assessment of GH secretion

The usual indication for the assessment of GH secretion is a growth disorder. Growth velocity appears to be related to GH secretion, particularly to the amplitude of endogenous GH pulses. However, the spectra of normal variation with both growth and GH secretion are very wide. Pathological *GH deficiency* and *GH hypersecretion* are rare disorders. Any engagement into the assessment of GH secretion of an individual child should be underbuilt by an auxological evaluation and a complete pediatric examination. *Hypothyroidism, celiac disease* and *psychosocial deprivation* are well known causes of growth failure and inappropriate GH secretion but need a different diagnostic and therapeutic approach. GH is measured in plasma, usually by radioimmunoassay. An instructive but laborious way to assess endogenous GH secretion is to measure GH in consecutively obtained plasma samples over 24 hours or during sleep overnight. In view of the short half-life of GH, intermittent sampling, at intervals of maximum 20 minutes, is required to detect major GH peaks accurately. GH profiles obtained with continuous withdrawal methods are less informative because GH pulses are lost or smoothed by the addition of lower basal concentrations which contribute around 80 percent of the levels measured over a 24 hour period. The latter also explains the poor diagnostic value of GH measurements in randomly obtained plasma samples. This diagnostic value increases when the sampling occurs after a vigorous physical effort (exercise test) or during the onset of slow wave sleep.

The classic and less difficult approach of assessing GH secretion is to verify whether a GH pulse can be elicited by standard provocative stimuli applied either separately or in combination. The β-adrenergic receptor blocker propranolol and the amino acid arginine normally evoke a burst of GH release by inhibiting the hypothalamic secretion of SRIF. The same mechanism is thought to be activated by insulin-induced hypoglycemia and by the relative hypoglycemia following glucagon-induced hyperglycemia. In contrast, the α-adrenergic precursor L-dopa and the α-adrenergic receptor agonist clonidine appear to provoke GH release through stimulation of hypothalamic GHRH secretion. A definite GH response in these controlled circumstances strongly suggests functional integrity of the hypothalamo–pituitary somatotropic axis, but offers no guarantee for normal spontaneous GH secretion. Some children, fulfilling the auxological criteria of *GH deficiency*, respond normally to provocative stimuli but fail to secrete sufficient GH spontaneously (so-called *neurosecretory GH dysfunction*). Conversely, normal subjects may occasionally fail to respond to a pharmacological stimulus. Therefore, the diagnosis of true GH deficiency cannot be based on a single test. The administration of GHRH may be helpful to localize the origin of *GH deficiency* in the hypothalamus (GH response to GHRH present) or at the pituitary level (GH response absent). In childhood, *GH deficiency* is most often of hypothalamic origin. GH hypersecretion during childhood, resulting in *gigantism*, is excessively rare and most likely due to a *pituitary adenoma*. In these cases, plasma GH levels are continuously elevated, nonsuppressible by hyperglycemia and responsive to stimulation with thyrotropin releasing hormone.

Developmental aspects

The fetus and newborn

GH does not pass the placenta. GH appears in fetal plasma at about 10 weeks of gestation and is exclusively of fetal pituitary origin. The fetal somatotropes secrete large amounts of GH in response to hypothalamic GHRH and appear to experience little inhibitory effect from SRIF and IGF-I. Around mid-gestation, this results in markedly elevated plasma GH levels (> 100 ng/ml) with intermittent GH pulses of an exaggerated amplitude. Inhibitory influences on the somatotropes become more effective towards term and certainly after birth, resulting in a gradual decrease of GH baseline levels and GH pulses. In the newborn, the GH pulse frequency approximates one per hour. GH secretion is relatively increased in premature infants and is decreased in the newborn with *hypopituitarism* or *primary hypothyroidism*. Paradoxically, glucose infusion elicits a GH response in the newborn, whereas dopamine inhibits GH secretion. Sleep-associated GH release develops shortly after the neonatal period. Placental GH, a GH variant synthesized by the placenta by a separate gene to pituitary GH, is not secreted into the fetal circulation but only into the maternal compartment. Plasma GH binding protein levels are low in the fetus and increase during early infancy, possibly reflecting an increase in GH-receptor number postnatally (see p. 176).

Puberty

At the end of the prepubertal period, GH secretion may be transiently low, particularly when the onset of puberty is delayed. GH secretion during midpuberty is two- to threefold increased compared to childhood. This change consists principally of an increase in GH burst amplitude. It is provoked by the circulating sex steroids and is probably mediated by an augmented hypothalamic GHRH release. After puberty, GH secretion decreases slowly throughout adult life. Because sex steroids increase GH secretion, sex steroid priming has been used in the evaluation of GH secretion when puberty is delayed.

Pregnancy

The secretion of GH by the pregnant woman decreases with advancing gestation, due to increased inhibition of GH release at the pituitary level by placental lactogen and placental growth hormone. The pulsatile presence of pituitary GH in the maternal circulation is gradually replaced by constantly elevated levels of placental GH.

GH actions (see p. 174)

GH acts through ubiquitously distributed GH-membrane receptors. These receptors are structurally related to prolactin receptors. The principal actions of GH are metabolic and growth promoting. The effects of GH on intermediary metabolism are complex and depend in part on the age, the nutritional status, and the endocrine equilibrium of the considered individual. GH appears to have net anabolic effects on protein metabolism and has insulin-antagonizing effects on lipid and carbohydrate metabolism, as GH has lipolytic, glycogenolytic and gluconeogenic characteristics. The growth-promoting properties of GH are thought to be mediated by IGFs and to be facilitated by thyroid hormones. GH is currently recommended to be administered subcutaneously, once daily, in the evening. Although this practice results in a single, large, plasma GH peak during the night—a profile differing markedly from the physiological pulsatile pattern—the resulting GH effects appear to mimic closely the effects of normal GH secretion. The classic indication for treatment with exogenous GH is *GH deficiency* during infancy, childhood and adolescence. However, the metabolic and growth-promoting properties of GH are increasingly explored in a variety of conditions associated with growth failure or catabolic status.

Selected reading

de Zegher F. Endocrine development of the fetus and the newborn: growth hormone and prolactin. In Bertrand J, Rappaport R, Sizonenko PC, eds. *Pediatric endocrinology*. Baltimore, USA: Williams & Wilkins, 1993.

Tannenbaum GS. Neuroendocrine control of growth hormone secretion. *Acta Pediatr Scand Suppl* 1991; **372**: 5.

D. Prolactin

P D Gluckman

The biological significance of prolactin (PRL) in man remains poorly defined. PRL stimulates milk secretion, provided the mammary gland has been primed with other hormones including estrogens. In hyperprolactinemic states (e.g. *pituitary microadenoma*), galactorrhea is frequently the presenting symptom. Pituitary infarction (*Sheehan syndrome*) is associated with lactational failure. Hyperprolactinemia inhibits the human gonadotropic axis. PRL secreting tumors are rare in childhood but may present in adolescence as delayed puberty or amenorrhea.

PRL may be associated with specific functions in the perinatal period, including effects on lung maturation and fluid and electrolyte homeostasis. The latter may reflect a similar role for PRL in amphibia and fishes.

Biochemistry

PRL is a single chain peptide of 198 amino acids evolutionarily related to growth hormone (GH) and placental lactogen. It is secreted from storage granules by the lactotrope, an eosinophilic adenohypophyseal cell. In the fetus a small proportion of PRL is secreted by a somatolactotrope, a cell that can secrete both GH and PRL and may be the precursor to both mature somatotrope and lactotrope forms of eosinophilic cells.

Regulation

Pituitary PRL, unlike other anterior pituitary hormones, is under a tonic inhibitory hypothalamic influence (Fig. 7.4). Thus, following hypothalamic–pituitary functional disconnection (e.g. *trauma, hypothalamic tumor*), PRL secretion is maintained or increased. Only if the pituitary itself is destroyed (e.g. *congenital pituitary aplasia*), is PRL secretion diminished.

Dopamine, the major PRL inhibitory neurohormone, originates in tuberoinfundibular neurons with cell bodies in the hypothalamic arcuate nucleus and secretes into the primary hypophyseal–portal plexus. Thus dopaminergic antagonists including many psychotropic agents (e.g. chlorpromazine, reserpine, angel dust) increase circulating PRL concentrations. Dopaminergic agonists (e.g. bromocriptine) reduce PRL secretion. The primary hypothalamic stimulatory factor is thyrotropin releasing hormone (TRH) which also stimulates thyrotropin (TSH) release. Thus in *primary hypothyroidism,* hyperprolactinemia may result from this overlap. Putative peptidergic specific PRL-releasing and inhibitory factors have been suggested.

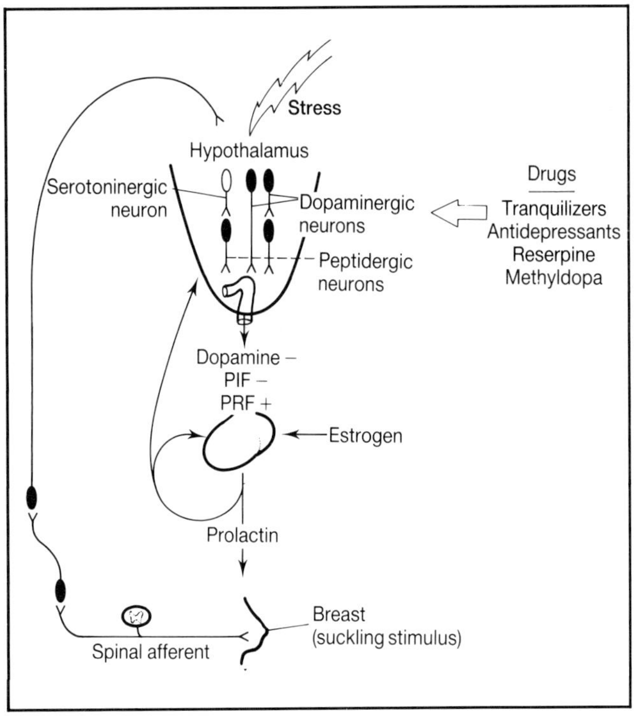

Fig. 7.4. Hypothalamic regulation of PRL secretion. The predominant effect of the hypothalamus is inhibitory, an effect mediated principally by dopamine secreted by the tuberohypophyseal dopaminergic neuron system. One or more prolactin releasing factors (PRFs) probably mediate acute release of PRL as in suckling and stress. There are several candidate PRFs, including TRH and VIP. Estrogen sensitizes the pituitary to release PRL. PRL feeds back on the pituitary to regulate its own secretion (short loop feedback). Short loop feedback is probably mediated indirectly by modifications of hypothalamic catecholamine secretion and turnover. Direct ultrashort feedback inhibition probably also occurs. (Modified from Reichlin S. Neuroendocrinology. In Wilson JD, Foster DW, eds. *Williams textbook of endocrinology*. Philadelphia: WB Saunders Co., 1992: 174. Reprinted with permission of WB Saunders Co.)

PRL is considerably influenced by other neurotransmitter and neuropeptidergic systems. Most operate through alterations in the secretion of the relevant neurohormones (dopamine and TRH). However, direct secretion of some, such as vasointestinal peptide (VIP), into the portal circulation and intrapituitary paracrine mechanisms provides greater complexity of control. PRL secretion is very sensitive to external stimuli. Stress of any type including, pain, exercise, or fear, elevates PRL secretion hindering interpretation of random samples. PRL secretion probably follows a diurnal rhythm in man, increasing in the early morning.

The other major influence on PRL secretion is estrogen, which stimulates PRL release by a number of actions at both hypothalamic and pituitary levels; these include inhibition of dopamine release and action, and an increase in mRNA coding for PRL synthesis. PRL levels surge at ovulation.

Actions

Prolactin acts via cell membrane receptors, but the signal transduction system is not known. These lactogenic receptors have a long extracellular portion, a short single transmembrane domain, and a relatively short intracellular region. Alternate splicing appears to give rise to different intracellular domains in different tissues. The extracellular region has high homology to the somatotropic (GH) receptor; therefore, GH has weak affinity for the lactogenic receptor and vice versa. In contrast, the intracellular region of the somatogenic receptor is not homologous, providing the basis for the different spectra of activities.

Evaluation of PRL secretion

PRL is measured by radioimmunoassay. In childhood there is little clinical indication for the measurement of PRL. Hypersecretion is determined from random measurement in nonstressed patients, by an enhanced response to TRH or dopaminergic antagonists and by incomplete suppression in response to bromocriptine. Pathophysiological hyperprolactinemia is most likely due to *pituitary microadenoma*. Hyposecretion is seen as a deficient response to TRH. This is useful in *neonatal hypopituitarism* to distinguish *pituitary agenesis* (an autosomal recessive condition) from more common, sporadic hypothalamic causes.

Specific developmental aspects

Fetal life

PRL does not pass the placenta. PRL is first detectable in fetal plasma at about 10 weeks of gestation. After 30 weeks concentrations rise progressively, peaking at delivery with levels 20-fold above adult values. This developmental hyperprolactinemia is likely secondary to high circulating estrogens of placental origin in the fetal circulation. A diurnal rhythm in fetal PRL levels, perhaps due to transplacental melatonin, is seen experimentally.

Changes at birth

PRL concentrations are very high in umbilical cord blood. They decline rapidly over the first neonatal week, then more slowly over the next 2 months, perhaps as residual effects wane.

Pregnancy and amniotic fluid

PRL concentrations also rise in the mother throughout pregnancy, presumably secondary to the estrogenic influences. This rise plays a part in mammary development. PRL remains elevated into the puerperium and can be maintained by suckling.

The endometrium, which in the pregnancy becomes the decidua, is a further source of PRL. Unknown local factors regulate decidual PRL which enters aminiotic fluid but not the blood stream. It may influence amniotic fluid volume and osmolality by affecting fluid and electrolyte transfer across the amnion and possibly the fetal skin. Decidual PRL may also play a role in inhibiting myometrial contractility.

The role of PRL in the fetal and neonatal period

PRL may be important in regulating fetal fluid balance through antidiuretic actions on the fetal kidney. The

reduction in total body water after birth may reflect the decline in PRL secretion. Most interest has focused on the role of fetal PRL in maturation of the pulmonary surfactant system. Cord blood PRL concentrations are low in infants who develop *respiratory distress syndrome*.

While PRL alone has little effect on fetal pulmonary maturation, in conjunction with glucocorticoids and thyroid hormones it has pronounced effects experimentally. Because TRH crosses the human placenta and stimulates both PRL and thyroid hormone release *in utero*, clinical trials of TRH have started.

Selected reading

Gluckman PD, Bassett NS. The development of hypothalamic function in the perinatal period. In Meisami E, Timeras P, eds. *Handbook of human growth and developmental biology*. Vol. II, Part A. Boca Raton: CRC Press, 1989: 3.

Gluckman PD, Grumbach MM, Kaplan SL. The neuroendocrine regulation and function of growth hormone and prolactin in the mammalian fetus. *Endocr Rev* 1981; **2**: 363.

E. The Hypothalamic–Pituitary–Thyroid Axis

J Sack

The secretion and metabolism of thyroid hormones are controlled by an autoregulated, negative feedback system that involves the central nervous system (CNS), hypothalamus, pituitary gland, thyroid and peripheral tissues. The system is initiated by CNS activation of the hypothalamus to release thyrotropin releasing hormone (TRH) to stimulate thyrotropin (TSH) secretion which in turn, provides the signal for synthesis and secretion of thyroid hormones from thyroid follicular cells (Fig. 7.5).

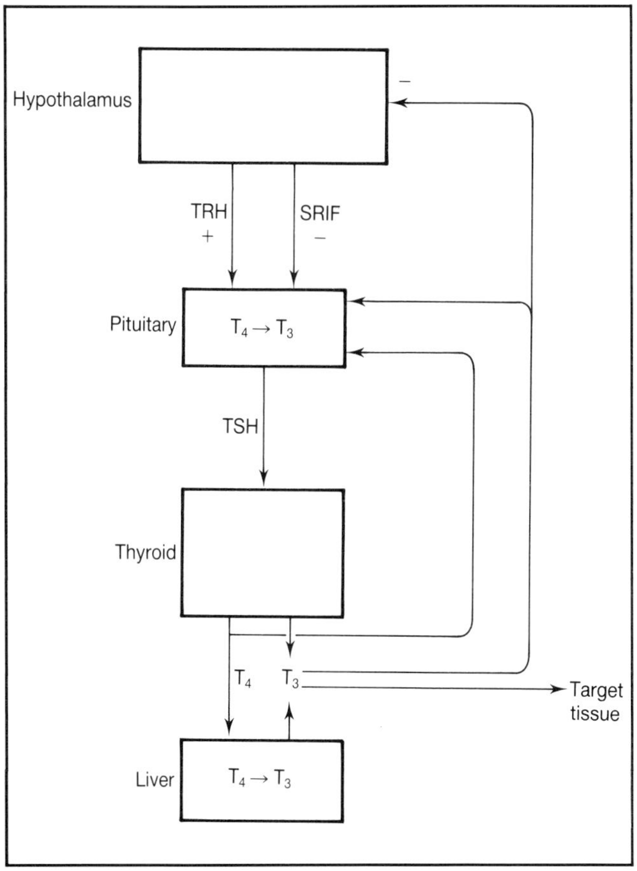

Fig. 7.5. Schema of the hypothalamic pituitary thyroidal axis showing the major factors regulating the generation of T_4 and T_3. TSH stimulates thyroidal secretion of T_4 and some T_3. However, 85 percent of circulating T_3 is derived from hepatic and other peripheral deiodination of T_4. Circulating T_3 and T_4 inhibit pituitary TSH release. The T_4 acts after intrapituitary conversion to T_3. T_3 may also exert negative feedback at hypothalamic level either by inhibiting TRF release or stimulating SRIF release.

Thyrotropin releasing hormone (TRH)

TRH is a tripeptide, (pyro) glu-His-Pro(NH_2), derived from a prohormone that undergoes extensive post-translational processing. It is secreted in response to neural stimulation into the adenohypophyseal–portal circulation. Somatostatin, norepinephrine and dopaminergic drugs have been reported to increase TRH release.

TRH is widely distributed throughout the nervous system. Some studies have shown an association between TRH administration and mood elevation, suggesting that this tripeptide may act as a neurotransmitter in addition to regulating TSH and prolactin (PRL) secretion by actions on the thyrotrope and lactotrope respectively.

TRH belongs to the group of G-protein-linked cell-surface interacting hormones. The binding of TRH to its receptor in the cell-surface membrane activates the guanine nucleotide binding regulatory proteins of the receptor. This binds guanine triphosphate (GTP), which in turn binds to the phospholipase C, and activates the enzyme which catalyzes the hydrolysis of phosphoinositol-4,5-biphosphate. This hydrolysis generates two intracellular mediators, inositol triphosphate and 1,2-diacylglycerol in the target cell, resulting in a rapid rise in the concentration of free calcium ions in the cell cytoplasm. The sudden elevation of the free calcium ions activates the movement of secretory granules to the cell surface and their fusion with the cell-surface membrane, followed by exocytosis and TSH release. The simultaneous activation of protein kinase C by 1,2-diacylglycerol leads to phosphorylation of proteins involved in exocytosis, that mediates the sustained phase of secretion.

TRH has a profound stimulatory effect on TSH secretion and is the major positive regulator of TSH secretion. Exogenous administration of TRH results in an increase in serum TSH and PRL, with a peak at 10–15 minutes. Intravenous administration of TRH is the only test available to distinguish between *pituitary* (secondary) and *hypothalamic* (tertiary) *hypothyroidism*. In *pituitary hypothyroidism* the TSH response to TRH is decreased or

absent while in *hypothalamic hypothyroidism* TSH response to intravenous TRH is adequate, but often with a delayed peak response because of an abnormal inhibitory control. This test can be used diagnostically as early as the neonatal period.

Fetal life

TRH is detectable at 9–10 weeks of gestation in the hypothalamus, at a time when the hypothalamic–hypophyseal–portal vascular system is functioning. By the thirteenth week of gestation, TSH-producing cells are identified.

Thyroid stimulating hormone (TSH)

The pituitary glycoprotein hormone TSH is synthesized and secreted by the thyrotropes in the anterior pituitary. TSH acts on the thyroid gland to increase the production of the thyroid hormones thyroxine (T_4) and triiodothyronine (T_3) which then act on organs throughout the body to modulate growth and various metabolic effects.

Biochemistry

TSH is a pituitary derived glycoprotein of 28–30 kDa. It is composed of two noncovalently linked subunits. The α-subunit is a glycoprotein: the protein core is identical to that of the α-subunit of pituitary LH and FSH and chorionic gonadotropin but with different glycosylation. The β-subunits of these hormones are also glycoproteins and show considerable homology. Unlike most glycoproteins, the oligosaccharides of TSH appear to play vital functional roles. Precursor forms of the oligosaccharides allow nascent subunits to fold properly during biosynthesis, and prevent degradation and aggregation of the subunits. The structure of the oligosaccharides may be regulated by endocrine factors during TSH biosynthesis, so that qualitatively different forms of TSH are secreted in different physiological states. TSH is more sialated in *hypothyroid* patients than in euthyroid patients. The biological activity or significance of free α-subunits is unknown, but the abundance of α-peptide has led to the speculation that regulation of TSH β-subunits is the limiting step in modulating hormone levels. Production of the intact hormone involves the coordinated synthesis of TSH β- and α-subunits.

Regulation

Negative feedback by thyroid hormones is the most important physiological regulator of TSH levels. High levels of thyroid hormones act at the level of the pituitary to suppress synthesis and secretion of TSH. T_3 treatment decreases the TSH response to TRH, an effect which may be at least partially due to the decreased numbers of pituitary TRH receptors. T_3-mediated feedback also regulates both TSH subunits. The β-subunit, which is responsible for the distinctive biological effect of TSH, is more closely and rapidly inhibited by T_3 than is the α-subunit.

Circulating TSH levels are also modulated, by neurotransmitters released by the hypothalamus. The most prominent are TRH which is stimulatory, and somatostatin (SRIF) and dopamine which are inhibitory. The effect of TRH on TSH can be modified by the thyroid state with more pronounced stimulatory effects in *hypothyroidism*. TRH administration to *growth hormone deficient children* is associated with a greater response of TSH. This effect can also be explained by lower somatostatin tone in GH deficiency. Increased responsiveness to TRH can also be induced by estrogens. This may be due to an increase in the concentration of TRH receptors in the pituitary.

Actions of TSH

TSH binds to specific receptors on the thyroid plasma membrane. TSH activation of adenylate cyclase leads to increased cAMP formation, and in turn to the activation of protein kinase. In the rare condition of *TSH unresponsiveness* there is a defect in coupling the receptor to cAMP generation.

TSH has been thought to stimulate growth as well as differentiation of the thyroid. This may be indirect via intermediary growth factors, like IGF-I, IGF-II and epidermal growth factor.

Although it is known that TSH stimulates iodine uptake by the thyroid follicular cell, the mechanism of iodine ion transport across the thyroid cell membrane is as yet speculative. Iodine transport from the extracellular fluid

into the thyroid cell is an energy-requiring process which concentrates iodine against an electrochemical gradient and involves oxidative metabolism and phosphorylation. Concentration gradients of iodine across the cell membrane higher than 20:1 are achieved by TSH stimulation. The response to TSH is known to be biphasic, iodine transport first decreasing then increasing, and the involvement of new protein synthesis in this process has been demonstrated. Iodine transport mechanisms which are independent of TSH stimulation have been observed in the gastric mucosa, salivary and mammary glands, the choroid plexus and the placenta.

Human chorionic gonadotropin (hCG)

Chorionic gonadotropin shares structural similarity with pituitary TSH. It is also a glycoprotein hormone with an identical α-subunit and a similar β-subunit (see p. 317). In patients with *trophoblastic tumors* with very high levels of circulating hCG, *thyrotoxicosis* may occur. Even in the absence of hyperthyroidism, changes in thyroid function have been noted. hCG has been shown to bind to, and compete with, TSH for receptor-binding sites, and to stimulate the membrane-bound adenylate cyclase. The potency of hCG as a thyroid stimulator is relatively low: however, hCG may be a regulator of the thyroid gland in early pregnancy.

The thyroid gland

The thyroid gland is unique among the endocrine glands because of its large store of preformed hormone. It is the first endocrine gland to appear in embryonic development. It appears at the third week of gestation as a single median endodermal placode in the primitive pharynx, caudal to the oropharyngeal membrane, between the first and the second branchial arches. This placode is lined by epithelium which forms the primordia of the thyroid gland and the thyroglossal duct. The placode evaginates into the vertical mesoderm. Then the opening in the pharynx closes and the duct elongates. At this stage the primordial thyroid is located close to the developing heart. The relatively high incidence of *congenital heart defects* found in many epidemiological studies on screening for *congenital hypothyroidism* may be explained by the anatomical proximity of the developing thyroid to the fetal heart.

During subsequent downgrowth there is bifurcation of the thyroid into two lobes. At about 5 weeks the thyroglossal ducts atrophy, the thyrocytes are arranged in epithelial cords and the follicular structure begins to form. At 10 weeks the colloid in the follicle appears. At this stage the thyroid gland can accumulate iodine, organify it and secrete thyroglobulin (Tg) into the colloid. Defects in the embryogenesis of the thyroid are not uncommon, leading either to *congenital hypothyroidism* associated with hypoplasia/atresia. Thyroglossal duct remnants may persist.

Secretion of the thyroid hormones
(see Fig. 7.6)

The first step in thyroid hormone synthesis is iodide trapping by the thyroid gland. This is a rate-limiting energy-dependent process and accumulates iodide against a marked concentration gradient. Similar mechanisms exist in the salivary gland, mammary gland, placenta and gastric mucosa. Rare *iodide trapping defects* are reported.

Thyroglobulin (Tg) is synthesized in the thyroid follicular cells. Its tyrosol residues are iodinated by the enzyme thyroid peroxidase (TPO). The iodide must be oxidized in the presence of H_2O_2 before it is organified. *Congenital peroxidase deficiency* causes goitrous hypothyroidism or cretinism. Iodide also transiently blocks this step and is the basis of the therapeutic use of iodide in acute *thyrotoxicosis*. The iodinated tyrosyl residues within the thyroglobulin are coupled to form triiodothyronine (T_3) and thyroxine (T_4). Congenital defects of coupling enzymes also cause goitrous hypothyroidism. Then vesicles containing Tg fuse with the cytoplasmic lysosomes that contain enzymes which degrade Tg to amino acids, diiodothyronine (T_2), mono-iodothyronine (T_1) and T_4 and T_3. The T_2 and T_1 are deiodinased to recycle iodine. *Deiodinase defects* cause goitrous hypothyroidism due to inability to efficiently conserve iodine. Following hydrolysis, T_4 and T_3 migrate toward the basal surface of the follicle, where they are secreted into the circulation. Excess iodide also inhibits this step. *Defects in Tg synthesis or transport* present as familial goitrous hypothyroidism.

Thyroxine is the major thyroid hormone released by the thyroid gland and while T_3 is the active thyroid hormone only a small portion of T_3 is secreted by the gland, the rest being formed by deiodination from T_4. The peripheral

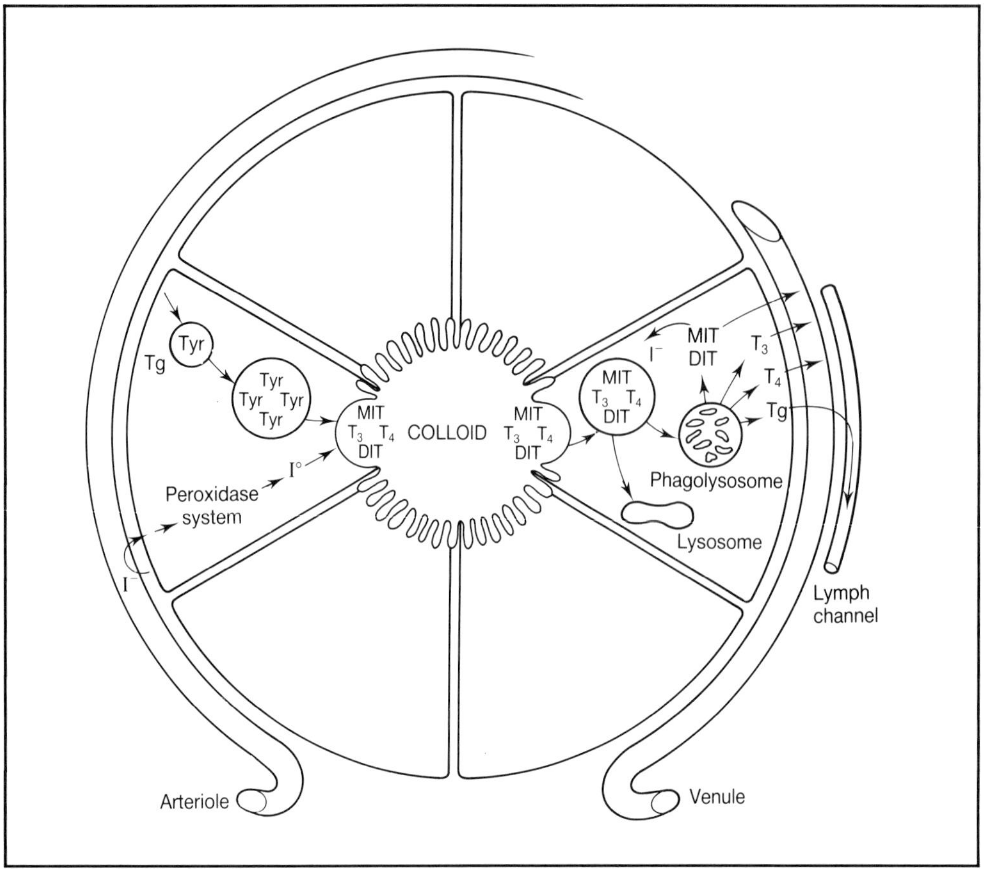

Fig. 7.6. Thyroid hormone synthesis and secretion by thyroid follicular cells. Synthesis and secretion are shown separately, but occur in the same cell. The thyroid follicular cells form spherules with a storage pool of colloid in the center; this drawing shows a cross-section of a spheroid follicle (Tg, thyroglobulin; I^-, iodide; I•, oxidized, reactive iodine; Tyr, tyrosine; MIT, monoiodotyrosine; DIT, diiodotyrosine; T_3, triiodothyronine; T_4, thyroxine). Thyroglobulin containing tyrosine residues is synthesized within the cell and transported to the luminal membrane, where it is exposed to oxidized, reactive iodine. The exposed tyrosine molecules within the Tg are iodinated to MIT or DIT and those MIT and DIT molecules are spatially oriented for coupling to form T_3 or T_4 molecules. The iodinated thyroglobulin is stored as colloid. Activation of secretion by TSH stimulates colloid endocytosis. Infolding colloid droplets fuse with cell lysosomes to form phagolysosomes within which thyroglobulin is degraded to release iodotyrosines T_3 and T_4. Some thyroglobulin escapes from the cell to the circulation, predominantly via lymphatics. (From Fisher DA. The thyroid. In Kaplan SA, ed. *Clinical pediatric endocrinology*. Philadelphia: WB Saunders Co., 1990; 87. Reprinted with permission from WB Saunders Co.)

turnover (half-life) of the two major iodothyronines T_4 and T_3 is relatively slow, at 7 days and 1 day respectively, due to the tight binding of the hormones to circulating plasma proteins. Approximately 99 percent of the T_4 is bound to three major binding proteins: thyroxine binding globulin (TBG), T_4 binding prealbumin, transthyretin (TTR), and albumin. About 77 percent of the T_4 is strongly bound to TBG, 15 percent is bound to TTR, and 10 percent is loosely bound to albumin. As regards T_3, about 99 percent is bound to the plasma proteins: 75 percent to TBG and some 25 percent to albumin. The bound hormone may serve as a reservoir or pool of hormone, available to the peripheral tissues for metabolic action and metabolism. Many drugs can interfere with the binding of thyroid hormones to these binding proteins. These include salicylates, sulfonylureas and Dilantin. The concentration of binding protein is increased by estrogens, and inhibited by androgens and gluco-

corticoids. In addition, genetic *hyper-* or *hypo-TBGemia* may occur. Thus the interpretation of abnormal thyroid hormone concentration depends on first elucidating the bound versus free hormone and secondly assessing for evidence of abnormal thyroidal function (e.g. altered plasma TSH, altered response to TRH).

Once secreted, T_4 is metabolized by several pathways including deiodination, deamination, decarboxylation, conjugation of metabolites, and ether link cleavage. The most important pathway is deiodination, which may account for 80 percent of T_4 metabolism.

Postnatally, 70–90 percent of the circulating T_3 is derived from peripheral monodeiodination of the outer phenolic ring of T_4. Monoiodination of the inner tyrosyl ring of T_4 produces reverse T_3 (rT_3), an inactive metabolite. Over 85 percent of circulating T_3 is derived by peripheral deiodination of secreted T_4 rather than by direct secretion of T_3. About 30 percent of T_4 secreted each day is converted to T_3. The most important sites are the liver and kidney and in the newborn, brown fat. In addition deiodination occurs in the central nervous system and in the pituitary gland; the latter is key to the negative feedback by thyroxine on TSH release. Many syndromes are associated with a decreased conversion of T_4 to T_3. These include starvation, use of glucocorticoids, chronic or acute illness: e.g. *burns, diabetic ketoacidosis*. They produce the *'low T_3'* or *'euthyroid sick'* syndrome. This can be differentiated from true hypothyroidism by the normal T_4 and often an elevated rT_3. Generally the circulating T_4 concentration is sufficient to prevent clinical hypothyroidism. A particularly confounded situation is the sick premature neonate when, for ontogenic reasons, T_4 and T_3 are lower than in term infants.

Degradation of T_3 and rT_3 produces three separate diiodothyronines (T_2): further metabolism leads to the formation of two monoiodothyronines (T_1), and finally terminal deiodination yields thyronine. Peripheral *deiodinase deficiency* may be isolated or be associated with *thyroidal deiodinase deficiency* and lead to goiter. The monodeiodination of T_4 can be affected by a multitude of physiological conditions, clinical disorders and pharmacological agents. Inhibition of the conversion of T_4 to T_3 may be a protective mechanism as it reduces the level of active T_3 hormone. Pregnant women have increased levels of T_2 and T_1, probably because of high TBG levels. Newborn infants have low T_3 and high rT_3 levels.

Thyroglobulin

Thyroglobulin is an important precursor protein for the synthesis of the thyroid hormones. It is a 660 kDa glycoprotein, composed of two identical subunits and containing about 10 percent carbohydrate. It can be found in the blood in low but detectable concentrations: its physiological role outside the thyroid gland is unknown. Elevated levels are observed with increased TSH stimulation of the thyroid gland. In subjects receiving suppressive doses of thyroid hormone, or in children who have ingested high doses of L-thyroxine, serum Tg may be undetectable (less than 3 ng/ml). In congenital hypothyroidism secondary to *thyroid atresia* Tg in the serum is undetectable. In patients with congenital hypothyroidism due to a small *ectopic thyroid gland*, Tg can be detected many years after the initiation of treatment with L-thyroxine. Tg is also found in the serum of children with *congenital hypothyroidism* resulting from dyshormonogenesis.

Thyroid hormone action

Nuclear level

A full understanding of the nuclear site of initiation of thyroid hormone action depends on the recognition that T_3 is the active hormone and that T_4 serves largely as a precursor. There is now general agreement about the nature of the high affinity, low capacity nuclear receptors and which are the primary sites of T_3 action. Extranuclear binding sites for T_3 have been identified, but there is no convincing evidence to date that the binding results in recognized hormonal action.

Recently it was demonstrated that c-*erb*-A proto-oncogenes encode a high affinity receptor for T_3 and T_4. The c-*erb*-A gene products are related to the superfamily of steroid hormone receptors (see p. 290). Each of these receptors is characterized by a carboxyl terminal ligand binding domain, and by a highly conserved cysteine-rich, DNA binding domain situated closer to the amino terminus. The DNA binding domain is characterized by a cysteine-rich amino acid sequence that is believed to chelate zinc. These structures are therefore referred to as zinc fingers and are the DNA binding regions. By analogy to other transcription factors, these receptors are also

likely to contain activation domains which interact with cellular transcription machinery. Three distinct thyroid receptors (TRs), α1, β1, and β2, are expressed in cultures of pituitary cells. TR α1 is a product of the c-*erb*-A α gene. The c-*erb*-A β gene encodes TR β1 and TR β2 which differ from one another only in their amino terminus. The human TR cDNA isolated from the placenta is designated β1, and the pituitary specific form, β2.

Although the existence of multiple TRs and their differential expression suggests unique biological roles for each, studies have not revealed important functional differences. The syndrome of *generalized resistance to thyroid hormone* is characterized by high serum levels of free thyroid hormones in the absence of increased basal metabolism and TSH suppression and provides evidence of the tissue distribution of α- and β-receptors. Such patients have high T_4 levels with persistently elevated TSH values. They may present with mixed clinical signs of hypo- and hyperthyroidism. There are both autosomal dominant and recessive modes of inheritance. In severe homozygous patients where there is a major deletion in both c-*erb*-A β-alleles resulting in the absence of β-receptor, there are signs of severe resistance leading to a delay in brain development and skeletal maturation, while persistent tachycardia and lack of weight gain suggest hyperthyroidism. Thus the β-receptor appears to have a crucial role in the pituitary, the brain, and bone, whereas the α-receptor may be more significant in mediating thyroid hormone action in cardiac tissue.

Action at the cell, tissue and organ level

A large volume of information has accumulated concerning the effects of thyroid hormones on target tissues. These data derive mostly from clinical and experimental observation on the effects of the excess or deficiency of thyroid hormones. However, much of the molecular basis for the clinical symptoms in *hypo-* and *hyperthyroidism* remains unexplained. In general, thyroid hormone effects resemble those of catecholamines: increase in the basal metabolic rate, in oxygen consumption and in thermogenesis.

Although the exact mechanism involved in the maintenance of constant body temperature is unknown there is no doubt that T_3 plays a critical role (see p. 357). It has been suggested that thyroid hormone exerts its thermogenic effect by stimulating futile biochemical cycles. The synthesis of fatty acid requires high energy phosphate, and since such high energy phosphate can be obtained in large part from that released in the course of fatty acid oxidation, the fatty acid synthesis–degradation cycle appears to be the thermogenic futile cycle stimulated by thyroid hormone action. It has also been suggested that the increase in thermogenesis by thyroid hormones occurs partly by increasing the metabolic response to catecholamines: thyroid hormones increase primarily the basal metabolic rate, while catecholamines increase the metabolic rate above the basal rate in response to environmental stimuli.

The abnormalities associated with thyroid hormone deficiency also involve retardation of body growth, and retarded maturation of individual cells and tissues. Thyroid hormone appears to function both by stimulation of growth and by accelerating the differentiation of specific cell types. Thus whereas in adult onset *hypothyroidism* most of the effects of thyroid hormone deficiency can be easily reversed, this is not the case in neonates.

Thyroid hormone and the CNS

Specific nuclear T_3 receptors are present in the fetal, neonatal and adult brain. From studies in the rat it has been shown that in the neonatal *hypothyroid* brain there is a reduction in the branching of dendrites and axons, as well as a deficiency in axonal myelin formation. The primary effect of thyroid hormone in the brain is probably to switch the cells from a proliferative to a differentiative state. Some of its effects may be mediated by stimulating nerve growth factor and other neurotropic factor production.

After the introduction of neonatal screening for *congenital hypothyroidism*, preliminary studies of the outcome in affected fetuses were very encouraging. However, evidence is now accumulating that not all the effects of fetal hypothyroidism are reversed by early postnatal treatment, and some neurological deficit may persist. Thus, complete prevention of neurological damage may be achieved only if hypothyroidism is diagnosed *in utero*, and treatment initiated either by intra-amniotic or cord injections of T_4 before birth.

Thyroid hormone and the skeleton

The absence of femoral, tibial and cuboid bone nuclei epiphyses in *hypothyroid infants* stresses the importance of thyroid hormone in bone maturation. Lack of thyroid hormone in the fetus and neonate also causes a depressed nasal bridge and delay in the closure of the fontanelles, while *hyperthyroidism* can cause craniosynostosis and premature closure of the skull sutures. Thyroid hormones are known to stimulate endochondrial ossification and bone cell maturation, and also influence increased cartilage cell proliferation via stimulation of growth hormone secretion and IGF-I function. *Hypothyroidism* can therefore cause the most extreme bone age retardation as seen on X-ray, while in *hyperthyroidism* there is acceleration of bone age. *Hyperthyroidism* increases and *hypothyroidism* decreases bone turnover. The hypercalcemia observed in the hyperthyroid state is the result of increased bone destruction as well as increased calcium absorption in the gut. In a recent study it was shown that a short-term increase in T_4 administration in *congenital hyperthyroid* children was followed by hypercalciuria, probably due to increased formation of 1,25-dihydroxyvitamin D from its precursors.

Thyroid hormone and the heart

The cardiovascular effects of thyroid hormone are very similar to those of catecholamines. However, it has been shown that in the hyperthyroid state, there is no increase in circulating catecholamines. An increase in the number of β-adrenergic receptors, and a concomitant increase in the heart muscle response to catecholamines has been suggested as an explanation. β-Adrenergic blockers are very effective in the amelioration of *hyperthyroidism*.

Effects on carbohydrate, lipid and protein metabolism

Thyroid hormone stimulates both glycolysis and gluconeogenesis. Key gluconeogenic enzymes phosphoenolpyruvate carboxykinase, pyruvate carboxylase and glucose 6-phosphatase, are stimulated by thyroid hormones.

Thyroid hormones also increase the secretion of mitochondrial enzymes, thus increasing pyruvate to glucose conversion. In the muscle there is also an increase in lactate formation and conversion to glucose. The glycogen content in the liver is diminished in both hyper- and hypothyroidism: in *hyperthyroidism* this is due to increased degradation, while in *hypothyroidism* the rate of synthesis is lowered.

Thyroid hormone increases lipogenesis and fat tissue lipolysis. Again, these effects may involve changes in catecholamine action via the cAMP pathway. Clinically, in *hypothyroidism* the best known changes in the serum are the hypercholesterolemia and increased low-density lipoproteins (LDL). The concentrations of both are low in *hyperthyroidism*.

Thyroid hormone normally increases body growth and induces a net positive nitrogen balance. In *hyperthyroidism*, thyroid hormone causes weight loss and a net negative nitrogen balance.

Thyroid function during development

Changes during fetal life

Maternal serum levels of thyroid hormones are higher than those in non-pregnant adults. This increase in thyroid hormone concentration is primarily due to the elevation of thyroxine binding globulin levels in the serum. In the mother hCG has a thyrotropic effect, probably contributing to the increase in total T_4 and T_3 concentrations. The placenta is impermeable to TSH. Maternal T_4 and T_3 do not cross the placenta in sufficient quantity to maintain fetal euthyroidism. This is most probably due to the presence of an active inner ring iodothyronine deiodinase, which deiodinates T_4 to inactive reverse T_3 (rT_3) and deiodinates T_3 to inactive T_2. The fetus is therefore dependent upon its own pituitary hormones and thyroid. Thus, the fetal pituitary–thyroid axis develops independently of the maternal system.

While TRH is not normally found in the circulation in significant amounts, TRH if given to the mother, will cross the placenta and stimulate fetal TSH and prolactin release. This has been used therapeutically to promote lung maturation.

TRH can be detected in the fetal pituitary and hypothalamus from about 10 weeks of gestation, and thyroxine and thyrotropin appear in the circulation from 12 weeks. Recently, studies of the fetal serum obtained by

percutaneous umbilical blood sampling have confirmed that the fetal pituitary secretes thyrotropin and the thyroid secretes T_4 as early as 12 weeks of gestation.

Significant increases in fetal serum concentrations of T_4, free T_4 (FT_4), TSH, TBG and albumin between 12 and 36 weeks of gestation have been demonstrated, while the maternal levels of these hormones and binding protein do not change significantly during pregnancy. Fetal T_4 increases throughout gestation, although at 28 weeks the levels of T_4 are still lower than the adult range, suggesting that the fetal thyroid gland is as yet immature. On the other hand, FT_4 was shown to reach concentrations within the normal adult range as early as 28 weeks of gestation. The difference between the changes in T_4 and FT_4 concentrations is probably due to changes in serum binding proteins.

Although circulating T_4 and FT_4 concentrations reach adult levels by 36 weeks of gestation, fetal serum T_3 and free T_3 (FT_3) concentrations are always less than 50 percent of the maternal levels. These low levels of T_3 and FT_3 are most probably due to low conversion of T_4 to T_3, or increased rapid degradation of T_3 to T_2 by the placenta.

In the *hypothyroid fetus* although a little T_4 may pass across the placenta from the mother, persistently low T_4 concentrations nevertheless lead to a rise in TSH. This in turn stimulates thyroid growth as shown by the goiter that sometimes develops in infants with defects of thyroid hormone biosynthesis (e.g. *organification defects*) or in the presence of excess iodide or goitrogens. The insufficient transfer of maternal T_4 to the fetus is also reflected by more severe manifestation of clinical hypothyroidism in infants with *agenesis of the thyroid gland*.

The rising concentration of fetal T_4 and TSH in late gestation suggests immaturity of the negative feedback loop. This deficient inhibition of TSH levels by T_4 in the fetus associated with FT_4 concentrations within the adult range suggests that the fetal pituitary is relatively insensitive to negative feedback. After birth T_3, produced mainly by intrapituitary local monodeiodination of T_4, is responsible for suppression of TSH concentrations. It is possible that because of the low circulating T_3 and FT_3 levels, the negative feedback threshold is never reached *in utero*. Delayed maturation of intracellular mechanisms for the conversion of T_4 to T_3, or of T_3 receptor/postreceptor mechanisms in the pituitary, may be other possible explanations.

Changes at birth

TSH levels are low in the umbilical cord after birth, and after the cord is cut there is a rapid excretion of TSH which results in peak serum values of 50–100 mU/l about 10–15 minutes after birth. This surge of TSH may constitute an adaptive mechanism to the cooler environment outside the uterus.

In a recent study, the lipolytic effect of several hormones on isolated human adipocytes obtained at different donor ages was examined. In neonates, norepinephrine and epinephrine had an insignificant lipolytic effect, while TSH had a significant effect in physiological concentrations. TSH may thus be an important lipolytic hormone during the neonatal period, and the TSH surge after birth may be essential for lipolysis during this period of life. During childhood and in adults the lipolytic effect of TSH gradually decreases.

In response to the rapid surge in TSH at birth after the umbilical cord is cut, T_4 and T_3 secretion from the thyroid gland are stimulated. T_4 peaks at 48 hours; T_3 rises abruptly between 1 and 4 hours after birth. A further progressive increase in T_3 levels occurs between 4 and 24 hours, because of augmented conversion of T_4 to T_3 in peripheral tissues resulting from accelerated increase in hepatic 5′-monoiododeiodinase (outer ring deiodinase) activity. Cord cutting and the separation from the placenta and its active enzyme iodothyronine deiodinase may also contribute to the abrupt rise in T_3. Brown fat is also rich in 5′-monoiododeiodinase activity leading to increased T_3 levels in brown fat, thus promoting thermogenesis.

Because the biological half-life of T_4 in the neonatal period is considerably shorter than the half-life in older children and adults, the T_4 requirement in the neonate per kg body weight is five times higher than in adults. Reverse T_3 production by fetal and neonatal tissues decreases by 1 month at which time serum rT_3 concentrations fall to the childhood and adult values.

Thyroid function in the premature infant

In the premature infant the hypothalamic–pituitary–thyroid axis is immature at birth. The early TSH rise and the postnatal increase in T_4 and T_3 concentrations in the

neonatal period are lower than in term infants. Using a sensitive immunoradiometric assay in premature infants (25 weeks), the mean TSH concentration increases from a very low value of <1 mU/l at 5 days to 6 mU/l by 5 weeks of age. The thyroid hormone feedback control of pituitary TSH release in the extremely premature infants begins to mature after 6 weeks of postnatal life, suggesting a delay in maturation of the axis. Thus, the maturational pattern of the thyroidal axis in premature infants is similar to that of the intrauterine fetus. The relatively hypothyroid state of premature infants is probably due to the immaturity of the hypothalamic–pituitary–thyroidal axis, relatively low activity of the outer ring deiodinase enzyme system, and resultant reduced conversion of T_4 and T_3. As discussed earlier, the interpretation of T_3 levels in the sick neonate is further confounded by systemic factors which may compromise peripheral conversion of T_4 to T_3.

Thyroid function in children

In healthy boys and girls serum TSH concentrations remain essentially constant from 1 month of age throughout childhood. On the other hand, serum T_4 and T_3 concentrations decrease progressively with increasing age. It appears that the decrease in serum T_4 and T_3 is due to the decrease in the serum TBG concentration which falls by about 30 percent between 1 and 15 years. The progressive decrease in the serum concentration of thyroid hormones during childhood is not associated with changes in serum TSH levels. As there is a progressive and proportionate increase in the absolute size of the thyroid gland during childhood this might suggest a decrease in TSH responsiveness with age would be likely. This could be due to a progressive decrease in TSH receptors per cell or to a decrease in the thyroid follicular cell response to TSH or to cAMP.

Thyroid function during puberty

Only a few studies correlate the thyroid hormone concentrations and the stage of puberty. Estrogen is known to increase the concentration of serum TBG while testosterone lowers it. On the other hand, serum T_4 concentrations decrease during puberty in both boys and girls. Serum T_3 does not change significantly during the pubertal stages, but toward adulthood it decreases.

Selected reading

Lazar MA, Berrodin TJ. Thyroid hormone receptors form distinct nuclear protein dependent and independent complexes with a thyroid hormone response element. *Mol Endocrinol* 1990; **4**(11): 1627.

Lever EG, Medeiros-Neto GA, De Groot LJ. Inherited disorders of thyroid metabolism. *Endocr Rev* 1983; **4**(3): 213.

Oppenheimer J. Tissue and cellular effects of thyroid hormones and their mechanism of action. In Burrow GN, Oppenheimer JH, Volpe R, eds. *Thyroid function and disease*. Philadelphia: WB Saunders, 1989: 90.

Shupnik MA, Ridgway EC, Chin WW. Molecular biology of thyrotropin. *Endocr Rev* 1990; **10**(4): 459.

Thorpe-Beeston JG, Nicolaides KH, Felton CV, *et al.* Maturation of the secretion of thyroid hormone and thyroid stimulating hormone in the fetus. *N Engl J Med* 1991; **324**: 532.

F. The Gonadotropic–Gonadal Axis

G E Richards

The hypothalamic–pituitary–gonadal (HPG) axis is responsible for some aspects of sexual differentiation and for orchestrating an orderly progression toward sexual maturity and reproductive capacity. This section reviews the physiology of the gonadotropic axis in the male and female. For further discussion refer to the section on puberty (p. 145).

The gonadotropic axis (see Fig. 7.7)

The control of gonadatropin release

Several neurotransmitters within the central nervous system (such as norepinephrine, dopamine and endogenous opiates) modulate the pulsatile release of gonadotropin releasing hormone (GnRH) from neurons which are located primarily in the medial preoptic area and the arcuate nucleus of the hypothalamus. The precise role of these CNS signals under physiological conditions is not well understood. GnRH is cleaved from its prohormone to yield GnRH and GAP (gonadotropin releasing hormone associated peptide). The biological significance of GAP, which stimulates gonadotropin secretion and inhibits prolactin *in vitro*, is not clear.

GnRH, a peptide of 10 amino acids also known as luteinizing releasing hormone (LHRH), is discharged from nerve terminals in the median eminence into the hypothalamic portal system by which it reaches pituitary gonadotropes and binds to specific receptors. GnRH stimulates both gonadotropin synthesis within the cell and also gonadotropin release from the pituitary into the general circulation. Pituitary gonadotropes may contain LH, FSH or both gonadotropins. In *Kallmann syndrome* of isolated gonadotropin deficiency the GnRH neurons are deficient: it is associated with olfactory bulb abnormalities. GnRH deficiency may also be part of a more extensive defect in *congenital hypothalamic hypopituitarism*.

GnRH containing neurons are found primarily in the periventricular nucleus, arcuate nucleus and the medial

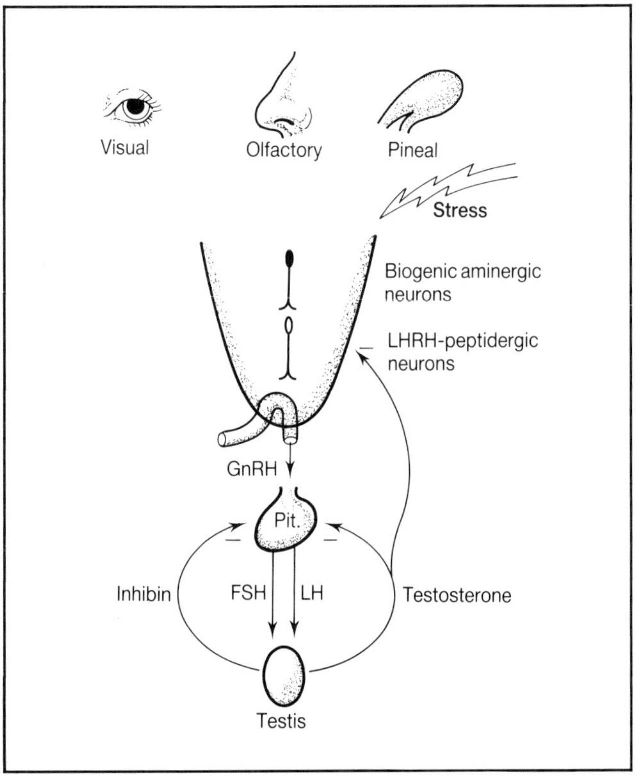

Fig. 7.7. Regulation of gonadotropin secretion in the human male. Schematic diagram of gonadotropin control system in the male, showing the interaction of neural and hormonal feedback controls. Pituitary and testis are connected by a negative feedback link. Secretion of testosterone by the testis is stimulated by LH, whereas maturation and growth of the tubule cells are stimulated by FSH. The secretion of testosterone in turn inhibits the secretion of LH and FSH. Inhibin is secreted by Sertoli cells and exerts a direct inhibitory effect on FSH secretion. The LHRH peptidergic neurons are in turn regulated by a biogenic aminergic system that links gonadotropin regulation to the remainder of the brain. Through this system a wide variety of impulses can be exerted on reproductive function. Stimuli affecting male gonadotropic secretion have been well demonstrated in experimental animals, although they are not as well worked out in the human. Visual influences include light-induced changes in seasonal breeders such as domestic cattle, deer and birds. Olfactory signals in male rats influence gonadal function. The pineal gland in many species of animals inhibits gonadotropin secretion by direct effects of pineal secretions on either the hypothalamus or the pituitary. The role of the pineal in human reproduction control has not been established. (Modified from Martin JB, Reichlin S, Brown GM. Neuroendocrinology of reproduction. In *Clinical neuroendocrinology*. Philadelphia: FA Davis, 1977: 93.)

preoptic area of the hypothalamus. These neurons provide a pulse of GnRH to the pituitary, by means of the hypophyseal–portal system, approximately every 90 minutes. The GnRH receptor is G-protein linked. If the pituitary is stimulated by more frequent pulses or continuous administration of GnRH, a decrease in gonadotropin secretion occurs as a result of desensitization of GnRH receptors. Similarly, pharmacological agonists of GnRH, which remain bound to the GnRH receptor longer than native GnRH, have a suppressive effect on gonadotropin secretion. This explains the apparently paradoxical use of GnRH superagonists in *central precocious puberty*.

LH and FSH reach the gonads through the general circulation and bind to specific receptors to exert their effects. These gonadotropins are dimeric glycoproteins. Each contains an α-subunit of 89 amino acids that has a molecular weight of 14 kDa and is identical to the α-subunit of TSH and hCG. The β-subunits of 115 amino acids determine the specific function of the molecule. The complete molecular weight of each gonadotropin is about 29 kDa. These weights are approximate because of the extensive and variable carbohydrate side-chains which complete the glycoprotein structure.

Gonadal function

The gonads have specific gonadotropin receptors, through which the gonadotropins stimulate sex steroid production and gamete maturation. Both LH and FSH receptors are G-protein linked and act via increased cAMP production. GnRH receptors are also present in the gonads but their significance is uncertain. In general LH stimulates steroid biosynthesis and FSH is responsible for gamete maturation but there are complex interactions which prevent complete separation of the function of the two gonadotropins. The gonads complete the feedback loop by signaling the hypothalamus and pituitary, and possibly higher brain centers, in both a negative and positive feedback fashion, the sensitivity of which is developmentally regulated.

The testis

In the male testosterone production is from the Leydig cell, the Sertoli cell producing inhibin and, in fetal life, anti-Müllerian hormone (see p. 129). The Leydig cell responds to LH by increasing testosterone release. In early fetal life hCG performs the same function. A defect in the common LH/hCG receptor is one cause of *male pseudo-hermaphroditism*. The seminiferous tubules which are the main site of FSH action are comprised of Sertoli cells and germ cells; spermatocytes mature from the latter. However, FSH may have indirect effects on testosterone production via increasing Leydig cell maturation or by increasing the number of LH receptors on Leydig cells.

The Leydig cell utilizes both *de novo* synthesis of cholesterol and cholesterol of low-density lipoprotein origin as the substrate for testosterone synthesis. The rate-limiting step, as for cortisol synthesis, is side-chain cleavage to form pregnenolone. The primary pathway is the Δ^5 pathway via 17-hydroxyprogesterone to DHEA to androstenediol to testosterone (see Fig. 7.8). Defects of the side-chain cleavage, enzyme 17-hydroxylase or 3β-hydroxysteroid dehydrogenase lead to rare forms of *adrenogenital syndrome* with incomplete virilization in the male (see p. 326). Defects in the other synthetic enzymes are restricted to the testosterone synthetic pathway and in the male are associated with *male pseudohermaphroditism* (see p. 134).

The ovary

Ovarian steroid production is more complex and depends on the developmental stage of the female and, if mature, the stage of the menstrual cycle. Ovarian follicles are embedded in the stroma of the ovarian cortex. Only a few are recruited each cycle. The primordial follicle is composed of an oocyte surrounded by a single layer of granulosa cells surrounded in turn by a basement membrane. Follicular development in the first instance is the formation of a primary follicle by the proliferation of granulosa cells associated with maturation of the oocyte which enlarges and secretes a glycoprotein coat (zona pellucida). FSH is responsible for this proliferation perhaps operating via local IGF-I production. Further granulosa cell proliferation occurs and the surrounding stroma begins to organize into the theca interna and externa to form first a secondary then tertiary follicle as the theca further organizes and an antrum appears in the granulosa cell. Gap junctions form between the granulosa and thecal cells which may be essential for the coordinated synthesis of estrogens and progesterone. A further rapid increase in follicular size leads to formation of the graafian follicle. Only one or two recruited

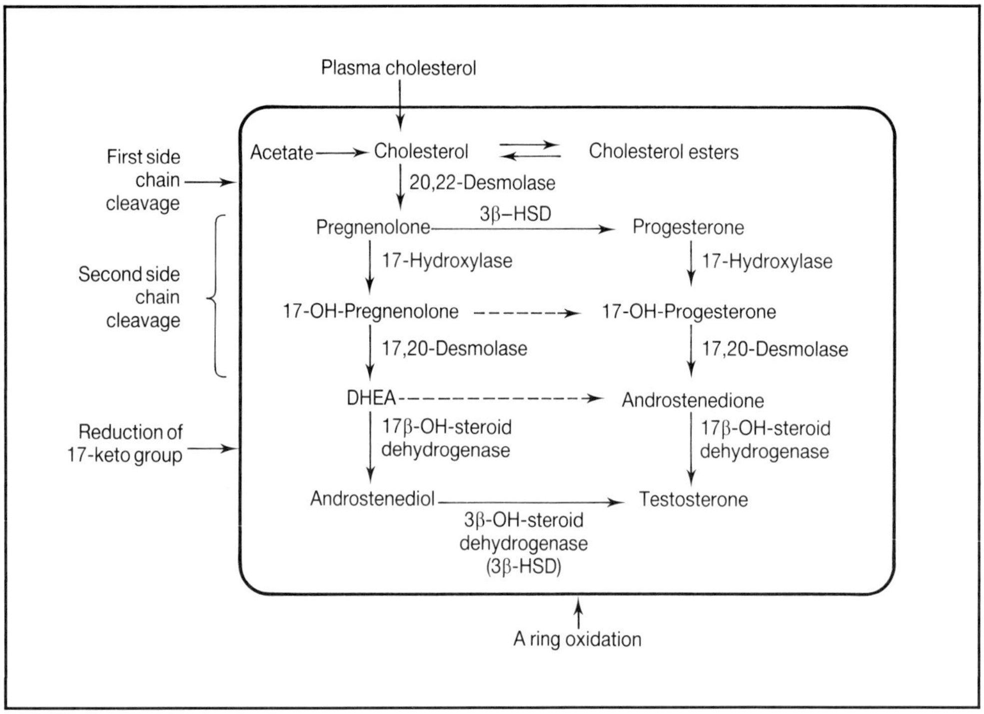

Fig. 7.8. Pathways of testosterone synthesis in human testis. The three potential sources of cholesterol for testosterone synthesis are (1) plasma cholesterol; (2) cholesterol synthesized within the cell; and (3) cholesterol stored in the form of cholesterol esters. The first side-chain cleavage of cholesterol to pregnenolone is the rate-limiting reaction in the process and is probably the process that is regulated by luteinizing hormone. Conversion of pregnenolone to testosterone can take place by two theoretical pathways—one in which side-chain cleavage and reduction of the 17-keto group are accomplished before A ring oxidation Δ^5 pathway, left-hand pathway), and the other in which this sequence is reversed (Δ^4 pathway, right-hand pathway). (From Griffin JE, Wilson JD. The testis. In Bondy PK, Rosenberg LE, eds. *Metabolic control and disease*. 8th ed. Philadelphia: WB Saunders Co., 1980: 1535. Reproduced by permission of WB Saunders Co.)

primordial follicles per cycle fully mature; the remainder become atretic at an earlier stage.

Estrogens are the major product of the granulosa cell. The primary estrogen is 17β-estradiol, but estrone and estriol are also formed. Both thecal and granulosa cells produce progesterone, but granulosa cell progesterone is largely used as a substrate for conversion to estrogen. Some androgens are also secreted by the ovary but, except in enzyme disorders, these are of minor significance. The primary source of ovarian steroid production is uptake of LDL cholesterol. There are two alternate pathways for steroid production utilizing the same enzymes in different order (Fig. 7.9). In the Δ^5 pathway, 17-hydroxylation of pregnenolone is the first step which then proceeds to DHEA and androstenediol and then to testosterone for aromatization to estradiol. The Δ^4 pathway involves first conversion by 3β-hydroxysteroid dehydrogenase of pregnenolone to progesterone and thence via 17-hydroxypregnenolone, androstenedione and testosterone to estradiol. In the ovary both pathways are utilized to different extents by granulosa, thecal and luteal cells such that the granulosa cell produces primarily estrogens, the luteal cells produce primarily progesterone and the thecal cells and stroma produce androgens. LH primarily stimulates the initial conversion of cholesterol to pregnenolone whereas FSH has a major effect on aromatase, the enzyme that converts testosterone to estradiol. It has therefore been suggested that FSH and LH act in concert on the thecal and granulosa cells to maximize estradiol production: LH stimulates androstenedione production by the thecal origin which is provided to the granulosa cell for FSH stimulated aromatization.

The corpus luteum regresses from the eighth day after

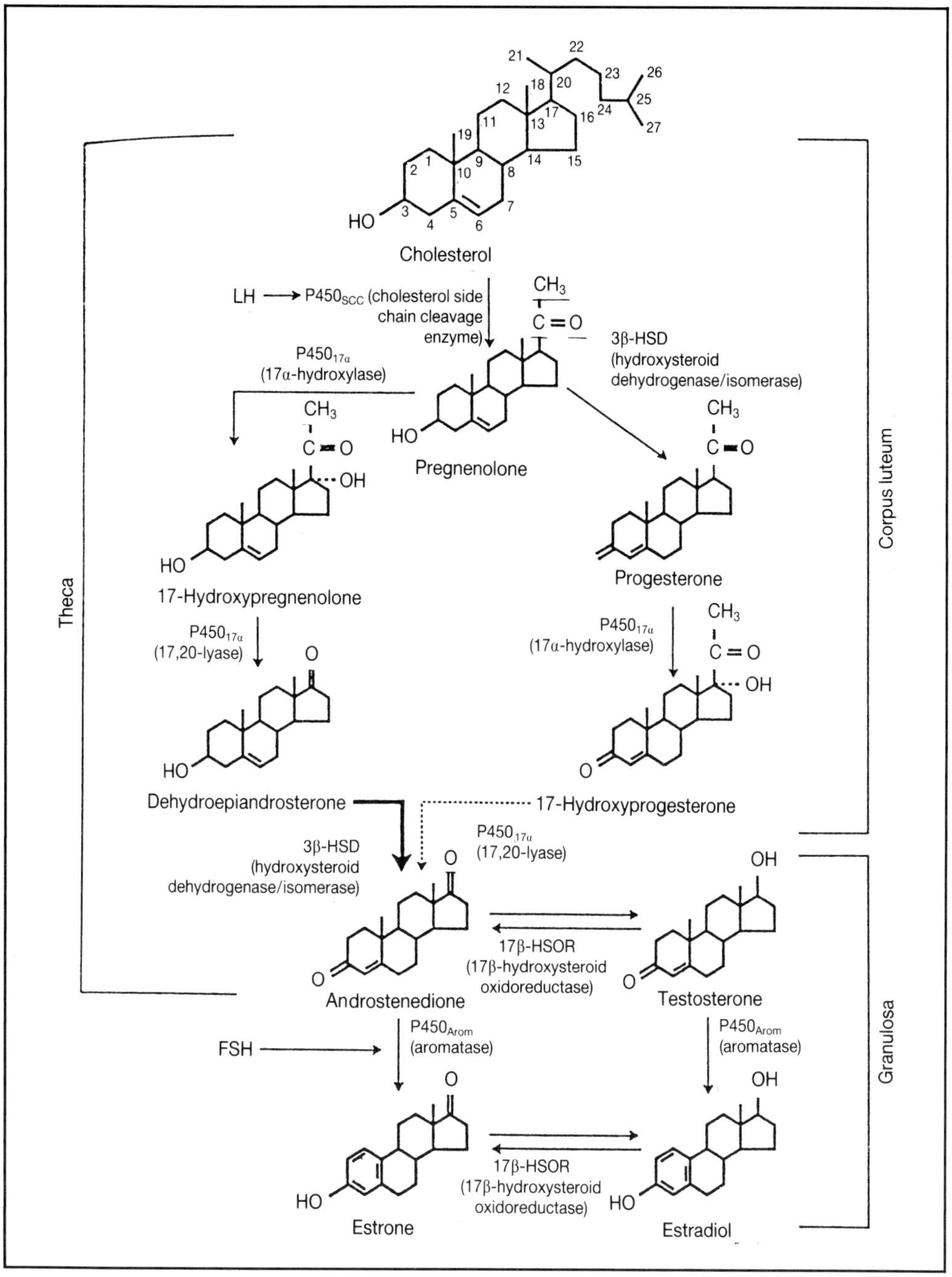

Fig. 7.9. Principal pathways of steroid hormone biosynthesis in the human ovary. Although each cell type of the ovary contains the complete enzyme complement required for the formation of estradiol from cholesterol, the amounts of the various enzymes and consequently the predominant hormones formed differ among the cell types. The major enzyme complements for the corpus luteum, theca, and granulosa cells are shown in parentheses; these cells produce predominantly progesterone and 17-hydroxyprogesterone (corpus luteum); androgen (theca), and estrogen (granulosa). The major sites of action of LH and FSH in mediating this pathway are shown by the horizontal arrows. The dotted line emphasizes that the metabolism of 17-hydroxyprogesterone is limited in the human ovary. (From Carr BR. Disorders of the ovary. In Wilson JD, Foster DW, eds. *Williams textbook of endocrinology*. 8th ed. Philadelphia: WB Saunders Co., 1992: 745. Reproduced by permission of WB Saunders Co.)

ovulation. The progesterone arising from the corpus luteum is responsible for preparation of the endometrium for implantation and for reducing uterine activity to maintain pregnancy.

Inhibin and activin

In addition to sex steroid mediated feedback, both the testis (Sertoli cell) and ovary (granulosa cell) produce inhibin, a heterodimeric protein which selectively

decreases FSH secretion. The β-subunit of inhibin has homology with transforming growth factor β and anti-Müllerian hormone (see p. 129). The placenta also produces inhibin: this may be one mechanism by which the maternal gonadotropic axis is suppressed during pregnancy. In addition, two covalently linked β-subunits of inhibin form activin; this has reciprocal actions to those of inhibin at both the pituitary and gonadal level. Activin stimulates pituitary FSH secretion and inhibits gonadal steroid production and cell multiplication. Inhibin, by contrast, stimulates gonadal steroidogenesis and cell proliferation in the gonad. Activin is also formed in the central nervous system where it is neurotropic and in the bone marrow where it is a potent stimulator of erythropoiesis.

Gametogenesis

The ultimate goal of the HPG axis is the production of functional gametes. In the male, germ cells increase in number under the influence of FSH facilitated by LH mediated testosterone production in nearby Leydig cells. At the time of puberty maturation of spermatogonia to spermatozoa occurs in coordinated groups of contiguous cells over a period of about 70 days such that about 200 million sperm are produced each day. Further development during epididymal passage, a process requiring 12–21 days, results in improved motility by changes in both nuclear chromatin and tail organelles. Although the dependence of spermatogenesis on gonadotropins is known, the molecular control mechanisms are uncertain. The hormonal requirements for initiation of spermatogenesis differ from those required for its maintenance. *Klinefelter syndrome*, or seminiferous tubule dysgenesis, is an example of failure of spermatogenesis which results from an extra X chromosome.

The ovary, by contrast, generates oogonia from primordial cells during gestation, with a maximal number of 6 or 7 million around mid-gestation. Germ cell numbers decrease rapidly through atresia so that about 1 million are present at the time of birth. These primary oocytes undergo meiosis, but division is arrested in the diplotene phase of the first meiotic division, to be continued only as ovulation occurs in later years. By the time of menarche further atresia has occurred so that only about 400 000 germ cells are present. Follicular growth and atresia occurs constantly during childhood, a phenomenon which may be responsible for the common occurrence of transient breast development in prepubertal girls.

The menstrual cycle

The pubertal process (see p. 145) results in a mature HPG axis, which functions in a cyclic fashion in females. The cycle involves orchestrated changes in gonadotropins and sex steroids, ovarian and endometrial structure as summarized in Fig. 7.10. During the early follicular phase, the ovary is stimulated by FSH to recruit follicles for the next cycle. Eventually one follicle is selected as the dominant or ovulatory follicle; the others undergo atresia. As this follicle grows, estrogen secretion increases. At a critical concentration and duration of estrogen secretion,

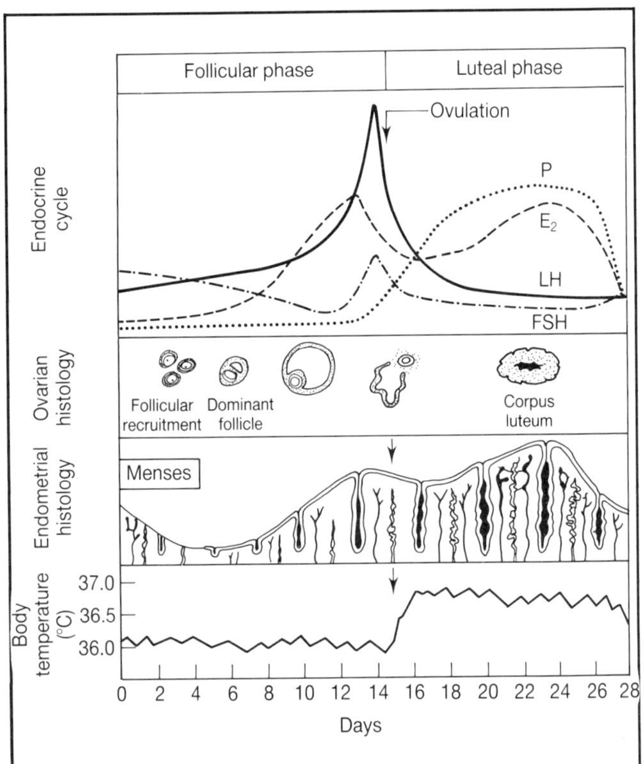

Fig. 7.10. Hormonal, ovarian, endometrial, and basal body temperature changes and relationships throughout the normal menstrual cycle. (From Carr BR, Wilson JD. Disorders of the ovary and female reproductive tract. In Braunwald E, Isselbacher KJ, Petersdorf RG et al., eds. *Harrison's principles of internal medicine*. 11th ed. New York: McGraw-Hill, 1987: 1818. Reproduced with permission of McGraw-Hill Inc.)

positive feedback results in a burst of gonadotropin secretion and ovulation. After ovulation the follicle changes its steroidogenic characteristics and begins to function as the corpus luteum, producing large amounts of progesterone as well as estradiol. These high steroid concentrations cause gonadotropins to decrease. Eventually, in the absence of pregnancy, the corpus luteum undergoes luteolysis. The withdrawal of hormonal support triggers shedding of the endometrium at the time of menses. The cycle begins again with increases in FSH secretion and follicle recruitment for the next cycle even as estradiol and progesterone concentrations reach their lowest concentrations before menses occur. It is very common for follicular development to be inadequate at the ends of the reproductive spectrum of midpuberty and the premenopausal years.

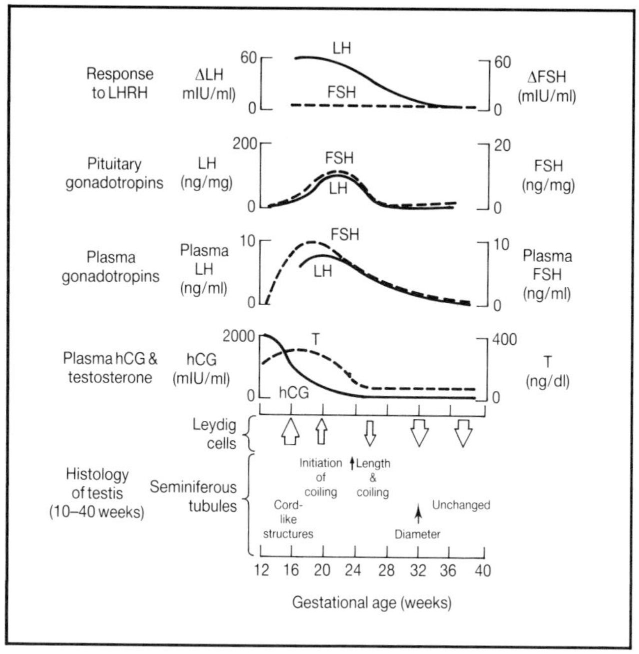

Fig. 7.11. Comparison of the pattern of change of serum testosterone, hCG, and serum and pituitary LH and FSH levels in the human male fetus during gestation in relation to the morphological changes in fetal testis. The top graph illustrates the regression curve for the increment (Δ) between a baseline plasma LH and FSH level and the 15 minute response to administration of GnRH to the male fetus plotted as a function of gestational age. The scale masks the slight increase in plasma FSH. The evidence supports the hypothesis that the hypothalamic GnRH pulse generator is functional early in gestation and mediates the rise in serum concentration of fetal pituitary gonadotropes. (From Grumbach MM, Styne DM. Puberty: ontogeny, neuroendocrinology, physiology, and disorders. In Wilson JD, Foster DW, eds. *Williams textbook of endocrinology*. 8th ed. Philadelphia: WB Saunders Co., 1992: 1157. Reproduced by permission of WB Saunders Co.)

Developmental aspects

The hypothalamic–pituitary–gonadal axis undergoes several developmental phases. Each phase can be thought of in a teleological sense as accomplishing a purpose to convey an evolutionary advantage.

Intrauterine phase (see Figs 7.11 and 7.12)

The tasks accomplished during the intrauterine phase of development of the HPG axis are sexual differentiation (see p. 127) and establishment of a sexually dimorphic regulatory system which has certain programmed aspects but retains the ability to respond to internal and external environmental conditions.

Gonadotropin releasing hormone (GnRH) is detectable in the hypothalamus by 8 weeks of gestation. The anatomical conditions necessary for regulation of the HPG axis are established in the fetus by 11–12 weeks of gestation. By this time, luteinizing hormone (LH) and follicle stimulating hormone (FSH) are detectable in the pituitary gland, implying that some form of relationship has been established. Regulation of pituitary secretion by the hypothalamus at this time could include an ultra short loop or paracrine mechanism as the hypophyseal–portal system becomes fully functional. Hypothalamic GnRH increases, as do pituitary and serum LH and FSH until mid-gestation (weeks 20–24). By this time, there is evidence for sexual dimorphism in the regulation of this axis. Female fetuses have higher serum FSH concentrations than males, a pattern which persists, at least in response to GnRH. Evidence from animal studies indicates that castration of a male fetus during gestation results in decreased serum testosterone and increased LH and FSH, whereas ovariectomy does not have the same consequence. Thus a difference in sensitivity of the feedback mechanism between male and female fetuses can be inferred.

By early in the third trimester the ovine fetus has established pulsatile gonadotropin secretion, responsiveness of gonadotropes to GnRH and GnRH superagonists, confirming the presence of a regulated system. Changes in the sensitivity of the feedback set points seem to be important to the phenomena observed in this and

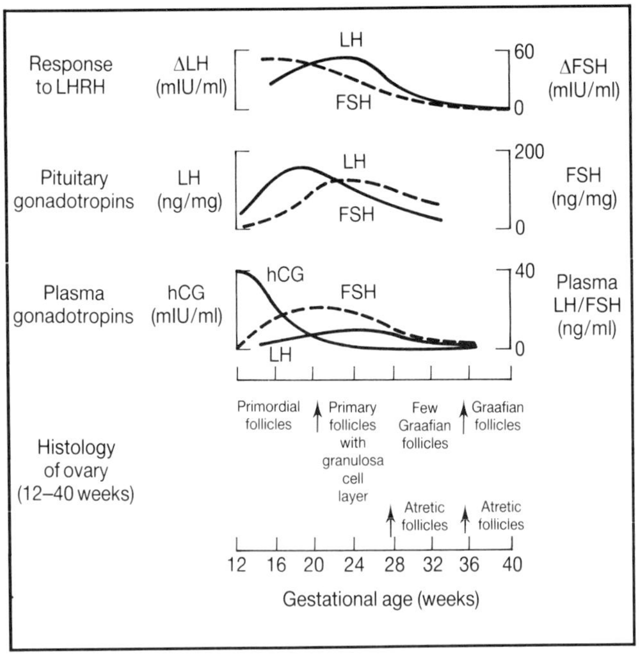

Fig. 7.12. Pattern of change of serum FSH, LH and hCG levels; concentration of pituitary FSH and LH; and increment (Δ) between baseline FSH and LH and the 15 minute response to administration of GnRH in human female fetus during gestation with the development of the fetal ovary. (From Grumbach MM, Styne DM. Puberty: ontogeny, neuroendocrinology, physiology, and disorders. In Wilson JD, Foster DW, eds. *Williams textbook of endocrinology*. 8th ed. Philadelphia: WB Saunders Co., 1992: 1157. Reproduced by permission of WB Saunders Co.)

subsequent phases of development. As gestation progresses, GnRH content of the hypothalamus, LH and FSH content of the pituitary and serum LH and FSH decrease.

Gonadal function is not entirely dependent upon the integrity of the fetal HPG axis, as human chorionic gonadotropin (hCG), produced from the beginning of gestation, can stimulate LH receptors on the gonad which in turn stimulate sex steroid synthesis. Thus by 6–8 weeks of gestation, Sertoli and Leydig cells are both present and testosterone synthesis begins. Within the testis, testosterone content is maximal at 12–14 weeks of gestation. The fetal ovary, in contrast, has very little activity of the steroidogenic enzymes and lacks hCG receptors.

Testicular cords with germ cells are present by 6–7 weeks of gestation. The germ cells may undergo meiosis and, like ovarian germ cells, remain in meiotic arrest until puberty. Ovarian development occurs later in gestation than the testicular development of analogous structures and functions. Although primitive germ cells in the female undergo mitotic division in the first month of gestation, the ovary is not organized until about 11–12 weeks. The number of oocytes is not maximal until about 20 weeks of gestation. Primary follicles appear around the sixteenth week, and preantral follicles, containing oocytes which have undergone meiotic prophase and include increasing numbers of granulosa and theca cells, reach a maximal number at term. In contrast to testes, ovaries have minimal capacity to synthesize sex steroids during intrauterine life.

In addition to sex steroids, other products of gonads which have been demonstrated include insulin-like growth factors (I and II), inhibin, activin, interleukin-1, transforming growth factor β, transferrin and androgen binding protein. The ontogeny and role of these factors in developmental physiology is not yet clear.

Neonatal phase

Serum LH and FSH are low in cord blood, presumably because a sufficiently sensitive negative feedback system has developed to respond to the high estrogen concentration of the intrauterine environment. Released from this estrogenic inhibition, LH and FSH increase for a few months and subsequently decrease. Thus infants in the first few months of life can have gonadotropin and sex steroid concentrations in plasma and pulsatile secretory patterns that are comparable to pubertal individuals. During this time, the gonadotropin response to exogenous GnRH is also comparable to the response seen at the time of puberty.

Gonadotropins and sex steroids decrease to very low concentrations, generally by 6–12 months of age. This decrease is thought to be due to both intrinsic development of central nervous system factors which restrain puberty, and to increasing sensitivity of the negative feedback loop to small concentrations of sex steroids.

A schematic representation of postnatal gonadotropin secretion patterns is described in Fig. 7.13.

Juvenile pause

After the neonatal increase in activity of the HPG axis, the entire system subsides into a period of apparent

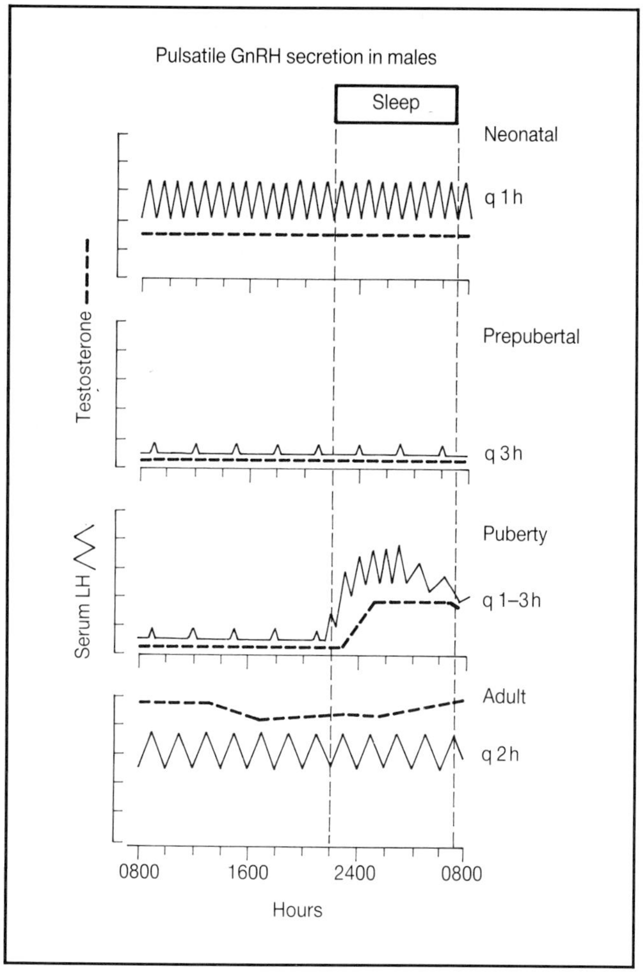

Fig. 7.13. Schematic diagram of presumed changes in the pulsatile secretion of GnRH as inferred by the pulsatile secretory patterns of LH throughout male sexual maturation. (From Kelch RP, Foster CM, Kletter GB *et al.* Neuroendocrine regulation of puberty in boys. In Aubert ML, Sizonenko PC, eds. *Developmental endocrinology*. Serona Symposia, vol. 67. New York: Raven Press, 1990: 104. Reproduced by permission of Raven Press, New York.)

quiescence which lasts until the hormonal changes of early puberty occur. The length of this juvenile pause is extremely important in an evolutionary sense. This time of prolonged dependence with freedom from reproductive pressures is thought to correlate with the ability of a species to provide extensive education to its young.

The physiological reasons for the juvenile pause are elusive. The occurrence of precocious puberty when portions of the brain are damaged by tumor or other pathology provides evidence that the central nervous system somehow restrains puberty. The search for a hormonal mediator of this period of restraint has not yielded results that are directly applicable to humans.

Puberty

Puberty is a period of several years during which the transition from sexual immaturity to reproductive competence occurs. This process involves changes in the activity of each level of the HPG axis. For details refer to p. 145.

Selected reading

Burger HG, de Kretser DM, eds. *The testis*. 2nd ed. New York: Raven Press Ltd, 1989.

Gluckman PD, Grumbach MM, Kaplan SL. The human fetal hypothalamus and pituitary gland. In Tulchinsky D, Ryan KJ, eds. *Maternal–fetal endocrinology*. Philadelphia: WB Saunders, 1980: 196.

Grumbach MM, Styne DM. Puberty: ontogeny, neuroendocrinology, physiology and disorders. In Wilson JD, Foster DW, eds. *Williams textbook of endocrinology*. Philadelphia: WB Saunders Co., 1992: 1155.

Kelch RP, Foster CM, Kletter GB, Marshall JC. Neuroendocrine regulation of puberty in boys. In Sizonenko PC, Aubert ML, eds. *Developmental endocrinology*. New York: Raven Press, 1990.

Ravinovici J, Jaffe RB. Development and regulation of growth and differentiated function in human and subhuman primate fetal gonads. *Endocr Rev* 1990; **11**: 532.

Richards JS, Jahnsen T, Hedin L, *et al.* Ovarian follicular development from physiology to molecular biology. *Recent Prog Horm Res* 1987; **43**: 231.

G. THE ADRENAL CORTEX

G1. The Hypothalamic–Pituitary–Adrenal Axis

W S Cutfield

Embryology and anatomy

The adrenal cortex arises from mesoderm of the mesonephros during the fifth week of fetal development. This corticoadrenal anlage is then penetrated by ectoderm from the neural crest to form the adrenal medulla (see p. 341). The adrenal cortex of the fetus and young infant consists of two distinct layers. The inner layer develops first to become the fetal cortex which rapidly increases in size from the seventh month of fetal life to occupy 80 percent of the adrenal cortex by birth. The adult or definitive cortex forms a thin, irregular outer layer and contains the zona glomerulosa and zona fasciculata. The fetal and adult cortices have quite different steroid synthetic capacities and functions. The differentiation and development of function of the adrenal cortex is influenced by the fetal pituitary.

The outer zone of the adrenal cortex is the zona glomerulosa and comprises 10 percent of the cortex during childhood. The zona fasciculata occupies the remainder of the definitive cortex until the development of the zona reticularis which first appears in early childhood. The zona reticularis, which is the primary source of androgen secretion in adrenarche, forms the inner zone of the adrenal cortex. It ultimately occupies 10 percent of the cortex by the end of puberty, at which time the adrenal cortex is fully mature.

Fetal adrenal cortex

The fetal adrenal cortex and placenta are termed the 'fetoplacental unit' as these two organs interact to produce essential hormones for mother and fetus. The fetal adrenal has two unique functions: to provide precursors for maternal estrogen production and to facilitate fetal organ enzyme maturation. 3β-Hydroxysteroid dehydrogenase is functionally inactivated in the fetal zone of the fetal adrenal cortex, partly by placental estrogen. The inactivation of this enzyme provides control by the placenta over the steroids produced by the fetal zone of the adrenal. Placental progesterone and pregnenolone are the major substrates for adrenal steroidogenesis by the fetal adrenal cortex. From approximately 8 weeks of gestation pregnenolone is converted principally to dehydroepiandrosterone sulfate (DHAS) which is hydroxylated in other fetal tissues, particularly the liver, to 16-hydroxyDHAS which then passes to the placenta to form estriol. The fetal adrenal therefore has an essential role in the maintenance of pregnancy by contributing to the dramatic estrogen production that occurs particularly during late pregnancy and which influences uterine growth and blood flow.

Late in gestation fetal ACTH and cortisol plasma levels rise, influencing the maturation of a number of enzyme systems in the lungs and gastrointestinal tract, including the liver and pancreas. The primary source of fetal cortisol production is the definitive cortex with a small contribution from the fetal zone. It appears that 3β-hydroxysteroid dehydrogenase is present in the fetal pituitary and activated in late gestation. This enzyme converts cortisol in the pituitary gland to less active metabolites and thus reduces negative feedback on ACTH release. The fetal adrenal is primarily under fetal hypothalamic–pituitary control with both ACTH and AVP playing an interactive role in its regulation. The placenta also secretes corticotropin releasing hormone (CRH) into the fetal circulation; however it is unclear whether placental CRH regulates fetal pituitary ACTH release.

Biosynthetic pathways of the adrenal cortex

Steroidogenesis occurs in all three zones of the definitive adrenal cortex, with each zone principally responsible for producing a single steroidal class. Mineralocorticoids are produced in the zona glomerulosa, androgens in the zona reticularis and glucocorticoids in the zona fasciculata. The zona fasciculata/reticularis and zona glomerulosa are regulated differently, may arise

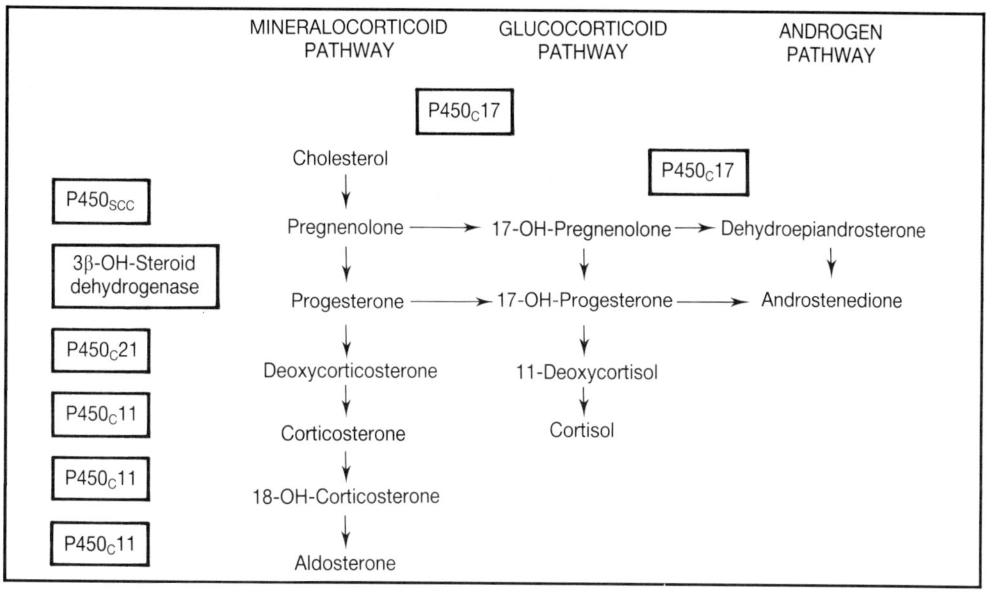

Fig. 7.14. Pathway of adrenal steroidogenesis divided according to class of steroid end product.

from different stem cells, and can be considered functionally separate glands housed within the same organ.

All adrenal steroid hormones are formed from cholesterol derived mainly from low-density lipoprotein (LDL) (see p. 290). Steroid biosynthesis is complex with intermediates sequentially formed in several sites within the cell (Fig. 7.14). Cortisol synthesis is under the control of adrenocorticotropic hormone (ACTH) which increases cholesterol ester hydroxylase activity (Fig. 7.14) through adenyl cyclase activation. The larger parent molecule, cholesterol, is hydroxylated twice and then oxidatively cleaved down in three steps to form pregnenolone. All three steps are catalyzed by the single enzyme side-chain cleavage, $P450_{scc}$, previously known as cholesterol desmolase (Fig. 7.15). This complex sequence is the rate-limiting step in adrenal steroid synthesis. $P450_{scc}$ is part of the mitochondrial cytochrome P450 oxygenase family, together with the majority of steroid biosynthetic enzymes. These enzymes are produced in the mitochondria and microsomes of the endoplasmic reticulum.

Pregnenolone passes from the mitochondria to the endoplasmic reticulum where dehydrogenation of the three hydroxyl groups by 3β-hydroxysteroid dehydrogenase yields progesterone. This is not a cytochrome P450 enzyme.

In the zona fasciculata most of the progesterone synthesized undergoes 17α-hydroxylation by another cytochrome P450 enzyme, $P450_c17$ to produce 17-hydroxyprogesterone. $P450_c17$ has a second, less important role to cleave 17,20 two-carbon side-chains (17,20 lyase activity) to yield androstenedione. This dual role enables this single enzyme to direct steroid precursors to glucocorticoid or androgen synthesis. This latter function becomes important in disorders such as 21-hydroxylase deficiency when $P450_c17$ redirects 17-hydroxyprogesterone to androgen synthesis. 17-Hydroxyprogesterone is in turn 21-hydroxylated to 11-deoxycortisol by $P450_c21$. 11-Deoxycortisol then passes

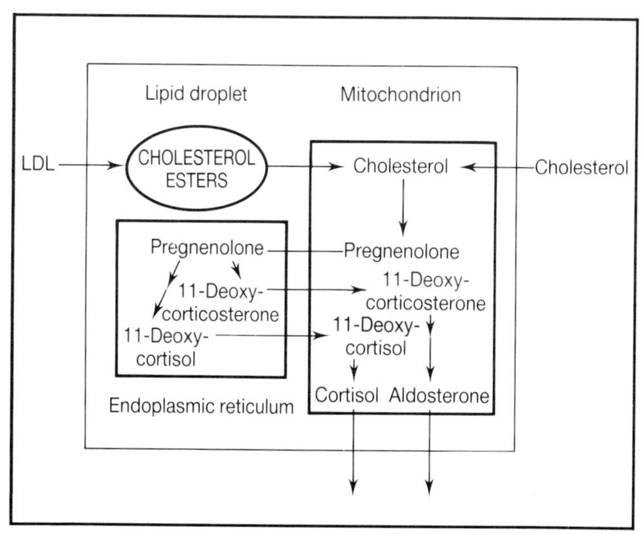

Fig. 7.15. Sites of steroidogenesis within the cell.

back to the mitochondria to be 11-hydroxylated by $P450_c11$ to cortisol.

Aldosterone, the principal mineralocorticoid, is produced under the control of the renin–angiotensin system. The enzymatic pathway of aldosterone biosynthesis is the same as the cortisol pathway except that $P450_c17$ is inactive in the zona glomerulosa, ensuring that aldosterone is the only steroid end product produced in this zone. Cholesterol is cleaved to form pregnenolone, dehydrogenated to progesterone and then sequentially hydroxylated to deoxycorticosterone and corticosterone. 18-Hydroxylation of corticosterone to 18-hydroxycorticosterone is catalyzed in mitochondria by the enzyme $P450_c11$ by means of its corticosterone methyl oxidase (CMO 1) activity. 18-Hydroxycorticosterone is in turn oxidized by CMO 2 resident on the same $P450_c11$ enzyme to aldosterone. Although the $P450_c11$ enzyme is present in the zona fasciculata, an unidentified inhibitor prevents CMO 2 activity.

Adrenal androgen production is confined to the zona reticularis and is insignificant until late childhood. Following puberty, DHA and DHAS are the most abundant steroids produced by the adrenal. Adrenal androgen synthesis follows the cortisol pathway until the intermediates 17-hydroxypregnenolone or 17-hydroxyprogesterone are reached. The presence of P450 reductase activity in the zona reticularis (which is not present in the zona glomerulosa) enables $P450_c17$ to exhibit 17,20-lyase activity. This enables 17-hydroxyprogesterone to be converted to DHEA and to a far lesser extent 17-hydroxyprogesterone to androstenedione. These two 19-carbon steroids serve as weak androgens or as precursors to more potent androgens formed peripherally.

The adrenal steroid hydroxylases are cytochrome P450 monooxygenases which are part of a family of heme-containing oxidative enzymes. They receive electrons from NADPH, through an electron transfer chain, to reduce molecular oxygen and insert it into the steroid substrate. The location and sequence of the genes of several of these enzymes in recent years has greatly increased understanding of adrenal enzyme deficient disorders such as *congenital adrenal hyperplasia* (CAH). Several of these enzymes (e.g. $P450_c11$) have more than a single function presumably localized to different active sites in the tertiary structure of the protein. Thus one enzyme may have a defect restricted to a single site, leaving other activity intact, or there may be inhibitors that act solely on one or other of the sites located in the enzyme.

$P450_c21$ is the most extensively studied of the adrenal cytochrome P450 enzymes. Deficiency of this enzyme results in the commonest form of *congenital adrenal hyperplasia*. 3β-Hydroxysteroid dehydrogenase is likely to be a composite of two separate isoenzymes. The pathophysiology of defects in adrenal steroidogenesis is discussed separately (see p. 326). A number of drugs that inhibit steroidogenesis are used in evaluating adrenal function or treating adrenal disorders. Metyrapone inhibits $P450_c11$, thus causing accumulation of cortisone and deoxycorticosterone. The latter metabolite prevents mineralocorticoid deficiency. Metyrapone is frequently used to test the integrity of the HPA axis and has been used to treat *Cushing syndrome*. Aminoglutathiamide blocks $P450_{scc}$. Ketoconazole inhibits both $P450_c11$ and $P450_c21$ and has been used in the treatment of *Cushing syndrome* and *testotoxicosis*.

Adrenal steroid regulation and rhythms

Regulation of cortisol secretion

The hypothalamus, pituitary and adrenal cortex comprise a neuroendocrine axis that controls cortisol secretion. Corticotropin releasing hormone (CRH), a 41 amino acid peptide, is primarily produced by neurons of the paraventricular nuclei located in the hypothalamus. Hypothalamic CRH is also found elsewhere in the brain where it has neurotransmitter function. CRH is released by the median eminence into the hypophyseal portal circulation to reach the anterior pituitary to stimulate ACTH production and release. ACTH release is not only regulated by CRH, but is also significantly stimulated by vasopressin (AVP) and to a lesser degree by other hypothalamic hormones. AVP and CRF have a synergistic effect on ACTH secretion. The role of AVP may be particularly important in the rise in ACTH release late in fetal life. ACTH also inhibits its own secretion. Both CRH and AVP have important roles in mediating the biological response to stress. CRH can be stimulated by neural stimuli from higher CNS centers, typically in response to stress, whether physiologically or pharmacologically induced. Excitatory neurotransmitters are serotoninergic, cholinergic and noradrenergic. The opioid system also influences ACTH release.

The major regulatory factor for ACTH release is the

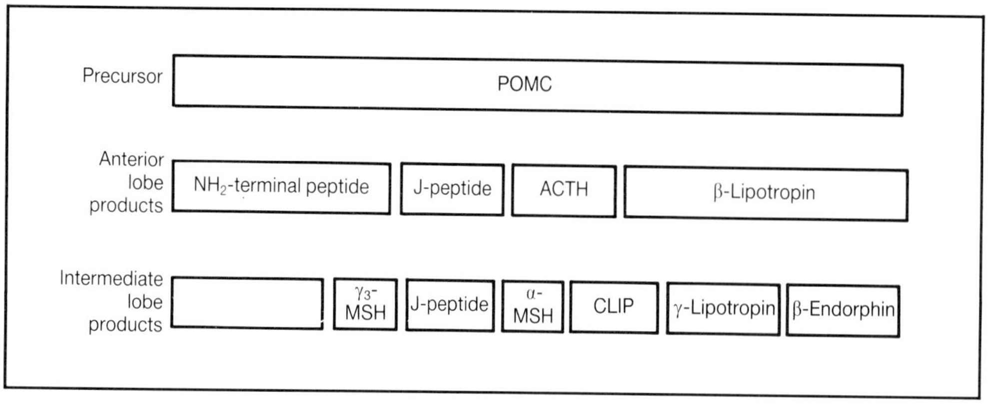

Fig. 7.16. Pituitary POMC and peptide hormone products.

level of negative feedback by circulating cortisol. Cortisol acts both at the hypothalamic level by inhibiting both CRH and AVP neurons and at the pituitary corticotrope. These are both short- and long-term latency feedback mechanisms. While the latter involves suppression of CRH, AVP and ACTH mRNA, shorter term feedback may involve direct steroidal effects on neuronal membranes to affect axonal discharge. It would appear that the efficiency of negative feedback is altered during the day such that in the morning a higher level of cortisol is needed to inhibit ACTH release. This allows the diurnal rhythm in cortisol to be exhibited.

ACTH is cleaved from a large prohormone, proopiomelanocortin (POMC) which contains the sequences of several other peptide hormones (Fig. 7.16). The gene is located on chromosome 2. The cleaved peptide products of POMC differ between the anterior and intermediate lobes of the pituitary, suggesting different cleavage enzymes between the two sites. The intermediate lobe only plays a significant role during fetal life and pregnancy. Aside from ACTH most of the pituitary POMC products do not yet have identified physiological roles. β-Lipotropin (βLPH) has weak steroidogenic and lipolytic activity and may have melanotropic activity. The amino terminal peptide and its products may potentiate ACTH action and act as adrenal growth factors. The intermediate lobe peptides are not normally produced in appreciable amounts; consequently while they are biologically active *in vitro*, they are unlikely to have significant biological effects. The melanocyte stimulating hormones (MSHs) stimulate melanocytes to produce melanin. Corticotropin-like intermediate lobe peptide (CLIP) has a weak stimulatory effect on pancreatic endocrine (β-cell) and exocrine function. The β-cell effects of CLIP may be mediated through the putative hormone, β-cell tropic hormone, an 18 amino acid fragment of CLIP. β-Endorphin has potent CNS opiate activity.

ACTH is a 39 amino acid peptide with a biological half-life of 4–8 minutes. The first 18 amino acid segments at the amino end of the molecule are necessary for biological activity. ACTH is essential for normal steroidogenesis and has a facilitatory role in maintaining normal adrenal size. ACTH has a weak melanocyte stimulating effect; however, in pathological states associated with chronically elevated ACTH levels (e.g. *Addison disease*), marked hyperpigmentation may occur. ACTH binds to a specific G-protein-linked receptor on the adrenal cell surface with the assistance of extracellular calcium. Intracellular effects of ACTH are mediated through cAMP. ACTH has both acute and chronic effects on adrenal steroidogenesis. Acutely, ACTH accelerates the conversion of cholesterol to pregnenolone. Chronic exposure to elevated levels of ACTH results in increased synthesis of all of the cytochrome P450 enzymes involved in steroidogenesis.

Circadian rhythm of cortisol secretion

During the first 2 days of life cortisol levels are continuously elevated. From 2 days to 2 months of age cortisol secretion exhibits free running oscillations without evidence of a circadian rhythm. At 3 months of age infants develop a diurnal rhythm to cortisol secretion similar to that seen in adults. The circadian rhythm control center is likely to either be located within, or signal through, the suprachiasmatic nucleus of the hypothalamus (see p. 254). The normal diurnal rhythm of cortisol secretion is due to increased amplitude of the pulses secreted of ACTH which peak between the last few hours of sleep and the first few awake hours. The frequency of ACTH pulses does not change through a 24 hour day. Pulses of cortisol secretion quickly follow and parallel pulses of ACTH secretion.

Control of aldosterone secretion

Aldosterone is the major circulating mineralocorticoid. Several precursors including deoxycorticosterone (DOC), corticosterone and 18-hydroxycorticosterone, possess weak mineralocorticoid activity. As considerably more DOC and corticosterone are synthesized in the zona fasciculata than the zona glomerulosa, production is principally driven by ACTH. However, aldosterone is exclusively produced in the zona glomerulosa and is principally regulated by the renin–angiotensin system. Prolonged elevation of ACTH leads to only a transient increase in aldosterone production. Aldosterone secretion, unlike cortisol, is not regulated by a significant circadian rhythm. Factors that influence aldosterone secretion are listed in Table 7.1. The renin–angiotensin system is reviewed on p. 334.

Aldosterone production is regulated at two points in its biosynthetic pathway: the early step of conversion of cholesterol to pregnenolone and the late step of conversion of corticosterone to aldosterone. Angiotensin II and III bind to a high affinity receptor on the zona glomerulosa and stimulate the activity of both these enzymes.

Table 7.1. Factors that influence aldosterone secretion

Stimulation: major factors	
	Renin–angiotensin
	Hypokalemia
Stimulation: minor factors	
	ACTH
	Hypernatremia
	Serotonin
	Metabolic acidosis
	ADH
	Vasointestinal polypeptide
Inhibition	
	Dopamine
	Atrial natriuretic factor
	Somatostatin

Plasma steroid binding proteins

Steroid hormones are predominantly protein bound in the circulation. The two major specific steroid binding proteins are corticosteroid binding globulin (CBG) and testosterone binding globulin (TeBG), also known as sex hormone binding globulin. These carrier proteins have high affinity, but limited capacity for steroid binding. The other major steroid carrier is albumin which is of high capacity and low affinity.

CBG is a member of the serine protease inhibitor superfamily which includes thyroxine binding globulin and angiotensinogen. CBG, which is mainly produced in the liver, binds up to 97 percent of normal levels of cortisol. Most remaining circulating cortisol is bound to albumin. CBG binds poorly to synthetic steroids with the exception of prednisolone. Only 60 percent of aldosterone is protein bound, the majority to albumin. The stress-induced high levels of cortisol saturate CBG, displace aldosterone from CBG and also increase the free cortisol fraction. CBG levels are markedly lower in the fetus than the adult, facilitating transplacental transfer of glucocorticoids from mother to fetus. In late gestation CBG levels rise under the control of the fetal adenohypophysis. CBG levels further increase considerably during childhood, falling to adult levels during puberty.

The adrenal androgens DHEA, DHEAS and androstenedione are predominantly bound to albumin, with minimal binding to TeBG. TeBG levels are high during childhood, fall to adult levels during puberty and rise again only in pregnancy.

Steroid metabolism

Glucocorticoid metabolism principally occurs in the liver by a variety of different enzymatic processes. Reduction of the Δ^4 double bond is the rate-limiting step in cortisol metabolism and is mainly catalyzed by 5β-reductase and 3α-hydroxysteroid dehydrogenase. Cortisol and cortisone may also be reduced by 20α- and 20β-hydroxysteroid dehydrogenase. Seventy percent of cortisol metabolites are catalyzed by these four enzymes. Ultimately the C-19 and C-21 cortisol metabolites are conjugated with glucuronic acid or sulfate and excreted in the urine. Cortisol is also metabolized in the kidney by 11β-hydroxysteroid dehydrogenase to cortisone. This conversion prevents cortisol binding to the mineralocorticoid receptor and blocking aldosterone action. This enzyme complex is also capable of catalyzing the reverse reaction. The cortisol to cortisone ratio is markedly lower in the fetus, indicating reductive conversion of cortisone to cortisol is less common in the fetus when compared to the adult. The higher circulating cortisone levels in the fetus are thought to protect against glucocorticoid effects as cortisone is less potent than cortisol.

Aldosterone, like cortisol, is reduced and conjugated in the liver and then excreted in the urine. DHEA is converted to androstenedione and then reduced, conjugated and excreted in urine and stool. DHEAS can be excreted directly into urine.

Adrenal steroid receptors (see also p. 24)

The glucocorticoid and mineralocorticoid receptors are a receptor superfamily which includes all steroid, thyroid hormone and retinoic acid receptors. All members when ligand bound are then capable of binding to DNA and regulating gene transcription. The central DNA binding domain of these receptors contains a highly conserved 'zinc finger'. Glucocorticoids and mineralocorticoids, which are both relatively lipophilic, enter target cells by passive diffusion. The site of hormone to receptor binding has not been clearly elucidated, occurring either in the cytoplasm or nucleus (Fig. 7.17). The hormone–receptor complex then binds to regulatory DNA sequences located near the promoter region of target genes. Glucocorticoid receptors are found within every organ in the body; consequently glucocorticoids display a wide array of biological effects.

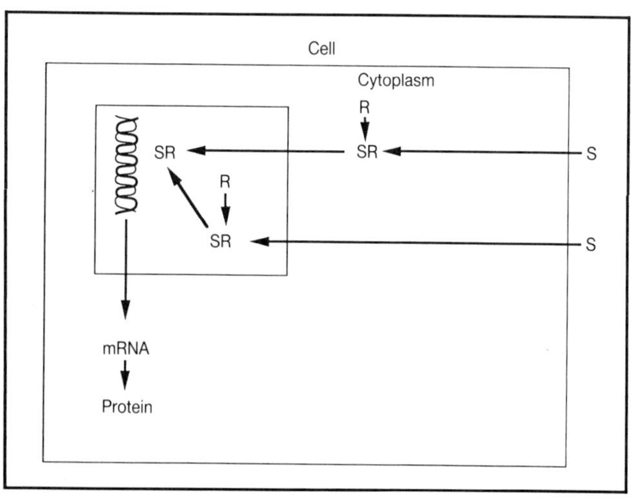

Fig. 7.17. Two possible mechanisms in which steroids (S) bind to target receptors (R) and intiate gene transcription and protein synthesis.

Aldosterone is able to bind to two distinct receptors in the kidney. Although the type I receptor mediates aldosterone action, it displays surprisingly little specificity for aldosterone. Cortisol is able to bind to the type I receptor with the same affinity as aldosterone. Local conversion of cortisol to cortisone protects the type I receptor from cortisol binding (see p. 337). The type II receptor has a high affinity for cortisol and a low affinity for aldosterone and is therefore thought to be a glucocorticoid receptor. Type I receptors are found predominantly in the kidney, gut and salivary glands, but are also present in the brain, pituitary, liver and circulating mononuclear cells.

Steroid sites of action and function

Glucocorticoids

Glucocorticoids were named after the effects that cortisol has on carbohydrate metabolism. Glucocorticoids act at many sites to optimize circulating levels and stores of glucose. Gluconeogenesis is achieved through two separate glucocorticoid effects; first, extrahepatic gluconeogenic amino acids are mobilized, principally from skeletal muscle. Secondly, conversion of these amino acids to glucose is increased in the liver. Other gluconeogenic hormones are ineffective without the permissive effect of glucocorticoids. Glycogenesis is promoted by glucocorticoid activation of glycogen synthetase and inhibition of glycogen phosphorylase. Glucocorticoids also inhibit peripheral glucose utilization by reducing glucose uptake. Although glucocorticoids acutely stimulate lipolysis from adipocytes, chronic glucocorticoid exposure leads to redistribution of body fat by an unknown mechanism.

The effects of glucocorticoids on the immune system, inflammatory processes, skeleton and connective tissue are only seen in states of prolonged glucocorticoid excess and therefore are unlikely to constitute normal physiological responses. Prolonged, excessive glucocorticoid exposure invariably occurs as part of a treatment regimen for severe chronic illness. During childhood the greatest adverse effect of this therapy is on the skeleton. The two major effects seen are impairment of normal bone formation and inhibition of bone growth. Reduced osteoblastic activity with concomitant increased osteoclastic activity leads to reduced new bone formation and osteopenia. There is also reduction of available mineral for bone with reduced calcium absorption from the gut, increased renal calcium excretion and direct stimulation of parathyroid hormone secretion. The mechanism of glucocorticoid inhibition of bone growth remains unclear. Unlike adults, growth hormone secretion is minimally impaired by glucocorticoids. The most likely mechanisms include inhibition of insulin-like growth factor I action and impairment of procollagen production. Inhibition of collagen and hyaluronidate synthesis results in poor wound healing.

Immunological and inflammatory responses are markedly suppressed by excessive glucocorticoids. Circulating lymphocytes (T and B cells) are reduced, due to relocation in extravascular sites. B-cell, T-cell and macrophage differentiation, proliferation and actions are also inhibited. Glucocorticoid suppression of inflammation occurs through inhibition of histamine action, prostaglandin synthesis and plasminogen activators. Plasmins stimulate kinin production, leading to vasodilatation and increased capillary permeability.

The mechanisms through which glucocorticoids maintain vascular integrity during stress are poorly understood. Glucocorticoid excess leads to hypertension, whereas glucocorticoid deficiency is associated with hypotension, suggesting that glucocorticoids have either a direct or indirect effect on vascular tone. Glucocorticoids inhibit AVP and increase ANF synthesis. Consequently in glucocorticoid deficient states, AVP and ANF levels are elevated, leading to increased sodium and water retention limiting the degree of hypotension.

Mineralocorticoids

Mineralocorticoids are essential for life. Severe mineralocorticoid deficiency, as seen in CAH, results in death due to hyperkalemia within weeks. Aldosterone accounts for 90 percent of mineralocorticoid activity with most of the remaining 10 percent provided by cortisol. The function of aldosterone is to enhance sodium absorption and potassium excretion across epithelium to maintain electrolyte balance and a normal circulating volume. Aldosterone promotes increased sodium reabsorption in exchange for increased potassium, and to a lesser extent, hydrogen ion excretion in the distal tubule and collecting ducts of the kidney. Aldosterone essentially has the same effect on salivary and sweat glands as on the kidney.

Normal adrenal steroid secretion

Neonatal

Many circulating adrenal steroid precursor levels are higher in preterm when compared to term infants although cortisol levels tend to be lower. Elevated DHEAS levels are due to reduced 3β-hydroxysteroid dehydrogenase activity in the fetal zone which comprises most of the adrenal cortex in late gestation. Increased 17-hydroxyprogesterone and 17-hydroxypregnenolone levels are most consistent with relative immaturity of the $P450_c11$ enzyme in the underdeveloped definitive cortex. The 17-hydroxyprogesterone levels are inversely correlated with gestational age and weight. Term infants also have increased levels of these steroid precursors in comparison to older children. After 2 days of age, cortisol levels are decreased, reaching adult levels by 2–3 months. However, accurate cortisol production rates have not been established for neonates and infants.

Despite elevated plasma renin and aldosterone levels in both preterm and term infants, hyponatremia is commonly observed in preterm infants during the first few weeks of life. This observation is presumed to be due to *transient pseudohypoaldosteronism* (see p. 337).

Childhood

During most of infancy and childhood DHEAS levels remain low. At approximately 8–10 years of age DHEAS and androstenedione levels rise, reaching adult levels in late puberty. The initiation of the rise in adrenal steroids prior to puberty is termed **adrenarche**. Throughout childhood and puberty there are no sex differences in DHEAS levels. Androstenedione and testosterone levels are also low and do not exhibit sex differences prior to puberty. Recently cortisol production rates for children and adolescents have been accurately determined at 6.8 ± 1.9 mg/m^2 per day, irrespective of age and sex.

Adrenarche

Adrenarche is the increase in adrenal androgen production that occurs in both sexes between the ages of 8 and 10 years. Adrenarche ultimately leads to the development of pubic hair (pubarche). The progressive increase in adrenal androgen production in late childhood and adolescence matches the growth of the zona reticularis with full development and adrenal androgen production during late adolescence. Prior to adrenarche the zona reticularis is poorly developed. The mechanism activating adrenarche and the development of the zona reticularis has not been elucidated. It is likely to involve a separate adrenal stimulating factor that may originate in the pituitary as a component of the POMC molecule.

Adrenarche and puberty are independent events controlled by separate mechanisms. Adrenarche precedes puberty by several years and is not essential for the onset of puberty. There are a number of disorders such as *primary adrenal insufficiency* and *precocious puberty* where these two events are discordant. Adrenal androgens do not normally contribute significantly to the adolescent growth spurt.

Selected reading

Brooks RV. Biosynthesis and metabolism of adrenocortical steroids. In James VHT, ed. *The adrenal gland*. New York: Raven Press, 1979: 67.

Carson-Junca MA, Schrader WT, O'Malley W. Steroid receptor family: structure and function. *Endocr Rev* 1990; **11**: 201.

Miller W. Molecular biology of steroid hormone biosynthesis. *Endocr Rev* 1988; **9**: 295.

Pepe GJ, Albrecht ED. Regulation of the primate fetal adrenal cortex. *Endocr Rev* 1990; **11**: 151.

G2. Pathophysiology of Adrenal Steroidogenesis

MI New

The pathways of steroid hormone synthesis in the adrenal gland are depicted on p. 320. A defect at a step may be manifested clinically not only because cortisol and other steroid hormones are not synthesized sufficiently, but also because precursor steroids proximal to the blocked step accumulate and are shunted into other metabolic pathways, particularly those of androgen biosynthesis.

The diseases that affect adrenal steroidogenesis include syndromes of hypoadrenocorticism, primarily the various forms of *congenital adrenal hyperplasia* (CAH), but also conditions caused by malfunction of the adrenals such as *congenital adrenal aplasia* or *hypoplasia*, *adrenal hemorrhage*, *congenital adrenocortical unresponsiveness to ACTH*, Addison disease (chronic hypoadrenocorticism as a result of damage to the adrenal which may occur by infection, or any destructive process); *hypopituitarism*; or *end-organ unresponsiveness to adrenal hormones*. Hyperadrenocorticism results primarily from neoplasms and manifests as *Cushing syndrome* (excess cortisol secretion), *virilization* (elevated adrenal androgens), *feminizing syndrome* (elevated estrogen secretion), or *hyperaldosteronism*.

Congenital adrenal hyperplasia

The term *congenital adrenal hyperplasia* (CAH) refers to a family of disorders that result from an inherited defect in any of the five enzymes required to synthesize cortisol from cholesterol:

1. 21-hydroxylase ($P450_c21$) deficiency (salt-wasting, simple virilizing, and nonclassic forms);
2. 11β-hydroxylase ($P450_c11$) deficiency (hypertensive virilizing CAH) (classic and nonclassic forms); special variants with additional corticosterone methyl oxidase deficiency (types I and II) also have salt-wasting;
3. 3β-hydroxysteroid dehydrogenase deficiency (classic and nonclassic forms);
4. 17α-hydroxylase ($P450_c17$) deficiency with 17,20-lyase deficiency;
5. Cholesterol desmolase ($P450_{scc}$) deficiency (lipoid hyperplasia).

21-Hydroxylase deficiency

In the overwhelming majority of cases, 90–95 percent, CAH is due to deficiency of 21-hydroxylase (21OH) or $P450_c21$. *Classic 21OH deficiency* is the result of total or near total blockage of hydroxylation of progesterone and 17-hydroxyprogesterone at the 21 position. Shunting of cortisol precursors into the pathways of androgen synthesis produces abnormally high levels of androgens, which have prenatal and postnatal effects on sex steroid-responsiveness tissues. A severe 21OH defect can also block aldosterone synthesis. About 75 percent of persons with classic 21OH deficiency have the aldosterone-deficient 'salt-wasting' form; about 25 percent are 'simple virilizers'. *Nonclassic* (NC), or milder and later-onset, *21OH deficiency* results from partial enzyme defects. The symptoms of nonclassic forms of CAH are more subtle versions of those of classic CAH. Masculinizing symptoms can appear at any time postnatally with a wide range of severity; they never occur prenatally.

Adrenocortical function begins in the third week of gestation. When 21OH is deficient, the fetus is exposed to excess androgens during the time of sexual differentiation. As a result, a female born with classic CAH will have an enlarged clitoris and labial fusion, which at times may lead to wrong sex assignment. Affected males look entirely normal at birth, which puts them at special risk for the consequences of undertreated salt-wasting crisis in the first weeks of life. Neonatal screening for 17α-hydroxyprogesterone (17OHP) is therefore recommended.

Postnatally, untreated androgen excess causes progressive virilizing changes and accelerated growth and development in both sexes. Continued androgen excess through adolescence, however, leads to premature closure of the epiphyses and short final height. The high levels of androgens also affect the hypothalamic–pituitary–gonadal axis in both sexes, impeding fertility. In females, high blood levels of progesterone in the follicular phase may interfere with the ability of estradiol to stimulate the luteinizing hormone surge, resulting in absent or irregular menses. In males, high levels of adrenal androgens may suppress the secretion of gonadotropins. Thus, although total circulating androgens are elevated, testosterone level in the testes may be low and spermatogenesis impaired. Fertility in both sexes is restored by treatment with glucocorticoids.

Molecular genetics of 21-hydroxylase deficiency

Reduction in, or loss of, function of the 21OH enzyme has been shown to result from a wide range of types of mutation in the gene coding for the enzyme (CYP21). Mutations include point mutations in coding regions (causing amino acid substitutions or termination), point mutations in introns (affecting mRNA splicing), short deletions/insertions (causing shift of the reading frame and early termination), and also large-scale DNA deletions, causing removal of the entire gene.

The gene locus for the 21OH enzyme is carried within the HLA major histocompatibility complex, which defines important transplantation antigens and is located on the short arm of chromosome 6. Its closest linkage is with the loci for the antigens encoding HLA-B and DR. Typing for these antigens provides a reliable means of tracking normal and CAH 21OH alleles in family studies. A number of types of 21OH deficiency have been found to be associated with specific HLA antigens or combinations of antigens ('haplotypes') in various populations.

In immediate proximity to the structural gene encoding $P450_c21$ is a very closely related, nonfunctional pseudogene (CYP21P) (Fig. 7.18). These 21OH genes alternate with the genes that encode the two forms of the fourth component of serum complement (C4B and C4A). As a result of the complex duplicated, alternating arrangement C4A-CYP21P-C4B-CYP21, misalignment of the pairing homologous chromosomes can occur during meiosis, producing complementary gametes with absence or further duplication of these genes. Unequal pairing with complete deletion of the CYP21B gene sequence causes the severe CAH haplotypes. A second cause of mutations is gene conversion, or replacement of segments of the active gene with the corresponding nucleotide sequence of the very similar pseudogene without reciprocal transfer of the true active gene segment. The mechanism of this event is not completely understood.

11β-Hydroxylase deficiency

Classic 11β-hydroxylase deficiency accounts for 5–8 percent of CAH in Europe and North America. In Israel, 20 percent of CAH is due to 11β-hydroxylase deficiency, an incidence of about 1 in 60 000 live births.

In this disorder, 11-deoxycortisol is not converted to cortisol. Ambiguous genitalia in the genetic female occur as in 21OH deficiency because of similar shunting into the pathways of androgen biosynthesis. The 11β-hydroxylase defect in the pathway of aldosterone synthesis leads to accumulation of deoxycorticosterone, whose mineralo-

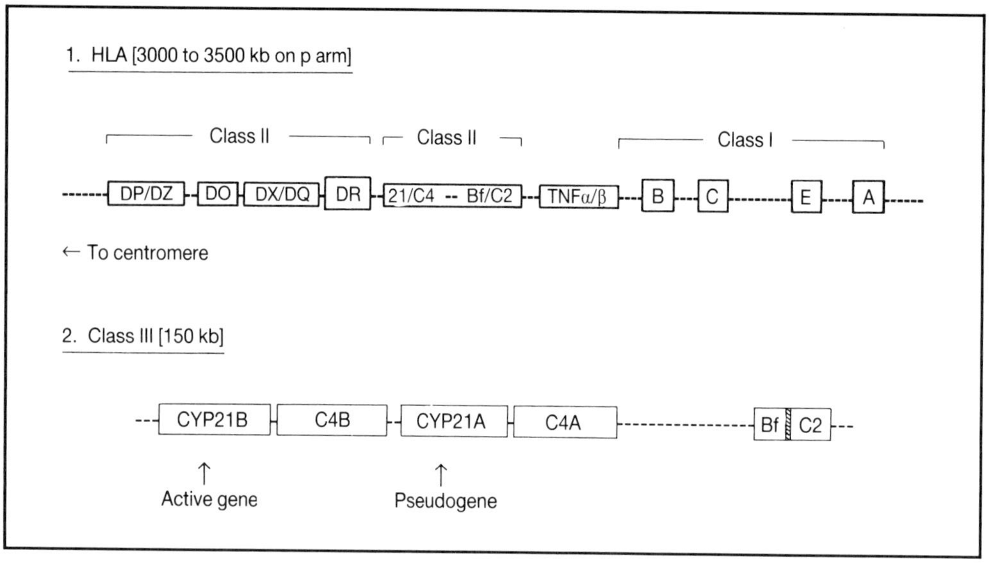

Fig. 7.18. (1) HLA region of chromosome 6. (2) Arrangement of 21OH active and pseudogenes.

corticoid activity may cause hypertension and hypokalemia. As with 21OH deficiency, there is considerable clinical heterogeneity in 11β-hydroxylase deficiency. The severity of hypertension is not strictly correlated with deoxycorticosterone levels.

A mild nonclassic form of this enzyme disorder, with mild symptoms of androgen excess like those of nonclassic 21OH deficiency and usually without hypertension, has been documented.

Two copies of the 11β-hydroxylase gene are found on the long arm of chromosome 8. There is 95 percent homology in the two genes. The first identified mutation was a single base substitution, or point mutation, in exon 8, codon 448, causing a substitution of histidine for arginine in the 11β-OH enzyme. Four mutations have now been identified in the B_1 gene in patients with classic and nonclassic 11β-hydroxylase deficiency.

Other CAH enzyme disorders

Diagnoses of all the remaining three enzyme defects account for less than 1 percent of reported cases of CAH. Mild or partial defects may occur more frequently.

3β-Hydroxysteroid dehydrogenase (3βHSD) deficiency

This disorder affects the synthesis of all classes of steroids. Levels of Δ^5-17-hydroxypregnenolone and dehydroepiandrosterone (DHEA) are elevated. While DHEA, a weak androgen, cannot be converted to androstenedione or testosterone in the adrenal of patients with 3βHSD, it is peripherally converted to bioactive androgens, suggesting that peripheral enzymes are under different genetic control.

In this enzyme disorder, while females may be slightly virilized because of peripheral conversion of DHEA, it is males who may suffer from genital ambiguity because of incomplete masculinization owing to feedback inhibition of synthesis of testosterone. In severe cases, salt-wasting occurs because of aldosterone deficiency. A nonclassic defect similar to NC21OH deficiency might be responsible for mild virilization of females.

17α-Hydroxylase deficiency

In the rare disorder 17α-hydroxylase deficiency, progesterone cannot be converted to 17α-hydroxyprogesterone, so that synthesis of cortisol is impaired. The $P450_c17$ enzyme has two functions. Its second action (called 17,20-lyase activity) is an essential step in sex steroid synthesis. It plays a vital role in sex steroid synthesis in both the adrenal and the gonads. As a result of 17α-hydroxyprogesterone deficiency, therefore, males are incompletely masculinized and adolescent females exhibit primary amenorrhea. The disorder presents to the clinician as hypertension in persons of either sex at any age and as primary amenorrhea in females at puberty.

Steroid 17α-hydroxylase appears to be coded for by a single-copy gene, located on chromosome 10. At least eight deviations from the normal coding sequence have been identified. Patients with this disorder, like those with 11-hydroxylase deficiency, have elevated deoxycorticosterone levels, hypokalemia and hypertension; they are distinguished by their high serum levels of corticosterone.

Lipoid adrenal hyperplasia

This disorder involves failure of cholesterol desmolase ($P450_{scc}$) activity, the first step in the common steroid biosynthetic pathway. The result is inhibition of all adrenal and gonadal steroidogenesis. Males are incompletely masculinized.

Selected reading

New MI, White PC, Pang S, *et al*. The adrenal hyperplasias. In Scriver CR, Beaudet AL, Sly WS, Valle D, eds. *The metabolic basis of inherited disease*. 6th ed. New York: McGraw-Hill, 1989: 1881.

Speiser PW, Laforgia N, Kato K, *et al*. First trimester prenatal treatment and molecular genetic diagnosis of congenital adrenal hyperplasia (21-hydroxylase deficiency). *J Clin Endocrinol Metab* 1990; **70**: 838.

H. Vasopressin and Oxytocin

P D Gluckman

The neurohypophyseal system

Anatomy

The two posterior pituitary hormones, arginine vasopressin (AVP), or antidiuretic hormone, and oxytocin (OT) are the neurosecretory products of hypothalamic neurons whose axons terminate in the posterior lobe and secrete directly into the systemic circulation. The cell bodies of these neurons lie within the paraventricular nucleus (PVN) and supraoptic nuclei (SON). Their axons traverse the inner zone of the median eminence to reach the posterior lobe. Also found within the posterior pituitary are glial-like small pituicytes. This direct neurosecretory system is in marked distinction from the hypothalamic control of anterior pituitary secretion (see p. 291).

The neurohypohyseal neurons arising in these two nuclei are very large as is the neurohypophyseal system, thus often termed the magnocellular system. Both OT and AVP staining neurons are found in both nuclei. While essentially all SON neurons are magnocellular and project to the posterior lobe, there are multiple cell types in the PVN including corticotropin releasing factor (CRF) neurons and small (parvicellular) AVP containing neurons that project to the median eminence. This subgroup of AVP neurons are believed to function in a manner analogous to other hypothalamic neurons regulating anterior pituitary function. These may costain for CRF and there is good evidence that AVP and CRF both interact in the control of ACTH release particularly in fetal life. Some AVP staining neurons are also found in the organum vasculosum of the lamina terminalis (OVLT), one of the circumventricular organs lying outside the blood–brain barrier (see p. 269).

Biochemistry

In man the only two neurohypophyseal hormones are AVP and OT. These are both nonapeptides with cysteines at positions 1 and 6 forming an N-terminal loop by a disulfide bond. Both hormones are synthesized as large prohormones which are transported in neurosecretory granules to the posterior lobe. Final post-translational modification occurs within these granules by proteolytic cleavage to release AVP or OT from the N-terminal. The large (10 kDa) other peptide derived from the prohormone is termed a neurophysin. The prohormones for OT and AVP are different. That for AVP is termed propressophysin and gives rise to AVP and neurophysin II; prooxyphysin gives rise to OT and neurophysin I.

Neurosecretion

There is good evidence that OT and AVP are secreted in response to specific firing patterns of the two respective classes of neurosecretory neurons. The AVP neurons generate action potentials leading to calcium-dependent exocytosis of the granules from the nerve terminals in a manner analogous to neurotransmitter release. Such action potentials are stimulated by hyperosmotic stimuli but the osmoreceptors are at least one synapse removed from the magnocellular neuron. Acetylcholine may be the critical intermediate neurotransmitter as nicotinic agents directly stimulate and muscarinic agents inhibit AVP release. This would explain the well known antidiuretic effect of smoking. While the neurophysins are coreleased with AVP or OT their biological significance remains uncertain. Other vasopressinergic neurons project from the PVN to the brainstem and limbic system. Vasopressin has thus been implicated as a neurotransmitter involved in a variety of functions including memory. Vasopressin is also secreted into the CSF from the suprachiasmatic nuclei in a diurnal rhythm—this may provide a wide ranging cue to the nervous system of the temporal state.

Vasopressin

Regulation of secretion

The most important stimulus to AVP release is an increase in plasma osmotic pressure. Osmoreceptors are concentrated in the anterior hypothalamus close to, but not within, the SON. They may be located outside the blood–brain barrier in the OVLT. These osmoreceptors appear to have a critical set point. Below an osmotic threshold of 280 mmol/kg, the secretion of AVP is low but above this point there is a steep rise in secretion (see Fig. 7.19). The sensitivity of this relationship may vary. The system is more sensitive to solutes such as sodium and mannitol and has little response to glucose and urea. This may reflect the different rate of solute transfer into the cell and thus differential effects on osmoreceptor cell volume.

Vasopressin release is also affected by changes in blood volume and blood pressure via baroreceptor reflexes. The afferent limb thus passes via the IXth and Xth nerves to the brainstem. The relationship between hypotension and AVP release is not linear, requiring at least a 10 percent fall before AVP release is enhanced. Any factor which alters blood volume or blood pressure may thus lead to changes in AVP secretion. These include posture, hemorrhage, changes in the renin–aldosterone system, catecholamine release, etc. In addition, the central angiotensin pathway stimulates AVP release. As angiotensin II is present both in the circumventricular subfornical organ and in the magnocellular nuclei, this neurotransmitter may be an important aspect of the link between peripheral fluid status and AVP release.

Nausea stimulates AVP release by a specific medullary pathway. Stress is also a potent stimulus—whether these effects are primary or mediated by the other mechanisms (e.g. the nausea pathway) or by central catecholaminergic mediated stimulation of AVP release is not certain.

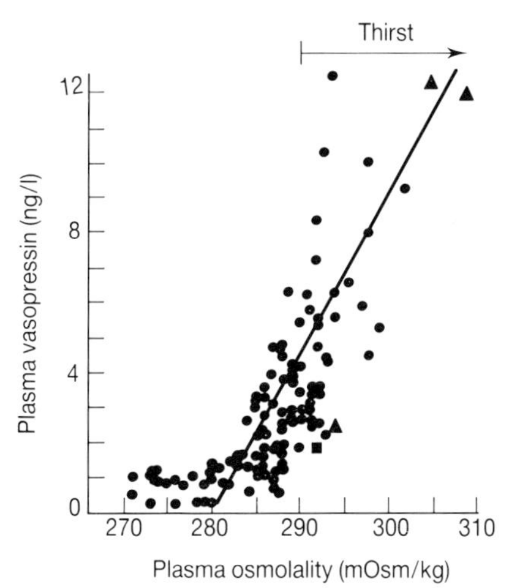

Fig. 7.19. The relationship between plasma osmolality and plasma AVP level. To convert AVP values to picomoles per liter, divide by 1.1. (Adapted from Robertson GL, Berl T. Pathophysiology of water metabolism. In Brenner BM, Rector FC. *The kidney*. Philadelphia: WB Saunders Co., 1991: 686. Reprinted with permission from WB Saunders Co.)

Actions of vasopressin

There are three classes of AVP receptor. The V_{1a} receptor is involved in pressor responses, the V_{1b} receptor in control of the corticotrope, and the V_2 receptor in control of water retention. The V_2 receptor is linked to a G_s-protein and acts via stimulation of cyclic AMP. The major action of AVP is to conserve water by promoting the absorption of solute-free water in the distal and collecting renal tubules. This system is intimately dependent on the countercurrent system of the loop of Henle and the interstitial osmotic gradient of the renal medulla, thus in *primary polydipsia* the efficiency of AVP is reduced (see p. 723). It is believed that AVP acts in the collecting ducts to stimulate the formation of 'water channels' on the apical surface of the cell. In the absence of AVP these channels reside intracellularly in endosomes and AVP stimulates their incorporation into the cell membrane.

AVP has extrarenal actions which include the stimulation of vascular smooth muscle constriction. This effect appears particularly important in the redistribution of blood flow in the fetal response to asphyxia. This pressor action is mediated by V_{1a} receptors. In the adenohypophysis AVP stimulates ACTH release and this appears to be an important aspect of the control of fetal ACTH release late in gestation where it is synergistic with corticotropin releasing factor (see p. 321).

Thirst (see also p. 261)

The related hypothalamic mechanism to preserve osmolality is thirst. This is stimulated by osmoreceptors in the OVLT and neighboring areas. However, they appear to be a distinct population from that involved in AVP regulation. The central angiotensin II pathway again appears to be a mediator of the effects of stimulating these osmoreceptors to promote thirst. Satiation of thirst is complex but depends primarily on restoring osmolality. The thirst mechanism is sufficiently powerful that in *diabetes insipidus* hypertonicity will not develop if there is free access to water. If, however, the *diabetes insipidus* is secondary to a lesion (e.g. *hypothalamic astrocytoma*) impinging on the thirst mechanism, the risk to the individual is severe.

Regulation of total body water and osmolality (see also p. 723)

AVP and thirst interact to maintain osmolality. Abnormalities in serum osmolality are more often a consequence of derangements in water balance rather than in sodium homeostasis. Normally when osmolality falls below 280 mmol/kg, AVP secretion is minimalized and the urine is maximally dilute and thirst is suppressed. The ability to excrete free water is such than an adult can ingest 20 l/day without water intoxication. As osmolality increases AVP secretion rises, leading to a reduction in free water clearance and thirst is driven. Thirst is only stimulated above an osmolality 290 mmol/kg. Thus a standardized water deprivation test is the easiest way of examining the AVP axis. Water deprivation should lead to an increase in AVP once plasma osmolality increases above 280 mmol/kg and urinary osmolality should consequently rise. Failure to increase urinary osmolality may be a reflection of *central diabetes insipidus*, of *nephrogenic diabetes insipidus*, which may be hereditary due to an X-linked defect in V_2 receptors or rarely acquired secondary to some drugs (e.g. methoxyflurane), or secondary to other electrolyte disturbances (hypercalcemia, hypokalemia), which affect the ability of the renal tubule to respond to AVP. Where renal medullary solute concentrations are reduced, as in *psychogenic polydipsia*, maximal urinary osmolality is also reduced. In *nephrogenic diabetes insipidus*, plasma AVP levels will be elevated.

Increases in plasma osmolality are primarily associated with elevations in plasma Na^+ which does not cross cell membranes. In *diabetes mellitus* the lack of insulin means that glucose entry is reduced and thus can lead to hyperosmolality. The major causes of hypernatremia are abnormalities of thirst (e.g. *hypothalamic tumors*), excessive fluid loss via the kidney (*diabetes insipidus*), skin (*burns*) or gut (*diarrhea*). Increased solute load, as in *diabetic ketoacidosis* or iatrogenic Na^+ loading, can cause hyperosmolality.

Decreases in plasma osmolality can occur if water intake is in excess of the maximal renal excretory capacity (*primary polydipsia*), or more frequently because the kidney is unable to excrete a maximally dilute urine. This can occur in the syndrome of *inappropriate ADH secretion* where AVP release escapes osmotic control. This may be due to cerebral disorders or ectopic tumor production. Hyponatremia can also be associated with a reduction in sodium delivery to the renal medulla. This may be associated with either increased or reduced extracellular fluid volume. The former can occur in advanced *heart failure* or *cirrhosis*. The latter may occur with loop diuretic abuse but in pediatrics the most important cause is *adrenal insufficiency* leading to volume depletion and thus elevated AVP levels, as well as reducing renal sodium retention. Extrarenal losses of solute via the skin (burns, sweating) or gut can also cause hyponatremia.

Developmental aspects

The neurohypophyseal system is anatomically mature by the end of the first trimester and AVP is present in the fetal pituitary by 12 weeks. The importance of AVP to fetal cardiovascular hemostasis is reviewed on p. 337. Hypoxemia is a potent stimulus to fetal AVP release and AVP has major effects on the redistribution of fetal blood flow. AVP, while active in the fetal kidney, is less effective because of the reduced medullary osmotic gradient and the low glomerular filtration rate. AVP levels are high immediately after birth. This may be important both to cardiovascular homeostasis during the physiological asphyxia of birth and may also promote fetal lung fluid resorption. While regulatory mechanisms appear fully mature at birth the ability to maximally concentrate urine is relatively reduced as a consequence of the immaturity in renal medullary osmotic gradient.

Oxytocin

Regulation of secretion

The regulation of OT secretion is coupled tightly to its specific reproductive related functions. Sucking of the nipple leads, via a neural reflex, to OT release. Similarly, vaginal or cervical distension leads to OT release. The consequent patterns of oxytocinergic neuron firing and thus of OT release differ between these two stimuli. Other factors can impinge on OT release. For example, opioids inhibit OT release, perhaps giving an explanation of how stress can interfere with effective lactation.

Actions

Oxytocin acts at specific membrane located receptors which probably act via cyclic AMP activation. OT receptors in the myometrium are increased late in pregnancy by estrogens. Until labor is imminent the uterus is insensitive to OT. The role of OT in the late phase of labor remains controversial. It is likely that its role is largely limited to the expulsive phase. There are interactions between the OT system and the prostaglandins. These may increase uterine sensitivity to OT and OT acts on the decidua to stimulate PG production. There is a rapid decline in uterine OT receptors after birth to reduce uterine sensitivity while maintaining mammary sensitivity. OT receptors in mammary myoepithelial cells are essential to milk ejection. OT receptors are found in other sites and OT itself is synthesized within other tissues such as the gonads, where a number of possible paracrine roles have been suggested. For example, testicular OT has been suggested to play a role in seminiferous tubule contraction. OT in pharmacological doses can be antidiuretic leading to water intoxication if used inappropriately in the induction of labor.

Developmental aspects

OT is present in the fetal pituitary by the end of the first trimester. Its levels are markedly elevated in cord blood: the biological significance is unknown.

Suggested reading

Reeves WB, Andreali TE. The posterior pituitary and water metabolism. In Wilson JD, Foster DW, eds. *Williams textbook of endocrinology*. 8th ed. Philadelphia: WB Saunders, 1992: 311.

Soloff MS, Fuchs A, Fuchs F. Oxytocin receptors and the onset of parturition. In Albrecht E, Pepe G, eds. *Perinatal endocrinology*. Ithaca: Perinatalogy Press, 1985: 289.

I. Hormonal Regulation of the Cardiovascular System, Fluids and Electrolytes

H S Iwamoto

Cardiovascular, fluid, and electrolyte homeostasis are effectively maintained by precise monitoring and regulation of blood pressure, blood volume, and plasma osmolality. A considerable array of systemic and local, sensory and effector mechanisms participate in these functions. Systemic sensory mechanisms include arterial and cardiopulmonary receptors, which monitor blood pressure and volume, and osmoreceptors located in the central nervous system. Input from these and other sensory mechanisms, and from the central nervous system, converges on centers in the hypothalamus and medulla. Output from these centers regulates neural efferent activity and hormone secretion. The response depends upon the degree to which neurohormonal stimulation is modified by the action of other neurotransmitters and hormones and by a complex network of sensory, metabolic, growth and paracrine factors local to epithelial cells and blood vessels. The net response to an abnormality in blood volume, blood pressure, or plasma osmolality is an integration of the action of a number of systemic and local response mechanisms.

Integration is not confined to the level of the target organ. Within the central nervous system, there is complex interaction of sensory inputs and integration among neuropeptide systems. Nerves containing angiotensin II, vasopressin, and atrial natriuretic peptide and receptors specific for these neuropeptides are located in areas of the brain that have been implicated in cardiovascular and fluid regulation. Centrally administered neuropeptide agonists and antagonists alter blood pressure, blood flow, heart rate, renal function, thirst, baroreflex sensitivity, and the secretion of other neuropeptides. Many of these responses result from interactions among neuropeptide systems and interactions with the sympathetic and parasympathetic nervous systems.

Blood pressure, volume, and osmolality are affected in large part by changes in blood vessel caliber or by changes in epithelial cell permeability to water or Na^+. Because over 30 distinct substances can modify one or many of these processes, redundancy is a prominent characteristic among mechanisms that regulate cardiovascular and fluid homeostasis. This redundancy helps to ensure that blood pressure and volume and plasma osmolality are maintained within narrow limits. Although redundancy is an important feature of homeostatic mechanisms, one should keep in mind that redundancy and compensatory actions make it virtually impossible to define the entire role for each regulatory mechanism.

The discussion in this section is limited to vasopressin, the renin–angiotensin–aldosterone system, and atrial natriuretic peptide (ANP). Additional mechanisms that affect cardiovascular and fluid and electrolyte homeostasis, i.e. other hormones, neuropeptides, local factors, prostaglandins (PGs), and peripheral and central nervous system function, are covered elsewhere (see p. 451).

The renin–angiotensin–aldosterone system

The renin–angiotensin–aldosterone system is generated by a number of components in a cascade of enzymatic reactions (Fig. 7.20). Renin is a highly specific aspartyl protease that converts angiotensinogen, an α_2-globulin, to angiotensin I, a decapeptide. Carboxypeptidase converting enzyme or angiotensin converting enzyme (ACE) or kininase II, a single-chain polypeptide anchored in plasma membranes, cleaves two amino acid residues from angiotensin I to form the octapeptide angiotensin II (AII). AII stimulates zona glomerulosa cells of the adrenal cortex to produce aldosterone. The classic systemic renin–angiotensin system is generated in blood from renin synthesized by juxtaglomerular cells in the kidney, angiotensinogen synthesized by the liver, and converting enzyme residing in endothelial cells, particularly in the lung. Additional complete systems reside within the brain, kidney, uterus, adrenal, ovary, testes, submaxillary gland,

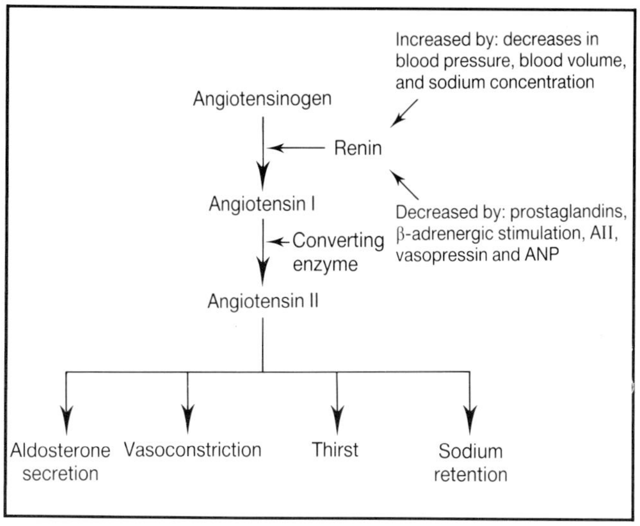

Fig. 7.20. Basic components of the renin–angiotensin system. See text for details.

and blood vessels and are believed to act locally near the site of AII generation.

The systemic renin–angiotensin–aldosterone system is regulated by a number of factors. Renin secretion is increased by decreases in systemic and renal arterial blood pressures, salt intake, and sodium chloride delivery to the macula densa of the kidney, by increases in PGE_2 and PGI_2 concentrations, β_1-adrenergic stimulation, and renal nerve stimulation, and by hypoxia, perhaps by a mechanism independent of adrenergic stimulation. Renin secretion is decreased by AII, vasopressin, and ANP. Angiotensinogen is available in excess in the adult; however, in pregnant women and preterm and term neonates, renin appears to be available in excess and angiotensinogen, rather than renin, may be rate limiting. Angiotensinogen secretion is increased by AII, adrenocorticotropic hormone (ACTH), estrogens, glucocorticoids, and thyroxine. AII is the primary regulator of aldosterone secretion, but additionally, ACTH stimulates, and ANP, high plasma Na^+, and low K^+ inhibit aldosterone secretion (see p. 323).

The active components of this system are AII and aldosterone. AII is a potent cardiovascular agent that increases blood pressure, heart rate, and myocardial contractility. AII mediates some cardiovascular effects through direct action on the heart (increased Ca^{2+} transport) and blood vessels (vasoconstriction), but also exerts actions via the sympathetic nervous system by facilitating catecholamine release by the adrenal medulla and sympathetic nerve terminals and by activating neural pathways in the central nervous system, which increase sympathetic outflow. AII increases extracellular fluid volume by stimulating thirst and aldosterone secretion, and by promoting Na^+ reabsorption in the proximal and distal renal tubules. Recently AII has been shown in a variety of tissues to have potentially important growth-promoting effects mediated by increasing expression of genes and proto-oncogenes (c-*myc*, c-*fos*, c-*jun*) for epidermal growth factor and platelet derived growth factor. Aldosterone promotes reabsorption of Na^+ and secretion of H^+ and K^+ in the distal renal tubule and alters ion transport in salivary glands, intestine, and sweat glands.

The actions of AII are mediated by at least two specific membrane receptors, AT1 and AT2. AT1 is the most abundant receptor type in the adult, is located in vascular smooth muscle, adrenal, and brain. Activation of AT1 receptors activates G_p-protein, which increases phosphatidylinositol turnover, and G_i-protein, which inhibits adenylyl cyclase. AT1 receptors are believed to mediate most of the cardiovascular and fluid actions of AII. The second receptor type, AT2, the most abundant receptor type in the fetus and newborn, is present in many organs including skeletal muscle, brain, skin, stomach, and duodenum and is localized mainly in mesenchymal tissue. At present, specific actions mediated by AT2 are unknown. However, because AT2 is widely distributed and because receptor numbers decrease precipitously after birth, AT2 may be important for cellular differentiation and fetal development.

Developmental aspects

Fetus

The renin–angiotensin system is more active during the perinatal period than later in life. Young animals have a superior ability to maintain blood pressure after hemorrhage that is dependent upon intact kidneys but not intact arterial baroreceptors. In contrast, fetal and neonatal renal responses to aldosterone are less active than in the adult. The components of the renin–angiotensin system in the fetus are derived from fetal sources. Plasma renin activity (PRA), the quantity of angiotensin I generated upon incubation of plasma, which is dependent upon renin and angiotensinogen concentrations, is significantly higher and more variable in the fetus than in the adult. Fetal nephrectomy decreases basal levels of PRA and AII concentrations and abolishes responses to furosemide in the fetus but not the mother.

The renin–angiotensin–aldosterone system develops early in fetal life. In the human fetus, renin immunoreactivity in the kidney is detectable by 5 weeks of gestation. In fetal rats, renin immunoreactivity and gene expression are initially detectable in the afferent interlobular and arcuate arteries. In the neonate, renin is located only in the afferent arterioles, and by 90 days after birth the amount of renin-specific mRNA decreases and is confined to the juxtaglomerular apparatus. A notable exception occurs in the adult when renin secretion is elevated secondary to converting enzyme inhibition, at which time renin gene expression expands to the arcuate arteries to recruit additional renin-secreting cells. Angiotensinogen immunoreactivity and gene expression are much lower in the fetus than in the newborn and adult. During the latter portion of gestation in sheep, hemorrhage, hypotension, bilateral carotid occlusion, β-adrenergic stimulation, and hypoxemia stimulate the renin–angiotensin system and increase PRA and AII concentrations. Cortisol inhibits renin release.

Although fetal concentrations of renin and angiotensin exceed those in pregnant and nonpregnant humans or animals, whether the renin–angiotensin system normally regulates fetal cardiovascular function remains undecided. When PRA is elevated slightly, AII in part maintains arterial blood pressure and blood flow to the umbilical–placental circulation. When PRA is low, AII appears to exert little or no cardiovascular effect.

The renin–angiotensin system plays an important role in maintaining fetal cardiovascular homeostasis in response to hemorrhage. Rapid removal of 15–20 percent of the circulating blood volume produces hypotension and bradycardia, and decreases combined ventricular output and blood flow to the umbilical–placental, peripheral, pulmonary, and renal circulations. When AII is inhibited, hemorrhage decreases heart rate, arterial blood pressure, combined ventricular output, and blood flow to the umbilical–placental and renal circulations dramatically. Some of these actions may not be direct, but rather mediated via the sympathetic nervous system as AII increases baroreceptor sensitivity in fetal sheep and may influence sympathetic nerve transmission.

Aldosterone has minimal effects in the fetus. Aldosterone administration to fetal sheep decreases the urinary Na^+/K^+ ratio, a measure of aldosterone action. Inhibition of endogenous aldosterone action with spironolactone produces the opposite effect. Although these data indicate that aldosterone modifies fetal renal function, the effects are small relative to those in the adult. The possible reasons for the smaller response in the fetus are: (1) fetuses have high concentrations of placental progesterone and deoxycorticosterone that compete for the aldosterone receptor; and (2) the fetal kidney does not retain as great a proportion of filtered Na^+ as does the adult kidney (see p. 706).

Neonate

PRA, AII, and aldosterone concentrations increase at birth and fall to low levels within 1–3 weeks. The increase at birth is magnified by prematurity, labor, vaginal delivery, and Na^+ depletion. Factors responsible for the normal increase at birth include stress of labor and delivery, sympathetic stimulation, hypotension, a decrease in metabolic clearance rate, an increase in prostaglandins, low glomerular filtration rate, and renal glomerulotubular imbalance. The increase in PRA may be due, in part, to an increase in hepatic angiotensinogen gene expression stimulated by the prenatal surge in fetal cortisol secretion, although this is not resolved. The increase in aldosterone concentration is not related to plasma AII concentration and may be regulated by another factor such as ACTH.

The renin–angiotensin system appears to be important at birth because captopril, an inhibitor of converting enzyme, reduces arterial blood pressure, glomerular filtration rate, and renal blood flow, increases renal vascular resistance, and causes fetal death. Although AII may contribute to the increase in blood pressure after birth, it does not sustain blood pressure in the infant as basal concentrations decrease while arterial blood pressure remains constant. Aldosterone increases Na^+ reabsorption by the newborn kidney, but overall effectiveness is limited by the relative immaturity of the renal tubule and Na^+ transport mechanisms. If aldosterone is not available after birth, plasma K^+ and PRA increase. After 2 weeks of aldosterone deprivation, so much Na^+ is lost that vasopressin and urine osmolality increase, and hyponatremia, hyperkalemia, and acidosis can result. The most common causes of neonatal hypoaldosteronism are associated with *adrenogenital syndrome* but isolated *disorders of aldosterone synthesis* involving the enzymes 18-methyl oxidase I or II, the enzymes involved in converting corticosterone to aldosterone (see p. 326), may also occur. *Pseudohypoaldosteronism* is a rare salt-losing syndrome of infancy: these infants appear to have defects in the mineralocorticoid receptor.

The mineralocorticoid receptor has high affinity for both aldosterone and cortisol. Specificity of aldosterone action is achieved by the presence of an enzyme in the kidney, 11β-hydroxysteroid dehydrogenase, which converts cortisol to low affinity metabolites. *11β-Hydroxysteroid dehydrogenase deficiency* may cause low renin hypertension as cortisol acts in this situation like aldosterone. Similarly licorice appears to cause hypokalemia by interfering with this enzyme. In the 11β-hydroxylase deficiency form of *adrenogenital syndrome* the increased 11-desoxycorticosterone acts at the mineralocorticoid receptor and may induce hypertension.

Vasopressin

Vasopressin, or antidiuretic hormone, or arginine vasopressin (AVP) is synthesized by magnocellular and parvocellular neurons in the supraoptic and paraventricular hypothalamic nuclei and by parvocellular neurons in the suprachiasmatic nucleus. Magnocellular neurons have nerve endings in the posterior pituitary and release vasopressin into the blood primarily in response to volume depletion, hyperosmolality, and stress. Parvocellular neurons project to several areas of the central nervous system, including the nucleus of the tractus solitarius, an important site in the cardiovascular regulatory pathway. Vasopressin secretion is increased by increased stretch of cardiopulmonary afferents and increases in plasma osmolality. Further details about the biosynthesis and regulation of vasopressin are provided elsewhere (see p. 330).

Vasopressin plays important roles in cardiovascular and fluid homeostasis. Vasopressin exerts its actions by interacting with at least three receptor types, V_{1a}, V_{1b}, and V_2. The V_2 receptors, located in the collecting duct and thick ascending limb in the kidney, are linked to adenylyl cyclase. Activation of these receptors in the collecting duct increases cAMP generation and promotes aggregation of proteins into water channels in the cell membrane. This permits water to move down its concentration gradient from the tubular lumen to the hypertonic medullary interstitium and decreases free water clearance. Activation of V_{1a} receptors activates Ca^{2+}-dependent inositol phosphate turnover, which constricts vascular smooth muscle and increases glycogenolysis in hepatocytes. The vasoconstrictor action is not particularly significant under normal conditions, but becomes important when blood volume or blood pressure is reduced or when other regulatory mechanisms are impaired. V_{1b} receptors are located on anterior pituitary cells and influence ACTH secretion by the anterior pituitary. Other actions ascribed to vasopressin include inhibition of renin secretion, sensitization of baroreceptor input, and increases and decreases in sympathetic nervous activity. The receptor subtypes and intracellular messengers that mediate these responses have not been clearly defined.

Developmental aspects

Fetus

Vasopressin is detectable in the human fetal hypothalamus as early as 11 weeks of gestation. Immunocytochemical studies in sheep during the last third of gestation show that AVP-containing neurons in the paraventricular and supraoptic nuclei project a network of fibers to the posterior and anterior pituitary glands and the median eminence.

Fetal vasopressin secretion is increased by hyperosmolality, hypovolemia, hypotension, epinephrine, vena caval obstruction, hypoxemia, and acidemia to an extent that increases with gestational age.

Under basal conditions vasopressin plays little role in circulatory regulation because inhibition of V_1 receptors does not alter fetal heart rate, arterial blood pressure, or organ blood flow. However, vasopressin does play an important role in the fetal response to acute intrauterine stress. Producing physiological concentrations of vasopressin in fetal sheep leads to cardiovascular changes similar to those caused by acute hypoxemia. Vasopressin infusion increases arterial and venous blood pressures and decreases heart rate in a dose-dependent fashion. Vasopressin also decreases blood flow to the intestine and skeletal muscle and increases the proportion of blood flow to the placenta, heart, and brain. This redistribution of blood flow accounts for the increases in oxygen delivery to the fetus and in fetal blood oxygen saturation observed during vasopressin infusion. Inhibition of V_1 receptors in hypoxemic fetuses decreases blood pressure and blood flow to the brain and heart, increases heart rate and blood flow to the placenta and intestine, but does not change blood flow to muscle and bone. However, it is not clear whether these responses were due solely to V_1 inhibition or to the local effects of hypoxemia and acidemia. Vasopressin participates in the fetal response to hypotensive hemorrhage by maintaining arterial blood pressure and increasing catecholamine secretion. Vasopressin also increases ACTH and cortisol secretion.

Fluid and electrolyte regulation

Vasopressin administration to fetal sheep elicits a prompt decrease in free water clearance. The degree to which urine is maximally concentrated in the fetus is about a quarter that in the adult. This is not related to an inability to respond to vasopressin, but rather is a measure of the low GFR and filtration fraction and shallow medullary interstitial osmotic gradient of the fetal kidney.

Vasopressin influences the acquisition of fluid by the fetus via both placental and extraplacental transfer mechanisms. Fetal vasopressin infusion increases amniotic fluid vasopressin concentrations and osmolality. Intra-amniotic infusion increases fetal blood vasopressin concentrations. Vasopressin in the amniotic fluid is derived from endogenous fetal sources and recirculates to the fetal circulation in biologically active form. The physiological significance of these actions appears to be related to fluid homeostasis.

Perinatal vasopressin treatment has been reported to decrease the number of renal vasopressin receptors and increase the sensitivity of isolated aortic strips later in life. These effects extend into adult life and support the concept that intrauterine stress may have long-lasting consequences that are mediated by vasopressin, a concept that should be investigated in more detail.

Newborn

Plasma vasopressin concentrations increase after the onset of labor and are greater following vaginal than cesarean delivery. Hypoxemia and acidemia or epinephrine secretion secondary to labor contractions, umbilical cord compression, and head compression may be responsible for the increase. The increase in vasopressin concentrations may play a role in lung fluid reabsorption at birth, which is necessary for the initiation of breathing and lung gas exchange. Vasopressin infusion has been shown to decrease lung fluid production in late gestation fetal sheep and goats. However, epinephrine is more important in this regard.

At birth, the kidneys assume responsibility for regulating fluid excretion, and total body and extracellular fluid volumes decrease. During the first few days of life, natriuresis and diuresis normally occur. The extent to which vasopressin mediates these changes is unknown. Vasopressin, along with epinephrine, may increase hepatic glycogenolysis after birth.

In the newborn, vasopressin has both pressor and antidiuretic activity. The action of vasopressin in the newborn does not differ from that in the adult, although maximal responses may be lower due to immaturity of receptors or of ability to activate intracellular response cascades. The increase in plasma vasopressin concentrations at birth may be responsible, in part, for the increase in arterial blood pressure that occurs at birth. However, plasma concentrations decrease within 2 days after birth, whereas blood pressure continues to rise.

Atrial natriuretic peptide

In 1981 cardiac atria of adult mammals were found to synthesize a substance that produces natriuresis, diuresis, and vasorelaxation and decreases intravascular volume. Although this substance is also synthesized by other tissues (brain, aortic arch, lung, anterior pituitary, adrenals, thyroid), and produces actions in addition to natriuresis, and appears not to be a single peptide but a family of peptides, this substance is commonly referred to as atrial natriuretic peptide (ANP, the term used in this section) or atrial natriuretic factor. In the human, plasma ANP is synthesized as preproANP, a 151 amino acid precursor, which is cleaved to proANP (1–126), the storage form. The active cardiac form is ANP (99–126), also termed ANP (1–28), which is formed upon secretion. There are minor species- and tissue-specific variations in structure, but common to all members of this hormone family is a structure that contains a 17 amino acid loop formed by an intramolecular disulfide linkage.

ANP secretion is increased by atrial stretch secondary to hypervolemia or tachycardia. ANP is increased also by glucocorticoids, hyperosmolality, hypernatremia, hypoxia, acetylcholine, thyroid hormone, epinephrine, vasopressin, and AII. Plasma concentrations are increased considerably prenatally, postnatally, and in pregnancy, three periods when plasma volume is expanded. ANP is also increased in patients with congenital heart disease in which there is volume loading and congestive heart failure, e.g. *patent ductus arteriosus* or *ventricular septal defect*, in *systemic hypertension* and in fetuses with *immune hydrops*.

ANP influences cardiovascular and fluid homeostasis by a variety of mechanisms. ANP dilates afferent renal arterioles and constricts efferent arterioles, resulting in increased GFR and filtration fraction. ANP also decreases reabsorption of Na^+ in the proximal tubule and collecting duct by direct and indirect means. These actions significantly increase sodium chloride excretion by the kidney. ANP produces diuresis as a consequence of the natriuresis and also because ANP decreases vasopressin secretion. ANP decreases arterial blood pressure by relaxing vascular smooth muscle, and by decreasing cardiac output. Physiological amounts of ANP inhibit thyroid hormone, renin, and aldosterone secretion and alter sympathetic nerve transmission. Thus ANP modulates responses of the renin–angiotensin system, vasopressin, and adrenergic mechanisms and local vascular modulators.

The biological actions of ANP result from interaction of ANP with one of at least three receptors, ANPR-A, ANPR-B, and ANPR-C. Each of these receptors has a conserved extracellular domain and transmembrane portion. Up to 95 percent of ANP receptors are of the third type, ANPR-C. The ANPR-C lacks a long intracellular portion, and intermediates in the response to ANPR-C activation have not been clearly defined. Because the ANPR-C binds ANP and ANP fragments with equal affinity (a feature not shared with the other receptors) and does not have a significant intracellular domain, the idea has been proposed that ANPR-C are important for clearing ANP from the circulation. Their abundance probably accounts for the short circulation half-life (2–4 minutes) of ANP. ANPR-A and ANPR-B both have intracellular portions consisting of kinase and guanylyl cyclase domains. Interaction of ANP with ANPR-A and ANPR-B activates particulate guanylyl cyclase and increases accumulation of cGMP. This stimulates cGMP-dependent protein kinases and increases protein phosphorylation. This interaction also results in dephosphorylation of myosin light chains and decreases intracellular Ca^{2+}, an obligatory step in vasorelaxation. ANP may also exert its actions by inhibiting adenylyl cyclase (a potential mechanism by which cAMP-dependent hormone actions are modulated) and decreasing intracellular Ca^{2+}. Specific receptors have been identified in the kidney, adrenal, blood vessels, brain, eye, hepatocytes, colon, and lung, but their function has not been entirely delineated.

Developmental aspects

Fetus

ANP is detectable in cardiac atria and ventricles soon after organogenesis is complete. The concentration of immunoreactive ANP and abundance of ANP-specific mRNA is higher in the cardiac ventricles than in the atria. During the neonatal period, ANP content gradually declines in the ventricles and increases in the atria, reaching adult levels by about 2 weeks after birth. The significance of this postnatal adjustment is not clear but may be related to an important change in ANP function in the perinatal period. A decrease in right ventricular production following the postnatal decrease in afterload may contribute.

ANP is detectable in fetal blood in concentrations greater than those in maternal samples obtained simultaneously or in the nonpregnant adult. The source of ANP in the fetus is primarily myocardial; synthesis is particularly high in the right atrium and ventricle as evidenced by high ANP concentrations in pulmonary arterial blood as compared with carotid arterial and descending aortic blood. Stimuli that increase fetal ANP concentrations include expansion of the blood volume by saline infusion in sheep fetuses, blood transfusion in human fetuses, and blood volume expansion secondary to spontaneous or experimentally induced hydrops. Fetal ANP also increases in response to hyperosmolality, hypoxemia, atrial hypertension secondary to pulmonary artery occlusion, ventilation with oxygen, and birth.

Specific binding sites for ANP have been identified in fetal blood vessels, brain, lung, and liver. When ANP is infused at rates that increase plasma concentrations to values observed following volume expansion, ANP has only minimal effects on renal function, arterial blood pressure, and heart rate but produces significant increases in blood protein concentration and hematocrit and decreases in fetal blood volume. ANP in larger amounts increases GFR and urinary excretion of Na^+, K^+, Cl^-, Ca^{2+}, and free water. ANP also constricts the umbilical–placental vascular bed and decreases umbilical–placental blood flow and combined ventricular output. Systemic ANP decreases renal blood flow velocity and increases renal vascular resistance by an action attributable not to a direct effect of ANP on the renal vasculature, but rather to activation of compensatory vasoconstrictor mechanisms.

Attempts to determine the role of endogenous ANP during fetal life have been hampered by the absence of a specific inhibitor of ANP action. Recently, however, endogenous ANP has been neutralized by administration of polyclonal antibodies directed against ANP. Plasma ANP concentrations decreased and remained low following antibody injection. The effects were mostly renal; urine flow rate decreased, as did Na^+, K^+, and Cl^- excretion, and blood volume increased. There were transient increases in heart rate and arterial blood pressure, probably due to transitory compensation by another cardiovascular regulatory mechanism such as AII.

Newborn

At birth, ANP concentrations in plasma increase and remain high for about 10 days. In children with *patent ductus arteriosus* or other *congenital heart disease* with elevated atrial pressures, ANP concentrations remain elevated for an extended period of time. This is probably related to the effects of preload or afterload on right atrial and ventricular production of ANP. In fetal sheep, occlusion of the pulmonary artery increases right atrial pressure and ANP secretion. ANP may play a role in decreasing pulmonary vascular resistance at birth. In fetal sheep, plasma ANP concentrations increase during rhythmic pulmonary ventilation with oxygen, and intrapulmonary infusion of ANP decreases pulmonary vascular resistance and increases pulmonary blood flow. Further studies are required to determine whether ANP is an important regulator of pulmonary blood flow at birth.

Perinatal increases in ANP may also be responsible for the natriuresis that commonly occurs after birth and for the redistribution of body water and electrolytes in the newborn, but further investigation is required to establish this relationship.

Selected reading

Ervin MG. Perinatal fluid and electrolyte regulation: role of arginine vasopressin. *Semin Perinatol* 1988; **12**: 134.

Gomez RA, Chevalier RL, Carey RM, Peach MJ. Molecular biology of the renal renin–angiotensin system. *Kidney Int* 1990; **38**: S18.

Reid JL, Rubin PC. Peptides and central neural regulation of the circulation. *Physiol Rev* 1987; **67**: 725.

Smith FG, Sato T, Varille VA, Robillard JE. Atrial natriuretic factor during fetal and postnatal life: a review. *J Dev Physiol* 1989; **12**: 55.

Symonds EM. Renin and reproduction. *Am J Obstet Gynecol* 1988; **158**: 754.

J. The Adrenal Medulla

J F Padbury

Embryology and development

The adrenal medulla is composed of hormone-containing cells and neuronal cells which arise early (8 mm stage in man) in fetal development from neural crest anlage. These neural crest precursors migrate to scattered retroperitoneal locations throughout the abdomen. Primordial neural crest cells are capable of differentiation along primary endocrine (chromaffin) or neuronal (sympathetic) lines. *Neuroblastoma* arise from these primitive neural crest cells. The chromaffin reaction, a traditional designation, refers to the characteristic appearance of catecholamine-containing cells on dichromate staining under light microscopy. The eventual location and local endocrine milieu of these neural crest precursors determines in great measure their final phenotypic expression. Cells residing within the confines of the adrenal and exposed to the high local concentrations of glucocorticoids express the endocrine phenotype and eventually contain high concentrations of epinephrine. Cells located more centrally within the medulla, and also scattered throughout the medullary tissue, retain neuronal characteristics, are capable of elaborating neurites and do not contain epinephrine.

In the majority of mammalian species, during fetal and early neonatal life there are additional collections of chromaffin-positive cells scattered throughout the retroperitoneum. These extra-adrenal chromaffin cells are unique to early development and involute spontaneously during postnatal life, e.g. by 1 year of age in the human. In some species, e.g. human and rabbit, these cells are discrete glandular structures known as extra-adrenal glands, para-aortic tissue or the organs of Zuckerkandl. The extra-adrenal glands, as distinct from adrenal medullary chromaffin cells, contain high concentrations of norepinephrine but do not express the enzyme phenylethanolamine *N*-methyltransferase (PNMT) and thus neither synthesize nor contain epinephrine.

Biochemistry

The catecholamines dopamine (DA), norepinephrine (NE) and epinephrine (E) are synthesized and stored in subcellular organelles known as granules or vesicles. Postganglionic sympathetic neurons, also derived from neural crest, contain small, 'dense' noradrenergic vesicles whereas epinephrine-containing adrenal medullary granules are larger and lighter by electron microscopy. The biosynthetic pathway for catecholamines is shown in Fig. 3.5 (p. 75). Tyrosine hydroxylase is the rate-limiting enzyme in catecholamine biosynthesis. PNMT is the final enzyme in the pathway and catalyzes the conversion of norepinephrine to epinephrine. PNMT is only expressed in adrenal medullary cells and in a few specific nuclei within the brainstem and central nervous system. While adrenal medullary chromaffin cells are differentiated along a final pathway for synthesis and secretion of catecholamines, they also contain other neurotransmitters/neuropeptides. The relative content of each of the other neurotransmitters, neuropeptides, proteins, purines and other molecules from adult bovine tissue is shown in Table 7.2. Thus while *pheochromocytomas* which are chromaffin cell tumors primarily secrete norepinephrine and epinephrine, they may also secrete many other bioactive substances.

During fetal development there are important maturational changes in the relative abundance of the primary catecholamines. PNMT is not expressed until after maturation of the adrenal cortical tissue and production of high local glucocorticoid concentrations. The adrenal epinephrine content is thus a relative marker for maturation and does not become the primary amine until 0.8 gestation in the sheep, 0.7 gestation in the rabbit, 0.8 in the rat. In the human, limited studies suggest that it is comparable to these other species. In contrast, the epinephrine/norepinephrine ratio of extra-adrenal tissue does not exceed 0.1 unless epinephrine synthesis is induced by exogenous glucocorticoid administration.

There are relatively few developmental studies of the content of the other neurotransmitters/peptides. As seen

Table 7.2. Relative molecular content in a single chromaffin granule

Constituent	Content
Total catecholamines (DA, NE, E)	1000
Purine nucleotides (ATP, adenosine)	310
Calcium	30
Ascorbic acid	40
Chromogranin A	1.6
Chromogranin B	0.03
Total enkephalin (ENK) immunoreactivity	1.3
Free ENK (penta, hexa, hepta, octapeptides)	0.09
Neuropeptide Y	0.1
Dynorphin	0.003
Neurotensin	0.0003
Substance P	0.00015
Dopamine β-hydroxylase	0.05

Adapted from Winkler, 1986.

in Table 7.2, proenkephalin derived peptides are the most abundant of the adrenal medullary neuropeptides. In the developing rabbit, the low molecular weight (penta-octapeptide) forms of enkephalin represent 40–50 percent of the total enkephalin immunoreactivity until postnatal life, then the percentage decreases into adulthood when it drops to less than 10 percent. In sheep, a more precocial species, the low molecular weight pentapeptides increase in relative abundance with advancing gestation. There are no comparable developmental studies in the human. In adults of most species the adrenal medulla and brain striatum contain the highest quantities of enkephalin peptides. The brain content is highly processed (>90 percent) to the low molecular weight forms and the adrenal contains predominantly the prohormone proenkephalin. Interestingly, proenkephalin derived peptides are co-localized with catecholamines predominantly within cells which express PNMT and contain high quantities of epinephrine. The physiological role of these neuropeptides has not been extensively studied. One of the documented important roles of opiate peptides, including enkephalins, is neuromodulation of sympathoadrenal system activity. Opiate receptor blockade during diverse forms of stress, e.g. circulatory shock, hypoglycemia, greatly augments sympathetic neuronal activity and adrenal medullary catecholamine release.

Physiology

Intrauterine life

Adrenal medullary catecholamine release occurs during the fetal/neonatal period in response to diverse stimuli including hypoxia, hypoglycemia, hypothermia, hemorrhage and at the time of labor and delivery. The adrenal medulla is innervated by splanchnic nerves which arise from the celiac ganglion. Immature fetuses, which lack intact splanchnic innervation, cannot activate catecholamine release by the usual neuronal cholinergic mediated mechanism. They are able, however, to release catecholamines in response to some direct stimuli like hypoxia. This direct, non-neuronal response results largely in norepinephrine secretion. Later, when splanchnic innervation has been established and epinephrine is the predominant adrenal amine, the response to hypoxia is greater and there is an increase in the proportion of epinephrine released. Splanchnic innervation and acquisition of neuronal control of adrenal epinephrine secretion occurs between 120 and 125 days of gestation in the fetal sheep where term gestation is 150 days. Similar findings have been described in neonatal rats where loss of the direct, non-neurogenic response and development of neural control of catecholamine release occurs after the first postnatal week. In calves and foals, development of neural control of catecholamine release and secretion of epinephrine as the predominant amine also occurs postnatally. Humans are presumed to resemble calves more than fetal sheep, with development of splanchnic innervation occurring at or near term gestation. However, direct studies in the human are unavailable.

In addition to the absence of glucocorticoid induction of PNMT, extra-adrenal chromaffin tissue differs from adrenal medullary tissue in that it is not innervated by cholinergic neurons. Secretion is thus solely by direct stimulation. Hypoglycemia and hypoxia both result in depletion of para-aortic norepinephrine content. Thus, this uniquely fetal/neonatal tissue is viewed as a source of catecholamines at a developmental time when dependence on circulating catecholamine levels may be greatest and assures the availability of high circulating levels of catecholamine during fetal and/or neonatal stress.

Blockade of catecholamine release or blockade of adrenergic receptors in a well unstressed fetus has little significant effect. In contrast, either receptor blockade or blockade of catecholamine secretion during intrauterine fetal stress (distress) is associated with significant physiological impairment and even death. This observation has been demonstrated most convincingly in animal models but is also recognized increasingly in human fetuses whose mothers had been treated for hypertensive disease with β-receptor blockers.

Role of catecholamine release in adaptation to extrauterine life

The immediate transition to extrauterine life is associated with remarkable alterations in a variety of important organ systems. These include: closure of fetal vascular shunts and increases in cardiac output and blood pressure; the resorption of lung water and the release of pulmonary surfactant to support the onset of effective pulmonary gas exchange; the onset of effective central control of breathing; and important metabolic changes including the mobilization of energy substrates during the early postnatal period. This time period is also associated with a remarkable increase in the levels of several circulating neuroendocrine mediators (catecholamines, angiotensin, vasopressin). For several of these agents the levels associated with this transition period are higher than observed under any other physiological circumstance throughout development and/or adult life. This is particularly true of catecholamines. Plasma catecholamines begin to rise during the last 2–3 hours of spontaneous labor in the chronically catheterized fetal sheep. Following delivery there is a further marked increase in circulating catecholamines. This increase in circulating epinephrine and norepinephrine levels represents a generalized increase in sympathoadrenal system activity, with release from postganglionic sympathetic neurons, as well as adrenal medullary secretion. This 'surge' in catecholamines at birth has been most carefully investigated in animal models. The precise stimulus for catecholamine release is not clear but probably represents an integrated response to compression, mild asphyxia, vestibular and tactile stimulation, hypothermia and a sudden increase in baroreceptor afferent impulse activity after cord cutting. This results in a sudden, generalized increase in centrally mediated sympathoadrenal activity and adrenal medullary secretion as well as increased postganglionic sympathetic neuronal activity and increased plasma spillover of synaptic norepinephrine.

The increase in sympathoadrenal system activity at birth is vital to successful neonatal adaptation. Adrenergic mechanisms significantly regulate many of the important physiological events at birth including: increased myocardial contractility; increased peripheral vascular resistance; secretion of pulmonary surfactant; resorption of lung water; onset of nonshivering thermogenesis; mobilization of glucose and free fatty acid energy substrates; secretion of vasopressin, atrial natriuretic peptide, glucagon and other important hormones. Abolition of the epinephrine surge at birth following fetal adrenalectomy or blockade of adrenergic receptors severely impairs postnatal cardiovascular, pulmonary, metabolic and endocrine responses.

Thus adrenal medullary secretion and the increase in circulating catecholamines during fetal and neonatal life exhibit unique importance compared to adults. In older animals and adults circulating catecholamines are accepted as a qualitative 'index of sympathetic activity'. In fetal/newborn animals adrenal medullary secretion and the maintenance of high circulating plasma catecholamine concentrations support vital adaptive physiological responses.

Selected reading

Lagercrantz H, Marcus C. Sympathoadrenal mechanisms during development. In Polin RA, Fox WW, eds. *Fetal and neonatal physiology*. Vol. I. London: WB Saunders, Harcourt Brace Jovanovich Inc., 1992: 160.

Padbury JF. Functional maturation of the adrenal medulla and peripheral sympathetic nervous system. *Baillière's Clin Endocrinol Metab* 1989; **3**: 689.

Slotkin TA, Seidler FJ. Adrenomedullary catecholamine release in the fetus and newborn: secretory mechanisms and the role in stress and survival. *J Dev Physiol* 1988; **10**: 1.

Winkler H, Apps DK, Fischer-Colbrie R. The molecular function of adrenal chromaffin granules: established facts and unresolved topics. *Neuroscience* 1986; **18**: 261.

K. Minerals and Bone

R D G Milner

In order to have a balanced appreciation of the relative importance of Ca^{2+}, Mg^{2+} and phosphate in the body it is desirable to know how much of each is present and where. Such information is available for the adult only and is shown in a simple form in Table 7.3 to give a sense of perspective. Almost every doctor has been confused at some time or other by divalent ionic concentrations expressed in mg/100 ml, mEq/l or mmol/l (see Table 7.3). All concentrations in this section are expressed as mmol/l.

Hormones of mineral metabolism

Vitamin D

Vitamin D permits normal bone growth, and deficiency results in disturbed Ca^{2+} homeostasis leading to *rickets* or *osteomalacia*. The term vitamin D refers to cholecalciferol (vitamin D_3) and ergocalciferol (vitamin D_2) each of which are produced nonenzymatically by ultraviolet irradiation of 7-dehydrocholesterol. 7-Dehydrocholesterol is the last intermediate in the synthesis of cholesterol from acetate and in most cells the transition takes place rapidly, but in the skin 7-dehydrocholesterol accumulation occurs in the deeper layers of the epidermis. The wavelength (290–320 nm) responsible for photo-oxidation is the same as that causing sunburn. The season, the latitude and skin pigmentation are the most important determinants of vitamin D formation. From a practical viewpoint a few hours of summer sunbathing are enough to protect from vitamin D deficiency for several months. In excess sunlight, biologically inactive compounds are synthesized, thus avoiding vitamin D intoxication.

Both forms of vitamin D occur in the diet and are absorbed in the upper intestine with the help of bile salts. The metabolism and biological potency of the two forms of vitamin D are identical in man. Being steroids the vitamins are transported initially in chylomicrons via the lymphatics. Vitamin D and all related metabolites in the blood travel on an α_2-globulin of hepatic origin, vitamin D binding protein (DBP) which has a molecular weight of 52 kDa. The binding protein is present in excess so that it binds approximately 99 percent of the vitamin D and acts as a buffer against vitamin D toxicity. DBP synthesis increases during pregnancy and under the influence of oral contraceptives. It is degraded by many different tissues and has a half-life of 1.7 days.

Vitamin D is biologically inactive until it has been hydroxylated (Fig. 7.21). The first step is 25-hydroxylation, which occurs predominantly in hepatic microsomes, but may also take place in the intestine and kidney. 25-OH vitamin D, 25(OH)D, is the major circulating D metabolite and its concentration is directly proportional to that of vitamin D. The 25-hydroxylation step is high capacity, but the second hydroxylation which occurs in the mitochondria of the proximal renal tubule to produce $1,25(OH)_2D$, the active D metabolite, is low capacity and tightly controlled. A defect in this enzyme leads to *vitamin D dependent rickets type I* which is

Table 7.3. Representative values for normal body content and distribution of divalent cations

	kg	%BW	Ca^{2+}		P		Mg^{2+}	
			(mmol)	%	(mmol)	%	(mmol)	%
Bone	7	10	31 350	99.5	19 000	85	600	68
Muscle	32	45	50		1900	9	170	19
Other	31	45	100		1300	6	112	13
Total	70		31 500		22 200		882	

%BW, Percentage body weight.
Note: for Ca^{2+} 1 mmol/l = 2 mEq/l = 4 mg/100 ml.

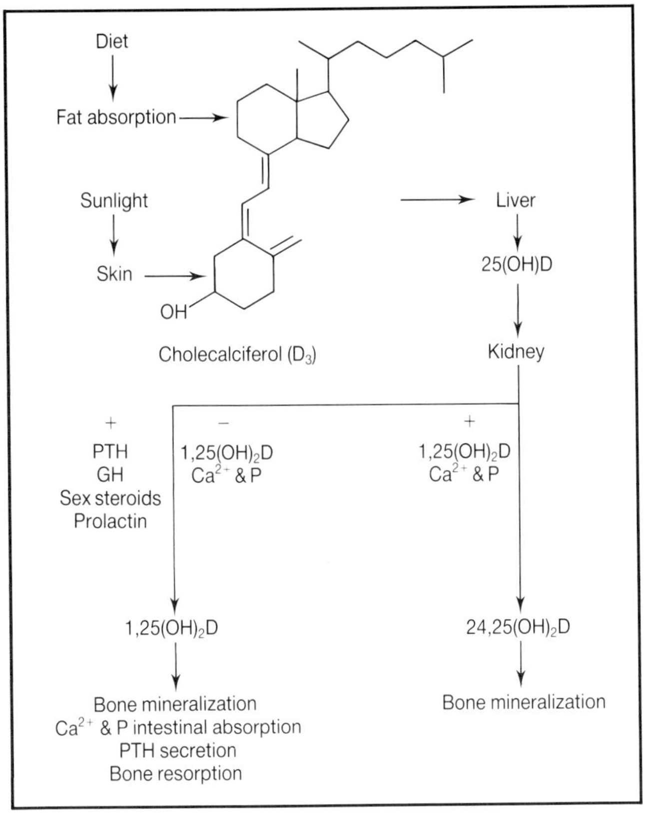

Fig. 7.21. The major steps in vitamin D metabolism and the actions of its metabolites.

usually autosomally recessive. The alternative renal hydroxylation of 25(OH)D is to $24,25(OH)_2D$ which has much less biological activity. $1,25(OH)_2D$ can also be synthesized in placenta, bone cells and granulomatous tissues. During growth, pregnancy and lactation the 1-hydroxylase is stimulated and more $1,25(OH)_2D$ produced. Normal serum levels of 25(OH)D vary with diet and exposure to sunlight, but the concentration of $1,25(OH)_2D$ is not so affected. The average serum concentration of $1,25(OH)_2D$ is about one thousandth that of 25(OH)D. The half-life of circulating $1,25(OH)_2D$ is measured in hours and of 25(OH)D in days. Vitamin D catabolism takes place in the liver and many biologically inactive metabolites are excreted in the bile.

Vitamin D deficiency remains a clinical problem even in societies where there is supplementation of milk with the vitamin. This is thought to be the result of marginally low Ca^{2+} intake, possibly related to dietary phytate and fiber, resulting in mild secondary hyperparathyroidism and increased production of $1,25(OH)_2D$ which effectively inhibits the formation of 25(OH)D in the liver. The same mechanism is responsible for vitamin D deficiency in a variety of conditions characterized by hyperparathyroidism or Ca^{2+} malabsorption such as *gastrointestinal* and *chronic liver disease*. *Hypervitaminosis D* results from excess vitamin D intake resulting in elevated 25(OH)D but normal $1,25(OH)_2D$. In these circumstances the 25(OH)D exerts a pharmacological action and causes hypercalcemia, soft tissue calcification, vomiting and diarrhea.

So many factors influence the activity of the renal 1-hydroxylase and thereby $1,25(OH)_2D$ production that it seems unlikely that all have a physiological regulatory role. $1,25(OH)_2D$ appears to have two actions in the body: one in Ca^{2+} homeostasis and the other as a modifier of cell function in a wide range of cell types. The action of $1,25(OH)_2D$ on Ca^{2+} homeostasis is to stimulate target cells in the intestinal mucosa, renal tubules and bone to increase Ca^{2+} transport with the net effect of raising the blood Ca^{2+} level. $1,25(OH)_2D$ reacts with a specific nuclear receptor protein which is a member of the steroid receptor superfamily (see p. 290). In *vitamin D dependent rickets type II* the defect is apparently at this level as plasma $1,25(OH)_2D$ levels are elevated. Activation of the vitamin D receptor initiates the synthesis of certain proteins which modify the cellular handling of Ca^{2+}. One such is Ca^{2+}-binding protein (CaBP) which has a weight of 8.6 kDa. This increases the capacity for intestinal Ca^{2+} absorption. $1,25(OH)_2D$ increases the activity of osteoclasts and suppresses the activity of osteoblasts. Osteoclasts do not have receptors for the vitamin and its action may be to increase osteoclast production from stem cells in the bone marrow.

Other proteins that are $1,25(OH)_2D$ dependent are osteocalcin in bone and intestinal alkaline phosphatase. The exact way in which they play a part in Ca^{2+} homeostasis is not yet clear. The nuclear $1,25(OH)_2D$ receptor is present in a wide range of cells and the spectrum of action of vitamin D includes depression of growth, initiation of differentiation, and of hormone secretion from endocrine cells. For example, there are $1,25(OH)_2D$ receptors in the brain and on the pancreatic B cell and $1,25(OH)_2D$ may be involved in immunoregulation and in the differentiation of a variety of cells including monocytes. The relative importance of these different actions to whole body physiology remains unclear.

The most prominent influence on $1,25(OH)_2D$ formation is parathyroid hormone (PTH). A fall in extracellular Ca^{2+} causes PTH stimulation which in turn activates the 1-hydroxylase enzyme. $1,25(OH)_2D$ has an important autoregulatory role by increasing the accumulation of 7-dehydrocholesterol in the skin, inhibiting PTH secretion, hepatic vitamin D 25-hydroxylase and renal 25(OH)D-1-hydroxylase and by inducing renal 25(OH)D-24-hydroxylase. All these should be viewed as coarse control mechanisms with the fine control being in the regulation of $1,25(OH)_2D$ receptors on the target cells. Receptors are increased by estradiol and decreased by glucocorticoids. If PTH is seen as the primary link in a simple feedback loop involving $1,25(OH)_2D$ and Ca^{2+}, the role of other putative 1-hydroxylase regulators becomes secondary.

Parathyroid hormone

PTH controls the extracellular fluid (ECF) Ca^{2+} concentration by actions on the transfer of Ca^{2+} from bone, glomerular filtrate and gut to the extracellular fluid. PTH is made in the chief cells of the four parathyroid glands. The parathyroids are derived from the endoderm of the third and fourth branchial pouches; the lower pair develop in close association with the thymus from the third branchial pouch and the upper pair come from the fourth pouch and remain stationary to end up dorsolateral to the thyroid at the level of the isthmus. *DiGeorge syndrome*, which is an embryonic failure of the third and fourth pouches, may cause thymic aplasia, parathyroid aplasia and cardiovascular defects.

PTH is a single polypeptide of 84 amino acids and a molecular weight of 9.5 kDa. Full biological activity lies in the 34 amino acids at the amino terminus. The PTH gene is on the short arm of chromosome 11 very close to the insulin gene. PTH is produced from a 115 amino acid precursor, preproPTH, by two sequential enzymatic cleavages during transport of the nascent peptide into the cisternal space of the endoplasmic reticulum and packaging into granules in the Golgi apparatus. Multiple forms of PTH are found in the circulation but the biologically active molecule is exclusively PTH (1–84). PTH is inactivated by cleavage between amino acids 33–43 by cathepsin-like enzymes found in the parathyroids, liver and kidney.

Two major mechanisms control the secretion of PTH: intracellular Ca^{2+} concentration and cAMP, of which Ca^{2+} is the more important. Secretion increases as extracellular Ca^{2+} falls and vice versa. The close link between extracellular and intracellular Ca^{2+} is shown by the fact that Ca^{2+} agonists are potent inhibitors of secretion and Ca^{2+} channel blockers interfere with the control mechanism. Mg^{2+} has a dual effect: hypermagnesemia is inhibitory but less potently so than Ca^{2+}, but profound hypomagnesemia can also block PTH release. Stimulants of the adenyl cyclase–cAMP system cause PTH release. These include β-adrenergic agents, secretin, dopamine and prostaglandins of the epinephrine series. Conversely prostaglandin F and α-adrenergic catecholamines are inhibitory.

Hyperparathyroidism in childhood is usually inherited. Three forms are recognized: *autosomal recessive parathyroid hyperplasia, autosomal dominant benign hypocalciuric hypercalcemia*, and *autosomal dominant hyperparathyroidism with hypercalciuria*. *Autosomal recessive parathyroid hyperplasia* begins before birth and there is marked hypercalcemia in the neonatal period resulting in anorexia, vomiting, constipation, renal insufficiency and hypertension leading to death within months unless the diagnosis is made and appropriate action taken. In contrast, *autosomal dominant benign hypocalciuric hypercalcemia* is usually asymptomatic and detected accidentally as a result of measuring serum Ca^{2+} for another reason, or by family studies after identification of a proband. Again by contrast, *autosomal dominant hyperparathyroidism* with hypercalciuria is characterized by symptoms that are likely to relate to renal stones or kidney failure. Investigation reveals hypercalcemia and hyperparathyroidism in the propositus and family members. Genetically determined hyperparathyroidism may also occur as part of *multiple endocrine adenomatosis* (MEN) *type I or II*. *Humoral hypercalcemia of malignancy* (HHM) must be distinguished from hyperparathyroidism with which it shares many clinical features. HHM is characterized by a low plasma Cl^- and $1,25(OH)_2D$, hypokalemia and an equivocally raised plasma immunoreactive PTH concentration. The actual hormone inducing the hypercalcemia is not PTH itself but a PTH-related protein. There are several of these which are produced by alternate splicing of a gene evolutionarily related to the PTH gene. Solid tumors may produce other stimulants of bone resorption such as TGFα.

Hypoparathyroidism may be due to inadequate release of PTH or resistance to PTH. Inadequate release may be permanent or transient as in *neonatal hypopara-*

thyroidism. If permanent it may be congenital as in *DiGeorge syndrome* or acquired as in *autoimmune* or *idiopathic hypoparathyroidism*. Activation of the PTH receptor initiates the adrenal cyclase/cAMP cascade via a guanine nucleotide regulatory (coupling) protein G_s. Resistance to PTH is found in *pseudohypoparathyroidism types I and II,* and secondary to disorders of vitamin D metabolism. The molecular defect in *pseudohypoparathyroidism type Ia* is a deficiency of the α-subunit of G_s. In type Ib, the abnormality in the receptor has not been defined but PTH cannot induce cAMP production. In pseudohypoparathyroidism type II, PTH can induce cyclic AMP production but there is a more distal end-organ resistance.

Calcitonin

Calcitonin is a 32 amino acid peptide made by the parafollicular, or C cells, of the thyroid gland. The C cells arise embryologically from the fifth branchial pouch and produce the ultimobranchial body which becomes incorporated into the parafollicular interstices of the thyroid. Biological activity of calcitonin depends on the integrity of the molecule. The calcitonin/CGRP gene is located on chromosome 11, as is the gene for PTH, and consists of six exons separated by five introns. Coding for calcitonin involves four of the six exons. Another protein, calcitonin gene related peptide (CGRP) is expressed by five of the six exons by alternate splicing and is found predominantly in the central nervous system where its physiological significance is uncertain. CGRP is vasodilatory and may play a part in autoregulation of the cerebral and other vasculatures. Expression of the gene in the C cell results in the synthesis of a large precursor polypeptide which is then cleaved to yield three peptides: N-terminal peptide, calcitonin and carboxy-terminal peptide.

Calcitonin secretion, like that of PTH, is controlled by intracellular Ca^{2+} and cAMP. A rise in extracellular Ca^{2+} concentration causes an increase in C-cell calcitonin concentration as well as in secretion. The adenylate cyclase–cAMP system is activated by a number of gut hormones including gastrin, cholecystokinin and glucagon. These may play a part in damping potential postprandial surges of Ca^{2+}. Calcitonin receptors are found on osteoclasts, and in the medullary ascending thick limb of the nephron. Calcitonin causes hypocalcemia primarily by inhibition of osteoclast activity in bone and by blocking the action of PTH. These actions may be mediated by blocking cAMP. Associated with this are a reduction of alkaline phosphatase and pyrophosphatase activity and inhibition of hydroxyproline production. Hypophosphatemia occurs as a result of increased phosphate entry into bone and phosphaturia.

Calcium

Ca^{2+} is the most abundant electrolyte in the body because of the skeleton. Ninety-nine percent of skeletal Ca^{2+} is unavailable for immediate homeostasis and only 0.1 percent total body Ca^{2+} is in the plasma and extravascular fluid. Ionized Ca^{2+}, both in the plasma and in the cytosol, plays a central part in the regulation of cellular activity, being involved in muscle contraction, nerve conduction, initiation of mitosis and microtubular contraction as well as enzyme action. Among circulating ions Ca^{2+} is the second most tightly controlled after sodium. The normal plasma Ca^{2+} concentration is 2.2–2.6 mmol/l. Approximately 40 percent is bound to protein. Of the protein bound Ca^{2+}, 60–90 percent is associated with albumin and the remainder with other globulins. Ca^{2+} binding to albumin is strongly pH dependent, being inversely proportional to the H^+ concentration. Nonprotein bound Ca^{2+} is a mixture of low molecular weight Ca^{2+} complexes and ionized Ca^{2+}. The major fraction of the ultrafilterable Ca^{2+} is ionized and represents about 45–50 percent of the total Ca^{2+} in normal individuals. Ca^{2+} in other extracellular fluids is technically difficult to measure. There is no reason to assume that the concentration of Ca^{2+} in the interstitial fluid of different organs reflects the circulating Ca^{2+} concentration and there is evidence that local tissue Ca^{2+} kinetics have an important influence on the Ca^{2+} in the extracellular fluid.

The mineralization of bone is poorly understood. Osteoblasts are important regulators and promote Ca^{2+} and phosphate precipitation first in an amorphous form and then as hydroxyapatite crystals. Crystals grow *in vivo* in a similar manner to their behavior in a homogenous salt solution, by nucleation and surface apposition. Bone matrix collagen has a staggered orientation that may provide nucleation sites and a bone-specific phosphorylated collagen α_2 chain has been identified. Other proteins are found in bone which have a high affinity for both collagen and apatite, the most avid of these being osteonectin which has the capacity to initiate mineralization on type I collagen fibers. Bone also contains a number of molecules that may inhibit mineralization. These include glycosaminoglycans, proteoglycans and pyrophosphate, but the most common, making up 1–2 percent bone protein, is osteocalcin. Osteocalcin is synthesized and secreted by osteoblasts under the action of $1,25(OH)_2D$. It appears after mineralization and binds to and stabilizes apatite crystals. Genetic defects resulting in abnormal collagen formation are responsible for diseases such as *osteogenesis imperfecta* and *Ehlers–Danlos syndrome*.

Calcium homeostasis

The major sites of Ca^{2+} transport in and out of the body are the intestinal tract, the kidneys and to a lesser extent the sweat glands. In the healthy adult renal Ca^{2+} excretion equals the net intestinal Ca^{2+} absorption, but in the growing child there is a net accumulation by bone. Normally about 20 mmol are ingested each day; 8 mmol are absorbed and 4 mmol are secreted into the gut lumen, resulting in a fecal loss of 16 mmol. The other 4 mmol are excreted in the urine. A schematic summary of Ca^{2+} balance is shown in Fig. 7.22. The fractional Ca^{2+} absorption increases as the absolute Ca^{2+} ingested decreases; a net positive Ca^{2+} balance can be maintained with a Ca^{2+} intake as low as 5 mmol/day. Fractional Ca^{2+} absorption is greater in childhood and adolescence than in adulthood, apart from pregnancy and lactation.

Ca^{2+} absorption takes place in all parts of the intestine distal to the pylorus and is fastest in the duodenum and jejunum but also significant in the ileum because of its greater length. Ca^{2+} transport is both passive (paracellular) and active (transcellular); the majority of the paracellular Ca^{2+} movement being controlled largely by solvent drag and electrochemical potential differences. Transcellular Ca^{2+} transport varies with both the structure and function of the intestinal and renal epithelium. Since cytosolic Ca^{2+} concentrations are known to be important in the regulation of other transport mechanisms, such as water and sodium, it is likely that more Ca^{2+} enters or leaves the body via the paracellular route than by the transcellular one, but the transcellular route may be the more important in fine tuning whole body homeostasis. The most important regulator of Ca^{2+} uptake by the gut is $1,25(OH)_2D$ which is operative from the early neonatal period. The mechanisms of Ca^{2+} transfer to the fetus are discussed on p. 140.

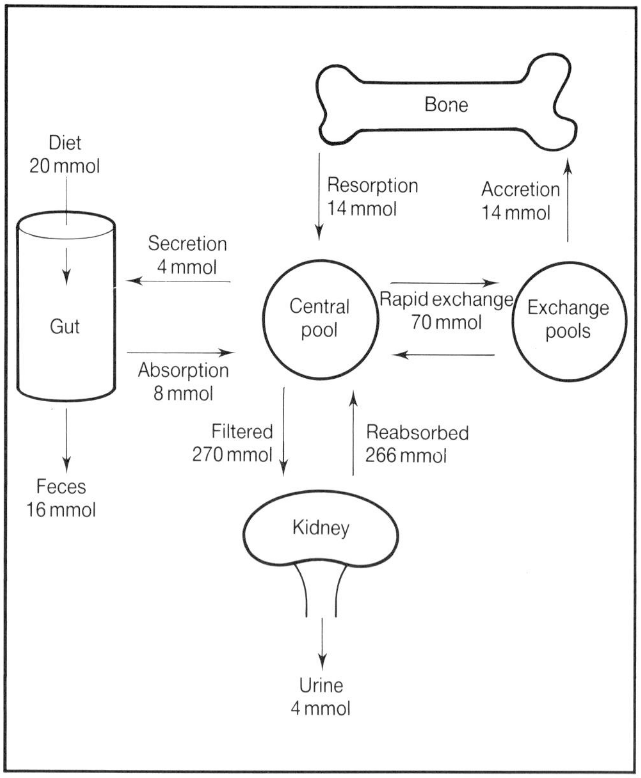

Fig. 7.22. Calcium balance in a normal 70 kg man.

Inhibitors of Ca^{2+} uptake include cellulose, phosphate, phytates, anticonvulsants and glucocorticoids. Cellulose and phytate bind Ca^{2+} in the lumen, whereas anti-convulsants interfere with vitamin D metabolism as well as having, together with glucocorticoids, a direct effect on the intestinal epithelial transport mechanism. The pool of circulating Ca^{2+} in the adult is approximately 25 mmol, but when Ca^{2+} is injected, it rapidly equilibrates with a much larger mass, the central miscible pool. Analyses of Ca^{2+} kinetics by pool modeling that are mathematically satisfying tend to lack physiological application and only the simplest model is of direct clinical relevance (Fig. 7.22).

Intracellular Ca^{2+} concentrations vary from 0.02 mmol/kg cell water in cells with no organelles, such as erythrocytes, to 5–10 mmol/kg cell water in muscle. In contrast to extracellular Ca^{2+}, intracellular Ca^{2+} is 99.9 percent bound to a large number of specific binding proteins mainly within the nucleus, mitochondria, endoplasmic reticulum and other special vesicles. The cytosolic concentration is about 10 mmol/l of which only about 0.1 mmol/l is ionized. This is achieved partly by active transport into the intracellular organelles, but more importantly by energy-dependent pumping of Ca^{2+} out of the cell. Three mechanisms are important: a Ca^{2+} Mg-ATPase, a Na^{+}-Ca^{2+} pump, and a Ca^{2+}-H^{+} pump. The Ca^{2+} Mg-ATPase is the principal pump at rest, and the Na^{+}-Ca^{2+} pump operates during cell activity or injury.

Hypocalcemia occurs commonly as a transient phenomenon in the newborn, particularly in the premature, *the infant of a diabetic mother*, or the asphyxiated baby. Hypocalcemia may also occur towards the end of the first week of life in infants fed cows' milk with a high phosphate content. In older children the commonest association with hypocalcemia is hypoalbuminemia. In these circumstances the ionized Ca^{2+} is normal and no action regarding Ca^{2+} therapy is indicated. Conditions marked by hyperphosphatemia, such as *chronic renal failure*, parenteral nutrition and *renal tubular acidosis* are all associated with hypocalcemia which resolves upon correction of the plasma phosphate. *Vitamin D deficiency* and *hypoparathyroidism* also cause hypocalcemia.

Hypercalcemia is less common and is most commonly seen in infants and children who have received excess vitamin D. The condition known as *idiopathic hypercalcemia of infancy*, which was diagnosed commonly in the UK but not in the USA, was probably the result of generous supplementation of cows' milk with vitamin D. *Williams syndrome* is characterized by mental retardation, supravalvular aortic stenosis and elfin facies and may be associated with hypercalcemia, but the nature of the link is a mystery. Vitamins D and A are fat soluble and therapeutic preparations often contain both. *Vitamin A toxicity* also causes hypercalcemia as a result of increased osteoclast activity, lysosomal disruption, the release of hydrolytic enzymes and increased bone resorption. If hypercalcemia is discovered unexpectedly, hyperparathyroidism or malignancy should be suspected. Hypercalcemia associated with malignancy may arise from osteolytic metastases or ectopic hormone production.

Magnesium

Mg^{2+} is the fourth most abundant cation in the body and, after K^{+}, the second commonest in the intracellular fluid (ICF). Intracellular Mg^{2+} plays a critical role in many metabolic processes including the production and utilization of energy. It is also necessary for a large number of enzymatic reactions including those involving DNA transcription, RNA aggregation and protein synthesis. Extracellular Mg^{2+} is involved in neuronal activity, neuromuscular transmission and cardiovascular tone. The availability of intracellular Mg^{2+} appears to be the determining factor in Mg^{2+} homeostasis, cellular Mg^{2+} being maintained at the expense of the ECF and bone.

The normal adult body contains about 900 mmol Mg^{2+}, of which two-thirds is in bone and one-third in the ICF with only 1 percent in the ECF. The normal ratio of Ca^{2+} to Mg^{2+} in bone is 50:1. Most bone Mg^{2+} is complexed to the apatite crystal rather than to the bone matrix. The normal intracellular Mg^{2+} concentration varies between 4 and 8 mmol/l and much of it is complexed to proteins and organophosphates. The normal plasma Mg^{2+} is 0.7–1.0 mmol/l, about half of which is ionized.

Magnesium homeostasis

The normal adult ingests about 12 mmol Mg^{2+} per day and absorbs half of this (Fig. 7.23). The absorbed Mg^{2+}

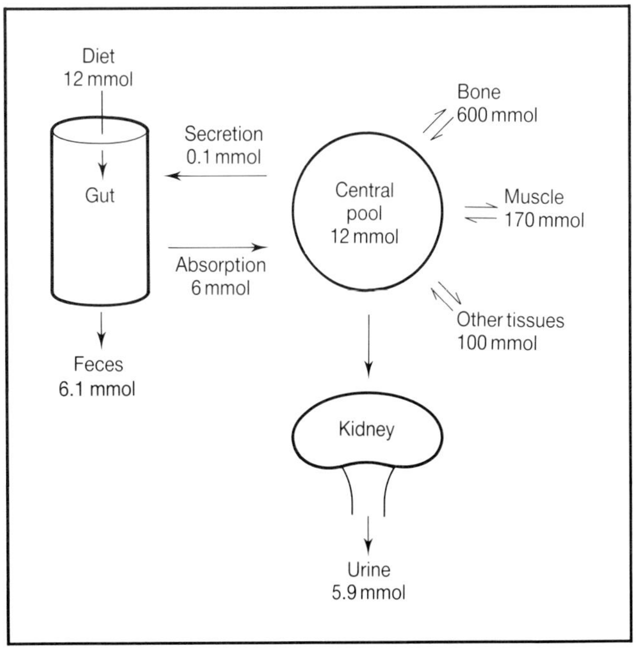

Fig. 7.23. Magnesium balance in a normal 70 kg man.

enters an extracellular pool containing 12 mmol Mg^{2+} which is in equilibrium with bone (600 mmol), muscle (170 mmol) and other tissues (100 mmol). Under stable conditions most of the absorbed Mg^{2+} is excreted in the urine and a small amount is secreted into the gut. Mg^{2+} is absorbed throughout the small bowel but most importantly in the ileum. Mg^{2+} deficiency may occur following *small bowel resection*.

Absorption takes place by both transcellular and paracellular routes and is appropriate to bodily needs, but the mechanisms controlling the process are not well understood. Both PTH and vitamin D have been alleged to augment Mg^{2+} absorption. Although Ca^{2+} and Mg^{2+} are influenced by similar controls, their pathways of absorption are thought to be independent. Approximately 80 percent of the plasma Mg^{2+} is filtered at the glomerulus. In the proximal convoluted tubule about 25 percent of the filtered Mg^{2+} is reabsorbed. Reabsorption occurs in parallel to that of Na^+ and Ca^{2+} but at a lower rate, suggesting that the proximal tubular cells are relatively impermeable to Mg^{2+} and the intraluminal concentration rises along the length of the tubule. A further 15 percent is reabsorbed in the straight proximal tubule which is also relatively impermeable to Mg^{2+}. Fifty percent Mg^{2+} is reabsorbed in the thick ascending limb of the loop of Henle via an active transport process which is apparently not saturable. About 80 percent of the delivered load is reabsorbed at all levels of luminal Mg^{2+} concentration, but reabsorption is inversely proportional to the serum Mg^{2+}. Mg^{2+} excretion is increased by increased renal perfusion or filtration, as occurs in volume overload or the use of osmotic diuretics. It is also increased by hypermagnesemia, hypercalcemia, loop diuretics, metabolic acidosis and phosphate depletion. It is decreased by the converse changes and also by PTH and *hypothyroidism*.

Because Mg^{2+} is principally an intracellular ion the plasma concentration and body level do not correlate well; Mg^{2+} depletion can occur in the presence of normomagnesemia and hypomagnesemia does not necessarily reflect a loss of Mg^{2+} stores. However, it is prudent to assume if a patient has hypomagnesemia there will be some degree of whole body magnesium depletion. The reduced dietary intake of Mg^{2+} seen in *protein-calorie malnutrition* results in both magnesium depletion and hypomagnesemia and the latter may be aggravated on refeeding when there is redistribution of total body Mg^{2+} into the intracellular compartment. Any condition characterized by *chronic diarrhea* or *chronic diuretic therapy* may be associated with Mg^{2+} losses that are not always reflected in the plasma concentration. The metabolism of Mg^{2+} and K^+ are closely interrelated and Mg^{2+} is important in K^+ homeostasis. Mg^{2+} deficiency is always associated with K^+ deficiency and the latter cannot be corrected by K^+ alone. It is a good idea to think of Mg^{2+} when considering problems of hypokalemia.

Inborn errors of Mg^{2+} metabolism occur in both the gut and kidney. *Hypomagnesemia* may result from a defect in the intestinal transcellular absorptive pathway with preservation of the paracellular mechanism. Mg^{2+} depletion and hypomagnesemia occur under normal conditions but can be corrected by the administration of Mg^{2+} salts that would otherwise be purgative. Two types of renal Mg^{2+} loss are known: an *isolated Mg^{2+} leak*, and a *combined Mg^{2+} and K^+ leak*. It is not understood if the isolated defect of renal Mg^{2+} conservation and intestinal Mg^{2+} absorption coexist.

Hypermagnesemia occurs rarely. It may be encountered in *azotemia* and in the newborn infant of a mother treated with intravenous magnesium for eclampsia.

Phosphate

The physiologically important circulating phosphate is orthophosphate which is present as $H_2PO_4^-$ and HPO_4^{2-}. At pH 7.4 the ratio of $H_2PO_4^-$ to HPO_4^{2-} is 4:1. Since plasma phosphate is a mixture of monovalent and divalent species it has an intermediate valency of 1.8. Plasma phosphate concentration is measured chemically as phosphorus and when expressed as weight the normal value of 31 mg/l is equivalent to 1 mmol/l. The normal plasma phosphate is 1.4–2.3 mmol/l. The terms plasma phosphorus and plasma phosphate are often used interchangeably, which makes it important to think and work in molar terms to avoid mathematical errors in calculation. Under normal conditions about 15 percent of plasma phosphate is protein bound.

Phosphate homeostasis

Dietary phosphate is both organic and inorganic and most of the organic phosphate is hydrolyzed in the gut lumen to yield inorganic phosphate for absorption, but some organic phosphate is absorbed as phospholipid. Most phosphate is absorbed in the jejunum and in normal subjects net phosphate absorption is a linear function of dietary intake and is approximately two-thirds. Phosphate absorption differs from Ca^{2+} absorption in a number of ways. Over a normal range of intake net phosphate absorption is linear, whereas net Ca^{2+} absorption is curvilinear, decreasing with increasing absolute Ca^{2+} load. Net phosphate absorption is about double that of Ca^{2+}: two-thirds compared to one-third. Intestinal phosphate absorption, like that of Ca^{2+}, is both paracellular and transcellular and under normal circumstances is almost entirely diffusional. $1,25(OH)_2D$ stimulates the active absorption of both phosphate and Ca^{2+}, but by separate mechanisms, and the effect of vitamin D on phosphate absorption is quantitatively unimportant. PTH has no direct effect on phosphate absorption. Since most diets contain an abundance of phosphate the quantity of phosphate absorbed always exceeds requirements.

Phosphate excretion takes place by filtration and fractional reabsorption; there is no phosphate secretion by the renal tubule. Reabsorption takes place principally in the proximal convoluted tubule and more occurs at the beginning than further down. PTH reduces phosphate reabsorption via a mechanism in the straight part of the proximal tubule involving cAMP. This represents the most important physiological effect on renal phosphate excretion and is the major determinant of plasma phosphate concentration. Vitamin D and its metabolites have no direct effect on renal phosphate reabsorption, but influence it profoundly by their overall action on mineral metabolism in different circumstances, being either phosphaturic or antiphosphaturic. Growth hormone (GH) causes phosphate retention by increasing both intestinal and renal absorption of phosphate, resulting in hyperphosphatemia. GH has a direct effect on the kidney but the site of action is not clearly defined. Thyroid hormones also have a direct action to stimulate renal phosphate reabsorption but this is masked by their overall effects on phosphate metabolism and their interactions with other hormone systems. Certain *mesenchymal tumors* and *neurocutaneous dysplasias* may be associated with phosphaturia which resolves on removal of the tumor. This has led to the hypothesis that there is a factor released by the pathological tissue which blocks phosphate reabsorption.

Plasma phosphate homeostasis is fundamentally controlled by intestinal phosphate absorption and renal phosphate excretion, with phosphate exchange between the plasma and skeleton and soft tissues playing a secondary role. Whereas the gut intermittently floods the ECF with phosphate, the kidney continuously regulates plasma phosphate and overall phosphate homeostasis by precisely excreting that which is in excess of the body's need. This balance is maintained independently of PTH. There is a pronounced diurnal rhythm in phosphate excretion with a nadir during the morning and a peak in the late evening. This does not appear to be tightly bound to food intake; it may be linked to diurnal changes in glucocorticoid secretion. Increased urine production, for whatever reason, is usually accompanied by increased phosphate excretion. The only diuretics that are not phosphaturic are the distal K^+-sparing ones such as triamterene, amiloride and spironolactone. Alkalinization of the urine causes phosphaturia.

Whole body phosphate homeostasis is directed more towards the needs of soft tissues than bone. Dietary phosphate restriction is followed immediately by virtual elimination of phosphate from the urine and a sharp reduction in fecal phosphate. Growth stops, thereby reducing the need for phosphate and phosphate is mobilized from bone to satisfy the needs of the soft tissues. Dietary phosphate deficiency may be responsible for *rickets* such as that seen in preterm infants fed unsupplemented breast milk. Any movement of phosphate into the intracellular compartment or bone can result in hypophosphatemia which may be symptomatic or even life threatening. This happens most abruptly during glucose or fructose infusion but is more likely to be serious during total parenteral nutrition if the hyperalimentation fluid is inadequately supplemented with phosphate. Phosphaturia can cause hypophosphatemia and this occurs most commonly as a result of acidosis. The hypophosphatemia of *disorders of vitamin D metabolism* is due to reduced intestinal absorption of Ca^{2+} and hypocalcemia leading to *secondary hyperparathyroidism* which causes increased renal excretion of phosphate. Increased renal phosphate loss also occurs in *primary tubular disorders* such as the *Fanconi syndrome, renal tubular acidosis*, and *familial X-linked hypophosphatemic rickets*.

Hyperphosphatemia occurs whenever the entry of phosphate into the circulation exceeds the renal capacity for phosphate excretion. If renal function is impaired hyperphosphatemia may occur in the face of normal or even reduced phosphate intake. Excess phosphate enters the circulation as a result of ingestion of phosphate-containing enemas, antacid preparations or laxatives, but more commonly in childhood from *vitamin D intoxication* stimulating both intestinal phosphate absorption and bone resorption. Acidosis, both metabolic and respiratory, causes hyperphosphatemia. Conditions associated with cellular breakdown, such as *tumor lysis syndrome* or *rhabdomyolysis*, release phosphate into the circulation with predictable results.

Bone

Mature bone is either cortical or trabecular. Cortical bone forms the outer surface of all bones; its principal component is mature mineral and its principal function is physical support. It is also referred to as compact or lamellar bone because it is made up of concentric lamellae of mineral penetrated by a fine network of interconnecting osteocytes. Cortical bone is being constantly remodeled. Trabecular or spongy bone makes up the center of most bones and is composed of a meshwork of thin plates of 200 mm thickness with a large area to volume ratio. The space between trabeculae is occupied by marrow which may be fatty or hemopoietic. Trabecular bone, because of its large surface area, turns over more rapidly than cortical bone.

Bone contains three morphologically distinct cell types: osteoblasts, osteoclasts and osteocytes. In addition there are flat surface-lining cells and marrow cells which are thought to be functionally important. The osteoblast is a typical protein synthesizing cell with a large Golgi apparatus and abundant rough endoplasmic reticulum. Osteoblasts synthesize and secrete type I collagen and also alkaline phosphatase which hydrolyzes pyrophosphate, an inhibitor of calcium phosphate crystal growth. When inactive the osteoblast is thought to become an osteocyte on the surface or inside the bone where it may modulate Ca^{2+} flux between bone and the ECF. The osteoclast is a multinucleated giant cell characterized by a ruffled border which is a pleated segment of plasma membrane structurally analogous to the brush border of the intestine and kidney. The ruffled border is in contact with resorbing bone and is the site of carbonic anhydrase production responsible for the acid needed to facilitate crystal resorption. A selective deficiency of carbonic anhydrase II is associated histologically with a lack of ruffled borders in osteoclasts and results in *osteopetrosis*.

Osteoblasts are responsive to PTH, but not calcitonin, and have intracellular receptors for $1,25(OH)_2D$. Osteoblast alkaline phosphatase is inhibited by PTH but may be stimulated or inhibited by $1,25(OH)_2D$ depending on the state of cellular differentiation. Both PTH and $1,25(OH)_2D$ inhibit osteoblast collagen production. Bone formation is not directly stimulated by the calciferols whose antirachitic actions are mediated mainly by their effects on Ca^{2+}, phosphate and PTH homeostasis. The direct stimuli of bone formation are insulin, prostaglandins and growth factors, all of which promote protein synthesis in a nonselective manner. Osteoclasts contain calcitonin receptors. Calcitonin inhibits osteoclast motility and causes the ruffled border to disappear.

Development and modeling

Primary bone is made in the embryo by either intramembranous or endochondral ossification. The clavicle and most skull bones are formed by intramembranous ossification which is initiated in membranous mesenchymal plates where some of the mesenchymal cells differentiate to osteoblasts with subsequent formation of organic bone matrix (osteoid). As osteoid calcifies and grows, previously active osteoblasts are incorporated as osteocytes and the bone becomes either cancellous or dense. Collagen fibers are initially randomly oriented, but become remodeled later.

The remainder of the skeleton is formed by endochondral ossification in which bone is laid down in preexisting hyaline cartilage. The primary ossification centers in tubular bones are most often in the mid-diaphysis. Growth in length comes from calcification of these plate-like structures and growth in diameter takes place in the periosteum, which is formed from the primitive perichondrium and has osteogenic properties in its deeper layers. Mineralization occurs rapidly during the third trimester of fetal life. Approximately 8 mmol Ca^{2+} are accumulated each day and a term infant contains 700 mmol Ca^{2+}. Over the next 20 years a further 20 000 mmol are added at a rate which varies from a nadir of 1–2 mmol/day in mid-childhood to a peak of 10 mmol/day during the pubertal growth spurt.

After primary formation, bones undergo continuous modeling to produce the final gross structure. In long bones this involves longitudinal and transverse growth and adaptation of shape. Longitudinal growth results from cartilage proliferation and the formation of primitive trabeculae at the growth plate. At the same time as transverse growth occurs at the periosteal surface, the marrow cavity is expanding due to resorption at the endosteal surface. Bone is continuously remodeled throughout life to maintain viability of the cells and to optimize its strength. Remodeling takes place by a group of osteoclasts being activated and eroding a canal through existing cortical or trabecular bone. The forward movement of activated osteoclasts is conical because resorption occurs frontally and centrifugally; the leading edge of resorption is called a cutting cone. The process of resorption continues for about 1 month and is then replaced by osteoblast activity which forms new concentric layers of lamellar bone: the closing cone. The total time for remodeling one site is about 3 months. The amount of bone turned over by a remodeling process is termed a basic structural unit, or osteon, and the cells involved are a basic multicellular unit. The osteons of cortical bone are nearly circular in cross-section and those of trabecular bone crescentic. Remodeling occurs at three anatomical surfaces: the periosteal, Haversian and endosteal surfaces.

Osteoclast precursors are activated to become osteoclasts and initiate resorption by prostaglandins or lymphokines released by surface cells or adjoining lymphocytes. Activation occurs at any one site about every 2 years. This time interval is called the activation frequency. The humoral signal for activation is complex and not completely understood. $1,25(OH)_2D$ stimulates the transformation of mononuclear cells of the monocyte–macrophage line to multinucleated osteoclasts. Calcitonin inhibits osteoclasts directly, but PTH only stimulates them in the presence of osteoblast-like cells. Normally there is a balance between bone resorption and formation which is referred to as coupling. The term decoupling is used when either resorption or formation is initiated independently or when there is an imbalance between resorption and formation. The normal fraction of trabecular bone involved in resorption is 4–5 percent and is a function of the life span of the resorptive sites and their activation frequency. The normal resorption period is 45 days. In *hyperparathyroidism* the surface area involved in resorption is increased due to increased activation frequency. In *hypo-* and *hyperthyroidism* there is little net effect on resorption surface area because of opposite effects of both diseases on activation frequency and the life span of the absorptive site.

Bone formation occurs as a result of osteoblasts laying down osteoid. In the normal activated osteon osteoid seams cover about 20 percent of the trabecular bone surface and are about 10 μm thick. The interval between osteoid formation and its mineralization is about 20–25 days. The normal cycle for remodeling lasts about 4–5 months and the mean osteoid thickness is an indicator of the speed of bone turnover. In humans about 5 percent cortical bone and 20–40 percent trabecular bone are replaced each year. In *osteomalacia* there is a marked increase in the osteoid formation time and a lag in mineralization which combine to produce a gross excess of osteoid.

Altered kinetics of remodeling may arise from a change in the activation frequency or the amount of bone resorbed or formed in each osteon. Bone mass may be decreased by either a change in the activation frequency or by decoupling. If the activation frequency increases, but bone resorption and formation remain synchronous, the number of active osteons per unit mass and thereby bone porosity increase. As the activation frequency slows, the canals refill with bone and density returns to normal. This is an example of reversible bone loss. In contrast, if decoupling occurs and resorption takes place without formation, irreversible bone loss occurs and this may be compounded if the activation frequency increases at the same time. Another way bone can be weakened is if the activated osteon moves across the thickness of the trabecular plate. The average trabecular thickness is about 150 mm, but is very variable The average resorption cone is 65 mm long, but it can be much longer. In some circumstances, particularly associated with increased activation frequency, resorption cones perforate the plate, leaving no anatomical basis for subsequent bone formation. If sustained this weakens the trabecular lattice.

Bone which is not weight bearing is made up of a honeycomb of uniform trabecular plates which combine maximum strength with minimum mass. Weight-bearing trabecular bone is made up of thick plates and columns oriented in the direction of the compressive forces and supported by thinner trabecular struts in the non-load-bearing plane. As a function of aging the thick load-bearing plates are successively perforated and converted into columns by remodeling and the thinner non-load-bearing trabeculae become disconnected and may disappear. The overall effect is to weaken the bone and at a critical point buckling or crush compression occurs.

Bone homeostasis

Bone homeostasis can be disturbed by alterations in bone turnover, osteoid mineralization or osteoid formation. Bone turnover is altered most in *hypo-* and *hyperthyroidism* and *hyperparathyroidism*. In *hypothyroidism* there is a balanced slowing of the total remodeling cycle, resulting in a normal or slightly increased amount of trabecular bone and a low serum alkaline phosphatase, osteocalcin and renal hydroxyproline excretion. *Hyperthyroidism* is characterized by increased serum levels and renal excretion of both Ca^{2+} and phosphate. Vitamin D metabolism is affected with reduced levels of $1,25(OH)_2D$ and increased levels of $24,25(OH)_2D$ in the presence of a normal serum 25(OH)D. The switch in vitamin D metabolism may be due to hyperphosphatemia. The fractional intestinal Ca^{2+} absorption is reduced in consequence. Bone turnover is increased with a slight imbalance between formation and resorption, resulting in gradual decrease in bone mass. These changes are reflected biochemically in a raised alkaline phosphatase, calcitonin and increased renal excretion of hydroxyproline. In *primary hyperparathyroidism* there is an increased serum concentration and renal excretion of Ca^{2+} with suppression of serum phosphate. $1,25(OH)_2D$ is increased despite normal concentrations of 25(OH)D leading to increased intestinal absorption of Ca^{2+}. Serum alkaline phosphatase and calcitonin are raised together with hydroxyproline excretion. Bone remodeling is faster than normal and is associated with a slight negative Ca^{2+} balance. This is confirmed by histomorphometry which shows increased porosity but relatively normal osteons.

Osteomalacia is caused by a lag in osteoid mineralization resulting in thickened osteoid seams. Appropriate Ca^{2+} and phosphate concentrations at the mineralization site are a prerequisite for normal bone formation, and a defect in their homeostasis as in *X-linked hypophosphatemic rickets* or *congenital hypophosphatasia* may lead to *osteomalacia* because of an inability to achieve a critical concentration. If malabsorption involves Ca^{2+} the resulting mild hypocalcemia leads to a *secondary hyperparathyroidism*. Despite a low 25(OH)D possibly from the malabsorption, $1,25(OH)_2D$ is normal or raised due to stimulation of the renal 1α-hydroxylase by PTH and hypophosphatemia. Serum alkaline phosphatase and renal hydroxyproline excretion are increased. Bone turnover is increased but mineralization is normal early in malabsorption, whereas in more advanced cases there is breakdown of biochemical homeostasis with a fall of serum Ca^{2+} and $1,25(OH)_2D$ despite secondary hypoparathyroidism. This leads to a lag in mineralization and an increase of osteoid in both thickness and surface area. In full-blown *osteomalacia* there is a slowing of bone turnover due to osteoclasts failing to penetrate the osteoid which continues to proliferate.

The bone disease of *chronic renal failure* comes from impaired renal phosphorus excretion leading to hyperphosphatemia and reduced $1,25(OH)_2D$ formation due to loss of renal parenchyma and hyperphosphatemia. Secondary hyperparathyroidism also occurs and the complicated interaction of mineral, vitamin D and PTH metabolism produces a spectrum of bone changes which range from osteopenia to osteosclerosis. In *mild renal failure* the characteristic bony finding is increased turnover due to secondary hyperparathyroidism resulting in increased porosity, disturbance of structure and marrow fibrosis. If the failure becomes long standing the bone becomes frankly osteomalacic due to defective mineralization. Similar changes may occur during *renal dialysis* in which the pathology is further complicated by the possible accumulation of aluminum from dialysis fluid and the ingestion of oral phosphate binders. Aluminum is deposited at the mineralization sites from which it can be removed by chelating agents, such as desferrioxamine, with clinical benefit.

Bone pathology resulting from a decrease in bone mass is seen mainly in the elderly, but a chronic catabolic state at any age will cause a reduction of bone mass. This may be seen in children with *chronic neurological disease*, *chronic inflammatory bowel disease* and those taking pharmacological doses of glucocorticoids. In all these cases osteopenia results from a decreased rate of bone formation in the presence of normal resorption, yielding a thin bone.

Selected reading

Martin TJ, Raisz LG, eds. *Clinical endocrinology of calcium metabolism*. New York: Marcel Dekker, 1987: 410.

Maxwell MH, Kleeman CR, Narins RG, eds. *Clinical disorders of fluid and electrolyte metabolism*. 4th ed. New York: McGraw-Hill, 1987: 1268.

Nordin BEC, ed. *Calcium in human biology*. London: Springer Verlag, 1988: 481.

8 • *Thermoregulation*

Associate editor: Tania R Gunn

A. Thermoregulation

J McIntyre, D Hull, J Nedergaard and B Cannon

Chemical reactions provide the energy for growth, activity, thermal control, maintenance and repair. As a consequence heat is produced. In most animal species (poikilotherms) this heat is dissipated from the surface of the body and the body temperature remains similar to that of the surroundings, whether water or air. When mammals developed, they acquired two properties which gave an evolutionary advantage: the ability to breast-feed their young, and the ability for extra heat production when necessary by facultative nonshivering thermogenesis. The latter allowed mammals to defend an elevated and constant body temperature and thus their activity became independent of ambient temperature: early mammals could therefore be active at night when no other predators or competitors were around, thus providing an evolutionary advantage.

Facultative thermogenesis is the distinctive outcome of the metabolism of brown adipose tissue. The earliest mammals were small, and in these small animals brown adipose tissue and a high thermogenic capacity probably persisted throughout life. However, as larger mammals, including man, developed, the need for extra heat production in the adult diminished because loss of heat to the surroundings decreases more rapidly with increasing size than does the resting metabolic rate. However, the smaller size of infants still requires extra heat production; thus neonates rely on brown adipose tissue to remain euthermic.

Homeothermy has been more strictly defined as 'a pattern of temperature regulation in which cyclic variation in core temperature, either diurnally or seasonally, is maintained within narrow limits, despite much larger variations in ambient temperature'.

Physical heat exchange

Heat is a form of energy and is thus subject to the laws of thermodynamic conservation which state that 'energy cannot be created or destroyed but only converted from one form to another'. Heat produced by metabolic processes in the body (M) must therefore either be stored in the tissues (S) or dissipated to the environment. The channels for dissipating heat are radiation (R), convection (C), conduction (K) and evaporation (E). The heat balance can be expressed as

$$M = E + C + K + R + S$$

Radiation (R)

Energy exchanged by this mode is in the form of electromagnetic waves, ranging from the short wave radiation of the visible spectrum to the long wave infra red radiation. In 'natural' environments solar radiation is the main source of short wave radiation (0.3–3.0 μm). In bright sunlight solar radiation can be the largest single factor in the heat balance equation and the exogenous provision of heat may be as much as ten times metabolic heat production. Indirect radiation from scattered sunlight and reflections can increase the net solar radiation flux.

Radiation of a longer wavelength (around 10 μm) is emitted by objects such as people, plants and buildings. At these longer wavelengths energy exchange can result in heat loss or gain depending on the temperature of the body and of the surrounding surfaces. The main factors determining radiant heat exchange are: (1) the surface temperature of the two objects, exchange being proportional to the difference to the fourth power of the surface temperatures, (2) the respective areas and orientation of the two objects, (3) their emissivity and reflectivity. Normal intact skin has an average emissivity of 0.97–0.98, irrespective of color or pigmentation and thus for practical purposes the human body can be considered to behave like a black body over most of the thermal spectrum.

Convection (C)

This describes the transference of heat by the movement of a liquid or gas from a warmer to a cooler region. In still air, free convection occurs in which the air in contact with the body is warmed, becomes lighter and so rises to be replaced with cooler air. The moving air provides an insulation and in the upright position this may be several centimeters thick by the time it reaches the face. The thicker the boundary layer, the lower the convective loss. Large differences in flow patterns and hence insulation can be produced by changes in posture; for example, when lying down the insulating properties of a thick boundary layer are largely lost. When the body is exposed to moving air the natural convective air streams are displaced, disrupting the boundary layer, and heat is lost by forced convection. Prediction of heat loss is difficult; the main determinants of convective heat exchange are the temperature difference between skin and air, air movement across the surfaces and the surface area exposed.

Conduction (K)

When two bodies are in direct contact thermal energy can be transferred from molecule to molecule: this is called conduction. The transference of heat will depend on the temperature gradient between the two objects, the area of contact and the heat capacity and conductivity of the materials. In practice the role of conductive heat exchange in humans is small, rarely exceeding 3 percent of the total.

Evaporation (E)

When evaporation occurs from the skin or respiratory tract the latent heat of vaporization represents a loss of heat from the body. Evaporative heat exchange is determined by the gradient of absolute humidity. Two processes are involved in evaporative heat loss from the skin. Transepidermal loss is due to the continuous evaporation of water that has been released following passive diffusion through the outer dead layers of the skin. This loss is driven by the difference between the vapor concentration below the epidermis and that in the ambient air. The stratum corneum is the main barrier to diffusion and provided this is intact, transepidermal water loss is a relatively small source of heat loss in the normal indoor environment.

The second process is sweating. In warm environments where non-evaporative heat loss is decreased large amounts of heat can still be lost by secretion of sweat that evaporates from the skin surface. The heat loss will depend on the rate at which the body can secrete sweat and the environmental humidity. Sweat rate can be adjusted over a wide range of climatic conditions and rates of heat production. It may be as high as 1.5 l/h in unacclimatized adults and up to 4 l/h in someone fully acclimatized.

Storage (S)

Heat is stored in, or released from, body tissues when their temperature changes. Clearly, over a long period, the mean rate of change of heat storage is zero but it can be an important short-term component of heat balance.

Developmental aspects

In fetal life there is a continuous exchange of heat between the fetus and its environment. The maternal arterial blood temperature is the single most important determinant of fetal temperature. The heat generated by fetal metabolism is readily transferred to the placenta by the umbilical arteries. Thus the temperature of the fetus is a little higher than that of the mother but remains close to it at all times.

The capacity of newborn mammals to control their body temperature varies between species. In the newborn of small mammals, the task of maintaining thermal control in the natural environment of their parents would place too great a demand on their energy reserves even if it were biologically possible. The small naked newborn hamster lacks obvious thermal control at birth, thermotaxis appears at around 8 days, behavioral thermoregulation 2 or 3 days later and thermogenesis at around 16 days of age. For such mammals, nests, huddling or cuddling are essential for survival. In the larger newborn mammals, like the lamb, the thermoregulatory capacities are well developed and their responses match, or might even be considered to exceed, those of adults. However, given their smaller size and shorter hair they are still vulnerable to cold conditions that can be weathered by their parents.

The mature newborn human infant has a modest

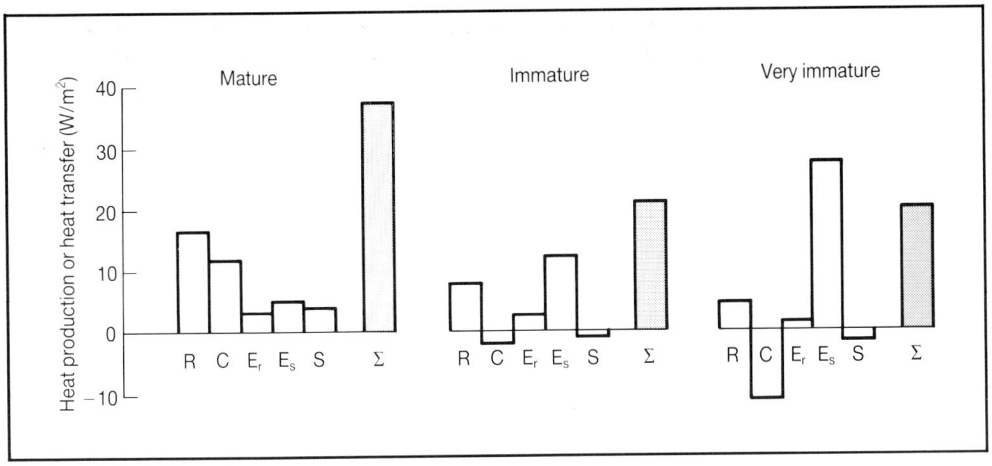

Fig. 8.1. Physical heat exchanges in term and preterm infants. The heat exchange in full-term, 32 week and under 28 week prematurely born infants nursed in an incubator. R, radiation; C, convection; E_r, evaporation from respiratory tract; E_s, evaporation from skin surface; S, heat storage; Σ, net sum of heat exchange.

capacity to modulate heat exchange by both behavioral and autonomic responses. Obviously changes in posture and vasomotor control will influence the characteristics of physical heat exchange as well as the characteristics of the environment. Figure 8.1 illustrates the modes of heat exchange of mature, preterm and very preterm infants nursed in incubators in a thermoneutral environment, that is, at a temperature where the infant need not make any attempt at thermal control. The main external variables are the difference in temperature between the infant's body and the environment, the velocity of air flow, the relative humidity and the area exposed for heat exchange. It will be seen that the size and maturity of the infant are important factors which influence heat flow. In the very preterm infant, the heat exchange is powerfully influenced by transepidermal water loss because the skin of infants under 28 weeks of gestation in the first weeks of life is only a few cells thick, with a very decreased stratum corneum, and is not watertight. This heat flow is determined by the humidity in the surrounding air. It is difficult to maintain 100 percent humidity in an incubator though it is important to keep it as high as possible. The use of adhesive semipermeable dressings markedly decreases transepidermal water loss. It is impossible to control the humidity surrounding infants nursed under radiant heaters. This is the main disadvantage of radiant heaters as the heat source for the care of the very preterm infant in temperate climates.

Heat production

A relatively constant internal environment allows cellular chemical reactions to proceed at a steady rate. Thus the homeotherm can maintain a high level of performance despite wide variations in environmental conditions. Such an advantage is expensive in energy terms.

Direct calorimetry measures the heat flux from the subject. Systems have been developed to make such measurements in both children and adults. This approach is technically demanding; it depends on many measurements and requires calculations for which some assumptions have to be made. Indirect calorimetry measures oxygen consumption and carbon dioxide production of the subject. Heat production can be calculated by measurements of respiratory gas exchanges and making assumptions about the energy content of nutrients. This is the usual method for measuring energy expenditure and substrate utilization in man.

Heat production varies widely depending on energy expenditure and environmental conditions. Thus to make useful comparisons between individuals the index used is the basal metabolic rate (BMR) which, strictly defined, is 'the rate of metabolic free energy production calculated from measurements of heat production or oxygen consumption in an organism in a rested, awake, fasting and thermoneutral state'. Such a state is often difficult to achieve in children since, if resting, they are usually postprandial and asleep. Thus the measured values are often the resting metabolic rate which is not a true BMR.

Under similar conditions a larger body will generate more heat per hour than a smaller one. Heat production can be expressed as watts per kilogram (W/kg), that is, in terms of body weight and this is appropriate when calculating nutritional requirements. However, as heat loss is determined in part by surface area the metabolic

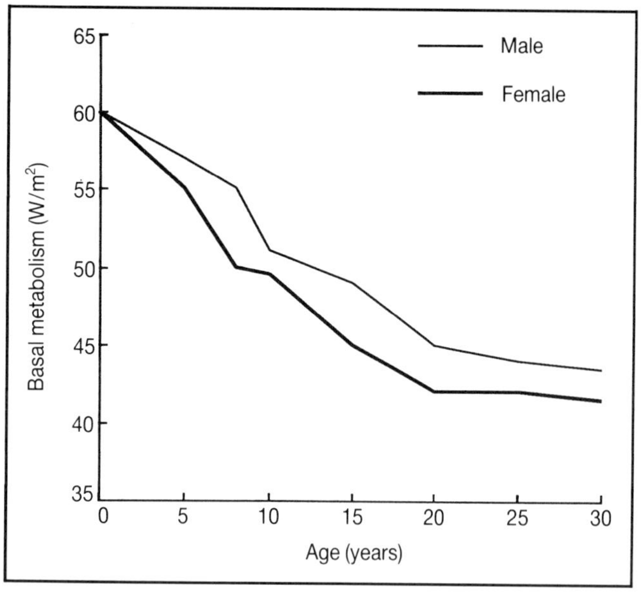

Fig. 8.2. Basal metabolic rate at different ages. (From Guyton AC. *Textbook of medical physiology*. Philadelphia: WB Saunders, 1986: 847, with permission.)

rate is usually expressed per unit surface area in W/m^2, when considering heat exchanges. The data on metabolic rates in infancy and childhood are limited. From the commonly quoted data it can be seen that from birth to sexual maturity there is a steady decline in BMR (Fig. 8.2). The newborn infant has a BMR per unit surface area nearly twice that of an old person. The BMR of males is higher than comparable females. This might be explained by the different amounts of body fat. Body shape affects the BMR: a lighter individual will have a higher metabolic rate per kg body weight than a thicker set person of the same height. This is because BMR depends on active tissue mass and a fat person will have a relatively smaller lean body mass. There are important hormonal influences on BMR. In the *hyperthyroid* state the BMR may increase by 40–80 percent and in *hypothyroidism* it may fall 40–50 percent. The BMR also fluctuates over 24 hours. Metabolism and body temperature are greatest during the day and fall during the night. This circadian rhythm appears to develop in the first 4 months of life. Ingestion of food also alters BMR; this so-called specific dynamic action can increase BMR by 6–10 percent.

Cold conditions and activity have far more impact on energy requirements and heat exchange than the factors that modify basal metabolic rate. The relationship between the metabolic rate and the environmental

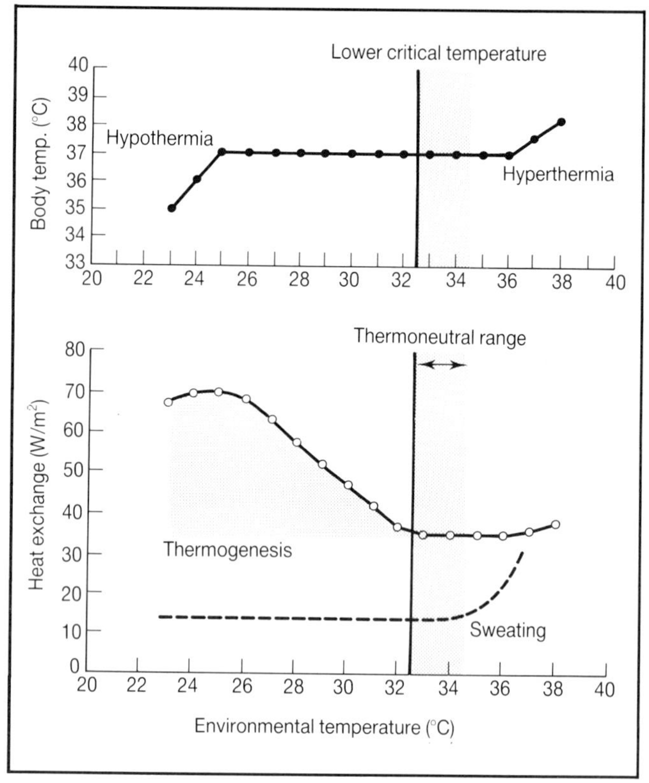

Fig. 8.3. The relationship between metabolic rate and environmental temperature.

temperature is illustrated in Fig. 8.3. When the environmental temperature lies in the zone of least thermoregulatory effort, that is the 'neutral thermal environment', metabolism is minimal. As the temperature falls below this, heat production increases until it reaches a maximum—the cold limit. Cooling beyond this results in a fall in metabolic heat production that, if continued, will cause hypothermia and death. When temperatures exceed the heat dissipating capacity, the hot limit, the metabolic rate will inevitably rise, causing hyperthermia and death unless cooling occurs.

The regulation of body temperature

The central body temperature is normally maintained within narrow limits. To achieve this, with continuously and rapidly changing rates of heat loss and heat production, requires complex interaction between sensing, integrating and effector units. Thermal sensors are located in the skin, central nervous system and several other locations.

Thermoreception

Humans can perceive temperature gradations of cold and heat progressing through painful (cold), icy, cold, cool, neutral, lukewarm, warm, hot, painful (hot). Thermoreceptors can be defined in physical terms as nerve endings excited only or preferentially by thermal stimuli. This definition holds for any thermosensitive structure irrespective of whether its excitation correlates with temperature sensation. The general properties of specific cutaneous thermoreceptors have been described as follows: (1) they have a static discharge at constant temperature, (2) they show a dynamic response to temperature change with either a positive temperature coefficient (warm receptors) or a negative coefficient (cold receptors), (3) they are not excited by mechanical stimuli and (4) activity occurs in the nonpainful range. Cutaneous thermoreceptors have been divided into warm and cold receptors based on these properties. It has been shown that cold receptors are fairly evenly distributed over the whole body surface. However, the density of warm receptors is more variable with, for example, a high density on the face and hands. The axons of cutaneous thermoreceptors run within the afferent cutaneous nerves to the segmental spinal ganglia and the dorsal root of the spinal cord. Spinal thermosensitive afferents are mainly conveyed in the contralateral spinothalamic tract, giving off collaterals to the midbrain reticular formation and to the hypothalamus.

Much of our current knowledge on central receptors is based on animal studies and may not apply to man. Local warming and cooling of the hypothalamus elicits thermoregulatory responses. These thermosensitive neurons are concentrated in the preoptic anterior area of the hypothalamus. There is also evidence for thermosensitive neurons in the midbrain, medulla oblongata and the spinal cord. Thermosensors are also present in deep tissues; for example, in blood vessels, the abdominal cavity, and carotid baroreceptors and chemoreceptors.

Elucidating how thermoregulatory pathways are integrated is difficult. It appears that the brainstem, from the septal preoptic region to the caudal posterior hypothalamus, participates in sensing temperature, integrating the message from different pathways, and organizing efferent pathways. The posterior hypothalamus seems of particular importance and single neurons in this region have been shown to respond to thermal signals from the anterior hypothalamus and to those arriving from the spinal cord and skin.

Effector systems

In addition to the classical physiological thermoregulatory mechanisms, homeotherms also regulate body temperature by behavioral means involving coordinated and voluntary motor activity. Seeking appropriate thermal environments, shelter and clothing are important in maintaining body temperature but this represents modification of thermal environment, not of the subject.

The concept of a 'set point' has to be used to understand how body temperature is maintained in a narrow range. Temperature control mechanisms or effector systems continually attempt to bring back the body temperature to this set point when a deviation is sensed. The temperature regulated or 'controlled variable' was formerly thought to be the deep body temperature best represented by the hypothalamic temperature. However, a more appropriate model may be the multiple input system in which the temperature regulated is a function of several local temperatures; that is an integrated body temperature. The set point can be thought of as this integrated body temperature that is maintained when output signals from the controller to effector systems are zero. At this point the mechanisms of heat loss and heat production are not being activated. Changes sensed as a deviation from this set point activate thermoregulatory effector systems to return the temperature field towards zero. The short-term control actions of temperature regulation are initiated via nervous pathways. The main effector systems are either behavioral or autonomic. The autonomic systems that respond in sequence from warm to cool are sweating, the vasomotor system, postural adjustments and thermogenesis.

Sudomotor system (sweat glands)

In conditions where non-evaporative heat loss is limited, sweating becomes the major channel for dissipating heat. Sweat glands are widely distributed over the body. Secretion of sweat is initiated and controlled by the activity of efferent cholinergic sympathetic nerves. It is an eccrine process involving transfer of fluid across the intact cell membrane. The apocrine sweat glands in the axillary and pubic areas are not involved in thermal sweating. The forehead has a particularly high sweating rate. Local skin temperature variations can also appreciably change the rate of eccrine sweat secretion in a small area.

Vasomotor

A major determinant of heat exchange is the skin temperature and it is the rate of blood flow to the skin that determines its temperature. The blood flow can be altered by changing the diameter of the arterioles, vessels with a thick muscle coat, which can contract or relax in response to nerve impulses. In warm conditions arterioles dilate, allowing warm blood to flow through the skin capillaries, warming the skin and dissipating heat. This effect is enhanced by returning blood flowing in the superficial veins close to the skin surface. In cold conditions skin blood flow and hence heat loss is minimized by vasoconstriction, conserving heat to the deeper parts of the body. Furthermore, returning blood flows in the deep veins that lie close to the arteries, a mechanism that helps reduce the temperature gradient across the skin surface. The control of peripheral blood flow varies regionally and three functionally different regions have been identified: (1) the extremities, hands, feet, ears, lips, nose, (2) trunk and proximal limbs and (3) head and brow.

Blood flow through the extremities is under noradrenergic sympathetic control. An increase in sympathetic tone causes vasoconstriction and a decrease in tone vasodilation. In the trunk and proximal limbs vasodilation induced by heat is an active process. It is mediated by the release of bradykinins from the sweat glands. Thus cutaneous regions where this active process occurs are the same as those in which pronounced thermal sweating occurs. On the forehead, vasomotor nerves have only a slight effect. With cold exposure there is very little vasoconstriction. In response to heat, however, vasodilatation and sweat production do occur.

Thermogenesis

Heat production is increased by shivering and nonshivering thermogenesis, both of which are under the control of nervous pathways. In adults the first response to cooling is an increase in muscle tone with muscle units firing out of phase and at different frequencies. This explains the feeling of stiffness on cold exposure. Further cooling causes the discharges to become more synchronized, creating a tremor and eventually frank shivering. The overall heat production can be five to six times the resting rate, but this can only be maintained for a few minutes. Over a period of an hour or more body heat production may be raised about 50–100 percent. It is more efficient than voluntary contractions in terms of heat production. Shivering is controlled through the descending tracts of the 'shivering pathway' that leave the posterior hypothalamus and run caudally through the midbrain tegmentum and pons. Here they contact the supraspinal motor pathways that make synaptic contacts on the motor neurons in the anterior horns of the spinal cord and activate muscles via the motor nerves.

In the newborn infant heat is generated on cold exposure but shivering does not appear to occur. Over the first year of life the relative contribution of this nonshivering thermogenesis declines to be replaced by shivering thermogenesis (Fig. 8.4). From animal models it is suggested that these two thermogenic effector mechanisms form an interlocked control system. It is thought that under natural conditions shivering will only occur after nonshivering thermogenesis has been evoked to its full extent.

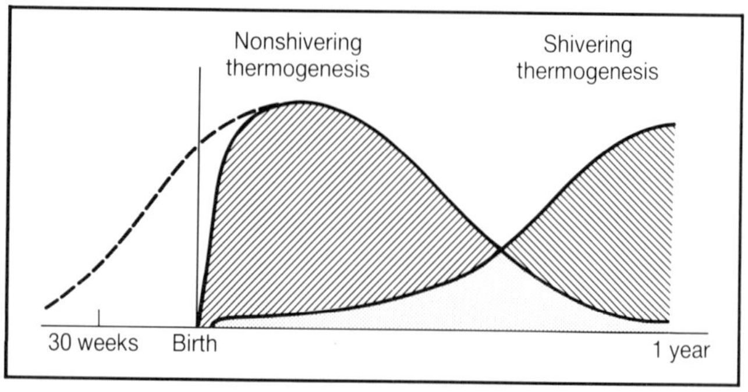

Fig. 8.4. Shivering and nonshivering thermogenesis.

Brown adipose tissue and nonshivering thermogenesis

Brown adipose tissue is found in several depots in the newborn, but the interscapular and perirenal depots are the most significant (Fig. 8.5). Heat production in brown adipose tissue is a facultative event: heat is only produced when it is needed to maintain the temperature of the newborn. The activity of brown adipose tissue is controlled by centers in the hypothalamus. These include

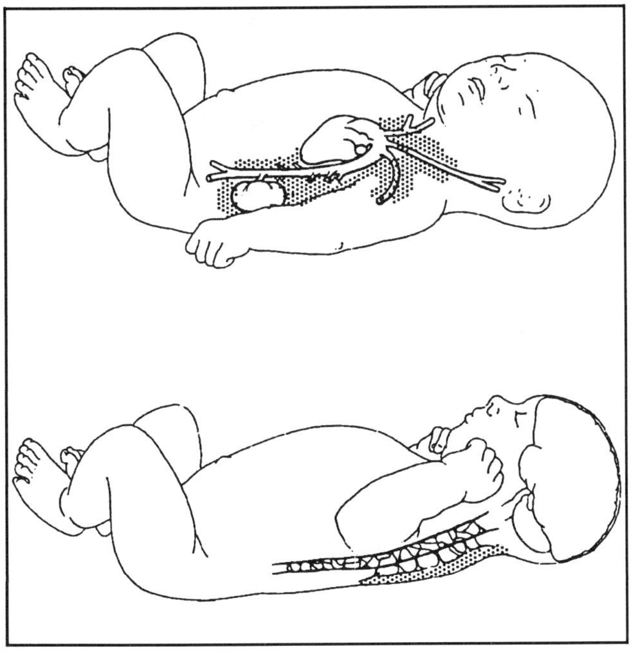

Fig. 8.5. The distribution of brown adipose tissue as identified by multilocular adipocytes.

regions around the optic chiasma, responsible for the integration of thermal signals and for the maintenance of body temperature, as well as centers in the ventromedial hypothalamus (VMH) and lateral hypothalamus (LH), responsible for feeding behavior and energetic control.

Physiological stimulation of each of these centers leads to a wide array of effects in the newborn. The temperature centers and the VMH have an inhibitory effect on lower centers which are specifically responsible for stimulating brown fat activity. Thus, when this inhibition is removed the thermogenic function of brown adipose tissue is induced. The signals are transmitted through the sympathetic nervous system. The nerve cell bodies directly responsible for control of brown fat activity are found along the sympathetic chain and especially in the sympathetic ganglia. It is likely that all brown fat depots are activated in parallel. As stimulation of brown adipose tissue occurs via the sympathetic nervous system, the tissue may be stimulated in a stress situation. However, activation of brown adipose tissue should normally be considered a specialized and distinct activation of the tissue through dedicated pathways.

Adrenergic receptors

Norepinephrine released from the sympathetic fibers within brown adipose tissue interacts with adrenergic receptors on the brown fat cell membrane. The dominant stimulatory pathway proceeds via the recently described β_3-receptors. These receptors respond to norepinephrine, as do all other β-receptors, but they have a different pharmacology, e.g. the classical β-adrenergic inhibitor propranolol is a weaker (10- to 100-fold) antagonist on them than on β_1- and β_2-receptors. For thermogenic action α_1-receptors are also positively involved, although α_1-stimulation proceeds via pathways different from those described below and only causes a minor fraction of the heat production. α_2-Adrenergic stimulation inhibits thermogenesis.

Cytosolic events

The initial intracellular responses in the brown fat cell to β-adrenergic stimulation are not different from those in white adipose tissue (Fig. 8.6). There is first an increase in cyclic AMP which activates intracellular protein kinase, which in its turn activates the hormone-sensitive lipase by phosphorylating it on a serine residue. When the lipase is activated, it breaks down the triglycerides in the cytoplasmic fat droplets to fatty acids and glycerol. The released fatty acids have two options: they may be combusted in the brown fat cell itself, as described in more detail below, or they may be exported from the cell and become metabolized in other tissues, e.g. as an energy supply for shivering thermogenesis in muscles.

Continued use of triglycerides for thermogenesis in the newborn rapidly leads to exhaustion of the supply available in the tissue, and therefore ultimately to cessation of thermogenesis. Replenishment of the triglycerides is therefore necessary to ensure thermogenesis. Brown adipose tissue has a comparatively active fatty acid synthesis pathway, but it is doubtful whether this pathway is active during thermogenesis (it is inhibited by norepinephrine and is thus probably mainly active in refilling the triglyceride droplets during periods without thermogenic demand on the tissue). Rather, the major influx of new substrate for thermogenesis comes from the activity of lipoprotein lipase. Lipoprotein lipase is regulated in a unique way in brown adipose tissue: it is stimulated by norepinephrine, via a β-adrenergic, cAMP-

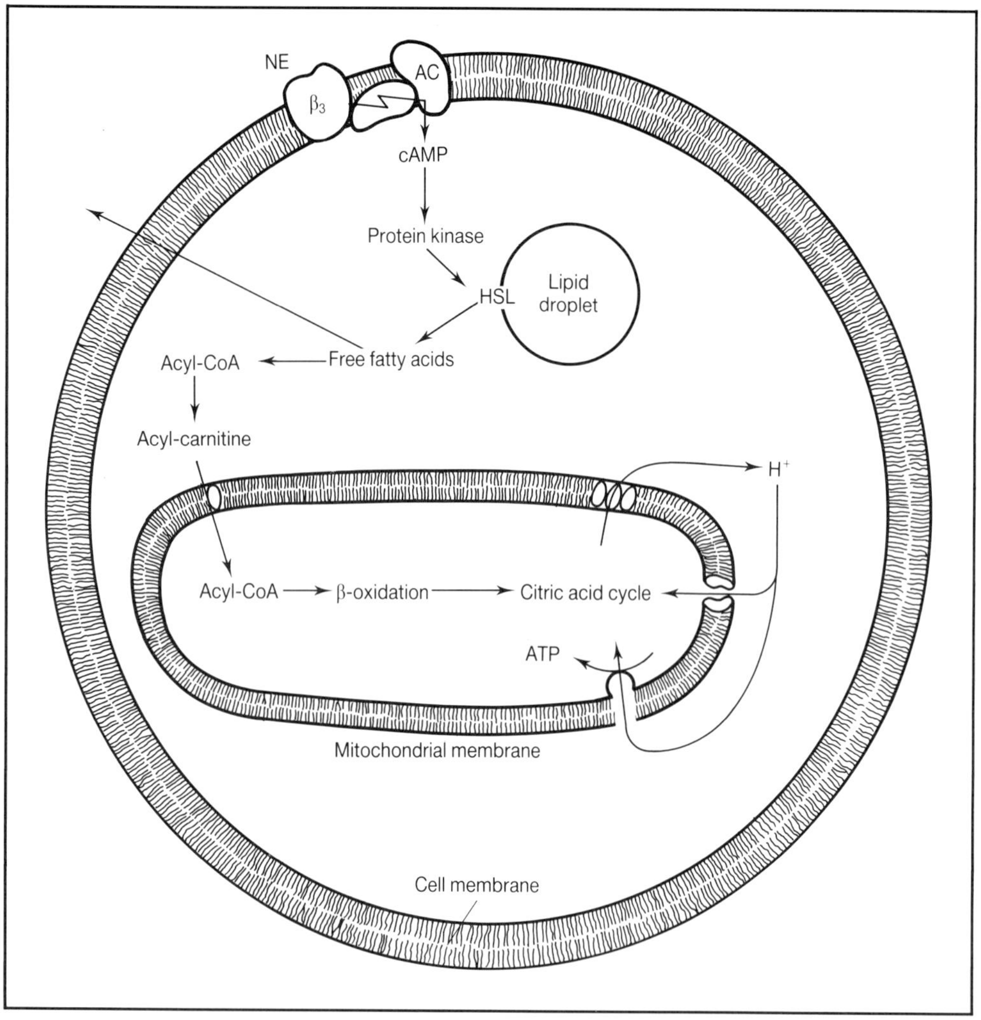

Fig. 8.6. The cytosolic events in the brown fat cell following β_3-adrenergic stimulation by norepinephrine (NE). AC, adenylyl cyclase; HSL, hormone-sensitive lipase. For details on mitochondrial function, see Fig. 8.7.

dependent pathway. The regulation of lipoprotein lipase activity occurs at the transcriptional level. The increased lipoprotein lipase activity in brown adipose tissue is induced via two pathways: when the newborn has an acute need for heat (via the norepinephrine pathway) and also when there is a fresh supply of food, after nursing (via an insulin pathway similar to that found in white adipose tissue).

The uncoupling protein thermogenin and mitochondrial thermogenic events

The combustion of the fatty acids released from the triglycerides takes place in the mitochondria. The fatty acids are first converted on the cytosolic side of the mitochondria to acyl-CoA; they are then transported in the form of acylcarnitine derivatives over the mitochondrial membrane, and on the inside, re-formed acyl-CoAs are degraded to acetyl-CoA moieties by going through the necessary number of rounds of so-called β-oxidation (see p. 89). The acetyl-CoA formed enters the citric acid cycle, CO_2 is released and the electrons from NADH and $FADH_2$ are transported to oxygen through the electron transport chain of the mitochondria, all this just as in other fat-metabolizing tissues. Here, however, ends the similarity with other mitochondria.

The unique properties of brown fat mitochondria are due to the presence of the uncoupling protein thermogenin. As seen in Fig. 8.7, the transport of electrons through the mitochondrial electron transport chain (or 'respiratory chain') is coupled to pumping of H^+ out from the mitochondria, into the cytosol. Through this, a proton electrochemical potential is built up; the size of this

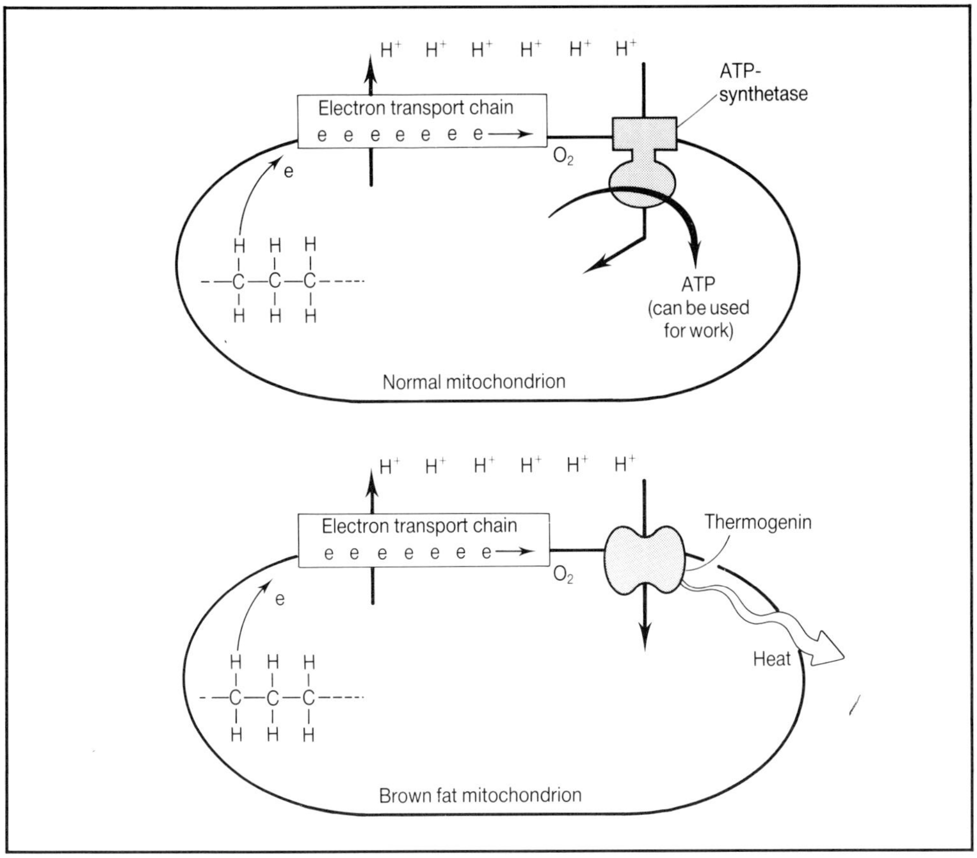

Fig. 8.7. The mitochondrial events: a comparison of the ATP-producing function of 'normal' mitochondria with the heat-producing function of brown fat mitochondria. For structural details of thermogenin, see Fig. 8.8.

potential increases, until it is equal to the energy available from electron transport. Then respiration ceases (no electrons are any longer transported to oxygen). In all mitochondria other than brown fat mitochondria the energy stored in the proton electrochemical potential is primarily utilized when H^+ re-enter the mitochondrial matrix through the ATP synthetase complex and the energy is captured in the form of ATP.

In brown fat mitochondria, thermogenin (Fig. 8.7) allows protons to re-enter the mitochondrial matrix, without capturing the energy in the form of a chemical bond. The function of thermogenin is thus to short-circuit the protonic circuit, and just as is the case when an electrical circuit is short-circuited, all energy is now released as heat. Thus, the energy which was released when electrons were transported from their high potential in fatty acids via NADH and $FADH_2$ to oxygen, and which was temporarily stored in the form of the proton electrochemical gradient, is now released in the form of heat. Thus the introduction of this single protein totally changes the purpose of the organized fatty acid degradation pathway to become energy-dissipative instead of energy-conserving.

The uncoupling protein thermogenin is exclusively found in brown adipose tissue and thus exclusively in mammals. Thermogenin has a monomeric molecular weight of 32 kDa, but it is likely that it is active in a homodimeric state. When the sequence of about 300 amino acids is analyzed, it becomes clear that thermogenin has developed from three repeats, each with a length of about 100 amino acids. As thermogenin is a membrane protein, it would be expected that stretches of hydrophobic amino acids should be observed; however, this is not the case. This paradox can be resolved if the structure is analyzed for amphiphilic α-helices: in each 100 amino acid sequence, two such amphiphilic sequences are found; they are characterized as being α-helixes which are hydrophilic on one side and hydrophobic on the other side. It is therefore believed that thermogenin has the structure sketched in Fig. 8.8.

When it is in its active state, thermogenin transports H^+ through the mitochondrial membrane. How this is

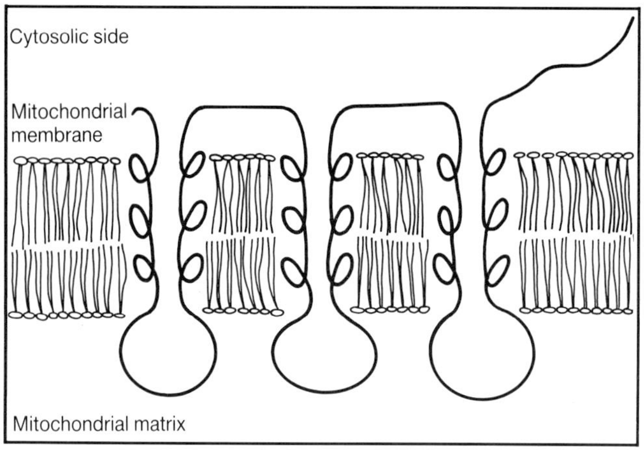

Fig. 8.8. Some of the accepted structural and functional characteristics of the uncoupling protein (see text).

accomplished molecularly is not known; it is most likely that thermogenin functions as a transporter on which only one H^+ can be transported at a time, i.e. not as an open channel with mass flux. Thermogenin is not constantly active, as this would lead to brown fat thermogenesis being permanently switched on, a physiologically unwarranted situation. Rather, thermogenin is endowed with a binding site for purine nucleotides; this binding site can bind ATP, ADP, GTP and GDP with high affinity (this binding site is often referred to as 'the GDP binding site'). Binding of, for example, ATP to this site leads to a conformational change in the thermogenin molecule, including a total inhibition of thermogenin H^+-transporting activity. Due to the high affinity of the site for ATP and to the high cytosolic concentration of ATP, it is likely that in the resting state, the site is always occupied and thermogenin activity is fully inhibited. Activation of thermogenin is thus by overcoming this inhibition but the mechanism is not yet clear. Based mainly on the fact that free fatty acids added to isolated brown fat cells can elicit thermogenesis without norepinephrine stimulation being necessary, most investigators favor postlipolytic hypotheses in which the activation occurs as an effect of fatty acids being released from the triglycerides.

Thermogenin has homology to the ATP/ADP carrier of the mitochondrial inner membrane. It appears that it belongs to a family of mitochondrial proteins, all of which are found in the mitochondrial inner membrane and all of which function as transporters of specific compounds over the mitochondrial membrane. For thermogenin, the transported species would thus be H^+. It can be imagined that these proteins, probably at least 15 different ones, have all developed from an ancestor which developed in free-living bacteria to help take up substrate (food) from the surroundings.

The recruitment process

Brown adipose tissue is particularly adaptable and responds to an increased demand for its activity by rapidly and extensively increasing its capacity for heat production in two ways: by acquiring more brown fat cells and/or by making 'better' cells (cells in a more recruited state). Mammalian species differ in this respect. The relative importance of these two mechanisms in the human neonate is uncertain.

The number of brown fat cells with which a child is born is probably established early during fetal development. Even in experimental animals it is not known whether there is a postnatal increase in the total number of brown fat cells. However, in adult rats during adaptation to cold the increase in thermogenic capacity mainly corresponds to an increase in the number of brown fat cells. Initiation of division of brown fat cell precursors (brown preadipocytes or stem cells) demands the presence of classical growth factors, but experiments indicate that such growth factors are not physiologically regulatory. Rather it would seem that norepinephrine, released when heat production is needed, can also initiate cell division, but in contrast to thermogenesis, the receptors involved are β_1-receptors. The undifferentiated cells which can respond in this way do not possess the more specialized β_3-receptors.

As thermogenin is the rate-limiting step for thermogenesis, an increase in the total amount of thermogenin in the tissue is the only way to increase thermogenic potential. It has been established that norepinephrine, working through β_3-receptors, induces thermogenin gene expression. Thermogenin can only function if its increased expression is accompanied by an increased amount of mitochondria in the tissue, with an ensuing higher capacity for the combustion of fatty acids. Mitochondrial recruitment is not directly under norepinephrine control; rather, the whole differentiation process of the brown fat cells is promoted by norepinephrine, and the lipid-metabolizing enzymes are induced as an effect of advanced general differentiation, not as a direct and specified effect.

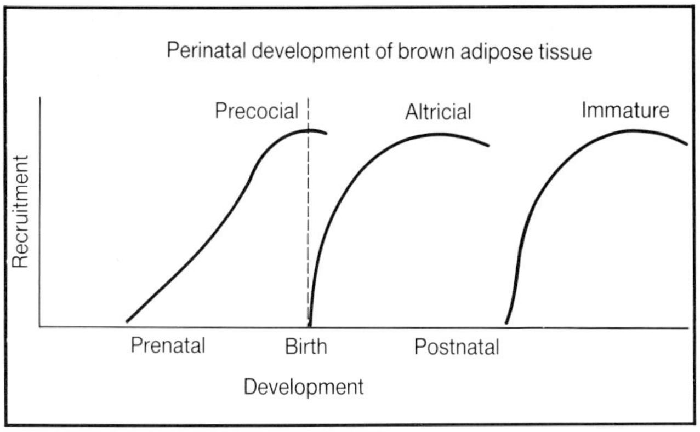

Fig. 8.9. Perinatal brown fat recruitments in immature, altricial and precocial mammals.

Perinatal recruitment

Both the acute thermogenic response and the recruitment process are stimulated by norepinephrine. In many physiological situations this makes good sense, since an increased demand for heat production suggests a requirement for increased total capacity. There are, however, physiological situations in which this relationship does not seem optimal. One of these is found during perinatal recruitment.

The principal patterns of brown fat recruitment in different types of mammalian newborn are shown (Fig. 8.9). The postnatal recruitment in **altricial** species is most easily understood. These species, e.g. rats and mice, are born blind and hairless, the pups huddle in the nest and are often warmed by the dam. Recruitment takes place as a response to a demand for thermogenesis as the pups are gradually exposed to the cold. In the *immature* newborn, e.g. hamsters, recruitment does not occur until a considerable time (weeks) after birth; this can be explained by an initial absence of sympathetic innervation to the brown adipose tissue and when the synapses are established, recruitment proceeds. However, many mammalian newborn are **precocial** and are well developed at birth; this is the case for newborn calves and lambs, and indeed for most larger mammals. These newborn can not only walk around soon after birth but they also have well developed brown adipose tissue at birth, and their acquisition of this represents a regulatory dilemma. *In utero*, there is no demand for thermogenesis, the fetus is even warmer than in its later free-living condition. Nonshivering thermogenesis cannot be demonstrated in fetal sheep cooled *in utero*. However, it can be induced following supplemental oxygenation and umbilical cord occlusion. It may therefore be suggested that a physiological inhibitor of fetal cAMP-dependent pathways present. It is likely that such an inhibitor exists, e.g. in the form of prostaglandins or adenosine produced by the placenta. However, such inhibitors would also inhibit the part of the β-adrenergic pathway which stimulates recruitment, and *in utero* recruitment thus remains unexplained in such species.

After birth, separation from the placenta would remove the placental inhibitor and so allow rapid brown fat thermogenesis to facilitate neonatal adaptation.

The human baby is considered to be 'typed' between altricial and precocial: newborn babies possess a 'basic' amount of active brown adipose tissue, but this can be markedly increased as a response to a cooler environment.

Developmental and pathological aspects

At birth the neonate experiences a dramatic change in thermal environment, from a tightly regulated one controlled by the mother to a less predictable one in which the responses of its own thermoregulatory system are essential for survival. Immediately after birth the deep body temperature falls. In the human infant under normal conditions it may fall to below 36°C 3 hours after birth, if care is not optimal, but by 8 hours it has usually returned to the adult range. Following this, the average level of body temperature is approximately the same as in adults. The human baby has limited thermal insulation due to a decreased thickness of body shell and a large body surface/volume ratio. As body mass increases to adult size the overall insulation increases by a factor of 1.8. On the first day of life control can be exercised over the peripheral vasomotor tone to effect a threefold change in tissue insulation, although this may still be inadequate insulation. Therefore additional thermal insulation is of great importance. Simply wrapping the baby in a blanket can alter the thermoregulatory range from 36–26°C to 30–10°C. Covering the head is of particular importance as it forms a large proportion of the baby's exposed surface area.

Regulation of temperature by active sweating can occur in babies born at term. About 400 sweat glands per cm^2 have been found on the thigh, six times as many as in adults, although each gland produces sweat at only a third of the rate. With earlier gestation, however, fewer infants sweat and below 32 weeks of gestation sweating has not been demonstrated.

Soon after birth the newborn is able to respond to a cool environment by an increase in metabolic rate and hence heat production. This takes place without shivering or physical activity, the heat being generated mainly from brown adipose tissue. The resting metabolic rate of immature infants per kg body weight is similar to term infants. Their thermogenic response to cold exposure is more difficult to determine. A breakthrough in the management of preterm infants came with the realization that keeping them in a thermoneutral environment improved survival. While preterm infants have a higher surface/volume ratio, implying more rapid heat loss than term infants, an additional reason for the higher susceptibility to hypothermia is incomplete development of brown adipose tissue which has a limited thermogenic capacity. There is certainly evidence of brown adipose tissue at 28 weeks of gestation; it is unclear whether this can lead to increased heat generation. Further, if nutritional support is inadequate, the brown adipose tissue may encounter a lack of substrate which will hamper the ability of the tissue to produce sufficient heat. Thus, in *malnutrition* the lack of sufficient food may lead to hypothermia in infants. This problem is not restricted to temperate latitudes; the baby relies on its brown fat thermogenesis to remain warm, even at tropical latitudes.

During neonatal surgery, problems with hypothermia are often encountered. This is usually explained as being due to the unfavorable surface/volume ratio of the newborn and to an inhibition of central thermoregulation. However, halothane has a profound inhibitory effect on brown fat thermogenesis, and newborn infants who are dependent on this heat production therefore cool rapidly when anesthetized.

The full-term human baby is born with a large amount of brown adipose tissue, and during early postnatal life the tissue probably becomes further recruited. The tissue remains metabolically important for several years, but with time it tends to become atrophied. It is not known whether this decrease in metabolic significance is an obligatory postnatal event, but extrapolation from other mammals indicates that the decrease does not occur if the young are under constant exposure to comparatively cold conditions. Thus, differences in acute tolerance to lower temperatures may reflect the extent to which the child has been protected from, or exposed to, comparative cold during early years.

As brown fat activity can also be induced via a dietary stimulus, it can be implied that the so-called specific dynamic effect of food, the increased metabolism seen after a meal, should be higher in the small child due to brown fat combustion. The lower efficiency (calories gained per calorie eaten) in small children may therefore not only be due to their generally higher rate of metabolism, but may also, to some extent, reflect brown adipose tissue activation.

There may be an increased amount of brown adipose tissue in the victims of the *sudden infant death syndrome* (SIDS). It is likely this is a secondary effect of hypoxic events which have occurred chronically in the prospective victim. This hypoxia would lead to a chronic sympathetic activation which in its turn would recruit the tissue. As an alternative hypothesis, it has been suggested that a subgroup of the babies diagnosed as SIDS victims in reality have died of hyperthermia, and that a high brown fat thermogenesis, evoked, e.g. by minor cold, has caused a fatal rise in body temperature in babies who have been too well insulated.

Selected reading

Clark RP, Edholm OG. *Man and his thermal environment*. London: Edward Arnold, 1985.

Gunn TR, Gluckman PD. The endocrine control of the onset of thermogenesis at birth. *Baillière's Clin Endocrinol Metab* 1989; **3**: 869.

Hensel H. *Thermoreception and temperature regulation*. London: Academic Press, 1981.

Lean, MEJ, James NPT. Brown adipose tissue in man. In Trayhurn P, Nicholls DG, eds. *Brown adipose tissue*. London: Edward Arnold, 1986: 339.

Nedergaard J, Connolly E, Cannon B. Brown adipose tissue in the mammalian newborn. In Trayhurn P, Nicholls DG, eds. *Brown adipose tissue*. London: Edward Arnold, 1986: 152.

B. Fever and Antipyresis

E Zeisberger

Although body temperature is tightly controlled, the thermoregulatory capacity can be exceeded. At the extremes of climatic conditions, hypothermia or hyperthermia can result. Furthermore, heat production may exceed heat loss, resulting in a rise in body temperature. In *malignant hyperthermia*, for example, there is a state of uncontrolled heat production by peripheral cells. Fever differs from hyperthermia. It can be defined as a body temperature regulated in a resting subject above the range of normal. It is brought about by active thermoregulation and is generally associated with a pathological condition.

Fever is now regarded as part of a complex immunological response to different antigenic stimuli including infections caused by bacteria, viruses and fungi, antigen–antibody complexes, neoplasms, delayed-type hypersensitivity reactions and other stimuli inducing inflammation. In homeotherms the thermoregulatory mechanisms behave during fever as if they were adjusted to maintain body temperature at a higher than normal set range. Depending on ambient temperature the heat loss is reduced, and in a cold environment the heat production is additionally increased until the new thermoregulatory set range is reached. Fever is the most universally known symptom of infectious disease and inflammatory responses.

The febrile response may be beneficial given that it evolved long ago in the phylogeny and persisted as a response to infections. It may facilitate the activation of the immune defence since antibody production and T-cell proliferation are more efficient at higher body temperatures than at normal levels. Moreover, many microorganisms grow best within a relatively narrow temperature range so that a rise in temperature inhibits their growth. Some poikilothermic lizards can resist bacterial infections at elevated ambient temperatures, but will die of the same infection in a cool environment. In man fevers were artificially induced before the advent of antibiotics for the treatment of *neurosyphilis* and proved to be beneficial. Hyperthermia seems to slow the growth of some tumors and has been found to benefit individuals with some bacterial, viral and fungal diseases.

Very high temperatures are harmful. When the central body temperature exceeds 41°C for prolonged periods, some permanent brain damage may result. At temperatures over 43°C *heat stroke* develops, frequently leading to death. Since the body temperature normally does not exceed 41°C during fever, it has been proposed that the elevation in body temperature is controlled and limited by the actions of endogenous antipyretic substances liberated within the brain during fever. The endogenous antipyresis is thus a normal constituent of the febrile response.

Mediators of fever

There is increasing evidence that the immune system and the central nervous system (CNS) are functionally connected and interacting. This bilateral communication is mediated by signal substances (Fig. 8.10). Lymphocytes, macrophages and other cells involved in immune responses communicate, in part, by hormone-like chemical messengers called cytokines (see p. 672). In addition to the immunomodulatory actions, cytokines

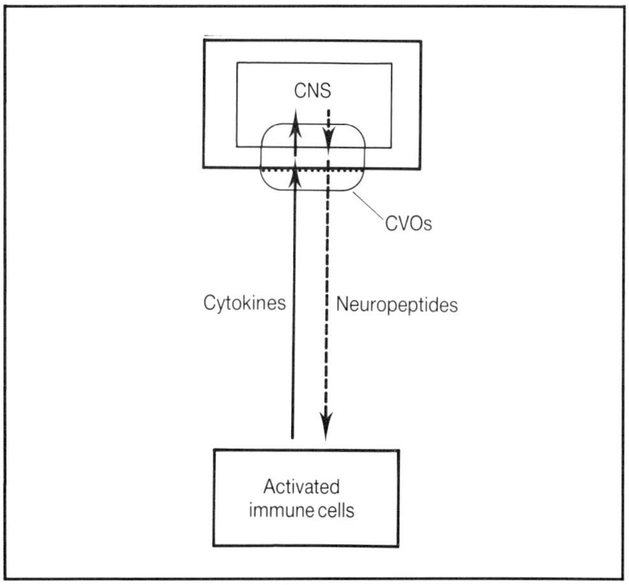

Fig. 8.10. Bilateral communications between immune and central nervous systems (circumventricular organs, CVOs).

exert effects on blood vessels, skeletal muscles, the liver and the brain. The effects on the central nervous system include anorexia, increased secretion of corticotropin releasing hormone (CRH), increased slow wave sleep and fever. The pyrogenic cytokines are also called endogenous pyrogens and include interleukin-1α (IL-1α), interleukin-1β (IL-1β), interleukin-2 (IL-2), interleukin-6 (IL-6), interferon-β2, tumor necrosis factor (TNF, cachectin), tumor necrosis factor β (TNFβ, lymphotoxin), interferon-α (IFN-α), interferon-γ (IFN-γ) and colony stimulating factors (CSF). The steps in the production of a fever are shown in a simplified form in Fig. 8.11.

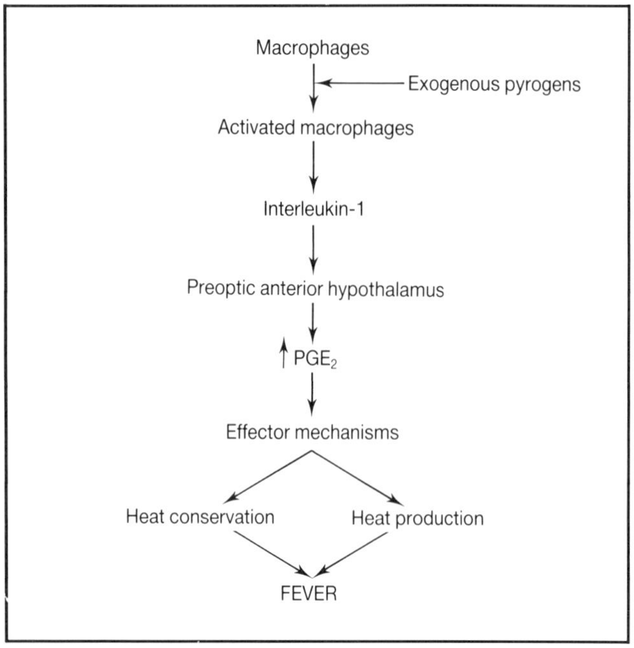

Fig. 8.11. Steps in production of a fever (simplified).

The metabolic effects of cytokines, resulting from their actions on liver and muscle, appearing simultaneously with a febrile rise in body temperature are called an acute-phase response. They include increased synthesis of hepatic proteins, increased sodium excretion, increases in ceruloplasmin-copper concentrations, decreases in serum iron and zinc concentrations, negative nitrogen balance, and aminoaciduria. It is accompanied by some hematological effects such as an increased number of circulating neutrophils and decreased number of circulating lymphocytes, increased secretion of colony stimulating factors and by inhibition of lipoprotein lipase.

It is possible to evoke fever by injections of endotoxins which are complex lipopolysaccharides derived from bacterial walls. They are recognized by immune cells as foreign and induce the immune defence reactions resulting in the release of endogenous pyrogens. After intravenous injection of bacterial endotoxin, fever develops after a 30 minute latent period, the time needed by the organism to release endogenous pyrogens like IL-1. In most laboratory animals the normal febrile rise of body temperature peaks about 3 hours after the injection of bacterial endotoxin. At this peak the increase of body temperature amounts to between 1 and 2°C, and it takes another 3 hours before the temperature returns to the original level. The entire febrile response to an intravenous injection of bacterial endotoxin lasts thus about 6 hours and after large doses the shape of the fever curve is biphasic. Repeated intravenous injection of endotoxin makes the recipient tolerant, i.e. no response occurs to further injections of endotoxin. There is evidence for both a peripheral immunological component to tolerance and also for central mechanisms (increasing activation of antipyretic systems and septal release of vasopressin). Endogenous pyrogens like IL-1 evoke fever after 5–15 minutes even in endotoxin tolerant recipients. IL-1 does not induce tolerance when administered repeatedly, and its activity is speeded and augmented when it is injected directly into the hypothalamus.

The pyrogenic effects of endogenous pyrogens are mediated by local release of prostaglandins. They are released from inflamed tissue. They also are found in the brain and may alter the release or effects of neurotransmitters. Circulatory levels increase after injection of pyrogens, probably because IL-1 can stimulate muscle proteolysis during fever by increasing production of prostaglandin E_2 (PGE_2). Anti-inflammatory steroids, such as cortisol, inhibit the release of arachidonic acid from phospholipid stores and thus block the formation of all eicosanoid products (see p. 103). Nonsteroidal anti-inflammatory drugs such as aspirin and indomethacin inhibit cyclooxygenase and thus block only the formation of prostaglandins, prostacyclin and thromboxanes, leaving the lipoxygenase pathways intact.

Injections of bacterial endotoxin, endogenous pyrogens or prostaglandins into the brain initiate fevers most promptly from special sites, such as the cluster of neurons in the organum vasculosum laminae terminalis (OVLT), the preoptic region in the limbic system, and the anterior hypothalamus. Also direct mechanical injury or application of chemical substances into the OVLT may release the endogenous PGE_2 which results in fever. Neurons and glial cells from these pyrogen-sensitive sites can produce and release PGE_2. Some of these cells and others in the hypothalamus can also produce IL-1. Many hypothalamic neurons have receptors for IL-1 and other endogenous pyrogens. In perfusates from these regions increased levels of IL-1, IL-6, TNF and PGE_2 can be found during the peripherally induced fever. However, it is very improbable that these increased levels derive from the blood as these molecules are too large to pass the intact blood–brain barrier. How can the peripheral mediators of fever influence the hypothalamic regulatory circuits?

The transduction mechanisms are poorly understood and largely hypothetical. The endogenous pyrogens can enter the perivascular space of circumventricular organs such as OVLT and bind to specific receptors on the surface of the parenchymal microglia and astrocytal end feet. They activate these cells to produce PGE_2 and other mediators and release them at the brain side of the barrier. The PGE_2 in turn activates neurons in the OVLT which transmit, via their axons, this excitation to neurons and glia at other central sites, e.g. in the preoptic area or anterior hypothalamus. These structures are responsible for simultaneous central release of endogenous pyrogens. They stimulate the local release of PGE_2, which can influence the activity of thermosensitive preoptic neurons and thermointegrative hypothalamic neurons, resulting in a change of the thermoregulatory set range with increases of both heat production and heat conservation and thus a fever.

Developmental aspects

Newborn infants can have severe infections, such as *meningitis* or *septicemia*, without increasing body temperature. Since the thermoregulatory system is operative at birth, this observation is sometimes ascribed to an immunological defect or inability to form IL-1. However, there is evidence that a febrile response does develop soon after birth and the lack of fever may reflect either a limited thermogenic capacity or the environmental temperature at which they are nursed. Pregnant ewes and guinea-pigs show a progressive loss of fever response to bacterial endotoxins before and after giving birth. Newborn of both species show similarly reduced febrile responses in the first few days of post-uterine life in spite of their fully developed abilities to produce endogenous pyrogens and to regulate their body temperature. Such lines of evidence suggest the activation of antipyretic systems. The biological significance of this fever suppression in the near-term human and newborn animal is not known.

Activation of endogenous antipyresis

The febrile signals transduced into the CNS result in a local release of PGE_2 in the anterior hypothalamus. This release activates parvocellular neurons in the paraventricular nucleus (PVN) to release mainly CRH from the terminals in the median eminence into the portal hypophyseal blood. CRH stimulates the secretion of ACTH and other proopiomelanocorticotropin derivatives from the corticotropes of the anterior lobe of pituitary (see p. 321). ACTH activates the release of cortisol which has suppressive effects on the immune system to inhibit the production of IL-2 by T lymphocytes and thus effectively stop the lymphocyte proliferation. Glucocorticoids have anti-inflammatory and antiallergic effects and also antipyretic actions because they inhibit phospholipase A, with a consequent reduction in the release of arachidonic acid and all its products including prostaglandins. They also inhibit the release of IL-1 from granulocytes.

Free glucocorticoids inhibit ACTH secretion at both the pituitary and the hypothalamic level. As a consequence the composition of the transmitter cocktail produced by parvocellular neurons in the PVN changes such that instead of CRH they produce arginine vasopressin (AVP). One part of the AVP-immunoreactive neurons does not project to the median eminence but to different areas of the limbic system, including the septum and amygdala. These systems are activated during the fever rise. Exogenous MSH (a metabolite of ACTH) and AVP microinjected or microinfused into the septum reduce or prevent fevers evoked by bacterial endotoxins, endogenous pyrogens or by intraventricular application of prostaglandins. The antipyretic site can be identified in a small area located ventrally to the lateral septum. The released AVP stimulates the septal neurons via V_1 receptors (see p. 331). This excitation is then transmitted via septofugal fibers to the hypothalamic thermoregulatory structures, where it cancels the changes induced by pyrogens. Another antipyretic mechanism, also mediated by AVP, has been found in the OVLT.

Thus endogenous antipyresis can be mediated by at

least three mechanisms. The first one is a neuronal pathway from the septum to the hypothalamic thermo-integrative neurons which can block the changes induced by pyrogens. The second is the disseminated AVP perivascular system in the OVLT, which is functionally interconnected with the antipyretic septal area. AVP released from this system may influence the permeability or the binding of endogenous pyrogens to their receptors. It can thus change the local production of PGE_2, transforming the immune signals into neuronal messages. The third mechanism is peripheral. It is based on the action of some hormones on immune cells. They may act as selective inhibitors of production of endogenous pyrogens and thus reduce the immune signals.

Selected reading

Brück K. Neonatal thermal regulation. In Polin RA, Fox WW, eds. *Fetal and neonatal medicine—physiology and pathophysiology*. Philadelphia: WB Saunders Co., 1991.

Zeisberger E. The role of septal peptides in thermoregulation and fever. In Bligh J, Voigt K, eds. *Thermoreception and temperature regulation*. Berlin, Heidelberg: Springer-Verlag, 1990.

9 ◆ *The gastrointestinal system and nutrition*

Editors: Colin D Rudolph and James E Heubi

INTRODUCTION

C D Rudolph and J E Heubi

Most animal behaviors have evolved primarily for the purpose of efficiently obtaining and selecting food. This process is directed by the central nervous system. An infant cries to signal the mother that it is time to feed. Adults either hunt food, grow food, or go to work to make money that they exchange for food. All these activities result in the ingestion of liquid and solid nutrients, which are transported to the stomach, where mixing and storage occurs. Complex hormonal and neural feedback mechanisms inform the central nervous system that adequate nutrients have been ingested prior to the nutrient absorption. The gastrointestinal system processes complex foodstuffs, providing sustenance to the entire body. Ingested foods are initially lubricated, mechanically ground, and chemically digested into an emulsion in the mouth and stomach. This emulsion, chyme, slowly passes from the stomach to the small intestine, where enzymes and bile secreted by the pancreas and liver further digest complex molecules into simpler carbohydrates, peptides, and fats for absorption into the blood stream. Subsequent metabolic processing and storage occurs in the liver. Non-absorbed electrolytes, water, and nutrients are salvaged by the colon before waste products are excreted as feces.

The initial sections of this chapter describe the ontogeny of the structural components of the gastro-intestinal tract, including the specialized epithelia, smooth muscle, hormonal, neural, and immunological tissues and blood vessels. Subsequent chapters describe the development of coordinated functions, such as propulsion of luminal contents and the digestion and absorption of fluids, electrolytes, and nutrients. For clarity, liver development and function are discussed separately. Nutrient requirements of the growing human are summarized in the final section.

A. Embryology and Anatomy of the Gastrointestinal Tract

M L Epstein and C D Rudolph

The gastrointestinal tract receives tissue contributions from all three germ layers. The primitive gut first forms as a cavity lined by endoderm, which gives rise to the entire epithelial lining of the digestive tube. Most digestive glands including the liver, gallbladder, and pancreas arise as buds from this endodermal lining. As a result of lateral folding, the splanchnic mesoderm comes to lie adjacent to, and eventually to surround the endodermal-lined gut tube, forming the connective tissue and muscular walls. Later the neural tube derived from the ectoderm gives rise to neural crest cells. These cells migrate from the neural tube and invade the mesodermal portion of the gut tube, where they form the neurons and glial cells intrinsic to the gastrointestinal tract.

Morphological development

The timetable of morphological development of the human gastrointestinal tract has been described in a number of texts and therefore is reviewed here only briefly (Fig. 9.1). The foregut and hindgut are first identifiable as blind, endoderm-lined pouches surrounded by mesoderm. The midgut represents the region opening to the yolk sac and is the last region to be invested with mesoderm. Several key morphological events occur as the gut grows. The respiratory primordium separates from the foregut so that the trachea is distinct from the esophagus. The foregut undergoes differential growth and rotates so that the stomach assumes its adult shape and position. The liver, gallbladder, and ventral pancreatic bud develop from an endodermal outgrowth appearing distal to the stomach, while the dorsal pancreatic bud arises from a different outgrowth. Rotation of the duodenum and migration of the ventral pancreatic bud result in both the juxtaposition, and ultimately fusion of the pancreatic buds to form a single pancreas, and the unification of the pancreatic and bile ducts. As the gut elongates, the peritoneal cavity becomes too small to accommodate the midgut, and the gut expands into the extraembryonic

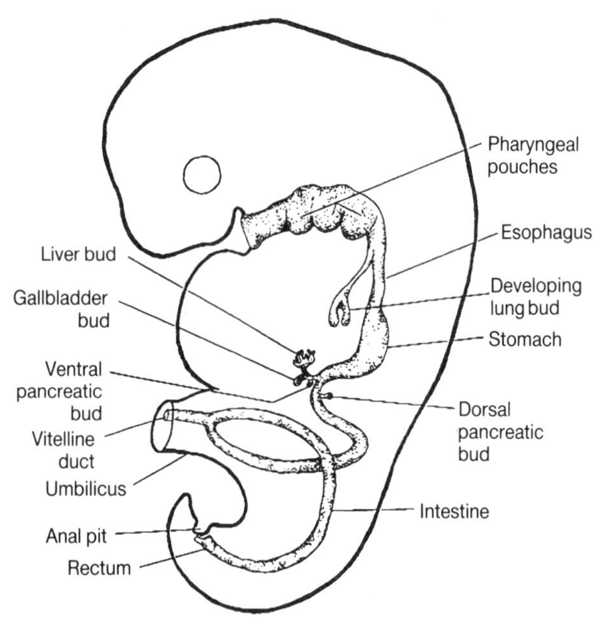

Fig. 9.1. Schematic representation of the morphological development of the human gastrointestinal tract at 5 weeks of gestation.

celom within the umbilical cord. During this herniation, the gut rotates 90° about the axis of the superior mesenteric artery; upon the return of the midgut to the peritoneal cavity, an additional 180° counterclockwise rotation occurs. The net result of this rotation is to position the cecum in the right lower quadrant of the peritoneal cavity. The mesenteries fuse to the parietal peritoneum, fixing the ascending and descending colon in place. The connection between the yolk sac and the gut is the vitelline duct, which can persist as an out-pocketing of the ileum, also called Meckel's diverticulum. The cloaca is divided by the urogenital sinus and eventually separates into the urinary bladder and rectum, which fuses with the overlying ectoderm to form the anus. At the site of the rectum is a depression in the ectoderm called the anal pit; this pit breaks down to permit continuity between the endodermal lining of the rectum and the ectodermal lining of the anus.

Mucosa and muscle development

The gastrointestinal wall is composed of external muscle layers, neural plexi, and mucosa throughout the gastrointestinal tract (Fig. 9.2). Differentiation of the epithelial lining of the gastrointestinal tract, the mucosa, confers specialized functions to each region. Variations in the geometric arrangement of the muscle layers may also confer specialized contractile functions. Whereas the esophageal mucosa has the relatively simple function of providing a lubricated conduit for bolus passage and a barrier to infection, the stomach and intestinal mucosa have additional complex secretory, digestive, and absorptive tasks. The maturation of mucosa proceeds from a proximal to distal direction. The entire bowel is initially lined by a multilayered epithelium with numerous vacuolizations. In man, the epithelium of the esophagus becomes ciliated at 10 weeks of gestation. Replacement by stratified squamous epithelia begins at the fifth month with patches of ciliated epithelium occasionally persisting until birth. In many mammals, especially those such as rodents and ruminants, which eat coarse vegetable foods, the esophageal mucosa undergoes keratinization.

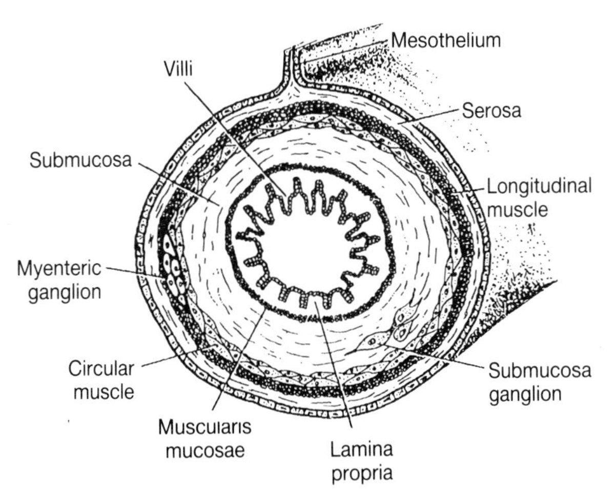

Fig. 9.2. Schematic representation of a cross-section of the small intestine, demonstrating the layers of the intestinal wall.

The mature mucosa of the stomach is lined by tall columnar cells that have an overlying mucous coat. Glandular pits contain acid-secreting parietal cells, pepsinogen-secreting chief cells, and goblet-shaped mucus-secreting cells. Slender flask-shaped cells with slender processes extending to the luminal surface known as enterochromaffin cells secrete hormones. Parietal cells are found in the fetal mucosa by 9 weeks of gestation. By 10 weeks enterochromaffin cells can be identified (see Section 9C), and by 13 weeks cells resembling chief cells are present. By 16 weeks mucus-secreting cells are present. Although peptic activity has been demonstrated in the human stomach by 16 weeks, chief cells cannot be demonstrated to contain pepsinogen until term. Parietal cells contain intrinsic factor by 14 weeks of gestation. The parietal cells do not secrete acid until after birth. The functional development of gastric acid secretion and barrier function are described in Section 9E.

Finger-like protrusions known as villi project into the lumen of the small bowel, markedly increasing the surface area available for digestion and absorption. Columnar intestinal cells with a microvillus luminal membrane occupy most of the surface of these villi, further increasing surface area. Transport proteins and digestive enzymes are present on the luminal membrane of these cells (see Section 9F). The various types of villous lining cells are thought to be formed from multipotent stem cells located in the crypts at the villous base. The cells differentiate during migration to the villous tip where they are shed into the bowel lumen. Migration times are longer in the fetus than in the adult. Columnar cells and mucus-secreting goblet cells become recognizable between 8 and 10 weeks of gestation in the human. By 10–12 weeks villi have appeared and enterochromaffin cells are present. A separate population of pyramidal-shaped mucosal cells with prominent secretory granules and little or no turnover, known as Paneth cells, are located at the base of the crypts in humans, monkeys, and ruminants but not in dogs, cats, or raccoons. These cells appear at 11–12 weeks of gestation. Their functional role is unknown. Aggregations of lymphocytes in the jejunum and ileum called Peyer's patches first appear at 5 months of gestation in the human.

The mucosal development of the large intestine follows the development of the small intestine. Villi are present at 10–12 weeks of gestation but disappear during later fetal life. The mucosa contains specialized absorptive cells, a large number of mucus-secreting cells, and enterochromaffin cells.

Layers of smooth muscle develop in the mesenchymal layer surrounding the mucosa in a craniocaudal pattern parallel to the rest of the components of the bowel. Circular muscle layers develop in the esophagus and stomach during week 5 of human gestation and are present in the ileum by 8 weeks. Longitudinal muscle layers are not present until 8 weeks and appear in the ileum by week 10. The thin layer of smooth muscle that separates the mucosa and submucosa, the muscularis mucosa, is not fully developed until 20 weeks. The development of smooth muscle has been more extensively studied in the developing chick embryo. In any given region of muscle, the cells develop at approximately the same rate. In the chicken gizzard, actin appears to be expressed on embryonic day 5, whereas myosin is not expressed until day 7. The quantity of each contractile protein increases through gestation. Gap junctions increase in number and size until they approach mature-sized junctions by 7 days after hatching. Myoglobin appears only at the time of hatching. In contrast to skeletal muscle, mitoses occur in smooth muscle cells even when the contractile apparatus is mature and cell-to-cell junctions are present.

Neural innervation

To study the formation of the enteric nervous system has been difficult in mammalian, let alone human preparations. Because the chick embryo can be readily manipulated and observed, studies in this preparation have substantially enhanced our knowledge regarding neural innervation of the intestine. Chickens hatch after 21 days of incubation; the gut is fully operative at hatching. Experiments with avian embryos have elucidated the source for enteric neuron precursors. These experiments involved either ablation of neural folds or replacement of portions of chick neural tube with comparable portions of quail neural tubes. The quail neural crest cells that migrated into the gut were identified by the unique appearance of quail nucleolar DNA. These experiments indicated that neural crest cells from the hindbrain region (rhombencephalic or vagal neural crest) populate the entire gut. In addition, a second source of crest cells arising posterior to somite 28 and termed sacral crest give rise to cells that populate the postumbilical gut. These findings have been confirmed in the chicken by the injection of cellular tracers such as the fluorescent dye DI or a replication-deficient retrovirus. After neural crest cells migrate to the bowel, the subsequent increase in neural cell numbers could arise either by migration of late-arriving crest cells or, more likely, by cell division. Cells continue to migrate along the gut and reach the ileocecal junction by embryonic day 5.5 in the chicken, roughly 2 days after entry into the foregut. The sacral crest appears to leave the spinal cord on day 2 to enter the hindgut.

A large body of indirect evidence in a variety of species supports the idea that as in the chicken, neural crest cells enter the gut at both anterior and posterior sites, although earlier workers reported a single craniocaudal migration of neuroblasts in the human fetus. Studies of two neuronal markers, neuron-specific enolase and substance P, demonstrated that neuronal differentiation in the pylorus was more advanced than the colon but that the ileum was least advanced. In the mouse, explant cultures from the embryonic foregut and hindgut reveal that neuronal precursors are present in both the proximal and distal portions of the gut at about the same time. Furthermore, the expression of neuronal phenotype markers, NADPH diaphorase and calcitonin gene-related peptide (CGRP), a peptide neurotransmitter, appeared at the ends of the gut before they appeared in the middle, an observation consistent with two sources of enteric precursors. More convincing is the finding of fluorescent cells in the fetal mouse hindgut after injection of fluorescent dye into the sacral neural tube. The mouse is of special interest because of the lethal spotted mutant, which develops congenital megacolon. Neural crest cells are unable to migrate into the terminal bowel of these mutants. This inability to enter the bowel may be related to an overabundance of laminin and type IV collagen. How well this model describes *congenital megacolon* in the human remains to be determined.

A number of important questions remain about two sources of enteric neuroblasts. Although two sources of enteric neuroblasts probably exist in the human, they have not been described to date. In the chick and mouse, where sacral crests have been found to enter the hindgut, it is unknown whether the sacral crests form neurons. Finally, the possible role of defects in sacral crest in congenital megacolon remains to be evaluated. Does the loss of the sacral crest lead to the absence or reduction in neuron numbers in the terminal hindgut?

Neuronal differentiation

Mature enteric neurons exhibit a number of transmitter phenotypes including acetylcholine, serotonin, GABA, a large number of neuropeptides, and combinations of these molecules. In the adult gastrointestinal tract, groups of chemically distinguishable neurons are associated with specific functions or targets, a relationship termed neurochemical coding. Neural crest cells migrate off the neural tube and enter the primitive gut. Once within the gut the crest cells appear to migrate, divide, and aggregate into small clusters of cells. In the chicken, these clusters of cells become connected in a network, increase in size, and take on the appearance of nascent ganglia between embryonic days 5 and 10. Within these nascent ganglia, crest-derived cells begin to express the different transmitter phenotypes found in the gut including acetylcholine, vasoactive intestinal peptide (VIP), somatostatin, enkephalin, and substance P.

The factors controlling phenotypic differentiation are unknown; however, the appearance of neurotransmitters varies with the region of the gastrointestinal tract and with the time of development. This process has been studied most extensively in the mouse. Choline acetyltransferase activity and serotonin uptake are present on embryonic day 9 of gestation, before elements with the morphological characteristics of neurons are recognizable. Cells transiently produce catecholamines on days 10–12, then the catecholamines disappear. Whether these transient catecholaminergic (TC) cells die or change their phenotype is not clear. TC cells, which have not been found in avian gut, also contain a number of neural markers including neurofilament protein, peripherin, GAP43, and MAP5. The TC cells also proliferate, indicating they are not yet neurons, which are defined as postmitotic cells. However, when day 10 gut explants were grown in culture, many of the TC cells also showed neuron-specific enolase, a marker for mature neurons. These results indicate that at least some of the TC cells are able to develop into mature neurons under culture conditions and suggest TC cells may give rise to mature enteric neurons *in situ*. At day 12 neuropeptide Y, at day 14 substance P and VIP, and at day 17 CGRP-immunoreactive neurons are found, while at day 18 serotonin is present. Thus expression of the different transmitter phenotypes follows a pattern in that acetylcholine appears early followed by peptides and serotonin.

Extrinsic nerves reach the gut at later times. In the developing chicken gut, sympathetic neurites reach the duodenum on embryonic day 12. Sympathetic fibers are functional in the rat small bowel by postnatal day 3, and fibers are found in the myenteric ganglia at that time.

Selected reading

Epstein ML, Poulsen KT, Thiboldeaux R. Formation of ganglia in the gut of the chick embryo. *J Comp Neurol* 1991; **307**: 189.

Furness JB, Costa M. *The enteric nervous system.* New York: Churchill Livingstone, Inc., 1987.

Gershon MD, Rothman TP. Neuronal determination in the enteric nervous system. In Edelman GM, Gall WE, Cowan WM, eds. *Molecular bases of neural development*. New York: Neurosciences Research Foundation, Inc., John Wiley and Sons, 1985: 213.

B. Intestinal Blood Flow

O R Velasquez and K D Crissinger

The intestinal circulation provides the energy substrates and O_2 necessary to support the digestive, propulsive, and transport activities of the bowel and carries absorbed nutrients, electrolytes, and fluids from the gastrointestinal tract to the different tissues of the body. The physiological processes of assimilation of nutrients and the rapid growth of fetal and neonatal intestine increase the blood flow and oxidative demands relative to those of the adult.

Basic concepts

Blood flow to the splanchnic organs is regulated by changes in the diameter of muscular arterioles controlled by extrinsic and intrinsic regulators. Terminal arterioles and precapillary sphincters control the number of capillaries perfused in a specific region, altering the local delivery of O_2 and substrates. O_2 diffuses from the capillary to the cell, where it is utilized for oxidative metabolism. Substrates and absorbed fluids and nutrients also exchange across the capillary bed. In the adult, intestinal O_2 uptake remains constant over a wide range of blood flows (Fig. 9.3). O_2 uptake is compromised only when blood flow reaches a critically low level, at which point O_2 uptake becomes flow-dependent and falls linearly with further reductions in blood flow. Usually, the resting intestinal blood flow exceeds the critical level at which O_2 uptake becomes blood flow-dependent. Modulation of arteriolar tone in small- to medium-sized arterioles changes blood flow, matching blood flow to the O_2 demands of the tissue. Stimulation or inhibition of oxidative metabolism shifts the plateau of the blood flow–O_2 uptake curve upward or downward, respectively (Fig. 9.3).

Terminal arterioles and precapillary sphincters modulate the number of capillaries perfused at any given moment, increasing local flow in the face of reduced

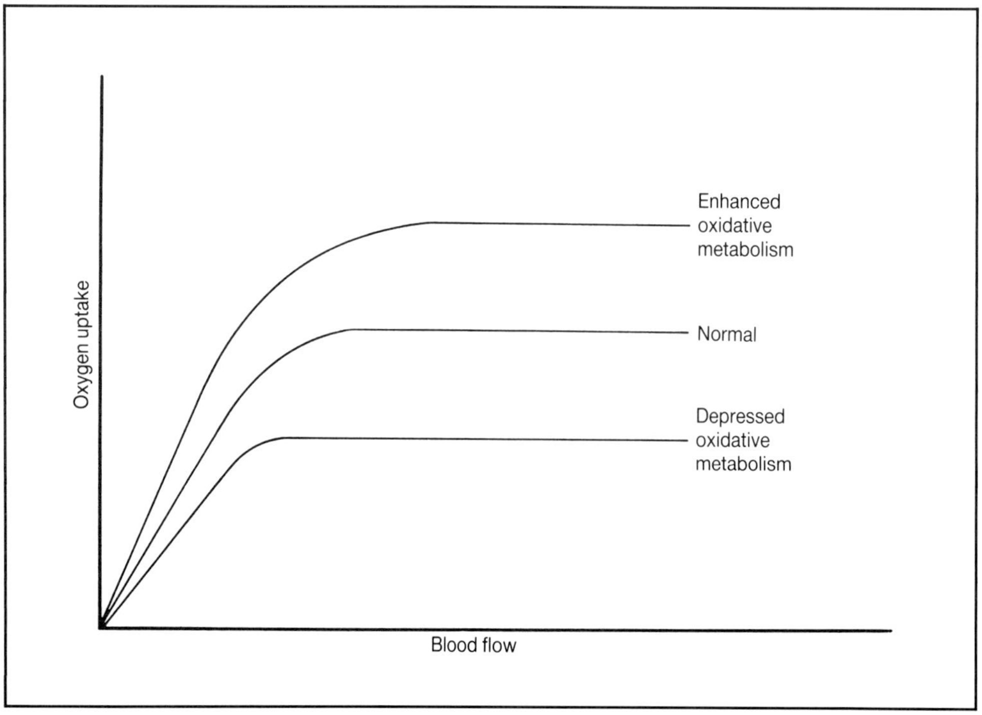

Fig. 9.3. Relationship between blood flow and O_2 uptake under normal conditions and during stimulation or inhibition of oxidative metabolism. (From Kvietys PR, Granger DN. *Am J Physiol* 1982; **243**: G1, with permission.)

capillary Po_2, thereby increasing O_2 delivery. Figure 9.4 shows the expected influence of capillary density on the relation between blood flow and O_2 uptake. If capillary density within an organ is increased, then the level of blood flow required to maintain O_2 uptake is reduced (i.e. the curve is shifted to the left) due to an increased capillary surface area and a reduced capillary-to-cell diffusion distance. In the adult intestine, changes in flow and numbers of capillaries perfused provide a wide margin of safety against development of tissue hypoxia when metabolic needs increase. In contrast, in the newborn intestine, reductions in blood flow in the normal physiological range result in reductions in O_2 uptake (Fig. 9.5).

The variables that determine cellular Po_2 are summarized in the following equation:

$$Po_2 \text{ cell} = Po_2 \text{ capillary} - (Vo_2/N)$$

where Vo_2 is the intestinal O_2 uptake and N is the number of perfused capillaries. Normal resting cellular Po_2 is above the critical level required to maintain oxidative metabolism, and stepwise reductions in blood flow do not produce concomitant reductions in cellular Po_2 until the capacity of the tissue for capillary recruitment is overwhelmed. In contrast, this relationship shows that when the rate of O_2 extraction is maximized and blood flow cannot increase, cellular Po_2 falls below the critical level required to maintain normal intracellular metabolism. The relation between O_2 uptake and cellular Po_2 has not been established in developing intestine; therefore, information is lacking about the critical cellular Po_2 at which O_2 uptake and oxidative metabolism become compromised.

Extrinsic regulation of intestinal blood flow

Neurohumoral factors are important regulators of blood flow and O_2 consumption within the intestine. During reductions in blood pressure due to hypovolemia or shock, gastrointestinal flow is markedly reduced in order to redistribute blood flow and O_2 to the heart and central nervous system. Extrinsic regulatory mechanisms assure the appropriate response of the intestinal circulation in the preservation of systemic circulatory homeostasis. Sympathetic noradrenergic nerves play a major role in neural control of intestinal blood flow. α-Adrenergic receptors decrease intestinal flow, whereas β-adrenergic and dopaminergic receptors increase flow. The net effect

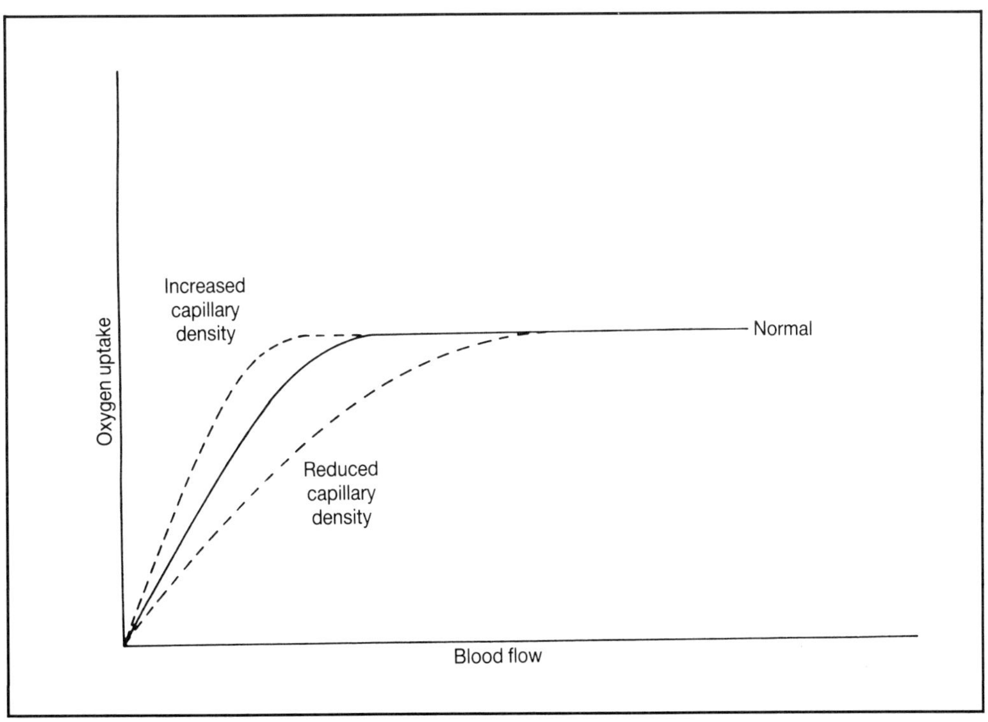

Fig. 9.4. Relationship between blood flow and O_2 uptake under conditions of increased or reduced perfused capillary density. (From Kvietys PR, Granger DN. *Am J Physiol* 1982; **243**: G1, with permission.)

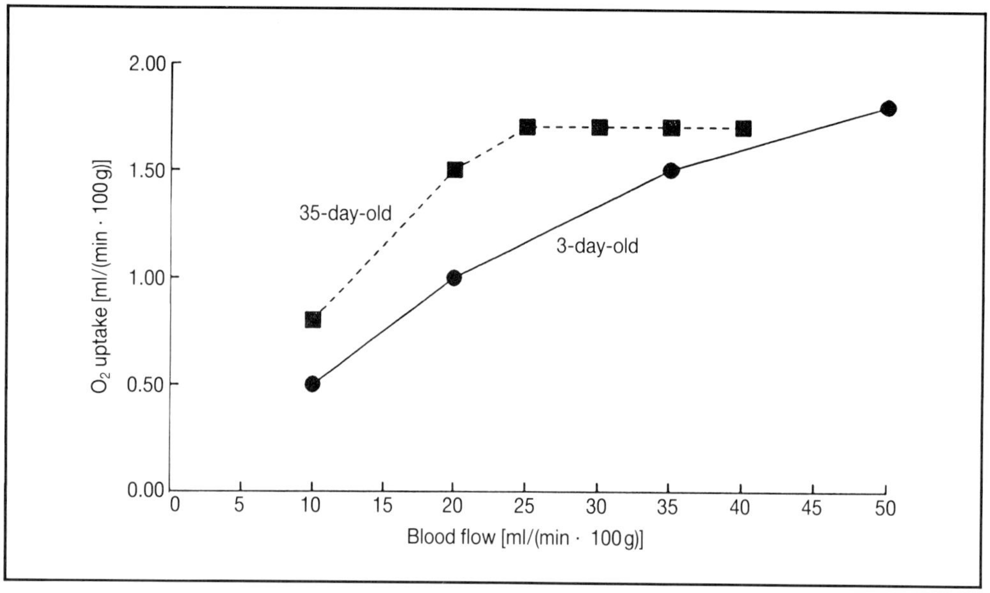

Fig. 9.5. Relationship between blood flow and O_2 uptake in *in vitro* ileal loops from 3- and 35-day-old swine. (Adapted from Nowicki PT, Miller CE. *Am J Physiol* 1988; **254**: G189, with permission.)

of sympathetic stimulation is to decrease intestinal blood flow.

Intestinal blood flow decreases in response to sympathetic stimulation in the ovine fetus. At birth, the blood flow to the intestine increases two- to threefold. The intestinal circulation appears to be under tonic sympathetic vasoconstrictor control. Adrenergic responses of the intestinal circulation are relatively active in newborns and continue to mature postnatally. The immature intestinal circulation appears less capable of vasodilation, suggesting that the neonatal intestine may be at metabolic risk during stresses involving increased sympathetic discharge.

Intrinsic regulation of intestinal blood flow

Adult intestine has the capacity to regulate its own blood flow after elimination of all nervous and hormonal influences. These local, or intrinsic, microvascular control systems allow the microcirculation to respond to the specific needs of the tissue that it subserves and result in the maintenance of the flux of O_2 and nutrients to the parenchyma. Several mechanisms of intrinsic vascular regulation probably play a role in this response. The metabolic hypothesis suggests that a reduction in blood flow or an increase in parenchymal cell activity causes a decline in tissue Po_2 and accumulation of metabolites, dilating arterioles and relaxing precapillary sphincters. The myogenic hypothesis proposes that arteriolar tension receptors modulate vascular smooth muscle tone in response to change in microvascular transmural pressure. Resistance vessels dilate when vascular transmural pressure is decreased, while an increase in transmural pressure causes arteriolar vasoconstriction and increased vascular resistance.

Intrinsic vascular regulation by the intestine has been studied after altering arterial and venous pressure, after altering arterial O_2 concentration, and during periods of increased metabolic demand. The adult intestine autoregulates blood flow, maintaining a constant flow with variations in arterial pressure. The pressure range over which intestinal autoregulation is effective is much narrower than that observed in tissues such as the kidney or brain, where autoregulation is the primary factor controlling blood flow. The effectiveness of intestinal autoregulation improves during periods of increased metabolic activity. In the newborn, the intestine has a blunted autoregulatory response that does not improve with increased metabolic activity. Autoregulatory responses of the intestinal circulation improve with advancing postnatal age.

The response of the intestinal vasculature to venous pressure (P_v) elevation is an important criterion for determining whether metabolic or myogenic mechanisms dominate in local vasoregulation. Studies of the stomach, small intestine, and colon in adult animals indicate that vascular resistance rises in response to P_v elevation, findings consistent with a myogenic mechanism. This typical myogenic response can be abolished or reversed by increasing the O_2 demands in adult intestine, suggesting that the response to P_v elevation is also influenced by the metabolic state of the intestine. In newborns, the intestinal circulation dilates, rather than constricts, in response to acute elevation of mesenteric P_v so that intestinal O_2 uptake is not compromised. This indicates that metabolic factors are dominant in the already metabolically active neonatal intestine.

Arterial hypoxemia increases blood flow and elicits capillary recruitment in adult intestine. Decreased vascular resistance and increased capillary density minimize the reduction in O_2 uptake induced by limited O_2 availability. This response is comparatively reduced in developing intestine. Only a modest vasodilation can be elicited in response to perfusion with hypoxic blood ($Pa{O_2}$ $\approx$35 mmHg; 4.65 kPa), whereas older subjects exhibit a more significant fall in intestinal vascular resistance and rise in blood flow. O_2 uptake also falls to a greater extent in developing intestine during arterial hypoxemia than in older animals. These observations indicate either that the intrinsic mechanism responsible for hypoxic vasodilation (i.e. the response to a vasodilator substance) develops postnatally or that the intestinal vessels are already dilated due to increased metabolic activity so that the ability of the neonatal intestinal vessels to dilate further during hypoxia is less than in the adult.

Ingestion of a meal increases blood flow to the splanchnic circulation, a phenomenon known as postprandial hyperemia. Intraluminal nutrients increase the metabolic demands of the intestinal parenchyma in adult animals and lead to an increase in intestinal blood flow and O_2 uptake. Newborns increase O_2 uptake postprandially by increasing O_2 extraction without a change in total intestinal blood flow. Mucosal blood flow, however, does increase at the expense of muscularis/serosa flow. This unique response rapidly changes to the adult response within 24 hours. Thus, O_2 extraction and mucosal blood flow appear to be near maximal during feeding.

In summary, the ability to regulate local blood flow and oxygenation in the developing intestine appears to improve as a function of postnatal age. The intestine of young animals increases O_2 extraction to meet metabolic demands, whereas the intestine of mature animals increases both blood flow and O_2 extraction. During periods of decreased O_2 delivery due to hypotension or hypoxemia, the newborn intestine may be at increased risk for tissue hypoxia and subsequent mucosal injury.

The immature capability to regulate intestinal blood flow may be important in the pathogenesis of *necrotizing enterocolitis* (see also Section 10G3). Many factors, including infectious agents, enteral alimentation, and mesenteric ischemia, have often been invoked as primary initiators of this disease. Efforts directed toward increasing the capacity of developing intestine to meet the oxidative demands of the tissue by increasing O_2 delivery while simultaneously minimizing these metabolic demands (e.g. by altering the composition of infant formula) ultimately may result in decreasing the incidence of necrotizing enterocolitis.

Selected reading

Crissinger KD, Granger DN. Gastrointestinal blood flow. In Yamada T, Alpers DH, Owyang C, Powel DW, Silverstein FE, eds. *Textbook of gastroenterology*. Philadelphia: JB Lippincott Co., 1991: 447.

Nowicki PT. Neonatal intestinal circulation. In Schultz SG, Wood JD, Rauner BB, eds. *Handbook of physiology. The gastrointestinal system 1*. Bethesda, MD: American Physiological Society, Waverly Press, 1989: 1597.

C. Gastrointestinal Hormones

T E Adrian

Gastrointestinal hormones play a key role in the control of alimentary functions. Regulatory peptides, such as vasoactive intestinal polypeptide (VIP), substance P, bombesin, and the enkephalins, function as neurotransmitters or neuromodulators, not as blood-borne hormones. The integration of neural and hormonal signals controls the digestion and absorption and subsequent metabolism of ingested nutrients. Furthermore, some of the gastrointestinal hormones and other peptides, such as epidermal growth factor (EGF), appear to play a major role in maintaining the growth and integrity of the alimentary tract.

Biochemistry, physiology, and molecular biology

Most gastrointestinal hormones fit into one of three major peptide families: the gastrin/cholecystokinin family, the secretin/glucose-dependent insulinotropic peptide/glucagon/enteroglucagon family, which also includes neurotransmitter relatives (VIP and PHM) and pituitary relatives (growth hormone releasing hormone), and the pancreatic polypeptide/peptide YY family, which has neuropeptide Y as its neural cousin. More distant relationships between motilin and gastrin, somatostatin and secretin, and neurotensin and PYY are suggested by some degree of sequence homology.

The gastrointestinal hormones and their neuropeptide cousins appear to have evolved from common ancestors by the process of gene duplication. Current examples of this evolutionary mechanism include the co-secretion of enteroglucagon and the glucagon-related peptides I and II from the same gene, and neurotensin from the same gene as neuromedin N. Several gastrointestinal hormones exist in multiple molecular forms with differences either in length or side-chain modification such as sulfation. Many have a C-terminal amide group that renders them resistant to carboxypeptidase activity.

Ten enteric peptides act on the alimentary tract via the circulation. The endocrine cells synthesizing these peptides, with the exception of those producing somatostatin, are of the open type, with luminal processes that presumably respond to nutrients and other factors such as pH within the lumen to stimulate their secretion. The biochemistry, anatomical localization, and physiological actions of each hormone are discussed below. The site of secretion and major actions are also listed in Table 9.1.

The gastrin family includes members with different chain lengths all sharing a biologically active C-terminus. The important molecular forms of gastrin have either 17 amino acids (little gastrin) or 34 amino acids (big gastrin). Both are important in the control of gastric acid secretion. About half our gastrin molecules are sulfated, but this modification does not affect biological activity. Gastrin is produced mainly in the gastric antrum, but some is also secreted from the duodenum. The role of gastrin in the control of gastric acid secretion is discussed in Section 9E. In addition to being an acid secretagogue, gastrin exhibits a potent trophic effect on the gastric mucosa, an action probably of profound importance in the newborn infant.

Cholecystokinin (CCK) shares the last five amino acids in the C-terminal end with the gastrins. This property leads to pharmacological overlap in the actions of these peptides. CCK exists in chains of different lengths including 83, 58, 39, 33, 22, 12, and 8 amino acids. All forms of CCK are sulfated, a modification necessary for its biological activity; the larger forms predominate in the circulation. Biological activity of all forms resides in the common, amidated, C-terminal end of the CCK molecule. CCK is responsible for postprandial pancreatic enzyme secretion and gallbladder contraction. CCK is released from the duodenum and upper jejunum by the presence of fat and protein in the small bowel. Recent evidence suggests a complex mechanism for the release of this peptide involving luminal releasing peptides.

Secretin is a 27 amino acid peptide with a C-terminal amide group. The whole molecule is required for biological activity. Secretin shares considerable sequence homology with the hormones glucagon and glucose-dependent insulinotropic peptide, as well as with several neuropeptides as mentioned above. A hormonal peptide localized to the duodenal mucosa, secretin stimulates

Table 9.1. The circulating gastrointestinal hormones and changes in concentrations in the newborn

Hormone	Localization	Major physiological actions	Observed changes in neonates
Gastrin	Gastric antrum	Stimulates gastric acid secretion	Hypersecretion at birth, remains elevated without increased acid secretion
Cholecystokinin (CCK)	Duodenum	Stimulates pancreatic enzyme secretion and contracts gallbladder	Marked postnatal surge, concentrations higher than in adult
Secretin	Duodenum	Stimulates pancreatic bicarbonate and hepatic bile secretion	Higher than adult in first week of life even without enteral feeding
Glucose-dependent insulinotropic peptide (GIP)	Upper small intestine	Potentiates glucose-stimulated release of insulin from the pancreas	Low concentrations in first days of life then adult pattern develops
Motilin	Upper small intestine	Triggers MMCs, speeds gastric emptying	Massive postnatal surge of pre-feed concentrations, post-feed fall in concentrations more marked than in adult
Neurotensin	Distal ileum	Stimulates mucosal growth, inhibits gastric function	Large postnatal surge and development of marked post-feed response
Enteroglucagon	Ileum and colon	Stimulates mucosal growth, inhibits gastric function	Massive postnatal surge and development of marked post-feed response
Peptide YY (PYY)	Ileum and colon	Inhibits gastric acid, slows gastric emptying and intestinal transit	High concentrations at birth, massive postnatal surge
Pancreatic polypeptide (PP)	Pancreas	Inhibits exocrine pancreas and relaxes gallbladder	Small postnatal surge of basal concentrations, post-feed response smaller than adult
Somatostatin*	Stomach, pancreas, small and large bowel	Inhibits release of all above hormones, inhibits secretions and motor effects	Not reported

* Note: May act locally (i.e. paracrine peptide). Somatostatin is also found in enteric nerves.

pancreatic and hepatic bicarbonate secretion. Secretin is released when acid chyme passes through the pylorus into the duodenal bulb. The ensuing bicarbonate secretion rapidly neutralizes the pH of the duodenum. This affords protection to the duodenal mucosa and provides a neutral environment for the activity of pancreatic enzymes.

Glucose-dependent insulinotropic peptide (GIP) is a 42 amino acid member of the secretin family; a larger molecular form exists, but its relative biological potency is unknown. Gastric inhibitory peptide was GIP's original name because of its property of inhibiting acid secretion; however, this effect is only seen at supraphysiological concentrations. GIP releases insulin from the pancreas, although to do this it requires a small elevation of blood glucose concentrations (approximately 1 mM), like that seen after the ingestion of food. Hence the peptide was renamed glucose-dependent insulinotropic peptide (retaining the acronym GIP). The secretion of intestinal GIP from the upper small intestine may account in part for the greater insulin response observed in the bowel after equal amounts of glucose are administered into the bowel and intravenously, previously described as being due to a peptide, 'incretin.'

As has been known for many years, glucagon-like peptides (enteroglucagon) are produced by the gut but these differ chemically as well as in biological actions and mechanism of release. Now that the sequence of preproglucagon has been derived from the gene sequence, it is clear that the same gene is transcribed in both gut and pancreas. The post-translational processing of the glucagon precursor differs in these sites, however, giving rise to quite separate products. The glucagon gene encodes for three similar sequences, glucagon and the glucagon-like peptides I and II (GLP I and II). The glucagon molecule itself is flanked by both C-terminal and N-terminal peptides. In the pancreas, the glucagon sequence is cleaved from these flanking peptides, whereas GLP I and II are secreted uncleaved as a single peptide. In contrast, in the gut two peptides containing the glucagon sequence are produced, the major one (glicentin) extended by both flanking peptides and the minor one (oxyntomodulin) extended only in the C-terminal end. The glucagon-like peptides are cleaved and secreted separately in the gut (GLP I 7–37 and GLP II). The antibodies used to measure 'enteroglucagon' are really N-terminally directed glucagon antibodies that cross-react with enteroglucagon (glicentin and oxyntomodulin). Glucagon concentrations, measured using specific C-terminally directed antisera, are subtracted from those measured using the nonspecific antibody, leaving a derived enteroglucagon concentration.

Enteroglucagon is released by carbohydrate and fat in the intestine, whereas these nutrients inhibit the release of glucagon from the pancreas. Although enteroglucagon has not been purified in sufficient quantities to undertake full physiological studies, a mass of circumstantial evidence points to a trophic role for this peptide. A patient with an endocrine tumor producing enteroglucagon had marked villus hypertrophy in the small bowel. Enteroglucagon concentrations are increased, like those of neurotensin, in any situation associated with malabsorption, such as celiac disease or after small bowel resection. Enteroglucagon concentrations correlate remarkably with crypt-cell hyperplasia in these conditions. In addition, partially purified enteroglucagon stimulates DNA synthesis *in vitro*. Enteroglucagon could, therefore, be considered to be the growth hormone of the intestinal mucosa. It should be emphasized, however, that the evidence linking enteroglucagon and mucosal growth is rather circumstantial. Furthermore, the co-released glucagon-like peptides might be involved in these trophic effects.

The recently discovered peptide YY (PYY) and pancreatic polypeptide (PP) are both 36 amino acid, tyrosine-rich, straight-chained polypeptides that are amidated at the C-terminal end. It is now clear that at least two receptor subtypes exist for PYY and neuropeptide Y (NPY). Structure/activity studies suggest that both ends of these peptides are involved in binding and activity at one receptor subtype, whereas C-terminal fragments are sufficient to bind to the other. PP, which is localized to the islets of Langerhans of the pancreas, inhibits pancreatic enzyme secretion and relaxes the gallbladder. As PP concentrations remain high long after concentrations of other hormones, such as CCK, have returned to basal, it has been suggested that PP may play a role in conserving bile and pancreatic enzymes in readiness for ingestion of the next meal. In the adult human PYY is found in the ileum but is more abundant in the colon, with highest levels in the sigmoid colon and rectum. Blood concentrations of PYY increase after ingestion of food, and the magnitude of the response reflects the size of meal ingested. PYY infusion in man at doses that achieve concentrations within the physiological range has potent inhibitory effects on gastric secretion and emptying and causes a marked delay in small bowel transit. These effects appear mediated by inhibition of presynaptic cholinergic transmission. PYY enhances net fluid absorption in the small intestine by inhibition of crypt cell cAMP-mediated Cl^- secretion. At higher concentrations, PYY infusion in animals also inhibits pancreatic secretion.

Neurotensin is a 13 amino acid peptide that circulates in low concentrations. The endocrine cells secreting neurotensin are localized to the terminal ileum; release of neurotensin is effected whenever nutrients reach the distal portion of the small bowel. Thus, in normal adult man, meals have little effect on neurotensin release. However, if unabsorbed nutrients pass through the distal small intestine, as in malabsorption due to celiac disease or in patients with post-gastrectomy symptoms of dumping, circulating neurotensin concentrations increase. The actions of neurotensin include inhibition of gastric acid secretion and slowing of the rate of gastric emptying. Neurotensin also reduces blood pressure, but this effect is not seen at physiological concentrations.

Motilin is a straight, 22 amino acid peptide secreted from the upper small intestine. A larger molecular form of motilin is also found in the circulation in man. The whole sequence of motilin appears important for biological activity. Motilin has powerful motor actions on the gut, including formation of the interdigestive migrating motor complexes. Motilin also accelerates gastric emptying and increases colonic motility. Macrolides, such as erythromycin, are agonists for the motilin receptor, explaining the motor effects of these drugs, which recently have been used clinically in a variety of motility disorders. Somatostatin (SRIF) exists in two molecular forms: a 14 amino acid cyclic peptide (SRIF-14), and a 28 amino acid peptide, which has the SRIF-14 sequence at its C-terminus. Biological activity resides within the ring, and a potent, long-acting analog is now available for clinical use. Somatostatin is found in endocrine cells of the gastric fundus and antrum, in the islets of Langerhans of the pancreas, and throughout the intestinal tract. Although evidence suggests that somatostatin has some actions through the blood stream, the cells producing this peptide have processes extending to other endocrine and exocrine cells, suggesting a paracrine action. Somatostatin is also found in enteric nerves of the myenteric and submucous plexi.

Fetal development of gastrointestinal hormones

Cells secreting gastrin, somatostatin, motilin, and GIP are detectable at 8 weeks of gestation, gastrin and somatostatin cells being most numerous. By 14 weeks, all of the endocrine cell types are present in the intestinal mucosa, although the anatomical distribution is somewhat different from that seen in the adult. For example, gastrin cells are found in the ileum, neurotensin cells in the duodenum, PP cells in the colon, and PYY cells in the pancreas early in the second trimester. By the end of the second trimester, however, the cellular distribution resembles that of the adult. Peptidergic nerves are first demonstrable in the myenteric plexus at about 12 weeks of gestation, correlating with the known developmental pattern of enteric nerve plexi. After 3 months, the enteric nerves migrate through to the submucous plexus. By the third trimester all of the regulatory peptide systems appear well developed, although tissue content of some, notably gastrin, rises dramatically just before birth. In early fetal life, large molecular forms of peptides such as GIP and motilin predominate, suggesting that the post-translational enzymic processing pathways may be immature. At birth the molecular forms of the gastrointestinal regulatory peptides and their distribution in the gut are similar to those of the adult.

Several alimentary hormones can be detected in umbilical blood, collected at fetoscopy in the second trimester. Moreover, some endocrine cell types are functional, because several hormones such as enteroglucagon, PYY, and GIP are found in higher concentrations in blood from the umbilical artery and vein than in the maternal circulation at 18–21 weeks of gestation. Other peptides, such as gastrin, glucagon, and PP, are also found in the fetal circulation, but at concentrations below those in the maternal blood. Even these hormones show evidence of activity during fetal life as they are found in substantial quantities in amniotic fluid, which is swallowed by the fetus and probably plays a role in gut development. It is tempting to speculate that trophic peptides, such as gastrin, in amniotic fluid play an important role in gastrointestinal development even before luminal nutrition begins at birth.

Neonatal development of gastrointestinal hormones

Early neonatal life brings marked functional changes in the alimentary tract, as well as substantial growth, for which surges of gut hormones appear to be responsible. Gastrointestinal hormone secretion changes substantially during this early neonatal period, triggered by the switch from intravenous to enteral feeding. Each of these changes is considered in the following sections. Table 9.1 summarizes the major changes seen in early infant life.

At birth, cord blood concentrations of gastrin are already four or five times higher than those in the adult, and prefeed basal concentrations remain elevated for several weeks. Furthermore, gastrin concentrations increase in response to the first milk feed. After 3 or 4 weeks of life, basal gastrin concentrations decline, accompanied by development of marked feeding responses. Gastric acid is detectable in the stomach at birth and reaches a peak in the first day or two. Thereafter, acid output decreases for about a month despite the hypergastrinemia and rapid growth of the stomach. It has been suggested that the lack of responsiveness could be due to a lack of receptors in the oxyntic gland mucosa. However, a more likely explanation may be that secretion is suppressed by some inhibitor, such as PYY or neurotensin, thus enabling gastrin to stimulate growth of the gastric mucosa without hyperstimulation of acid secretion.

PYY concentrations are elevated in cord blood and rise postnatally to a peak within the first 2 weeks postpartum. At their peak, the plasma PYY concentrations are about 50 times higher than fasting concentrations in normal adults. Evidence suggests that gastric emptying and intestinal transit are rapid during the first week of life, both in term and preterm infants. The triggering mechanism for the ensuing changes is as yet unknown, but factors such as PYY likely play a role. In addition, the very potent inhibitory effect of PYY on gastric secretion may account for the prevention of hypersecretion of acid during the early neonatal period despite the marked hypergastrinemia.

CCK has marked trophic effects on the adult pancreas and appears responsible for regeneration following resection or acute pancreatitis. The observed postnatal surge of plasma CCK concentrations therefore may be of importance in stimulating growth of this organ.

Basal plasma secretin concentrations are higher at birth than in adults, and during the first 3 weeks of life a more marked postprandial response develops. As secretin is considered to be a major factor in triggering the neutralization of acid chyme entering the duodenum, the increase in circulating secretin concentrations may be of considerable importance in mucosal protection during this period. Notably, the postnatal surge of secretin, unlike that of the other alimentary hormones, occurs even in the absence of feeding, indicating the importance of this mucosal cytoprotective function.

Basal GIP concentrations are low at birth and increase gradually throughout the first month of life, along with the development of a marked post-feeding GIP response similar to that seen in the adult after ingestion of a mixed meal. The development of the GIP response to feeding in neonates is mirrored by the postprandial insulin response, which increases through the first month of life to maintain glucose homeostasis.

Plasma enteroglucagon concentrations show a very marked postnatal surge that peaks within the first week and is associated with the development of a marked postprandial response. As the rate of small intestinal mucosal growth is known to increase during this period, one may speculate that the increase of this trophic hormone is important in neonatal alimentary maturation. The resulting mucosal growth increases the absorptive area for uptake of nutrients from the gut.

Concentrations of PP, which at birth are lower than those of the adult, show a small postnatal surge that is particularly evident in preterm infants. During the first weeks of life, postprandial PP responses develop, but these are smaller in magnitude than those seen in the adult. Overall there is little evidence of a major developmental role for this peptide.

Plasma neurotensin concentrations are higher in the neonate, and an enhanced postprandial response develops in the first month of life. Both reduced gastric secretion and slowing the rate of gastric emptying decrease the rate at which acid chyme enters the duodenum and, therefore, result in a more steady absorption of nutrients from the gut. Thus neurotensin may be important in the adaptation of the neonate to enteral nutrition.

Motilin concentrations are low in cord blood, but preprandial basal concentrations show a massive, 10-fold postnatal surge that is particularly evident in preterm neonates. The peak occurs at around 2 weeks of postnatal life. As basal concentrations increase, a fall in motilin concentrations following milk feeding becomes evident, which is more like the pattern seen in the normal adult after a mixed meal. The relationship between maturation of the migrating motor complexes and the late postnatal surge of motilin in the preterm neonates is not clear at present.

Feeding and the development of gastrointestinal hormonal responses

Clearly, marked changes in gastrointestinal physiology accompany the introduction of enteral feeding in the infant. It is therefore of considerable interest that the postnatal surges of gut hormones are not seen in infants who have never received enteral feeding. Concentrations of all of these hormones, with the exception of secretin, remain low in babies receiving only parenteral nutrition. The composition of food as well as the mode of administration are also important in the development of gastrointestinal hormonal responses. This can be demonstrated as early as the first feed in infants, when dextrose elicits a different response than milk. Also, there are differences in hormonal responses between breast- and bottle-fed infants.

Influence of different feed types on gastrointestinal hormones

The first feed of human milk given 4–6 hours after full-term birth is associated with a marked rise in circulating concentrations of gastrin and enteroglucagon, whereas GIP concentrations are unaffected. The composition of the feed is important, however, as a first feed of glucose has no effect on enteroglucagon although the increment of gastrin is similar to the milk feed.

Substantial differences in gastrointestinal hormone responses are seen between infants fed human breast milk and formula-fed babies. By day 6, preprandial concentrations of the small intestinal hormones motilin, GIP, and neurotensin were much higher in bottle-fed infants, who also had greater postprandial changes in concentrations of insulin, motilin, neurotensin, enteroglucagon, and PP. Possible explanations for these alterations include the differences between the composition of human milk and cows' milk formula (despite attempts to humanize it) and the reduced milk intake of breast-fed infants during the first days of life, as lactation is developing. One should note, however, that by day 6 of life milk intake was similar in both groups. The differences in composition include the greater absorbability of fat in human milk and the higher total fat and branched-chain amino acid content of formula. Other factors may include the presence of active lipase and other enzymes as well as hormones in human breast milk. The presence of growth factors, such as EGF, in human milk may also be of profound importance in neonatal gut development.

Several other regulatory peptides have been reported in human milk including gastrin, neurotensin, PYY, VIP, PHM, and bombesin. Of these peptides, bombesin, which has trophic effects in a number of tissues, was present in higher concentrations in breast milk than in plasma.

The differences in hormone responses between breast- and bottle-fed infants may be of considerable practical importance. The enhanced insulin response in bottle-fed infants despite a similar degree of glycemia may result from increased circulating concentrations of branched-chain amino acids or GIP, both of which enhance glucose-stimulated insulin secretion. Because insulin enhances cellular glucose uptake and inhibits lipolysis, the greater insulin release may explain the increased deposition of subcutaneous fat seen in bottle-fed infants. Differences in motilin concentrations may account for the well known differences in stool frequency between bottle- and breast-fed infants. As enteroglucagon is likely to exert a major trophic effect on the small bowel mucosa, changes in concentrations of this hormone may influence postnatal gut development.

Comparison of continuous infusion feeding with intermittent boluses on gut hormones

Preterm infants receive gastric milk feeds either as continuous feeds or intermittent boluses; however, information is scant concerning the influence of these feeding modes on gastrointestinal hormones and gut development. Both groups show similar increases in plasma motilin, neurotensin, enteroglucagon, and PP concentrations. By 13 days, infusion-fed infants have higher concentrations of insulin, gastrin, and GIP. While both methods of feeding result in progressive changes in circulating enteroinsular hormone concentrations, the development of postprandial increases in response to bolus feeding is absent in infusion-fed infants. The absence of meal-stimulated gut hormone responses may have effects on the developing alimentary tract, but does not appear to influence body weight gain, which is similar between the two groups.

Practical significance of minimal enteral feeding on gut hormones

The relationship between the quantity of milk ingested and the development of postnatal surges of gut hormones has been investigated in infants recovering from hyaline membrane disease. Six-day-old infants who had been exclusively fed parenterally showed no postnatal elevation of gastrin, motilin, GIP, neurotensin, or enteroglucagon. In contrast, infants who had received restricted enteral feeding over this period had similar hormone surges to those seen in healthy infants on full enteral feeds. Substantial elevations of gastrin, GIP, and enteroglucagon were seen after a cumulative enteral feed volume of only 24 ml had been consumed since birth. By the time infants had received a cumulative intake of 96 ml, the hormone surges had reached maximal concentrations, which were identical to those of enterally fed healthy infants. Greater feed volumes were required to induce the normal surge of motilin and neurotensin, but even these were considerably lower than those required for full enteral feeding. These observations suggest that minimal enteral feeding may have an important therapeutic role in maintaining functional gastrointestinal integrity in infants undergoing prolonged parenteral nutrition.

Selected reading

Adrian TE. Gastrointestinal hormones. In Wyllie R, Hyams JS, eds. *Pediatric gastrointestinal disease: pathophysiology, diagnosis, management*. Philadelphia: WB Saunders, 1992.

Aynsley-Green A. The adaptation of the human neonate to extrauterine nutrition: a prerequisite for postnatal growth. In Cochburn F, ed. *Fetal and neonatal growth*. New York: John Wiley and Sons, 1988: 153.

D. Food Ingestion and Gastrointestinal Motility

C D Rudolph

Appetite

Food intake is regulated by complex interaction between centers in the hypothalamus, other regions of the central nervous system, and the gastrointestinal system. Although poorly understood, the factors controlling food ingestion and satiation at each mealtime are better understood than homeostatic regulation of caloric intake over longer periods of time, i.e. weight control. Stimulation of the lateral hypothalamic area results in hunger and food-seeking behavior. Damage to this area results in starvation due to a lack of nutrient ingestion. Stimulation of the ventromedial nucleus of the hypothalamus results in satiety. Gastric distension inhibits continued food ingestion before nutrients are absorbed into the blood stream. Distension of the stomach inhibits food intake, whereas when food is allowed to drain from the stomach through a fistula, animals will continue eating for long periods of time. Blood-borne nutrients and hormones may also affect satiety. Glucose infusion in the portal vein decreases food intake. Similarly, injection of cholecystokinin, to mimic the pattern of hormone release after feeding, decreases food intake.

Taste

Taste buds are located primarily on the walls of the tongue, with a few located throughout the palate, pharynx, and proximal larynx and esophagus. Taste-bud response to different stimuli varies with the region of the tongue: sweet and salty at the tip, sour on the sides, and bitter on the soft palate and posterior tongue. Microelectrode recordings indicate that most taste buds respond to two or three different chemical stimuli. Integration of these stimuli occurs in the central nervous system. Taste impulses pass through the chorda tympani of cranial nerves VII, IX, and X to the nuclei of the tractus solitarius. Within the brain, taste stimuli pass through the brainstem to the thalamus and cortex, paralleling the somatic pathways from the tongue.

Taste preferences vary tremendously between individuals and species and with age. For example, humans have a 'sweet tooth', whereas cats show no preference for sweets. Interestingly, opioid antagonists reduce the preference for sucrose in humans, suggesting that the pleasurable sensation enjoyed by sweet-lovers is mediated by opioid transmitters. Specific taste aversions develop in a wide variety of species when ingestion of a particular taste is linked to an unpleasant experience. Thus, nausea or other discomfort linked to the ingestion of a particular food leads to future avoidance of that food.

Although taste buds are present in mid-gestation, the number and maturity of taste buds increase postnatally in all species studied. Human infants' taste preferences change during development. Newborn infants prefer sweet tastes. Infants less than 4 months of age show no salt preference; however, between 4 and 24 months children prefer salty solutions. By 30 months children tend to reject saline solutions. Subsequent development of specific taste preferences depends largely on social and cultural factors.

Gastrointestinal motility: introduction

The muscle coat of the gastrointestinal tract is composed of an inner circular layer and an outer longitudinal layer. Contraction of these muscles results in alterations in the pressure and shape of the lumen, which grinds the food in the stomach and then transports it through the intestine, ensuring adequate mixing and exposure to the absorptive surface. The intrinsic gastrointestinal nervous system and extrinsic neural inputs act in concert to alter movement of food by changing the rate and spatial distribution of muscle contractions. In this section the mechanism of contraction of smooth muscle will be discussed initially.

Development of coordinated control of muscular contractile activity in each region of the gastrointestinal tract will then be summarized.

Smooth muscle contraction

A detailed discussion of smooth muscle electrophysiology and mechanics exceeds the scope of this chapter. A resting cell membrane potential is maintained by active extrusion of Na^+ in exchange for K^+. As in other tissues, the electrochemical gradient generated by the Na^+-K^+-ATPase pump is directed strongly inward, allowing its use as an energy source for transporting other ions or molecules against their electrochemical gradients. Low intracellular concentrations of Ca^{2+} are maintained by Ca^{2+} extrusion into the extracellular space and sequestration in intracellular organelles by an ATP-dependent pump.

Gastrointestinal smooth muscle undergoes a cyclic variation in basal membrane potential described as 'slow waves', 'basic electrical rhythms', or 'pacesetter potentials'. These waves are not associated with smooth muscle contraction, but rather represent changes in the excitability of the muscle cell. During the repolarization phase of the slow wave, the muscle cell is not excitable; thus the slow wave rate determines the maximal frequency of contraction of a particular smooth muscle. Which cells are responsible for initiating these spontaneous depolarizations is unclear. Various studies suggest that the interstitial cells of Cajal, which are located on the outer layer of the circular muscle and have gap junction connections to the smooth muscle cells, may be responsible.

The frequency, plateau, and repolarization rates of slow waves vary in different bowel regions and in different species. For example, in the dog the rate decreases from 18/min in the duodenum to 11/min in the ileum. The slow wave appears to propagate around the circumference of the circular muscle at a rapid rate, resulting in a synchronized contraction of a ring of smooth muscle that can increase luminal pressure. Superimposed on the slow wave are action potentials that result in contraction of the smooth muscle (Fig. 9.6). Action potentials can only be initiated during the crest of the slow wave. Depolarization of the membrane opens channels that allow the influx of Ca^{2+}, as in skeletal muscle. The membrane is rapidly repolarized due to the outward movement of K^+. An increase in the free cytoplasmic Ca^{2+} concentration results in the binding of Ca^{2+} to calmodulin (in skeletal muscle Ca^{2+} binds troponin), which activates myosin light chain kinase. The myosin and actin then interact, forming an ATPase system leading to mechanical contraction. Action potentials are only propagated for approximately 5 mm. Therefore, any coordination of peristalsis requires that action potentials be initiated in each segment of the bowel. If action potentials occur on the peak of every slow wave, a tonic contraction can occur. Some smooth muscles, particularly those associated with sphincters, maintain some contractile activity in the absence of clear action potentials. The electrical events associated with changes in baseline muscle tone are not well described. Patterns of coordination of contractile events in different regions of the gastrointestinal tract are discussed in the following sections.

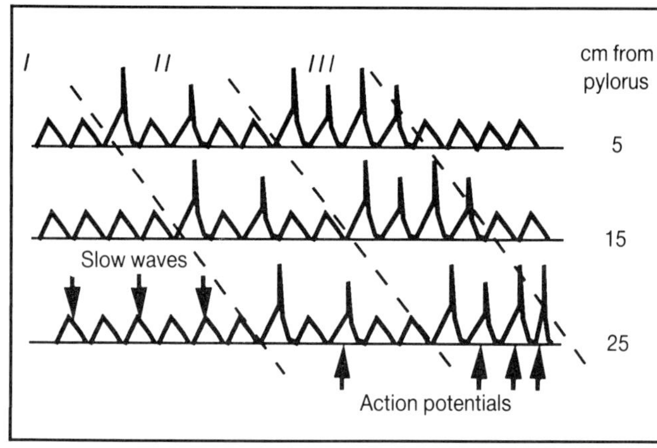

Fig. 9.6. Electrical activity of smooth muscle in the small intestine. This recording demonstrates the regular cyclic slow wave and overlying action potential. The aboral progression of the phases of the organized migrating motor complexes is also shown. During phase I there are no action potentials. Phase II has irregular action potentials at the slow wave peaks. Phase III is characterized by the presence of action potentials superimposed on each slow wave.

Swallowing

Swallowing of secreted saliva occurs constantly during the day. In the adult human, swallowing is composed of four phases (Fig. 9.7). Coordinated contraction of 32 pairs of skeletal type muscles is required for the preparatory, oral, and pharyngeal phases of swallowing. During the oral phase the food is ground and lubricated to form a

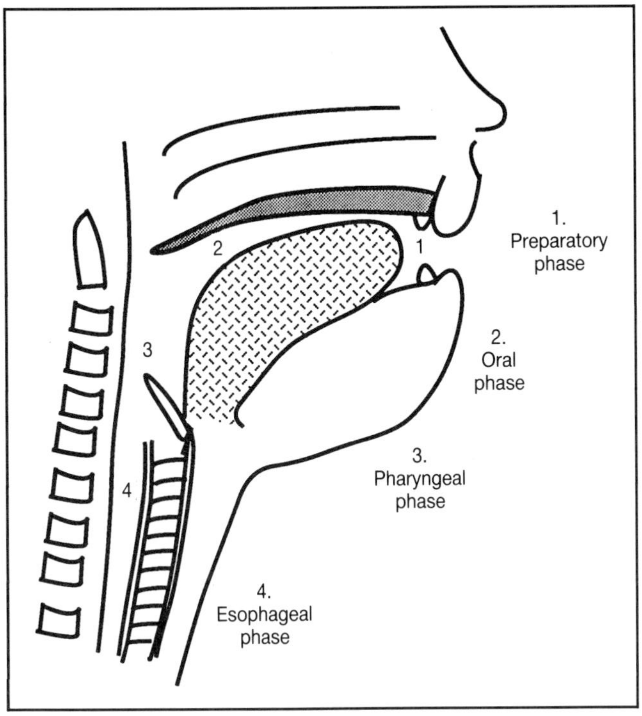

Fig. 9.7 The phases of swallowing in the adult human.

bolus. The bolus is then transferred to the pharynx by a sweeping contraction of the tongue against the hard and soft palates. In preparation for bolus passage, the soft palate closes against the posterior pharynx, sealing the nasopharynx; the larynx elevates and the vocal cords close while the upper esophageal sphincter relaxes. Presence of the food bolus or oral secretions in the upper pharynx initiates a swallow reflex, and peristaltic contractions through the pharynx and esophagus propel the bolus into the stomach. The bolus passes around the airway to enter the esophagus. Sensory feedback via cranial nerves V, IX, and X alters the amplitude and timing of the peristaltic contractions as bolus size and consistency change. Cranial nerves V_2, VII, X, and XII control the muscles required for swallowing. Anatomical defects such as palatal or laryngeal clefts, or neuromuscular disease alter the normal swallow and frequently result in aspiration of food into the lungs.

Infants ingest food only in a liquid form as milk. The infant does not chew food in the oral cavity. The lips are sealed over the nipple, and the tongue closes the region between the oral cavity and pharynx. Lowering the tongue then produces a negative pressure greater than 100 mmHg in the oral cavity, sucking milk from the bottle or breast. Rhythmic burst of sucks at a rate of one per second are followed by cessation of breathing and transfer of the liquid bolus into the pharynx, where swallowing proceeds as in the adult. Mature sucking patterns are first noted at about 35 weeks of gestation. Swallowing of pharyngeal contents is seen as early as 11 weeks of gestation. As the fetus or premature infant approaches term, the length of the bursts of sucking increases, as does the magnitude of the negative pressure produced in the oral cavity, and the coordination of the suck and swallow mechanism gradually improves. Non-feeding infants often are comforted by sucking on a thumb or pacifier. 'Non-nutritive' sucking is characterized by its rapid rate (~2/s). At 24 weeks the most primitive non-nutritive suck is observed.

As the infant matures the anterior oral cavity enlarges. Between 4 and 6 months of age the tongue begins to transfer soft solids from the oral cavity to the pharynx. Over the next year teeth develop and the tongue and oral muscles develop coordinated movements that transfer solid foods laterally into the buccal pouches for chewing, grinding, and lubrication by saliva. This masticated bolus is then transferred into the pharynx and swallowed as in the adult.

The esophagus

The esophagus is a conduit between the pharynx and the stomach with muscular sphincters at either end, the upper and lower esophageal sphincters. In humans, the upper quarter of the esophagus is composed of skeletal type muscle, and the remainder is smooth muscle. When a food bolus enters the esophagus, rings of circular muscle contract sequentially from the top to the bottom of the esophagus. This 'primary peristaltic wave' propels the bolus down into the stomach. The lower esophageal sphincter relaxes to allow bolus passage into the stomach. Stretching of the esophageal wall stimulates a 'secondary peristaltic wave', initiated just above the site of distension, which progresses down the esophagus in a similar fashion. Propagation of the peristaltic wave depends on the intrinsic myenteric plexus and on vagal afferents. Even in the absence of vagal input, peristaltic waves can be initiated in the smooth muscle portion of the esophagus and transmitted by the intramural myenteric plexus. Abnormal peristalsis results in food impaction and pain. The limited information regarding maturation of esophageal peristalsis indicates that peristalsis is poorly coordinated until after 32 weeks of gestation, suggesting that coordinated contractions are not present until several days after birth even in the term infant.

The lower esophageal sphincter prevents the acid contents of the stomach from constantly refluxing into the esophagus. Incompetence of the lower esophageal sphincter allows acid to reflux from the stomach, causing inflammation of the mucosal wall and pain. A disorder known as *achalasia,* caused by a lack of relaxation of the lower esophageal sphincter, results in massive esophageal distension and malnutrition due to an inability to eat. These clinical problems have made the lower esophageal sphincter the focus of tremendous investigative effort. The lower esophageal sphincter is characterized by its ability to remain tonically contracted. A 2–4 cm zone in the lower esophagus maintains a pressure of approximately 30 mmHg in the adult human. This tonic contraction appears to be a property of the smooth muscle itself. Neural blockade with tetrodotoxin does not affect the tonic pressure. Esophageal or gastric distension or vagal stimulation all cause relaxation of the sphincter muscle. The relaxation of the sphincter elicited by swallowing is mediated by the vagus. The relaxation due to distension is mediated by the intramural neural plexus. Non-cholinergic, nonadrenergic neurons appear to be responsible for these reflex relaxations. A variety of substances including vasoactive intestinal peptide, calcitonin gene related peptide, peptide histidine isoleucine, and nitric oxide all may play a role in this relaxation response. Although pharmacological doses of many gastrointestinal hormones have been shown to alter lower esophageal sphincter tone, the physiological role of these hormones remains controversial. Recent evidence indicates that the lower esophageal sphincter relaxes transiently in the normal human. Some reflux of acid into the esophagus is a normal event. Secondary peristaltic waves combine with the buffering activity of swallowed saliva to clear the refluxed acid from the esophagus rapidly. Thus disorders of esophageal clearance may be more important in the pathogenesis of esophageal damage from gastroesophageal reflux than simple incompetence of the sphincter muscle.

Two factors other than the intrinsic smooth muscle tone appear to contribute to competence of the lower esophageal sphincter. In the normal human, a short segment of the esophagus located below the diaphragm is constricted when intra-abdominal pressure increases, helping to prevent reflux into the esophagus. In addition, contractions of the crura of the diaphragm, which wrap around the lower esophagus, contribute to the pressure barrier to gastroesophageal reflux during inspiration.

Regurgitation of food is common in infants. The lower esophageal sphincter region of the infant is shorter than in the adult. In addition, the anatomical relationship of the stomach and diaphragm is different in the infant so that a relatively shorter segment of esophagus than in the adult lies within the abdominal cavity. At 26 weeks of gestation, the lower esophageal sphincter resting pressure is only 4 mmHg; this increases to 18 mmHg by term. The increased abdominal cavity pressure associated with straining or coughing overcomes this pressure barrier relatively easily, resulting in reflux of gastric contents or regurgitation. Despite an increased tendency toward gastroesophageal reflux, esophageal mucosal damage is rare in infants because refluxed acid is efficiently cleared from the esophagus. Similarly, infants rarely aspirate refluxed material because inspiration ceases and the airway closes until the refluxed material is cleared from the pharynx by swallowing.

Gastric and small intestinal motility

The stomach grinds and emulsifies food and then serves as a reservoir, gradually emptying nutrients into the intestine for absorption. The fundus and antrum differ in their functional roles. The upper body and fundus of the stomach relax with distension, maintaining a relatively constant intraluminal pressure with variations in volume. This receptive or adaptive relaxation allows the fundus to serve as a reservoir for a large volume of food. The pressure difference between the fundus and duodenum is the most important factor regulating liquid emptying. Adaptive relaxation is mediated by noncholinergic, nonadrenergic inhibitory vagal neurons. After vagotomy, the reservoir function of the stomach is disturbed and liquids empty rapidly, causing *'dumping' syndrome.*

The tonic contractions of the fundus and body drive liquid and solid food to the antrum. Strong contractions of the antrum mix liquids and grind solid food. The liquid passes easily through the pylorus, whereas the solid particles are retropelled back into the body of the stomach. This antral mill grinds the solids into a size small enough to pass through the pylorus (~2 mm). The rate of gastric emptying of solids and liquids is controlled by the central nervous system and by feedback from the intestine. Emotional stress decreases gastric emptying. The presence of acid, fat, carbohydrates, or amino acids (especially tryptophan) in the duodenum decreases gastric emptying. Intramural nerves, vagal pathways, and gastrointestinal hormones, in particular cholecystokinin, all appear to have a role in the feedback regulatory process.

The liquid emulsion that enters the small intestine, chyme, slowly passes from the duodenum to the ileum. In the adult human this occurs over 1–3 hours. Distension of the small intestinal wall results in an aboral peristaltic contraction as in the rest of the bowel. The pattern of constant churning with continual slow movement of the food down the intestinal tract that characterizes the period after feeding is poorly understood. Complex interactions between the luminal contents and intestinal smooth muscle wall result in this integrated pattern. This process is independent of extrinsic innervation. Recordings of isolated regions of contractile activity in the fed bowel indicate that there are frequent contractions, but a clear, coordinated pattern is difficult to discern. In contrast, in the fasted human a cyclic pattern of antral and intestinal contractile activity, called a migrating motor complex (MMC), migrates from the antrum to ileum. Periods of no contractile activity (phase I) are interrupted by irregular contractions (phase II). In phase III, regular contractions occur at the same rate as the slow wave. The cycle repeats itself every 45–90 minutes. Similar patterns are noted in other species. In the rat, cycles recur at intervals of 15–30 minutes. The MMC removes indigestible substances, i.e. ingested foreign bodies, from the bowel and sweeps bacteria out of the small intestinal lumen into the large intestine, preventing bacterial overgrowth of the bowel. In most mammals, feeding interrupts the MMC pattern. In weaned ruminants, an MMC pattern persists throughout the day. The movement of intestinal contents occurs during phase II of the MMC.

The factors that control gastric emptying appear to be similar in term infants and adults. Studies of the development of gastric emptying in preterm infants indicate that although the mechanisms controlling emptying are similar, the rate of emptying may be slower than in term infants. Small intestinal contractile patterns are similar in the adult and term infant. In fetal lambs disorganized sporadic contractions are seen from 0.6 to 0.8 of gestation. From 0.8 to 0.95 of gestation, clustered rhythmic bursts of activity are noted, which propagate aborally and orally. The mature MMC pattern appears after 0.95 of gestation. In dogs the clustered burst pattern persists until 15 days after birth, when MMC patterns appear. Therefore, although the presence of an MMC pattern indicates that bowel neuronal maturation has occurred, food can be adequately propelled and absorbed before this activity pattern develops. In the human premature infant, analogous patterns of intestinal activity are evident. Prior to 30 weeks of gestation, contractile patterns are of low pressure, sporadic, and nonpropagative. Clusters of rhythmic contractions appear at 30 weeks, then increase in rate of propagation and amplitude over the next several weeks. By approximately 37 of weeks gestation the mature MMC pattern is evident.

Colonic motility and defecation

The smooth muscle wall and innervation of the colon are essentially similar to those of the small intestine. The longitudinal muscle does not extend around the entire circumference of the colon, and the neuronal phenotypes differ with location and species. In contrast to the small bowel, propulsion of contents through the colon is slow, being measured in hours or days rather than in minutes. Movement of the luminal contents in the colon has been subjected to extensive study only recently. Distension appears to stimulate contractions. Bursts of contractions occur intermittently and are propagated in aboral and oral directions. The proximal and transverse colon have regions of stasis, allowing absorption and bacterial fermentation of their contents. The distal colon appears to mold and form the stool bolus, which is transported into the rectum. The anorectal region temporarily stores the feces until it is convenient to defecate. Like the proximal stomach, the rectum serves as a reservoir, accommodating increased volume with little change in luminal pressure. After meals, rectal tone increases. Large, high-amplitude, aborally propagated bursts of contraction sweep through the colon, moving a large segment of the luminal contents into the next region. These contractions are associated with defecation. Control of defecation is an important skill learned by toddlers during the toilet-training years. Achievement of normal control of defecation is viewed as a major milestone in social development, whereas loss of bowel control results in social censure. Continence of stool is maintained by the anal sphincter, which is composed of a smooth muscle 'internal sphincter' and a striated muscle 'external sphincter'. The internal sphincter is responsible for anal continence at rest and is not under voluntary control. Passage of stool or gas into the rectum distends the wall of the rectum. An intramural reflex mediated by vasoactive intestinal peptide (VIP), the 'rectoanal inhibitory reflex', relaxes the internal sphincter when the rectal wall is stretched as stool or gas enter from above. Infants spontaneously pass the stool. Older children and adults sense the need to defecate but voluntarily contract the external sphincter to prevent the passage of stool or gas until they reach a socially acceptable place and time. The rectum accommodates the increased volume, and the internal sphincter contracts, allowing relaxation of the external sphincter. During straining to stool, the resting tone of the external anal sphincter decreases, allowing defecation. Passage of flatus alone is achieved when pressure in the rectum increases due to gaseous distension and a small opening in the anal sphincter permits gas, but not feces to be passed.

Distension of the rectum with a balloon elicits the anorectal inhibitory reflex relaxation of the internal sphincter in normal individuals. In the newborn and premature infant, the magnitude of the resting internal anal sphincter pressure is reduced, but the anorectal inhibitory reflex is intact. In *Hirschsprung disease,* the anorectal inhibitory reflex is absent due to the lack of normal intramural neural pathways.

Selected reading

Milla PJ, ed. *Disorders of gastrointestinal motility in childhood.* Chichester, NY: John Wiley & Sons, Ltd, 1988.

Schultz SG, Wood JD, eds. *Handbook of physiology, Section 6: The gastrointestinal system, Vol. 1: Motility and circulation.* Bethesda, MD: American Physiological Society, 1989.

E. Gastric Acid Secretion and Gastroduodenal Mucosal Defense Mechanisms

A R Euler

Gastric acid secretion

One of the major physiological functions of the stomach is the secretion of hydrochloric acid by oxyntic gland parietal cells. Gastric acid secretion occurs in three phases: cephalic, gastric, and intestinal. Secretion occurs prior to ingestion of any food. Simply the smell or thought of food can stimulate gastric acid secretion during the cephalic phase. Entry of food into the stomach or intestine further stimulates gastric acid secretion.

Gastric glands containing parietal cells are branched, tubular, coiled structures located within the deeper mucosal layers of the gastric fundus and body. In addition to producing hydrochloric acid, which denatures protein, converts pepsinogen to pepsin, and is bacteriostatic or bactericidal for most microbes, these cells also secrete intrinsic factor and small amounts of bicarbonate. The parietal cell contains a network of secretory canaliculi that extend from the luminal surface of the cell through the body of the cell. These canals expand when acid secretion is stimulated.

The synthesis and secretion of hydrochloric acid by parietal cells has been studied intensively. H^+ ions are secreted to obtain a pH of 1.0 when intracellular pH is 7.1–7.2, achieving a two-millionfold concentration gradient. The mechanisms by which this is achieved are summarized in Fig. 9.8. Carbonic anhydrase catalyzes the formation of HCO_3^- and H^+ ions from CO_2 and H_2O. H^+-K^+-ATPase, an enzyme located on the parietal cell luminal surface, secretes H^+ ions across the apical membrane in exchange for K^+ ions. By a separate pathway, K^+ and Cl^- ions are secreted into the canalicular space, down their concentration gradient with H_2O following. Thus electrochemical and osmotic balance are maintained across the apical membrane. Secretion of this large amount of acid into the lumen requires that an equivalent amount of base be secreted from the basolateral surfaces of the parietal cell to maintain the intracellular pH in the physiological range. Cl^- ions are exchanged for OH^- (HCO_3^-) ions. The Na^+-K^+-ATPase,

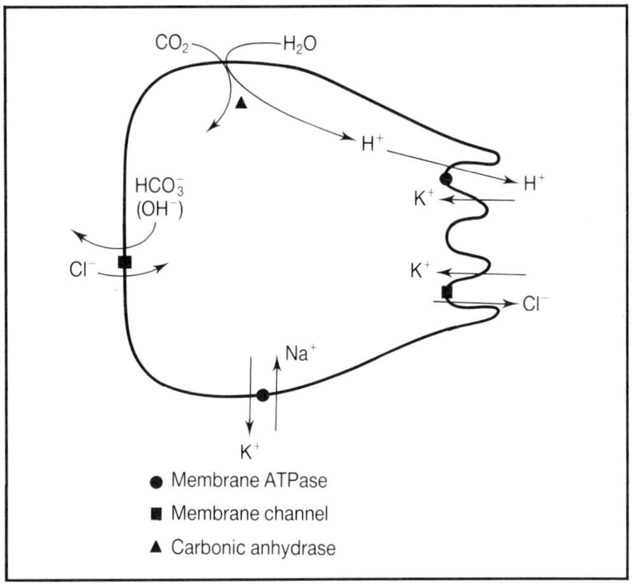

Fig. 9.8. Schematic representation of the mechanism of H^+ ion secretion by the gastric parietal cell. H_2O and CO_2 are converted to H^+ and HCO_3^- by carbonic anhydrase (CA). HCO_3^- is exchanged for Cl^- across the basal membrane through a membrane channel. Na^+ and K^+ are exchanged by an energy-requiring ATPase on the basal membrane. H^+ is exchanged for K^+ on the apical membrane surface. The net effect is to secrete HCl from the apical surface and $NaHCO_3$ from the basal surface.

located on the basolateral membrane, maintains the higher intracellular K^+ concentrations that are necessary to drive K^+ ion into the lumen.

Secretion of H^+ ions by the parietal cell is stimulated by neurocrine, endocrine, and paracrine pathways through three receptors located on the cell-surface membrane: H_2-histaminergic, M_2-cholinergic, and gastrinergic. The parietal cell may also express receptors for somatostatin and epidermal growth factor. When histamine from adjacent mast cells occupies H_2 receptors on the parietal cell, intracellular cAMP increases. When acetylcholine from the vagus occupies cholinergic receptors, membrane permeability to Ca^{2+} ions increases, allowing an influx of Ca^{2+}. Intracellular Ca^{2+} interacts with calmodulin, which probably acts as the second messenger in this pathway. There is conflicting evidence regarding the mechanism of gastrin action on the parietal cell. In some species, gastrin stimulates the mast cell with histamine, secondarily stimulating the parietal cell. In others, the gastrinergic receptor seems to affect acid secretion in a manner similar to that found after cholinergic stimulation, by increasing intracellular Ca^{2+}.

Development of gastric acid secretion

Only the gastric and intestinal phases of gastric acid secretion have been evaluated during the neonatal period. Enterally, or enterally plus parenterally nourished infants have significantly higher basal and maximal gastric acid secretory rates than those receiving only parenteral nutrition. Enteral feedings are therefore necessary for optimal parietal cell function in these infants. The gastric phase is discussed below.

In mammals the upper gastrointestinal mucosa develops early in fetal life, with parietal cells appearing by week 14. Parietal cells have a pink, granular cytoplasm with dark, centrally located nuclei and are usually round or triangular in shape. In the fetal rat, the stomach responds to pentagastrin on day 20. Similar data are not available for the human fetus, although the human newborn is known to have elevated serum gastrin concentrations, which are not of maternal origin. These increased gastrin concentrations are not associated with significantly increased gastric acid secretion relative to the older child or adult. This situation is identical to that in the rat, where even 5-day-old pups did not respond to pentagastrin with significant acid secretion. The genes regulating the synthesis of carbonic anhydrase and H^+-K^+-ATPase appear to be coordinately regulated during acid secretion. The activity of these proteins is diminished in young animals, potentially contributing to the lack of responsiveness of the newborn to secretagogues. mRNA coding for these enzymes is present at levels similar to those in the adult rat, suggesting that mRNA translation or post-translational processing is decreased.

In many mammals, maternal milk prostaglandin E_2 (PGE_2) content may play a role in regulating acid secretion as these PGs are known to suppress gastric acid secretion. Solid foods also have an effect on acid secretion, stimulating greater gastric acid secretion than liquid nutrition. All of these associations have been discovered in animals. One such association has also been confirmed in human neonates; enteral feedings are associated with greater acid secretion than parenteral. This effect may result from specific amino acids contained in the feeds and occurs without a concomitant increase in serum gastrin. This acid secretory response to oral feedings also increases with increasing age, with an approximately twofold elevation between 1 and 2 weeks of life.

Gastric secretory studies are performed either during fasting conditions (basal acid output [BAO]) or after a stimulus (maximal acid output, [MAO]), e.g. pentagastrin, histamine, or food. Neither type of secretory study has been reported in the human fetus; however, in the 1-week-old premature infant, BAO was 12 mmol/(kg·h) increasing to 30 mmol/(kg·h) at 4 weeks of age. MAO after pentagastrin stimulation was 21 mmol/(kg·h) and 44 mmol/(kg·h) at 1 and 4 weeks of age, respectively. These increases were not associated with increases in serum gastrin concentrations. Also using pentagastrin as a stimulus, BAO on days 1 and 2 were nearly identical, 0.110 and 0.114 mEq/(kg·h), while the MAO on the same days was 0.122 and 0.133 mEq/(kg·h), respectively. Serum gastrin concentrations were elevated in these newborns, indicating a relative lack of response by the parietal cells to this supraphysiological stimulus early in life. In a different study, betazole (Histalog®), which stimulates the histamine H_2 receptor on the parietal cell, increased MAO. Secretory rates were approximately 10 times greater at 8 weeks of age than on day 1. This indicates that histamine is a more potent stimulus during the neonatal period than gastrin. When acid secretion was stimulated with a meal (5 percent glucose plus an elemental formula), newborns responded in a manner similar to older infants (age >6 months), but their response was quantitatively different. Specifically, BAO in the newborn and older infants was 0.038 and 0.067 mmol/(kg·h), respectively, while MAO after the meal was 0.011 and 0.149 mmol/(kg·h), respectively.

Intrinsic factor (IF), a peptide that is important for absorption of vitamin B_{12}, is also secreted by the parietal cell. In rat pups, IF mRNA content changes in parallel with the developmental change in H^+-K^+-ATPase levels noted above. Similar rates of secretion of IF have been documented in premature and full-term infants (10.9 and 6.3 ng/(kg·h), respectively). In term infants, IF levels increase from 7.1 ng/(kg·h) on day one to 31.2 by day 28. Normal adult levels (118 ng/(kg·h)) are not achieved until 3 months of age. Pepsinogen is secreted by the chief cells in the gastric mucosa. Pepsinogen secretion is reduced in the premature versus full-term infant. The combination of lower acid output and decreased pepsinogen release may place premature infants at considerable disadvantage in gastric proteolysis. Therefore, providing a protein hydrolysate formula rather than intact proteins may facilitate nitrogen uptake. Pepsinogen and gastric proteolysis are discussed in Section F.

Gastroduodenal mucosal defense mechanisms

Upper gastrointestinal mucosal damage is believed to result when mucosal destruction by hydrochloric acid, pepsin, or bile salts overcomes the mucosal defense mechanisms. Gastric acid hypersecretion (due to *Zollinger–Ellison syndrome* or *mastocytosis*) results in mucosal ulceration. More commonly, gastric mucosal destruction is due to inadequate mucosal defense. The important role played by these mucosal defensive factors was unappreciated until Andre Robert described a process termed **cytoprotection**. Cytoprotection is defined as the ability of certain substances, especially PGs, to protect the deeper layers of the mucosa, below the surface epithelium, from being injured when exposed to various noxious agents such as strong acids (0.6 M HCl). Cytoprotection occurs with doses of exogenous agents that do not affect gastric acid secretion. This observation has led to an entirely new area of investigation involving the mechanisms of gastrointestinal mucosal protection.

Complex mechanisms underlie the gastroduodenal mucosal defensive barrier. The gastroduodenal mucosa has a well defined layer of mucus overlying the surface epithelial cells. Bicarbonate is secreted into this mucous layer by the surface epithelial cells, forming the 'mucobicarbonate barrier'. Mucus is secreted primarily by cells located in the neck segments of gastric glands. These mucus-producing cells have pale foamy cytoplasm, basal nuclei, and large amounts of para-aminosalicylic acid (PAS)-positive mucus. Somatostatin, vasoactive intestinal peptide (VIP), acetylcholine, and particularly PGE_2 stimulate mucus secretion, while PGE_2, vagal efferents, and gastric acid stimulate bicarbonate secretion. Neither mucus nor bicarbonate alone is a very effective defense mechanism, but the two combined form a substantial barrier when the gastric luminal pH is >2–3. When the intraluminal pH is <2 or when noxious agents other than acid are present, the mucosa must enlist other protective mechanisms.

One of the most important alternative mechanisms is maintenance of mucosal blood flow and microcirculation. Severe gastroduodenal mucosal damage occurs whenever the vascular supply is compromised because adequate O_2 and energy substitutes are not available to support intracellular aerobic metabolism. As a result the mechanisms that underlie normal cellular acid–base balance cannot be maintained. These deleterious effects can be avoided by maintaining mucosal blood flow. Endogenous PGE_2 increases mucosal flow and increases the resistance of the individual mucosal cells to damage. The mechanisms underlying this increased cellular resistance are unknown. Surface-active phospholipids, which repel water-soluble irritants, are also an important component of mucosal defense. These phospholipids are present as a thin film adhering to the epithelial cells and are stimulated by PGs.

The most important component of the mucosal defensive mechanisms is surface epithelial cellular renewal. It is a slower responding mechanism but is essential for maintenance of the epithelium. Soon after injury to an area of the surface epithelium, cells can be observed moving out of gastric pits onto the surface. Very rapidly they re-establish integrity of the mucosal surface, as can be documented with more negative potential difference (PD) measurements. With injury, PD becomes less negative. While repair is underway, subsequent injury is also prevented by secretions from uninjured epithelial cells, which result in a mucoid cap over the area undergoing repair. Prostaglandins and epidermal growth factor stimulate these less immediate defensive parameters.

Development of mucosal protective mechanisms

Research into the development of gastroduodenal mucosal defense has not involved human newborns or neonates. Limited information has been derived from animal studies. In the rat, the intrinsic ability of the gastric mucosa to protect itself against acid-induced damage does not develop until 14–21 days. The natural time course of development seems to depend on endogenous PGs and glucocorticosteroids. Exogenous hydrocortisone can accelerate this development. Also in the rat, surface hydrophobicity, which results from the actions of surface-active phospholipids, cannot be consistently induced by exogenous PGs until the third week of life. This development is not influenced by corticosteroids or thyroxine. Combined, these studies indicate that the gastroduodenal mucosal defensive barrier evolves during the neonatal period and is not fully developed at birth. The exact mechanism(s) underlying the development of the mucosal defense barrier in the human neonate is unknown. Circulating PG concentrations during the first month of life are greater in both the premature and full-term infant than in adults. These concentrations may result from endogenous production by the infant, PGs in breast milk, or both sources. Physiologically significant concentrations of PGs are present in breast milk. These PGs are absorbed from the infants' gastrointestinal tract and may have significant influences on many gastrointestinal functions including the development of various mucosal defensive components.

Selected reading

Malinowska DH, Sachs G. Cellular mechanisms of acid secretion. *Clin Gastroenterol* 1984; **13**: 309.

Schubert ML, Shamburek RD. Control of acid secretion. *Gastroenterol Clin North Am* 1990; **19**: 1.

Shorrock CJ, Rees WD. Overview of gastroduodenal mucosal protection. *Am J Med* 1988; **84**: 25.

F. Intraluminal Digestion and Absorption in the Small Intestine

R J Shulman

The primary role of all organs of the gastrointestinal system is to digest complex forms of ingested nutrients into simpler components that are easily absorbed and utilized for energy and growth by the organism. This section summarizes the process of digestion and absorption of carbohydrates, fats, proteins, and minerals.

Carbohydrates

Digestion of carbohydrates

The primary carbohydrate in the diet of the breast-fed human infant is lactose, which is also the carbohydrate in most infant formulas. Alternative carbohydrates used in infant formulas include sucrose or complex carbohydrates in the form of glucose polymers (molecules of glucose linked almost exclusively by α-1,4 bonds in a linear formation). Complex carbohydrates, such as those found in cereals, amylopectins, contain α-1,6 bonds as well as α-1,4 bonds.

Lactose is digested by the enzyme lactase, which resides in the brush border of the small intestinal mucosa. The K_m for lactase is 18 mM and the optimum pH is 6.0. The products of hydrolysis are glucose and galactose. In adults the rate of hydrolysis is the rate-limiting step in the absorption of lactose. The rate-limiting step in infants is unknown. Lactase activity is highest in the jejunum and decreases progressively toward the ileum; this gradient is established by the eleventh week of gestation. At the beginning of the third trimester, lactase activity is approximately 25 percent of the amount found at term. Some lactase activity is demonstrable in the colon in early fetal life, but is undetectable by 28 weeks of gestation. In many individuals, lactase activity decreases as age increases. This process, which is genetically determined, begins between 3 and 5 years of age. The decrease in lactase activity appears to be caused by a reduction in synthesis of the protein, possibly because of altered transcriptional and/or post-transcriptional processing. In humans, lactase activity is not inducible by dietary lactose. Despite high lactase activity at birth, most studies suggest that full-term, and especially premature infants digest and absorb lactose incompletely. In older individuals with low lactase activity, ingestion of lactose may cause diarrhea, flatulence, or cramping (i.e. *lactose intolerance*). Congenital absence of lactase has been reported, but is extremely rare.

Digestion of complex carbohydrates is accomplished by a number of enzyme systems. The quantitative contribution of each to complex carbohydrate digestion remains poorly defined. Salivary and pancreatic amylase (secreted by the salivary glands and pancreas, respectively) have identical actions: hydrolysis of starch at interior α-1,4 bonds. They are not active against those located next to α-1,6 bonds or those at the reducing end of the starch molecule. The end products of digestion by amylase are maltose, maltotriose, and α-limit dextrins. Salivary amylase is present in premature infants, and its activity may increase with increasing gestational age. However, the role of salivary amylase in the digestion of complex carbohydrates remains poorly defined. Although salivary amylase is rapidly inactivated at pH <4, the inability of some premature infants to generate significant gastric acidity may permit the enzyme to remain active. Additionally, some evidence indicates that complex carbohydrates themselves may offer some protection of salivary amylase against destruction by gastric secretions. Pancreatic amylase activity is extremely low in premature and full-term infants. Pancreatic amylase secretion in newborns does not appear to respond to pancreozymin and secretin stimulation. Pancreatic amylase activity does not begin to increase until 4–6 months of age, and adult values are not achieved until 1–2 years of age.

The enzyme glucoamylase resides in the brush border of the small intestine. It has activity against complex carbohydrates, primarily those that are nonbranched (i.e. only 1–4 bonds), with greatest activity against amylose with a degree of polymerization between 5–9 glucose units. It hydrolyzes α-1,4 bonds from the nonreducing end of the molecule. Thus, the product of glucoamylase activity is glucose. Small intestinal glucoamylase activity is detectable by 20 weeks gestational age, and activity in infants of 28–30 weeks gestational age is approximately half that found at 36–38 weeks. Glucoamylase, like lactase, is present in low levels in the colon only early in fetal life. Glucoamylase activity in the small intestine of young infants is similar to that found in older children and is approximately half that found in adults. Because pancreatic amylase activity is low, glucoamylase is the primary determinant of complex carbohydrate digestibility in newborns. Short-chain units of amylose (between 5 and 9 glucose units) appear to be absorbed and digested more easily than longer-chain units. Overall, however, digestion and absorption of complex carbohydrates in the small intestine is incomplete. Rice cereals, for example, contain small amounts of protein, but consist primarily of amylopectin. Recent studies suggest that approximately 30 percent of rice cereal is not absorbed in the small intestine of infants 1–2 months old.

The disaccharidase sucrase–isomaltase (sucrase-α-dextrinase) is found in the small intestinal brush border; its K_m is 1–4 mM and its pH optimum is ~6. Sucrase–isomaltase is synthesized as a 230 kDa precursor. The molecule is hydrolyzed into sucrase and isomaltase at the brush border by the action of pancreatic proteases, although cleavage is not required for activity. In a pattern similar to that of lactase, a proximodistal gradient of activity is present by the end of the first trimester. Sucrase–isomaltase activity develops early in gestation, and by 20 weeks of gestation achieves levels approximately one-half to three-quarters those found in term newborns and adults. Sucrase–isomaltase activity remains high throughout life. Maltase activity is provided mostly by the sucrase–isomaltase complex. A *deficiency of sucrase–isomaltase* can be transmitted as an autosomal recessive trait.

Not only does sucrase–isomaltase hydrolyze sucrose to its components glucose and fructose, it is also important during the final steps of the hydrolysis of complex carbohydrates. As with glucoamylase, sucrase–isomaltase is capable of hydrolyzing α-1,4 bonds. The hydrolysis of α-1,6 bonds occurs by means of isomaltase activity. Sucrase–isomaltase activity appears to be inducible by sucrose and fructose in the diet. Few data are available on the ability of infants to digest sucrose. Studies in adults suggest that more than 95 percent of dietary sucrose is digested in the small intestine.

Absorption of carbohydrates

After hydrolysis, the final step in the assimilation of carbohydrates is the absorption of the component monosaccharides, i.e. glucose and galactose in the case of lactose, glucose and fructose in the case of sucrose, and two molecules of glucose in the case of maltose. Active transport of glucose is demonstrable *in vitro* by 10 weeks gestational age. The maximal absorption rate of glucose increases with age through gestation and after birth to adulthood. Infants less than 37 weeks gestational age have a lower K_m for glucose than full-term infants. Infants who are small for gestational age have a lower apparent K_m than those who are appropriate for gestational age. Recent studies suggest that a high-affinity transport system exists throughout the small intestine with a low-affinity system limited to the proximal small intestine. These systems are present by 17–20 weeks gestational age. The transport of glucose involves movement of the molecule across the brush border and basolateral surfaces; glucose is actively transported at the brush border with two molecules of Na^+. Energy is provided by Na^+-K^+-ATPase at the basolateral membrane surface.

Thus, the absorption of glucose facilitates the absorption of Na^+, which is the rationale for adding glucose to rehydration solutions. Glucose absorption can also occur passively down a chemical gradient. Glucose movement across the basolateral surface out of the cell is by facilitated diffusion, which is Na^+-independent. Galactose is believed to be transported by the same system as glucose, although recent evidence suggests that there may be two systems with overlapping specificities. In contrast, a separate Na^+-independent transport system exists in the brush border for fructose. The ontogeny of galactose and fructose absorption in the human is unknown. Less than 0.1 percent of an ingested disaccharide is absorbed intact through passive diffusion.

Fats

Digestion of fats

Fats not only are a major energy source for newborn infants, but also are integrally involved in normal brain development, are components of cell membranes, and act as vehicles for the absorption of fat-soluble vitamins. In contrast to proteins and carbohydrates, fats are water-insoluble molecules that must be solubilized before they can be digested and absorbed.

Most dietary fats (triglycerides) consist of long-chain fatty acids ($\geqslant C_{16}$) and are thereby hydrophobic. The digestion of dietary fats primarily involves processes to increase their water solubility. The initial process in fat digestion is emulsification, which begins with the mechanical grinding action of the stomach and small intestine. Dietary proteins and the products of fat digestion, fatty acids, monoglycerides, and lecithin, further the emulsification process and stabilize the fat particles. The emulsified particles of fat, which are less than 1.0 µm in size, are further stabilized by bile salts, which are synthesized by the liver and secreted in bile. The emulsion is stable at neutral pH. The term 'mixed micelles' refers to these spherical particles of bile salts, hydrolysis products, phospholipid, and cholesterol. For micelles to be formed, bile salt concentration must be above the 'critical micellar concentration', which is determined by a number of factors including the properties of the individual bile salts. The major enzymes involved in the digestion of fats are the lipases (lingual, gastric, pancreatic). Although pancreatic lipase is the primary enzyme involved in small intestinal fat digestion, it requires the action of pancreatic colipase to anchor lipase to the fat droplet. The products of these actions are mono- and diglycerides, fatty acids, and glycerol. Because medium-chain triglycerides (C_{10}-C_{14}) are water soluble, they are absorbed directly through the stomach and the small intestine without the need for emulsification by bile acids.

The lipases undergo dramatic developmental changes. Although lingual lipase is demonstrable at birth, its contribution to lipid digestion is small in contrast to gastric lipase, which is released from the gastric fundus. Lingual and gastric lipases appear before 26 weeks of gestation and have high activities at birth. Newborns can digest 80–90 percent of ingested fat despite the fact that pancreatic lipase activity is extremely low at birth. Gastric lipase activity is similar in infants and adults. The underdeveloped gastric acid production of premature and full-term newborns provides an optimal milieu for enzyme activity. Approximately 10–30 percent of dietary fat is estimated to be hydrolyzed in the stomach of full-term infants. Presumably, the relative pancreatic insufficiency of newborn infants results in a lower duodenal pH, which enables lingual and gastric lipases to retain activity and continue fat digestion in the duodenum. Lingual and gastric lipases hydrolyze short- and medium-chain triglycerides more rapidly than long-chain triglycerides. Consequently, the triglyceride profile of the diet fed to newborn infants determines, in part, the digestibility of fat. Pancreatic lipase production is limited even in full-term newborn infants. Neither premature nor full-term infants have lipase-secreting response to pancreozymin or secretin at birth or at 1 month of age. The lipolytic activity of the duodenal contents is also low during the first year of life. The possible effect of diet composition on the development of lipase activity is a subject of debate. The developmental profiles of the individual lipolytic enzymes, lipase–colipase, phospholipase A_2, and cholesterol esterase, remain to be determined.

The cholic acid synthesis rate and the cholic acid pool are fourfold less in premature infants between 32 and 36 weeks of gestational age than in full-term infants. Full-term infants have values approximately half those found in adults. Developmental changes in bile acid secretion are discussed in Section 9N. Reduced duodenal concentrations of bile salts and pancreatic lipase activity decrease the capacity of infants to digest and absorb lipid. Fat is absorbed more easily from human milk than from formula, which may be the consequence of the presence of a bile salt-sensitive lipase present in human milk. Human milk-fed infants aged 31–36 weeks gestational age do not change fat absorption with increasing postnatal age. Ninety-four percent of ingested fat is absorbed by the breast-fed infant at 33 days after birth. In contrast, fat absorption in formula-fed infants is correlated with postnatal age and the duodenal concentration of bile acids. In general, the greater the fatty acid chain length and saturation, the poorer the absorption of fat.

Absorption of fats

Micelles *per se* are not absorbed into the small intestinal epithelial cells. However, because products of lipolysis are fat soluble, they encounter little difficulty traversing the lipoprotein membrane of the epithelial cells. Uptake of fatty acids occurs by passive diffusion and is concentration dependent. Most absorption of fatty acids and monoglycerides occurs in the duodenum and upper jejunum. Bile salts are absorbed primarily by active transport in the terminal ileum. Once fat digestion products have entered the cell, they are resynthesized into triglycerides. They are assembled with cholesterol, phospholipids, and apolipoproteins into chylomicrons, which are then discharged into the intercellular space and enter the lymphatic system.

Ileal uptake of cholic acid conjugated with taurine (taurocholate) is less shortly after birth in both premature and full-term infants than at 8 months. When bile acid uptake is reduced, the bile acid pool available for micellar formation presumably is decreased. The duodenal concentrations of bile acids in full-term infants are roughly one-tenth those found in adults. Premature infants appear to have greater fecal losses of bile acids than older infants, and the loss is greater for infants fed cows' milk formulas than for those fed human milk.

Proteins

Digestion of proteins

Protein digestion is a complex process requiring hydrolysis of many different peptide bonds. Absorption of the varied products of hydrolysis requires multiple transepithelial transporters. Protein digestion begins in the stomach. Acid denatures proteins, and pepsin I and II begin the process of hydrolysis. The development of gastric acid secretion is covered in Section 9E. Gastric peptic activity is low in premature infants but increases in proportion to gestational age. Although the stimulated value, corrected for body weight, increases after birth, at 1 month of age it is still approximately one-third that found in the adult. In 3–4-week-old premature infants (mean age 31 weeks of gestation at birth), meal-stimulated pepsinogen secretion was 5–10 percent that found in full-term infants 1–6 months of age. Thus, both pepsin(ogen) production and activity are diminished in premature infants. Activity is low, in part, because gastric pH must be <5 for these enzymes to be activated. Pepsin activity increases approximately twofold between infancy and adulthood. These studies indirectly support the data suggesting that protein digestion in the stomach of full-term newborns is limited.

The activity of enterokinase, the enzyme responsible for the activation of trypsinogen into trypsin, appears only after 26 weeks of gestation. Its activity at term is approximately 10 percent of that found in adults. Trypsin in turn activates the other pancreatic proteolytic enzymes. Most studies suggest that pancreatic trypsin levels are substantial in both premature and full-term infants. Trypsin and chymotrypsin activity have been demonstrated *in vitro* at approximately 25 weeks gestational age in the presence of enterokinase. The amount of trypsin secreted in response to pancreozymin and secretin stimulation has been reported to be similar at birth in premature (32–34 weeks of gestation) and term infants. By 1 week of age, this response reaches approximately 15–30 percent of that in children aged 9 months to 13 years. In premature infants (28–34 weeks gestational age) trypsin activity (units/mg protein secreted) increases twofold between birth and 1 month of age. Despite these differences, the trypsin activity level and concentration in duodenal fluid is similar at birth and at 2 years of age.

Recent studies have focused on the development of other pancreatic peptidases. The responses of chymotrypsin and carboxypeptidase B to pancreozymin and secretin are blunted in the same manner as those of trypsin in newborn and 1-month-old premature infants. Little change in activities occurs over the first month of life in premature infants of 28–34 weeks of gestation. Activities are approximately one-half those found at 2 years of age. Trypsin, chymotrypsin, and elastase are demonstrable in fetuses at 20 weeks gestational age, with no differences found in histochemical staining when compared with full-term infants. The lower activity of pancreatic proteases found in newborn and premature infants compared with full-term infants does not appear to limit protein digestion significantly. Serum albumin is absorbed to a similar extent in premature and full-term newborns during the first month of life. The ability to digest casein does not appear to be age related; no apparent change occurs in casein digestion (total proteolytic activity) from 2.5 months of age through adulthood. The action of the luminal proteases produces free amino acids (approximately 30 percent of ingested protein in adults) and peptides (two to six amino acid residues in length).

Many proteases are present in the brush border and cytoplasm of the small intestine. The activity of many of the peptidases is detectable between 10 and 16 weeks of gestation. The activity of dipeptidases is similar in infants, children (2 months to 14 years), and adults. Aminopeptidase activity in infants at 28–30 weeks gestational age is approximately one-half that found at 36–38 weeks. By 22 weeks gestational age, γ-glutamyltranspeptidase, aminopeptidase A, dipeptidylaminopeptidase IV, and carboxypeptidase are detectable, and except for aminopeptidase A, their activities are similar to those in adults. In contrast, γ-glutamyltranspeptidase activity decreases with increasing gestational age. Aminopeptidase activity is also found in the colon of both premature and full-term infants, but at levels approximately one-half of those found in the small intestine. The contribution of these enzymes to digestion in the premature and full-term infant, however, remains unclear.

Absorption of protein

Amino acid transporters are generally classified on the basis of their Na^+ dependence, affinity for the amino acid transported, and their possible inhibition by other amino acids. There are at least four different Na^+-dependent systems for neutral amino acids. Dibasic and some short-chain polar amino acids also have Na^+-dependent transport systems. Na^+-dependent transport is facilitated by the energy derived from Na^+-K^+-ATPase at the basolateral cell surface. The movement of Na^+ across the brush border enables Na^+-coupled transporters to use the energy for amino acid uptake. Na^+-independent (through facilitated diffusion) transport involves some neutral amino acids, cysteine, glutamine, and, in part, alanine. The enzyme γ-glutamyltranspeptidase may also be involved in amino acid transport. In some cases, transport of amino acids out of the cell across the basolateral membrane appears to occur through a Na^+-independent system. There is some overlap between the systems for amino acid transport in the small intestine and systems in the kidney; the overlap is defined by genetic disorders of amino acid transport that are common to both organs. The reader is referred to the selected reading at the end of this section for a more complete discussion of the types of amino acid transporters and their specificities.

Di- and tripeptides can be transported directly into the enterocytes. Peptides larger than three amino acids must be hydrolyzed before they can be absorbed (i.e. by brush border peptidases). Some amino acids are absorbed more rapidly as di- and tripeptides than as free amino acids. The absorption of amino acids from a protein hydrolysate is faster than from a mixture of the individual amino acids. The transport systems for peptides are poorly characterized, but are not those that transport amino acids. Peptide transport can be independent of, or dependent on, Na^+. Most of the peptides within the cell appear to be hydrolyzed by cytoplasmic peptidases, although some peptides are transported intact across the basolateral membrane. Little information is available about the transport of amino acids and peptides by the developing human small intestine. Amino acid transport appears to have developed by the end of the first trimester. Peptide transport has been demonstrated by the beginning of the second trimester.

Minerals

Ca^{2+} and phosphorus are the major minerals found in bone. At least 99 percent of the Ca^{2+} and phosphorus in the body are found in bone. Little is known about age-related changes in Ca^{2+} and phosphorus absorption in the human.

Calcium absorption

Ca^{2+} absorption is controlled by two processes: active transport and nonsaturable diffusion. Active transport of Ca^{2+} appears to occur through the transcellular route, whereas diffusion occurs through a paracellular pathway. Gastric acidity appears to enhance Ca^{2+} absorption by means of ionization. Most Ca^{2+} absorption occurs in the jejunum, primarily through active transport, although transport is most efficient in the duodenum. K_m values increase aborally along the small intestine, whereas V_{max} is lowest in the jejunum. Absorption of Ca^{2+} via diffusion occurs throughout the small intestine and decreases aborally. Most evidence suggests that little Ca^{2+} absorption occurs in the colon. Vitamin D ($1,25(OH)_2D$) stimulates the active absorption of Ca^{2+} across the brush border, the intracellular movement of Ca^{2+}, and the exit of Ca^{2+} across the basolateral membrane (through Ca^{2+},Mg^{2+}-ATPase). In this regard, there is a strong correlation between the concentration of calbindin in the intestine and the rate and efficiency of Ca^{2+} absorption. Calbindin appears to facilitate the intracellular movement of Ca^{2+}. Calmodulin, however, may alter the permeability of the cell to Ca^{2+}. Calbindin, but not calmodulin, is vitamin D responsive. At high luminal concentrations, Ca^{2+} is absorbed through vitamin D-independent diffusion. Movement of Ca^{2+} out of the enterocyte is mediated through a Na^+-Ca^{2+} exchange system and is facilitated by calmodulin; it is dependent on ATP and magnesium. Some evidence suggests that Ca^{2+} can also be translocated in vesicles by an energy-dependent mechanism (endocytosis and exocytosis).

Ca^{2+} absorption appears to decrease with age, i.e. absorption in premature infants is approximately 50 percent, whereas in adults it is closer to 30 percent. The nature of a diet can affect Ca^{2+} absorption; phytates and cellulose decrease Ca^{2+} absorption, whereas carbohydrates which can be digested and absorbed facilitate Ca^{2+} absorption. Steatorrhea also diminishes Ca^{2+} absorption. Active absorption of Ca^{2+} varies inversely with dietary Ca^{2+} intake.

Phosphorus absorption

Phosphorus appears to be absorbed both actively and passively. Both absorption routes are more active at pH 6.1 than at pH 7.4. Active transport appears to be the result of a Na^+-phosphate cotransport system located at the brush border. The transporter accepts both $H_2PO_4^-$ and HPO_4^{2-}. Each phosphate molecule is cotransported with two Na^+ ions. As in the case of Ca^{2+}, vitamin D ($1,25(OH)_2D$) increases active phosphorus transport. Passive diffusion of phosphorus occurs predominantly in the duodenum. In contrast to Ca^{2+}, thyroid hormone increases phosphorus absorption. Studies in animals suggest that phosphorus absorption decreases with age. The movement of phosphorus out of the cell appears to occur by means of a Na^+-phosphate carrier that is ATP-dependent.

Iron absorption

Absorption of iron is the primary mechanism whereby the content of total body iron is controlled. Most iron absorption occurs in the duodenum and proximal jejunum. Ferrous iron remains more soluble at the pH of the intestinal lumen and is better absorbed than ferric iron. Iron absorption is also affected by the composition of the diet; absorption is increased by some amino acids and vitamin C and decreased by carbonates and phosphate, which form insoluble precipitates. Hemoglobin iron is absorbed better than non-heme iron. Iron within the cells may come from either the diet or body stores. Because iron is known to bind to receptors on enterocytes, it is believed that when body stores of iron are adequate, the receptors are occupied by the endogenous iron, leaving few receptors available to bind dietary iron. In humans, iron uptake appears to be an active, carrier-mediated process that is mediated, in part, by a membrane protein and free fatty acids. The roles of transferrin and endocytosis in iron uptake by enterocytes have yet to be established.

Iron absorption in animals decreases with age. During a condition of iron deficiency, the uptake of other divalent metals (e.g. lead) is increased, presumably because iron and lead share a common transport mechanism. Iron leaves the enterocyte to enter the portal circulation. Iron absorption may be regulated at the brush border as well as at the basolateral membrane.

Selected reading

Argiles JM, Lopez-Soriano FJ. Intestinal amino acid transport: an overview. *Int J Biochem* 1990; **22**: 931.

Cross HS, Debiec H, Peterlik M. Mechanism and regulation of intestinal phosphate absorption. *Miner Electrolyte Metab* 1990; **16**: 115.

Flanagan PR. Mechanisms and regulation of intestinal uptake and transfer of iron. *Acta Paediatr Scand* 1989; **S361**: 21.

Johnson LR, ed. *Physiology of the gastrointestinal tract.* New York: Raven Press, 1987.

Walker WA, Durie PR, Hamilton JR, *et al.*, eds. *Pediatric gastrointestinal disease.* Philadelphia: BC Decker Inc., 1991.

Wasserman RH, Fullmer CS. On the molecular mechanism of intestinal Ca^{2+} transport. *Adv Exp Med Biol* 1989; **249**: 45.

G. Absorption and Secretion of Electrolytes and Fluid by the Intestine

M B Cohen

The intestine is the primary organ of water and nutrient absorption. The intestine also plays an important role in maintaining fluid and electrolyte balance, and intestinal secretory mechanisms aid in the digestion of food. Disorders of intestinal fluid and electrolyte absorption or of intestinal secretion have profound impact on health.

Water transport

Fluid and electrolytes are reabsorbed along the entire length of the gastrointestinal tract; however, the distal segments are more efficient than the proximal segments in their ability to absorb water. The absorptive efficiency of the entire human intestine for H_2O and Na^+ is 95–99 percent. This means that only 1–5 percent of the water load presented to the upper intestinal tract is actually excreted by the colon. Nonetheless, the human colon is usually not required to absorb fluid to its maximal capacity. In the adult, the human colon can compensate for up to a 50 percent reduction in small intestinal absorption before there is a change in stool volume.

Sodium absorption

Na^+ represents the major driving force for absorption of fluid in the intestine. Furthermore, as fluid progresses to the distal intestine, there is an increasing ability to absorb Na^+ against a high concentration gradient (≥100 mM). The human colon can reduce the intraluminal Na^+ concentration to <15 mM under normal conditions and to 3 mM when required by water and salt deprivation.

Na^+ enters the intestinal cell both by diffusion and by active transport. Active transport of Na^+ involves two distinct steps. First, there must be carrier- or channel-mediated transport of Na^+ across the apical cell membrane. Next, Na^+ must traverse the enterocyte and be pumped out by a basolateral membrane Na^+ pump. A number of transport mechanisms permit entry of Na^+ into the enterocyte through the apical membrane (Fig. 9.9). These include Na^+-Cl^- cotransport (Na^+-H^+ and Cl^--bicarbonate exchange), Na^+-glucose (or galactose) transport, Na^+-amino acid cotransport, volatile fatty acid-stimulated Na^+ transport, and aldosterone-stimulated Na^+ transport. Whereas there are several mechanisms for Na^+ entry through the apical membrane, there is a single active mechanism of Na^+ exit through the basolateral membrane. The basolateral Na^+ pump, Na^+-K^+-ATPase, is present in sufficient quantity to accommodate the influx of Na^+ resulting from the multitude of apical transport systems.

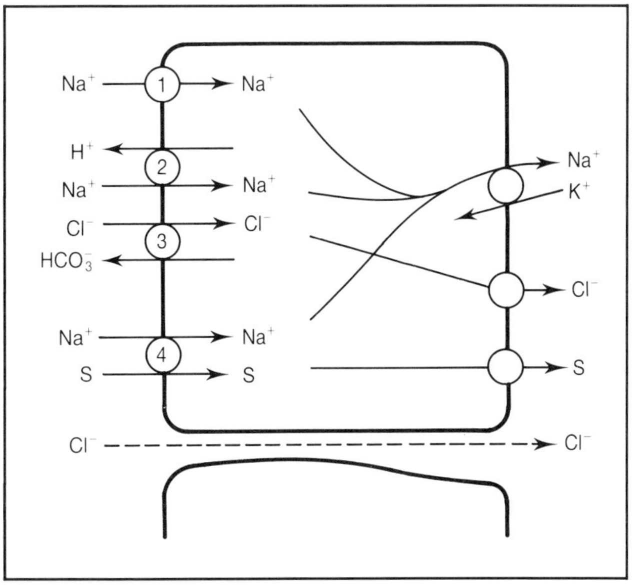

Fig. 9.9. Major intestinal electrolyte transport systems. Na^+ is transported actively across the apical membrane by a number of different processes: (1) through an electrogenic conductance channel, (2) through an intestinal cation exchanger, (3) through an intestinal anion exchanger, and (4) coupled with organic solutes (S) including glucose, galactose, amino acids, and volatile fatty acids. The diagram also shows Cl^- being transported through the paracellular pathway as a result of the electrochemical gradient generated by transport processes 1 and 4. Na^+ is excreted through the basolateral membrane via Na^+-K^+-ATPase. (From Guandalini S. *Drugs* 1988; **36** (Suppl 4): 26–38, with permission from Adis International.)

Bicarbonate-stimulated Na^+ transport

The jejunum absorbs both Na^+ and bicarbonate, which results in electrically neutral absorption of both ions. This process begins with the equimolar exchange of Na^+ and H^+. The H^+ that is liberated into the intestinal lumen is dissipated by combination with bicarbonate. This results in the formation of carbonic acid, which dissociates into H_2O and CO_2. CO_2 is reabsorbed into the cell and combines with a hydroxyl group to form bicarbonate, which then diffuses across the basolateral membrane.

Chloride-bicarbonate exchange

An important mechanism of Na^+ absorption in the ileum and distal colon is electrically neutral absorption of Na^+ with Cl^-. In the ileum, Cl^- is actively exchanged for bicarbonate by the Cl^--bicarbonate anion exchanger. The increase in the luminal concentration of bicarbonate drives the intestinal cation exchanger to absorb Na^+ in exchange for H^+. This double ionic exchange model provides a mechanism whereby volatile fatty acids might also stimulate Na^+ and Cl^- transport via fatty acid-bicarbonate exchange.

Glucose- and amino acid-stimulated sodium transport

Glucose and galactose have a dramatic effect on both Na^+ and H_2O absorption via a specific Na^+-glucose cotransporter. The maximal stimulatory effect occurs in the range of 50–100 mM glucose. The effects of amino acids on Na^+ and H_2O absorption are additive to those of monosaccharides, demonstrating the existence of a separate amino acid-Na^+ transporter. These observations led to the use of glucose-containing oral electrolyte solutions for treatment of *dehydration* and have also resulted in the preparation of 'super' oral rehydration solutions that contain polymeric monosaccharides (starch) and protein for maximal stimulation of Na^+ and H_2O absorption.

Volatile fatty acid-stimulated sodium transport

Volatile fatty acids are produced by the normal fecal flora as a result of bacterial metabolism of undigested starch and fiber. These volatile fatty acids stimulate colonic Na^+ and H_2O absorption (see Section 9H). Although the mechanism by which these volatile fatty acids exert a stimulatory effect is unclear, there is some evidence for a Na^+-fatty acid cotransporter. Alternatively, fatty acids may stimulate both Cl^- and Na^+ absorption via fatty acid-bicarbonate exchange. Thus, the fatty acids produced by anaerobic fermentation in the colon serve a beneficial role, augmenting Na^+ and H_2O salvage in the colon in addition to the role they play in the colon as a useful energy supply. In circumstances where there has not been adequate establishment of the colonic flora, e.g. in the newborn, or where the colonic flora have been drastically reduced, e.g. antibiotic therapy, there may be inadequate production of volatile fatty acids and an inability to achieve maximal absorption of water and electrolytes that have passed through to the colon. In contrast, excess production of volatile fatty acids can result in the clinical phenomena of cramping and osmotic diarrhea.

Aldosterone-stimulated sodium transport

Several lines of evidence suggest an alternative mechanism of Na^+ entry through the apical cell membrane, by way of channels that open and close. These Na^+ conductance channels are inhibited by the diuretic amiloride or its analogs and can be operationally defined as amiloride-sensitive Na^+ channels. During dehydration or states of Na^+ depletion, aldosterone increases, which may increase the number and/or sensitivity of the amiloride-sensitive Na^+ conductance channels. In addition mineralocorticoids increase the amount of Na^+-K^+-ATPase on the basolateral membrane, which may ensure the rapid export of absorbed Na^+. Glucocorticoids also increase Na^+ absorption by stimulating amiloride-sensitive Na^+ transport and Na^+-K^+-ATPase activity. The response of the colon to aldosterone is not as significant as is that of the kidney. Nonetheless, aldosterone-stimulated Na^+ transport may play an important role in

Na^+ homeostasis in circumstances of Na^+ deprivation or excess loss, e.g. patients with an ileostomy.

Potassium absorption and secretion

The intestine plays an important adjunctive role to the kidney in the maintenance of normal plasma K^+ concentrations. K^+ is both absorbed and secreted. In the small intestine, K^+ is passively absorbed. In the proximal colon K^+ is normally secreted, whereas in the distal colon K^+ is absorbed. However, under the appropriate stimuli, both the proximal and distal colon can be made to secrete K^+.

Intestinal K^+ secretion results from K^+ absorption across the basolateral membrane through the action of Na^+-K^+-ATPase and subsequent diffusion across the apical membrane through conductance channels. Intestinal K^+ absorption results from K^+ transport across the apical membrane via K^+-H^+-ATPase to achieve a net increase in the intracellular concentration of K^+. K^+ will then move through the basolateral membrane based on an electrochemical equilibrium. Administration of corticosteroids or an elevation in plasma K^+ increase the basolateral membrane Na^+-K^+-ATPase. This results in increased K^+ secretion. Intestinal diseases that result in inflammation or in elevated levels of cAMP will also increase intestinal K^+ secretion, possibly by increasing the apical membrane K^+ conductance.

Acid–base homeostasis

Bicarbonate absorption and secretion

The major mechanism of bicarbonate absorption in the proximal intestine is through bicarbonate-stimulated Na^+ transport as described above. Bicarbonate is secreted in the ileum and colon predominately by bicarbonate-Cl^- exchange. Bacterial toxins, such as *cholera* toxin and *E. coli* heat-labile toxin, as well as other substances that elevate intracellular cAMP, cause an increase in bicarbonate secretion in the distal ileum and colon. The increased stool losses of bicarbonate caused by these agents can result in severe acidosis.

Systemic acid–base balance

Volatile fatty acids that can be absorbed in the colon and metabolized to bicarbonate make a significant contribution to systemic acid–base balance. Stool electrolyte excretion is significantly altered by conditions of acidosis or alkalosis. Na^+ absorption increases during acidosis and decreases during alkalosis. In addition, intestinal bicarbonate secretion increases during periods of high blood bicarbonate concentrations (metabolic alkalosis and respiratory acidosis) and decreases during periods of low blood bicarbonate concentrations (metabolic acidosis and respiratory alkalosis).

Intestinal secretion

Intestinal fluid secretion is important to the digestive process. By diluting foodstuffs, the intestine is able to maintain a relatively isotonic environment. In addition, formation of a liquid suspension facilitates the mixing and movement of luminal contents. Another important postulated role for intestinal secretion is that of cleansing the intestine of infectious agents and antigens.

A number of agents have been shown to inhibit intestinal water and electrolyte absorption or to stimulate intestinal secretion. These agents include acetylcholine, vasoactive intestinal polypeptide, secretin, bile salts, and bacterial enterotoxins as well as a number of inflammatory response mediators and other neurotransmitters. These agonists presumably bind to an enterocyte receptor that, when activated, increases the intracellular concentration of a secondary mediator such as cAMP, cGMP, or ionized Ca^{2+}. These secondary signal transducing agents result in inhibition of coupled Na^+ and Cl^- absorption and/or stimulation of Cl^- secretion. Both of these processes result in increased net intestinal secretion (Fig. 9.10).

Paracellular secretion and absorption

The active transport of Na^+ and other ions in the intestine occurs via specific transporters on the apical membrane of the enterocyte. Another mechanism for ion movement is passive diffusion, especially through the paracellular space (Fig. 9.11). The paracellular or intercellular space is marked by the zonula occludens

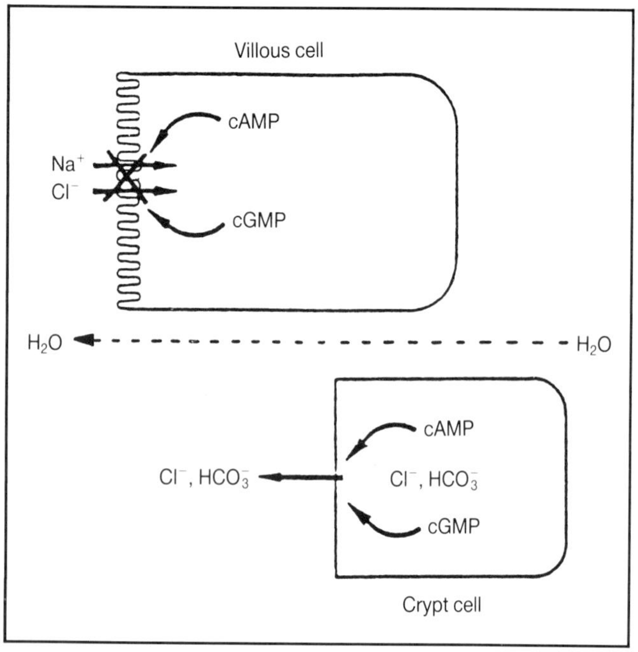

Fig. 9.10. Scheme of action of cyclic nucleotides on intestinal electrolyte and water transport. cAMP and cGMP inhibit the coupled entry of Na^+ and Cl^- into villous cells and stimulate the secretion of Cl^- and bicarbonate from crypt cells. Both of these effects result in net water transport being reversed from absorption to secretion. (From Guandalini S. *Drugs* 1988; **36** (Suppl 4): 26–38, with permission from Adis International.)

region, which may be viewed as a functional and physical barrier to the passive flow of molecules. However, the zonula occludens may also contain specific ion channels to accommodate the paracellular movement of solutes such as Na^+. The paracellular pathway works in cooperation with the active transcellular pathway to couple ion transfer effectively. For example Na^+, which is actively transported across the apical cell membrane, can passively diffuse into the paracellular space. This sets up a transepithelial potential difference across the zonula occludens and drives the passive absorption of Cl^-. In fact this particular schema seems to work better in reverse where paracellular Na^+ secretion is coupled to transcellular Cl^- secretion as in the case of *secretory diarrhea.* Recently, a zonula occludens toxin produced by *Vibrio cholerae* has been identified. Thus, disruption of the normal actions of the paracellular pathway may be important in the pathophysiology of some diarrheal diseases.

Secretory diarrhea

Bacterial toxins

Secretory diarrhea is most commonly associated with infections caused by toxin-producing bacteria such as *Vibrio cholerae* and toxigenic *E. coli*. These organisms produce toxins that activate adenylyl cyclase (cholera toxin, *E. coli* heat-labile toxin) or guanylyl cyclase (*E. coli* heat-stable enterotoxin) and increase the intracellular concentrations of the cyclic nucleotides, cAMP or cGMP (Fig. 9.10). This results in increased secretion of Na^+ and Cl^- from intestinal crypt cells and/or inhibition of the

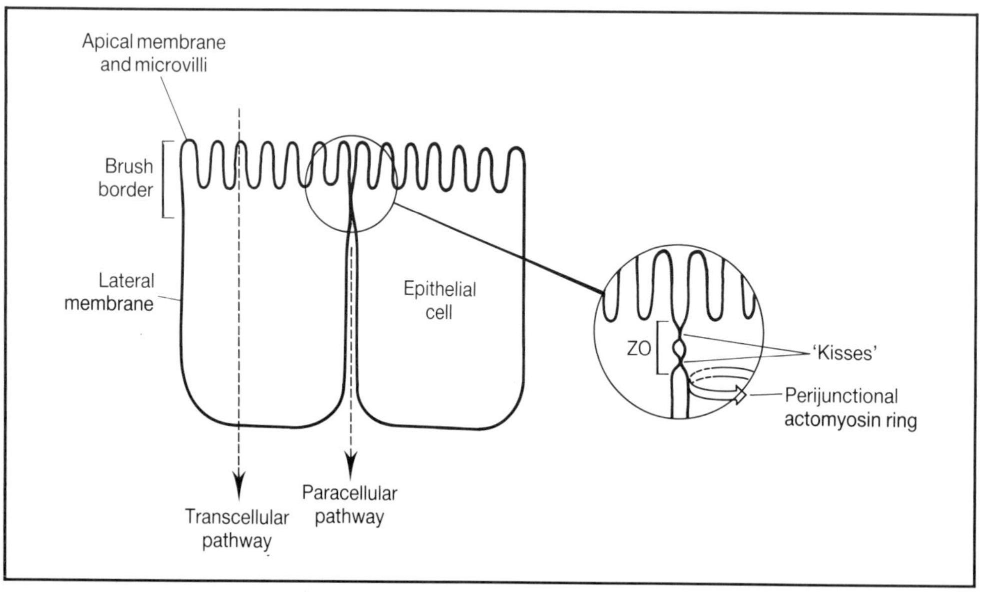

Fig. 9.11. Schematic representation of intestinal epithelial cells demonstrating transcellular and paracellular pathways. The enlargement of the zonula occludens (ZO) depicts the architecture of this region as it is seen by routine electron microscopy. (From Madara JL. *Cell* 1988; **53**: 497, with permission. © Cell Press.)

reabsorption of Cl^- by villous cells. The net result of derangement of the normal absorptive process is an outpouring of fluid and electrolytes resulting in secretory diarrhea. The immature intestine may be more sensitive to some of these processes. For example, immature rats have an increased response to *E. coli* heat-stable enterotoxin. This may be explained by the presence of an increased receptor number in the immature intestine and/or an inability of the immature intestine to inactivate the toxin. Furthermore, the immature colon may be less able to compensate for increased small intestinal secretion.

Bile acids

Other examples of secretory diarrhea include *bile acid-induced diarrhea.* Bile acid diarrhea may occur when an increased bile acid load is presented to the colon. Bile acids may alter the net fluid and electrolyte absorption by increasing mucosal cAMP levels, by increasing cytosolic ionized Ca^{2+} levels, and by alterations in prostaglandin metabolism.

Hormone-secreting tumors

Secretory diarrhea can also result from *hormone secreting tumors.* The term WDHA (watery diarrhea, hypokalemia, and achlorhydria) or *pancreatic cholera* was coined to describe a syndrome in which there is massive watery diarrhea related to a non-islet cell pancreatic adenoma. This term is now applied to any condition in which there is a tumor producing vasoactive intestinal peptide (VIP). VIP produces net secretion of Cl^- and Na^+ by raising intracellular cAMP levels.

Congenital transport defects

Another mechanism for secretory diarrhea is the presence of a congenital electrolyte transport defect. These defects include *congenital Cl^- diarrhea,* which results from defective Cl^--bicarbonate exchange, and congenital Na^+-H^+ exchange, which results in *congenital Na^+ diarrhea.*

Oral rehydration

The laboratory observation that glucose increases intestinal salt and water absorption via the Na^+-glucose cotransporter has been applied directly to the care of patients. The addition of glucose to oral rehydration solutions has improved their efficacy, saving millions of children with dehydrating diarrheal disease. Further improvements in this safe, effective, and inexpensive therapy may result from future additional understanding of the intestinal mechanisms of absorption of fluid and electrolytes. For example, to maximize the Na^+-glucose cotransporter further, as well as to take advantage of the separate amino acid-Na^+ cotransporters, recent studies have used cereal-based oral rehydration solutions. This approach allows the use of several times as many cotransporting molecules of glucose (as starch) and peptides (as amino acids) while still maintaining a low osmolar solution. Amino acids (L-alanine or glycine) and dipeptides (glycyl-glycine) have also been added to glucose-containing solutions to maximize intestinal absorption of Na^+ and H_2O further in the treatment of cholera diarrhea.

Selected reading

Hirschhorn N, Greenough WB. Progress in oral rehydration therapy. *Sci Am* 1991; **264**: 50.

Lebenthal E, Duffy ME, eds. *Textbook of secretory diarrhea.* New York: Raven Press, 1990.

Powell DW. Intestinal water and electrolyte transport. In Johnson LR, ed. *Physiology of the gastrointestinal tract*. Vol. 2. New York: Raven Press, 1987: 1267.

H. The Nutritional Role of the Colon

R D Murray

The primary functions of the colon are the absorption of electrolytes and water and the storage of fecal material. Recently, a role for the colon in nutrition has also been recognized. Carbohydrates that are not absorbed by the small intestine pass across the ileocecal valve. Malabsorbed carbohydrates from sloughed cells, secretions, and mucus as well as from exogenous sources including dietary starch, undigestible sugars, and fiber enter the colon. Bacteria digest these carbohydrates and produce metabolic end products that are readily absorbed, preventing *osmotic diarrhea.*

In the healthy adult, the colon absorbs 2 liters of fluid and nearly 275 mmol of Na^+ per day. Absorption of fluid changes the liquid material in the cecum into formed feces as the luminal contents are moved from the ileocecal valve to the anus. Bacteria are critical to normal colon physiology. Normally bacteria digest osmotically active substrates into diffusible anions. When bacteria are prevented from colonizing the large intestine, many morphological and physiological changes occur. The intestinal wall becomes thinner, especially the mucosa. The plasma cells, one of the primary constituents of the lamina propria, become sparse. The typical columnar cells of the colon change to a cuboidal shape. Cell turnover slows. This results in a drastic reduction in absorption from the germ-free colon. The cecum enlarges and fills with a hypotonic solution that is low in diffusible anions and is high in the osmotic particles that are usually digested by bacteria. As a result, fluid absorption decreases, while fluid secretion increases. In this setting, even minor malabsorption of carbohydrates by the small intestine results in osmotic diarrhea. Clearly, the presence of a healthy bacterial flora fosters the conditions that allow the colon to perform its important absorptive functions.

Bacterial metabolism

Daily fecal weight on a Western diet normally ranges from approximately 35 g in newborns to 400 g in adults; 10^{11} bacteria are present in each gram of feces. Thus, to replenish this massive daily bacterial loss requires substrate, almost exclusively provided by luminal carbohydrates. Under the strict anaerobic conditions of the colon, the flora metabolize CHO to short-chain fatty acids (SCFA) (i.e. acetate, butyrate, and propionate) and gases (i.e. CO_2, H_2, and methane). SCFA are absorbed by the colonic mucosa, salvaging nutrient energy that would otherwise be lost. In addition, SCFA stimulate salt and water uptake, increase cell turnover and repair, and serve as substrates for colonocytes.

Neonatal carbohydrate malabsorption

Lactose is the sole carbohydrate in breast milk and in the most commonly used infant formulas. The newborn infant ingests 12.6 g/kg per day of lactose when taking a 120 cal/kg per day diet. Studies have shown that intestinal lactase (β-galactosidase) activity is insufficient to digest this daily load of lactose. Although the enzyme lactase is detectable as early as 12 weeks of gestation, it accumulates so slowly that by 34 weeks its activity is only 30 percent of a term infant, and by 37–38 weeks, only 70 percent. Calculation of carbohydrate malabsorption using breath H^+ measurements suggests that extensive malabsorption occurs in both the premature and term newborn. Because H_2 is a product of bacterial fermentation, its presence in breath can be used as a semiquantitative measure of malabsorbed carbohydrate. Multiple studies on term and premature infants have revealed breath H_2 at concentrations of up to 250 ppm, which is well beyond the level observed in physiological malabsorption ($<$10 ppm). Colonic absorption of H_2 is more avid in newborns than adults, partially accounting for higher breath values in infancy. Studies suggest that up to 15–20 percent of ingested lactose is not absorbed in the small bowel. Doubling the infant's lactose intake doubles the pulmonary excretion of H_2 but does not increase stool carbohydrate losses, suggesting that increased colonic salvage can occur if necessary.

Bacterial colonization of the colon

Although the colonic flora is likely to be an important factor for the energy balance of the newborn, its contribution appears limited in the first days of life. The colon is sterile at birth, acquiring an aerobic flora (*E. coli*, streptococci), then a mixed aerobic and facultative anaerobic flora (*Lactobacillus*), and finally a strictly anaerobic flora (*Bifidobacterium, Bacteroides*) gradually over the first few weeks of life. During this time, the SCFA products of bacterial metabolism are modest. Changes in the bacterial flora affect the products of colonic carbohydrate digestion. Lactose infusion into the colonic lumen of piglets during the first postnatal week produces lactate as the primary product of bacterial digestion. After the fourth day of life, lactate production declines, while SCFA production becomes predominant.

Immediately after birth, the colonic mucosa can directly absorb the dissacharide lactose without bacterial or mucosal enzymatic digestion. Perfusions of the newborn colon showed a 20-fold greater absorption of lactose than of its constituent monosaccharides, glucose and galactose. Na^+ and water uptake were stimulated by lactose absorption. Thus, in neonates, lactose substitutes for SCFA in stimulating salt and water absorption. The mechanism of lactose absorption was not found to be saturable at concentrations between 15 and 240 mM. When colonic tissue was mounted in Ussing-type lucite chambers that isolate the solutions bathing the mucosal and serosal sides of the colon, lactose was found to traverse the tissue from mucosa to serosa as a disaccharide, without prior digestion. Molecules that are similar in size to lactose did not cross the mucosa, suggesting that solvent drag through the tight junctions cannot explain this phenomenon. Lactose may be absorbed from the colonic lumen by the process of endocytosis, a transcellular pathway that is open to the movement of proteins and lipids in the first days of life.

A true symbiosis exists between the human host and the colonic bacterial flora. The colonic flora salvage malabsorbed carbohydrate that would otherwise be lost in feces, preventing both diarrhea and caloric deficit. Yet even in neonates when the flora is attenuated, the colon seems to have a compensatory mechanism for direct lactose assimilation that prevents potentially life-threatening carbohydrate losses.

Selected reading

Fleming SE, Arce DS. Volatile fatty acids: their production, absorption, utilization, and roles in human health. *Clin Gastroenterol* 1986; **15**: 787.

Murray RD. Effects of bacterial fermentation end products on intestinal function: implications for intestinal dysfunction. *J Pediatr* 1990; **117**: S59.

Potter GD. Development of colonic function. In Lebanthal E, ed. *Human gastrointestinal development*. New York: Raven Press, 1989: 545.

I. Gastrointestinal Immunology

B K Wershil

The gastrointestinal tract develops in a sterile environment *in utero*, but becomes exposed to a vast array of foreign antigens immediately after birth. The neonatal gastrointestinal tract adapts to this change in environment by developing mechanisms both to limit antigens from crossing the intestinal epithelium, **the mucosal barrier**, and to control the systemic immune response to foreign antigens, **oral tolerance**.

The mucosal barrier

The gastrointestinal tract is in continuity with the external environment. A variety of non-immunological processes (Table 9.2) act in concert with the mucosal immune system to prevent the attachment and penetration of antigens through the mucosal surface, thus limiting the development of adverse inflammatory reactions.

Thick mucus overlies the epithelial surface and acts as a physical barrier that inhibits the attachment of antigens. Certain parasitic and microbial infections stimulate additional production and secretion of mucus, increasing the thickness of the layer. Mucus also interferes with bacterial adhesion through direct interaction with specific carbohydrate moieties on bacteria that act like receptors for epithelial cells. The binding of mucus to these recognitions sites on the bacteria prevents bacterial adhesion and penetration of the intestinal wall.

Table 9.2. Components of the mucosal barrier to antigens

Non-immunological
Intraluminal
Gastric barrier
Proteolysis
Peristalsis
Mucosal surface
Mucosal coat
Microvillus membrane
Immunological
Secretory IgA
Secretory IgM
Combination of immunological and non-immunological
Immune complex-mediated mucus release of goblet cells
Immune complex-facilitated mucosal surface proteolysis
Kupffer cell phagocytosis of immune complexes

The composition of the intestinal microvillus membrane is another factor affecting bacterial adhesion. The enterocyte cell membrane changes as the cell migrates from crypt to villus. The composition and functional properties of the enterocyte membrane also change during development. These changes may determine antigen attachment sites. Microvillus membranes isolated from newborn animals bind certain bacteria enterotoxins and protein antigens more avidly than membranes isolated from adult animals. This may be due to the lower protein/phospholipid ratio in the newborn membranes compared with adult membranes. These developmental changes in membrane composition may explain the different response to diarrhea-causing enteric pathogens.

Secretory IgA (sIgA) is a major component of the mucosal immune system that plays an important role in barrier function. sIgA constitutes the largest component of the humoral immune system in man. Approximately 3 g of sIgA is transported into the adult intestinal tract each day. IgA-secreting plasma cells develop from precursor cells that mature under the influences of accessory cell populations and T-cell-derived cytokines, which produces an immunoglobulin isotype switch to predominantly IgA-bearing B cells. These cells deliver polymeric IgA into the submucosa of the intestinal tract, where it is taken up by epithelial cells, covalently linked to secretory component, and secreted into the intestinal lumen. sIgA performs its barrier function by binding to intraluminal microbes and antigens, inhibiting their uptake.

The liver also plays a role in mucosal barrier function through its participation in IgA metabolism. Hepatocytes can remove polymeric IgA from the peripheral circulation and transport it into the bile, thus delivering a significant amount of IgA into the intestinal lumen. In addition, as much as 50 percent of the IgA in bile is newly synthesized from plasma cells within glands near the large hepatic ducts. The liver can also take up small circulating IgA immune complexes, which may be an important route for the elimination of absorbed antigens.

The mucosal immune system

The gut-associated lymphoid tissue (GALT) is distinct from the systemic immune system. It is composed of three compartments: organized lymphoid tissues, or Peyer's patches, diffuse lymphoid tissues of the lamina propria, and intraepithelial lymphocytes. In humans, Peyer's patches are found predominantly in the ileum and are organized into a germinal center and a parafollicular area composed primarily of B cells and T cells, respectively. These areas underlie specialized epithelia known as M (microfold) cells. M cells appear to function in the uptake and sampling of luminal antigens. Stimulation of GALT occurs when particulate antigens are taken up by M cells and transported into the Peyer's patch (Fig. 9.12). These antigens are processed and presented to T cells, resulting in activation of lymphoid cells within Peyer's patch. Stimulated T and B cells egress from Peyer's patch into the lymph, then pass into the peripheral circulation. Next these lymphocytes 'home' to the lamina propria of the gut and other exocrine tissues via specific receptors on intestinal vascular endothelium. The B cells mature to plasma cells producing polymeric IgA or IgM. T lymphocytes that reside in the lamina propria are predominantly of the $CD4^+$ (helper) phenotype, while

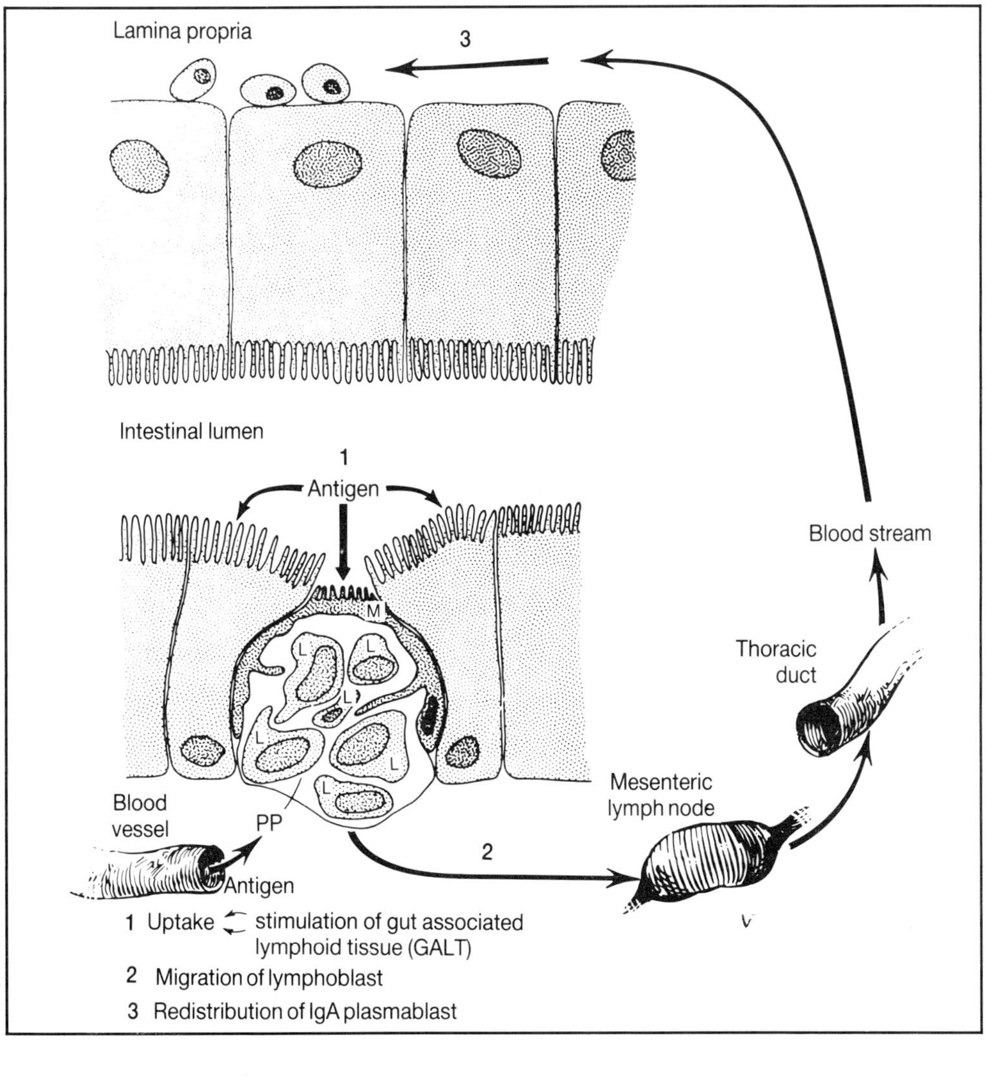

Fig. 9.12. Lymphocyte migration. Schematic representation of the cell cycle of an IgA-producing plasma cell. Lymphocytes derived from the bone marrow take residence in GALT tissues such as the Peyer's patch (PP). Stimulation of lymphoid tissues occurs when antigens are taken up via M cells from the intestinal lumen (1). Lymphoblasts migrate to mesenteric lymph nodes (pathway 2), then enter the systemic circulation to redistribute along intestinal mucosal surfaces (pathway 3) and produce secretory IgA antibodies in response to absorbed antigens. (From Walker WA, Isselbacher KJ. *N Engl J Med* 1977; **297**: 767, with permission.)

most of the lymphocytes that migrate into the epithelium are CD8+ (cytotoxic/suppressor) cells, known as intraepithelial lymphocytes. In addition to T and B cells, the lamina propria contains large numbers of macrophages, mast cells, and eosinophils.

Intraepithelial lymphocytes (IELs) have several phenotypic characteristics that distinguish them from other T lymphocytes. In mice, 25–50 percent of IELs express a T-cell receptor (TcR) made from γ and δ chains, while the remainder express a TcR pattern of α and β chains, as is commonly seen in peripheral T cells. In humans, 2–30 percent of IELs express γ and δ chains, although the proportion of TcR$\gamma\delta$ cells can increase significantly in certain inflammatory conditions such as celiac disease. This suggests that TcR$\gamma\delta$-positive T cells either preferentially localize or mature in the epithelium. The functional significance of these phenotypic variations is not known.

One possible mechanism of IEL activation is presentation of luminal antigens in association with either class I or class II molecules of the major histocompatibility (MHC) locus. Macrophages, other accessory cells, and intestinal epithelial cells express class II antigens and may play a role in antigen presentation to IELs and other cells. Alternatively, certain enterotoxins, termed superantigens, bind directly to the MHC class II molecule and can activate many T cells. The function of the IEL is not known, but they may be involved in mucosal immunity in several ways. Some IELs contain cytoplasmic granules and have been shown to have cytotoxic functions, which would act to limit microorganism invasion. IELs can secrete a variety of cytokines, which can have protective effects on epithelium and may modulate epithelial cell growth. Finally, it has been suggested that IELs function in the development of oral tolerance.

Oral tolerance, a unique aspect of the mucosal immune system, is a specific immunological state of unresponsiveness induced by the prior feeding of an antigen. For example, the single feeding of a soluble protein antigen can suppress **systemic** IgM, IgG, and IgE antibody production as well as cell-mediated immune responses such as delayed-type hypersensitivity. The complex mechanisms involved in the development of oral tolerance have not been defined completely. Oral tolerance has been shown to be principally due to T-cell unresponsiveness, while B cells remain potentially active. Animals fed protein antigens develop active immune suppression mediated through T-suppressor cells, but the precise immunoregulatory mechanisms are unclear. It is generally accepted that the development of oral tolerance prevents hypersensitivity reactions to soluble antigens while maintaining active immunity to particulate antigens such as invasive organisms.

Development of the gastrointestinal immune system

Immune development occurs in an **antigen-independent stage** prenatally and an **antigen-dependent stage** beginning after birth when luminal antigens are present. During *in utero* development, columnar epithelium and intestinal villi are present at 9–10 weeks of gestation. Before 11 weeks, only macrophages are found in the lamina propria, but by 11 weeks intraepithelial lymphocytes are identifiable. By 17–19 weeks IELs increase to about half the levels seen in postnatal intestines, and approximately half of these cells are TcR$\gamma\delta$ positive. At 14 weeks small clusters of CD4+ (helper) phenotype T lymphocytes are present in the lamina propria, but virtually no B cells or plasma cells are seen until after birth. By 16 weeks the secretory component for IgA is detectable, and this increases substantially at 20 weeks. Eosinophils are present in the lamina propria at 19 weeks. Peyer's patches are not identifiable until 24 weeks of gestation, then increase in size and density until birth. Within Peyer's patch, the T cells are mainly CD4+ and the B cells are IgM+ and IgD+; there is no cellular zonation, and almost every cell is class II MHC positive. The intestinal epithelium becomes class II positive between 18 and 22 weeks of gestation.

By birth the mucosal immune system is well developed. Further postnatal development appears to be antigen driven. Germinal center formation in Peyer's patch occurs. The lamina propria is populated by B cells, and the T-cell population in the lamina propria expands. The numbers of intraepithelial lymphocytes increase, and there is a shift in relative numbers of T cells with $\gamma\delta$- and $\alpha\beta$-receptors. Ultimately, the fate of the mucosal immune system is directed by the antigens and pathogens present in the gastrointestinal tract.

Selected reading

Brandtzaeg P, Nilssen DE, Rognum TO, Thrane PS.

Ontogeny of the mucosal immune system and IgA deficiency. *Gastroenterol Clin N Am* 1991; **20**: 397.
MacDonald TT, Spencer J. Ontogeny of the mucosal immune response. *Springer Semin Immunopathol* 1990; **12**: 129.
Mowat M. The regulation of immune responses to dietary protein antigens. *Immunol Today* 1987; **8**: 93.
Walker WA. Pathophysiology of intestinal uptake and absorption of antigens in food allergy. *Ann Allergy* 1987; **59**: 7.

J. Development and Function of the Exocrine Pancreas

J W Adelson

The exocrine pancreas is the major organ of digestion; its primary tasks are the production of large quantities of alkaline fluid and digestive enzymes, which are secreted into the intestinal lumen. The enzymes function to hydrolyze complex dietary substrates. The fluid neutralizes gastric acid and creates an appropriate alkaline pH milieu for the function of the enzymes.

Morphological development

The pancreas originates as two separate buds from the differentiating intestine, one dorsal, the other ventral. The dorsal bud is destined to form the greater portion of the gland, including the main body and tail. The ventral bud originates at the origin of the common bile duct and gallbladder, which explains how the pancreatic–biliary ductular system arises. As pancreatic differentiation and organ enlargement occur, the dorsal bud rotates around the intestinal axis to lie directly next to, and cephalad to, the ventral bud. The buds then fuse. The dorsal and ventral buds each contain their own main axial ducts, which in most cases fuse together. Subsequent development of the duct draining the ventral bud results in the formation of the major pancreatic duct, the duct of Wirsung. The dorsal bud's duct will usually drain the head of the pancreas into the ventral or main duct, but not infrequently a separate accessory duct, the duct of Santorini, drains the dorsal pancreatic region into the intestine through its own papillus. This variant, known as *pancreas divisum,* is a debatable contributor to some cases of *pancreatitis,* presumably because of problems in the drainage via the accessory duct. Aberrant fusion of the buds results in an *annular pancreas* in which the intestine is encircled with pancreatic tissue; this can lead to variable degrees of duodenal obstruction. The commonest presentation occurs at birth with complete obstruction. This anomaly occurs sporadically in the general population and relatively commonly with *trisomy 21.*

Other primary problems with pancreatic development are occasionally reported. These include hypoplasia or complete *agenesis of the pancreas*. Excess pancreatic material, known as pancreatic rests, can occur at ectopic locations elsewhere in the gastrointestinal tract, especially the stomach. A complex syndrome, variously named *Schwachman syndrome* or the *Schwachman–Diamond syndrome,* is the second commonest cause of pancreatic insufficiency in childhood. This recessively inherited syndrome results in the complete replacement of pancreatic acinar tissue (but not the ductular or endocrine portions) with adipose tissue. These patients present as infants with failure to thrive, steatorrhea, and a normal sweat test. Other accompanying manifestations of the syndrome are noted with varying frequency, including metaphyseal dysostosis, a developmental abnormality of bone, immunodeficiency, short stature, dwarfism, and anemia with cyclic neutropenia.

The histological generation of the pancreas is exemplified by the usual progression from undifferentiated precursor cells without specialized organelles to the highly specialized cells of the mature organ, which can be divided into three functional types: the acinar cells, the ductular elements, and the endocrine subset comprising the islets of Langerhans. The acinar cells, organized into connective tissue-surrounded lobules, constitute the great bulk of this relatively homogeneous-appearing gland. Differentiation of the acinar cells proper occurs such that at about 12 weeks of gestation there are recognizable secretory zymogen granules. The fully differentiated acinar cell is capable of a great degree of protein synthesis, storage, and secretion, nearly all of which is devoted to the production of pancreatic enzymes. In fact, the pancreas is so specialized in protein secretion that it was the gland upon which were conducted the original, classic studies on the intracellular route of protein synthesis, processing, storage, and secretion. The pyramid-shaped acinar cells are organized into small round groups or short tubes of cells surrounding a central lumen; the groups are celled acini (Fig. 9.13). The

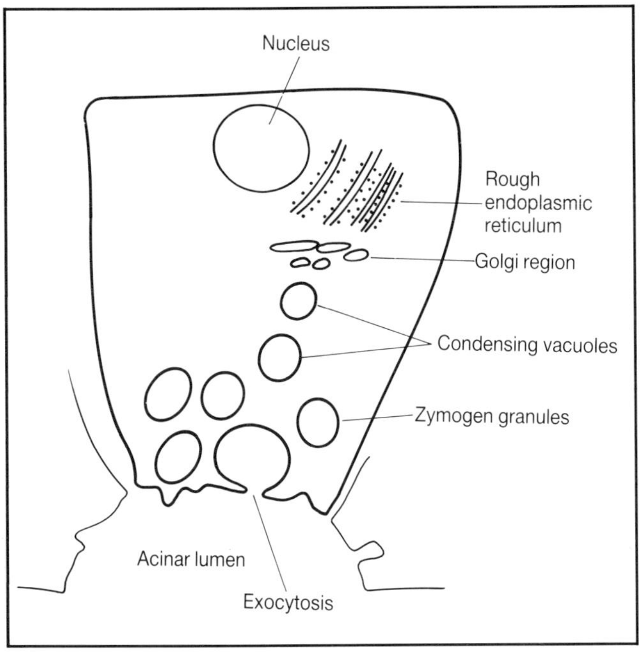

Fig. 9.13. Generalized schematic of pancreatic acinar cell. Newly synthesized secretory proteins are formed by the rough endoplasmic reticulum, glycosylated in the Golgi region, and packaged in the condensing vacuoles, which mature into zymogen granules. The granule contents are expelled following fusion of the zymogen granule membrane with the plasma membrane.

secretory granules are located at the apical or luminal pole of the cell. A massive amount of rough endoplasmic reticulum is present in each acinar cell and is primarily devoted to the production of the exportable digestive enzyme. The endoplasmic reticulum is located in the basal portion of the cytoplasm, as is the nucleus. The Golgi region lies apical to the endoplasmic reticulum, above the secretory granule-containing region. Near the Golgi, and apparently budding off from it, are immature or condensing vacuoles, which are thought to be the direct precursors to the zymogen granules.

During embryogenesis, the digestive enzymes are found at first in extremely low amounts, then appear in greater and greater quantities in what appears to be a preset sequence, dependent upon the set of genetic instructions with which this organ is endowed. In a singularly revealing experiment in transgenic mice, the 'upstream' or 5′ control region for mouse chymotrypsinogen was fused with the DNA sequence for human growth hormone and implanted in the transgenic mouse ovum. Following fertilization, implantation, and development, the end result was a mouse that secreted human growth hormone through the pancreatic duct into the digestive lumen! This shows that the placement of a tissue-specific secretory protein into the 'right' place at the 'proper' time in the differentiation process is due to the information contained in the upstream control region for the structural gene in question.

Fluid secretion

Pancreatic fluid is alkaline in composition due to the presence of a high concentration of bicarbonate ion. The ionic composition of the secretion is rate-dependent; more bicarbonate occurs at higher flow rates, while at lower rates, the secretion contains relatively more Cl^-. The fluid is secreted by the ductular system, which begins at the entrance to the acinar lumen proper; the cells at the acinar opening are centroacinar cells. Ductular secretory cells then continue as a tubular epithelial lining of the pancreatic ducts of increasing caliber, which ultimately drain into the main duct. One of the main pathophysiological manifestations of *cystic fibrosis,* a well known genetic disease, appears to be due to a malfunction of a Cl^- channel present in these ductular cells. A failure of pancreatic fluid and electrolyte secretion occurs in cystic fibrosis, which results in the inability to wash the secreted digestive enzymes from the level of the pancreatic acinus into the intestinal lumen. This results in a secondary, severe pancreatic enzyme deficit that cripples the digestive process, resulting in the loss of fat and other digestive substrates in the stool. The exact relationship between the inability to secrete Cl^-, which is characteristic of several tissues in cystic fibrosis, and the bicarbonate secretory defect has not been completely worked out, but is possibly due to failure of a transport system that exchanges Cl^- for bicarbonate, or that transports both of these anions.

Endocrine pancreas

The third element of the differentiated pancreas is the islets of Langerhans. These originate from the general exocrine primordium, not, as became fashionable to suppose a few years ago, from the primitive neural crest tissue in the so-called APUD system. The embryological and morphological relationships between the endocrine and exocrine pancreas are important. A mini-portal system of capillaries leaves the endocrine islets and enters the peri-insular acinar tissue before finally joining the portal vein drainage. Possibly as a result of hormonal influences from the 'insular–acinar axis', the acinar cells immediately surrounding the islets are distinct from the remaining acinar cells with respect to enzyme composition, cell size, and size of the secretory granules.

Enzyme secretion

Exocrine pancreatic digestive function has been appreciated for several hundred years, and is still a very active area of investigation. The pancreas synthesizes, and stores for secretion, large quantities of digestive enzymes, making it the body's largest protein secretor with the exception of the lactating mammary gland. The gland produces both exo- and endoproteases, various lipases and phospholipases, nucleases, and amylase; a number of the enzyme species are isoenzymes, alternative enzyme structures differing little from each other in function. Many of the enzymes require activation by various agents before they reach full function. All of the proteases are activated by the hydrolysis of a peptide from the pro-enzyme form; the cleavage is performed primarily by trypsin. Trypsin itself is activated from trypsinogen by enteropeptidase, a proteolytic enzyme secreted by the duodenal mucosa, possibly in response to cholecystokinin (CCK) release, and by autocatalysis by already activated trypsin. Lipase is activated by another molecule secreted by the gland called colipase.

Development of pancreatic enzyme secretion

The development of the enzymatic secretory capacity of the pancreas during human gestation is not well studied for obvious reasons. The bulk of secretory function is present from birth, and full-term newborns as well as more developed premature infants have quite adequate pancreatic function. With respect to the ultimate capacity of the pancreas to handle fats, newborns frequently exhibit a mild steatorrhea; although a fat absorption coefficient of about 95 percent is expected in the older child or adult, newborns and young infants frequently absorb less fat; the acceptable norm is 85 percent or more. Similarly, amylase secretion is not fully developed at birth, and only becomes so after several months. However, there is no indication that infants cannot digest starch polymers, and it may be that the intestinal enzyme glucoamylase is responsible for handling starches when they are fed in infancy.

Stimulus-secretion coupling

In general, the intracellular stimulus-secretion coupling systems found in the pancreas resemble those found in most other secretory tissues. The basolateral membranes of the acinar cell contain receptors that are highly specific for CCK and cholinergic agonists. Similarly, duct cells have secretin receptors. Numerous other receptors are also found on the cell surfaces; their roles are not presently clear, but perhaps the interaction of the receptors with the several ligands that bind to them serves to modulate various aspects of enzyme secretion.

Following binding of a secretagogue to its receptor, a long chain of events ensues, beginning with transmission of information across the cellular membrane by deformation of the receptor itself, which causes activation of a coupling G-protein, which exchanges GTP (guanosine triphosphate) for GDP (guanosine diphosphate). This membrane-related event initiates a further intracellular series of events, dependent on which specific G-proteins have been activated. In the acinar pancreas, both CCK and cholinergic stimuli appear to be connected to the final secretory effectors through the G-proteins by pathways involving the metabolism and intracellular production of inositol phosphates and diacylglycerol, as well as via a pathway which leads to the mobilization of Ca^{2+} from stores within the acinar cell. Less is known about stimulus-secretion coupling in the ductular cell, but the pathway there appears to involve activation of adenylyl cyclase by the secretin receptor with the formation of cAMP. The ultimate activation of the secretory effectors involves the phosphorylation of specific proteins involved in the secretory events in the cell membranes leading to the fusion of the zymogen granule membrane with the plasma membrane.

Variations in enzyme secretion

The enzyme composition of the pancreatic zymogen granules and the pancreatic juice can be made to vary with long-term dietary changes so as to more closely match the expensive daily investment in digestive enzymes to the actual substrate upon which these enzymes work. There has been long-standing controversy as to whether the composition of the digestive enzyme mixture can also be regulated over the short term, i.e. within the digestive time required by the processing of a single meal. Such regulation would be highly economical in terms of saving unnecessary enzymes, but because the zymogen granules were thought to all contain the full mixture of digestive enzymes, the release of their contents by exocytosis must result in a parallel discharge of each enzyme species. However, many examples of nonparallel secretion of digestive enzymes have been reported, and recent work has focused on the increasingly strong possibility that the exocrine pancreas may be a surprisingly heterogeneous organ, secreting digestive proteins from multiple distinct sources containing enzyme mixtures of differing composition.

Control of secretion

The control of pancreatic secretion, as with other digestive organs, is due to a mixture of hormonal and neural inputs. Neural stimulation is primarily via the vagus nerve, with stimuli originating in the digestive tract or higher centers in the brain, dependent on the stage of digestion. Most stimulation, whether neural or hormonal, appears to arise when digestive substrates arrive in the duodenum. The hormone primarily responsible for pancreatic stimulation is CCK, a close relative of the gastric stimulatory hormone gastrin. CCK and gastrin share a common sequence at their carboxyl termini, and overlap in actions when the doses administered are high enough. At physiological concentrations, CCK stimulates pancreatic enzyme release and gallbladder contraction. There is now some evidence that pancreatic secretion, at least in the interdigestive period, is cyclic in character.

Pancreatic enzyme secretion is not only stimulated by the nervous system or by the direct release of CCK from the duodenal mucosa into the blood stream in response to the presence of peptides in the digestive lumen. Pancreatic secretion is also caused by a CCK-releasing peptide present in the intestinal lumen, which appears to be derived from intestinal mucosal cells. The peptide is sensitive to proteolytic degradation by pancreatic enzymes, and can thereby act as a signal to the pancreas to secrete more enzyme because whenever luminal levels of proteolysis fall low enough, the CCK-releasing peptide will survive and signal for more CCK release from the mucosa into the blood stream. A second peptide called the monitor peptide is secreted in bile and appears to serve the same function. When food is present in the intestinal lumen, the CCK-releasing peptide is protected from degradation simply by competition with the foodstuffs that serve as a competitive substrate for proteolysis. Thus, during periods when a large amount of undigested protein is present in the lumen, the survival of the CCK-releasing peptide will ensure ongoing stimulation of the pancreas.

Stimulation of pancreatic fluid secretion also depends on neurological and hormonal influences. As with enzyme secretion, the neurological input arises at both the level of the intestine and in higher centers in the brain, dependent on the stage of digestion. The major hormone responsible for mediating fluid secretion is known by its elegantly simple name **secretin**, the first hormone ever discovered, by Bayliss and Starling early in this century. Secretin mediates pancreatic fluid secretion independently of the stimulation of enzyme secretion by CCK; however, the two hormones do augment each other's activities when administered together. Because conditions leading to CCK release into the blood stream—the presence of peptides and proteins in the duodenum—usually overlap directly with the major stimulus for secretin release, acidification of the duodenum, the usual result is the simultaneous arrival of both fluid and enzyme in the duodenum. As discussed briefly above, failure of fluid secretion secondarily leads to the insufficiency of pancreatic enzymes seen in *cystic fibrosis*.

Selected reading

Adelson JW. Pancreatic function in infancy and early childhood. In Heird WC, ed. *Nutritional needs of the six to twelve month old infant*. Carnation Nutrition Education Series, Vol. 2. New York: Raven Press, 1991: 19.

Adelson JW, Miller PE. Heterogeneity of the exocrine pancreas. *Am J Physiol* 1989; **256**: G817.

Miyasaka K, Guan D, Liddle RA, Green GM. Feedback regulation by trypsin: evidence for intraluminal CCK-releasing peptide. *Am J Physiol* 1989; **257**: G175.

Owyang C, Williams J. Pancreatic secretion. In Yamada T, Alpers DH, Owyang C, Powel DW, Silverstein FE, eds. *Textbook of gastroenterology*. Philadelphia: JB Lippincott Co., 1991: 294.

K. Embryology and Anatomy of the Liver

S S Kaufman

The liver of the human embryo begins to differentiate during the third to fourth week of gestation. A diverticulum of endodermal epithelium extends from the ventral surface of the posterior foregut to meet the adjacent primordial anterior diaphragm, the septum transversum. Primitive hepatocytes (hepatoblasts) mix with, and attach to, mesodermal mesenchymal cells of the septum. Hepatocytes aggregate into cords up to 10 cells thick. Cords are separated from one another by small blood vessels or sinusoids, which receive blood from the anterior vitelline vessels from the yolk sac. The vitelline vessels are progressively engulfed by the enlarging liver and ultimately evolve into the portal venous and hepatic venous systems. The primitive hepatocytes mature along two divergent lines. The majority eventually become mature hepatocytes, while the remainder form intrahepatic bile ducts. The functional differentiation of each of these cell types is described below. Pluripotent hematopoietic stem cells are recognizable as clusters between adjacent hepatocytes by the second month of gestation. These cells originate from septal mesenchyma. A discussion of fetal hematopoiesis is included in Chapter 12.

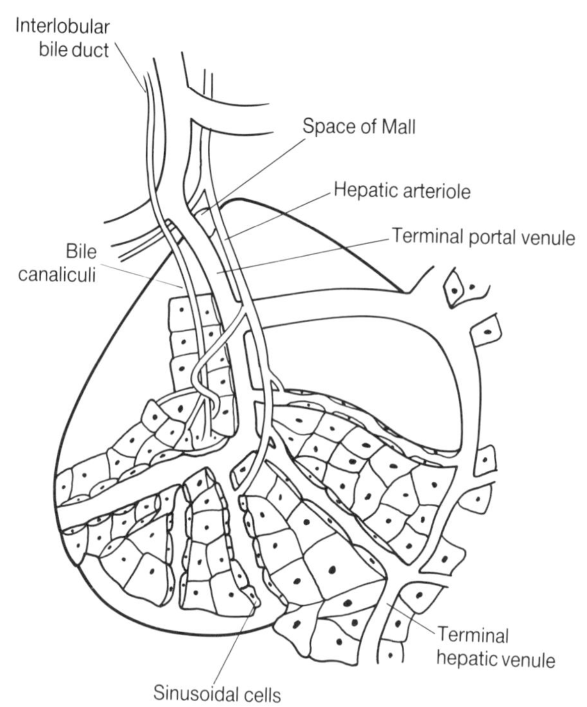

Fig. 9.14. The liver acinus is supplied with blood from a terminal portal venule and a terminal hepatic arteriole. Blood percolates through the sinusoid to a terminal hepatic venule. The hepatic venules flow into the hepatic veins and drain into the inferior vena cava. Bile is secreted into the bile canaliculus and flows opposite to the direction of blood flow, into the interlobular bile ducts. The interlobular bile ducts receive their blood supply from the hepatic arteries. The space of Mall is an extracellular space through which the hepatic arteriole and portal venule pass. Lautt and Greenway have postulated that the secretion of adenosine into this space plays a role in controlling hepatic arterial blood flow (see Section 9L).

Acinar organization

The basic functional unit of the liver is the acinus (Fig. 9.14). Acini are organized during the late second and third months of gestation, in concert with formation of constituent cells. The acinus encompasses the region perfused by a terminal portal venule, a branch of the portal vein and the terminal arteriolar branch of the hepatic artery. Blood flows centrifugally from these vessels through sinusoids emanating radially from each portal area. Drainage from sinusoids is accomplished by terminal hepatic venules positioned at intervals around the border of the acinus. Each hepatic venule receives sinusoidal blood from several adjacent acini.

In mature liver, major functions of hepatocytes vary depending on their position along the sinusoid. This zonal variation in function has been best demonstrated in regard to carbohydrate metabolism. Hepatocytes located closest to portal areas are primarily responsible for gluconeogenesis, containing the key enzymes of gluconeogenesis including phosphoenol-pyruvate-carboxykinase (PEPCK), fructose 1,6-biphosphatase, and glucose 6-phosphatase. In contrast, hepatocytes located near the hepatic vein predominantly contain the key enzymes of glycolysis, including glucokinase and pyruvate kinase, and also contain enzymes active in glutamate metabolism. Periportal hepatocytes are primarily responsible for extraction of bile salts from the sinusoidal circulation. Heterogeneity of other liver functions has not been well studied. Some of these regional differences may represent hepatocellular adaptation to regional variations in the O_2 or substrate composition of sinusoidal blood. Elegant studies by Jungermann and his colleagues have shown that hepatocytes express different phenotypes when cultured in varying O_2 or hormone concentrations. Other hormones, growth factors and innervation patterns may also play a role.

Metabolic zonation is not present until after birth. In newborn rats, zonal heterogeneity of cytosolic PEPCK develops during the first day of life. The heterogeneous distribution of PEPCK and succinate dehydrogenase is seen by the second week of life. Changes in hepatic O_2 and substrate delivery at birth likely explain the development of zonal heterogeneity.

Hepatocyte differentiation

Small quantities of characteristic hepatocellular proteins including α-fetoprotein, α_1-antitrypsin, and transferrin are expressed by the fourth gestational week. By 5–6 weeks of gestation, the rough endoplasmic reticulum and Golgi apparatus enlarge progressively. Selective distribution of proteins to specific regions of the plasma membrane defines the various plasma membrane domains. Each domain is endowed with its own group of receptors, transport enzymes, and other proteins. The canalicular domain borders the canaliculi. The lateral membrane region contains desmosomes and gap junctions between adjacent hepatocytes. The sinusoidal region has a microvillus surface whose increased surface area likely promotes exchange with sinusoids.

A basement membrane, whose framework is composed of type IV collagen, separates hepatocytes and sinusoidal cells. Laminin and another glycoprotein, fibronectin, attach collagen to hepatocytes via specific receptors on the sinusoidal subdomain. Strengthening the interaction of type IV collagen and these attachment glycoproteins are proteoglycans embedded within the hepatocellular plasma membrane, particularly heparan sulfate. The composition of the basement membrane and likely that of its adjacent hepatocyte basolateral domain change during development. *In utero*, the relative quantity of heparan sulfate is reduced and that of laminin increased. The basement membrane, via its interaction with hepatocyte plasma membrane receptors, appears to direct early hepatocellular differentiation during organogenesis. Several extracellular substances including liver cell-adhesion molecule (L-CAM) and the glycoprotein laminin facilitate attachment of hepatocytes to septal cells. Similarly, the basement membrane may maintain hepatocellular differentiation in the mature organ.

The canalicular domain is composed of transport proteins that exteriorize bile constituents to the canalicular lumen. Thus, the canaliculus is the initial site of free bile flow. It is formed by the circular joining of two to three canalicular domains of separate hepatocytes, each sealed with a tight junction. Well defined canaliculi appear during the second month of gestation. The canalicular region, like the sinusoidal region of the basolateral domain, has microvilli that increase the surface area available to form bile. Various membrane transport proteins appear at programmed times during development. The development of bile salt secretion, bilirubin metabolism, and the other metabolic functions of the liver are discussed elsewhere in this chapter.

Bile cells and bile ducts

Bile duct cells first evolve from hepatoblasts at the liver hilum during the second month of gestation. The hilum is the point at which the common bile duct, portal vein, and hepatic artery enter the liver. Just as the affinity of hepatoblasts for septal mesenchymal cells appears to be mediated by laminin, evolution of hepatoblasts to bile duct cells and the latter's affinity for portal vein branches are also mediated by laminin. At the hilum, hepatoblasts flatten to form a ductal plate of primordial biliary cells. The plate is reorganized into a series of cysts or tubules. Thereafter, tubules fuse into continuous ducts as the tubules progressively extend peripherally into the four partially separated lobes (right, left, caudate, quadrate). These ducts become interlobular bile ducts, remaining in close proximity to terminal portal venules, and are joined by terminal hepatic arteries. Collectively, these groups of three vessels surrounded by scant collagen define portal areas or triads.

Interlobular bile ducts receive bile from canaliculi via a series of intermediate tributaries penetrating the peripheries of portal areas. These tributaries, the canals of Hering, are also derived from hepatoblasts. Bile is conveyed from canaliculi to canals of Hering to interlobular ducts and then to larger channels, finally reaching the hilum. At the hilum, connection is made with the extrahepatic biliary system. The gallbladder and very proximal portions of the extrahepatic biliary system are derived from the cranial hepatic diverticulum. The remainder of the biliary system comes from the caudal aspect of the hepatic diverticulum. Formation of major biliary vessels is completed by about 10–12 weeks of gestation. Interlobular bile ducts do not completely extend to the hepatic periphery until late in the third trimester.

Sinusoidal cells

By 1 month following conception, hepatocytes are organized into multilayered cords. Sinusoids separating the cords have a noncontiguous endothelial lining. However, within a few weeks, hepatocellular cords thin to about three cells deep. Simultaneously, endothelial cells proliferate to become nearly continuous along the length of each sinusoid. Large numbers of vesicles are present within endothelial cytoplasm. This finding suggests that endothelium serves as a structural and functional filter between hepatocytes and the sinusoidal circulation. *In utero*, maturing erythroblasts migrate through perisinusoidal spaces for release into the sinusoidal circulation. During this migration, erythroblasts pass directly through, not between, endothelial cells. In mature liver, gaps in the endothelium, known as fenestrae, alter the size of molecules that penetrate the endothelial lining. The time at which endothelial fenestration occurs as well as the consequences of its early absence are unknown.

In addition to endothelial cells, two additional types of sinusoidal cells, Kupffer cells and Ito cells, can be identified from the beginning of sinusoidal morphogenesis. Kupffer cells are macrophages that ingest particulate materials passing through the sinusoids. The earliest embryonic Kupffer cells are carried into the liver from the yolk sac by the primordial portal venous system. Later on, Kupffer cells are derived from bone-marrow macrophages. Kupffer cell density is low through the first half of gestation. Cell densities typical of mature liver can be observed in the neonatal period. Some Kupffer cells are situated within the sinusoidal lumen. Others lie on the margins of sinusoids, connecting adjacent endothelial cells. Fetal Kupffer cells are similar both structurally and functionally to those present in mature liver. They are large, irregularly shaped, and contain pseudopodial projections. Fetal Kupffer cells also respond to stimuli with production of cytokines that include interleukin-1 and tumor necrosis factor α. In addition, fetal Kupffer cells phagocytose erythrocytes, their extruded nuclei, and other erythrocytic fragments as these cells emerge from the endothelium. Thus Kupffer cells may be final regulators of hematopoiesis, possibly preventing release of defective blood cells into the circulation.

Ito cells reside in the perisinusoidal space of Disse where they are attached to inner surfaces of endothelial cells. In mature liver, these cells, also known as fat storage cells or lipocytes, are thought to participate in hepatic vitamin A storage and to produce laminin basement membrane glycoprotein. Along with endothelial cells, they contribute to the synthesis of basement membrane type IV collagen. Embryonic Ito cells, unlike their mature counterparts, are capable of phagocytosis. Ito cells appear very similar to early fibroblast-like cells in the septum transversum and are thought to originate from those cells.

Whole-organ growth patterns

Following formation of the liver during the first trimester, the right lobe enlarges linearly through the remainder of gestation. Left lobar growth slows during the third trimester and, by birth, is about 10 percent smaller than the right. As with most developing tissues, initial liver growth results primarily from hepatocellular proliferation, i.e. cellular hyperplasia. Hepatocellular proliferation peaks during the second trimester. Hepatocellular levels of so-called proto-oncogenes, sequences that positively modulate mitosis by encoding various stimulatory growth factors, are at maximal concentration at this time. By the third trimester, mitosis slows, coinciding with repression of transcription of enzymes associated with DNA replication. These include thymidine kinase. Subsequently, enlargement of individual hepatocytes, i.e. cell hypertrophy, increasingly contributes to whole-organ enlargement. Hematopoiesis peaks by mid-second trimester and diminishes through the end of gestation. Liver growth continues until the end of the second decade after birth. Hepatocellular replication still contributes to postnatal growth. The neonatal liver has less than 20 percent of the hepatocytes present in the adult organ. Additional postnatal growth results from hepatocellular hypertrophy associated with attainment of polyploidy. Polyploid hepatocytes are randomly distributed in the acinus. They are enlarged compared to diploid cells in direct proportion to their increase in chromosome number. Polyploid hepatocytes are mostly 4N during childhood and 8N by early adulthood. Polyploidy may increase hepatocellular protein synthesis and bile production. However, only remaining diploid hepatocytes are capable of cell division.

Stimulation of hepatocellular hyperplasia is under the combined influence of endocrine, paracrine, and autocrine systems. Placental lactogen, insulin-like growth factors I and II (IGF-I, IGF-II), epidermal growth factor, and transforming growth factor α may all play a role in liver growth.

Selected reading

Andersen, B, Zierz S, Jungermann K. Perinatal development of the distributions of phosphoenol-pyruvate carboxykinase and succinate dehydrogenase in rat liver parenchyma. *Eur J Cell Biol* 1983; **30**: 126.

Enzan H, Hara H, Yamashita Y, *et al*. Fine structure of hepatic sinusoids and their development in human embryos and fetuses. *Acta Pathol Jpn* 1983; **33**: 447.

Ruebner RH, Blankenberg TA, Burrows DA, SooHoo W, Lund JK. Development and transformation of the ductal plate in the developing human liver. *Pediatr Pathol* 1990; **10**: 55.

Sell S. Is there a liver stem cell? *Cancer Res* 1990; **50**: 3811.

Traber PG, Chianale J, Gumucio JJ. Physiologic significance and regulation of hepatocellular heterogeneity. *Gastroenterology* 1988; **95**: 1130.

L. Liver Blood Flow

C D Rudolph

Blood from the gastrointestinal tract, pancreas, and spleen drains through the portal vein into the liver before mixing with the systemic circulation. This strategic anatomical arrangement allows the liver to cleanse the portal blood of absorbed toxins, process absorbed nutrients efficiently, as well as secrete bile acids in response to gastrointestinal hormonal stimulation. The splanchnic organs that drain into the portal vein utilize O_2 and thus the O_2 content of portal venous blood is reduced. The hepatic artery provides additional O_2-rich blood to the liver, assuring that adequate O_2 is available to perform the many energy-requiring functions. A similar pattern prevails in the fetus. Nutrients supplied from the placenta pass through the umbilical vein to the liver. However, in many species, a portion of this blood bypasses the liver, shunting through the ductus venosus to the systemic circulation.

Liver blood flow in the adult

The hepatic artery and portal vein arborize into small terminal vessels in the portal triad (Fig. 9.14). Both vessels supply blood to the liver parenchyma, emptying into the hepatic sinusoids. The hepatic artery provides the only blood supply to the intrahepatic bile ducts. Sphincters control the flow of portal venous and arterial blood into each liver sinusoid. The blood percolates through the sinusoids to the central vein, into the large hepatic veins, and then into the inferior vena cava. Twenty to 25 percent of the total cardiac output supplies the liver, providing a total flow of about 100 ml/(min·100 g). Approximately 75 percent of liver blood flow is provided by the portal vein and 25 percent by the hepatic artery. Hepatic arterial O_2 content is high compared to the portal vein; thus approximately equal portions of the O_2 supplied to the liver are derived from each vessel.

Portal flow increases after a meal and decreases during fasting. Hepatic arterial flow decreases or increases accordingly, maintaining a relatively steady blood flow and O_2 delivery to the liver. The intrinsic hepatic mechanisms underlying this 'hepatic arterial buffer response' have been elucidated by Lautt and Greenway. The hepatic arterioles and portal venules pass through an extracellular space, the space of Mall (Fig. 9.14), before entering the sinusoid. Adenosine is produced and released into this space at a constant rate. The concentration of adenosine washed out of the space of Mall varies with portal flow; reductions in flow result in the accumulation of adenosine. Adenosine is a potent arteriolar dilator. Thus as portal flow decreases, adenosine accumulates and dilates hepatic arterioles, increasing hepatic arterial flow. Specific adenosine antagonists suppress this response.

Extrinsic factors also regulate hepatic blood flow. Sympathetic stimulation reduces both portal venous flow and hepatic arterial flow by stimulation of α-adrenoreceptors. β-Adrenoreceptor stimulation reduces hepatic arterial resistance to flow. Other hormones including angiotensin II and vasopressin reduce hepatic flow.

The liver is a highly vascular organ, containing about 10 percent of the total blood volume. Thus, changes in liver volume could control the amount of blood in the systemic circulatory system. A sphincter has been described in the small hepatic veins between the sinusoid and main hepatic veins. Contraction of this sphincter with hepatic nerve stimulation or by hormonal stimulation presumably could alter intrahepatic pressure and blood volume.

Liver blood flow in the fetus

In the fetus liver blood flow is provided by the umbilical vein, portal vein, and hepatic artery (Fig. 9.15). The common umbilical vein passes towards the liver hilum under the left lobe of the liver. Branches arborize into the left lobe before the point where the umbilical vein gives rise to the ductus venosus, which shunts blood across to the inferior vena cava. The umbilical vein then passes into the right lobe of the liver and joins the portal vein. Branches supplying the right lobe of the liver arise in this region. As suggested by the anatomical description, more than 90 percent of the blood supplying the left lobe of the

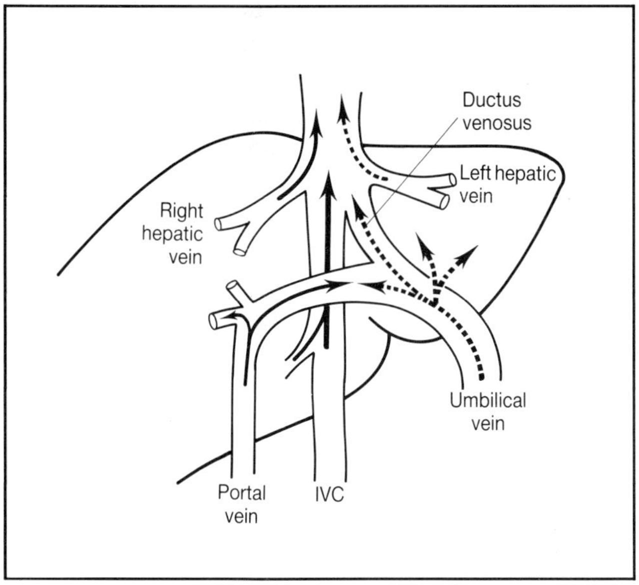

Fig. 9.15. Schematic representation of liver blood flow in the fetal lamb.

liver is derived from the umbilical vein. Less than 10 percent is supplied by the hepatic artery. The right lobe receives 60 percent of its blood supply from the umbilical vein, 35 percent from the portal vein, and 5 percent from the hepatic artery. Most mammalian species have a ductus venosus; however, it is absent in several including the horse, pig, and guinea-pig.

Total blood flow to the liver is more than four times greater in the fetus than in the adult, reaching values of approximately 400 ml/(min·100 g). The proportion of umbilical venous blood flow that bypasses the hepatic circulation by shunting to the inferior vena cava through the ductus venosus varies widely, but approximates 50 percent in the unstressed fetus. This highly oxygenated blood is preferentially distributed to the fetal heart and brain (see Chapter 10). Most of the blood from the portal vein is distributed to the right lobe of the liver with less than 10 percent passing through the ductus venosus.

The fetus responds to various stresses by altering hepatic blood flow and/or the portion of oxygenated umbilical venous blood shunted through the ductus venosus. Maternal hypoxemia results in a reduction in liver flow of about 20 percent with a corresponding increase in shunting of blood across the ductus venosus. Umbilical cord compression or hypovolemia result in an even more striking increase in the proportion of blood shunted across the ductus venosus with a corresponding large decrease in total hepatic blood flow and a resultant decrease in O_2 delivery to approximately 25 percent of control values. The proportion of blood flow passing through the ductus venosus versus the liver could be altered by changes in the resistance to flow of the liver or the ductus venosus. There appears to be a sphincter mechanism at the origin of the ductus venosus from the umbilical vein. Neural control of the ductus venosus is unlikely because administration of atropine to block parasympathetic neural activity or phentolamine to block α-adrenergic sympathetic neural activity does not alter ductus venosus flow. Isolated rings of ductus venosus relax upon exposure to prostaglandin (PG) E_2 and PGI_2 and contract when exposed to indomethacin, an inhibitor of PGs. Local autocrine regulators or other hormonal factors may control ductus venosus resistance.

Changes in the resistance of flow through the liver could also increase the proportion of blood distributed through the ductus venosus. Liver blood flow decreases dramatically in response to reductions in umbilical blood flow; however, there are not associated changes in umbilical venous or inferior vena caval pressure, suggesting that liver resistance increases and ductus venosus resistance decreases. The mechanisms controlling this change in liver resistance have not been elucidated. If presinusoidal resistance increases, the volume of blood contained in the liver would be redistributed to the central circulation, an appropriate response to hypovolemic stress.

Changes in liver blood flow at birth

At birth umbilical flow ceases and the liver receives all of its blood supply from the hepatic artery and portal vein, as in the adult. The ductus venosus can remain open for as long as 10 days after birth. Studies in newborn lambs demonstrate that blood flow to the liver abruptly falls to adult rates of approximately 100 ml/(min·100 g) and then rises slowly to approximately 300 ml/(min·100 g) over the first 10 hours of life. Similar flow rates have been demonstrated in 1-week-old fasted lambs. Changes in total liver blood flow, the proportion of flow provided by the hepatic artery or portal vein, and the intactness of the 'hepatic arterial buffer response' have not been well studied during infancy or childhood.

Selected reading

Lautt WW, Greenway CV. Conceptual review of the hepatic vascular bed. *Hepatology* 1987; **7**: 952.

Rudolph AM, Rudolph CD. Fetal and postnatal hepatic vasculature and blood flow. In Polin RA, Fox WW, eds. *Fetal and neonatal physiology*. Vol. II. Philadelphia: WB Saunders Co., 1992: 1095.

M. Development of Gallbladder Motility

J P Ryan

Bile salts stabilize pancreatic lipolytic enzymes and solubilize the products of lipolysis into micelles. Bile salts are produced by the liver and are secreted into the biliary ducts. The gallbladder stores and concentrates bile for secretion into the duodenum. Coordination of the motor activities of the gallbladder and the sphincter of Oddi assure that bile salts are released into the intestinal lumen when required for fat digestion. While there is no question that gallbladder emptying involves active contraction of the gallbladder, the dynamics at the sphincter of Oddi are much more controversial. In several species such as guinea-pig, rabbit, and opossum, the sphincter most likely serves the role of a pump and contributes to bile flow into the duodenum by increasing or decreasing the force of its characteristic peristaltic contractions. In other species, such as the human, the sphincter is believed to influence bile flow by serving as a variable resistor, with the magnitude of bile flow being inversely related to sphincter tone.

Emptying patterns in adults

In adults, gallbladder emptying occurs during both the interdigestive period and after ingestion of a meal (digestive phase). In adult humans bile flows into the duodenum during the interdigestive period in a cyclical pattern. During this period, water is removed from gallbladder bile because of solvent drag created by active NaCl transport by gallbladder mucosal cells. Mucus and IgA are also secreted into the gallbladder lumen. The periodic increase in bile delivery into the duodenum correlates closely with phase II of the migrating motor complex (MMC) discussed in Section 9D. The periodic increase in bile delivery into the duodenum during the interdigestive period involves cyclical changes in hepatic secretion of bile and periodic activation of gallbladder emptying, which involves gallbladder contraction and sphincter of Oddi relaxation. The physiological role of gallbladder emptying during the interdigestive period remains unsettled. A 'housekeeper' function has been proposed in which gallbladder emptying prevents the accumulation of microcrystals or debris in the concentrated bile during fasting. The periodic mixing and emptying of bile may serve to prevent gallbladder stasis during fasting and thus decrease the likelihood of gallstone formation.

The gallbladder empties promptly in response to ingestion of a meal, generally within 2 minutes. Characteristically, the gallbladder empties 60–70 percent of its fasting volume and does so with a half-emptying time of 10–20 minutes. The major stimulus for gallbladder emptying occurs during the intestinal phase of digestion and absorption. The gastric emptying of chyme into the duodenum, through the activation of neural and hormonal inputs, serves as the primary stimulus for the initiation of gallbladder emptying. Preduodenal factors also may contribute to gallbladder emptying during the cephalic and gastric phases of digestion. Excitatory cholinergic vagal fibers, activated by esophageal and gastric distension, input onto the gallbladder and lead to active contraction of the gallbladder smooth muscle.

Regulation of gallbladder emptying

The factors responsible for contraction of the gallbladder during the interdigestive period are unclear. Motilin, when given exogenously during the interdigestive period, increases the contractile activity of the stomach, small intestine, and gallbladder. Gallbladder contraction during the interdigestive period closely correlates with increased antral motility during phase II of the MMC.

Cholecystokinin (CCK) mediates the intestinal phase of gallbladder emptying in a number of animal species (including humans). A close correlation exists between plasma concentrations of CCK and changes in gallbladder volume after ingestion of a meal. Recent evidence indicates that CCK may stimulate gallbladder contraction via activation of excitatory vagal cholinergic fibers. Gallbladder contraction combined with a CCK-mediated decrease in sphincter of Oddi resistance (humans) leads to the prompt delivery of bile into the duodenum.

Developmental aspects of gallbladder function

The delivery of bile into the duodenum depends not only upon bile acid excretion as determined by hepatic function, but also upon the contractile ability of the gallbladder. Sufficient intraluminal pressure needs to be developed by active contraction of gallbladder smooth muscle to overcome resistances offered by the common bile ducts and the sphincter of Oddi.

The mechanical properties of the gallbladder, assessed by analyzing the pressure–volume relationship of the organ basally and following stimulation with CCK, indicate that the compliance of the unstimulated gallbladder is significantly less in the neonate than in the adult. When stimulated with CCK, gallbladders from adult animals show decreased compliance, whereas gallbladders from newborn animals have no change in compliance. The rise in gallbladder intraluminal pressure in response to CCK stimulation is less in newborn versus adult animals. The reduced gallbladder force-generating capacity in the neonate may result from the inability of gallbladder smooth muscle to generate significant active tension when stimulated with an agonist. The magnitude of gallbladder contractile response in adult animals is greater than that in preterm and term animals. The differences remain even when the contractile responses are normalized for differences in tissue cross-sectional area.

The contractile response to Ca^{2+} is concentration-dependent in gallbladder smooth muscle from newborn and adult guinea-pigs; however, at all concentrations examined, the contractile response from newborn animals was significantly less than from adults, supporting the hypothesis that basic differences exist between newborns and adults with respect to the ability of the contractile machinery to generate force in response to an agonist-mediated rise in intracellular Ca^{2+}. Recent evidence in vascular and tracheal smooth muscle indicates that postnatal changes in contractile protein content and/or isoforms, as well as changes in Ca^{2+} concentration and calmodulin sensitivity, might account for the decreased response to Ca^{2+}. Perhaps gallbladder smooth muscle exhibits a similar postnatal maturation of contractile machinery. Other possible explanations for the differences in neonatal versus adult gallbladder contractile activity include age-related differences in the mechanism of action of acetylcholine and CCK, or in the muscle fiber geometric arrangement in the gallbladder.

Sphincter of Oddi

The delivery of bile into the duodenum involves both gallbladder contraction and the efficient passage of bile through the sphincter of Oddi. The ability of the sphincter of Oddi region to serve as a pump is not fully developed in the newborn guinea-pig. Using intravital microscopy, the contractile activity of the sphincter upon ingestion of a meal is seen to be decreased in newborns compared with adults. Differences between sphincter smooth muscle or responses to specific agonists in newborns and adults have not been studied.

Limited animal data suggest that the contractile behavior of the gallbladder and the sphincter of Oddi is less in newborns than in adults. Should this also be true for humans, hypomotility of the gallbladder and sphincter may diminish the flow of bile into the duodenum, contributing to physiological cholestasis in the newborn. Although this is an attractive hypothesis, more data must be obtained before it can be expressed with confidence.

Selected reading

Cox KL, Cheung ATW, Lohse CL, *et al.* Biliary motility: postnatal changes in guinea pigs. *Pediatr Res* 1987; **21**: 170.

Denehy CM, Ryan JP. Development of gallbladder contractility in the guinea pig. *Pediatr Res* 1986; **20**: 214.

Lambert R, Ryan JP. Response to calcium of skinned gallbladder smooth muscle from newborn and adult guinea pigs. *Pediatr Res* 1990; **28**: 336.

N. Bile Acid Metabolism and the Enterohepatic Circulation of Bile Acids

J E Heubi

Normal physiology

Bile acids serve at least three major functions: (1) they stimulate bile flow during secretion across the biliary canaliculus; (2) in the upper small intestine, they form aggregates called micelles, which solubilize the water-insoluble products of lipolysis; and (3) they are major regulators of sterol metabolism. In health, the enterohepatic circulation of bile acids is localized to the liver and biliary tract, the intestinal tract, and the portal and peripheral circulations. In the liver, cholesterol is converted to the highly polar bile acids, cholic acid (3α,7α,12α-trihydroxy-5β-cholanoic acid) and chenodeoxycholic acid (3α,7α-dihydroxy-5β-cholanoic acid), which are termed primary bile acids (Fig. 9.16). The initial step of bile acid synthesis involves the 7α-hydroxylation of the sterol nucleus of cholesterol, which is effected by the rate-limiting enzyme of bile acid synthesis, cholesterol 7α-hydroxylase. This enzyme is regulated by a mechanism of feedback inhibition based on the quantities of bile acids returning to the liver via the portal vein. After hepatic synthesis, bile acids are conjugated with glycine or taurine as *N*-acyl conjugates. All but a small fraction of bile acids are conjugated before excretion by the hepatocyte.

Bile is a mixture of organic and inorganic materials. The major organic compounds include conjugated bile acids, phospholipids, cholesterol, and bile pigments. Proteins and hormones are present in low concentrations. Bile acid concentrations in adult bile ranges from 2 to 45 mM. Bile acids are amphipathic molecules forming micelles (macromolecular aggregates) above a critical micellar concentration (CMC), which in human bile is approximately 2–4 mM. Bile acids in hepatic and gallbladder bile greatly exceed the CMC. Therefore, bile acids in bile and the upper small bowel lumen are present as micelles with small amounts present as monomers. Bile acids are important in relation to the other organic compounds in bile because hepatocyte secretion of cholesterol and phospholipids depends upon bile acid secretion, and the solubility of cholesterol and phospholipids is largely dependent upon bile acids.

Bile acid-dependent bile flow, linked directly to bile acid transport through the hepatocyte and into the canalicular lumen, provides the major impetus for bile flow. The bile acid-independent component accounts for a smaller fraction of bile flow. Uptake of taurocholate into the hepatocyte from portal blood depends upon an inwardly directed Na^+ gradient, which may be diminished by other bile acids, amino acids, and furosemide. Transcellular passage of bile acids is facilitated by binding to intracellular carrier proteins. Canalicular transport carriers facilitate passage of bile acids into the canalicular lumen. Canalicular transport is via a Na^+-independent process driven by a negative transmembrane potential. The osmotic activity of transported bile acids leads to movement of water and other solutes into the canalicular lumen. Choleresis is stimulated by increasing the flux of bile acids across the hepatocyte.

During fasting, most of the bile acid pool is present in the gallbladder; however, some bile acids are always entering the intestinal lumen and produce basal intraluminal concentrations and small but measurable concentrations in the serum because of continuous intestinal absorption with less than complete hepatic extraction from portal blood. When a meal is ingested, the gallbladder contracts at least once, and most of the bile salt pool is emptied into the small intestinal lumen (Fig. 9.17). Within the upper small bowel, bile salts form mixed micelles with the lipolytic products, fatty acids and monoglycerides. Cholesterol, phospholipids, and fat-soluble vitamins are also solubilized within mixed micelles. The lipolytic products are absorbed; thereafter, bile acids are reabsorbed by two mechanisms. A Na^+-dependent, active transport system localized to the distal ileum is the principal pathway for reabsorption. Bile acids can competitively inhibit each other for transport across the ileal active transport system. Passive transport by nonionic diffusion may occur at any location along the length of the small and large intestine; however,

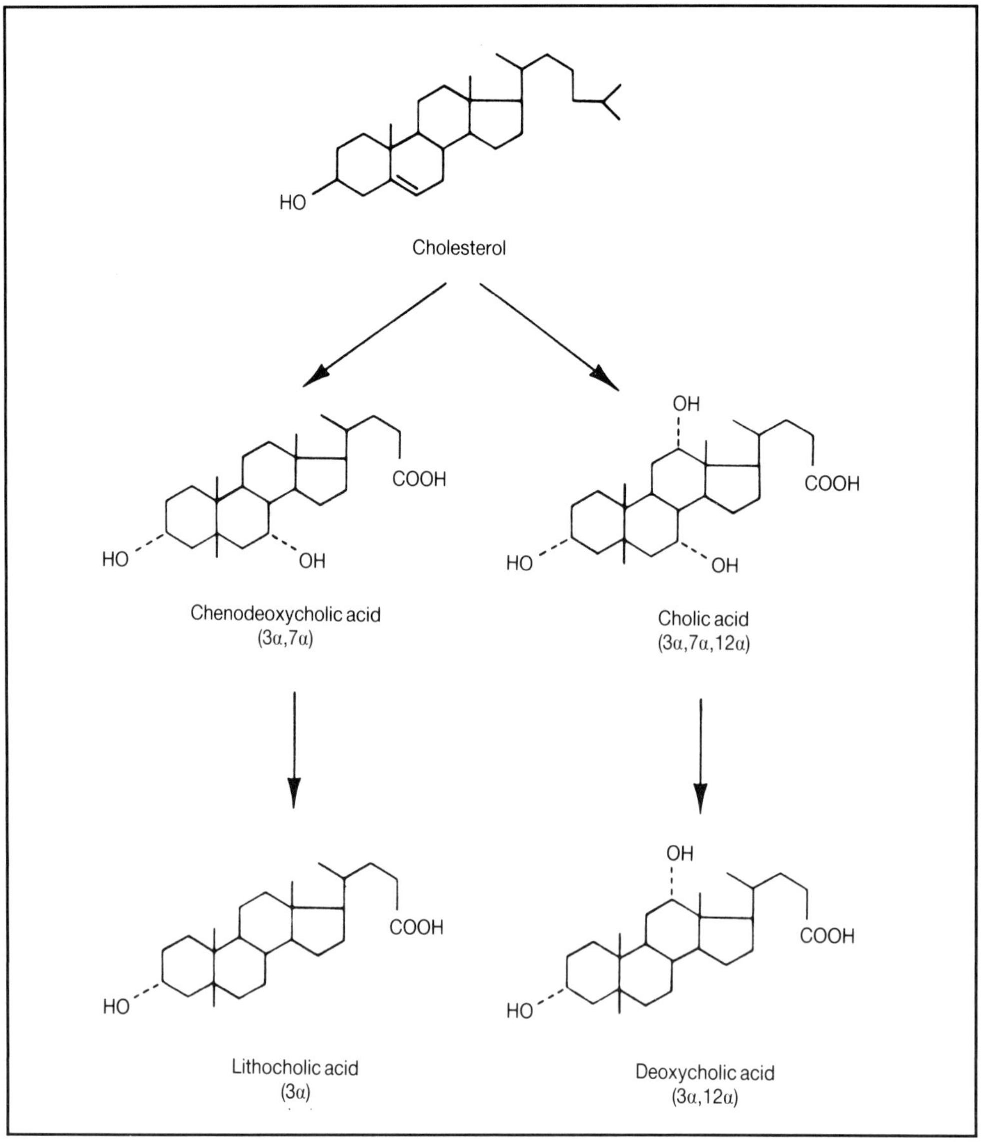

Fig. 9.16. Primary bile acids synthesized in liver from cholesterol and the secondary bile acids produced by bacterial 7α-dehydroxylation.

absorption is markedly curtailed for most bile acids because their pK_as are low and they tend to remain ionized at luminal pH. Only unconjugated bile acids and glycine conjugates of dihydroxy bile acids are likely to be nonionized and in a suitable state for passive absorption. In addition, luminal nutrients tend to inhibit passive uptake of bile acids.

After bile acids are transported out of the enterocyte, they are carried to the liver where transport systems efficiently remove them from the portal blood. A small fraction of the bile acids in portal blood spill over into the systemic circulation, leading to a predictable postprandial rise in serum bile acids during each of the 6–10 enterohepatic cycles of bile acids during the day.

Most of the conjugates of cholic and chenodeoxycholic acid excreted in the bile are reabsorbed without intraluminal bacterial alteration. Approximately one-fourth of the primary bile acids are deconjugated by bacteria in the terminal ileum and colon. Most of these free bile acids are reabsorbed and reconjugated in the liver with either glycine or taurine. Additional modifications to the steroid nucleus after deconjugation may also be made within the gut lumen. The most common biotransformation made by bacteria is 7α-dehydroxylation with the formation of secondary bile acids (Fig. 9.16). Deoxycholic acid (3α,12α-dihydroxy-5β-cholanoic acid) is formed from

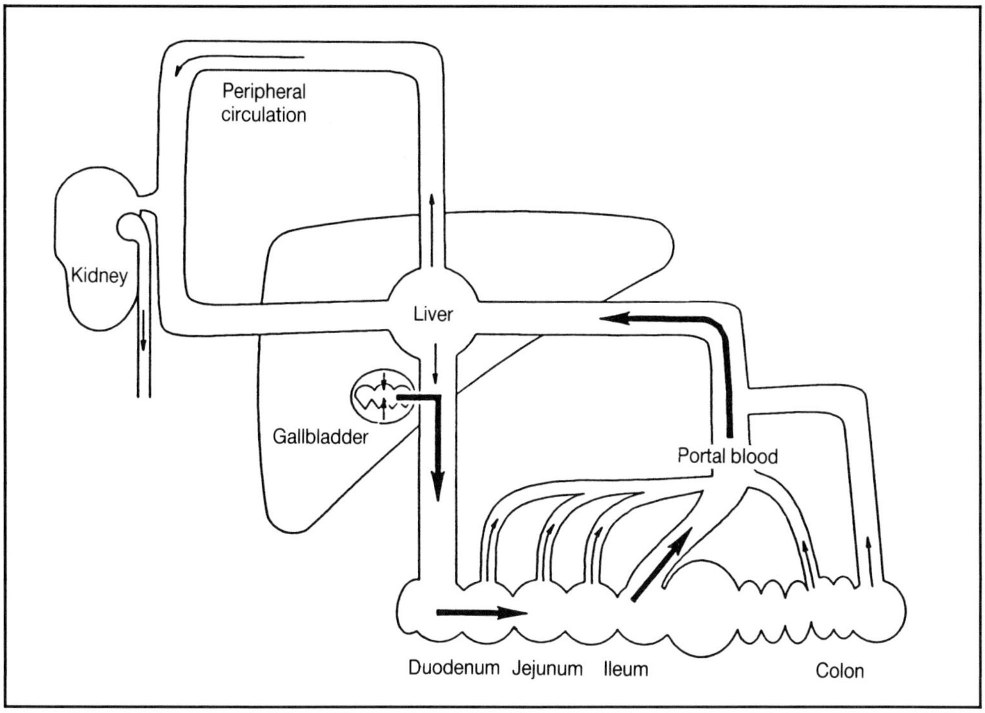

Fig. 9.17. The enterohepatic circulation of bile acids. With gallbladder contraction, bile acids are expelled into the duodenum. Passive intestinal absorption is depicted by small arrows; the large arrow in ileum depicts active uptake of bile acids. Bile acids return to the liver via the portal venous system. Despite efficient uptake of bile acids, a small fraction of the bile acids in portal blood spill over into the systemic circulation and may be filtered and excreted by the kidneys. (From Heubi JE. In: Banks RO, Sperelakis N, eds. *Essentials of basic science: physiology*. Boston: Little, Brown and Company, in press, with permission.)

cholic acid, and lithocholic acid (3α-hydroxy-5β-cholanoic acid) is formed from chenodeoxycholic acid. The produced deoxycholic acid is absorbed relatively efficiently and reconjugated, whereas lithocholic acid is absorbed poorly. If reabsorbed, lithocholic acid may be conjugated with glycine or taurine; however, the majority of conjugates are sulfated in the three position to form sulfated lithocholate conjugates. Sulfated conjugates are poorly absorbed and are excreted. Fecal bile acids are reflective of major bacterial transformation. The majority of bile acids are unconjugated and lack the 7α-hydroxyl group.

In adults, biliary bile acids are generally cholic (36 percent), chenodeoxycholic (36 percent), deoxycholic (24 percent) and lithocholic (1 percent) in a glycine-to-taurine ratio of 3–4:1. Each day about one-fourth to one-third of the cholic acid pool and one-fourth to one-fifth of the chenodeoxycholic acid pool is lost from the adult human enterohepatic circulation. This turnover of bile acids is commonly expressed as the fractional turnover rate (FTR). The bile acid pool is in a steady state in health so that losses of bile acids are replaced by hepatic synthesis by a carefully regulated mechanism of feedback inhibition of the rate-limiting enzyme of bile acid synthesis, cholesterol 7α-hydroxylase.

Developmental aspects of bile acid synthesis and the enterohepatic circulation of bile acids

The enterohepatic circulation of bile salts is immature at birth. Impairment of hepatic synthesis, secretion, and uptake, of intestinal conservation, and of gallbladder contractility (see Section 9M) all contribute to the reduced biliary secretion and intraluminal concentrations encountered in the neonate.

Bile acid biosynthesis is markedly reduced *in utero*; it is first observed near week 12 in the human fetus. A 30-fold increase in the biliary concentrations of cholic and chenodeoxycholic acids is observed between 16 and 20 weeks of gestation in the human fetus. The bile acids produced (and their metabolic pathways) during gestation are considerably different from those in the infant, child, and adult. The primary bile acids, cholic and chenodeoxycholic acids, make up less than 50 percent of the total bile acid pool in the fetus. The ratio of cholic to chenodeoxycholic acid is 0.85 between 16 and 20 weeks of gestation, in contrast to 2.5 in the neonate and 1.6 in the adult. This suggests immaturity of hepatic 12α-hydroxylation during development. The fetal liver possesses enzymes capable of synthesizing relatively large proportions of bile acids not found in older infants or healthy adults; however, these compounds are found in biological fluids from adults with cholestatic liver disease. These unique bile acids account for 5–15 percent of the total biliary bile acid of the human fetus. The physiological relevance of almost all of these compounds is unknown; however, they may be directly responsible for the development of cholestasis. Extremely low hepatic bile flow rates secondary to small primary bile acid pool sizes and the presence of an array of bile acids that are unique to the fetus and may be intrinsically cholestatic probably exaggerate the immaturity of hepatic excretory function.

The phenomenon of reduced fat absorption in the immediate neonatal period is referred to as *physiological steatorrhea*. Newborns share two common defects that lead to impaired fat absorption: reduced prandial-related intraluminal bile salt concentrations and diminished pancreatic lipase activity (see Section 9F). Both are consistently reduced and correlate with gestational and postnatal age. A progressive rise in both occurs in infants in the first few months. Term and preterm infants have markedly reduced primary bile salt pool sizes compared with adults on a surface-area basis. These reduced pools are accompanied by reduced intraluminal bile salt concentrations (Fig. 9.18). Initial studies suggested that compared with adults, the turnover rate for the primary bile salts in neonates might be increased due to impaired intestinal conservation, and synthesis rates reduced because of impaired regulation of the rate-limiting enzyme of bile salt synthesis, cholesterol 7α-hydroxylase. Breast-fed preterm infants, when compared with age- and weight-matched infants fed a proprietary formula, have larger bile salt pools and lower turnover rates (both cholic and chenodeoxycholic acids), higher intraluminal concentrations (4.8 vs 2.6 mM compared to the critical micellar concentration of 2.00), and better fat absorption efficiency (93 vs 82 percent) at age 11 days. By age 31–38 days, all infants have substantial reductions in the turnover rate for cholate and chenodeoxycholate and increases in cholate and chenodeoxycholate pools; however, synthesis rates for both bile salts remain unchanged. Concurrently, intraluminal bile salt concentrations increase from about 5 mM in breast-fed and about 3–4 mM in formula-fed infants, while fat absorption increases from 78 to 83 percent of dietary intake in both formula- and breast-fed infants. This finding suggests that breast milk may provide a stimulus to maturation of the enterohepatic circulation in the preterm infant.

Because bile acids are the major determinant of bile flow, their synthesis and the development of an adequate

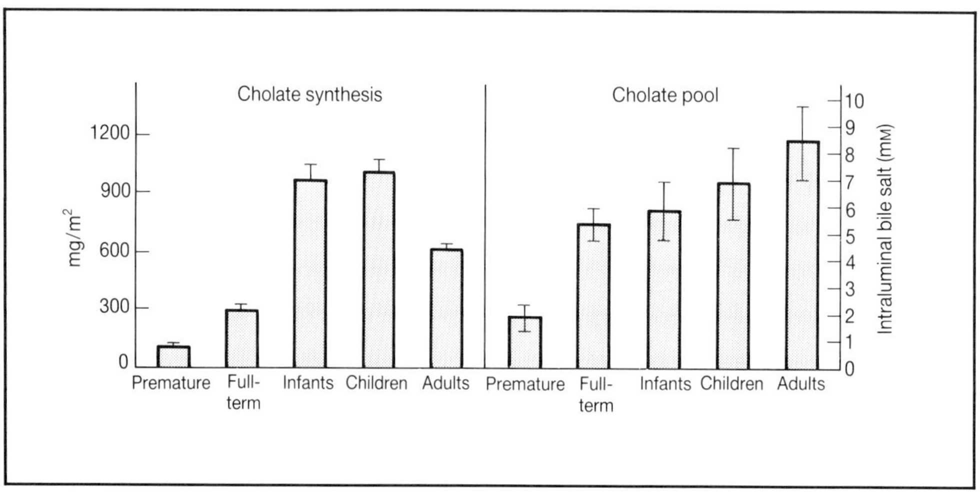

Fig. 9.18. Left panel: Comparison of cholate pool size (mg/m²) in preterm and term infants (studied by Watkins *et al. N Engl J Med* 1973; **288**: 431; *Gastroenterology* 1975; **69**: 706), infants and children (studied by Heubi *et al. Pediatr Res* 1980; **14**: 943; *J Lab Clin Med* 1982; **100**: 127), and adults (studied by Vlahcevic *et al. Gastroenterology* 1971; **61**: 85). Right panel: Comparison of meal-stimulated intraluminal bile salt concentrations (mM) in preterm and term infants (studied by Watkins *et al. N Engl J Med* 1973; **288**: 431; *Gastroenterology* 1975; **69**: 706), infants and children (studied by Heubi *et al. Pediatr Res* 1980; **14**: 943; *J Lab Clin Med* 1982; **100**: 127), and adults (studied by Porter and Sanders, *Gastroenterology* 1971; **60**: 997).

pool of bile acids in the neonatal period is essential to biliary excretion. Although unproved in the human neonate, it seems extremely likely that biliary excretory function is impaired in the first weeks of life. Despite a reduced load of bile acids returned from the intestine in the neonate compared with the adult, elevated serum bile acid concentrations are commonly encountered in preterm and term infants. In term infants, the elevated concentrations decline with postnatal age and normalize at about 6–12 months. This phenomenon has been termed 'physiological cholestasis'. The clearance of additional organic ions including sulfobromophthalein (BSP) is impaired in term and preterm infants with progressive improvement during the first month of life. The exact mechanism by which organic ion transport is compromised is unclear, but it likely relates to impaired hepatic uptake at the basolateral membrane, as well as alterations of blood flow and biliary excretion.

Studies on the ontogeny of the enterohepatic circulation in rats have helped to formulate a working model in the mammal that may improve our understanding of developmental physiology in the human. The rat is a particularly good model for comparison to the human premature infant because of its extreme immaturity at birth. In the newborn rat, the bile salt pool is very small and is localized predominantly in the liver and peripheral serum rather than the intestinal lumen, as observed in the adult. Bile acid synthesis begins in the fetal rat on days 15–17. Synthesis rates increase from 82 pmol/mg dry liver weight on day 18 to 1043 pmol/mg on day 21. Fetal bile acid synthesis can be enhanced *in vitro* by corticoid treatment. During the first postnatal weeks, hepatocyte bile salt uptake matures. The K_m for hepatic bile salt transport across the basolateral membrane remains unchanged with increasing age; however, the V_{max} increases fourfold between ages 1 and 8 weeks. This suggests that the transport process is present initially and the number of transport sites increases with postnatal age. Transport across the canalicular membrane appears to be similar in suckling and adult rats. Elevated serum bile acids in the suckling rat decline with increasing postnatal age, suggesting an improvement in the clearance mechanisms. Only passive intestinal bile salt transport is present in the suckling rat; however, during the third postnatal week, ileal active transport first appears with kinetic characteristics that are qualitatively similar to those of older animals. Corticosteroids and thyroxine in pharmacological doses have been shown to induce precocious development of the active transport mechanism. Concurrently, the pool size, initially located predominately in the liver, increases fivefold between 2 and 8 weeks of age, when it becomes largely localized to the intestinal lumen.

Extrapolating the observations made in laboratory animals to humans is difficult; however, fragmentary human data allow inferences regarding postnatal development of the enterohepatic circulation in neonates. Hepatic bile acid synthesis in the human is severely reduced, and alternative pathways for synthesis are present in the fetus as well as newborn term and preterm infants. Synthesis of the primary bile acids markedly increases in the first postnatal weeks. Hepatic uptake of bile salts is impaired at birth in term, and especially preterm infants, with subsequent improvement in the first year of life as indicated by high serum concentrations of total serum bile acids and conjugates of cholic and chenodeoxycholate, which decline to concentrations comparable to older children by 10 months. The turnover rate of bile salts is increased at birth, but declines postnatally. Because the turnover rate reflects biliary secretion rates, intestinal transit, gallbladder contractility and intestinal uptake of bile salts, it is impossible to dissect out exactly which process(es) is compromised at birth and matures with postnatal age. Neither biliary secretion, intestinal transit, nor gallbladder contractility has been directly examined in the human neonate. Results of *in vitro* studies in which ileal segments were incubated with bile salts suggest that ileal active bile salt transport is absent in human fetuses, with its first appearance in infants at age 8 months. However, bile salt kinetic studies in preterm and term newborns, infants, and children strongly suggest that ileal active bile salt transport is present at birth even in very premature infants.

Intraluminal bile salt concentrations increase postnatally coincident with pool size enlargement in formula-fed and mixed diet-fed infants and children (Fig. 9.18). Qualitative composition of duodenal bile in newborn infants changes dramatically with age. Although cholic acid and chenodeoxycholic acid predominate in neonatal bile, additional other bile acids, including 6-OH, 1-OH, and oxo-bile acids have been identified. With the appearance of intestinal microflora, secondary bile acids appear in the bile and other less commonly found bile acids disappear. During the first year, cholic acid constitutes 60 percent of duodenal bile acids, while chenodeoxycholic constitutes 36 percent. Small quantities of deoxycholic acid are detected between 6 and 10 months. The glycine-to-taurine ratio of bile in the preterm neonate is less than one but increases to 3.3 during the first year of life.

Fecal bile acids in the neonate consist of only primary bile acids, with no secondary bile acids detectable. With development of the gut microflora, secondary bile acids appear in the stool. Daily excretion by adults and children older than 18 months is eight to nine times greater than by children less than age 18 months; however, differences in excretion rates disappear when body surface-area differences or weights are taken into account. For all newborns and children, bile acid excretion is relatively consistent when based upon body weight (3–6 mg/kg per day) and is similar to that observed in adults.

Selected reading

Balistreri WF, Heubi JE, Suchy FJ. Immaturity of the enterohepatic circulation in early life: factors predisposing to 'physiologic' maldigestion and cholestasis. *J Pediatr Gastroenterol Nutr* 1983; **2:** 346.

Hofmann AF. Enterohepatic circulation of bile acids. In Schultz SG, Forte JG, Rauner BB, eds. *Handbook of physiology*. Bethesda, MD: American Physiological Society, 1989: 567.

Setchell KDR, Street JM. Inborn errors of bile acid synthesis. *Semin Liver Dis* 1987; **7**: 85.

Suchy FJ, Bucuvalas JC, Novak DA. Determinants of bile formation during development: ontogeny of hepatic bile acid metabolism and transport. *Semin Liver Dis* 1987; **7**: 77.

O. Perinatal Bilirubin Metabolism

G R Gourley

Bilirubin formation and structure

Bilirubin is formed when the protoporphyrin ring of heme-containing compounds is degraded. Hemoglobin is the largest source for the production of bilirubin, but other heme-containing proteins (e.g. cytochromes, catalases, tryptophan pyrrolase and muscle myoglobin) are also degraded to bilirubin. The first enzyme system involved in bilirubin formation is microsomal heme oxygenase, located primarily in the reticuloendothelial tissues, and also in tissue macrophages and intestinal epithelium. Heme oxygenase causes cleavage of the tetrapyrrole ring at one of the methine (=C–) carbon bridges, resulting in equimolar production of the excised carbon (carbon monoxide) and the linear tetrapyrrole, biliverdin. The central (C-10) carbon of biliverdin is then reduced from a methine to a methylene group ($-CH_2-$), by the cytosolic enzyme biliverdin reductase, thus forming bilirubin. Bilirubin is given the IX designation according to Fischer's protoporphyrin isomer groups, group IX being the physiological source of bilirubin. Although the tetrapyrrole ring can be cleaved at any of the four (α, β, γ, and δ) methine bridges, in the fetus, bilirubin IXβ is first produced and can be found in fetal bile at 14 weeks of gestation. The major human isomer, bilirubin IXα, appears in fetal bile at 16 weeks. Bilirubin formation, assessed by carbon monoxide production, indicates that the daily production rate of bilirubin is 6–8 mg/kg per 24 h in healthy term infants and 3–4 mg/kg per 24 h in healthy adults.

Bilirubin is not linear, but rather contains extensive internal H^+ bonding that shields the polar propionic acid groups and makes bilirubin poorly soluble in aqueous media (Fig. 9.19). The carbon–carbon double bonds at positions 4–5 and 15–16 can assume two different configurations depending on whether the higher priority atoms or groups (based on atomic number) are on the same (*Z*, zusammen, German: 'together') or opposite (*E*, entgegen, 'opposite') sides of the double bond. The naturally occurring form of bilirubin is 4*Z*,15*Z*-bilirubin IXα. The poor aqueous solubility of bilirubin requires binding to albumin while in the circulation and hepatic transformation to more water-soluble derivatives prior to excretion.

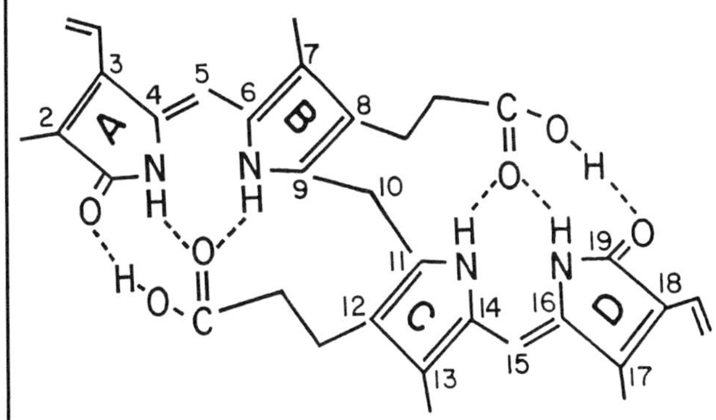

Fig. 9.19. 4*Z*,15*Z*-bilirubin IXα, the most prominent physiological isomer of bilirubin in humans.

Binding and transport

Each albumin molecule possesses a single high-affinity (7×10^7 M^{-1}) binding site for one molecule of bilirubin. This strong binding results in essentially all bilirubin being transported to the liver bound to albumin, with negligible amounts free to diffuse into other tissues. Secondary binding sites of lessor affinity also exist on albumin. Other substances (e.g. fatty acids, sulfonamides, ceftriaxone, and other drugs) are also bound to bilirubin and potentially can displace bilirubin.

Hepatic uptake

A receptor in the plasma membrane of the hepatocyte facilitates uptake of bilirubin and is competitively inhibited by bromsulfophthalein and indocyanin green. Once within the hepatocyte, bilirubin is bound by glutathione *S*-transferase B (GST), traditionally referred to as ligandin. The affinity of purified GST for bilirubin

($K_a = 10^6$), is less than that of albumin; however, GST is believed to be of importance in preventing bilirubin and its conjugates from refluxing back into the circulation.

Conjugation

Bilirubin is conjugated with glucuronic acid within the endoplasmic reticulum of the hepatocyte. Bilirubin glucuronosyltransferase (BGT) is the enzyme responsible for this conjugation. Uridine diphosphate glucuronic acid (UDPGA) is the glucuronic acid donor. Several different classes of glucuronosyltransferases, with different substrate specificity, have been described. Catalysis of bilirubin by BGT results in both mono- and diglucuronides of bilirubin. BGT activity for bilirubin can be induced by narcotics, anticonvulsants, contraceptive steroids, and bilirubin itself. Alternatively, BGT activity can be decreased by caloric and protein restriction. BGT is present in human fetal liver at levels approximately 0.1 percent of adult values. At 30 weeks of gestation BGT begins to increase and reaches approximately 1 percent of adult values by 40 weeks. BGT activity increases postnatally, and by 14 weeks plateaus at adult values.

Secretion, reabsorption and excretion

Following bilirubin conjugation, the bilirubin mono- and diglucuronides are secreted into bile via the biliary canaliculus. In normal adult duodenal bile, 70–90 percent of the bile pigments are bilirubin diglucuronide, and 7–27 percent are bilirubin monoglucuronides. Smaller amounts of other bilirubin conjugates are also seen. In infants excretion of bilirubin diglucuronide is decreased with a concomitant increase in monoglucuronides, consistent with decreased BGT activity. After the first week of life secretion of bilirubin conjugates by the hepatocyte is the rate-limiting step in bilirubin clearance. Canalicular secretion of bilirubin conjugates can be increased by choleretic agents (e.g. phenobarbital) and decreased by cholestatic agents (e.g. estrogens and anabolic steroids) or pathological conditions (e.g. liver disease).

Once bilirubin conjugates reach the intestine, several metabolic alternatives arise. In adults and older infants, intestinal bacteria hydrogenate various carbon double bonds in bilirubin to produce urobilinogens. Subsequent oxidation of the C-10 carbon produces the related urobilins. These reduction–oxidation products of bilirubin, known collectively as urobilinoids, are excreted in the feces. ***Clostridium ramosum*** is the most important bacterium for urobilinoid production, and ***Escherichia coli*** acts synergistically. The conversion of bilirubin conjugates to urobilinoids prevents the intestinal absorption of bilirubin known as the enterohepatic circulation. Because neonates lack intestinal bacteria, they are more susceptible to bilirubin reabsorption.

Alternatively, intestinal bilirubin conjugates can act as substrate for either bacterial or tissue β-glucuronidase. This ubiquitous enzyme cleaves glucuronic acid from bilirubin glucuronides, producing unconjugated bilirubin, which is more easily absorbed from the intestine. In the fetus, tissue β-glucuronidase, which is detectable by 12 weeks of gestation, is believed to play an important role in facilitating intestinal bilirubin absorption, which enables bilirubin to be cleared via the placenta. Bilirubin glucuronides are present *in utero* by 22 weeks of gestation. The effectiveness of bilirubin clearance via the placenta is shown by the fact that almost all infants are born nonicteric, even if they go on to develop severe hyperbilirubinemia in the first days of life. Lacking placental assistance, the neonate with increased intestinal β-glucuronidase is at risk for higher serum bilirubin concentrations.

Jaundice

Most, if not all infants will develop bilirubin concentrations greater than 1.4 mg/dl during the first week of life. This common observation has led to the term 'physiological jaundice'. Serum concentrations of bilirubin greater than 7 mg/dl result in visible jaundice or icterus, which develops in a cephalopedal manner. Moderate jaundice (bilirubin >12 mg/dl) occurs in at least 12 percent of breast-fed infants and 4 percent of formula-fed infants, while severe jaundice (>15 mg/dl) occurs in 2 percent and 0.3 percent of these feeding groups, respectively.

Total serum bilirubin includes two fractions: conjugated bilirubin (so-called 'direct' reacting because color development takes place directly without the addition of methanol in van den Bergh's test), and unconjugated bilirubin ('indirect' fraction). Traditionally the terms 'direct' and 'indirect' are used interchangeably with conjugated and unconjugated bilirubin, although it is now recognized that this is not quantitatively correct. Jaundice can result from elevation of either of these fractions. Serum bilirubin measurements are most commonly made with automated laboratory methods. Erroneously elevated direct fractions have been seen with high total bilirubin concentrations.

Neonatal jaundice can result if bilirubin is excessively produced or inadequately excreted. Recent reviews of this broad subject have been published elsewhere. Pathological neonatal jaundice is a concern because of the deleterious effects of high unconjugated bilirubin concentrations on the central nervous system known as *kernicterus* or *bilirubin encephalopathy*. Therapeutic options to lower serum bilirubin concentrations include phototherapy, exchange transfusion, interruption of the enterohepatic circulation, induction of BGT, interruption of breast-feeding, and inhibition of heme oxygenase. Phototherapy is effective because light produces isomers of bilirubin (lumirubin, and *E* isomers), which disrupt the internal H^+ bonding and allow direct excretion into bile without conjugation.

Selected reading

Gourley GR, Odell GB. Bilirubin metabolism in the fetus and neonate. In Lebenthal E, ed. *Human gastrointestinal development*. New York: Raven Press, 1989: 581.

Maisels MJ, ed. Neonatal jaundice. *Clin Perinatol* 1990; **17**: 245.

McDonagh AF, Lightner DA. 'Like a shrivelled blood orange'—bilirubin, jaundice and phototherapy. *Pediatrics* 1985; **75**: 443.

Odell GB, Schutta HS. Bilirubin encephalopathy. In McCandless DW, ed. *Cerebral energy metabolism and metabolic encephalopathy*. New York: Plenum Publishing Corp., 1985: 229.

P. Nutritional Requirements

B Specker

Nutrient requirements can be considered in three broad categories. First, **macronutrients** including carbohydrates, fats, and proteins serve as energy substrates. The proportion of total energy needs provided by each type of macronutrient varies tremendously in different cultures and socioeconomic groups. Second, **minerals** including Ca^{2+}, PO_4, and Mg^{2+} are required to synthesize bone. Third, specific components of foods that cannot be synthesized by the human body, **vitamins or trace metals**, are required in small amounts for synthesis of other structures, such as iron and hemoglobin, or to facilitate specific biochemical reactions. Water and electrolyte requirements are discussed in Chapter 14. Deficiencies due to inadequate intake, malabsorption, or inappropriate losses of these micronutrients result in the characteristic patterns of diseases discussed briefly in this chapter.

The macronutrient requirements for growth and development have been well established. However, the ideal ratio of carbohydrate, fat, and protein intake remains controversial. The Recommended Dietary Allowances (RDAs), which are set by the Committee on Dietary Allowances of the Food and Nutrition Board of the National Academy of Sciences, are defined as 'the levels of intake of essential nutrients, on the basis of current scientific knowledge, to be adequate to meet the known nutrient needs of practically all healthy persons'. These recommended values do not represent optimal or ideal intakes, but rather represent amounts required for the average American individual of a specific age and sex. Recommended micronutrient amounts, in fact, are set at a high value to provide a margin of safety, covering the range in the entire population. The values change with illness or other specific defects in absorption of specific nutrients. These nutrient requirements are readily available in several pediatric and nutrition textbooks.

Macronutrients

Energy requirements

Energy is supplied to the infant and child from protein, carbohydrates, and fat. The distribution of these macronutrients in the diet varies depending upon the food. The energy value of food is typically expressed in terms of heat units or **kilocalories (kcal)**; a kilocalorie is defined as the amount of energy necessary to raise the temperature of 1 kg of water by 1°C. The *Système International* (SI) unit of measure for energy is the **kilojoule** (kJ; 1 kJ = 0.24 kcal). During combustion, these energy sources are oxidized to CO_2 and water. The ratio of CO_2 produced/O_2 consumed is termed the respiratory quotient (RQ).

$$RQ = CO_2 \text{ produced}/O_2 \text{ consumed}$$

The amount of energy produced per liter of O_2 consumed is approximately the same for all three nutrients; the amount of energy produced per liter of CO_2 produced is higher for fats and lower for carbohydrates.

Indirect calorimetry, used to determine food energy utilization and requirements, involves measurement of O_2 consumption and CO_2 production following the ingestion of a known quantity of macronutrients. Studies using indirect calorimetry have been used to established energy requirements in infants and children. Energy requirements, which vary throughout infancy and childhood as a result of differing needs, are the sum of basal metabolism (resting energy expenditure, or REE), growth of tissues, physical activity, and thermic effect of ingested foods. During the first year of life, the energy required for growth exceeds that required for any other use. After the child reaches ~15 kg, the growth rate decreases and the REE accounts for the largest component of the total energy requirement. REE accounts for 30 percent of the total energy needs, followed by energy required for physical activity and growth.

Protein

Protein is essential for the synthesis of enzymes, transport proteins, and other structural components of cells. Proteins supply necessary nitrogen and amino acids. Nitrogen is not stored and must be replaced continuously.

Although the body can synthesize and interconvert many of the amino acids, nine cannot be synthesized by the human and must be supplied in the diet. These **essential amino acids** include histidine, isoleucine, leucine, lysine, methionine, phenylalanine, threonine, tryptophan, and valine. Taurine, an amino acid present in high concentrations in human milk, appears to have a low endogenous synthesis. Although taurine may be necessary for functional aspects of the brain, retina, heart, and liver, a deficiency state has not been identified and its essentiality has not been established.

Serum albumin, transferrin, thyroxine-binding prealbumin, and retinol-binding protein are often used to assess visceral protein status. However, these proteins are not always specific indicators of protein status; concentrations also are affected by altered metabolism from trauma, stress, sepsis, or hypoxia, by specific deficiency of plasma proteins caused by protein-losing enteropathy and liver disease, by capillary permeability changes, or by reduced synthesis from inadequate energy intake, electrolyte deficiency, trace element deficiencies (e.g. iron and zinc), or vitamin deficiency (e.g. vitamin A).

Although some studies have indicated that a deficiency of protein, rather than energy, is the most common factor limiting growth in infants and children, few objective criteria exist for assessing the adequacy of dietary protein and amino acids. The classic features of *kwashiorkor,* the clinical syndrome that results from dietary protein deficiency, include irritability, edema, hypoproteinemia, and hypoalbuminemia. Skin abnormalities also occur, including hyperpigmentation, hyperkeratosis, desquamation, and ulcerated lesions. Hair becomes sparse and depigmented. Subcutaneous fat stores are preserved and peripheral edema occurs, making it difficult to diagnose kwashiorkor from anthropometric measurements such as weight. *Marasmus,* or nonedematous protein energy malnutrition, is primarily a deficiency of total calories in which there is severe wasting with little edema.

Carbohydrate

Carbohydrates are needed for the synthesis of nucleic acids and glycoproteins. Twenty-four to 50 percent of the infant's energy needs are provided by dietary carbohydrates. Glucose, fructose, and galactose are produced by the digestion of dietary carbohydrates, as discussed in Section 9F.

Deficiency of carbohydrates does not occur in healthy human milk-fed or formula-fed infants. Incomplete absorption may occur with rapid transit time, impaired digestion (*disaccharidase deficiency* or *pancreatic insufficiency*), or reduced absorptive surface area (*mucosal atrophy* or *short bowel*). An osmotic diarrhea may occur if excessive amounts of carbohydrates are consumed, overwhelming the absorptive mechanisms.

Fat

Fats, the main energy source of the infant, are essential to normal development. Fatty acids are necessary for brain development and are an integral part of all cell membranes. Unlike proteins and carbohydrates, fat can be stored in the body in nearly unlimited amounts and is an important source of stored energy.

The major lipid classes consist of glycerides, phospholipids, sterols, and fatty acids. Glycerides are the result of esterification of glycerol and fatty acids. Three forms occur in nature: monoglycerides, diglycerides, and triglycerides. These compounds result from ester links between glycerol and one, two, or three fatty acids, respectively. Triglycerides, the most abundant lipid in animal tissue, serve as an important energy source. Phospholipids are found in all biological membranes and are important in oxidative phosphorylation, membrane transport, and electron transport reactions. Phospholipids may be subdivided into three classes: derivatives of glycerol 3-phosphate, sphingosine, and glycolipids. Sterols are alcohols with a cyclopentanoperhydrophenanthrene skeletal structure. Cholesterol is the principal sterol.

Fatty acids are a major energy source and serve as precursors of prostaglandins. Most naturally occurring fatty acids are straight-chained saturated or unsaturated acids containing an even number of carbon atoms. Palmitic acid and stearic acid are by far the most commonly occurring and widely distributed saturated fatty acids. The nomenclature of unsaturated fatty acids specifies the total number of carbon atoms and the total number of double bonds present. Families of unsaturated fatty acids are defined based on the location of the first double bond, counting from the methyl, or ω terminus. Oleic (ω9 family) and linoleic acid (ω6 family) are the most common unsaturated fatty acids. Linolenic (ω3 family) and linoleic acids are considered essential fatty acids and must be supplied in the diet. It has been estimated that 1–4 percent of total fat intake should consist of polyunsaturated fats from the ω6 family. An elevated triene/tetraene ratio (>0.4) is used as an indicator of essential fatty acid deficiency. The rationale for the use of this ratio is that although the ω9, ω6, and ω3 fatty acids all compete for the same desaturase enzymes in their respective metabolic pathways, ω6 and ω3 fatty acids have a greater affinity for the desaturase that forms tetraene than do ω9 fatty acids. Therefore, when the diet is deficient in linoleic acid (ω6 fatty acid), tetraene production is diminished and production of trienes from ω9 fatty acids is increased. Linolenic acid and its longer-chained derivatives (in particular docosahexaenoic acid) are important to brain development, cell proliferation, myelination, and retinal functions. The developing central nervous system incorporates significant amounts of polyunsaturated fatty acids of 20 carbons or greater; it has been speculated that preterm infants may not be able to desaturate and chain-elongate 18-carbon polyunsaturated fatty acids for several weeks to months following birth.

Water-soluble vitamins

Vitamin C (ascorbic acid)

Ascorbic acid is involved in the synthesis of neurotransmitters, may play an important role as an antioxidant, and is important in enhancing hydroxylation reactions of many biosynthetic reactions, such as *p*-hydroxyphenylpyruvic acid oxidase. Deficiency of ascorbic acid results in petechial hemorrhages and *scurvy*. Infantile scurvy may present with findings of tenderness, swelling, and pseudoparalysis of the lower extremities. Failure to thrive is a common characteristic of preterm infants with scurvy.

Ascorbic acid requirements of preterm infants may be greater than those of term infants due to the hyperoxic environment resulting from mechanical ventilation and transient tyrosinemia and/or relatively high protein intake. Ascorbic acid concentrations of milk are reduced by pasteurization and exposure to iron, copper, and O_2. High ascorbic acid intake may result in acidosis, decreased vitamin B_{12} absorption, and enhanced iron absorption.

Vitamin B_1 (thiamin)

Thiamin is absorbed by both passive and active transport in the small intestine and is phosphorylated in the intestinal mucosa to form thiamin pyrophosphate and adenylic acid. Thiamin functions as a coenzyme in the metabolism of branched-chain amino acids and of carbohydrates, such as the oxidative decarboxylation of α-keto acids and pyruvate and transketolase reactions of the pentose pathway.

Deficiency of thiamin during infancy results in *beriberi* and is accompanied by apathy, anorexia, vomiting, and restlessness, which can lead to dyspnea, cyanosis, and congestive heart failure. Thiamin is inactivated by alkaline solutions, heat, and ionizing radiation. No toxic effects have been noted with high oral doses of thiamin.

Riboflavin

Riboflavin, as part of the coenzymes flavin adenine dinucleotide (FAD) and flavin mononucleotide (FMN), is involved in metabolism of glucose, fatty acids, and amino acids. Riboflavin deficiency results primarily in abnormalities involving the epithelium (stomatitis, cheilosis, glossitis, seborrheic dermatitis), normocytic anemia, and vascularization of the cornea.

Biochemical riboflavin deficiency, without any clinical signs, has been reported in term infants fed human milk during phototherapy: riboflavin is inactivated by light, particularly that emitted from phototherapy. Toxicity of riboflavin is unlikely in term infants because excess riboflavin can be excreted by the kidney. This may not be the case in preterm infants because renal clearance of riboflavin may be inadequate.

Vitamin B_6 (pyridines)

Pyridoxine (pyridoxol), pyridoxal, and pyridoxamine are the three naturally occurring pyridines. Vitamin B_6 refers to these three pyridines, in addition to the phosphates of the latter two, pyridoxal-5-phosphate and pyridoxamine-5-phosphate, which are the major forms of vitamin B_6 found in blood. Vitamin B_6 is important in the biosynthesis of heme and prostaglandins, carbohydrate metabolism, immune development, and conversion of tryptophan to niacin and serotonin.

Vitamin B_6 deficiency in infants may result in hypochromic microcytic anemia, vomiting, diarrhea, failure to thrive, listlessness, hyperirritability, and seizures. *Pyridoxine-dependent seizures in the neonate, pyridoxine-responsive hypochromic microcytic anemia, xanthurenic aciduria, cystathioninuria,* and *homocystinuria* are syndromes that require pharmacological doses of vitamin B_6 for adequate function. High dietary protein intakes increase the need for vitamin B_6, which is destroyed upon exposure to light. Pyridoxine is used for fortification due to the sensitivity of pyridoxal and pyridoxamine forms to heat. Vitamin B_6 deficiency may occur during isoniazid treatment (binding of drug to vitamin) or when an infant is fed human milk from a vitamin B_6-deficient mother or exclusively breast-fed for extended periods of time (low vitamin B_6 content in milk). Although high doses of pyridoxine do not appear to be toxic, there is a report of sensory neuropathy in adults ingesting megadoses of pyridoxine.

Vitamin B_{12} (cobalamin)

Vitamin B_{12} is necessary for DNA synthesis and red blood cell formation. The initial release of cobalamin from dietary proteins is facilitated by gastric acid and pepsin. Cobalamin binds to R proteins (haptocorrin) in the stomach, because their affinity for cobalamin is greater than that of intrinsic factor. R proteins are found in saliva, gastric juice, and biliary secretions. Whether cobalamin binds to R proteins, however, depends upon the oral dose of cobalamin, gastric pH, and the amount of R proteins and intrinsic factor present. Pancreatic proteases degrade R proteins and release cobalamin, which then avidly binds to intrinsic factor and resists digestion by proteases. Intrinsic factor is synthesized by gastric parietal cells and protects cobalamin from bacteria within the intestinal lumen. The cobalamin-intrinsic factor complex binds to specific receptors in the distal small intestine, a process that requires Ca^{2+}, but not energy. The complex is believed to be taken up by the enterocyte and split intracellularly, although intrinsic factor is not absorbed into the blood. Cobalamin then binds to transcobalamin II either within or at the serosal surface and is released into plasma. Release may occur through receptor-mediated endocytosis. When large amounts of cobalamin are ingested, passive diffusion along the length of the small intestine can also occur. Studies in piglets suggest that sows' milk contains a cobalamin-binding protein that promotes cobalamin uptake in newborn piglets more effectively than intrinsic factor.

Vitamin B_{12} deficiency may result from congenital defect in absorption and metabolism (lack of intrinsic factor, inborn error of metabolism), surgical resection of terminal ileum (necrotizing enterocolitis, malformations), or bacterial overgrowth in the ileum. Nutritional deficiency occurs exclusively in infants fed human milk from strict vegetarian mothers. Manifestations of vitamin B_{12} deficiency include megaloblastic anemia and demyelinization of the spinal cord. In adults, administration of large doses of folic acid may mask vitamin B_{12} deficiency and cause irreversible neurological damage. Toxicity from vitamin B_{12} has not been reported.

Niacin

The term niacin refers to nicotinic acid and nicotinamide. Nicotinamide, the predominant form of the vitamin, is a component of the coenzymes nicotinamide adenine dinucleotide (NAD) and nicotinamide adenine dinucleotide phosphate (NADP). Niacin is involved in numerous metabolic processes including fat synthesis, glycolysis, and intracellular respiration. Because of the role of NAD and NADP in the respiratory chain, the allowances for niacin are related to energy expenditure. Approximately 3 percent of dietary tryptophan is converted to niacin in adults; however, there are no data on this conversion in infants.

Deficiency of niacin results in *pellagra,* which is characterized by a cutaneous inflammation, weakness, inflammation of mucous membranes, diarrhea, vomiting, dysphagia, and in severe cases, dementia. Excessive amounts of niacin may result in cutaneous vasodilation, reduced serum cholesterol concentrations, arrhythmias, abnormal liver function tests, jaundice, increased gastric acid secretion, and gastrointestinal hypermotility.

Biotin

Biotin is a coenzyme that is important in fat and carbohydrate metabolism as a component of several carboxylase enzymes. Under normal conditions, biotin deficiency is not common. Biotin is produced by intestinal bacteria, and the use of antibiotics may decrease biotin synthesis by intestinal flora. There are no reports of toxicity from biotin.

Folic acid

Folate is a coenzyme necessary for many of the reactions in the synthesis of nucleic acids and in the metabolism of some amino acids. Risk factors for folate deficiency are prematurity (rapid growth and decreased hepatic stores), hemolytic disease of the newborn (increased erythropoiesis), anticonvulsant therapy (interference with digestion), prolonged use of antibiotics (decreased production from intestinal bacteria), and any malabsorption syndrome. Manifestations of folate deficiency include, in order of appearance: low serum folate, hypersegmentation of neutrophils, low red cell folate, and macrocytic anemia. Poor growth has been found in some studies. No toxic effects have been reported for folate; however, theoretically, large amounts of folate may partially reverse the anticonvulsant effect of diphenylhydantoin and phenobarbital.

Pantothenic acid

The primary role of pantothenic acid is its incorporation into coenzyme A, the active factor required for metabolic acetylation processes. Deficiency of pantothenic acid is rare in the human, but may accompany severe malnutrition. Very high doses of pantothenic acid may result in diarrhea.

Fat-soluble vitamins

Fat malabsorption occurs due to a variety of defects including bile acid deficiencies due to liver disease or bacterial overgrowth of the bowel, pancreatic enzyme deficiencies, and disorders of mucosal function such as celiac disease. Fat-soluble vitamin deficiencies may occur in any of these clinical settings.

Vitamin A

Vitamin A exists in several isomeric forms: the basic component of vitamin A is all-*trans* retinol. Retinol is absorbed in the small intestine, incorporated into chylomicrons, and transported to the liver where it is stored and mobilized as a specific complex of retinol-binding protein. Retinol, following isomerization and combination with opsin to form rhodopsin, facilitates visual processing in the rod cells of the retina. Retinol also appears to have a role in regulation and differentiation of epithelial cells. The classic signs of deficiency (night blindness, dry cornea, and perifollicular dermatitis) have no practical value in the newborn because overt clinical signs have not been reported. Newborns at risk for vitamin A deficiency are those with any form of fat malabsorption (decreased absorption), those born preterm (low hepatic stores), those with bronchopulmonary dysplasia (possible increased requirements due to the healing process), and those on total parenteral nutrition (adherence of vitamin A to plastic intravenous tubings). There is no evidence of dietary deficiency of vitamin A with either formula or human milk feeding of term infants.

Toxicity from vitamin A may occur. Acute toxicity has occurred from single doses of 100 000 IU or more given to infants and includes bulging cranial fontanelles accompanied by nausea, vomiting, fever and neurological symptoms. Symptoms of chronic toxicity include dry skin, alopecia, and headaches. Continued high doses can lead to hepatotoxicity and death.

Vitamin D

Vitamin D is necessary for maintaining Ca^{2+} and PO_4 homeostasis. Vitamin D is transported to the liver where it is converted to 25-hydroxyvitamin D (25(OH)D), which is often used as an indicator of vitamin D status. 25(OH)D is further converted in the kidney to 1,25-dihydroxy-vitamin D ($1,25(OH)_2D$), which is the most biologically active metabolite of vitamin D. The conversion of 25(OH)D to $1,25(OH)_2D$ is dependent upon the Ca^{2+}, PO_4, and parathyroid hormone (PTH) status of the individual. $1,25(OH)_2D$ increases intestinal absorption and decreases renal excretion of Ca^{2+} and PO_4. In conjunction with PTH, $1,25(OH)_2D$ also results in release of Ca^{2+} and PO_4 from bone. Deficiency of vitamin D results in disturbances of Ca^{2+} and PO_4 homeostasis and ultimately in *rickets*.

Theoretically, vitamin D is not a vitamin because it can be produced endogenously in the skin; therefore, it is more appropriately considered a hormone. If not obtained through the diet, vitamin D is produced endogenously in the epidermis of skin upon exposure to ultraviolet radiation. Unlike other vitamins, vitamin D is not present in significant amounts in naturally occurring food items except oily fish; human milk concentrations of vitamin D also are low. Sunshine exposure results in a significant increase in serum 25OH vitamin D concentrations to well within the range in which vitamin D deficiency is not observed. Vitamin D supplementation of human milk-fed infants who are not receiving sunshine exposure appears to be necessary to maintain adequate vitamin D status.

Alterations in the metabolism of vitamin D have been proposed as factors in the development of hypocalcemia or rickets in preterm infants. The administration of the biologically active vitamin D, both orally and intravenously, for the prevention of hypocalcemia has been investigated. However, only pharmacological doses have been found to be effective, and these doses are not recommended until possible long-term or subtle biological effects are investigated.

Vitamin E

Vitamin E comprises a group of fat-soluble compounds (tocopherols and tocotrienols) with similar biological roles. α-Tocopherol, the most active of these compounds, accounts for more than 90 percent of the vitamin E in human tissues. Due to the different biological activities of the different forms of vitamin E, preparations have been standardized to International Units. The primary role for vitamin E is as an antioxidant. Vitamin E scavenges free radicals that are generated by the reduction of molecular O_2 and as normal byproducts of oxidative enzymes; thus vitamin E inhibits the naturally occurring peroxidation of polyunsaturated fatty acids in the lipid layers of cell membranes.

Vitamin E status is assessed by measurement of tocopherol in blood. Due to the influence of circulating lipids on tocopherol concentrations, it is preferable to express plasma α-tocopherol as a ratio to cholesterol or total lipid. Vitamin E requirements are increased with high intakes of polyunsaturated fatty acids as well as in infants or children with fat malabsorption. Vitamin E requirements also are increased in preterm infants due to limited tissue stores at birth, poor absorption of fat, and rapid postnatal growth.

Vitamin E is toxic at pharmacological doses. A syndrome of pulmonary deterioration, thrombocytopenia, and liver and renal failure in very-low-birth-weight infants was associated with the use of parenteral α-tocopherol (E-ferol) in preterm infants. The risk of sepsis and necrotizing enterolitis also may be increased in preterm infants receiving high doses of vitamin E. Thus, extreme caution should be taken in treating infants with pharmacological doses of vitamin E.

Vitamin K

Vitamin K is necessary for hepatic synthesis of coagulation factors II, VII, IX, and X and for the conversion of inactive precursors to the active form of clotting factors. Vitamin K_1 (phylloquinone) is synthesized by plants, while vitamin K_2 (menaquinone) can be synthesized in animals. In normal adults, up to 50 percent of the total supply might come from intestinal synthesis by bacterial flora. Because the human infant has a very low storage capacity for vitamin K and the vitamin has a rapid turnover, the time required to reach a deficiency state is deemed to be short.

Vitamin K deficiency is associated with *hemorrhagic disease of the newborn (HDN)*. HDN has recently subdivided the disease into three categories: (1) early HDN, occurring within the first 24 hours of life and usually associated with maternal anticonvulsant therapy; (2) classic HDN occurring between 1 and 7 days of life; and (3) late HDN, occurring after 2–4 weeks of life, which is presently the most common form. Common factors associated with HDN are a low intake of vitamin K (no supplementation at birth and breast-feeding) and, as with all other fat-soluble vitamins, any form of fat malabsorption. There are few data on the toxicity of vitamin K in the human. There appears to be no toxicity from phylloquinone since it has become available for use as a prophylaxis.

Minerals

Calcium, phosphorus, magnesium

Ca^{2+}, PO_4, and Mg^{2+} are essential for tissue structure and function. Mineral absorption is discussed in Section 9F. Hypocalcemia in the neonatal period may result in seizures; several studies in human infants have shown electroencephalographic seizures during clinically asymptomatic hypocalcemia. Chronic deficiency of Ca^{2+} and PO_4 results in bone demineralization or *rickets*. Toxicity of Ca^{2+} results in high circulating concentrations of these minerals and possible nephrolithiasis, nephrocalcinosis, bradycardia, and hypertension. Blood concentrations of Ca^{2+}, PO_4, and Mg^{2+} are maintained within physiological ranges through the combined effects of parathyroid hormone (PTH), 1,25-dihydroxyvitamin D (the biologically active metabolite of vitamin D), and calcitonin. Chronic deficiency of Mg^{2+} may result in an inability to maintain serum Ca^{2+} within physiological ranges due to the parathyroid gland's Mg^{2+} requirement for normal functioning.

Cow's milk-based formula feeding during the first week of life appears to result in a higher serum PO_4 and possibly a lower serum ionized Ca^{2+} concentration than those found in infants fed human milk. Although the clinical significance of these findings is not clear, these studies support the hypothesis that infants fed formula containing high phosphate may be at increased risk for late neonatal hypocalcemia; however, because this disorder is rare, additional risk factors apparently must be present.

Additional Ca^{2+} and PO_4 in formula-fed, preterm infants appears to improve net Ca^{2+} retention and bone mineralization, as indicated by increased bone mineral content and lower serum alkaline phosphatase concentrations in infants receiving high Ca^{2+} and PO_4 formula compared with infants fed standard formula.

Trace elements

Trace elements by definition constitute less than 0.01 percent of body mass. Those considered essential include iron, zinc, copper, selenium, chromium, manganese, molybdenum, iodine, fluorine, and cobalt. Other trace elements may include arsenic, lithium, nickel, silicon, vanadium, bromium, cadmium, lead, and tin.

Iron

Many iron-containing compounds, such as hemoglobin, the cytochromes, and iron–sulfur proteins, are involved in transport and utilization of O_2 for the production of cellular energy. Ferritin and hemosiderin contribute to maintenance of iron homeostasis. There are marked age-related changes in hemoglobin concentrations following birth: high hemoglobin concentrations at birth, resulting from a relative hypoxic *in utero* environment, are followed by 4–6 weeks of a marked depression in the rate of red blood cell production and a decline in hemoglobin concentrations. At about 2 months of age, hemoglobin concentrations begin to rise. They plateau at 12.5 g/dl at about 6 months; concentrations are maintained at this level through age 4 years.

Iron deficiency, defined as a lack of iron resulting in a restriction of hemoglobin synthesis, usually is due to an iron-poor diet and rarely develops before 4–6 months of age. Ingesting cows' milk early in infancy also may result in iron deficiency from blood loss in the gastrointestinal tract. Iron stores may become marginal in unsupplemented human milk-fed infants or in unfortified formula-fed infants around 6 months of age. Because preterm infants have a lower iron store at birth than term infants, iron supplementation or introduction of iron-fortified formula should occur at an earlier age in this population.

Measurement of hemoglobin concentrations is one of the most useful laboratory assessments for *iron deficiency anemia*. Red cell indices also are important: mean red cell volume (MCV) decreases with or without a low mean red cell hemoglobin (MCH) in iron deficiency. Confirmatory findings include a low serum ferritin (depressed only in iron deficiency), elevated erythrocyte protoporphyrin (also occurs during infection or lead toxicity), or a low transferrin saturation (serum iron–iron binding capacity, which also can occur during infection).

Zinc

Zinc is an essential cofactor for many enzymes such as DNA and RNA polymerases and alkaline phosphatase. Zinc deficiency results in reduced growth velocity, acro-orificial skin rash, hypoproteinemia, and generalized edema. An autosomal recessive disorder, *acrodermatitis enteropathica,* results from a selective defect in intestinal absorption of zinc. Long-term, exclusively breast-fed infants as well as children consuming vegetarian diets may be at risk for zinc deficiency due to low dietary zinc. Zinc toxicity results in copper deficiency and increased cholesterol concentrations.

Copper

Copper is a coenzyme for many oxidative enzymes involved in collagen and melanin synthesis. In plasma, copper is bound to ceruloplasmin. In the fetus, copper is accumulated mainly in liver during the last trimester of pregnancy. Although preterm infants have smaller copper stores than term infants, their hepatic stores are significant. In the normal infant serum copper concentrations are very low due to limited ceruloplasmin synthesis. Therefore, neither serum copper nor ceruloplasmin concentrations appear to be good indices of copper status. *Menke disease* is an inheritable, X-linked, recessive disorder of copper absorption. Abnormalities include hypopigmentation, bone changes, thrombosis, arterial rupture, progressive cerebral degeneration, and hypothermia. Both serum copper and ceruloplasmin concentrations are very low. *Wilson disease* is a disorder of copper balance. Copper absorption is thought to be normal, but biliary secretion is impaired and large amounts of copper accumulate in the body. Abnormalities include hepatitis, central nervous system impairment, bone demineralization, ophthalmic abnormalities, and hemolytic anemia. Copper toxicity is rare in humans.

Selenium

Selenium is an important part of the enzyme glutathione peroxidase (GSHPx), which is involved in protecting cells from oxidative damage by destroying cytosolic hydrogen peroxides. Selenium deficiency previously occurred in patients receiving total parenteral nutrition that was not supplemented with selenium and also occurs in free-living populations that reside in areas with low soil selenium concentrations. Clinical symptoms of deficiency include muscle pain and weakness predominantly in the extremities. *Keshan disease,* a selenium-responsive syndrome, has been found to occur in infants, young children and women of child-bearing age in rural China. The syndrome is characterized by necrosis and fibrosis of the myocardium resulting in acute or chronic heart failure. Erythrocyte fragility associated with low blood selenium concentrations also has been reported in orally fed preterm infants. Because selenium is highly toxic, blood concentrations are often monitored during supplementation; a concentration >800 ng/ml is considered hazardous to children. Symptoms of toxicity include loss of hair, roughening of nails, nausea, and fatigue.

Chromium

Chromium is important in glucose metabolism because it may potentiate the action of insulin at the cell membrane. Although very rare, chromium deficiency may result after long-term total parenteral nutrition when glucose is utilized as the major energy source. Chromium absorption is poor, and it is thought to be relatively nontoxic.

Manganese

Animal studies indicate that the most vulnerable period for manganese deficiency is during gestation and early infancy. Manganese is important in glycosoaminoglycan synthesis, carbohydrate metabolism, lipid metabolism, and central nervous system function. Clinical deficiency of manganese has not been observed in humans. Manganese homeostasis is regulated by the liver and large doses have been shown to cause mild intrahepatic cholestasis in animals.

Molybdenum

Molybdenum is involved in sulfur metabolism, where it is incorporated into three known enzymes: sulfite oxidase, xanthine oxidase/dehydrogenase, and aldehyde dehydrogenase. The most important, sulfite oxidase, catalyzes the oxidation of sulfite to sulfate, the terminal step in degradative sulfur metabolism. Molybdenum deficiency is uncommon, although there are several *inborn errors of molybdenum metabolism* (sulfite oxidase deficiency, xanthine oxidase deficiency, and combined deficiencies of sulfite and xanthine oxidases).

Iodine

The only known function of iodine is its integral part of the thyroid hormones. Iodine is readily absorbed and taken up by the thyroid gland where it is bound to thyroglobulin, an iodinated glycoprotein from which thyroxine (T_4) and triiodothyronine (T_3) are formed. The role of iodine in thyroid hormone synthesis is discussed in Chapter 7. *Iodine deficiency* is rare in regions where supplementation programs (addition to table salts) exist or where soil concentrations are high. Unfortunately, many areas of the world still have a high prevalence of dietary iodine deficiency resulting in goiter and neonatal deficiency. Excessive iodine results in *thyrotoxic goiter*; in the United States, goiter in children is now likely to be associated with higher-than-normal iodine intakes.

Fluoride

Fluoride is important in the prevention of *dental caries*; it strengthens dental enamel by substituting for hydroxyl ions in the hydroxyapatite crystalline mineral matrix of the enamel. Fluoride is incorporated into enamel during the mineralization stage, and the resulting fluorapatite is more resistant to both chemical and physical damage. Because the major source of fluoride is water, the need for supplementation will depend on the fluorine exposure of the child from the local water supply. Excessive fluoride results in fluorosis or mottling of the enamel. Acute ingestion of very large amounts of fluoride may cause cardiac and respiratory abnormalities and hypocalcemia.

Selected reading

Farrell PM, ed. Essentials of pediatric nutrition. In Rudolph AM, ed. *Rudolph's pediatrics*. 19th ed. Norwalk, CT: Appleton & Lange, 1991: 211.

Tsang RC, ed. *Vitamin and mineral requirements in preterm infants.* New York: Marcel Dekker, Inc., 1985.

Tsang RC, Nichols BL, eds. *Nutrition during infancy.* Philadelphia: Hanley and Belfus, Inc., 1988.

10 ♦ *Cardiovascular system*

Editor: Michael A Heymann

A. Vascular Physiology

A1. Vascular Growth

K R Stenmark, C L Cook and R A Majack

Vascular development begins early in embryogenesis. As morphogenesis of organs begins, vascular channels and capillary plexuses are established throughout stromal tissue, a process essential for continued development of the organ. Numerous studies have begun to elucidate the manner in which various tissues and organs are vascularized. Two separate processes of vascular development, resulting in apparently identical vessels, have been described (Fig. 10.1 schematically diagrams these processes). In the first model, termed **vasculogenesis**, pre-existing endothelial cell precursors or angioblasts are thought to assemble *in situ* to form primitive vascular channels. These channels remodel, giving rise to arteries, veins and lymphatics. The stimuli and information directing the angioblast to form a particular specialized channel apparently is contained within the surrounding mesenchyme at the site where vascular organization begins. The angioblasts, after organizing into a visible endothelium, either induce the expression of smooth muscle phenotype in the surrounding mesenchyme or recruit existing smooth muscle cells to the forming vessels. In the second model, termed **angiogenesis**, capillaries form by budding or sprouting from pre-existing venules or capillaries. The process of angiogenesis has received a great deal of attention both in embryogenesis as well as in physiological and pathophysiological states. Depending on the tissue studied, vasculogenesis and angiogenesis make greater or lesser contributions to the process of vascularization. There is a consensus that vascularization in the lung, pancreas, and spleen occurs by vasculogenesis, whereas angiogenesis is responsible for development of tissue vasculature in kidney, brain and retina.

As the organ, and thus blood vessels, continue to grow and develop, significant morphological, gene, protein, and functional changes occur in cells of the vessel wall. An understanding of the processes involved in normal vessel wall development is crucial because any external pathophysiological stimulus applied to this changing baseline will have a significant impact on the phenotypic expression of the vascular wall cell. Thus the characteristics of the vascular response to a given stimulus vary with age and state of vascular development at the time of onset of injury.

Normal vascular development: structure and function

Most studies of normal developmental changes in the vasculature have used rat aorta. In the rat embryo (term gestation 21–22 days), the tunica media develops around the endothelial tube at about 12.5 days of gestation when actomyosin filaments are first visible in a cell layer surrounding the endothelium. As development proceeds, cell proliferation continues, matrix protein synthesis begins, and lamellar units are established. While the basic structure of the rat aorta is developed by birth, growth of the aorta continues postnatally. Quantitative morphological analysis has indicated that the doubling of wall thickness that occurs in the rat aorta between 1 and 11 days of postnatal age is due to the combined effect of a nearly 2-fold increase in muscle cell volume, a 2.6-fold increase in the number of muscle cells, and 8- and 10-fold increases in the amount of elastin and collagen, respectively. The replication of **smooth muscle cells** within the aorta slows considerably between postnatal days 5 and 11 and declines to adult levels by 90 days. In normal adult animals, the replication index of smooth muscle cells in an uninjured vessel is only 0.06 percent per day. During normal development there is a progressive increase in the DNA ploidy of medial smooth muscle cells and the percentage of tetraploid (4N) cells reaches approximately 10 percent by 12 weeks of age. Virtually nothing is known concerning the significance of this developmental change in smooth muscle cell DNA content. There is a marked heterogeneity between the developmental responses of large and small vessels. Morphometric analysis of arteries less than 250 mm in outer diameter indicates that smooth muscle cell size, but not number, increases during postnatal development.

Extracellular matrix protein production by cells of the vascular wall also changes significantly during the course of normal development. The connective tissue elements of the vascular wall are complex and include molecules from virtually every class of extracellular matrix: elastin, collagens, proteoglycans, and structural and adhesive glycoproteins. The relative proportions of each matrix component appear to reflect either the physical and functional properties expected of a particular vascular segment or the forces to which that vascular segment is exposed. Vascular protein composition therefore changes significantly with development and with type and location of the vessel studied. For example, elastin is the most abundant protein in major arteries subjected to large pulsatile pressures generated by cardiac contraction. Elastogenic progenitor cells giving rise to at least some of the smooth muscle cells that constitute the aorta, and other elastic vessels, arise from mesenchyme adjacent to the myocardium. Elastogenic activity in these cells, at least in developing chick aorta, appears in an orderly, sequential proximal-to-distal deployment, beginning nearest the heart and advancing downstream into all nascent elastic vessels. The proportion of elastin in the vessel wall increases for a short and defined period after birth, then remains constant. No significant tropoelastin is produced by the normal adult vascular smooth muscle cells. As distance from the heart increases, a progressive decrease in the amount of elastin and a progressive increase in the amount of collagen are observed. Mature crosslinked collagen is much stiffer than elastin and thus confers different structural properties to the vessel wall. Collagens are an important family of structural proteins localized in the basement membrane and interstitial spaces of the vascular wall. Many excellent studies have evaluated accumulation of collagen in both systemic and pulmonary vessels during normal development. The amount of collagen in a vessel wall depends on both age and site of the vessel studied. Furthermore, the amount of this fibrous protein, like elastin, can be correlated with differences in vascular wall tension that normally occur in different arteries during growth.

Immunohistochemical studies have evaluated the appearance and distribution of various **collagen types** in the developing pulmonary artery. Particularly striking is the paucity of type I collagen in the newborn compared with the adult lung vessel. Little type I collagen is noted in either the media or adventitia of newborn vessel walls, whereas collagen types III and V were abundant. The interstitial collagens are deposited in the order of types V, III, and then I during embryonic development. The amount of types I and V collagen in pulmonary arterial media increases with age. Interesting functional implications can be drawn from these studies. Type I collagen is characterized by a high tensile strength; large quantities of this protein are prominent in tissues which are relatively indistensible. On the other hand, type III collagen is present in distensible connective tissue as is found in the uterus. The relative lack of type I collagen in neonatal pulmonary vessels may explain the plasticity of the pulmonary arteries in early life. Because not only do the cells composing the vessel wall change rapidly in shape and position during the first hours of life, but also the vessel walls themselves are continually remodeled with growth, these events may be facilitated by the lack of type I collagen. Although present in small amounts, type I collagen appears crucial for the maintenance of vascular integrity during normal development because mutant mice, deficient in type I collagen, die at about 15 days of gestation with ruptured major blood vessels.

Although it has been common to characterize all vascular smooth muscle cells as expressing a common secretory phenotype, the secretory properties of the smooth muscle cell may differ depending on location of the cell within the vessel wall. For instance, secretory properties of smooth muscle cells in small arteries differ from those in conducting vessels or in veins. Recent information suggests a complex heterogeneity of the secretory phenotype of smooth muscle cells at any particular location in the vessel wall. For instance, at certain stages of development in the pulmonary artery, some cells appear actively to produce elastin and collagen and demonstrate very little synthesis of contractile proteins, whereas other cells at the same vessel location express neither collagen nor elastin mRNA, but clearly produce contractile proteins (see Fig. 10.1).

Significant changes also occur in expression of **contractile and cytoskeletal proteins** during normal development. Morphological studies have demonstrated that the volume percentage of myofilaments in the aorta increased from 5 percent at birth to a maximum of 20 percent at 8 weeks of age. The noncollagenous, alkaline-soluble protein fraction of the vessel wall, which in part represents the contractile proteins, does not change after 10 weeks of age. Thus the net production of contractile protein increases during the first 10 weeks after birth and then remains constant. Biochemical studies demonstrating that neonatal rat aortic smooth muscle cells express primarily nonmuscle β-actin while adult smooth muscle cells express predominantly smooth

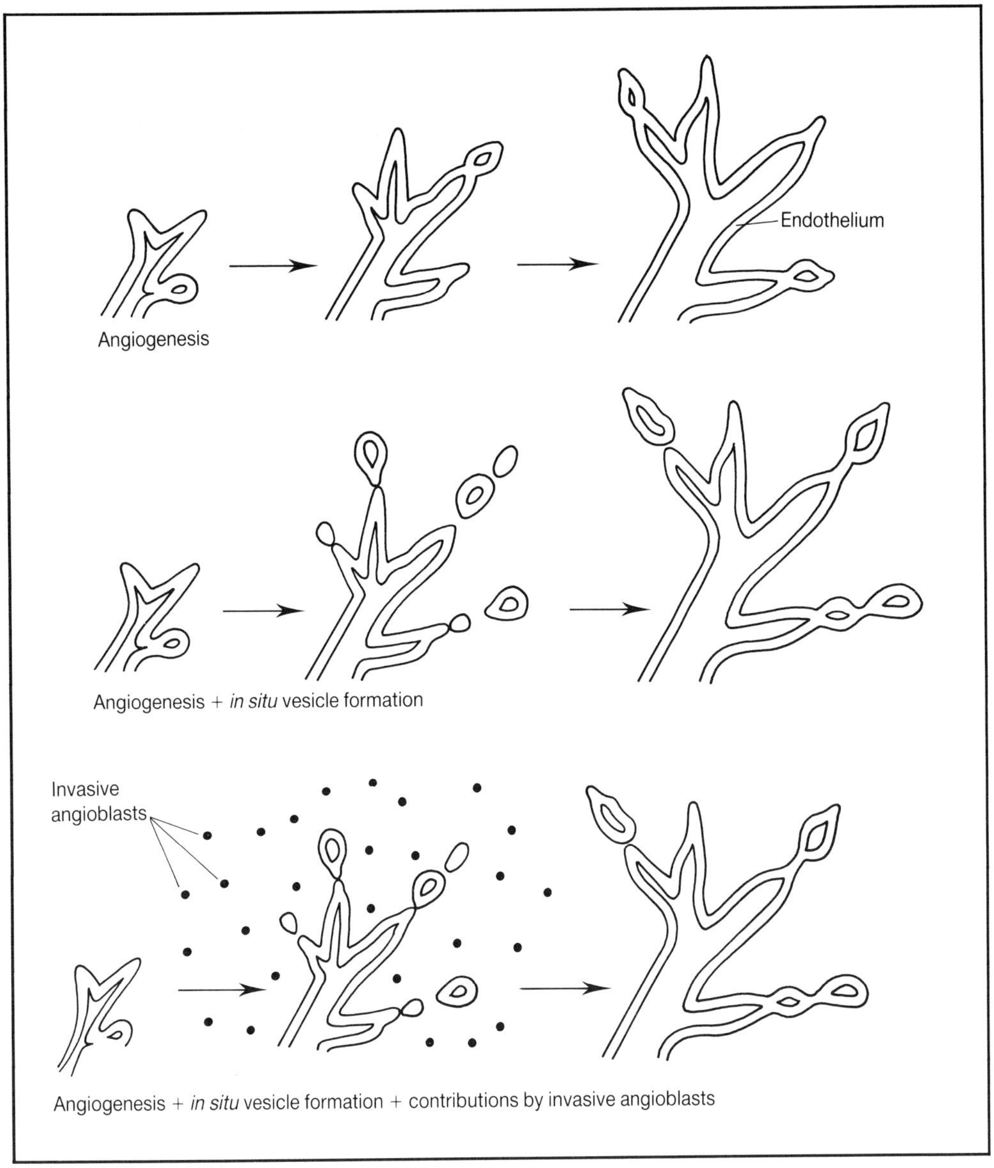

Fig. 10.1. Schematic representation of the processes by which embryonic blood vessels may develop. Angiogenesis results in the formation of sprouts and branches from existing branches. In some instances, endothelial vesicles form independent of existing vessels and subsequently all endothelial populations coalesce to form new channels. Developing vessels may be formed or receive contributions from invasive angioblasts (shown in black) that move throughout embryonic mesenchyme. (Redrawn from Noden DM, *Am Rev Respir Dis* 1989; **140**: 1097.)

muscle (SM)-specific α-actin isoforms confirm this observation. In addition to this shift from nonmuscle β-actin to the SM-specific form of α-actin during maturation, the cellular content of tropomyosin, vimentin, and desmin in aortic smooth muscle cells increases with age. Recently the SM2 isoform of SM-myosin heavy chain was found to be expressed only in adult blood vessels, while the SM1 isoform was found to be expressed earlier in development. Newborn rat aortic smooth muscle cells underexpressing α-actin isoforms exhibit a higher replication rate than α-actin positive cells, suggesting an inverse correlation between acquisition of the adult phenotype and cell replication.

Studies in the developing human aorta recently have evaluated expression of the regulatory contractile proteins, h-caldesmon and calponin, in conjunction with expression of α-SM-actin and SM-myosin heavy chain (SM-MHC). Actin and myosin are expressed far earlier in development than caldesmon and calponin, suggesting that these proteins, because they are involved in the regulation of contraction, may serve as markers of more highly differentiated smooth muscle cells. Interestingly, these investigations also confirm a heterogeneity of smooth muscle phenotypes even in the adult aortic vessel wall. In the subendothelial part of the adult tunica intima, smooth muscle cells expressed α-SM-actin and SM-MHC but lacked h-caldesmon and calponin, indicating a much less well differentiated phenotype of these cells. Neither the reasons for these differences nor the functional implications of the findings are known at present.

Clearly then, substantial differences exist in the proliferative, secretory, and contractile phenotypes of fetal and adult vascular wall cells. One may reasonably assume that many more such differences exist and that these differences may play pivotal roles in the control of smooth muscle cell replication and gene expression in the adult or fully differentiated vascular wall cell.

Significant changes also occur in the **functional responses** of the developing vessel to constrictor and dilator stimuli. Many of these changes are due to differences in ability to produce or respond to vascular wall constrictor and dilator stimuli. For instance, the maximum contractile response of vessel preparations demonstrates significant changes during development. Most work to date supports the hypothesis that the maximum contractile response, at least in conduit vessels, increases during early postnatal life and then either declines or remains unchanged at later ages. It has been suggested that in contrast to large vessels, small arteries do not undergo an increase in force-generating ability with development, though extensive work in this area has not been performed. Changes in maximum contractile response that occur during development are not due to changes in the active length–tension properties of the muscle. The increase in maximum response early in development might be explained in part by the increasing proportion of actomyosin. However, the decline in this response observed in older animals cannot be explained by a loss of contractile material. Different actin isoforms may interact differently with myosin, which could result in differences in force-generating ability. Also, the magnitude of change in maximum response with development depends on the contractile agent. This observation suggests that developmental changes in excitation, contraction, and coupling also occur. Changes in the ED_{50} value for various contractile agents have also been observed during development. Large vessels from young animals usually demonstrate a higher sensitivity.

Changes in the ability to contract may be significantly influenced by endogenous activity or locally produced products that control cAMP or cGMP levels in cells within the vessel wall. In ovine pulmonary vascular smooth muscle, for instance, basal adenylyl cyclase activity decreases markedly during the last trimester of fetal development. Further, but lesser, decreases are noted between late gestation and adulthood. Prostacyclin (PGI_2) production is threefold greater in late-gestation pulmonary artery than in the adult. Differences in the coupling of the β-adrenergic receptor to G-proteins (G_s vs G_i) in fetal versus adult smooth muscle have been identified. A predominance of G_i activity in fetal tissue, with resultant suppression of cAMP levels, has been observed. The ability of fetal endothelium to produce endothelial-derived relaxing factor (EDRF) is significantly less than the adult in response to at least certain agonists (e.g. acetylcholine). Changes in EDRF activity could account for some of the differences in response to agonists observed between fetal, neonatal, and adult tissues.

Factors influencing vessel growth and cell differentiation

Many factors contribute to regulation of new blood vessel growth. These factors influence cell number, production of extracellular matrix molecules, intracellular contractile proteins, and the state of cell differentiation. Among factors considered to have the strongest influence are growth factors, mechanical factors, the extracellular matrix, and intercellular interactions.

Regulation of cell proliferation

As stated above, active cell proliferation occurs during vascular development. For smooth muscle cells, this active replication state slows considerably at or about the time of birth, then virtually ceases under normal conditions. Thus two important concepts and the factors controlling them need to be described. First, the stimuli and factors responsible for cell proliferation must be characterized. Second, and very important for normal growth and development, are investigations of the mechanisms that regulate or suppress endothelial and smooth muscle cell replication once morphogenesis is complete.

Many studies have confirmed roles for various growth factors such as fibroblast growth factors (FGFs), type β transforming growth factors (TGFβs), the insulin-like growth factors (IGFs), platelet derived growth factors (PDGFs), and epidermal growth factors (EGFs) in influencing endothelial and smooth muscle cell proliferation *in vitro*; the *in vivo* roles of these factors during development have not been firmly established to date. However, because some of these growth factors play a role in vascular repair and disease, it is likely that they play a role in the developing vessel. Tables 10.1 and 10.2 list many locally produced and circulating factors known to influence vascular wall cell growth and matrix protein synthesis.

Fibroblast growth factors (FGFs)

Compelling evidence suggests a role for the FGF family in the control of vascular growth. The FGFs are a family of **mitogenic polypeptides** of which the prototypic members are the acidic and basic FGFs. There is a 53 percent sequence homology between basic and acidic FGF, and both are highly conserved among species. This group of growth factors was characterized and, in fact, initially purified on the basis of their strong affinity for the glycosaminoglycan heparin. A unique characteristic of acidic and basic FGFs is the absence of a consensus signal sequence for secretion; these factors therefore do not appear to be secreted from cells by conventional means. The majority of biologically active proteins in cells known to synthesize basic FGF remain cell associated or are deposited into the extracellular matrix. Immunohistochemical analysis has demonstrated the presence of basic FGF in basement membranes in the cornea and skeletal muscle, suggesting that extracellular matrix may serve as a reservoir for basic FGF.

The FGFs have a variety of actions on cells from both mesodermal and neuroectodermal origin. Both acidic and basic FGF are mitogenic and chemotactic for cells in the vascular wall, including large and small vessel endothelial cells, smooth muscle cells, and pericytes. FGF increases production of proteases by endothelial cells, a function probably important in the formation and remodeling of new blood vessels because movement of cells through the extracellular matrix requires breakdown of that matrix. Furthermore, a number of *in vivo* studies have demonstrated convincingly the ability of these factors to elicit the formation of new blood vessels. Both acidic and basic FGF are present in high amounts in the major vessels of embryonic rats by day 14 (by immunohistochemical staining) and continue to be expressed by vascular cells into adult life. In a transplanted rat embryo model, antibodies to basic FGF retarded growth of the

Table 10.1. Factors regulating vascular wall cell growth

Factors	EC	SMC	FIB
bFGF	↑	↑	↑
aFGF	↑	↑	↑
IGF-I	↑	↑	↑
IGF-II	↑	↑	↑
Insulin	↑	↑	↑
TGFβ*	↑/↓	↑/↓	↑/↓
TGFα	↑	ND	↑
PDGF	↔	↑	↑
EGF	↑	↑	↑
HB-EGF	↔	↑	ND
PD-ECGF	↑	↔	↔
V-EGF (VPF)	↑	↔	↔
Serotonin	↔	↑	ND
Histamine	↑	↑	ND
TNFα	↔	↓	↑
IL-1	↓	↑/↓	↑/↓
Heparan sulfates	↔	↓	↓
Interferons	↓	↓	↓
Prostaglandins (PGE_2, PGI_2)	↔	↓	↓
Leukotriene C_4 (LTC_4)	ND	↑	↑
PAF	ND	↑	↑

EC, endothelial cell; SMC, smooth muscle cell; FIB, fibroblast; ↑, stimulates cell growth; ↓, inhibits cell growth; ↔ no effect on cell growth; ND, effect not determined.
* The effects of TGFβ are complex and depend on age of cell and conditions of cell confluency under which experiment was done.

Table 10.2. Factors regulating vascular wall matrix protein synthesis

Factors	Elastin	Type 1 collagen
IGF-I	↑	↑
IGF-II	↑	↑
TGFβ	↑	↑
PDGF	ND	↑/↔
Leukotriene C_4 (LTC_4)	ND	↑
PAF	↑	ND
IL-1	↓	↑/↓ *
EGF	↓	↔
PGE_2	↔/↓	↓
Interferons	↓	↓
Protein kinase C activation	↓	↓

↑, stimulates matrix protein synthesis; ↓, inhibits matrix protein synthesis; ↔, no effect on matrix protein synthesis; ND, effect not determined.
* The effects depend on fibroblast type studied.

major vessels. In addition, these factors are important in *wound healing* and are associated with smooth muscle cells proliferation in *atherosclerotic plaque*. However, the mechanisms through which FGFs control vascular growth and differentiation remain to be determined.

Transforming growth factor β (TGFβ)

The TGFβ family contains nearly 20 members; evidence suggests that members of this family play an important role in the control of vascularization. TGFβ stimulates new vessel growth *in vivo*, yet can inhibit smooth muscle cell and endothelial cell proliferation *in vitro*. These two apparently divergent responses to TGFβ demonstrate the **importance of the microenvironment in which growth factors act** in determining the ultimate effect they have on cells. The angiogenic effect of TGFβ may be due to its extremely potent chemoattraction for monocytic cells that may mediate neovascularization by the release of other angiogenic factors. Thus *in vivo* TGFβ may induce new vessel growth through either a direct or indirect action on endothelial cells. Further evidence suggests that TGFβ is probably important during normal vascular wall development. These peptides are capable of controlling the proliferation, biosynthetic phenotype, and differentiation of a variety of cell types. The effects of TGFβ on vascular smooth muscle cells, for instance, are diverse and include control over gene expression, organizational behavior, connective tissue synthesis, cell hypertrophy, and cell proliferation. TGFβ is a bifunctional, density-dependent regulator of smooth muscle proliferation, the actions of which may be mediated through distinct receptor subtypes. In adult cells, TGFβ causes inhibition of growth in sparsely plated cells and stimulates growth in confluent cells. However, preliminary work suggests that TGFβ always causes inhibition of growth in neonatal cells.

Insulin-like growth factors (IGFs)

IGFs may play a role in vascular remodeling and, by analogy, in normal development of the blood vessel wall. IGF-I has mitogenic effects on aortic smooth muscle cells and significantly increases collagen and elastin production by smooth muscle cells as well as fibroblasts. Localization of IGF-I in the media by immunostaining varies with vascular load, suggesting that IGF-I expression is modulated by hemodynamic forces. IGF-I mRNA has been localized by *in situ* hybridization to adventitial areas of human fetal pulmonary arteries. Both porcine fibroblasts and aortic smooth muscle cells produce IGF-I *in vitro* and production by porcine aortic smooth muscle cells is stimulated by platelet derived growth factor. In addition to local production within the vessel wall, IGF-I is present in serum in concentrations up to 1000 ng/ml, and serum-derived IGF-I could have increased access to the vascular media in the presence of an altered endothelial barrier function. Importantly, vascular smooth muscle cells have receptors for IGF-I and IGF-II (type I and type II receptors), and receptor expression appears to vary during vessel development. Less is known regarding the role of IGF-II and blood vessel development. IGF-II expression precedes that of IGF-I in the developing vessel, and IGF-II recently has been shown to have significant effects on the proliferation of neonatal smooth muscle cells and fibroblasts, in addition to increasing elastin and collagen synthesis. The effects of IGF-II on vascular wall cells, however, appear to be mediated through the type I IGF receptor.

Platelet derived growth factor (PDGF)

PDGF, an extremely potent mitogen for vascular smooth muscle cells and fibroblasts, is a 30 kDa dimeric protein consisting of homo- or heterodimers of two distinct polypeptide chains (the A and B chains). Three isoforms, AA, AB, and BB, and two receptor subtypes have been described. The A chain recognizes the α-receptor, and the B chain, in contrast, binds to either the α- or β-receptor. The receptor protein is a glycoprotein with tyrosine kinase activity. The receptor kinase activity is believed to generate a mitogenic signal leading to DNA synthesis. PDGF is stored in platelets (α-granules), and PDGF-like molecules are known to be synthesized by endothelial cells, smooth muscle cells and activated macrophages. Growth factors, such as PDGF, produced locally in the vascular wall can act through separate receptors and signaling pathways to additively or synergistically effect cell proliferation. Figure 10.2 schematically diagrams the multiple pathways through which various stimuli can initiate cell proliferation.

A role for PDGF in regulation of vascular wall development is suggested by experiments documenting its effects on cultured smooth muscle cells. In addition to its potent mitogenic effects on mesenchymal cells, PDGF is chemotactic for a variety of cells including neutrophils,

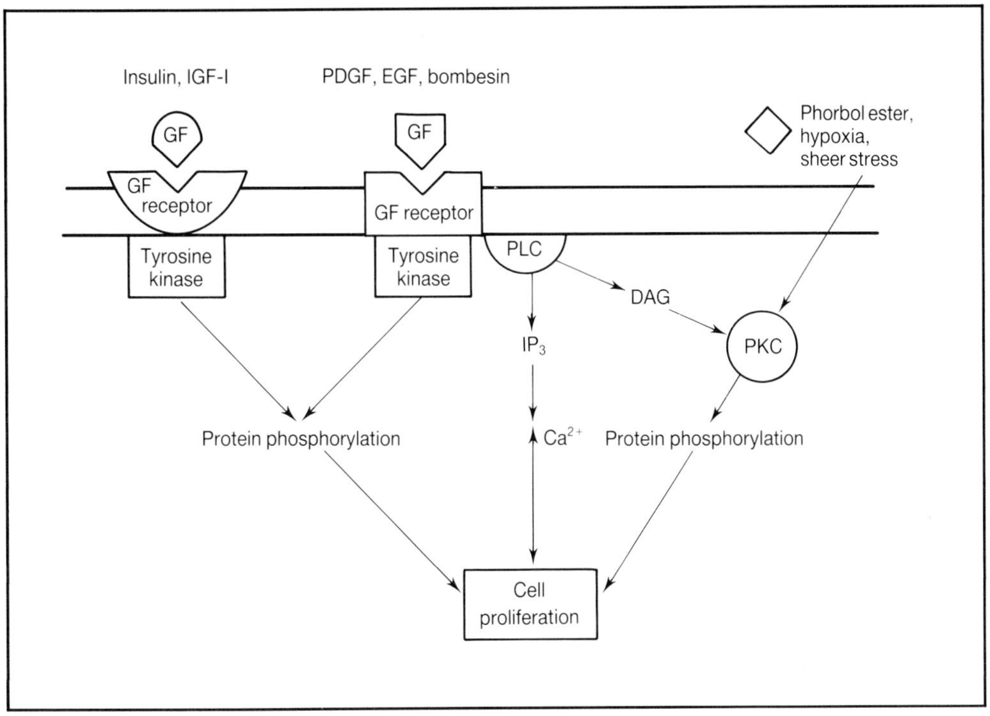

Fig. 10.2. Schematic representation of the multiple pathways through which growth factors and other stimuli can act to stimulate cell proliferation. For instance, IGF-I appears to stimulate cell proliferation through a PKC-independent pathway. When agents are present that activate PKC, marked enhancement of the IGF-I effects occurs.

monocytes, smooth muscle cells, and fibroblasts. These actions are not thought to be mediated through the tyrosine kinase receptor pathway. Furthermore a subtype of smooth muscle cells derived from neonatal rats express increased amounts of a PDGF-like mitogen. This neonatal smooth muscle cell subtype demonstrates autocrine growth characteristics, in contrast to the adult smooth muscle cells, suggesting a possible role for PDGF. Early mouse embryos express PDGF-AA and α-receptor mRNA. The appearance of the B receptor lags two days behind, and the PDGF-BB product still later in development. Therefore, there is evidence that PDGF is developmentally regulated and may play a role in the proliferative response of smooth muscle cells *in vivo* during normal and abnormal vascular growth.

Negative growth-control mechanisms

Cells in mature vessel walls normally exhibit a very low index of replication. In addition, smooth muscle cells in the vessel wall are highly resistant to tumor formation, suggesting that at least in these cells, potent growth suppressive activities exist. This suggests that strict growth-control mechanisms exist for smooth muscle cells of the adult vessel wall and that these mechanisms are largely absent in fetal (i.e. replicating) vessels or in neointima responding to atherosclerotic or other injurious mechanisms.

A variety of potential mechanisms (discussed below) may contribute to the establishment and/or maintenance of smooth muscle cell quiescence following development. Active growth arrest could occur in response to **inhibitors of smooth muscle cell replication** such as heparin-like glycosaminoglycans, TNFα, interferon-γ, or TGFβ. Further specific proteins from 'tumor suppressor' genes (e.g. p53 or the retinoblastoma gene) may be responsible for suppression of cell proliferation in adult cells. While smooth muscle cells are capable of expressing each of these factors, the timing and expression of these potential active growth inhibitors during development and the contribution of these factors to growth inhibition *in vivo* are not known. It is also clear that novel, as yet unidentified growth inhibitors, operative in the vessel wall, may also exist. Should growth arrest in the developing vessel wall be dependent on the induced synthesis of an active growth inhibitor, much further work will be required to determine the physical or biochemical signals (such as O_2 environment) underlying the induction of this factor.

Passive growth arrest might result from absence of growth stimulatory cytokines, growth factors, or their receptors. Little is known about the expression of growth factors, cytokines, or receptors during smooth muscle cell development and maturation. As mentioned above, cultured neonatal rat smooth muscle cells secrete a PDGF-like mitogen that is not secreted by cultured adult cells; however, the mRNAs for both chains of PDGF are not significantly different in neonatal versus adult vessels *in vivo*. As suggested above, IGF-II expression has been demonstrated in fetal, but not in adult arteries. Fetal smooth muscle cells have been suggested to grow in an autocrine fashion in culture. If early arterial development is characterized by autocrine smooth-muscle growth mechanisms, factors responsible for turning off expression of the autocrine factor must be identified.

Extracellular matrix-mediated growth arrest might occur indirectly as the result of alterations in the extracellular matrix, which collectively might constitute a growth-restrictive environment. Various studies have shown that the **extracellular matrix can exert significant effects on the replication of cells** in culture. Of particular relevance for the smooth muscle cells are thrombospondin (a growth factor-inducible matrix protein known to facilitate smooth muscle cell replication), heparin-like glycosaminoglycans (potent inhibitors of smooth muscle cell replication both *in vivo* and *in vitro*), and an uncharacterized heparin-inducible collagen, the synthesis of which correlates with heparin-regulated growth inhibition. In addition, immunolocalization studies have demonstrated that a heparan sulfate proteoglycan, potentially capable of inhibiting smooth muscle growth, is present in the endothelial basement membrane, thus placing this molecule in a strategic location to mediate endothelial–smooth muscle interactions during arterial morphogenesis.

Differentiation-mediated growth control might also play a role in the regulation of vessel wall growth. In many cell systems (e.g. skeletal muscle), terminal differentiation is accompanied by a complete loss of replicative ability. This does not seem to be true for vascular smooth muscle cells: following experimental arterial injury *in vivo*, fully 'differentiated' smooth muscle cells enter G_1 and S phase with kinetics comparable to cultured cells. G_1 and S are the first two stages of the cell cycle; thus 'differentiated' smooth muscle cells, in contrast to 'differentiated' skeletal muscle cells, can easily be induced to proliferate in response to many agonists. No consensus has yet emerged as to what constitutes a differentiated smooth muscle cell. Smooth muscle cells exist along a continuum from a relatively immature fetal state to a more mature adult state, but the functional significance of smooth muscle cell maturation in terms of growth control is not known. Interestingly, recent work has demonstrated that smooth muscle cells near the lumen even in adult vessels retain certain characteristics of fetal cells. It has been suggested that this may allow these cells to migrate more easily and replicate in response to injury. Possibly, maturation of the smooth muscle cell to an adult phenotype occurs concomitant with the acquisition of certain growth-restrictive characteristics conferred by the tunica media environment.

Regulation of connective tissue production

Elastin

In most mammalian tissues, the bulk of elastin production occurs during the fetal and neonatal periods and is essentially complete by the first decade of life. The temporal sequence of elastogenesis is unique in that elastic fibers are deposited during a defined developmental window, whereas many other extracellular matrix proteins are made and turned over continually. A number of factors have been demonstrated to participate in the normal regulation of tropoelastin expression. However, none has been definitively implicated in controlling elastin gene expression during normal vascular wall development.

The limited developmental expression of elastin indicates that a finely tuned and complex regulatory system controls production of this extracellular matrix protein. The microenvironment within which the elastin-producing cell exists certainly influences differentiation to the elastin phenotype and this induction involves signals which traverse to the cell surface. For instance, it has been shown that the developing elastogenic cell may have the capacity to create a microenvironment conducive to its own phenotypic differentiation by the production of an extracellular matrix which autocatalyzes the induction of elastogenesis. In addition, it has been shown that the mature elastic matrix can also stimulate tropoelastin synthesis by cells already producing elastin and can elevate the very low levels of elastin production noted in adult cells. Thus the tissue milieu influences both the start and maintenance of elastin production. In addition, cell–matrix contact is required for complete differentiation, suggesting strongly that a cell-surface molecule is involved as the instructive signal for elastogenesis.

Numerous other **factors** are **able to modulate elastin synthesis** in vascular wall cells. IGF-I stimulates tropoelastin synthesis and mRNA levels in neonatal arterial smooth muscle cells. IGF-I may be involved in embryonic production of elastin because the circulating concentration of and the hepatic mRNA levels for this cytokine correlate with tropoelastin synthesis in developing chick aorta. In addition, IGF-I mRNA levels in the embryonic chick aorta have been correlated with the onset of tropoelastin expression in this tissue. $TGF\beta_1$ has also been shown to enhance tropoelastin expression in neonatal arterial smooth muscle cells. No *in vivo* experiments have been done to confirm the role of $TGF\beta_1$ in normal vascular wall development, nor has it been convincingly demonstrated that $TGF\beta_1$ is required for the increased elastin deposition seen during vascular remodeling. During periods of elevated elastin deposition, increased expression of tropoelastin may be controlled by a soluble cytokine-like factor that may act in both an autocrine and paracrine fashion. This factor, called smooth muscle elastogenic factor (SMEF), is secreted by smooth muscle cells derived from the pulmonary arteries of calves with severe pulmonary hypertension. SMEF stimulates tropoelastin synthesis in actively producing cells and induces expression in pre-elastogenic cells. The biochemical properties of SMEF have not been characterized, although it is not thought to be one of the known cytokines capable of regulating elastin synthesis. Glucocorticoids have also been shown to increase elastin production and, notably, these compounds seem to be acting through age-specific mechanisms. Elastin-producing cells from the fetus or neonate demonstrate increased production of tropoelastin upon exposure to glucocorticoids. Glucocorticoids do not induce tropoelastin expression in pre-elastogenic cells or in fully differentiated adult cells.

Many factors have also been shown to down-regulate tropoelastin gene expression. Marked inhibition of tropoelastin synthesis and mRNA levels and elastin deposition in various cultured cells is mediated by epidermal growth factor, recombinant interleukin-1β (rIL-1), tumor necrosis factor α (TNFα), interferon-γ, 1,25-dihydroxyvitamin D_3 ($1,25(OH)_2D_3$) and the phorbol esters.

Thus, although both stimulators and repressors of tropoelastin production have been identified, the actual physiological action of these modulators is not known. Conditions such as the developmental stage, the composition of the extracellular matrix with which the cell interacts, the proliferative potential of the elastin-producing cells, the presence of migratory cells, and physical forces add to and complicate the influences affecting extracellular matrix gene activity.

Collagens

Factors controlling collagen formation during normal growth and development remain unclear. However, studies on cultured cells have provided some insights into factors that may be important in modulating at least type I collagen formation. TGFβ and insulin-related peptides are two substances that clearly can induce large increases in collagen formation by smooth muscle cells and fibroblasts in culture. Recent studies have also demonstrated that the potent inflammatory mediator leukotriene C_4 (LTC_4) can increase type I collagen formation. Many other molecules such as prostaglandin E_2 (PGE_2) and interferon-γ inhibit collagen accumulation. Thus the net accumulation of collagen, at least as it is controlled by cytokines, depends on the interaction of these and, of course, many other factors. Collagen accumulation and incorporation in the matrix is also limited by intra- and extracellular degradation of intact collagen fiber by enzymes. Newly synthesized collagen can be degraded intracellularly. Furthermore, although the assembly of collagen fibers involves the formation of crosslinks that render the collagen molecule relatively resistant to protease digestion, mature extracellular collagen can be degraded by several mammalian collagenases. $TGF\beta_1$, which stimulates the type I collagen gene, inhibits the expression of collagenase and transin/stromelysin, members of a family of matrix-degrading metalloproteinases. Also, $TGF\beta_1$ stimulates production of an inhibitor of the metalloproteinases (TIMP-1). The regulation of connective tissue synthesis and degradation within the vessel wall therefore appears to be well coordinated and controlled by a balance of stimulators, inhibitors, and degradation pathways of the collagen molecules.

Structural remodeling in vascular disease

Abnormal cell proliferation and connective tissue deposition by vascular smooth muscle cells characterizes both *atherosclerosis* and *hypertension.* Atherosclerotic lesions consist of a proliferation of smooth muscle cells in the intima of large vessels with concomitant lipid and connective tissue accumulation, producing enlargement of the atherosclerotic plaque and focal narrowing of the vascular lumen. In hypertension (pulmonary or systemic), cell proliferation and an increased connective tissue deposition can occur in any of the three vessel compartments (intima, media, or adventitia). The resulting increase in wall mass produces a diffusely narrowed lumen and a vessel with altered mechanical and functional properties. Common to both atherosclerosis and hypertension is a phenotypically altered smooth muscle cell that first appears to escape from its normal tightly controlled state of quiescence and then produces both more and different connective tissue components than do cells in the normal vessel.

Multiple changes in the phenotype of smooth muscle cells within the atherosclerotic plaque have been observed. Obviously these cells have escaped normal growth control mechanisms and have migrated and proliferated abnormally. Increases in elastin, collagen, and fibronectin synthesis have been documented by both immunohistochemical and *in situ* hybridization studies. Changes in the cytoskeletal and contractile phenotype of the smooth muscle cells within the atherosclerotic lesion have also been reported, with cells characterized as having 'fetal-like' characteristics.

A number of changes in the phenotype of the smooth muscle cell have also been documented during the development of *pulmonary hypertension* (Fig. 10.3). A newborn calf model of severe neonatal pulmonary hypertension induced by hypobaric hypoxia has demonstrated severe pulmonary vascular changes that mimic those found in forms of severe human neonatal pulmonary hypertension. A significant increase in smooth muscle cell and fibroblast proliferation occurs almost immediately after exposure of the newborn animal to hypoxia as opposed to cells in the normal developing pulmonary artery, which in the neonatal period have a low replication index. This marked hyperplastic response is seen in both large and small vessels of the hypertensive

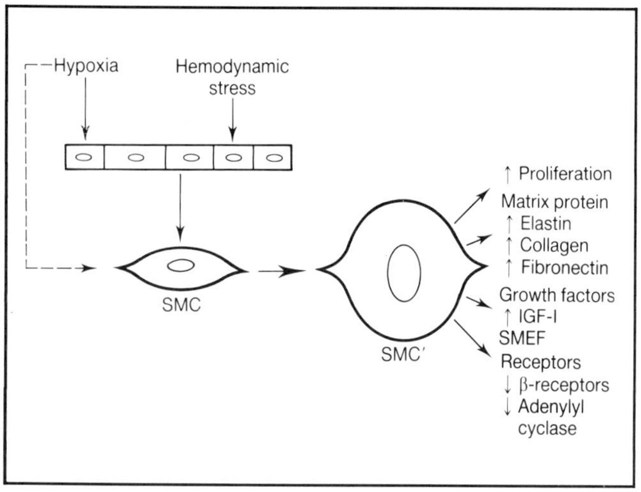

Fig. 10.3. Schematic representation of the phenotypic changes which occur in the pulmonary vascular smooth muscle cell (SMC) during the development of chronic hypoxic pulmonary hypertension. Hypoxia and/or hemodynamic forces act through the endothelial cell, or directly, to cause a 'transformation' of the smooth muscle cell. This cell exhibits several characteristics which are much different from the smooth muscle cell in the normal pulmonary artery.

pulmonary vascular bed. Moreover, when examined by *in situ* hybridization techniques, pulmonary arterial tissue from hypertensive calves exhibits a much different pattern of matrix protein gene expression than tissue from age-matched normal calves. In large vessels a marked decrease in tropoelastin mRNA expression occurs immediately after birth; this decrease in mRNA occurs in a radial fashion, progressing from the outer to the inner wall. In animals with severe neonatal pulmonary hypertension, on the other hand, the fetal and neonatal pattern of tropoelastin gene expression persists. This could have significant functional implications for the vessel wall and could also imply that other genes in the hypoxic pulmonary hypertensive animal may not undergo the same postnatal transition in gene expression that occurs during normal development. Animals developing severe neonatal pulmonary hypertension rapidly exhibit marked increases of type 1 collagen gene expression in the media and adventitia of the small pulmonary artery walls. As stated above, these rapid changes in collagen gene expression and collagen accumulation could have marked functional implications during this critical period of transition. A marked increase in wall stiffness would be expected, as well as an inability to adapt rapidly to the changes taking place in neonatal life. Interruption of the normal postnatal adaptation process by early injury may have long-lasting implications. Although on removal of the stimulus, the newborn vessels may return to a morphologically and functionally 'normal' state, upon re-exposure to the injurious stimulus (in this case, hypoxia) 6 weeks after apparent full recovery, animals that had been exposed to hypoxia in the neonatal period had greater vascular remodeling and higher pulmonary arterial pressures than animals that had adapted normally to extrauterine life.

The primary stimuli responsible for vascular remodeling remain unclear. Mechanical forces (increased wall tension and shear stress) and hypoxia have received considerable attention with regard to their effects on cell phenotype. Various models including vessel coarctation, venous to arterial autologous grafts, and *in vitro* preparations of stretched vessel wall or isolated vascular smooth muscle cells have been employed to evaluate the effects of increased load on vascular wall cells. In general, these studies have shown that increased tension or load stimulates an almost immediate increase in net protein production. Expression of connective tissue proteins increases before that of contractile proteins, and the amounts of specific proteins within individual classes can change independently. The effects of elevated strain on cellular hyperplasia are unclear and may depend on the age and type of vessel examined. Significant differences between the responses of veins and arteries have been observed, again suggesting a heterogeneous response to vascular load. Recent studies have documented both stretch-activated and stretch-inactivated ion channels within various cell types, including muscle. These voltage-dependent channels can lead to electrical polarization changes within the cell, perhaps directly activating second-messenger systems necessary for protein synthesis or cell proliferation. Changes in Na^+ can also stimulate protein production, and Na^+-channel blockers have been demonstrated to ameliorate the response to increased load. Cells may also sense deformation of the membrane directly via filaments connecting the cell surface to the nucleus. Complex cell–cell interactions are certainly important in this response as endothelial cells have been shown to modulate the response.

The effects of *chronic hypoxia* on vascular wall cells are especially important in the pulmonary circulation. Chronic hypoxic exposure is associated with significant pulmonary hypertension in most species, as well as changes in the vessel wall that include cell proliferation (predominately in the adventitial fibroblast) and significant increases in the production and deposition of elastin and collagen. The direct effect of hypoxia on these changes, however, is uncertain. Hypoxia alone has been demonstrated to decrease smooth muscle cell proliferation and elastin and collagen production in cultured neonatal smooth muscle cells. On the other hand, hypoxia has been shown to stimulate fibroblast proliferation. In addition, in certain cell types (including the endothelium), hypoxia has been demonstrated to enhance growth factor production and responsiveness. One possible hypothesis is that hypoxia induces cellular changes that make cells more responsive to mechanical and hormonal stimuli.

Recent studies have begun to evaluate some of the cytokine factors that may be involved in mediating the vascular remodeling process. Basic FGF seems to be involved in the proliferation of cells observed in the *atherosclerotic plaque* and in *restenosis* of the vessel after induced endothelial injury such as occurs during *angioplasty* procedures. In models of pulmonary hypertension, TGFβ, IGF-I, and IGF-II have been correlated in a temporal fashion with the changes in cell proliferation and matrix production that are observed. TGFβ, for instance, was found to be temporally and specifically related to areas in the vessel wall that were undergoing intense remodeling.

Characterization of the signals involved in initiating the vascular response to injury as well as of the mediators generated by endothelial, smooth muscle, and fibroblast cells during the vascular remodeling response require intense investigation. In addition, evaluation of the mechanisms responsible for cell activation and protein synthesis will be an important new direction for further research into the molecular and cellular mechanisms responsible for regulating cell proliferation and connective tissue synthesis in normal and diseased vessels.

Selected reading

Adair TH, Gay WJ, Montani J-P. Growth regulation of the vascular system: evidence for a metabolic hypothesis. *Am J Physiol* 1990; **259**: R393.

Carey DJ. Control of growth and differentiation of vascular cells by extracellular matrix proteins. *Annu Rev Physiol* 1991; **53**: 161.

D'Amore PA. Developmental aspects of vascular disease. In

Developmental mechanisms of disease in the newborn. Report of the 101st Ross Conference on Pediatric Research. Columbus, Ohio: Ross Laboratories, 1991: 95.

Mecham RP, Stenmark KR, Parks WC. Connective tissue production by vascular smooth muscle in development and disease. *Chest* 1991; **99**: 43S.

Mitchell JJ, Reynolds SE, Leslie KO, Low RB, Woodcock-Mitchell J. Smooth muscle cell markers in developing rat lung. *Am J Respir Cell Mol Biol* 1990; **3**: 515.

Noden DM. Embryonic origins and assembly of blood vessels. *Am Rev Respir Dis* 1989; **140**: 1097.

Stenmark KR, Majack RA. Response of the developing pulmonary circulation to injury. In *Developmental mechanisms of disease in the newborn. Report of the 101st Ross Conference on Pediatric Research.* Columbus, Ohio: Ross Laboratories, 1991: 102.

A2. Vascular Smooth Muscle and Endothelial Cell Function

L J Ignarro and G M Buga

Vascular smooth muscle function

Smooth muscle is a form of involuntary muscle composed of specialized cells that can generate force, produce movement, and maintain organ dimensions against applied loads. Thus, vascular smooth muscle must accommodate the load imposed by the blood pressure to regulate local blood flow. Specialized contractile and regulatory mechanisms are present to serve this function economically.

The contractile system

Vascular smooth muscle cells range in size from 100 to 500 μm in length and from 2 to 5 μm in width, and are embedded in a connective tissue matrix that limits distension of the tissue to lengths near the optimum for force development. Small contractile elements that are functionally equivalent to a sarcomere underlie the mechanical similarities between smooth and skeletal muscle. The sliding filament–crossbridge mechanism characteristic of skeletal muscle contraction also underlies vascular smooth muscle contraction. Contraction velocities are much slower in smooth muscle than in skeletal muscle; this is attributed to a **myosin** isoform with low ATPase activity in smooth muscle. Vascular smooth muscle contracts tonically (sustained partial activation); this is characterized by reduced rates of crossbridge cycling.

Smooth muscle cells contain **calmodulin** as the Ca^{2+}-binding regulatory protein but are devoid of troponin, which has a similar function in the thin filaments of skeletal and cardiac muscle. The link between Ca^{2+} and initiation of crossbridge cycling is not well understood. Vascular smooth muscle contains myosin kinase and myosin phosphatase, which phosphorylate and dephosphorylate the crossbridges, respectively. Crossbridge phosphorylation depends on the intracellular concentration of free Ca^{2+}. The active form of myosin kinase is a ternary complex of myosin kinase–calmodulin–Ca^{2+}. The calmodulin serves to facilitate the binding of Ca^{2+} to myosin kinase. Smooth muscle stimulation causes increased Ca^{2+} levels, which promotes crossbridge phosphorylation. Relaxation of vascular smooth muscle is associated with decreased Ca^{2+} levels, myosin kinase inactivation, and net dephosphorylation. The regulation of myosin phosphatase is not well understood.

Excitation–contraction coupling

Although vascular smooth muscle contains a sarcoplasmic reticulum, most neurotransmitters, hormones, and drugs that cause contraction are largely dependent on extracellular Ca^{2+} (influx) for maximal responses. Ca^{2+} influx depends on two types of channels (Fig. 10.4). One channel is a voltage-dependent slow channel that responds to changes in the membrane potential and leads to depolarization as a result of Ca^{2+} influx. Smooth muscle cell membranes do not possess fast channels. Many neurotransmitters, hormones, and drugs interact with selective receptor-operated Ca^{2+} channels to cause Ca^{2+} influx and thus elicit contractile responses, often without changing the membrane potential. Intracellular Ca^{2+} mobilization can also be involved, and the chain of

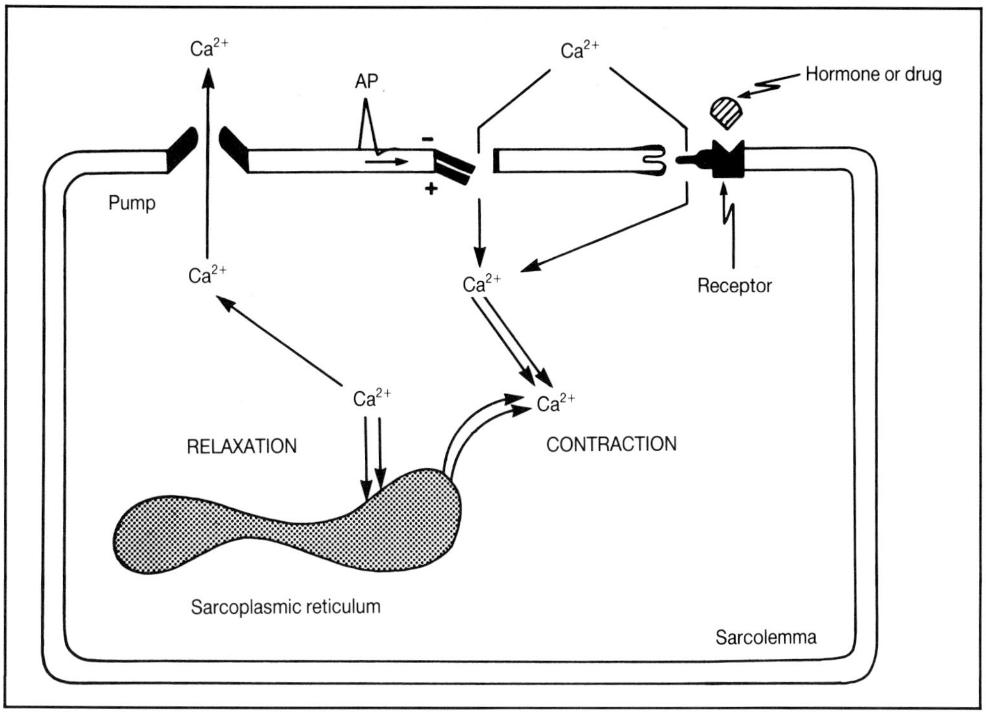

Fig. 10.4. Schematic illustration of the involvement of Ca^{2+} in vascular smooth muscle contraction. Extracellular Ca^{2+} can enter the smooth muscle cell via voltage-dependent or potential-activated (AP = action potential) slow Ca^{2+} channels and receptor-operated or receptor-activated channels. Intracellular free Ca^{2+} can increase via release from bound stores in the sarcoplasmic reticulum. Both processes lead to contraction. Movement of Ca^{2+} back into the sarcoplasmic reticulum and out of the cell via the active sarcolemmal pumps leads to relaxation.

events that takes place in the smooth muscle cell leading to contraction is termed pharmacomechanical coupling.

Relaxation of vascular smooth muscle is caused by a variety of hormones and drugs that stimulate the intracellular formation of cyclic AMP (**cAMP**) or cyclic GMP (**cGMP**). These second messengers activate distinct protein kinases, which results in phosphorylation of various enzymes with consequent modulation of their activities. Relaxation results from increased Ca^{2+} efflux and/or intracellular sequestration, presumably by phosphorylation of Ca^{2+}-binding proteins.

Functional adaptation

Because of the structural arrangement of vascular smooth muscle cells, a moderate shortening of smooth muscle can produce disproportionately large volume changes. The overall volume reduction is 30–40-fold for an arterial segment that undergoes a 50 percent cell shortening, and this can stop blood flow. Unlike skeletal muscle, vascular smooth muscle shows little dependence on extrinsic innervation for maintaining contractile activity.

During development and growth, the number of smooth muscle cells increases (hyperplasia). In adults, the tissue mass increases if the smooth muscle is subjected to a sustained increase in mechanical work (compensatory hypertrophy). A striking example of this principle is the thickening of the tunica media of arterioles in patients with *essential hypertension*. This may actually be attributed to cellular hypertrophy. Significant numbers of polyploid cells may result from chromosomal replication. The polyploid cells (with multiples of normal sets of chromosomes) synthesize more contractile proteins and increase in size with each chromosomal replication.

Control of vascular smooth muscle function

Vascular smooth muscle is the tissue responsible for the control of peripheral systemic and pulmonary vascular resistance, arterial and venous tone, and distribution of blood throughout the body. Contractile activity is elicited by either neuronal or humoral stimuli. Some blood vessels show spontaneous contractions; this is termed electrical–mechanical coupling. Most of the arteries and veins are innervated by sympathetic adrenergic fibers, which release norepinephrine as the neurotransmitter. Therefore, the predominant autonomic tone to blood vessels is sympathetic, and vasoconstriction or increased smooth muscle tone is the prevailing effect. Various hormones and drugs (humoral stimuli) cause smooth muscle contraction without evidence of electrical excitation. This is mediated by intracellular Ca^{2+}. Such chemical agents include catecholamines, acetylcholine, histamine, serotonin, angiotensin, certain eicosanoids, endothelin, and other endogenous substances.

Extrinsic control of vascular smooth muscle tone

The **sympathetic** division of the autonomic nervous system exerts a vasoconstrictor influence on arteries and veins, attributed to the action of norepinephrine on postsynaptic α_1-adrenergic receptors. Inhibition of the sympathetic nerves, either centrally or peripherally, causes passive vascular smooth muscle relaxation and vasodilatation. Although the major neuronal control of the peripheral blood vessels is provided by sympathetic adrenergic vasoconstrictor fibers, sympathetic cholinergic fibers innervate resistance arteries in the skeletal muscle and skin. These fibers release acetylcholine and cause vasodilatation, but the physiological role of these cholinergic fibers in the regulation of local blood flow is unknown. The cholinergic efferent fibers of the parasympathetic division innervate some blood vessels in the head and viscera, and their stimulation causes vascular smooth muscle relaxation and vasodilatation. The mechanism by which acetylcholine causes relaxation is attributed to an endothelium-dependent interaction resulting in the formation and release of **endothelium derived relaxing factor** or **EDRF** (discussed below, p. 469).

Studies indicate that nonadrenergic-noncholinergic (NANC) neurons innervate some but not all arteries. The arterial system in the gastrointestinal tract and corpus cavernosum of the penis are two striking examples. Electrical stimulation of NANC neurons causes vascular smooth muscle relaxation. Neither the NANC neurotransmitter nor the mechanism of relaxation is well understood, but the newly discovered autacoid, **nitric oxide (NO)**, appears to be involved (discussed below, p. 469).

Humoral factors such as circulating epinephrine released from the adrenal medulla affect vascular smooth muscle tone. Contraction or relaxation can occur depending on the tissue distribution of α_1- and β_2-adrenergic receptors. In the skeletal muscle vasculature, the predominant effect of epinephrine is relaxation due to interaction primarily with β_2-adrenergic receptors, whereas the principal effect of epinephrine in the skin is contraction due to the tissue predominance of α_1-adrenergic receptors. Locally synthesized bradykinin, histamine, and serotonin in certain species can cause local vasodilatation that is endothelium dependent and attributed to the generation of EDRF. The direct action of these endogenous substances on vascular smooth muscle is contraction, but this generally is not observed in normal, healthy blood vessels *in vivo*. Locally synthesized **eicosanoids** (prostaglandins [PGs], thromboxanes, leukotrienes [LTs]) can cause contraction or relaxation depending on the blood vessel, species, and eicosanoid. The current view by some is that the various autacoids, including bradykinin, histamine, serotonin, and eicosanoids, serve a pathophysiological role in modulating local blood flow at sites of inflammation and tissue injury or repair. Other chemical substances such as the potent vasoconstrictor angiotensin II (AII) serve a physiological role in regulating blood pressure and circulating blood volume. Endothelin is a newly discovered vasoconstrictor polypeptide synthesized by vascular endothelial cells, the function of which is yet unknown.

Intrinsic control of vascular smooth muscle tone

In a variety of tissues, the local blood flow is modulated or adjusted to the existing metabolic activity or functional state of the smooth muscle. For example, changes in local blood flow or perfusion pressure can result in changes in vascular resistance or vascular smooth muscle tone that tend to maintain a constant blood flow. The mechanism of this autoregulation of local blood flow is not well understood; multiple mechanisms likely exist.

The myogenic hypothesis states that the vascular smooth muscle contracts in response to stretch (sudden increase in local blood flow). Thus, the initial increase in flow is followed by a return of flow to prior control levels. The myogenic hypothesis may explain the vasoconstriction that occurs in the lower extremities when one changes position from lying to standing.

The metabolic hypothesis requires that local blood flow is regulated by the metabolic activity of the smooth muscle or a decrease in oxygen supply to the smooth muscle. This appears to occur in many tissues including the heart and skeletal muscle, where blood flow closely parallels metabolic activity. The metabolic hypothesis may explain the increase in local blood flow that occurs during exercise. Numerous chemical substances have been proposed as mediators of metabolic vasodilatation including adenosine, certain PGs (PGE_2 and PGI_2), and EDRF.

The flow hypothesis is based on the observation that if arterial inflow to a vascular bed is stopped for a few seconds or longer, the local blood flow increases immediately on release of the occlusion (Fig. 10.5). The mechanism of this reactive hyperemia is unknown but may be attributed to the increased local formation of EDRF that is triggered by an increase in intracellular Ca^{2+} levels in the affected smooth muscle. This situation may be analogous to the concept of flow-dependent vasodilatation, where a sudden local increase in blood flow causes a downstream vasodilatation to accommodate the increase in blood flow. Flow-dependent vasodilatation is an endothelium-dependent phenomenon. The stimulus for flow-dependent vasodilatation is increased shear forces or tangential forces imposed on the vascular endothelial cells by the increase in blood flow. The chemical agent that mediates the vascular smooth muscle relaxation appears to be EDRF, as the response can be abolished by inhibitors of EDRF synthesis.

Regulation of peripheral blood flow

Clearly, the direct changes in vascular smooth muscle tone brought about by neuronal influences are modified by the concomitant changes in the flow and pressure of the blood. Nevertheless, the control of vascular smooth muscle tone by both intrinsic and extrinsic mechanisms

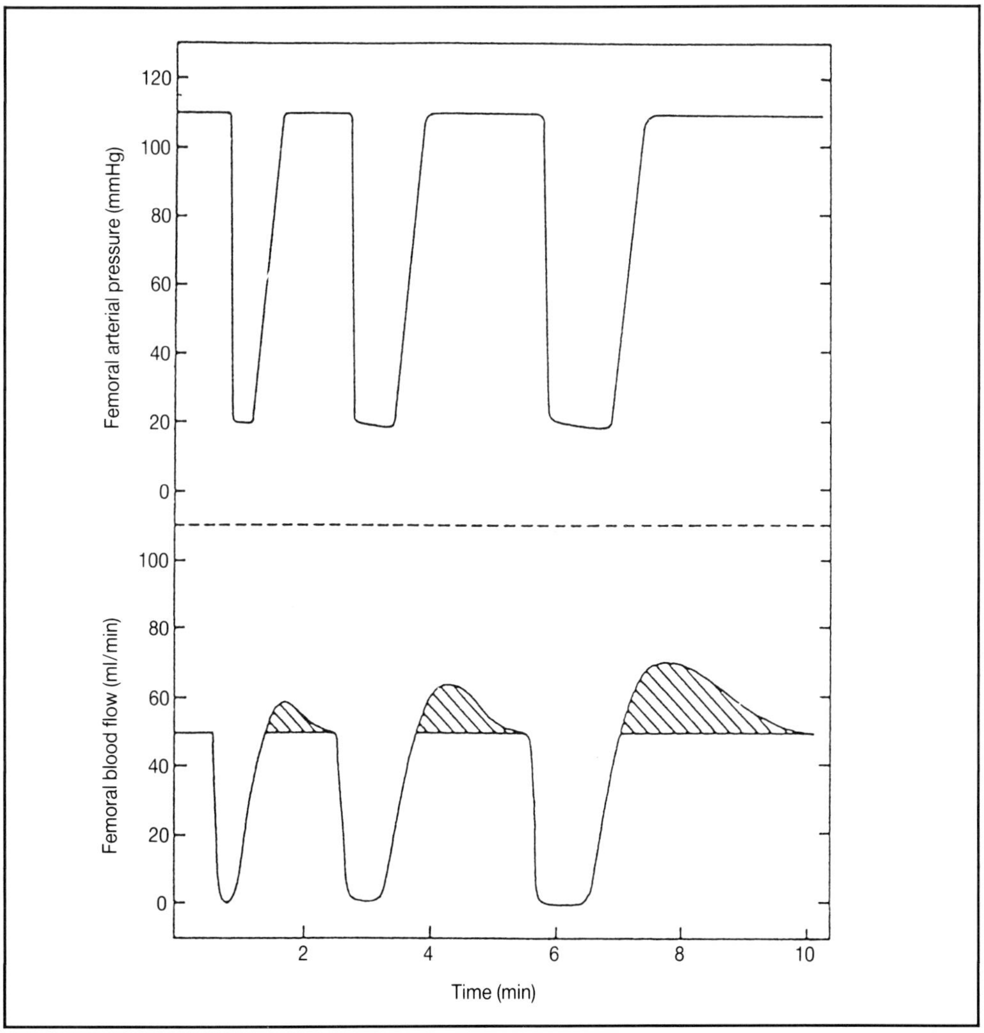

Fig. 10.5. Schematic of experimental tracings illustrating reactive hyperemia in the hind limb of the dog after 15-, 30-, and 45-second occlusions of the femoral artery. The hatched areas in the lower tracing represent the reactive hyperemia.

allows for vascular adjustments to provide changes in local blood flow as required under the prevailing conditions of metabolic organ function. Intrinsic flow-regulating mechanisms predominate in vital organs such as the heart and brain, and sympathetic nervous system activation during severe hemorrhage or shock has negligible effects on the arterioles within the heart and brain, whereas marked vasoconstriction occurs in the skin, renal, and splanchnic regions. Extrinsic flow-regulating mechanisms predominate in the skin, especially through reflex hypothalamic pathways to contribute to the regulation of body temperature. In skeletəl muscle there appears to be more of a balance between extrinsic and intrinsic flow-regulating mechanisms. For example, neuronal control (vaso-constriction) predominates in resting muscle, whereas intrinsic control (vasodilatation) predominates in exercising muscle. Moreover, mere anticipation of impending skeletal muscle activity results in a predominance of intrinsic over extrinsic mechanisms.

Second messenger functions of cGMP and cAMP

Cyclic GMP mediates the vascular smooth muscle relaxant effect of endogenous **EDRF** (identified as NO) as well as nitrovasodilator drugs such as nitroglycerin and nitroprusside. Vascular smooth muscle contains two isoforms of **guanylyl cyclase**. The cytosolic isoform contains heme and is activated markedly by NO and EDRF. Nitrovasodilators are converted in vascular smooth muscle cells to nitric oxide, which then activates guanylyl cyclase. The membrane-bound isoform is not influenced by NO but is activated by atrial natriuretic peptides or atriopeptins. Activation of either isoform of guanylyl cyclase results in intracellular cGMP formation and vascular smooth muscle relaxation. Cyclic AMP-mediated relaxation is caused by β-adrenergic agonists, certain PGs, adenosine, and other activators of adenylyl cyclase. **Adenylyl cyclase** is a membrane-bound enzyme that is coupled to extracellular or surface receptors via G-proteins. Interaction with β_2-adrenergic receptors, PG receptors, and receptors for other substances results in adenylyl cyclase activation, intracellular cAMP formation, and vascular smooth muscle relaxation. Both cyclic nucleotides lower the intracellular concentration of Ca^{2+} in vascular smooth muscle, thereby causing a decrease in tone. Cyclic GMP-dependent protein kinase in vascular smooth muscle is required for the Ca^{2+}-lowering action of both cAMP and cGMP. Evidence indicates that Ca^{2+}-ATPase activation by phosphorylation of phospholamban by cGMP-dependent protein kinase underlies the mechanism of action of both cAMP and cGMP.

Role of potassium channels in vascular smooth muscle relaxation

Vasodilatation is produced by the action of a variety of endogenous and exogenous compounds that are capable of hyperpolarizing the vascular smooth muscle cell membrane. Hyperpolarization appears to be attributed to increased inward K^+ conductance and accelerated Ca^{2+} efflux. Elevated intracellular K^+ also causes the voltage-dependent Ca^{2+} channels to close, thereby decreasing vascular smooth muscle tone. In blood vessels the prevailing types of K^+ channels involved in hyper-polarization are the Ca^{2+}-activated K^+ (K_{Ca}) channels, delayed rectifier channels, and ATP-sensitive K^+ (K_{ATP}) channels. Activation of these channels by specific agents causes vascular smooth muscle relaxation, whereas inhibition causes depolarization of the cell membrane and consequent smooth muscle contraction.

Vascular endothelial cell function

The vascular endothelium is a single layer of squamous epithelial cells on the intimal surface of all blood vessels. The **endothelium** is not merely a passive compatible lining for the containment of blood; rather, it is a metabolically active tissue that functions to maintain vascular homeo-stasis. The vascular endothelium serves to maintain vascular integrity and repair, produce and inactivate various chemical agents, regulate the function of platelets and other cells, and regulate vascular smooth muscle tone by releasing contracting and relaxing factors. The vascular endothelium is constantly exposed to the physical forces of flow and pressure. In maintaining endothelial integrity, the cells adhere firmly to the subendothelium, forming tight junctions with adjacent cells. The cells also adapt to changes in shear stress, pressure, and wall tension. Thus, the endothelial cytoskeleton is essential in maintaining the integrity of the endothelium exposed to hemodynamic stress.

Endothelial cell function is modulated by acute changes in physical forces, soluble chemical agents in the blood, the subendothelial matrix, and cell–cell and cell–platelet interactions. These modulating factors often induce cellular responses that involve a reorganization of the endothelial cell cytoskeleton, sometimes to the detriment of the cell.

Biochemical properties of endothelial cells

Vascular endothelial cells play an important role in modulating blood flow, coagulation, fibrinolysis, inflammation, lipoprotein metabolism, and macromolecular synthesis. The endothelial cell layer is coated with a carbohydrate-rich cell coat, the glycocalyx, consisting of glycosaminoglycans and polysaccharide side-chains of plasma membrane glycoproteins and glycolipids. The endothelium is in close contact with the underlying subendothelial matrix. This matrix can influence endothelial cell proliferation, migration, spreading, and cellular organization via specific cell-surface matrix-binding proteins.

Endothelial cells are capable of synthesizing matrix proteins and glycosaminoglycans including collagen, elastin, laminin, fibronectin, heparan and chondroitin sulfates, and von Willebrand protein of factor VIII. Endothelial cells influence coagulation and fibrinolysis by synthesizing thromboplastin (tissue factor, factor III) and coagulation factor V, by activating coagulation factor XII (Hageman factor), and by binding coagulation factor IX and IXa. In addition, endothelial cells can remove circulating adenosine, which is an inhibitor of platelet aggregation. Several anticoagulant mechanisms are active on the endothelial cell surface including coagulation factor Xa turnover, antithrombin III activity, thrombomodulin–thrombin interaction, and synthesis of protein S and plasminogen activator. Moreover, endothelial cells synthesize and release antiplatelet substances including prostacyclin (PGI_2) and NO (EDRF).

Vascular endothelial cells interact with neurotransmitters and vasoactive substances and participate in the inflammatory process and in immunological reactions. Angiotensin-converting enzyme (which is the same enzyme as bradykinin-degrading enzyme or kininase) is localized to the luminal surface of vascular endothelial cells. Various receptors are located on the extracellular surface of vascular endothelial cells, which can interact with various neurotransmitters and tissue hormones or autacoids. Most of the latter substances stimulate the formation and release of endothelium derived relaxing factors such as NO. Endothelial cells produce platelet activating factor (PAF), a phospholipid that increases the adherence of neutrophils to endothelial cells and activates platelets. Endothelial cells can also synthesize the third complement factor and convert LTA_4 to LTs B_4, C_4, D_4, and E_4.

Vascular endothelial cells are capable of synthesizing several different **growth factors** and **cytokines**. One is a platelet-derived growth factor that is mitogenic and chemotactic for fibroblasts and smooth muscle cells. Another factor is mitogenic for endothelial cells. Endothelium derived growth factor is another distinct growth factor. A heparin-like substance and a peptide inhibitor of vascular smooth muscle proliferation are produced by endothelial cells. Endothelial cells can be stimulated to produce at least three different hematopoietic growth factors, a granulocyte-macrophage colony-stimulating factor, and factors that stimulate the neutrophil respiratory burst reaction. Cytokines including interleukin-1, interleukin-6, and interleukin-8 are products of the vascular endothelial cell.

Endothelial cells participate in **lipoprotein metabolism** by taking up acetate and mevalonate and incorporating them into sterol, and by taking up and degrading LDL, including chemically modified LDL. The endothelial cell surface has distinct binding sites also for HDL but the reason for this is not well understood. A lipoprotein lipase that is active at the endothelial cell surface functions to hydrolyze triglyceride-rich lipoproteins. These observations indicate clearly that vascular endothelial cells are of great importance in certain disease processes involving atherosclerosis, thrombosis, hemostasis, fibrinolysis, and inflammation.

Endothelial cell communication

The vascular endothelial cell layer is strategically located at the interface of flowing blood and vascular smooth muscle. Thus, the endothelium is in a unique location for interaction with soluble and cellular elements of the blood on one side and with smooth muscle cells on the other side. Endothelial cells interact with neighboring cells by two general mechanisms, humoral and direct contact. In humoral communication, endothelial cells synthesize and release (by diffusion) a variety of vasoactive substances and agents that affect the activities of neighboring cells. Direct contact between endothelial and adjacent cells occurs primarily by the communicating gap junction.

Humoral mechanisms of communication

Vascular endothelial cells synthesize soluble molecules that leave the cell by diffusion. The endothelial products interact with selective receptors on the surface of the target cell. Some endothelial proteins are secreted into the extracellular fluid as a result of well defined steps regulated at the transcriptional, translational, and post-translational levels. Other endothelial products are rapidly synthesized and diffuse out of the cell. The latter include NO, endothelin and related contractile peptides, and PGI_2.

The discovery that endothelial cells synthesize and release chemical agents that relax or contract vascular smooth muscle led to the realization that the vascular endothelium plays an important role in regulating cardiovascular function. The two important endothelium derived relaxants were PGI_2 and the nonprostanoid substance EDRF. EDRF was later discovered to be NO or a closely related labile nitroso compound that liberates NO. The important endothelium derived contracting factor was isolated and identified as a 21 amino acid peptide termed endothelin.

Gap junction mechanisms of communication

Gap junctions are channels of communication between the cytoplasm of adjacent cells. Gap junctions can be observed by electron microscopy and freeze fracture. Such channels allow for the rapid diffusion of hydrophilic molecules up to a molecular weight of approximately 1000 Da. In addition to endothelial cell-to-cell communication, gap junctions exist between endothelium and smooth muscle cells, especially in the microcirculation. Endothelial cells may act as a receptor system for subendothelial cells by transferring small second messenger molecules through gap junctions. In addition, myoendothelial junctions may represent an electrically coupled system that influences smooth muscle tone. The precise physiological role of gap junctions, however, is not well understood. They may influence or modulate the formation of endothelial products, cell proliferation and transformation, and interaction with neighboring cells.

Secretory functions of the vascular endothelium

The endothelium contributes to the modulation of vasomotor tone by secreting two important vasodilator substances, PGI_2 and EDRF. Endothelial cells may also secrete certain other endothelium-dependent vasodilator substances such as acetylcholine, ATP, and substance P, as well as the vasoconstrictor peptide, endothelin. Endothelium derived vasoactive agents may be important in mediating the influence of flow on vasomotor tone, vascular geometry, and angiogenesis.

A second function of the endothelium is regulation of *thrombosis*. Thrombosis is promoted by secretion of platelet adhesion proteins including thrombospondin, fibronectin, collagen, and von Willebrand factor, but is prevented by secretion of PGI_2 and EDRF. The endothelium promotes coagulation via expression of tissue factor and secretion of factor V and plasminogen activator inhibitor (PAI), but inhibits coagulation via secretion of thrombomodulin and tissue plasminogen activator (TPA).

The secretion of mitogens and vascular smooth muscle growth inhibitors may be important in atherogenesis. Endothelial regulation of leukocyte extravasation by expression of adhesion proteins and secretion of interleukin-1 and platelet activating factor (PAF) also plays a role in influencing atherogenesis and the inflammatory process.

Endothelin

Endothelin is a 21 amino acid peptide that exists as four isoforms. Each isoform has a corresponding precursor or proendothelin, also termed big endothelin. Endothelin gene expression and translation into an active protein product has been studied in cultured endothelial cells. The induction of endothelin-1 isoform mRNA and the rate of peptide release are increased by thrombin, transforming growth factor β (TGFβ), AII, vasopressin, hemodynamic shear stress, interleukin-1, phorbol esters, and Ca^{2+} ionophores. Some of these inducers of endothelin production can promote Ca^{2+} accumulation and/or protein kinase C activation, which may act at the level of transcription and/or translation. Endothelin-converting enzyme (ECE) is a membrane-bound metalloproteinase that cleaves the bond between tryptophan and valine in converting big endothelin-1 to endothelin-1. Endothelin-1 is about 100-fold more potent than big endothelin-1 as a vasoconstrictor.

Endothelin may elicit autocrine, paracrine, and endocrine functions. A possible autocrine function of endothelin may be in the modulation of endothelial cell proliferation. Other possible autocrine functions include stimulation of the synthesis and release of PGI_2 and EDRF, as well as modulation of angiotensin-converting enzyme activity. Paracrine functions of endothelin include vascular smooth muscle contraction and mitogenesis. Indirect evidence for an endocrine function of endothelin is the presence of endothelin in the circulation, cerebrospinal fluid, and urine.

Functionally, endothelin causes contraction of the underlying smooth muscle and can stimulate the synthesis and release of endothelium derived relaxing factors. The latter effect may account for the vasodilator, antiplatelet, and anticoagulant properties of endothelin. Other functions of endothelin may include a centrally mediated increase in systemic blood pressure, stimulation of aldosterone biosynthesis in the adrenal cortex, inhibition of glomerular filtration rate, modulation of the renin–angiotensin system, and stimulation of release of atrial natriuretic peptide. More work is necessary before we can draw definitive conclusions about the physiological or pathophysiological role of endothelin in man.

Endothelium derived relaxing factor (EDRF)

Despite the knowledge that vascular endothelial cells displayed various synthetic, degradative, and secretory functions, the modulatory role of the endothelium on vascular tone remained unrecognized until 1980, when Furchgott and Zawadzki discovered **EDRF**. In this original study, acetylcholine-elicited relaxation of isolated rabbit aorta preparations was shown to be endothelium dependent and due to the release of an EDRF that was chemically unstable. An attractive hypothesis was offered that this relaxing substance might be a lipoxygenase product of arachidonic acid. Furchgott and co-workers went on to propose that EDRF is responsible also for the arterial relaxant responses to bradykinin, histamine, ATP, ADP, and Ca^{2+} ionophores.

About 13 years ago we discovered that bubbling **NO** gas into Krebs bicarbonate solution containing isolated strips of bovine coronary artery caused a rapid and marked, but transient, relaxation that was antagonized by hemoproteins and methylene blue. NO activated soluble guanylyl cyclase in coronary artery, and this was inhibited by hemoproteins and methylene blue. These observations were made before the discovery of EDRF. Shortly after the discovery of EDRF, we found that NO activated human platelet guanylyl cyclase, elevated platelet cGMP levels, and produced a profound inhibition of platelet aggregation. When we started to study the pharmacological properties of EDRF, we did not envision that EDRF could be NO, although we found that endothelium-dependent vascular smooth muscle relaxation was associated with marked tissue formation of cGMP, both of which were inhibited by the soluble guanylyl cyclase inhibitor methylene blue. Further studies revealed the remarkable similarities in biological properties between EDRF and NO and in 1986 we proposed that EDRF is NO or a labile nitroso precursor. The following year we and others provided chemical evidence for the identity of EDRF as NO.

Many studies were reported showing the similarities between EDRF and authentic NO. As had been shown for NO, EDRF activated purified soluble guanylyl cyclase by heme-dependent mechanisms and inhibited platelet aggregation and adhesion by mechanisms involving cGMP. Several inconsistencies were reported in which EDRF was suggested to be not NO, but rather a labile nitroso precursor. Definitive evidence has not been provided, however, to refute the well accepted concept that EDRF is NO.

EDRF or NO is released from artery and vein and appears to be involved intimately in the regulation of vascular smooth muscle tone. NO is responsible, at least in part, for the endothelium-dependent vasodilator action of acetylcholine, bradykinin, histamine, serotonin, ATP, ADP, substance P, and thrombin. These endogenous substances interact with selective receptors located on the extracellular surface of the vascular endothelial cell. Agonist–receptor interaction is coupled to the intracellular formation of NO via Ca^{2+}. Receptor occupancy by agonist results in the influx of Ca^{2+}, which combines with calmodulin to activate NO synthase, thereby stimulating NO production. The vascular endothelium is capable of modulating the tone of the underlying smooth muscle in arteries in response to local changes in shear stress, pressure, and other mechanical factors. The purpose of endothelial regulation is to adapt blood vessel diameter to sudden changes in tissue perfusion demands. Studies using isolated arterial segments and cultured arterial endothelial cells have shown that endothelium derived NO is likely responsible for shear stress-induced or flow-dependent vasodilatation, perhaps through a K^+ channel mediated mechanism. Thus, NO likely plays an important physiological role in the regulation or modulation of blood flow.

Endothelium derived NO plays a role in modulating the systemic blood pressure. *In vitro* studies have shown that inhibitors of NO synthesis (discussed below) cause endothelium-dependent contractions of isolated arterial preparations. *In vivo* studies have shown that the same inhibitors of NO synthesis cause a marked increase in peripheral vascular resistance and systemic blood pressure. Endothelium derived NO also plays a role in modulating platelet adhesion and aggregation, thereby endowing the vascular endothelium with the capacity to provide a thrombogenic-free surface. Local damage to the vascular endothelium can promote local vasoconstriction and blood clot formation. Figure 10.6 illustrates some of the important influences of the endothelium on vascular smooth muscle tone and platelet function.

NO is synthesized from **L-arginine** through a multistep oxidation reaction catalyzed by **NO synthase**. The second product of the reaction is L-citrulline (Fig. 10.7). N^G-substituted analogs of L-arginine including the methyl, nitro-, and amino-analogs are inhibitors of NO synthase, and inhibition can be prevented or overcome by addition of excess L-arginine. These inhibitory analogs of L-arginine have been shown to cause vascular smooth muscle contraction, vasoconstriction, hypertension, and thrombosis. The inhibitory analogs of L-arginine are being used by many investigators in widely diverging areas of research to assess the physiological and pathophysiological roles of endogenous NO formed in

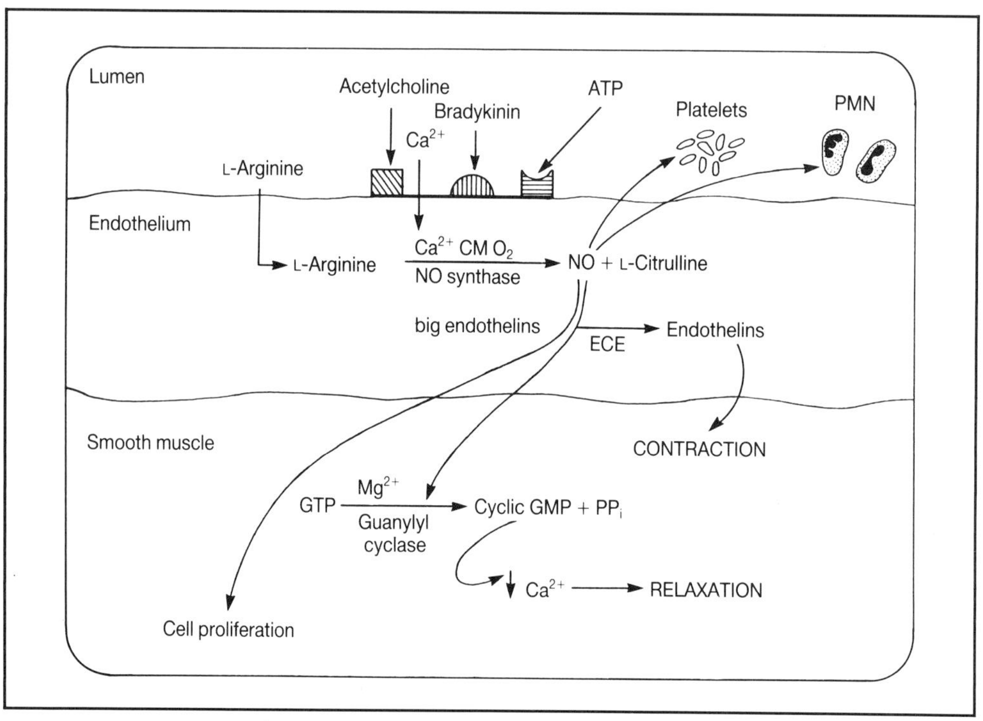

Fig. 10.6. Schematic illustration of the formation of NO and endothelin in the vascular endothelium and their subsequent actions on nearby target cells. Ca^{2+}, in the presence of calmodulin (CM) and O_2, activates NO synthase, thereby catalyzing the conversion of L-arginine to NO plus L-citrulline. NO diffuses into the underlying smooth muscle to activate cytosolic guanylyl cyclase, elevate cyclic GMP levels, decrease intracellular free Ca^{2+} levels, and cause relaxation. NO can also modulate smooth muscle cell proliferation. NO can diffuse out into the lumen and inhibit the adhesion of platelets and polymorphonuclear leukocytes (PMN) to the vascular endothelial surface. Big endothelins are converted by endothelin converting enzyme (ECE) to endothelins within the vascular endothelium. Endothelins diffuse out into the underlying smooth muscle to cause contraction.

many different cell types.

Acetylcholine is believed to cause endothelium-dependent vascular smooth muscle relaxation entirely by receptor-mediated mechanisms (muscarinic, M_1) involving NO production. Some studies indicate, however, that a portion of the endothelium-dependent relaxant action of acetylcholine may be attributed to the generation and release, by a different receptor-mediated mechanism (M_2), of an endothelium derived hyper-polarizing factor, which diffuses into the underlying smooth muscle to decrease in tone. Other endogenous endothelium-dependent relaxants do not appear to work by this mechanism.

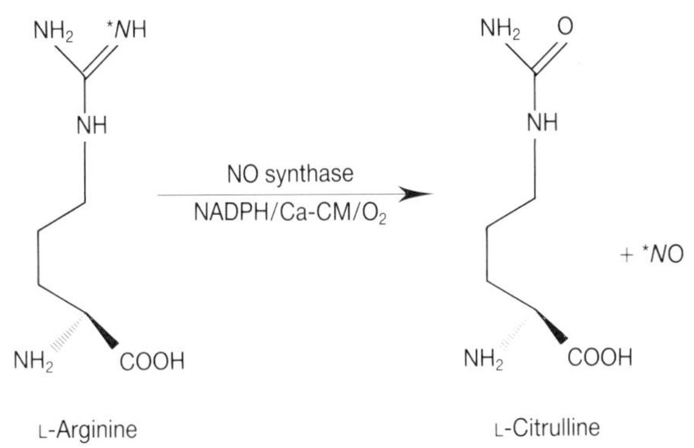

Fig. 10.7. Schematic representation of the biosynthesis of nitric oxide (NO) from L-arginine by the NO synthase pathway. Ca–CM signifies the Ca^{2+}–calmodulin complex. Although a single arrow depicting the reaction is shown, the enzymatic conversion of L-arginine to NO plus L-citrulline is a complicated, multistep oxidation process.

Conclusions

The vascular endothelium functions as a general endocrine gland by secreting diverse biologically active chemical substances that serve to regulate or modulate vascular smooth muscle function. Vascular smooth muscle receives its signal input not only from various neurons innervating the smooth muscle, but also from chemical agents generated in the adjacent endothelial cells. Thus, vascular smooth muscle function is critically dependent on normal endothelial cell function. Endothelial cell pathology contributes to conditions such as *atherosclerosis*, *hypertension*, *vasospasm*, *tissue inflammation*, *thrombosis*, *acute respiratory distress syndrome*, and perhaps *diabetes* and *tumor growth*.

Selected reading

Bassenge E, Busse R. Endothelial modulation of coronary tone. *Prog Cardiovasc Dis* 1988; **30**: 349.

Borsum T. Biochemical properties of vascular endothelial cells. *Virchows Arch [B]* 1991; **60**: 279.

Ignarro LJ. Biological actions and properties of endothelium-derived nitric oxide formed and released from artery and vein. *Circ Res* 1989; **65**: 1.

Ignarro LJ. Biosynthesis and metabolism of endothelium-derived nitric oxide. *Annu Rev Pharmacol Toxicol* 1990; **30**: 535.

Rubanyi GM, Parker Botelho LH. Endothelins. *FASEB J* 1991; **5**: 2713.

B. Cardiac and Myocardial Structure and Myocardial Cellular and Molecular Function

J Bristow

Anatomical development

The familiar four-chambered heart of mammals has its beginnings in the early embryo as two amorphous collections of cells. Not surprisingly, an extraordinary series of transformations is required to produce the configuration of the mature heart, and the complexity of this process has long fascinated embryologists. Driven by the wide spectrum of congenital heart defects occurring in children, an extremely detailed anatomical account of cardiac development has now been produced which provides a very useful framework for the categorization and understanding of many human congenital heart defects.

Normal development

The earliest heart cells can be recognized as a collection of cardiac progenitor cells located on opposite sides of the lateral plate of the presomite embryo (approximately 17 days after conception in the human). These cells form bilateral tubular structures that migrate to the midline and fuse to form the primitive cardiac tube by day 21 of gestation. Shortly after its formation, the cardiac tube commences beating. Although the regions of the early heart tube are not morphologically distinct, each portion of the tube is named according to the structure that will arise from it. Hence, the caudal portion of this tube is called the sinus venosus, followed sequentially as one

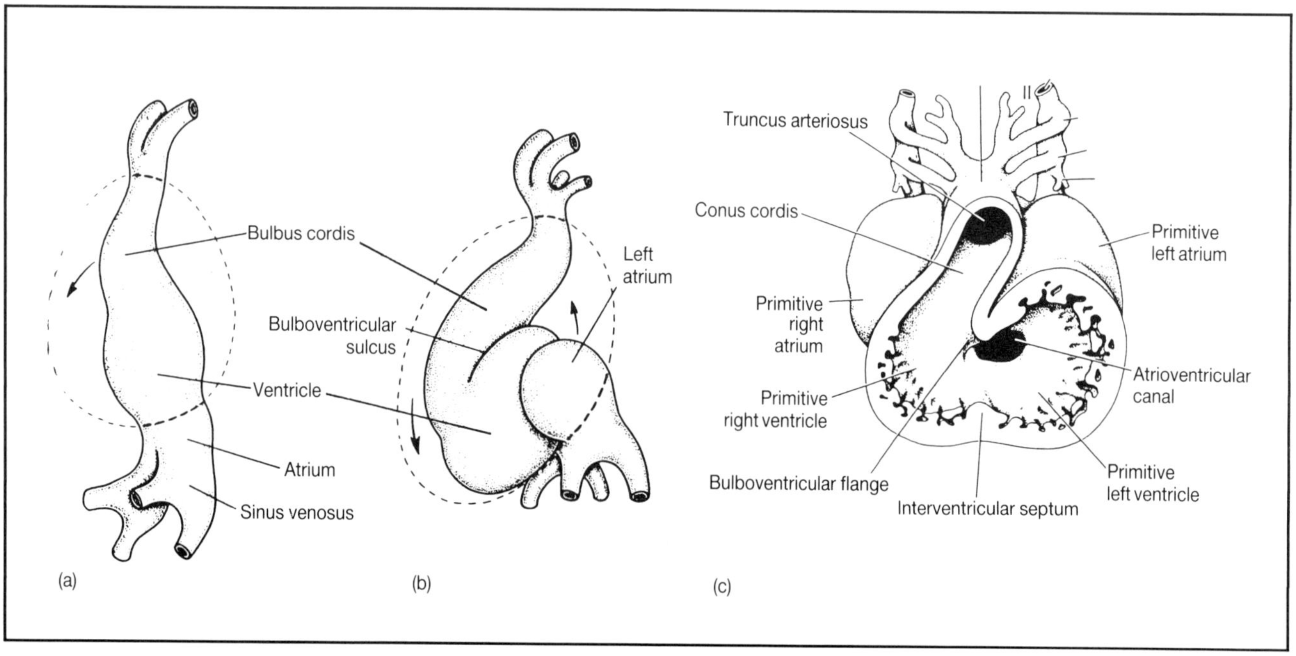

Fig. 10.8. Looping of the cardiac tube. (a) Regions of the cardiac tube before looping. (b) The cardiac tube after looping viewed from the left. (c) Frontal section of the heart shown in b. Note inlet is to the primitive left ventricle and outlet is from the primitive right ventricle. (From Langman J. *Medical embryology: human development—normal and abnormal*. 3rd ed. Baltimore: Williams and Wilkins, 1975, with permission.)

moves cephalad by the primitive atrium, ventricle, and bulbis cordis (Fig. 10.8a). At about 25 days of gestation, the cardiac tube bends and elongates, forming a loop anteriorly and to the right, the so-called D-loop (Fig. 10.8b). This process positions the atrial portion of the tube posteriorly, the proximal portion of the ventricular segment, which will form the left ventricle, leftward, and the distal portion, which will form the right ventricle, rightward. At this stage, a frontal section through the heart demonstrates division of the tube's lumen into the primordial cardiac chambers (Fig. 10.8c). The inlet from the posterior atrium into the left portion of the primitive ventricle is through the atrioventricular (AV) canal. Outlet is superiorly, from the right portion of the ventricle into the conus cordis, which will form the outflow tracts of both ventricles. The transverse portion of the loop between halves of the primitive ventricle contains a slight swelling, which marks the beginning of the interventricular septum that will eventually close this communication. Finally, the conus cordis is in continuity with the truncus arteriosus, which will give rise to pulmonary artery and the aorta.

In the 3 weeks following completion of looping, the atria, AV canal, ventricles, conus cordis, and truncus arteriosus must all be septated. Beginning at 38 days of gestation, the atrial septum is closed, first by upward growth of the primum septum from the endocardial cushions, then by downward growth from the roof of the atrium (Fig. 10.9a). A portion of this septum is then resorbed, and the hole thus produced is closed by growth of the secundum septum just to the right of the primum septum. The secundum septum does not completely close, but leaves a centrally placed hole, the foramen ovale, which is covered by a flap valve consisting of primum septum. At the same time as the atria are being septated, the AV canal must be divided into the tricuspid and mitral orifices. This occurs by upward and downward growth of the endocardial cushions located at the superior and inferior margins of the AV canal (Fig. 10.9b). This same process provides tissue to close the inlet portion of the

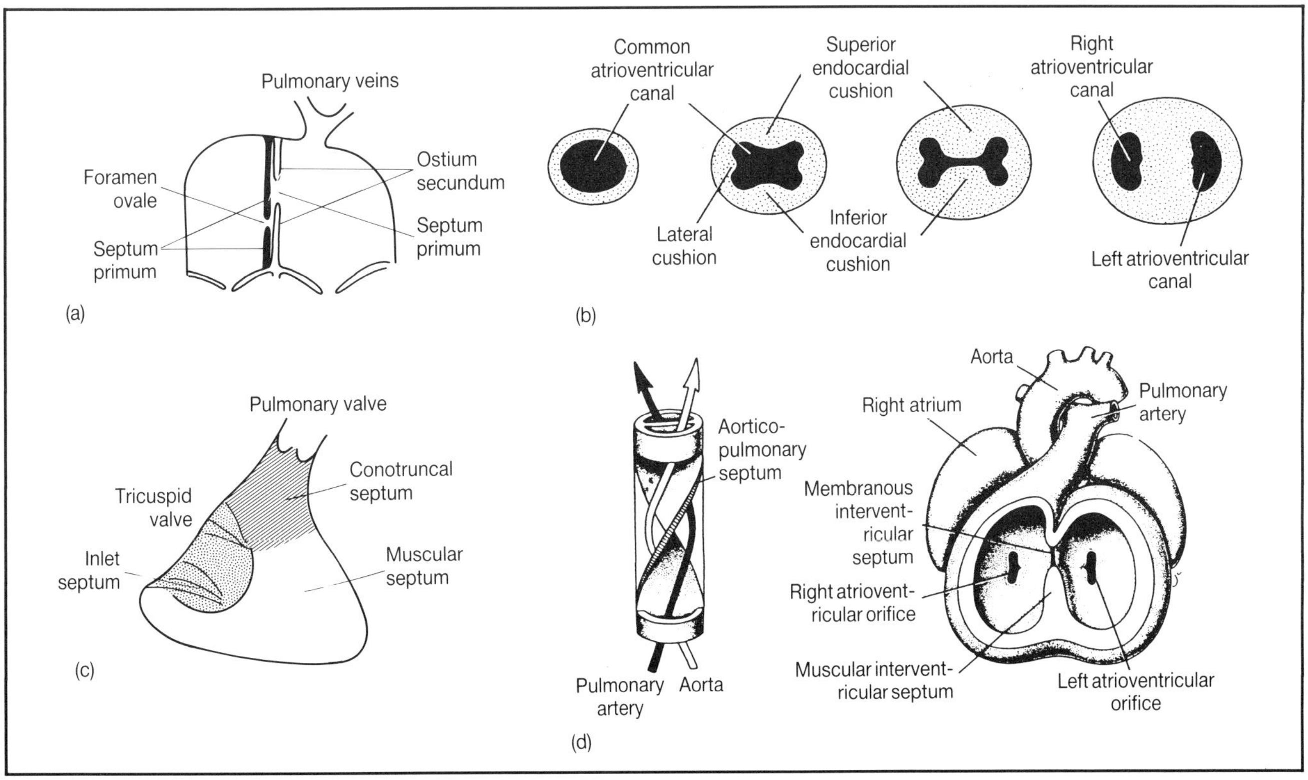

Fig. 10.9. Formation of cardiac septa. (a) Apposition of the primum and secundum septa closes the atrial septum, but leaves a communication, the foramen ovale. (b) Division of the AV canal into left and right atrioventricular orifices. The valve leaflets will form later. (c) View of the mature ventricular septum from the right ventricle showing the origin of its three parts. (d) Schematic view of the conotruncal septum, showing that the septum rotates within the conus cordis and truncus, leading to the mature configuration of the great vessels. (From Langman J. *Medical embryology: human development—normal and abnormal.* 3rd ed. Baltimore: Williams and Wilkins, 1975, with permission.)

ventricular septum. The remainder of the ventricular septum in turn is closed by tissues from two other regions (Fig. 10.9c). First, the muscular septum is formed by upward growth of ventricular muscle from the inferior margin of the primitive ventricle. Second, within the conus cordis a spiraling septum divides it into right and left ventricular outflow tracts. The inferior margin of this septum comes in contact and fuses with the muscular septum. Figure 10.8c demonstrates that if the conus cordis is to supply the outlet from both ventricles, it must move substantially to the left. This is accomplished by resorption of the bulboventricular flange (Fig. 10.8c). The truncus arteriosus is septated in concert with the conus cordis so that the anterior pulmonary artery is ultimately in continuity with the right ventricle and the posterior aorta is in continuity with the left ventricle (Fig. 10.9d).

Formation of the cardiac valves occurs immediately after septation of the AV canal and the truncus arteriosus (Fig. 10.10). Formation of the mitral and tricuspid valves begins with proliferation of undifferentiated cells surrounding both orifices, accompanied initially by growth of ventricular muscle below. Gradually the ventricular muscle below becomes hollowed out, leaving the tips of the nascent valve attached to the ventricular wall by muscular strands or chordae tendineae. The tissue in the chordae and the valve leaflets is eventually replaced by dense connective tissue, and the valves are complete. The semilunar valves are produced in similar fashion. After septation, three outpouchings grow from the wall of the aorta and pulmonary artery. In this case resorption of tissue above the valve and at the commissures between valve leaflets, combined with continued growth of the central portion, produces elongation and thinning of the valve leaflets. Resorption above the valve is complete so that the valve leaflets are attached to the vessel wall only at the hinge points.

By 55 days of human gestation the basic form of the heart has been attained. Hence the remaining 80 percent of gestation is used for growth and maturation of cardiac structures. During this time, myocardial cells proliferate in tandem with dramatic accumulation of contractile proteins and metabolic machinery required to meet the circulatory needs of the rapidly growing fetus.

Abnormal development

Not surprisingly, abnormalities in each of the morphogenetic transformations described above occur and give rise to characteristic congenital heart lesions. Many of these defects are best understood as arrested development producing abnormal mature configurations that closely resemble normal stages in cardiac development. Several common examples, beginning with cardiac looping, are illustrated in Fig. 10.11 and serve to illustrate this point. If the primitive cardiac tube loops to the left rather than to the right, the primitive ventricles will be right-left

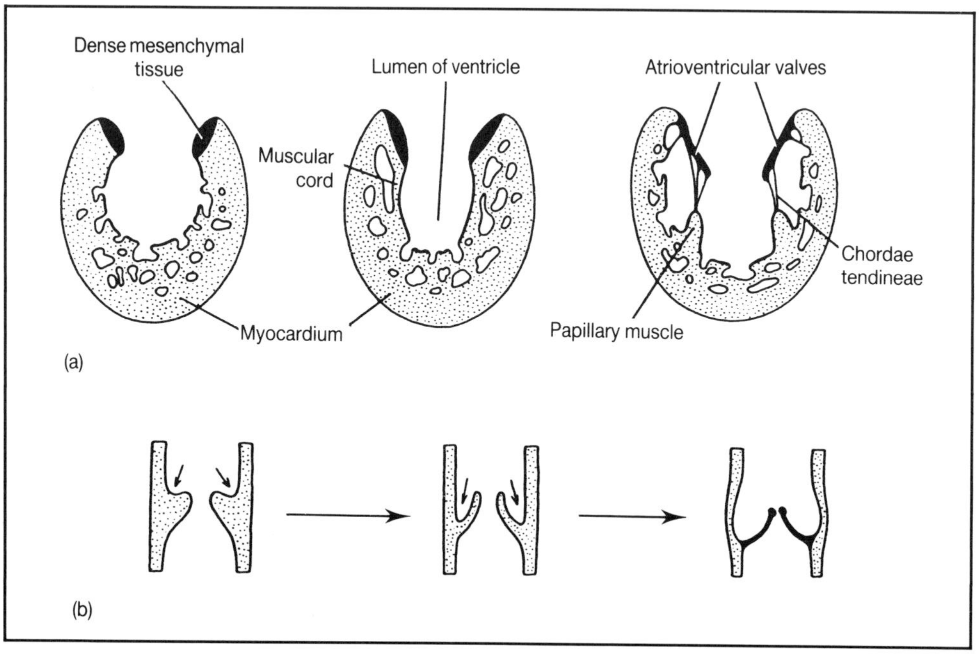

Fig. 10.10. Formation of cardiac valves. (a) The atrioventricular valves are formed by incomplete resorption of underlying myocardium, leaving papillary muscles and chordae tendineae attached. (b) The semilunar valves are formed by more complete regression of tissue from above the valve. (From Langman J. *Medical embryology: human development—normal and abnormal*. 3rd ed. Baltimore: Williams and Wilkins, 1975, with permission.)

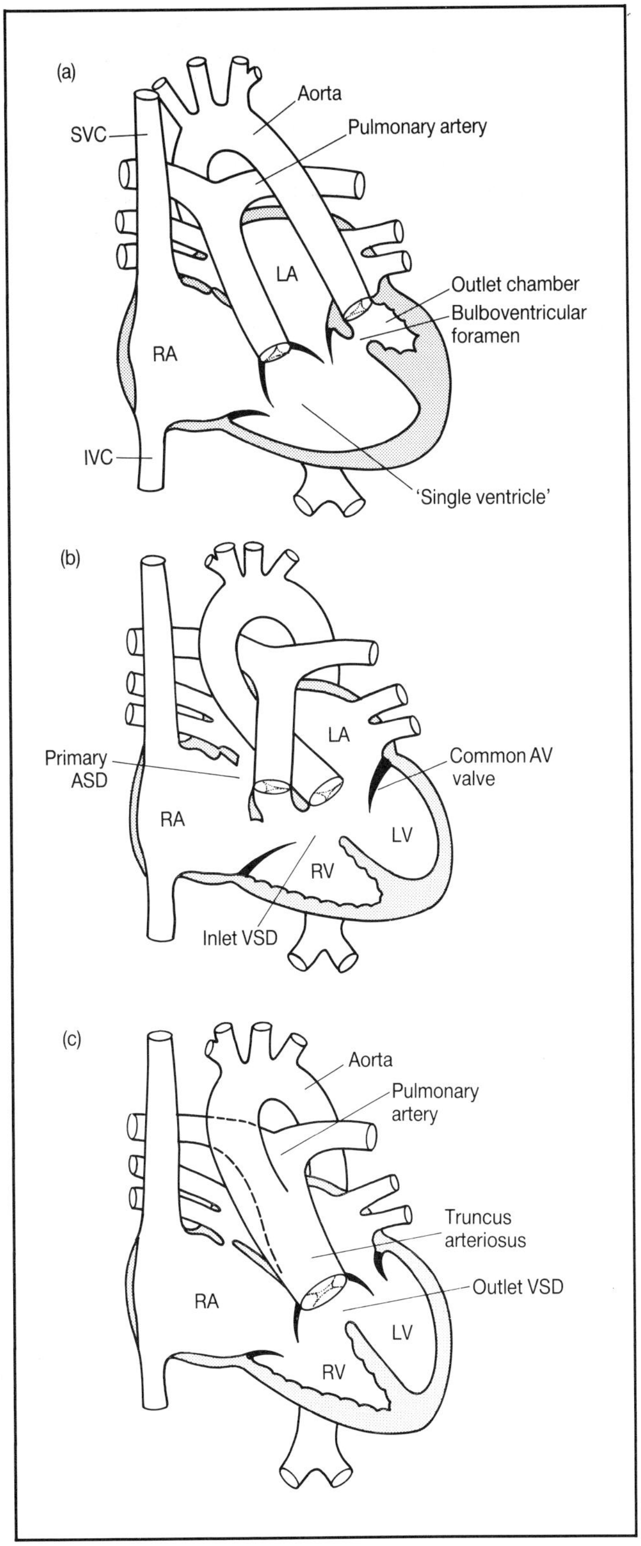

Fig. 10.11. Congenital heart defects arising from arrested maturation. (a) Single ventricle and L-transposition. Atrioventricular connection is to the left ventricle, which connects to an outlet chamber derived from conus cordis. (b) Complete AV canal defect. The AV canal was not septated, leaving a single atrioventricular orifice. Septal defects are present both above and below this orifice. (c) Persistent truncus arteriosus. Failure of conotruncal septation leaves a single outlet from the ventricles and leaves a defect in the outlet portion of the ventricular septum.

reversed. If the remainder of cardiac morphogenesis proceeds normally but also right-left reversed, a functionally normal, mirror-image heart will be produced, as is commonly seen in *complete situs inversus*. A functionally normal heart can also result after looping to the left if malrotation of the conus cordis establishes continuity between the left-sided 'right' ventricle and the aorta, and between the right-sided 'left' ventricle and the pulmonary artery. This rare malformation is called *congenitally corrected transposition of the great arteries* or *L-transposition* because the malrotation of the conus cordis corrects the abnormality in cardiac looping. More frequently, looping to the left is accompanied by arrest of ventricular septation giving rise to a *double-inlet single ventricle* (Fig. 10.11a). In this case the conotruncal septum forms but is malrotated so that the single ventricle gives rise to a posterior pulmonary artery while the aorta arises from the persistent bulbis cordis. Not surprisingly, septation of the AV canal may also fail. In this circumstance the atrial and ventricular anatomy is strikingly similar to that in Fig. 10.8c.

The most common cardiac defects arise from incomplete septation of the atria or ventricles and are termed *atrial septal defect* and *ventricular septal defect*, respectively. Predictably, defects in both the primum and secundum atrial septum and defects in each of the three components of the ventricular septum also occur. Occasionally, development of the endocardial cushions is abnormal, causing failure of septation of the AV canal as well as the inferior portion of the atrial septum and inlet portion of the ventricular septum. Clinically this is termed a *complete AV canal defect* (Fig. 10.11b) and is common in children with *Down syndrome*.

Abnormalities of conus cordis and truncus arteriosus development are commonly seen, and are usually grouped together as conotruncal malformations (Fig. 10.11c). If the conotruncal septum fails to form, one would predict the finding of *persistent truncus arteriosus*. This lesion is always found with a defect in the outlet portion of the ventricular septum because this portion of the ventricular septum is actually derived from the conotruncal septum. In each of these circumstances, the defect of the mature heart arises by persistence of normal embryological configurations. Not all congenital heart disease arises from arrested maturation, but analyses like that above have provided considerable information about the genesis of congenital heart lesions, and have suggested avenues for experimental inquiry.

Although much is known about the anatomical causes of various congenital heart defects, very little is known about the molecular and cellular basis for these defects. Both genetic and environmental factors contribute to cardiac malformations. The importance of genetic factors is suggested by the high incidence of heart defects in *human trisomies and deletion syndromes*, the occurrence of several rare, but well described autosomal dominant and recessive conditions producing congenital heart defects, as well as the recent demonstration that abnormalities of cardiac looping seen in the situs inversus mouse are due to a single gene locus. The importance of environmental factors is supported by the growing list of **cardiac teratogens** including drugs (alcohol, lithium, thalidomide), infectious agents (rubella), maternal environment (diabetes), and fetal environment (phenylketonuria). Much work remains in defining the cause of most congenital heart defects.

Microscopic organization and function of the heart

The developing heart, like the mature heart, is made up of several different cell types, including myocytes, specialized conducting cells, fibroblasts, neural cells, and vascular elements. During the process of cardiac morphogenesis, the heart also contains numerous undifferentiated cells, termed mesenchymal cells, that ultimately will differentiate into mature cardiac cells or may die (as we have seen in the formation of the cardiac valves). The predominant cell type in the mature heart is the myocyte, which can be identified by the numerous myofibrils that contain the contractile apparatus. Within each myocyte the myofibrils are arranged in parallel along the cell's long axis, giving the myocyte its characteristic striated appearance. In the embryonic heart the first myocytes appear in the primitive cardiac tube; however, these contain relatively few myofibrils, the arrangement of which is somewhat more random than in the mature heart. After the developing heart reaches the four-chambered adult configuration, cardiac mass increases rapidly by myocyte division (hyperplasia). The myofibrillar content of myocytes increases steadily through gestation (hypertrophy). After birth, most species, including humans, have relatively little capacity for hyperplasia, but myocyte hypertrophy continues.

The cardiac myocyte, a relatively large and highly

specialized cell, has a subcellular structure uniquely organized to carry out its contractile function. Myocytes are packed with myofibrils, each containing numerous sarcomeres, the fundamental contractile unit, linked end to end. Each myofibril is surrounded by a complex network of membranes called the sarcoplasmic reticulum (SR), which supplies calcium to activate the contractile apparatus for each contraction and removes calcium during cardiac relaxation. Also nearby are vast numbers of mitochondria, the site of oxidative phosphorylation, which supply the high energy phosphates necessary for cellular contraction and maintenance of cellular integrity. The transmission of tension from the contractile apparatus to the whole ventricle requires a series of links from the sarcomere to the fibrous supporting matrix. This function is assumed by the cytoskeleton and the extracellular matrix. Each of these several cellular components will be examined in detail.

The sarcomere

As noted above, the myocyte contains many myofibrils arranged in parallel, each in turn composed of many sarcomeres arranged in series. As seen in Fig. 10.12, the sarcomere consists of an array of partially overlapping thick filaments composed of myosin as well as thin filaments composed primarily of actin. The sarcomere has been divided into various regions according to its microscopic appearance, and the content of each region is now known with some precision. Hence the dark Z line is the fibrous end of the sarcomere to which the actin filaments are anchored. The I band corresponds to the proximal portion of the actin filament not overlapping with myosin, while the A band corresponds to the length of the myosin filament. A great deal is now known about the several components of the sarcomere, the precise mechanism of sarcomere shortening, and the expression of contractile proteins during development.

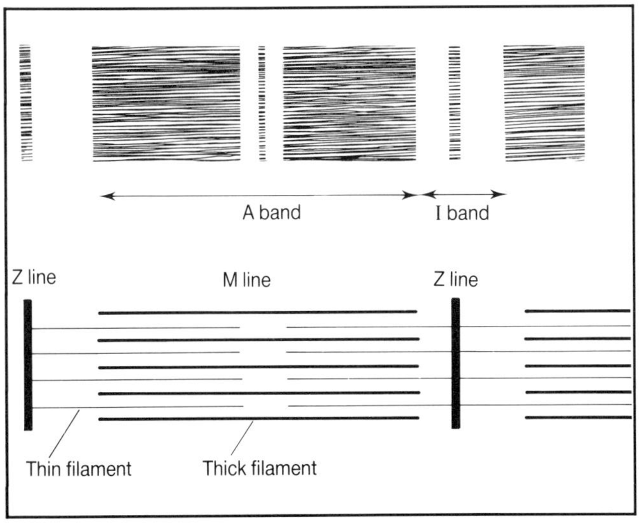

Fig. 10.12. The sarcomere is the fundamental contractile unit. Its appearance under the electron microscope (top) is produced by overlapping of thick filaments composed of myosin and thin filaments composed primarily of actin (bottom).

The thick filament is approximately 1.6 μm in length and about 10 nm in diameter at the center, but tapers toward each end. It is composed of overlapping double-stranded myosin heavy-chain molecules, each of which contains a rod-like portion and a globular head. The myosin heads are radially oriented, and attached to each is a myosin light-chain molecule. The head of the heavy chain contains the contractile ATPase. The thin filament is composed of a double-stranded helix of actin, through the center of which runs a third protein called tropomyosin. At regular intervals (0.3 μm), the troponin complex is found. Troponin comprises three proteins: troponin C, which binds calcium, troponin I, which inhibits intrinsic ATPase activity, and troponin T, which anchors the complex to the actin/tropomyosin chain. It is now generally accepted that the fundamental event in sarcomere shortening is the formation of crossbridges between the head of the myosin molecule and the thin filament, followed by rotation of the myosin head with consequent displacement of the actin filament by about 10 nm. Following displacement of the thin filament, the myosin head is released, and the cycle can be repeated. The details of this process are diagrammatically represented in Fig. 10.13. According to this model, the process is begun by the binding of Ca^{2+} to troponin C. This produces a conformational change in the thin filament that allows binding of the myosin heads, which are already charged with ADP and inorganic phosphate, the hydrolysis products of ATP. Once the myosin head is bound, its rotation is induced and the thin filament is displaced. After the stroke is completed, the ATP hydrolysis products are released and a new ATP molecule is bound before the myosin head is released from the thin filament. ATP is finally hydrolyzed in the process of restoring the activated conformation of the myosin heavy chain. One immediate consequence of this cycle arises

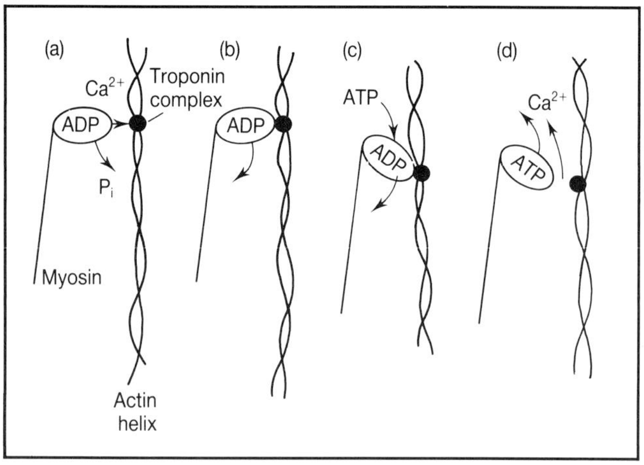

Fig. 10.13. The contractile cycle. (a) In response to increased Ca^{2+}, the myosin heads form crossbridges with actin thin filaments. (b) The myosin head rotates, thereby displacing the thin filament. (c) ADP and inorganic phosphate (P_i) are released and ATP is bound by the myosin head before the crossbridge is broken. (d) Ca^{2+} is removed and the crossbridge is broken. ATP is hydrolyzed, and the energy is stored as a change in conformation of the myosin head.

from the observation that ATP must bind to the myosin head before the latter is released from the thin filament. In circumstances that deplete ATP, myosin remains attached to the thin filament. In skeletal muscle this gives rise to rigor mortis, and in cardiac muscle it is a potential mechanism for impaired relaxation during periods of metabolic failure.

This model of sarcomere function has been greeted with enthusiasm because it provides an ultrastructural basis for several important physiological properties of the heart, the most important of which is Starling's law of the heart (see p. 499). Most simply stated, this law suggests that the heart is able to change the force of contraction as its initial size (or length) is changed. As seen in Fig. 10.14, this phenomenon can be explained based on the overlapping of thick and thin filaments. At a sarcomere length of 3.6 μm, there is essentially no force generation, because there is no overlap between thick and thin filaments. As the sarcomere is shortened, force generation increases due to increasing overlap of thick and thin filaments. At a sarcomere length of 2 μm, overlap and force generation are maximal. With further shortening, thin filaments begin to overlap each other, interfering with myosin crossbridge formation and force generation. The minimum sarcomere length corresponds to the length of the thick filament at which time the I band can be seen to disappear.

Over the past several years, intense interest has centered on the molecular biology of contractile proteins, the best studied of which are the myosin heavy chains. As has long been known, myosin heavy chains exist in three forms, denoted V1, V2, and V3, which differ in their relative rates of ATP hydrolysis. We now know that two myosin heavy-chain genes give rise to distinct isoforms called α and β. Dimerization of these isoforms yields the three V isoforms: V1 and V3 are α and β homodimers, respectively, while V2 is an αβ heterodimer. It is also known that in most mature mammals, ventricular muscle contains the V1 isoform with the highest ATPase activity. However, before birth the V3 isoform predominates. In human heart, ventricular muscle does not switch from V3 expression after birth, but whether contractile protein expression may be altered in some disease states is not known.

Switching of myosin heavy-chain genes occurs in many other muscles throughout the body, but not all switch from V1 to V3. This raised an interesting molecular question: why under the influence of thyroid hormone does one muscle switch from V1 to V3, while another will switch from V3 to V1 or V2? The basis of the neonatal myosin heavy-chain switching is now known to be due to the neonatal increase in thyroid hormone concentrations, and the answer to this question comes from knowledge of thyroid hormone receptors. This ever-expanding family of receptors binds thyroid hormone, and the complex can then bind to the regulatory regions of responsive genes either to enhance or to repress transcription of specific genes. The myosin heavy-chain genes contain several sequences upstream (5′ in DNA language) of the coding sequences that are capable of binding the thyroid hormone–receptor complex. Hence tissue-specific expression of myosin heavy-chain genes depends upon the thyroid hormone receptor(s) being expressed by each muscle at a particular time. This observation was very important in developmental biology because it demonstrated one way in which expression of a single gene can be independently regulated by the several tissues that must express the gene at one time or another.

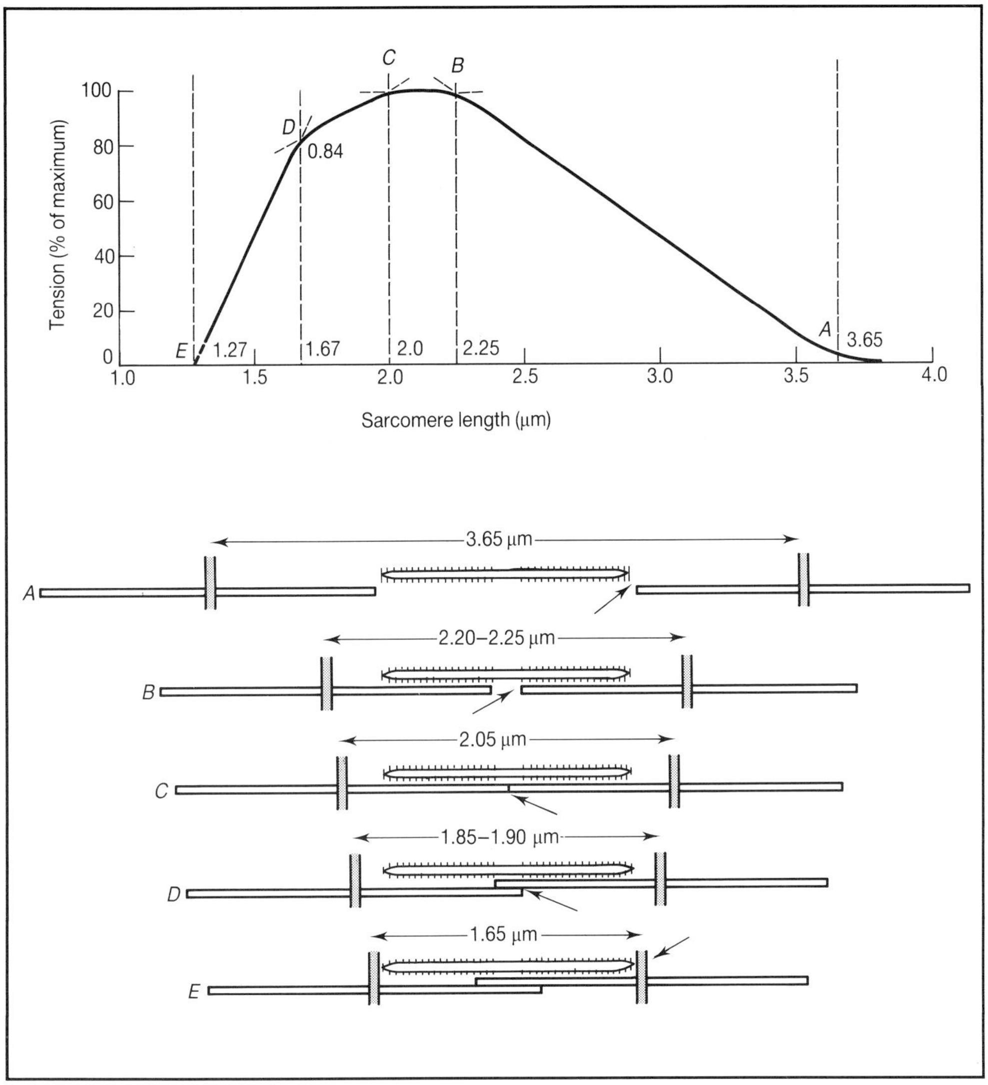

Fig. 10.14. The ultrastructural basis for Starling's law of the heart. Upper panel: Developed tension as a function of sarcomere length. Lower panel: Force generation is dependent upon initial sarcomere length which determines overlap between thick and thin filaments. Maximal tension occurs with optimum overlap (about 2 μm). (From Braunwald E, ed. *Heart disease, a textbook of cardiovascular medicine.* Philadelphia: Saunders, 1980, p. 427, with permission.)

Sarcoplasmic reticulum and excitation–contraction coupling

For the myocyte to contract and relax as frequently as three or four times per second, an extremely rapid mechanism must activate and deactivate myofibrillar contraction. The sarcoplasmic reticulum (SR) is now well known to play the central role in this process. The SR is a membrane-limited intracellular organelle that surrounds each sarcomere with longitudinal tubules. The SR alternately releases and sequesters intracellular calcium ions that are ultimately responsible for myofibrillar contraction. The cell membrane of the myocyte contains invaginations localized over the Z line of each sarcomere, and from these, further extensions called T tubules penetrate the myocyte. At some points the SR and T tubule lie very close (10 nm), and in these regions the SR flattens into sac-like structures called cisternae. One should remember that although the T tubule system and the SR are both membrane systems, they do not communicate directly. The T tubule system is in communication with the extracellular space, while the SR is an intracellular organelle. They are, however, closely coupled, as depolarization of the cell membrane is channeled through the T tubules, leading to a small increase in intracellular Ca^{2+} concentration during the plateau phase of the action potential. This increase in

Ca^{2+} is not sufficient to activate contraction, but does activate release of Ca^{2+} from the SR, which raises intracellular Ca^{2+} by 100-fold, which in turn activates myofibrillar contraction. This integrated process is termed 'excitation–contraction coupling.'

In mature myocytes the primary site of Ca^{2+} release and storage is the cisternae of the SR, where Ca^{2+} is sequestered by a binding protein called calsequestrin. Because of its central role in excitation–contraction coupling, Ca^{2+} concentration in the cisternae of the SR is believed to play an important role in determining the inotropic state of the myocyte. During relaxation, Ca^{2+} is actively transported into the SR by a Ca^{2+}-dependent ATPase and bound by a second Ca^{2+}-binding protein, phospholamban. Both the Ca^{2+}-dependent ATPase and phospholamban are confined to the longitudinal tubules. Because the sites of systolic and diastolic Ca^{2+} flux are different, it is not surprising that abnormalities of systolic and diastolic function are frequently separable.

Present evidence suggests that Ca^{2+} handling by the sarcolemma of immature myocytes is relatively well developed. Conversely, Ca^{2+} transport by the SR is less well developed. There are fewer cisternae in the SR, and Ca^{2+} uptake by the SR has been shown to be decreased due to a lower rate of ATP hydrolysis and a lower coupling ratio (moles Ca^{2+} pumped/mole ATP hydrolyzed). The first implication of these findings is that extracellular Ca^{2+} may be quantitatively more important for activation of the contractile apparatus in immature myocardium, which may explain its more pronounced Ca^{2+} sensitivity when compared with mature myocardium. Furthermore, the impaired Ca^{2+} uptake by SR may be responsible for altered diastolic function in the fetus. Finally, in mature myocardium, the availability of intracellular Ca^{2+} to the contractile proteins obviously is a major determinant of inotropic state. This is true for increases in inotropy due to increased heart rate, both following a premature extrasystole, and following administration of cardiac glycosides (digoxin). Because both release and uptake of Ca^{2+} by SR are reduced in the immature heart, it has been postulated that fetal cardiac function is impaired relative to the adult. Whether this speculation will be borne out in intact animals remains an open question.

Extracellular matrix and cytoskeleton

During each systole, individual myocytes obviously must shorten. It is equally true that for this to occur there must be a link between the myofibril and the cell wall and between the cell wall and the extracellular matrix. Individual myofibrils are linked together and to the cell wall through a complex network of microtubules and microfilaments. In recent years interest has grown in the connections of the cell with the extracellular matrix (ECM). For many years it was believed that the ECM was a static collection of structural elements that merely provided support for the cellular elements. While the ECM certainly fills this function, it is now known to be a dynamic mix of adhesive, structural proteins such as collagen, fibronectin, and laminin, antiadhesive proteins such as tenascin, SPARC, and thrombospondin, as well as a host of other regulatory molecules including growth factors and proteases. This is especially true during cardiac development. Indeed much of the interest in cardiac ECM has been stimulated by observations suggesting that the ECM plays important roles in cell migration, proliferation, and maturation during organogenesis in organisms as diverse as *Drosophila* and humans and in organs as diverse as skin and brain.

Cell migration is an integral part of cardiac morphogenesis, and the ECM plays a critical role in cell migration throughout cardiac development. The earliest cardiac progenitor cells appear to migrate along a fibronectin gradient on their way to forming the primitive cardiac tube. Experimental perturbations that disrupt the interaction between these cells and ECM components (especially fibronectin) completely prevent heart formation at this stage. Once formed, the primitive cardiac tube consists of a thick layer of ECM sandwiched between an epithelial layer of cardiac progenitor cells above and an endothelial layer below. It has long been suspected that the process of looping depends upon the presence and composition of the ECM. The ECM also plays a crucial role in the closure of the endocardial cushions. The endocardial cushions begin as acellular masses of ECM, into which mesenchymal cells must migrate, followed by proliferation and subsequent maturation. Alteration of the ECM has been shown to interfere with this process, leading to the hypothesis that the primary defect leading to endocardial cushion defects is an augmentation of cell adhesion to ECM. Finally, closure of the conotruncal septum has been shown to require the influx of migrating cranial neural crest cells. Although not shown directly for migration into developing heart, the migration of neural crest cells is known to require both adhesive and antiadhesive matrix interactions.

The precise mechanism of ECM interaction with cells is known for very few matrix elements; however, the interaction of fibronectin with cells is prototypic in this respect (Fig. 10.15). Fibronectin appears to bind to cells through a specific receptor or integrin. The fibronectin receptor is one of a large family of related receptors with overlapping affinities for ECM components. Fibronectin is a large molecule containing three different types of protein domains, each repeated several times. The different domains have affinities for cells or other matrix components. The primary binding of fibronectin to its receptor involves a very short amino acid sequence (Gly-Arg-Gly-Asp-Ser), and several other matrix proteins

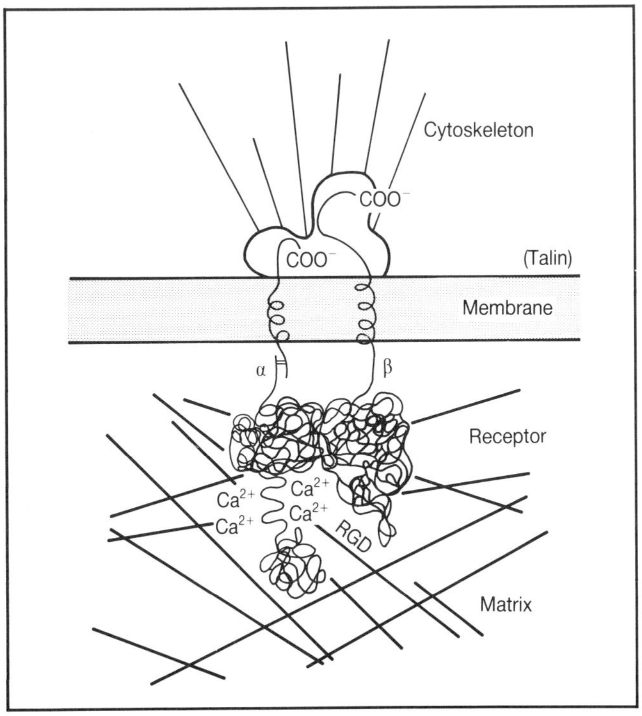

Fig. 10.15. Integrins establish a physical link between the cytoskeleton and ECM. The integrin receptor is composed of one α and one β chain. Binding of the sequence Arg-Gly-Asp (RGD) by the globular extracellular domain requires extracellular Ca^{2+}. Both integrin chains span the cell membrane and contact the cytoskeleton through the membrane-associated protein talin. This mechanism allows cells to flatten themselves by pulling on a rigid matrix or to deform the matrix if it is weak. (From Ruoslahti E, Pierschbacher MD. *Science* 1987; **238**: 496, with permission.)

appear to bind to integrin receptors using this short sequence. As one might expect from the discussion above, occupancy of the receptor may do more than anchor the cell to the ECM. The integrin receptor is coupled to the cytoskeleton through the protein talin, and in this way can dramatically affect cell shape. Remarkably, occupancy of the receptor can also lead to changes in gene expression, which in turn could stimulate or repress cellular proliferation or lead to the production of new proteins associated with the maturing myocyte phenotype. The mechanism(s) by which the ECM can turn on gene expression is unknown, but an intriguing hypothesis is that a change in cell shape also produces a change in nuclear shape, which alters expression of certain genes in some unknown fashion.

Evidence is accumulating that other ECM proteins also interact with cells through specific receptors, and one can easily envision that interaction with different receptors may produce quite different cellular behaviors. A useful model, although clearly oversimplified, defines cellular interactions with ECM as either adhesive or antiadhesive. How these interactions might be important in morphogenesis is best demonstrated by two relevant, but hypothetical examples. The first is the case of cardiac progenitor cells migrating to form the primitive cardiac tube (Fig. 10.16). It is considered axiomatic that to migrate, cells must adhere to ECM. As mentioned above, cardiac progenitor cells migrate along a path rich in fibronectin, the prototypic adhesive molecule. One can easily envision the cells sticking to such a matrix, but what allows them actually to move? One possibility is that the leading edge of migrating cells is firmly attached to the ECM, while the trailing edge is freed by competing antiadhesive forces. This may entail elaboration at the trailing edge of antiadhesive proteins (like tenascin) by the cell or weakening of the interaction of cell with matrix by proteolysis of the matrix. In some cell types, occupancy of certain integrin receptors with fibronectin fragments can induce expression of proteases that break down ECM proteins, including fibronectin. Hence a feed-forward loop is established that could rapidly free the trailing edge of the migrating cell. What then signals migrating cells to stop? Again at least two possibilities exist. Perhaps as the cells encounter a greater concentration of adhesive matrix components, the antiadhesive forces are simply overwhelmed. More likely, some new signal turns off the elaboration of antiadhesive proteins or proteases.

The interaction of adhesive and antiadhesive forces can

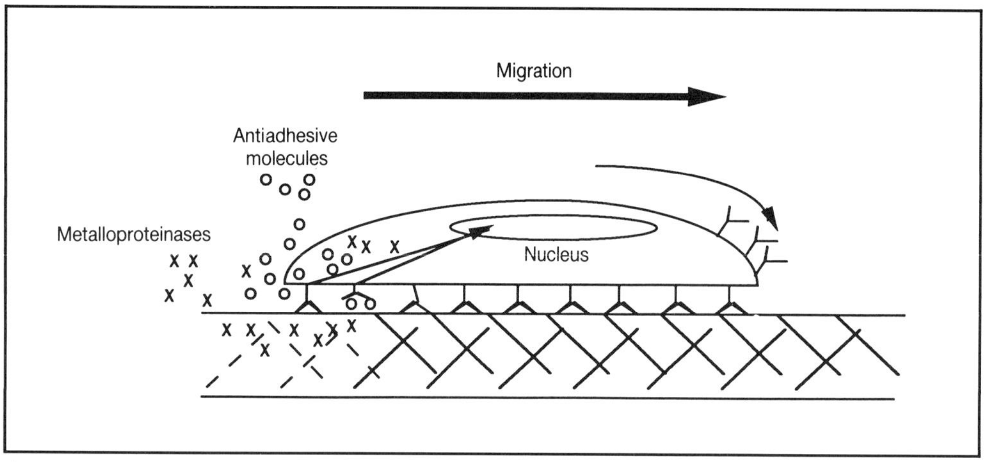

Fig. 10.16. Adhesive and antiadhesive effects are required for cell migration. During migration the leading edge of the cell is anchored while the trailing edge is freed by elaboration of antiadhesive factors. Migration ceases when the antiadhesive signal is interrupted.

also be invoked to explain changes in organ shape. The most energetically favorable cell shape is round, the shape assumed by myocytes when in solution rather than attached to ECM. The primitive cardiac tube is composed of a cardiac epithelium resting on a layer of ECM. When the tube is straight, the epithelial cells are flattened onto the matrix. If the matrix is weakened, e.g. by proteolysis, cells will seek a more energetically favorable conformation and will begin to deform the matrix as shown in Fig. 10.17. If the weakening of the matrix is radially asymmetric, the tube will begin to bend, with the weak matrix on the convex side. Cells on the convex side may need their interaction with the matrix to be weakened by anti-adhesive proteins that allow the matrix to be deformed without undue strain on the myocytes. Some experimental evidence supports this hypothesis: incubation of cardiac tubes with colchicine, which disrupts microtubules that are critical for maintenance of cell shape, prevents looping. This observation suggests that the energy to deform the tube is supplied by the cardiac cells rather than by deforming forces within the ECM.

Mitochondria and myocardial O_2 and energy metabolism

Heart muscle is unique among the body's tissues because of the frequency with which it must perform mechanical work. Mechanical work uses much more energy than metabolic interconversions or transport processes. This is demonstrated by the observation that the O_2 consumption of the resting heart is less than 20 percent that of the contracting heart. The primary determinant of myocardial O_2 consumption is wall tension or stress, although heart rate, contractility, and stroke volume are also important. The O_2 consumption of the fetal and adult heart are similar. However, because fetal blood O_2 content is substantially less than that of the adult, and because both fetal and adult hearts extract nearly all of the available O_2 from blood, fetal myocardial blood flow is roughly twice that of the adult. This is probably accomplished by a greater capillary density in the fetus than in the adult. For the first few months of postnatal life in most mammalian species, muscular growth of the ventricles (hypertrophy) is accompanied by growth of new blood vessels. The mechanism(s) responsible for new vessel growth during hypertrophy and its cessation with time are presently unknown.

As pointed out above, O_2 extraction by the heart is maximal under basal conditions, and therefore increased O_2 demands must be met with increases in blood flow. Normally, O_2 demand and coronary blood flow are closely coupled and both increase approximately fourfold with maximal exertion (see p. 493). The difference between basal and maximal coronary blood flow is termed coronary flow reserve, and because it is so large in infants and children, imbalances between myocardial O_2 demand and delivery are unusual. However, such an imbalance can occur in response to *severe aortic stenosis*. In this setting, left ventricular outlet obstruction causes muscular hypertrophy. During the first few months of life, this is accompanied by new blood vessel growth. Eventually, new vessel growth stops; at this point, blood flow to new muscle reduces coronary reserve. If hypertrophy becomes massive, or if additional stresses of hypoxemia, anemia, exercise, or tachycardia are added, O_2 demand may

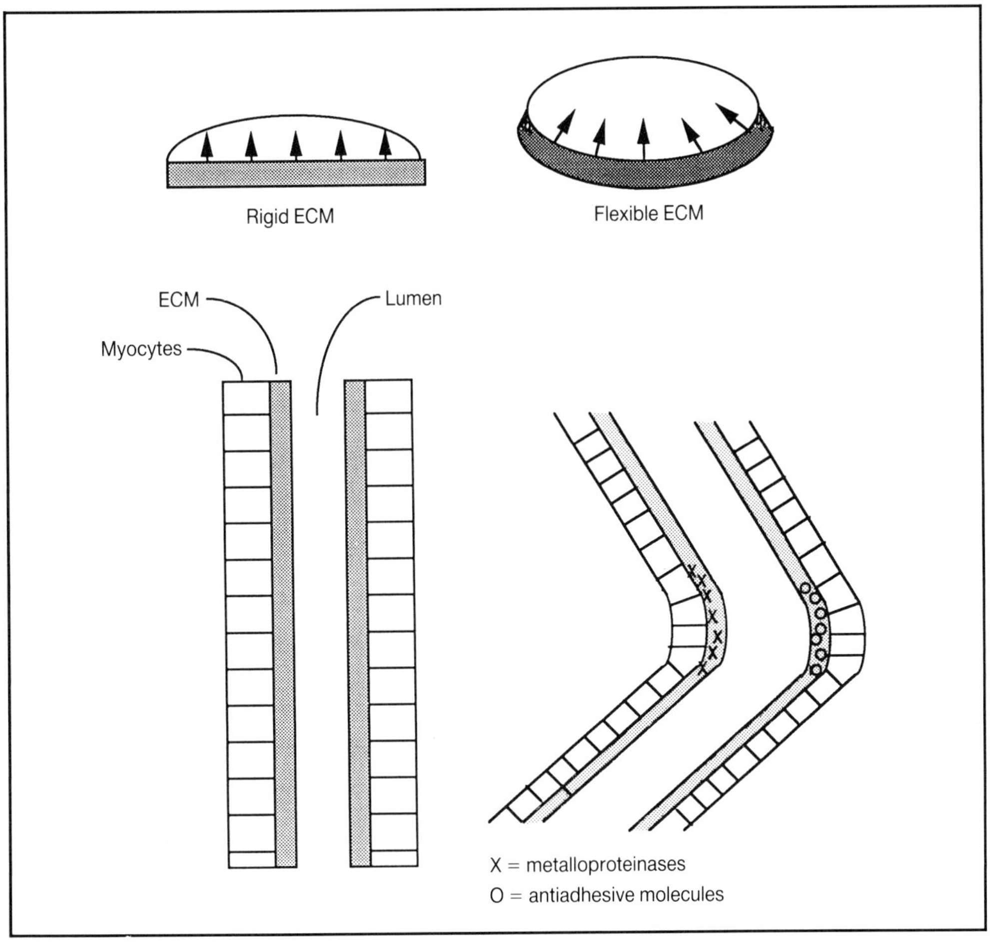

Fig. 10.17. Deformation of the cardiac tube. Upper panels: when adherent to a rigid matrix, myocytes are flattened. When the matrix is weakened, tension from the myocyte is transmitted across the sarcolemma to the ECM at points of attachment and the matrix is pulled up around the myocytes. Bending of the ECM allows myocytes to assume an energetically more favorable configuration. Lower panels: radially asymmetric weakening of the ECM, by the action of matrix degrading enzymes, will lead to bending of the tube.

eventually outstrip coronary flow reserve, and ischemia results, especially in the subendocardium, the deepest layer of the myocardium. During ischemia, myocardial concentrations of high-energy phosphates fall, interfering with contraction and eventually leading to myocyte death. It is not at all unusual to see patchy areas of fibrosis or necrosis in hearts of children with severe aortic stenosis, especially in the subendocardium, although this rarely produces a macroscopic myocardial infarction. With surgical relief of obstruction, hypertrophy gradually regresses and coronary reserve is returned to normal.

A second related circumstance is that of *familial hypertrophic cardiomyopathy.* In this autosomal-dominant disease, abnormal ventricular muscle accumulates progressively, leading to massive ventricular hypertrophy. Histologically this muscle is characterized by disorganization of myofibrils, and fibrosis (presumably due to myocyte death). Remarkably, the disorder has been found to be due to point mutations in the β-myosin heavy-chain gene in 50 percent of cases. Although the abnormal arrangement of myofibrils might be expected to result from such a defect, it is not known why this also leads to cellular hypertrophy. It is attractive to hypothesize that myocytes containing both normal and abnormal myosin initially have a mild defect in tension development, and that this leads to increased synthesis of contractile proteins. This is plausible because the normal response to increased wall tension is synthesis of contractile proteins and myocyte hypertrophy. Hence a mechanism must exist that transduces tension into synthesis of contractile proteins. As abnormal myosin accumulates, more myofibrils are affected and tension generation worsens, leading to further hypertrophy. This exciting observation promises to teach us much about the pathophysiology of myocardial hypertrophy in normal hearts.

Although O_2 consumption is similar in adult and fetal myocardium, the fuels used by the two are dramatically different. The adult heart preferentially uses fatty acids, while the fetal heart is an obligatory user of carbohydrates, burning about 35 percent glucose, 60 percent lactate, and 5 percent pyruvate in the fetal lamb. This observation is of some clinical importance; severe hypoglycemia can precipitate metabolic failure and seriously depress cardiac function in neonates, but is quite unlikely to do so in older children or adults.

The perinatal difference in myocardial fuel preference was initially felt simply to reflect substrate availability, i.e. comparatively low fatty acid concentrations in the fetus, and low lactate concentrations in the adult. However, it is now known that exogenous free fatty acids are not utilized by the fetal heart *in vitro* or *in vivo*. In fact, they are actually detrimental to fetal cardiac function. To gain insight into how myocardial fuel preference is regulated in the fetus and the adult, we must first understand something about the metabolism of energy substrates and the process of high-energy phosphate production in the heart.

Within the cell, the site of O_2 consumption and ATP production is the mitochondrion. Consistent with its role as the primary source of the high-energy phosphates required for contraction, cardiac mitochondria are tightly packed between adjacent myofibrils. They are also numerous, occupying as much as 30 percent of total myocyte volume. Mitochondria are bounded by an outer membrane and an inner membrane. Associated with the inner membrane are the enzymes of the citric acid cycle, which oxidizes two carbon fragments to CO_2 and supplies NADH and $FADH_2$ to the respiratory chain for generation of ATP (Fig. 10.18). The inner membrane is folded into numerous cristae, which greatly increase the surface area available for these reactions. ATP is not freely diffusible out of mitochondria. ATP is transported across the mitochondrial membrane in exchange for ADP by the adenine nucleotide antiporter. Once outside mitochondria, ATP is still not freely diffusible as it quickly transfers its high-energy phosphate to creatine using the enzyme mitochondrial creatine kinase. Creatine phosphate then diffuses to sites of ATP hydrolysis (such as the contractile apparatus) where the high-energy phosphate is transferred back to ADP by other creatine kinase isoforms. Regardless of the fuel used, these reactions represent the pathway for ATP production, so regulation of fuel preference clearly must be proximal to the citric acid cycle.

The counter-regulation of fuel substrates in mature myocardium is illustrated in Fig. 10.19. Fatty acids entering the cardiac cell are quickly esterified to coenzyme A, forming acyl-CoA. This is necessary because unesterified fatty acids can associate with and injure many of the cell's membranes. However, acyl-CoA is unable to cross the mitochondrial membranes for subsequent metabolism, so a specific transport mechanism is required. For transport, acyl-CoA is transesterified with carnitine to form acylcarnitine and free coenzyme A. A specific transport protein called carnitine-palmitoyl transferase 1 (or CPT 1) mediates this transfer. A second enzyme termed CPT 2 mediates transfer across the inner mitochondrial membrane and conversion back to acyl-CoA. The fatty acid then undergoes β-oxidation, liberating acetyl-CoA for entry into the citric acid cycle. The primary site of regulation in this pathway appears to be the entry of fatty acids into mitochondria, and this is accomplished through inhibition of CPT 1 by malonyl-CoA, the first committed intermediate in fatty acid synthesis. Concentrations of malonyl-CoA are lower in muscle than in liver (where fat synthesis is active), but muscle CPT is far more sensitive to malonyl-CoA inhibition than is liver CPT. Malonyl-CoA concentrations in turn are regulated by circulating concentrations of glucagon. After birth, glucagon concentrations surge, removing malonyl-CoA inhibition of CPT 1 and allowing fatty acid oxidation to begin.

The next question is how fatty acid oxidation feeds back to inhibit glucose utilization. In contrast to fatty acids, primary regulation of glucose metabolism occurs in the cytosol. As shown in Fig. 10.19, the glycolytic pathway splits glucose into two molecules of pyruvate. This initial phase of glucose metabolism nets only a small amount of ATP and is quantitatively unimportant for both fetal and mature myocardium. A much larger yield of ATP is produced when pyruvate enters the mitochondrion where acetyl-CoA is generated and oxidized by the citric acid cycle. It has been known for many years that when fatty acids are being oxidized, glucose utilization is limited by inhibition of the glycolytic enzyme phosphofructokinase (PFK1), which catalyzes the phosphorylation of fructose 6-phosphate (F-6-P) to fructose 1,6-bisphosphate (F-1,6-P) in an ATP-requiring reaction. This highly regulated enzyme has been the focus of many investigations through which more than a dozen different metabolites have been found to affect the activity of the purified enzyme *in vitro*. The most potent inhibitors of PFK activity are ATP and citrate. In isolated perfused hearts, the rise in cytosolic citrate accompanying fatty acid

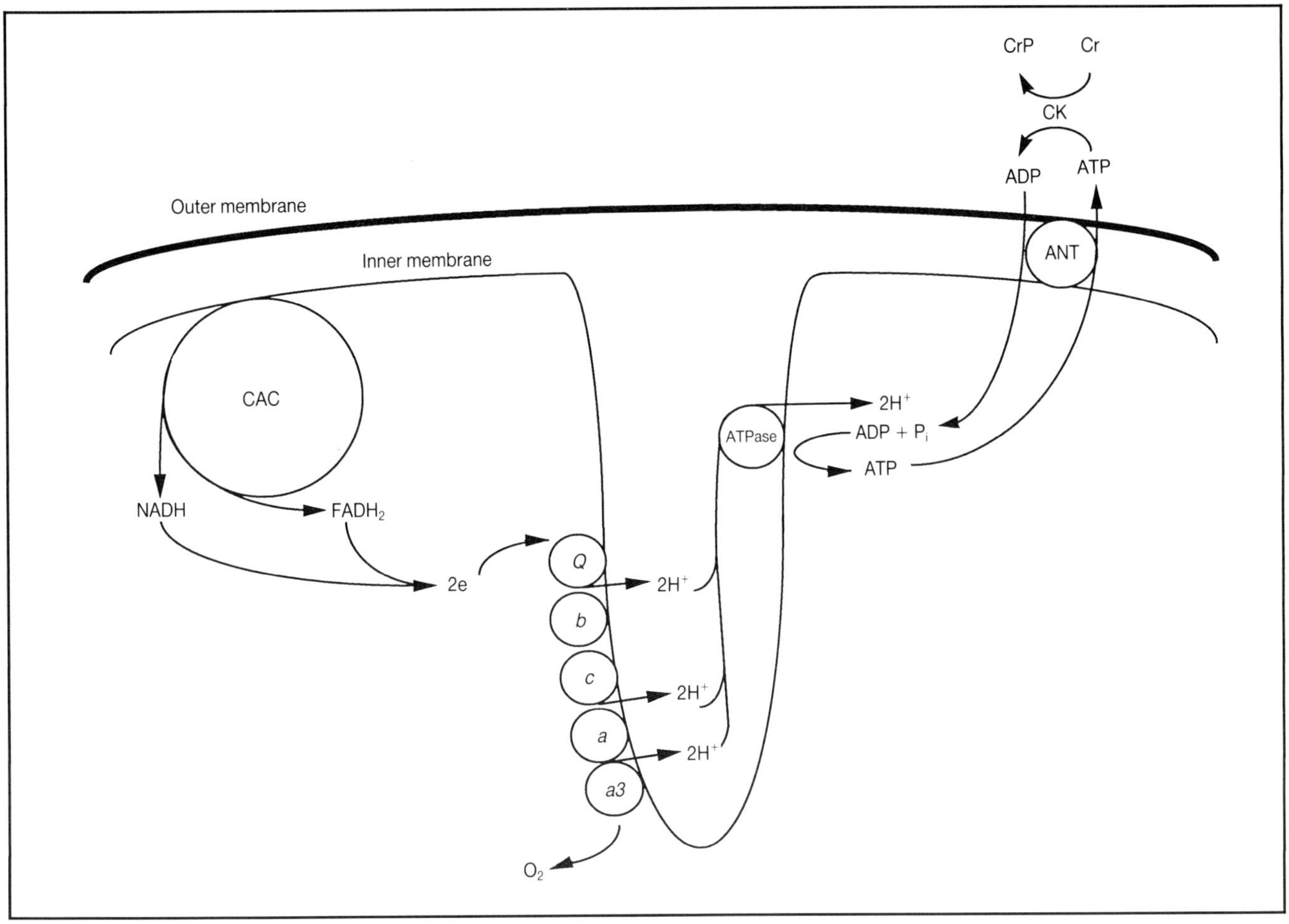

Fig. 10.18. Mitochondrial generation of ATP. The enzymes of the citric acid cycle (CAC) oxidize acetyl-CoA to CO_2, reducing NAD and FAD in the process. NADH and $FADH_2$ transfer their electrons (2e) to the respiratory chain where electron transport causes H^+ to be transported across the inner membrane. This creates a pH gradient. Movement of H^+ back across the inner membrane is coupled with phosphorylation of ADP to ATP. Finally, high energy phosphate from ATP is transferred to creatine (Cr) via the adenine nucleotide transporter (ANT) and creatine kinase (CK). CrP, creatine phosphate; Pi, inorganic phosphate; *Q*, *b*, *c*, *a*, *a3*, cytochromes; see text for remaining abbreviations.

oxidation probably is primarily responsible for inhibition of PFK. Indeed, citrate and ATP inhibition are so powerful that in the presence of physiological concentrations of its substrates and its numerous positive and negative effectors, there is no demonstrable PFK activity *in vitro*. How then does the cardiac cell metabolize glucose *in vivo*? Only recently a powerful new positive effector was discovered, capable of overcoming the inhibition produced by ATP and citrate. Its identity is fructose 2,6-bisphosphate (F-2,6-P_2), and it is formed by a second PFK enzyme (PFK_2), so named because it phosphorylates the 2 position of F-6-P and because it was the second PFK enzyme discovered. F-2,6-P_2 is present in both fetal and mature hearts at concentrations that activate PFK_1 sufficiently to account for glycolytic fluxes observed *in vivo*.

It seems likely that in heart, as in liver, glucose and fatty acid oxidation are regulated in parallel. In liver, both malonyl-CoA and F-2,6-P_2 concentrations are regulated by the circulating glucagon:insulin ratio, and it is likely that the same is true in the heart. In the fetus the insulin:glucagon ratio is high, malonyl-CoA and F-2,6-P_2 concentrations are both high, and CPT is inhibited, while PFK_1 is stimulated. After birth, the glucagon surge dissipates malonyl-CoA and F-2,6-P_2, releasing CPT inhibition and allowing fatty acid oxidation to proceed, while allowing citrate and ATP to inhibit PFK_1 and glycolytic flux. The extent to which the hormonal milieu

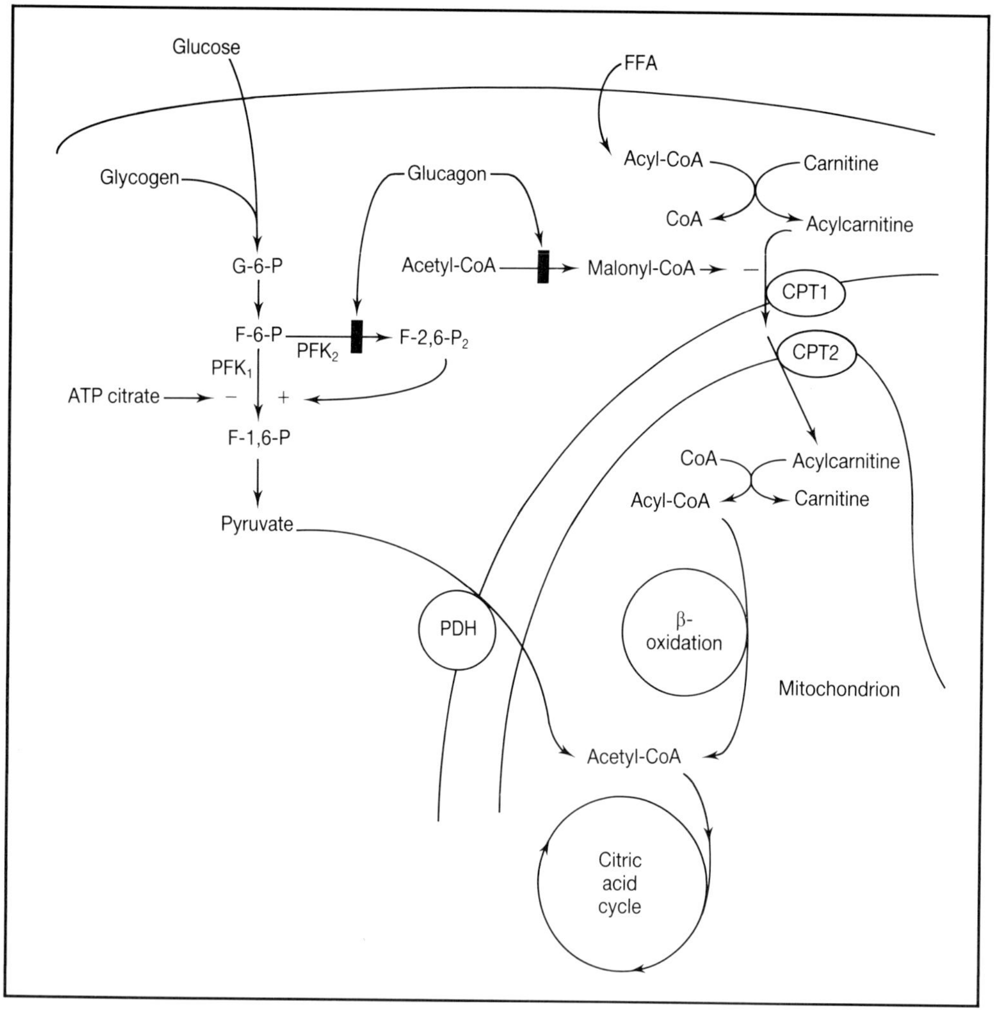

Fig. 10.19. The probable role of glucagon in the regulation of fatty acid and glucose utilization. The glycolytic pathway leading from glucose to pyruvate is regulated at the PFK_1 reaction. This reaction is potently inhibited by ATP and citrate and activated by F-2,6-P_2. The latter is formed by PFK_2, the activity of which is decreased by glucagon in a cAMP-dependent mechanism. Fatty acid oxidation is regulated at the level of acylcarnitine transport across the outer mitochondrial membrane, mediated by CPT 1. CPT 1 is inhibited by malonyl-CoA, which is synthesized from acetyl-CoA and HCO_3^- in the cytosol. Malonyl-CoA levels are also decreased by glucagon. The postnatal glucagon surge will decrease both F-2,6-P_2 and malonyl-CoA, allowing fatty acid oxidation, while inhibiting glycolysis. PDH, pyruvate dehydrogenase; see text for remaining abbreviations.

may influence myocardial fuel preference of adult hearts on a day-to-day basis is largely unexplored.

Selected reading

Anderson PAW. Immature myocardium. In Moller J, Neal WA, eds. *Fetal, neonatal and infant cardiac disease*. Norwalk, CT: Appleton & Lange, 1990: 35.

Damsky CH, Bernfield M. Cell-to-cell contact and extracellular matrix. *Curr Opin Cell Biol* 1991; **3**: 777.

Icardo JM. The growing heart: an anatomical perspective. In Zak R, ed. *Growth of the heart in health and disease*. New York: Raven Press, 1984: 41.

Van Mierop LH. Morphological development of the heart. In Berne RM, ed. *Handbook of physiology, Section 2: The cardiovascular system, Vol. 1: Circulation*. Bethesda, MD: American Physiologic Society, 1979: 1.

C. Myocardial Receptors

E Birk

Myocardial receptors and guanine nucleotide-binding proteins

Receptors can be defined as cellular macromolecules that, when bound to a discrete group of compounds, lead to a cascade of intracellular events. Many receptors reside in the plasma membrane and, when bound to an appropriate ligand, propagate its signal into the cell. The formation of a receptor–ligand complex leads to a cellular effect either directly or by inducing the release or synthesis of another regulatory molecule (the latter known as a second messenger). This chain of events eventually leads to biochemical and physiological responses.

Mammalian myocardium contains a variety of receptors. These receptors can be activated by neurotransmitters released from autonomic efferent nerve fibers, by hormones secreted from distant organs, or by autacoids produced locally by cardiac tissue.

Receptors elicit a cellular response through a series of steps. The activated receptor couples to a membrane-associated signal transducer, which in turn stimulates a response element (Fig. 10.20). A common succession of such a pathway (Fig. 10.21) begins with the coupling of a guanine nucleotide (GTP)-binding protein (G-protein) to an activated receptor. The G-protein is then coupled to a cellular response element, which is either an enzyme or an ion channel. Coupling to an enzyme produces a second messenger, which in turn leads to a physiological event either directly or via activation of other cellular enzymes.

G-proteins are a family of proteins; each one is formed by heterotrimers, consisting of α-, β-, and γ-subunits. The α-subunit is thought to be the actual signal transducer of the G-protein, interacting with the effector. It also serves as the activation-deactivation element of the G-protein by binding and hydrolyzing GTP, respectively. Once activated by a stimulated receptor, the α-subunit releases a GDP molecule and binds GTP instead; at the same time, the affinity of the α-subunit to β/γ-subunits is decreased, and a β/γ complex is released. Deactivation of the G-protein occurs by GTPase activity of the α-subunit (releasing a free phosphate from the α-subunit-bound GTP) and by

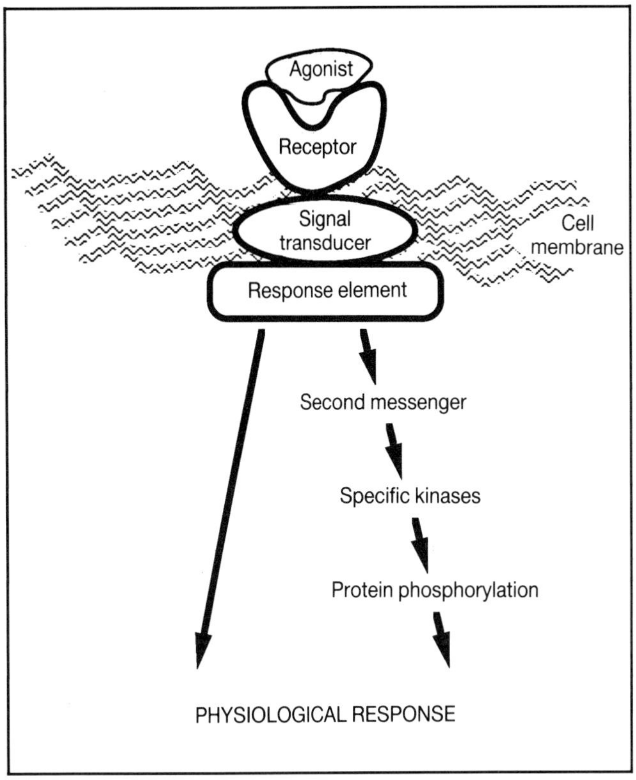

Fig. 10.20. Description of transmembrane signal transduction: an agonist activates a receptor, which in turn stimulates a signal transducer (e.g. G-protein). Once activated, the signal transducer stimulates a response element (e.g. ion channels, enzymes) that, either directly or via additional steps, results in a physiological response.

reassociation with the β/γ complex. G-proteins can have a stimulatory (G_s-protein) or an inhibitory (G_i-protein) effect on cellular response elements.

Several G-proteins may regulate myocardial function. Some appear able to interact with more than one receptor and with more than one cellular response element. Therefore, activation of different receptors may cause the same cellular response; on the other hand, activation of a single receptor group can stimulate various cellular responses.

Little information exists regarding developmental changes in the expression and function of cardiac G-proteins. There is an increase in the G-protein that

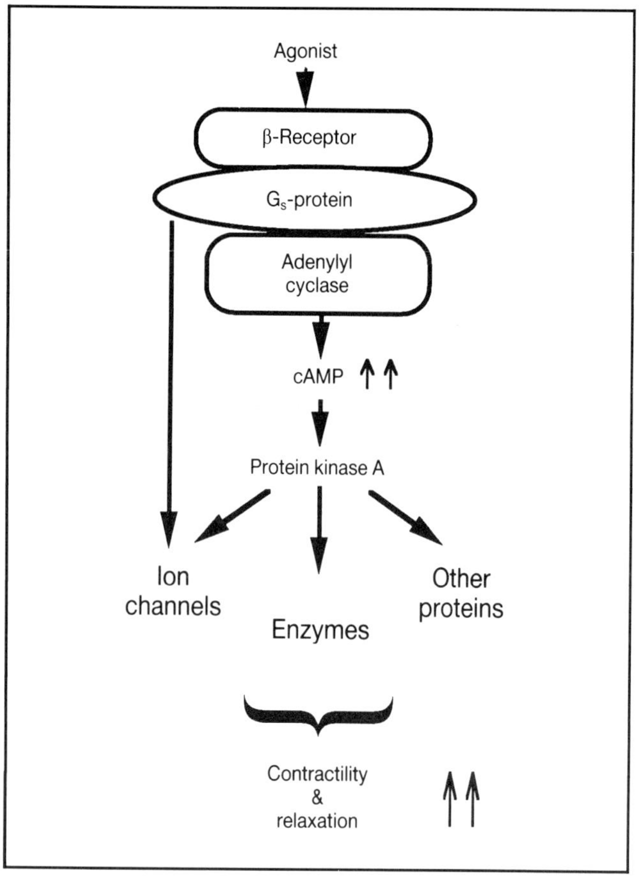

Fig. 10.21. The activation of a β-adrenergic receptor leads to a chain of events resulting in an increase in myocardial contractility and relaxation rate.

mediates α_1-adrenergic responses in developing neonatal rat myocytes. This increase was associated with developing myocardial innervation, and changed the chronotropic effect of α_1-adrenergic stimulation from a positive to a negative one. Ventricular $G_{i\alpha}$ decreases during development and aging in rat myocardium. However, the regulatory consequences of this process are not clear.

The G-proteins transmit the signals generated by hormone–receptor interactions to a diverse group of effectors, including adenylyl cyclase, phospholipase C, and ion channels.

Specific receptors and their signal transduction pathways

β-Adrenergic receptors

β-Adrenergic receptor activation provides a major means of regulating myocardial contractility: adrenergic agonists potentiate myocardial contraction and enhance the rate of relaxation.

β-Adrenergic receptors are glycoproteins located in the membrane bilayer. β-Adrenergic receptors are not uniform, and can be classified into two major groups: the β_1 subtype, which provide a major cardiac signaling pathway, and the β_2 subtype, which mediate signal transduction in smooth muscle cells. Most mammalian ventricular myocardium contains the β_1-receptor subtype almost exclusively; in humans, the β_1 subtype constitutes approximately 80 percent of the myocardial β-receptor population. Both subtypes are coupled to adenylyl cyclase and a positive inotropic response.

β-Adrenergic receptors utilize G-proteins in translating receptor occupancy into a biochemical response. The receptor interacts with $G_{s\alpha}$ to stimulate adenylyl cyclase mediated production of the second messenger cAMP. Next, cAMP activates its protein kinase. The activated enzyme, in turn, phosphorylates several key regulatory proteins of the cardiac muscle, including phospholamban and troponin I. $G_{s\alpha}$ can also stimulate mammalian cardiac Ca^{2+} channels and inhibit Na^+ channels in neonatal ventricular myocytes, both directly and via cAMP production (Fig. 10.21).

Maturation of β-adrenergic receptors, in terms of their ability to respond to an agonist with the production of a second messenger and their ability to elicit a physiological response, has been shown to occur early during fetal myocardial development. The pharmacological characteristics and function of the β-adrenergic receptors are similar in fetal, newborn, and adult myocardium.

The β-adrenergic receptor cascade appears to play a substantial role in compensatory mechanisms during fetal stress as well as in increasing heart rate and cardiac output during labor and delivery. Such an adrenergic effect can be modulated by changes in β-receptor agonist concentration, e.g. catecholamines, as well as by a change in receptor availability and function. Indeed, it appears that more than one mechanism regulates the β-adrenergic pathway.

Circulating catecholamine concentrations increase significantly during fetal stress (e.g. hypoxemia), as well as during birth and shortly thereafter; the latter has been shown both in humans and sheep. Moreover, the density of myocardial receptors is higher in neonates than in adults. Changes in myocardial adrenergic responsiveness during fetal and neonatal development are modulated by thyroid hormones. An increase or decrease in hormone concentrations results in a significant increase or decrease in β-adrenergic receptor number, respectively. In other systems, steroids modulate adrenergic receptor number.

α_1-Adrenergic receptors

α_1-Adrenergic receptors, found in mammalian and human myocardium, have both a chronotropic and an inotropic effect. However, their density is significantly lower than that of the β-adrenergic receptors, and their physiological role is not clearly understood. α_1-Adrenergic stimulation results in a negative chronotropic effect in the adult. Reports regarding myocardial mechanical responses to α_1-adrenergic stimulation have been conflicting; some have indicated a positive inotropic effect, while others have shown no effect on cardiac contraction.

α_1-Adrenergic receptors are coupled to hydrolysis of phosphatidylinositol to produce two second messengers: inositol triphosphate (IP_3) and diacylglycerol (DAG). IP_3 is linked to Ca^{2+} metabolism, and DAG is linked to the activation of protein kinase C, which has several myocardial substrates.

The ontogeny of α-adrenergic receptors and their role in myocardial development are not clear. One study describes a reduction in myocardial receptor concentration with advancing gestational age during the third trimester in fetal sheep. During early postnatal development, the chronotropic response to α_1-adrenergic stimulation changes from positive to negative in the rat and dog heart. As mentioned above, this change is associated with myocardial innervation, and with an increase in the G-protein that mediates α_1-adrenergic responses. α-Adrenergic mechanisms appear to play an essential role in regulating cardiovascular responses during stress in growth-retarded fetal lambs, because α-blockade during acute hypoxic stress resulted in death. However, the relative role of the myocardium in this process is not well established.

Another potential role for α-adrenergic mechanisms during growth and development may stem from their ability to induce myocyte hypertrophy in neonatal rats. Again, the importance of this mechanism in myocardial development remains to be elucidated.

Muscarinic receptors

Muscarinic-receptor activation has been associated with negative chronotropic and inotropic effects in adult hearts. Muscarinic receptors are not structurally and functionally uniform, and to date, at least five different receptor genes (M_{1-5}) have been cloned and pharmacologically characterized. They are expressed in a tissue-specific manner, and their affinity to cellular response elements varies. In most mammalian hearts, including human, the muscarinic subtype identified is M_2.

The presently known biochemical responses to muscarinic stimulation in the heart include a reduction in cAMP concentration, an increase in the hydrolysis of phosphoinositides, activation of K^+ channels, and interaction with Na^+ channels.

The inhibitory myocardial effects of muscarinic stimulation may be executed through coupling with G_i, leading to inhibition of adenylyl cyclase activity. Receptor interaction with a different G-protein, G_p, stimulates phospholipase C to cause phosphoinositide hydrolysis. The effect of the latter response is not clear; as stated above, the products of phosphoinositol hydrolysis are the two second messengers, IP_3 and DAG. IP_3 is linked to Ca^{2+} metabolism, and DAG is linked to the activation of protein kinase C, which has several myocardial substrates. Several recent studies have associated phosphoinositol hydrolysis with a positive inotropic effect (Fig. 10.22).

The ontogeny of myocardial muscarinic receptors and their physiological importance during myocardial growth and development are not clear. Prior to vagal innervation, the response of embryonic chick heart to muscarinic stimulation is low; following vagal ingrowth, this response increases, while no change in receptor density is detected. Later in gestation, myocardial muscarinic receptor concentrations in fetal myocardium appear to be significantly higher than in adults. The receptor signal transduction pathway in the fetus is intact, and is capable of mediating a cellular response. The physiological significance of this pathway in cardiac development is not clear.

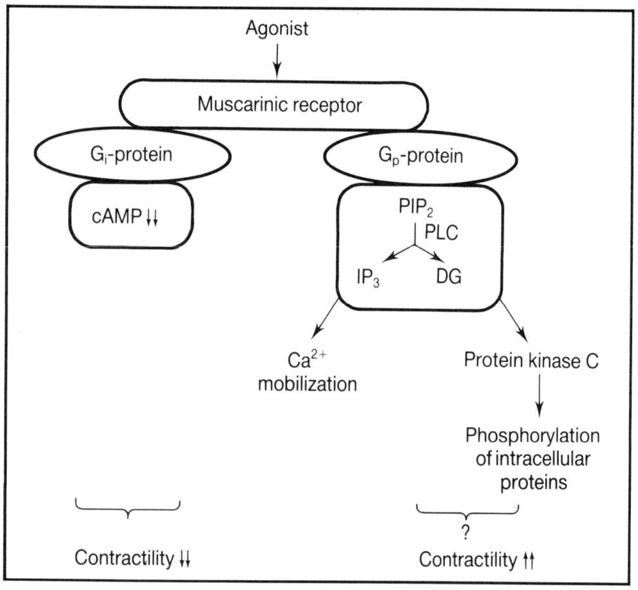

Fig. 10.22. T activation of a muscarinic receptor leads to a G_i-mediated reduction in cAMP and reduced contractility. G_p-mediated phospholipase C activation leads to the hydrolysis of phosphatidylinositol 4,5-bisphosphate (PIP_2). The latter reaction produces the two second messengers inositol triphosphate (IP_3) and diacylglycerol (DAG), leading to a cascade of intracellular events that may increase contractility.

Selected reading

Chen FM, Yamamura HI, Roeske WR. Ontogeny of mammalian myocardial β-adrenergic receptors. *Eur J Pharmacol* 1979; **58**: 255.

Cheng BC, Cornett LE, Goldfien A. Decreased concentration of myocardial α-adrenoceptors with increasing age in foetal lambs. *Br J Pharmacol* 1980; **70**: 515.

Cheng JB, Goldfien A, Cornett LE, Roberts JM. Identification of β-adrenergic receptors using [^{3}H]dihydroalprenolol in fetal sheep heart: direct evidence of qualitative similarity to the receptors in adult sheep heart. *Pediatr Res* 1981; **15**: 1083.

Galper JB, Klein W, Catterall WA. Muscarinic acetylcholine receptors in developing chick heart. *J Biol Chem* 1977; **252**: 8692.

Nedoma J, Slavíková J, Tucek S. Muscarinic acetylcholine receptors in the heart of rats before and after birth. *Pflügers Arch* 1986; **406**: 45.

Robishaw JD, Foster KA. Role of G proteins in the regulation of the cardiovascular system. *Annu Rev Physiol* 1989; **51**: 229.

Simpson P. Stimulation of hypertrophy of cultured neonatal rat heart cells through an α_1-adrenergic receptor and induction of beating through an α_1- and β_1-adrenergic receptor interaction. Evidence for independent regulation of growth and beating. *Circ Res* 1985; **56**: 884.

Whitsett JA, Pollinger J, Matz S. β-Adrenergic receptors and catecholamine sensitive adenylate cyclase in developing rat ventricular myocardium: effect of thyroid status. *Pediatr Res* 1982; **16**: 463.

D. Myocardial Nervous Innervation and Regulation

D F Teitel and J I E Hoffman

Developmental aspects

Adrenergic, muscarinic, and other receptors appear early and function before autonomic innervation occurs; parasympathetic innervation precedes sympathetic innervation in all species. The earliest viable human premature infants have rudimentary autonomic innervation. Innervation is most advanced in those species that are independent immediately after birth.

Anatomy and physiology

Cardiac sympathetic nerves come from cervical sympathetic ganglia and stellate ganglia, and from the upper four thoracic sympathetic ganglia. Right sympathetic nerves innervate the right and anterior portions of the heart, and left sympathetic nerves innervate the left and posterior portions of the heart. The efferent sympathetic nerve endings make and store dopamine, norepinephrine, and neuropeptide Y; the latter two are co-released with nerve stimulation. Vagal nerves from the medullary centers supply both atria and ventricles along with the proximal part of the bundle of His; the distal part of the bundle of His has only sympathetic nerve supply. Vagal nerve endings contain not only acetylcholine, but also vasoactive intestinal peptide (VIP) and somatostatin. Sympathetic and vagal afferents leave the heart and carry information from baroreceptors that are stimulated by high pressures in the ventricles and lower pressures in the atria, cavae, and pulmonary veins, and also by chemoreceptors that can be stimulated by an exogenous substance, veratridine, but also by locally produced substances such as bradykinin and prostaglandins. The cell bodies of the afferent unmyelinated nerves produce vasodilator peptides substance P, neurokinin A, and CGRP (calcitonin gene-related peptide), which are transported down the axon to the nerve endings and are co-released upon stimulation of the nerves.

The heart can function without cardiac nerves; cardiac function is normal after cardiac transplantation. However, the response to exercise in denervated hearts is slower than normal, and is due to increases in circulating catecholamines and the rise in body temperature. In intact animals and humans, β-adrenoceptor blockade blunts the heart rate increase with exercise and abolishes the inotropic response, as judged by the increase in dP/dt_{max}. **This effect is used to attempt to prevent dissection of the aorta in patients with *Marfan syndrome*.**

Sympathetic–vagal interaction

Neurogenic cardiac control varies with the state of consciousness and the basal level of sympathetic and parasympathetic tone. In conscious animals, resting sympathetic tone is low, and parasympathetic tone is high. Therefore, sympathetic blockade changes heart rate and myocardial contractility minimally, but vagal blockade causes significant tachycardia. In contrast, many anesthetics depress the sympathetic nervous system, and lead to impaired contractility and tachycardia. After **surgery**, patients often have high circulating catecholamine concentrations, and their myocardial function depends on the balance of catecholamine concentrations, stimulation of the sympathetic nervous system by pain, and the degree of myocardial depression by the drugs used for sedation.

Patterns of stimulation

With exercise and *hemorrhage,* plasma catecholamines and heart rate increase greatly, but inotropic responses differ. dP/dt_{max} increases up to 400 percent with exercise, but by only 30–50 percent with hemorrhage. The peripheral vascular bed dilates and cardiac output increases with exercise, whereas cardiac output falls and most vascular beds vasoconstrict with hemorrhage. Thus, the pattern of sympathetic neural stimulation, rather than circulating catecholamine concentrations, determines how the heart responds to these stimuli.

Vagal effects

Vagal stimulation changes heart rate, but may also have effects on myocardial contractility that depend on existing sympathetic tone. Vagal stimulation has little effect on myocardial contractility when there is little sympathetic tone, but markedly reduces the inotropic effects of increases in circulating catecholamines or sympathetic nerve stimulation. Conversely, blockade of muscarinic receptors can intensify the myocardial contractile response to sympathetic stimulation. **Vagal stimulation slows conduction through the atrioventricular node, an effect used in treating *supraventricular tachycardias*.**

Baroreceptors

Carotid and aortic baroreceptors respond to changes in arterial blood pressure. With normal low basal sympathetic tone, inhibiting sympathetic tone by raising aortic pressure has little effect on myocardial contractility. However, lowering arterial pressure reflexly increases sympathetic tone, and increases heart rate and contractility. Baroreceptor sensitivity increases throughout gestation in fetal lambs, but may decrease after birth. In fetal lambs, denervating the baroreceptors did not alter mean arterial blood pressure or heart rate, but increased their variability; in adult sheep, denervation increased variability of pressures, but not of heart rate. Denervation in the fetuses also decreased peripheral resistance.

Chemoreceptors (see p. 610)

Carotid and aortic chemoreceptors are stimulated by marked decreases of Po_2 and pH, and by marked increases of Pco_2, but the increase in myocardial contractility is modest; the fetus seems less sensitive than the adult to chemoreceptor stimulation. The bradycardia of severe hypoxemia is due to vagal stimulation.

Vascular innervation

The autonomic nerves innervate coronary vessels and interact with circulating and local hormones to regulate coronary vascular tone. Because of the major effect of metabolic regulators on coronary vascular tone, it is difficult to ascribe specific actions to the autonomic nerves, but α-adrenergic vasoconstriction is well recognized. **It may play a part in the onset of *angina pectoris* in patients with *coronary arterial disease*.**

E. Coronary Circulation and Myocardial Oxygen Consumption

D F Teitel and J I E Hoffman

Determinants of myocardial O_2 consumption

Pressure work

Pressure work by the heart consumes more O_2 than does volume work, and Sarnoff and colleagues found a good correlation between the area under the left ventricular pressure curve in systole (the tension time index) and left ventricular O_2 consumption. Later work showed that peak wall tension (or stress) was a better predictor of left ventricular O_2 consumption. Therefore, wall thickness and ventricular dimensions must be used in estimating myocardial O_2 consumption; this is why the tension time index, which ignores wall stress, is not the best predictor of myocardial O_2 consumption, particularly in abnormal hearts. Increased contractility or heart rate also increases myocardial O_2 consumption, but decreases ventricular size, and thus wall stress, so that the increased O_2 consumption is not as great as would be expected from studies in muscle strips.

Volume work

Stroke volume is an added predictor that must be considered. Suga and colleagues concluded that the best predictor of left ventricular O_2 consumption was the area in the pressure–volume loop plus the area representing end-systolic pressure energy (Fig. 10.23a); the total area was termed the pressure–volume area. By subtracting the contributions of basal metabolism and excitation–

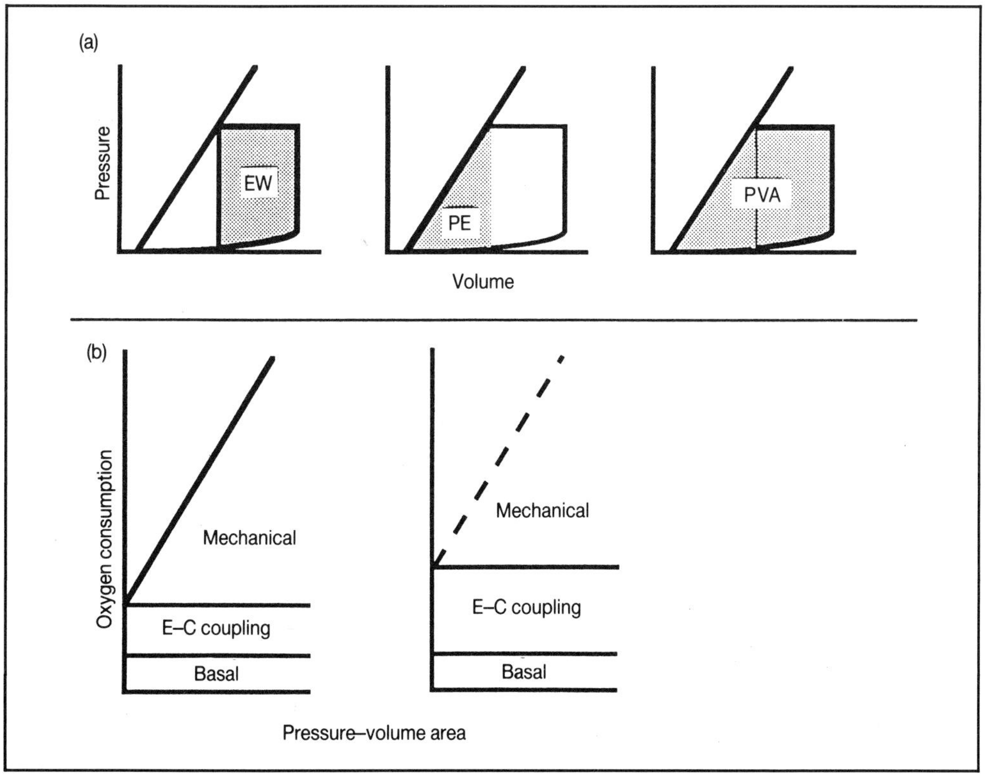

Fig. 10.23. Determinants of myocardial O_2 consumption. (a) Pressure–volume diagrams to show the component of external work (EW) on the left, of potential energy (PE) in the middle, and on the right, the combination of both to make up the pressure–volume area (PVA). The PVA is closely related to myocardial O_2 consumption. (b) Diagrams to show relation between myocardial O_2 consumption (vertical axis) and pressure–volume area (horizontal axis) at normal (left) and increased contractility (right). Increased contractility increases the component of myocardial O_2 consumption related to excitation–contraction coupling (E–C coupling) but not the other two, so that myocardial O_2 consumption and mechanical work remain proportional. (Adapted from the publications of Suga and his colleagues.)

contraction coupling, they were able to show that the O_2 consumption/pressure–volume area relationship was independent of contractile state (Fig. 10.23b).

Substrate effects

Because more O_2 is used oxidizing fats than carbohydrates, more O_2 should be used per unit of work when burning fatty acids. This has sometimes, but not always, been found, but has not been carefully studied. Because fetal myocardium uses mainly carbohydrate as substrate, rather than fatty acids as in the adult, this difference could be considered a mechanism for conserving O_2 in the fetus.

Structure and development of the coronary circulation

Embryology

In the early embryo, the primitive cardiac tube has an inner wall that is heavily trabeculated and derived from endothelium, whereas the myocardium is derived from mesoderm. Connective tissue grows out from the base of the truncus arteriosus to enter the muscle and form its connective tissue, and from this tissue the coronary arteries are formed. Initially, the inner layer of the myocardium is supplied with O_2 and substrates by diffusion from the cavity, but as the heart grows and its metabolic needs increase, the coronary arteries take over the role of supplying the actively growing and working muscle.

Anatomy

The human heart has two major extramural coronary arteries. The right coronary artery, which comes off the right anterior sinus of Valsalva, is dominant in two-thirds of people, i.e. it reaches the crux of the heart and gives off the posterior descending coronary artery, which supplies the posterior third of the ventricular septum and part of the adjacent left ventricular wall. The left coronary artery, which comes off the left sinus of Valsalva, is dominant in about 15 percent of people, i.e. it reaches the crux of the heart and gives off the posterior descending coronary artery, so that the left coronary artery supplies all the left ventricle and a small part of the right ventricle. In the remaining 18 percent of people, neither artery is dominant; these people are said to have a balanced circulation. The right coronary artery usually gives off the artery to the sinoatrial node, and the posterior descending artery supplies the atrioventricular node.

Microcirculation

The arteries penetrate the muscle and go towards the endocardium, giving off branches as they go and forming a subendocardial plexus. The major control of coronary vascular resistance lies in arterioles less than 400 μm in diameter. The myocardium of the left ventricle has a relatively large blood volume of about 15 percent of wall volume, and this can change substantially during contraction. In systole, blood is squeezed out of the left ventricular subendocardium and midmyocardium; some of this blood passes retrograde into the extramural coronary arteries, some into the coronary veins, and some actually passes into the subepicardial vessels, which therefore receive a dual blood supply: in systole from the subendocardium and in diastole from the extramural coronary arteries.

Myocardial O_2 demand–supply relationship; coronary blood flow

Basic features

The left ventricle extracts about 60–75 percent of the O_2 from the blood passing through the myocardium. Therefore, because it is impossible to remove the residual O_2 from hemoglobin without producing dangerously low O_2 tensions, increased myocardial O_2 demand must be met by increased myocardial blood flow. Normally, with maximal exertion, left ventricular O_2 consumption increases fourfold, and so does left ventricular blood flow. If coronary perfusion pressure does not change during exertion, the increased flow must be achieved by a decrease in coronary vascular resistance.

Coronary vascular resistance has three components: a basal low resistance in the arrested heart with maximally dilated vessels, an added resistance when vessels have tone, and a phasic resistance added whenever the ventricle

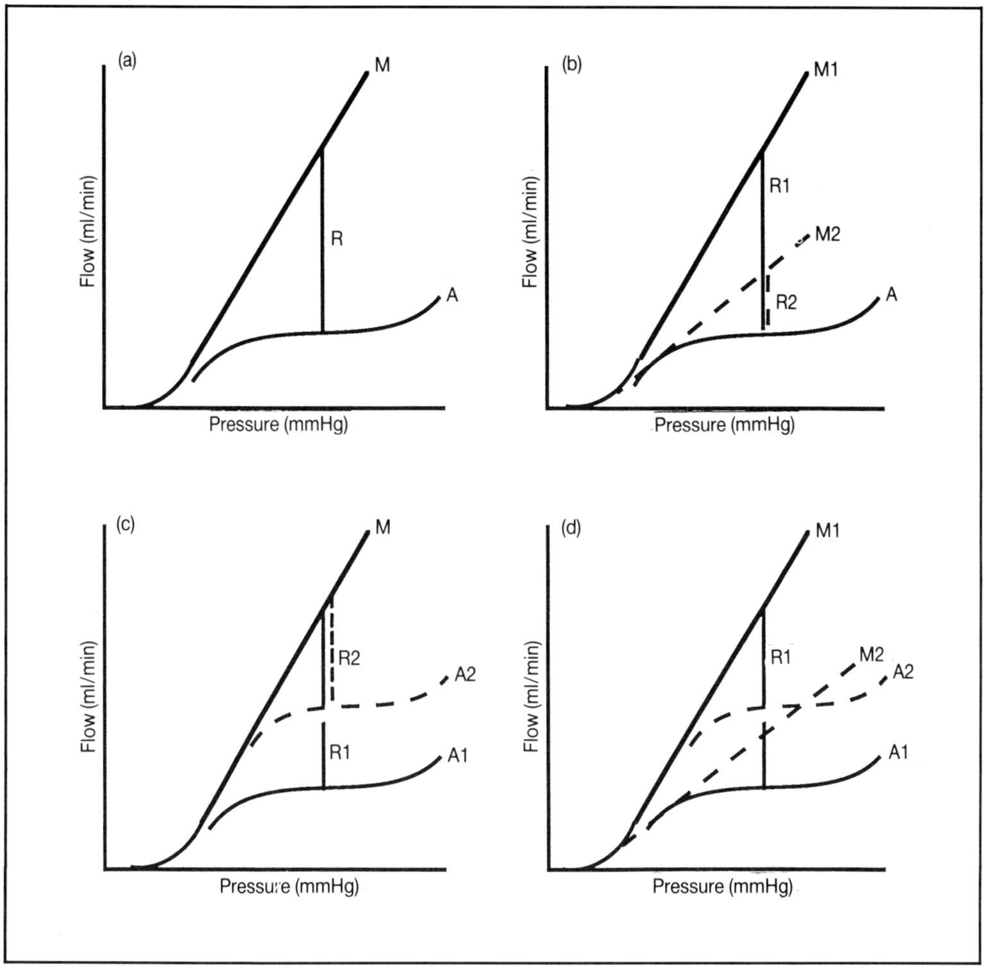

Fig. 10.24. Coronary flow reserve diagrams. (a) Coronary flow reserve diagram with autoregulation curve (A), pressure–flow line of maximal vasodilatation (M), and coronary flow reserve (R) at normal perfusing pressure. (b) Normal coronary flow reserve diagram that shows, in addition to the normal maximal pressure–flow line (M1), the dashed line of reduced maximal pressure–flow relation (M2). The normal flow reserve (R1) is reduced to R2 (short dashed line). (c) Normal coronary flow reserve diagram that shows, in addition to the normal autoregulating curve (A1), a curve showing autoregulation at an increased level of flow (A2). Once again, flow reserve is reduced from the normal value of R1 to a lower value of R2 (short dashed line). (d) Normal coronary flow reserve diagram with an abnormally high autoregulation curve (A2) and an abnormally low maximal pressure–flow line (M2). As can be seen, at a normal perfusing pressure there is no reserve left. This combination can occur with hypertrophy, polycythemia, and hypoxemia, as well as with other combinations of factors.

contracts. The second of these resistances can be abolished with vasodilator drugs; then perfusion of the left ventricular myocardium will produce a steep pressure/flow relation that is linear at higher flows but usually curvilinear at low pressures and flows (Fig. 10.24a). Because the vessels are maximally dilated, flow is uncoupled from metabolism and depends only on driving pressure and resistance. If heart rate is increased, the maximal flow at any perfusion pressure will decrease because the heart is in a relaxed state for a smaller proportion of each cardiac cycle.

Autoregulation

If coronary vessels have tone, then the pressure/flow relationship can be assessed at different perfusion pressures after cannulating the left coronary artery. Cannulation is necessary because when cardiac metabolism and blood flow are coupled, increasing aortic blood pressure will increase coronary flow by increasing myocardial O_2 demand. If perfusion pressure is raised or lowered from its control value, flow changes transiently in the direction of the change of pressure and then returns towards the previous steady state. There is a range over which there is almost no change in steady-state flow; a rise in pressure has caused vasoconstriction, and a fall in pressure has caused vasodilatation. This response, in which for a constant myocardial O_2 consumption, flow remains almost constant despite changes in perfusion pressure, is termed autoregulation. At perfusion pressures above the upper end of the range, flow increases, probably because the pressure overcomes the constriction. At pressures less than about 40 mmHg (5.3 kPa) (but varying—see below), flow decreases (Fig. 10.24a), indicating that some vessels are maximally dilated and can no longer decrease resistance to compensate for the decreased perfusion pressure. At these low pressures, flows are decreased in some small pieces of myocardium, particularly in the subendocardium, although adjacent small pieces of muscle may have normal flows. As pressures are lowered still further, more and more pieces of muscle develop low flows and become ischemic; the majority of the hypoperfused and ischemic pieces are in the subendocardium. Similar changes occur if the perfusion pressure is kept constant and the pressure in the left ventricle, systolic or diastolic, is greatly elevated, the heart rate is greatly increased, or the O_2 content of coronary arterial blood is decreased. In each of these circumstances, an imbalance between myocardial O_2 consumption and myocardial blood (and O_2) supply develops. **These changes have their counterparts in human disease; for examples, *subendocardial ischemia* and *patchy subendocardial necrosis* occur in *critical aortic stenosis*, *cyanotic heart disease*, *severe anemia* (especially if chronic), *carbon monoxide poisoning*, *extreme tachycardia*, *dilated cardiomyopathy*, or *coronary artery atheroma*.**

Role of vasoactive peptides and other vasoregulators

Although the control of tissue O_2 tensions seems to be the aim of the autoregulatory and other metabolic control systems, the mechanisms by which tissue O_2 is kept fairly constant are poorly understood. Adenosine, a powerful coronary vasodilator, is a prime candidate for a control mechanism. More cardiac work or decreased coronary perfusion results in increased breakdown of ATP to adenosine monophosphate; this is broken down by 5′-nucleotidase to adenosine, which could then dilate the vessels. On the other hand, less cardiac work or increased perfusion decrease the amount of adenosine produced, and so might lead to some vasoconstriction. Adenosine clearly is not essential for coronary regulation because a great decrease in its concentration produced by infusing adenosine deaminase does not affect autoregulation, and also because certain dynamic considerations do not fit the adenosine model. Nevertheless, it could play a role during ischemia.

Several powerful vasoactive peptides are known to affect the coronary circulation. Cardiac sympathetic afferent nerves can be stimulated by ischemia, perhaps by release of local bradykinin or eicosanoids. On stimulation, these nerve endings release substance P and CGRP, which are powerful coronary vasodilators. Once coronary flow is increased, the coronary endothelium is stimulated to release endothelial derived relaxing factor (EDRF), which is probably nitric oxide (NO), and this helps to maintain the vasodilatation. Coronary vasodilators such as acetylcholine and substance P act entirely through the release of EDRF. **Endothelial damage from *air embolism* or *atheroma* decreases or prevents EDRF release, and the absence of this potent vasodilator may explain some instances of coronary spasm.** Atrial natriuretic peptide (ANP) is released from atria (and to some extent from ventricles) when these are distended. ANP dilates renal vessels and aids diuresis, and also inhibits sympathetic tone. What part it plays in coronary vasomotion is not clear. Finally, recent studies have shown that ATP-dependent potassium channels are important in the coronary bed. Ischemia has been shown to activate these channels, and reactive hyperemia can be reduced by about 60 percent when these channels are inhibited.

There are also potent coronary vasoconstrictors. Norepinephrine released from sympathetic nerve endings activates α-adrenergic receptors and produces vasoconstriction, and so does neuropeptide Y, which is co-released with norepinephrine. The endothelium also produces endothelins, a family of powerful vasoconstrictors like some snake venoms. These are released by ischemia and appear in high concentration in patients with congestive heart failure, but their role in pathophysiology is not yet defined. Another vasoconstrictor hormone is vasopressin, which may also rise in concentration during congestive heart failure. Finally, some potent eicosanoids are vasoconstrictors, notably leukotrienes and thromboxane A_2. The latter is released from platelets activated during aggregation; the vasoconstriction and the platelet plug help to prevent hemorrhage from any break in the vascular wall. Coronary endothelial damage, by reducing local production of prostacyclin (PGI_2), encourages platelet aggregation, which together with thromboxane A_2 release may play a role in coronary spasm.

Coronary flow reserve

General principles

At any pressure, the difference between autoregulated and maximal flows is termed coronary flow reserve; this has the same units as the original flows, but a dimensionless ratio with similar implications can be obtained by dividing maximal by resting flow. Flow reserve depends greatly on perfusion pressure because of the steepness of the pressure/flow relation in maximally dilated vessels. Coronary flow reserve indicates how much added flow the myocardium can get at a given pressure to meet increased demands for O_2; if reserve is much reduced, then flow cannot increase sufficiently to meet demands, and myocardial ischemia occurs. Decreases in coronary flow reserve are always more profound in the subendocardium than in the subepicardium, so that myocardial supply–demand imbalance and ischemia will occur in the subendocardium before the subepicardium.

Decreased maximal flow

If autoregulated flow is normal but maximal flow is decreased (Fig. 10.24b), then coronary flow reserve will be reduced. Such a change can occur with marked *tachycardia;* a decrease in the number of coronary vessels due to small vessel disease, as in some *collagen vascular diseases,* especially *systemic lupus erythematosus;* increased resistance to flow in one or more large coronary vessels because of *embolism, thrombosis, atheroma,* or *spasm*; impaired myocardial relaxation due to *ischemia* or *hypothermia*; myocardial edema; a marked increase in left ventricular diastolic pressure; a marked increase in left ventricular systolic pressure if coronary perfusion pressure is not also increased, as in *aortic stenosis or incompetence*; and an increase in blood viscosity, most commonly seen with a hematocrit over 65 percent but also occurring with *macroglobulinemia* or very high white blood cell counts in *leukemia*.

Increased control (autoregulated) flows

Coronary flow reserve will also be reduced if maximal flows are normal but autoregulated flows increase (Fig. 10.24c). Myocardial flows increase above normal values with exercise, *tachycardia, anemia, hypoxemia, carbon monoxide poisoning,* leftward shift of the hemoglobin O_2 dissociation curve as in infants with a high proportion of fetal hemoglobin or certain *abnormal hemoglobins, thyrotoxicosis, acute ventricular dilatation* (because of increased wall stress), inotropic stimulation by catecholamines, and acquired ventricular hypertrophy.

Effects of ventricular hypertrophy

When hypertrophy occurs after about 4–6 months of age in lambs and swine, ventricular muscle mass increases without a concomitant increase in conducting coronary blood vessels. Ventricular hypertrophy returns wall stress to normal, and myocardial flow per minute per gram of muscle remains approximately normal. Total left ventricular flow is increased in proportion to ventricular mass, but because maximal flow per ventricle is usually unchanged, the coronary flow reserve is diminished. Often autoregulated flow is increased and maximal flows are reduced at the same time, e.g. with severe tachycardia or cyanotic heart disease with hypoxemia, ventricular hypertrophy, and polycythemia. Under these circumstances, coronary flow reserve can be drastically reduced or even absent at normal perfusing pressures (Fig. 10.24d).

Hypertrophy and angiogenic potential

Hypertrophy occurring in fetal life or very soon after birth, however, has been associated in experimental animals with an increased total number of conducting coronary vessels and no loss of coronary flow reserve. This angiogenic potential disappears within the first few months after birth.

Myocardial wall stress, O_2 consumption, and coronary flow reserve

Myocardial wall stress is regulated within a fairly narrow range, with or without myocardial hypertrophy. Consequently, myocardial blood flow per unit mass is fairly constant at about 1 ml/(min·g) of left ventricle at rest. There is a close relationship between left ventricular mass-to-volume ratio and peak wall stress in systole. If the heart dilates acutely, then the mass-to-volume ratio decreases, wall stress and myocardial O_2 consumption increase, and coronary flow reserve falls. This is particularly serious when there is hypertrophy in which coronary flow reserve is already reduced. Decreasing ventricular dilatation by afterload and preload reduction reverses these unfavorable events and is another reason for the value of this therapy.

Note from Fig. 10.24a–d that because the line of maximal pressure/flow relations slopes up and to the right, any decrease in that slope (Fig. 10.24b) or any increase in autoregulated flow (Fig. 10.24c) causes autoregulation to fail at pressures much higher than usually occurs.

Right ventricular myocardial flow

Right ventricular myocardial blood flow is governed by the principles described above, but there are differences due to the low right ventricular systolic pressure and because right ventricular pressure work is not changed by alterations in aortic and coronary pressures. Acute right ventricular hypertension, e.g. from *pulmonary embolism* or *severe pulmonary vasoconstriction*, if severe, will cause right ventricular failure; the increased wall stress increases right ventricular O_2 consumption, but the increased systolic pressure reduces the coronary flow, and right ventricular myocardial ischemia occurs because supply cannot match demand. If under these circumstances aortic perfusing pressure is increased mechanically or with α-adrenergic agonists, right ventricular myocardial blood flow will increase and restore right ventricular function to normal.

With chronic right ventricular hypertension and hypertrophy, as in severe *pulmonic stenosis*, many forms of cyanotic congenital heart disease, and some *chronic lung disease*, right ventricular myocardial blood flow behaves in the same way as left ventricular blood flow. If aortic pressure is lowered, however, left ventricular pressure decreases, as does left ventricular work and O_2 consumption, but in the right ventricle the workload may not be reduced, so that imbalance between myocardial O_2 supply and demand may occur. **The greatest imbalance occurs when right ventricular systolic pressure is maintained but coronary perfusing pressure decreases, as can happen in a child with *tetralogy of Fallot* who has too large an aortopulmonary anastomosis.** The right ventricular systolic pressure will be raised because of the systemic aortic and left ventricular systolic pressures, but the low diastolic aortic pressure due to the shunt lowers coronary perfusion pressure in diastole and can cause both left and right ventricular ischemia and failure.

Reperfusion injury

When a heart is ischemic for 15–20 minutes and is then reperfused, a transient period of impaired function may last for hours but function recovers completely; this phenomenon, known as stunning, is due to unknown biochemical processes. Periods of ischemia longer than 40–60 minutes lead to regions of cell death, predominantly in the subendocardium of the left ventricle. The reperfusion, rather than the ischemia, seems to cause much of the damage, because the use of certain experimental reperfusates may allow up to 6 hours of normothermic ischemia without any cell death. Cell death is preceded by overload of Ca^{2+} in the mitochondria and by loss of nucleotides from the cytosol, both of these being in part due to profound membrane damage. Some of this damage may be due to free radicals like superoxide and hydroxyl radicals, and recently, investigators have shown that EDRF released during reperfusion may generate peroxynitrite anions, which produce hydroxyl radicals. Possibly, oxygen free radical injury plays a particularly important role in the reperfusion after cardiac surgery of hearts of children with cyanotic heart disease.

Selected reading

Hoffman JIE. Coronary artery physiology. In Garfein OB, ed. *Current concepts in cardiovascular physiology*. New York: Academic Press, Inc., 1990: 289.

Strauer BE. Myocardial oxygen consumption in chronic heart disease: role of wall stress, hypertrophy and coronary reserve. *Am J Cardiol* 1979; **44**: 730.

F. Ventricular Function

D F Teitel and J I E Hoffman

Isolated muscle

General considerations

In addition to the components of individual myocytes, factors that affect the interaction between myocytes determine the force developed by a muscle strip. Relative concentration and organization of myocytes within a region affect force generation, as do the extracellular matrix and connective and vascular tissues. Developmental changes occur at all these levels. Contractile elements increase as a proportion of total volume throughout gestation, increasing the force generated per gram of tissue. Collagen, the major protein responsible for the complex network that connects myocytes and allows maximal force generation, changes greatly throughout development, from initially showing only small quantities of very disorganized material to becoming a well developed and structured framework to which the myocytes attach. Collagen type also changes over development, although the functional significance of the different types is not known. Other extracellular components, including fibronectin and growth factors, may have important effects on cardiac growth and development.

If a muscle is stimulated to contract, it develops force. Isometric contractions occur at infinite afterload so that no shortening occurs; the function of the isometrically contracting muscle can be described entirely by the extent and rate of force generation. If the muscle is allowed to shorten, the amount and rate of shortening are also parameters of function. In the extreme, a fully unloaded muscle reaches maximal velocity of shortening with no force generation. Thus indices of force generation and shortening have been applied to the study of isolated muscle strips in a variety of conditions and at different developmental stages.

Length–tension relationships in muscle strips

A basic property of cardiac muscle is defined by the **Frank–Starling relationship**: the greater the initial stretch (preload) of that muscle, the greater the force it generates upon contraction. At a sarcomere level, this phenomenon can be understood in terms of crossbridge units: the greater the length of a sarcomere before contraction, the more crossbridges are available for the myosin heads to shorten the sarcomere.

To study the Frank–Starling relationship in cardiac muscle strips, investigators have isolated small pieces of tissue, usually in papillary muscle with its nearly parallel fibers, but also in portions of the ventricular walls. The muscle strip is placed in a water bath, one end tied to a pivoted lever, the other attached to a force transducer (Fig. 10.25). Weights attached to the other end of the lever extend the muscle to any desired length before

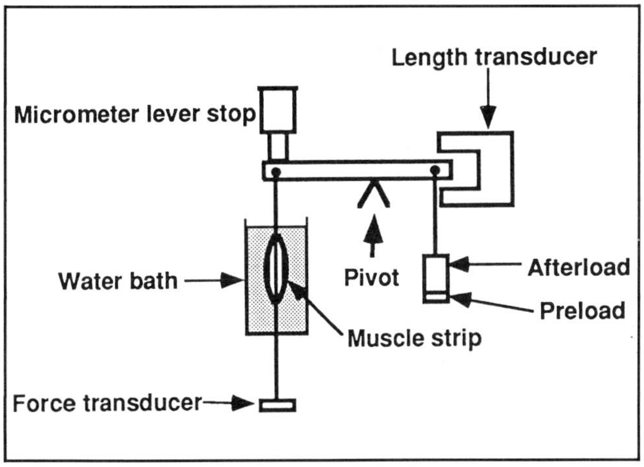

Fig. 10.25. Diagram of muscle bath. The muscle is in a water bath. One end of the muscle is suspended from a pivoted lever, and the other end is attached to a force transducer. The other end of the lever is attached to a length transducer. A weight (preload) attached to the lever stretches the muscle to an extent determined by the stop. Then another weight (afterload) is added, and the muscle is stimulated to contract by electrodes (not shown) in the bath.

contraction (**preload**); excessive stretching is prevented by a stop. Other weights added to the lever after initial length has been set affect the muscle only after contraction has begun, and are therefore termed the **afterload**. Muscle length and force can be measured before and during contraction. The muscle is stimulated to contract by an electrical impulse. Instruments to measure sarcomere length, Ca^{2+} entry, and many other functions can be added.

Active contraction is studied in two ways (Fig. 10.26, left panels). If cardiac muscle is stimulated to contract at different initial muscle lengths, but is not allowed to shorten (isometric contraction), no force is generated at the shortest lengths; the muscle remains slack. Then as sarcomere lengths increase, force is generated, and this force increases to reach a maximum at sarcomere lengths of about 2.2 μm. At longer sarcomere lengths, there may even be a decrease in force, because the sarcomere is overstretched so that the actin filaments are separated from the myosin filaments and efficient crossbridging cannot be achieved. If at any muscle or sarcomere length, passive tension is subtracted from the tension generated during isometric contraction, the resulting curve demonstrates active tension as a function of length. If afterload is small, the contracting muscle generates an appropriate force, and then shortens while force remains constant (isotonic contraction). The rate of shortening is fastest at the onset of shortening, and from it the velocity of shortening is measured (Fig. 10.26, right panels). The shortening velocity will range from zero when the load is so heavy that it prevents shortening to a maximum when the external load is zero; because of internal viscosity and

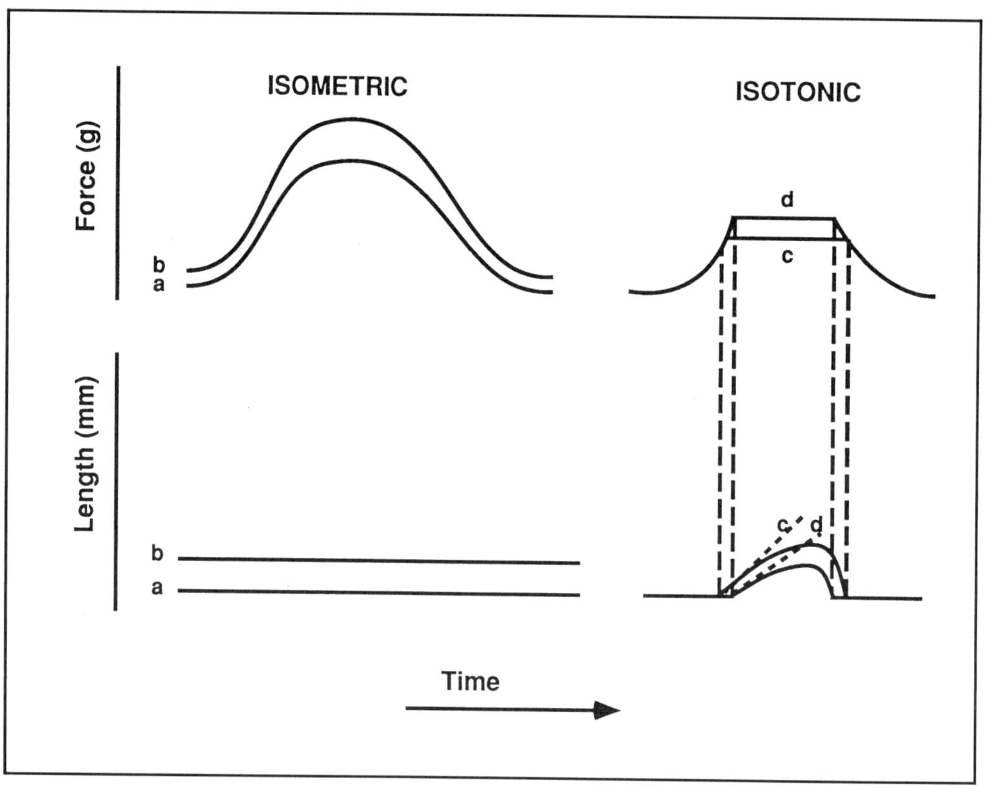

Fig. 10.26. Length–tension curves during isometric (left) and isotonic (right) contractions. Left panels: the isometric curves are made at two different initial muscle lengths (a and b) and show no shortening (below). The maximum force generated from the longer initial length (b) is greater than that generated by the shorter length (above). Right panels: isotonic curves are made at two different afterloads. As shown in the upper diagram, force rises until the afterload is reached, and then it remains constant at the afterloads of c and d, as shown by the intervals between the two sets of dashed lines, until relaxation begins. The corresponding shortening curves (below) show an initial rapid shortening; tangents to this initial rapid upstroke (dotted lines) are used to calculate the initial velocity of shortening. Note that for the higher afterload (d), it takes longer before shortening begins, the initial velocity of shortening is less, and relaxation begins earlier.

elastic forces, however, true zero loading is impossible. Increases in cytosolic Ca^{2+} increase the force generated during contraction, but have little effect on the maximal velocity of shortening.

Conceptually, the sarcomeres can be considered to have at least three functional components: an inelastic contractile element (CE) and two elastic elements, one in series with the contractile element (SE) and one in parallel with it (PE). These elastic elements were needed to explain the results of stretching the muscle passively, and of releasing it suddenly during contraction. The exact arrangement of these elements is still debated; in one popular model (Maxwell model), the parallel elastic element is parallel to both the CE and SE, which are in series, whereas in the other popular model (Voigt model), the PE is parallel only to the CE, and both are in series with the SE. In addition, there is internal viscosity that affects some of the changes noted in these experiments.

Force–frequency relationship

Another basic property of cardiac muscle is that force generation is altered by the frequency of contraction. If intrinsic contractility of a muscle is defined as the alterations in force generation or shortening caused by changes in either Ca^{2+} availability to or Ca^{2+} sensitivity of the sarcomere, then the force–frequency relationship can be considered a product of beat-to-beat changes in contractility. If the frequency of contraction changes suddenly from one steady rate to a higher frequency, there is an increase in contractility over several contractions until some maximum is attained. This increase is due to a greater influx of Ca^{2+} into the cells because of the greater duration of membrane depolarization per minute. Eventually Ca^{2+} influx and efflux equilibrate, but with a greater level of (releasable) intracellular Ca^{2+} that is responsible for the increase in contractile force. Transient analyses are based on the phenomenon of post-extrasystolic potentiation, namely that force is reduced during a premature beat but is supernormal after the compensatory pause. This phenomenon can be tested formally in muscle strips to obtain the force–frequency or the force–interval relationship. The muscle is stimulated to beat at a regular rate, and then every eighth stimulus is put in prematurely; this procedure is repeated with varying intervals between the last regular stimulus and the premature stimulus. In the second stage, a second premature stimulus is put in at varying intervals after the first premature stimulus. The maximal force achieved in each contraction is plotted against the interval between the last normal beat and the first or second premature beat. The force achieved is low at short interstimulus intervals, and rises to a maximum at an interval of about one second. The force is about twice as high after two premature stimuli as after one. The interpretation of this relationship is that when the muscle is excited to contract, Ca^{2+} enters the cytosol from outside and also from the sarcoplasmic reticulum. In diastole, Ca^{2+} is taken up by the sarcoplasmic reticulum, but is not available for release until some time has passed. Therefore, after a premature beat, a subnormal amount of Ca^{2+} is available to generate force, which is submaximal. After the compensatory pause, however, more releasable Ca^{2+} is in the storage sites and, when released, produces a supramaximal contraction. Thus, post-extrasystolic potentiation requires a well functioning sarcoplasmic reticulum and a condition in which Ca^{2+} availability is not maximal—that is, a low initial contractile state.

Developmental aspects

Active tension per mm^2 cross-sectional myocyte area at any given afterload is below adult values, but is proportional to the reduced number of myofibrils present; about 60 percent of adult cardiac muscle consists of contractile material, whereas this amounts to only 30 percent in the fetus. The extent and velocity of shortening are also reduced in fetal heart muscle, but correction for the amount of contractile machinery suggests that the intrinsic performance of fetal and adult actin-myosin filaments is similar. Some of the differences between fetal and adult cardiac muscle may be due to differences in collagen and cytoskeletal composition. The change from fetal to adult performance seems to occur fairly soon after birth, when myofibrillar array becomes regular and when the T tubules and the sarcoplasmic reticulum develop into their adult form. For this reason, prematurely born infants (and, to a lesser extent, full-term infants) have a much reduced ability to tolerate an increase in afterload, and are also unduly sensitive to reductions in serum Ca^{2+} concentrations. Early in fetal development, post-extrasystolic potentiation is limited because of immaturity of the sarcoplasmic reticulum. Post-extrasystolic potentiation increases in late fetal life in the sheep, but then after birth decreases again because of the high resting β-adrenergic state that exists following birth. With the increased catecholamine stimulation necessary to drive the increased O_2 demands of respiration and thermoregulation, Ca^{2+} influx to the cytosol is near maximal with each beat, so that the sarcoplasmic reticulum is limited in its ability to increase this further.

Integrated muscle function: intact ventricle

Systolic function

Factors determine heart function *in vivo* beyond those that determine the function of the isolated muscle; nevertheless, there are close correlations between what is found in muscle strips and in the whole ventricle. If one defines the contractile performance of the isolated muscle in terms of force developed and length, one can define the global systolic performance of the intact ventricle in terms of pressure and volume. The amount and rate of pressure developed and the amount and rate of blood volume ejected per beat can fully describe the performance of the heart as a pump. Thus evaluation of systolic performance is best made in the pressure–volume plane, which has been the primary direction of studies over the past 20 years.

In the adult heart, the four major determinants of systolic performance are preload, afterload, contractility, and heart rate. Clear definition of these determinants is important, because in many studies, the definitions have not been appropriately used.

Frank–Starling mechanism (preload effects)

The preload that stretches a muscle strip is equivalent to end-diastolic fiber length of the intact ventricle. This length can be measured readily by various devices in animals, but in the intact human ventricle, end-diastolic fiber length is best related to end-diastolic diameter or volume. Frequently, end-diastolic pressure has been used interchangeably with end-diastolic volume as an index of preload, but this can be misleading if the distensibility of the ventricle changes or if pressure outside the heart (pericardial or intrathoracic) rises. Furthermore, there is normally little rise in tension for a fairly considerable change of fiber length, so that similar end-diastolic pressures might coexist with very different fiber lengths. Now that ventricular volumes can be measured fairly accurately by modern imaging methods, there is no reason not to use length or volume to assess preload.

The Frank–Starling relationship is active in the intact ventricle as well as in isolated muscle. Increasing preload increases the pressure generated by an isolated ventricle that is not allowed to eject, as described over 100 years ago by Otto Frank. If the ventricle is allowed to eject, then increased preload allows the heart to eject the same stroke volume against an increased afterload, or else to eject a greater stroke volume against a constant afterload; this is what Ernest Starling showed. The Frank–Starling mechanism has been shown in fetal sheep as well as in the embryonic chick heart. The reserve to increase output, and the plateau pressure at which output is maximal, is significantly lower in fetal than in postnatal sheep. Thus, although intact, the Frank–Starling mechanism cannot be invoked to a great extent before birth to increase output in times of increased demand (see below).

Afterload effects

Afterload is more complicated in the intact ventricle than in isolated muscle strips. Frequently, aortic systolic pressure is equated with afterload. However, in the muscle strip, afterload represents the force exerted by the muscle during contraction, and pressure and force are not the same. The afterload against which the intact ventricle ejects includes the peripheral resistance of the systemic vascular bed, the impedance of the central vasculature, the inertia of blood, and the ventricular wall. Because the stress in the ventricular wall is equal to the force or afterload against which it is contracting, stress is the most accurate estimate of afterload. It is preferable to calculate circumferential or meridional wall stress, which at the midwall is a function of ventricular pressure, diameter, and wall thickness. Both peak systolic and end-systolic wall stress can be used in assessing ventricular function. Calculations of wall stress are based on the **Laplace relationship**:

$$\text{wall stress} = \frac{Pr}{2h}$$

where P is pressure, r is radius of curvature, and h is wall thickness. Because the left ventricle is not a regular sphere, particularly in systole, the Laplace formula is an oversimplification. A fairly simple and accurate formula for calculating meridional wall stress that incorporates the important variables was developed by Grossman and others:

$$\text{wall stress} = \frac{1.35Pd}{4h(1+h/d)}$$

where P is pressure, d is left ventricular minor-axis dimension, and h is wall thickness at the level of the minor axis.

Heart rate effects

Heart rate as a determinant of performance in the intact heart is more complex than in isolated muscle. The force–frequency relationship has been demonstrated in intact hearts, measuring ventricular minor-axis diameter with ultrasonic crystals, and using the two-stage procedure described above. The maximal rate of change of pressure (dP/dt_{max}) in the ventricles was similar to that found previously in muscle strips. In cats and dogs, after steady pacing, an optimal dP/dt_{max} occurred 720 ms after the last normal beat; this shortened to 560 ms during epinephrine infusion, and dP/dt_{max} increased if the control pacing rate was elevated. These findings can be explained by the effects of these maneuvers on Ca^{2+} stores and their release. Applying this technique to humans with normal or abnormal left ventricular function, the optimal RR interval is 800 ms. If two beats were given at optimal intervals after the premature stimulus, dP/dt_{max} of the first normal beat after the premature beat was potentiated because the extra Ca^{2+} introduced into the cytosol by the premature beat was available to potentiate the first beat after the premature stimulus. The second post-premature beat was also potentiated, but less so; the ratio of the potentiation of these two beats is used to calculate the fraction of Ca^{2+} recirculating from one beat to the next. This amount is constant in any one patient, but is much less in those with left ventricular dysfunction.

In addition to the force–frequency relationship, heart rate affects systolic performance by the Frank–Starling relationship by virtue of its effects on diastolic filling. At normal rates, the ventricle fills and ejects a normal stroke volume. As heart rate increases, stroke volume falls slightly at first because there is a decrease in filling time; however, the increase in contraction frequency may more than offset the decrease in stroke volume so that cardiac output is maintained or may increase. When heart rate increases further, diastolic filling is impaired enough that cardiac output falls. Similarly, as heart rate decreases, cardiac output is maintained through a certain range because of an increase in preload and thus stroke volume. When heart rate decreases further, the increase in preload is insufficient to maintain cardiac output. The range over which cardiac output is maintained is an index of the heart rate sensitivity; the wider the range, the lesser the sensitivity. The newborn and adult heart are relatively insensitive to changes in heart rate over a wide range. The fetal heart, however, is quite rate sensitive, and heart rate may be the major determinant of cardiac output under normal conditions. This is partly because the fetal ventricles are relatively less compliant than the postnatal ventricles, so that increasing diastolic filling time is not associated with compensatory increases in preload, and partly because the fetal heart is exposed to positive rather than negative extracardiac pressures. In addition to rate sensitivity, the filling of the ventricles is exquisitely sensitive to venous flow patterns, because the right atrial return is the main source of left ventricle filling as well. Thus, a change in the site of the pacemaker (left versus right atrium) has significant effects on relative right and left ventricular output as well as combined ventricular output.

Contractility

The last major determinant of systolic performance is contractility. This is the most difficult determinant of performance to define and yet it is the one most studied. Contractility perhaps can be defined best as the alterations in cardiac function that occur secondary to changes in cytosolic Ca^{2+} availability or sarcomere sensitivity to Ca^{2+}. Thus, β-adrenergic agonists or phosphodiesterase inhibitors, which increase cytosolic Ca^{2+}, and thyroxine, which alters myosin ATPase sensitivity to Ca^{2+} in some species by altering the dominant isoform, are positive inotropic agents. However, to quantify contractility in the intact heart or to assess the contractile effects of an intervention is very difficult because all presumed indices of contractility are in fact indices of overall performance. Insofar as the indices change with changes in the other determinants of performance (loading conditions and heart rate), they are not entirely specific for changes in contractility. For example, cardiac output is an excellent index of the systolic performance of the intact ventricle, but it is so sensitive to preload, afterload, and heart rate that it is not a useful index of contractility.

This has led many investigators to search for indices of performance that are load insensitive and thus specific for changes in contractility. Unfortunately, it has become increasingly clear that such a search is fruitless and in fact misdirected, because contractility is itself not independent of the other determinants of performance. For example, changes in contractility are not independent of changes in heart rate; as described above, the force–frequency relationship describes increases in contractility secondary to increases in heart rate. It is now apparent that changes in both preload and afterload also directly alter contractility. Direct preload effects on contractility have been clearly shown in the intact heart and at the sarcomere level by demonstrating length-dependent contractility likely secondary to increased Ca^{2+} sensitivity of the sarcomere at longer initial lengths. Afterload dependence has also been demonstrated; recent studies in the intact circulation have shown that acute increases in afterload acutely increase contractility independent of indirect effects of β-adrenergic stimulation. Some of this afterload dependence has been thought to be on the basis of beat-to-beat changes in Ca^{2+} flux related to shortening deactivation. Recently it has also been shown that ejecting beats can actually generate greater rather than lesser pressures than isovolumic beats, so that there appear to be subcellular processes which act in a direction opposite to shortening deactivation. Probably, these as-yet poorly defined processes that lead to pressure deficits and excesses in ejecting beats will be based on beat-to-beat alterations in Ca^{2+} flux and sensitivity.

Developmental aspects

In the immature heart, and particularly in the fetal environment, factors other than those described above may be important determinants as well. Most importantly, the right ventricle fills to a greater extent and under a higher pressure than the left, and it ejects more blood under the same pressure and against a greater impedance. Thus, the effects of the right ventricle on left ventricular performance (termed 'ventricular interaction') may well be another major determinant of left ventricular performance in the fetus, and must be considered. In addition, it is possible that the constraining effects of the pericardium and the uninflated lungs have a greater effect in the fetus than they will have postnatally. Finally, one must realize that the fetal circulatory environment is very different from the postnatal environment. Most importantly, the ventricles do not function strictly in series and the left ventricle is in physical continuity with a high-pressure right ventricle. Thus the right ventricle may have a far more significant direct effect on left ventricular filling and ejection in the fetus than postnatally. Such a significant effect of the right ventricle on left ventricular performance has been demonstrated in the setting of pulmonary hypertension in the adult dog, and large increases in maximal left ventricular output shown in fetal sheep during *in utero* ventilation support this hypothesis. Thus ventricular interaction, although only a minor determinant of left ventricular output postnatally, is likely a major determinant before birth.

In summary, the major determinants of fetal cardiac output may be quite different than those of postnatal cardiac output. Heart rate normally may be the major determinant of output; fetal bradycardia has a very detrimental effect on blood flow and O_2 delivery. The fetal heart can respond to increased preload (Frank–Starling law) with increased stroke volume, but this response is limited, perhaps because of a concomitant increase in afterload and the interactive effects of the right ventricle on left ventricular filling and ejection. The importance of inotropic stimulation in the fetus also appears limited. Conversely, whereas direct ventricular interaction appears to be a minor determinant in the postnatal state, it may be a major determinant of output in the fetus, and more importantly, alterations in ventricular interaction at birth may contribute substantially to the left ventricular ability to more than double its output after birth.

Indices of performance and contractility

If one clearly cannot evaluate myocardial contractility specifically because it is intricately dependent upon loading conditions and heart rate, one must rethink all the indices of systolic performance that in the past have been used to separate the effects of contractility from those of preload and afterload. It seems more appropriate to accept that all indices are reflections of global performance and, rather than try to dissect out the independent contributions of various determinants, to determine the nature and magnitude of their interaction (equivalent to the interaction of sarcomere length, Ca^{2+} dynamics, and frequency of contraction in the isolated myofibrils). Two general statements should precede a discussion of indices of performance. First, because different determinants of performance are more important at different phases of systole (e.g. preload during the isovolumic phase and afterload during ejection), it is worthwhile to divide the indices of systolic performance by the phase or phases of systole during which they occur. Second, because contractility is intricately related to load, any single beat index of performance is by necessity very load sensitive and thus of limited use in evaluating the contractile state of the heart. Thus any acceptable index of the contractile state of the heart should be obtained over a range of loading conditions. That is, a relationship of systolic performance over different loads would best describe the intrinsic ability of that heart to contract and eject blood.

Pressure–volume loops; ventricular elastance

Because the systolic function of the intact heart is to generate pressure and eject blood, many recent investigators have studied performance in the pressure–volume plane. If left ventricular pressure and volume are measured simultaneously, the resulting pressure–volume loop gives information about ventricular function and can be used to assess myocardial contractility in the intact heart. The modern approach to analyzing these loops is based on the elastance concept of Suga and Sagawa; by definition, elastance is the ratio of pressure change to volume change. Consider first an isolated ventricle containing a balloon that can be inflated to different volumes. At each volume the ventricle is stimulated to contract and generates a peak systolic pressure (Fig. 10.27a); as volumes increase, so do the peak systolic pressures generated, and the relationship is relatively linear. The line joining the peak pressures intercepts the volume axis at a positive value, termed V_0, that indicates the unstressed volume of the ventricle. The equation for this line is:

$$P_{es} = E_{es}(V_{es}-V_0),$$

where P_{es} is end-systolic pressure, E_{es} is the slope of the line, V_{es} is the end-systolic volume, and V_0 is the unstressed volume (the ventricular volume when the transmural ventricular pressure is zero). If contractility increases (more Ca^{2+} enters the cells), the ventricle can generate greater pressures at any given volume, thereby generating a steeper pressure–volume line (higher value of E_{es}), as shown by the dashed line C+ in Fig. 10.27a. If contractility decreases, the ventricle generates lower pressures at any given volume, and the pressure–volume line is less steep (lower value of E_{es}).

If the ventricle ejects in the intact circulation, the typical pressure–volume loops shown in Fig. 10.27b are seen. During diastolic filling, volume increases and diastolic pressure rises slightly due to the increase in passive tension. At the end of diastole, isovolumic systole occurs, and ventricular pressure rises with no change in volume. When ventricular pressure exceeds aortic diastolic pressure, the aortic valve opens, blood is ejected, and ventricular volume decreases. Then ejection ends, and pressure falls to diastolic levels as isovolumic relaxation occurs. The pressure and volume reached at the end of systole are those that would have been reached by the isolated ventricle at that same end-systolic volume; in other words, at a given volume, no higher pressure can be generated (loop 1, Fig. 10.27b). The decrease in volume during ejection is the stroke volume, which divided by the end-diastolic volume gives the ejection fraction; normally, ejection fraction is over 65 percent.

To evaluate contractility in the intact circulation, one needs to evaluate the index (here, end-systolic elastance) over changing load, as discussed above. This has been done with pressure–volume loops with increases (volume infusion) and decreases (inferior vena caval occlusion) in preload or increases (aortic occlusion) in afterload. For example, if afterload is increased by raising aortic pressure, the normal heart responds as shown in Fig. 10.27b, loops 2 and 3. In the first beat after the increase, the ventricle must generate a higher pressure before the valve opens. Then it ejects, but cannot eject a normal stroke volume because of the higher pressure that is required from the same end-diastolic length (preload). In fact, the end-systolic volume is that which is appropriate for the higher pressure. Because the ventricle has emptied incompletely, the next normal diastolic inflow increases end-diastolic volume, and this increase of end-diastolic volume continues until the ventricle ejects a normal stroke volume, but now at a higher end-diastolic volume (compare loops 1 and 2, and loops 2 and 3). The ventricle has adapted to the higher afterload by increasing

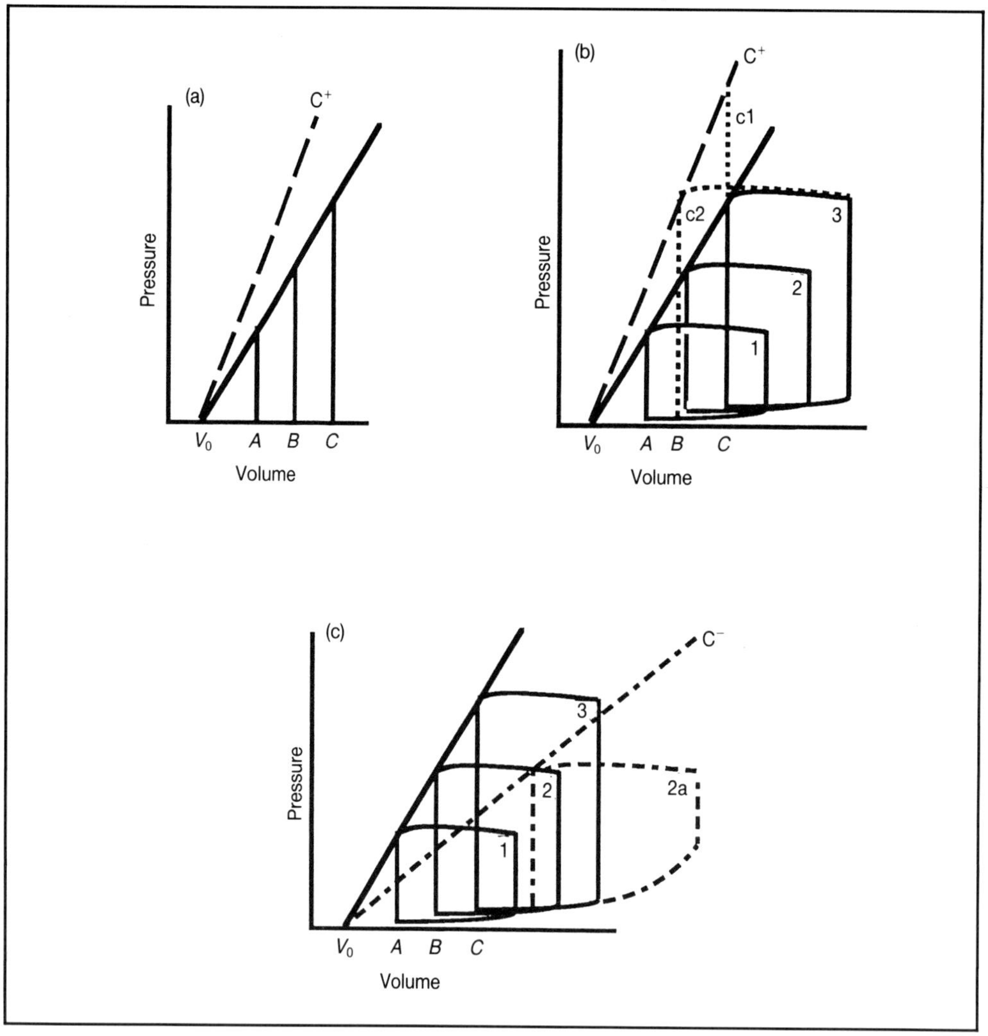

Fig. 10.27. Ventricular pressure–volume relations. (a) Pressure–volume characteristics of non-ejecting (isometric) ventricle. *A*, *B*, and *C* are three arbitrary ventricular volumes, and V_0 is the unstressed volume. The solid diagonal line is the pressure–volume relation of the normal ventricle, and the diagonal dashed line C+ is the corresponding relation when contractility is increased. (b) Pressure–volume characteristics of ejecting ventricles. Loops 1, 2, and 3 in solid lines represent three ejecting beats at three different aortic pressures. The diagonal solid line is the elastance line obtained at end-systole; it is usually the line of maximal elastance when afterload is measured accurately. The end-systolic volumes for loops 1, 2, and 3 are the same volumes *A*, *B*, and *C* as appeared in (a). When contractility is increased, as shown by the diagonal dashed line C+, the ventricle with pressure–volume loop 3 can either generate a higher pressure at the same stroke volume (extension c1) or else can expel a greater stroke volume at the same aortic pressure (extension c2). (c) Pressure–volume characteristics when contractility is greatly impaired. Loops 1, 2, and 3 are as in (b). Loop 2a indicates the pressure–volume loop during impaired contractility. Note that if the ventricle cannot dilate, as in restrictive cardiomyopathy, it can eject only a small stroke volume as shown by the vertical dashed line at end-systole for loop 2. If the ventricle can increase its end-diastolic volume, as in loop 2a, then it can eject a normal stroke volume, but at the expense of a very elevated end-diastolic pressure.

end-diastolic fiber length, a phenomenon described under the term 'preload reserve'. If different afterloads are used, the end-systolic pressure–volume points define a sloping line that is predicted to have the same slope as the line obtained in the isolated heart at those same volumes, the line of maximal ventricular elastance. This end-systolic pressure–volume relationship can then be described by its slope (E_{max}) and intercept (V_0); these indices have been used separately and together to describe changes in contractility in the intact animal and human. However, this theoretical relationship does not hold exactly in the intact circulation. First, there is no theoretical reason for the relationship to be linear. Secondly, ejecting beats, probably through beat-to-beat changes in contractility, can achieve either higher or lower pressures than isovolumic beats. For these reasons, both curvilinearity and load dependence have been demonstrated in the adult and young heart, particularly when studied over a wide range of loads or at very high or very low contractile states. In the physiological range of measurements, however, and particularly in the young animal, the relationship appears to be linear enough to ignore the adjustments of curvilinearity, and E_{max} appears to be reasonably sensitive to changes in contractility. However, because of curvilinearity in the far ranges of load, extrapolation to unstressed volumes is probably not valid. Thus, the positional index of the relationship generally used is a volume at a pressure in the range of measurement, such as V_{100} rather than V_0. One must note that the end-systolic pressure–volume relationship can be generated over load using a variety of techniques, and afterload increases are not necessarily the best, because of the rapid baroreflex response. Typically, the relationship is generated during inferior vena caval occlusion in most studies. This alters preload over an adequate range for one to define the slope and position of the relationship, but without large changes that would induce major and rapid neural responses to those changes.

Increased contractility and elastance

If ventricular contractility increases, then the ventricle can attain higher ejection pressures at any given volume, and the end-systolic pressure–volume points lie on a steeper line that lies above and to the left of the normal line, as shown by dashed line C^+ in Fig. 10.27b. Therefore, as shown by the dotted lines extending from loop 3, the ventricle can eject a higher stroke volume (see extension c2) at the same end-diastolic pressure (which is what happens during exercise) or can eject the same stroke volume at a higher pressure (see extension c1).

Decreased contractility and elastance

If ventricular contractility decreases, then the ventricle cannot generate normal pressures at any given end-diastolic volume, and the end-systolic pressure–volume line lies below and to the right of the normal line, as shown by the dashed line C^- in Fig. 10.27c. Note from this figure that the ventricle with impaired contractility either can eject a normal stroke volume at much increased end-diastolic volumes and pressures (loop 2a), or else can eject at a normal end-diastolic volume and pressure only by reducing its stroke volume drastically (loop 2). Any increase in afterload causes a further increase in end-diastolic volume, and this increase causes diastolic pressures to rise rapidly to high values that cause pulmonary congestion. The normal preload reserve has been used up in attempting to eject a reasonable stroke volume against a modestly increased afterload. In hearts that are still further depressed, the ventricle cannot handle even normal afterloads without getting a pathologically raised diastolic pressure in the ventricles or else a drastic decrease in stroke volume. In these hearts, because of the relatively flat slope of the maximal ventricular elastance line, a slight reduction of afterload produces a relatively large increase in stroke volume and a relatively large decrease in ventricular end-diastolic volume and pressure. This is one of the mechanisms for cardiac improvement with afterload reduction.

Ventricular function curves

Ejection phase indices

More classical evaluation of systolic performance during ejection is the use of ventricular function curves. Sarnoff and colleagues first measured left ventricular diastolic pressure and stroke work, then infused fluids and examined the relationship between these two variables. A pressure–stroke work curve (N) is shown in Fig. 10.28. If contractility increased (I), the curve shifted up and to the left; that is, at any end-diastolic pressure, a greater stroke work was achieved. If contractility decreased (D), the curve shifted down and to the right. Sarnoff recognized a major problem with this technique, namely that curvilinearity of the diastolic length–pressure relationship produced an S-shaped curve when relating stroke work to end-diastolic pressure, and at that time techniques for measuring fiber length or ventricular volume were inadequate. In addition, using pressure instead of fiber length or volume may lead to misinterpretations if there are substantial changes of pericardial or pleural pressures. Subsequent groups of investigators used similar function curves to examine the stroke volume–end-diastolic

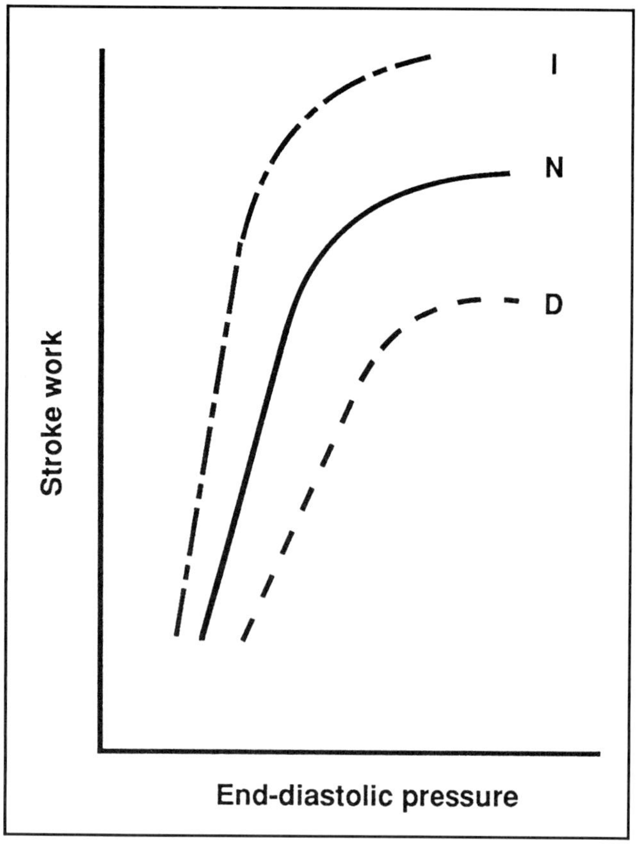

Fig. 10.28. Curves to illustrate the ventricular function curves introduced by Sarnoff and colleagues. Curve N is the normal relation which can be moved up and to the left by increased contractility (I) or down and to the right by decreased contractility (D).

pressure relationship; this is even less satisfactory because stroke volume is affected by increases of afterload.

In conscious dogs with autonomic blockade, the relationship of stroke work to end-diastolic fiber length or ventricular volume, termed preload recruitable stroke work, is linear and independent of changes in afterload. The line intercepts the length or volume axis at values close to the unstressed length or volume. Ca^{2+} infusion increases the slope of the line without changing the intercept on the length axis. In ischemic ventricles, depression of ventricular function shifts the stroke work–end-diastolic segment length relationship to the right (increases the intercept on the horizontal axis) and decreases the slope. These two effects can be evaluated simultaneously by calculating the area under the curve, termed the preload-recruitable stroke work area. These concepts and the ventricular elastance concept have much in common, and both give acceptable approaches to assessing myocardial function independent of changes in preload and afterload provided one can measure wall force, stroke work, ventricular volume, or minor-axis diameter and change these over a range so that the lines or areas defining these indexes can be obtained.

In addition to ejection phase analyses, it is possible and useful to evaluate performance during other phases of systole, and in other planes. The force–velocity relationship is another well described attribute of cardiac muscle, and can be evaluated prior to ejection (during isovolumic contraction). The concept of the maximal velocity of contraction against zero load (V_{max}) was once popular; this value in muscle strips was independent of muscle length but varied in the right way with inotropic changes. The principle, based on studies of skeletal muscle by A V Hill, was reasonable, but the complexity of the mechanics of cardiac muscle, with its mixture of contractile, series elastic, and parallel elastic elements as well as viscosity, made it difficult to assess what would have been the true index, namely the V_{max} of the contractile element alone. In practice too, one cannot abolish internal loading of the muscle fiber. Applying this concept to the intact heart was even more difficult.

As a substitute for V_{max}, investigators began to use dP/dt_{max} (the maximal rate of change of ventricular pressure). This index, however, is affected markedly by changes in afterload, and so must be used with care when afterloads are very different. A variant of this method is to measure dP/dt at a developed ventricular pressure of 40 mmHg (5.3 kPa), because this virtually guarantees that the aortic valve will still be closed when the measurement is made. Little has recently described an index of ventricular performance by varying load while measuring the change in dP/dt_{max}. The dP/dt_{max}–end-diastolic volume relation is similar to the end-systolic pressure–volume relation and to the preload recruitable stroke work index, is relatively linear, and varies with changes in contractility, but is less sensitive than are the other two indices.

Combined ejection and isovolumic phase indices

Combining ejection and isovolumic phase indices may be the best way to evaluate systolic performance. Such an index has been created in both adults and children by providing normal data for the relationship between end-systolic wall stress and velocity of shortening. As contractility increases, the relationship shifts upward. Unfortunately, the effect of decreasing afterload beyond the range of the normal data has not been carefully explored, and from early studies it appears that, just as would be predicted from the force–velocity relationship, such decreases in afterload also appear to increase the stress-corrected velocity of shortening.

Arterial and venous coupling

Arterial coupling

Because the heart is a mechanical pump that ejects blood into the arterial system and in turn is supplied with blood by the venous system, these three components interact. One way to evaluate this is to consider what would happen if we disconnect (uncouple) the heart from the rest of the circulation and consider each component separately. The heart's pumping ability can be tested by finding out how much it can eject against different afterloads, just as we can test how much force a muscle strip can exert by increasing the afterload. As the load against which the left ventricle pumps increases, the output decreases until, at some high load, the heart cannot eject. The relationship of load to output is approximately linear (Fig. 10.29a). Then we connect a pump to the aorta, and determine how much blood can be pumped through the system at different perfusing pressures; the higher the pressure, the more the flow through the system. For simplicity, this relationship is shown in Fig. 10.29b as linear, although the actual shape of the curve depends on many variables. Now in the intact

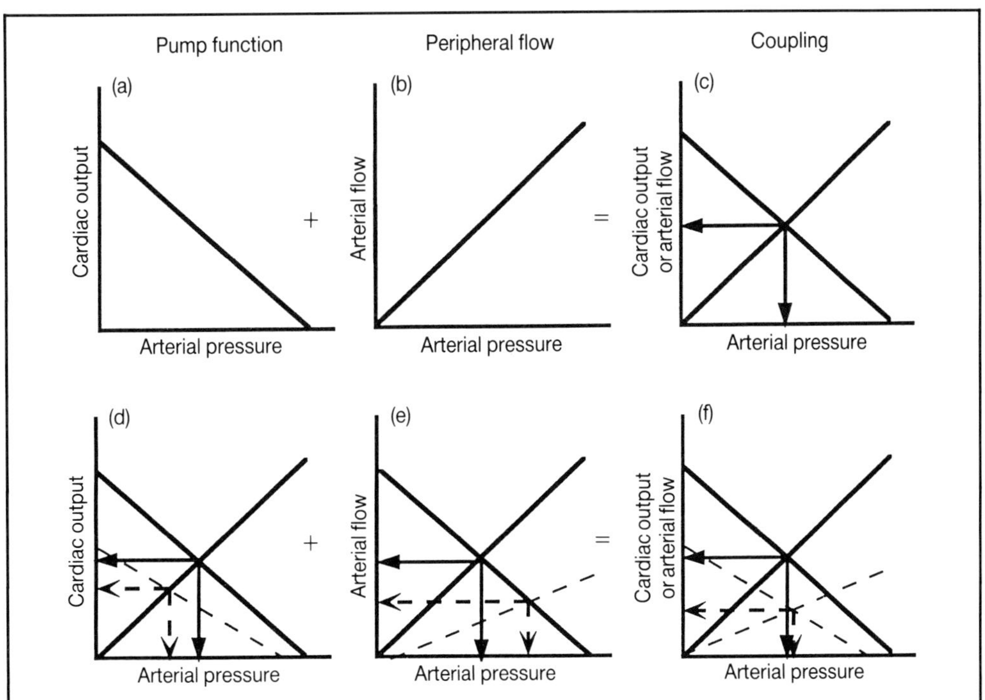

Fig. 10.29. Arterial coupling. (a) Pump function of heart shown by plotting pump (cardiac) output at increasing peripheral (arterial) pressures. As the afterload increases, the output decreases. (b) Arterial function shown by how much flow is obtained at different perfusing pressures. The slope of the line is the resistance. (c) Normally cardiac output and arterial flow are equal, and the values for these flows occur where the two function lines cross. The solid arrows show the normal operating flow and pressure. (d) With decreased pump function, the cardiac output afterload line is depressed (dashed line), and if peripheral resistance is normal, both output and arterial pressure will be low, as shown by the dashed arrows. (e) With normal pump function but an increased peripheral resistance (as shown by the decreased slope of the dashed pressure–flow line) cardiac output is also decreased, but arterial pressure may be increased, as shown by the dashed arrows. (f) With heart failure, both a decrease in pump function and an increase in peripheral resistance will occur (dashed lines). Therefore both cardiac output and arterial pressure will be reduced, the former more than the latter (dashed arrows).

circulation, there is an afterload for the ventricle, and a perfusion pressure that pushes blood around the body; both of these are in equilibrium, and cardiac output and peripheral flow will be equal and occur where the two pressure–flow lines intersect (Fig. 10.29c). With decreased contractility, the heart can pump less blood at any given pressure, so that we get the dashed line shown in Fig. 10.29d; where this crosses the (normal) peripheral resistance line gives the new equilibrium, and shows that both pressure and cardiac output will be reduced. If peripheral resistance is elevated without a change in contractility, then cardiac output will be low but arterial pressure can be normal (dashed lines and arrows in Fig. 10.29e). Usually, however, with severe heart disease, there is an increase in peripheral resistance as well as a decrease in contractility, so that the two function lines cross at a markedly reduced stroke volume, even though the arterial pressure may be fairly normal (Fig. 10.29f). Therefore, treatment by agents that reduce afterload or increase inotropy, or both, will raise the crossover point and increase stroke volume by raising the equilibrium point at which the two function lines cross.

Venous coupling

To study venous coupling, we first examine the relationship between ventricular output and atrial pressure (Fig. 10.30a). Increases in pressure cause a large increase in output at first (preload effect), and then at increasing atrial pressures, output rises less markedly because preload reserve is used up; that is, sarcomeres have reached or passed their optimal lengths. If, on the other hand, we examine the effects of changing atrial pressures on venous return (Fig. 10.30b), the venous return does not change for small increases in atrial pressure, but above atrial pressures of about 10–12 mmHg (1.3–1.6 kPa) the venous return decreases more or less linearly as atrial pressures increase. The point at which these two curves cross is the operating point for the normal circulation (Fig. 10.30c); this is normally on the plateau of the venous return curve. In the normal heart, decreasing venous return decreases cardiac output (Fig. 10.30d), as is seen transiently in the brief hypotension that occurs when suddenly standing up from a sitting position. In other words, cardiac output is normally limited by venous return and not by cardiac performance. In congestive heart failure, however, the venous system is overfilled and at high pressure. The crossover point occurs on the sloping portion of the venous return curve because cardiac output is now determined by the depressed cardiac function and is low, and because venous pressure is high; cardiac function is not limited by venous return (Fig. 10.30e). What happens to the circulation when sodium nitroprusside is given? Systemic venous capacity increases, and causes a shift of blood from the pulmonary to the systemic circuits. Left ventricular filling pressure is decreased, thus reducing left ventricular preload with resulting improvement in left ventricular function, partly by improving subendocardial blood flow. Therefore, cardiac output increases and the patient improves. Increased cardiac output from vasodilators also tends to lower venous pressure and increase venous return.

Diastolic function

Systolic function affects the force and rate of ventricular contraction and the amount of blood ejected with each beat; diastolic function concerns the rate and extent of ventricular relaxation. Many forms of heart disease manifest abnormalities of both systolic and diastolic function, but dysfunction of one or the other may predominate and determine the type of therapy needed.

Diastolic dysfunction is indicated by an increased ventricular diastolic pressure at normal ventricular volumes. Dysfunction may be caused by increased passive stiffness of the ventricles due to chronic infiltrates (e.g. *amyloid*), *myocardial scars*, *constrictive pericarditis*, or *diffuse myocardial fibrosis*. It can also be due to impaired relaxation. Normally, ventricular muscle relaxes rapidly in diastole, the primary mechanism being the rapid release of Ca^{2+} bound to troponin and its uptake by the sarcoplasmic reticulum. Removing Ca^{2+} allows actin-myosin crossbridges to dissociate and the sarcomeres to lengthen, so that the ventricle can dilate. Decreased Ca^{2+} removal because of abnormalities in major contractile proteins or transport processes decreases the rate and extent of relaxation. Ischemia is one major factor that impairs Ca^{2+} metabolism and diastolic ventricular function, but many other forms of heart disease have similar effects. Clinically, diastolic function is assessed by relating end-diastolic pressure and volume; by observing the rate of ventricular filling by angiography or by Doppler studies of the mitral valve inflow; by measuring the peak rate of fall of ventricular pressure (negative

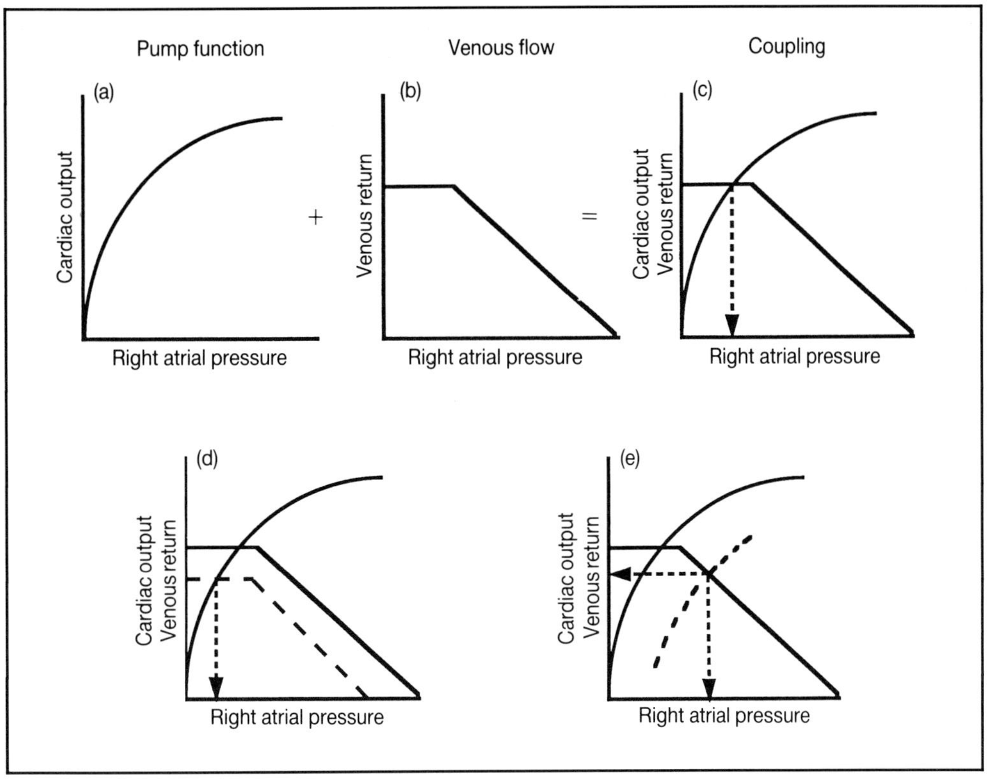

Fig. 10.30. Venous coupling. (a) Typical preload–flow relation of an atrium. (b) Typical normal venous return–right atrial relation. As right atrial pressure is increased from very low values, the venous return does not change because of the systemic venous waterfall. At higher pressures, raising right atrial pressure will lower venous return. (c) Where the right atrial pressure–cardiac output and the right atrial pressure–venous return curves cross will determine the venous return and right atrial pressure for that subject. As shown by the dotted arrow, this is usually on the plateau of the venous return–atrial pressure curve. (d) A sudden decrease in venous return, as occurs with standing up, decreases right atrial pressure and cardiac output. (e) With decreased cardiac contractility, right atrial pressure rises until it impedes venous return.

dP/dt_{max}); or by calculating the time constant of the fall in ventricular pressure.

Role of the pericardium

The parietal pericardium is a stiff membrane that surrounds the heart, separated from it only by a small amount of pericardial fluid. Normally, the pressure in the pericardial cavity is negative, due to the negative intrapleural pressure. Therefore, normally transmural diastolic pressure across the wall of the left ventricle is slightly greater than diastolic ventricular pressure. Pericardial pressure can become positive and may restrict dilatation of the left ventricle if there is a tense pericardial effusion (tamponade) or if the ventricles dilate acutely because of a sudden volume load or sudden myocardial depression. In some patients with acute myocardial ischemia, left ventricular diastolic pressure can be greatly increased without much change in ventricular volume because of tension in the pericardium. This mechanism makes it difficult to interpret changes in diastolic pressure–volume relations only in terms of myocardial stiffness.

It is important to realize that the pericardium can restrict ventricular dilatation even when pericardial cavity pressure is not positive. Imagine replacing the pericardium with a loose mesh of fibers resembling a tennis net. These fibers can press against the surface of the heart and exert a surface force that restrains the heart, but there can be no positive liquid pressure in the cavity because it is very leaky. The difference between surface and liquid pressures explains some of the discrepancies previously reported in the literature. Some investigators believe that the right atrial pressure is the closest approximation to pericardial surface pressure, so that it could be used when calculating transmural ventricular pressure, but caution is advised when doing this because there is not yet clear evidence that the surface pressures are identical at every part of the external cardiac surface.

Pericardial tamponade

The positive pericardial pressure of *pericardial tamponade* is the major cause of pulsus paradoxus (a fall in systemic arterial blood pressure of more than 6–8 mmHg with inspiration). It acts via two main mechanisms. One of them is that with inspiration the intrathoracic pressure decreases, and so do pressures in the pulmonary veins. Normally, left atrial pressure decreases to a similar extent with inspiration, and left atrial filling is changed little by inspiration. When, however, pericardial pressure is positive, left atrial pressure remains high during inspiration, and there may even be pressure gradient from left atrium to pulmonary veins that produces retrograde flow. Consequently, left ventricular filling is impaired and arterial blood pressure decreases. The second major mechanism is discussed below in the section on ventricular interaction.

Ventricular interaction

Because the left and right ventricles share the ventricular septum, distension of the right ventricle, e.g. in acute pulmonary embolism, pushes the septum to the left, thereby decreasing left ventricular volume and preload. The resulting decrease in cardiac output should not be taken to indicate left ventricular dysfunction. In fact, a lesser degree of this shift occurs with each inspiration, and is one of the mechanisms responsible for the slight fall of systemic arterial pressure that takes place with each inspiration. This mechanism is accentuated when there is pericardial tamponade, because the stiff pericardium does not allow the total intrapericardial volume to increase. Therefore, when the right ventricle dilates during the inspiratory increase in venous return, the left ventricular volume is much reduced and arterial pressure falls significantly. This is one of the major mechanisms responsible for the pulsus paradoxus that is the primary method of diagnosing pericardial tamponade.

Selected reading

Friedman WF. The intrinsic physiologic properties of the developing heart. In Friedman WF, Lesch M, Sonnenblick EH, eds. *Neonatal heart disease*. New York: Grune & Stratton, 1973: 21.

Hori M, Suga H, Baan J, Yellin EL, eds. *Cardiac mechanics and function in the normal and diseased heart*. Tokyo: Springer-Verlag, 1989.

Kass D, Maughan WL. From 'Emax' to pressure-volume relations: a broader perspective. *Circulation* 1988; **77**: 1203.

Ross J, Jr. Mechanisms of cardiac contraction. What roles for preload, afterload and inotropic state in heart failure? *Eur Heart J* 1983; **4**(Suppl A): 19.

Teitel DF, Sidi D, Chin T, *et al*. Developmental changes in myocardial contractile reserve in the lamb. *Pediatr Res* 1985; **19**: 948.

G. Specific Circulations

G1. Cerebrovascular Regulation

W J Pearce

At birth, the human brain is quite immature. Myelination is incomplete, synapses are still forming, and motor coordination is rudimentary at best. Correspondingly, the blood vessels of the brain are also immature at birth, particularly in preterm infants. At about 26 weeks gestational age, human cerebral blood vessels begin to grow rapidly, increasing in both density and diameter, and reach peak numbers and size by 35 weeks. Thereafter, the composition and function of the arteries begin to change most dramatically, while their numbers and size change relatively little.

A key maturational change in the **composition of cerebral arteries** is a progressive increase in mechanical stiffness after birth. This is primarily due to changes in connective tissue composition but also is associated with some reduction in extracellular water during the first few days of extrauterine life. Subsequently the arterial walls thicken due to the synthesis and extracellular deposition of collagen and elastin. As maturation proceeds, connective tissue turnover continues with the production of relatively more type III and less type I collagen, and increases in the collagen to elastin ratio, with the greatest increases in the largest arteries.

Accompanying these changes in stiffness and composition are important changes in cerebrovascular reactivity, many of which are coincident with the changes in circulating hormone concentrations that occur during the perinatal period. For example, plasma renin activity and concentrations of angiotensin II, arginine vasopressin, T_3, and T_4 are all higher in newborns than adults. Although a causal link between changes in circulating hormone concentrations and changes in cerebrovascular reactivity has yet to be demonstrated, the connection seems probable in light of the well documented ability of steroid hormones to change tissue levels of key enzymes such as Na^+-K^+-ATPase and guanylyl cyclase.

Cerebral artery reactivity

At all ages, the contractile characteristics of cerebral arteries are heterogeneously distributed throughout the cerebrovascular tree. Differences exist not only between arteries and veins, but also between large and small arteries, between arteries of the brainstem and those of the cortex, and between pial and parenchymal arterioles. Species differences further contribute to this heterogeneity. Thus, it is important to bear in mind both the species and the specific artery under study when considering cerebrovascular reactivity.

Perinatal studies of the cerebral circulation have chiefly employed puppies, piglets, and lambs. Of these, cerebral development at birth is least mature in puppies and most mature in term lambs. Nonetheless, certain characteristics are common to the cerebral arteries of all three species. First, maximum contractile force increases with advancing age. Secondly, sensitivity to the nitrogenous vasodilators, such as nitroglycerine and nitroprusside, is present at birth. Thirdly, sensitivity to the vasodilating effects of adenosine is also present at birth. In general, each of these characteristics is also present in cerebral arteries of all sizes from term human infants (Fig. 10.31).

Another characteristic common to most species is that the reactivity of the cerebral arteries to receptor-dependent agonists changes dramatically between fetal and newborn life. For example, cerebral artery contractile responses to serotonin are greater in term fetuses than in newborn lambs, and both are greater than in adult sheep. Similar differences have been reported in a wide variety of species for many agents including norepinephrine, acetylcholine, vasoactive peptides, and others. Such differences suggest that the type and number of receptors populating the cerebral arteries are dynamic and under developmental, and probably hormonal, control. Equally important, these populations appear subject to environmental modulation, as suggested by the finding of different patterns of receptor-dependent cerebrovascular reactivity in fetal lambs at sea level and those at high altitude.

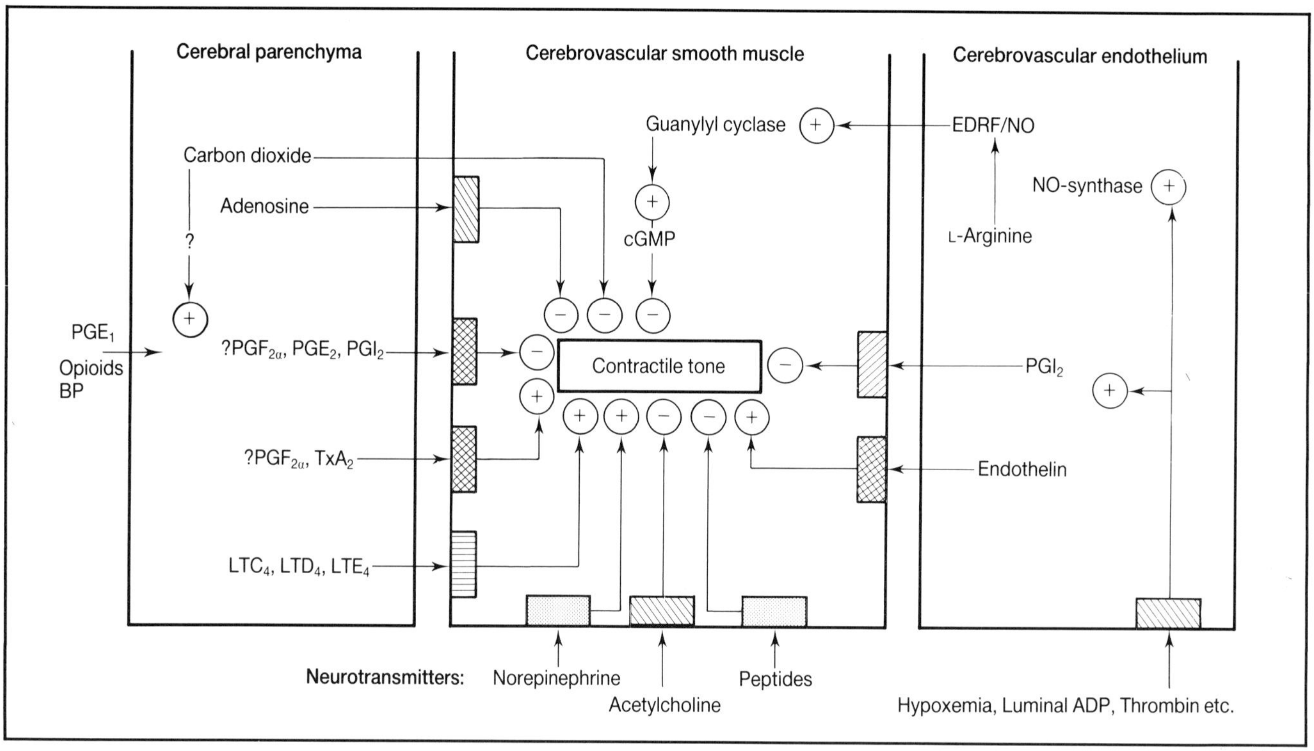

Fig. 10.31. Diagrammatic scheme of factors effecting cerebrovascular tone. See text for abbreviations.

Prostaglandins and the cerebral circulation

One group of receptor-dependent vasoactive compounds, the prostaglandins (PGs), plays an important role in the perinatal period, both by maintaining patency of the ductus arteriosus, and also by influencing vascular resistance in many organs, including the brain. They are synthesized perivascularly and act predominantly as mediators and/or modulators of adaptive responses to a variety of stimuli such as changes in blood pressure or hypoxia, and to some receptor-dependent agents such as opioids (see below). Total PG concentrations are higher in cortical subarachnoid cerebrospinal fluid than in either the cisterna magna or arterial blood, suggesting a cortical site of synthesis. PGs appear to be net cerebral vasodilators in the perinatal period, since indomethacin, an inhibitor of cyclooxygenase (a key enzyme in PG synthesis), produces a fall in cerebral blood flow (CBF) in almost all species. However, in the piglet, ibuprofen (another cyclooxygenase inhibitor) does not alter basal CBF, but actually widens the range of autoregulation so that it more closely approximates the range found in

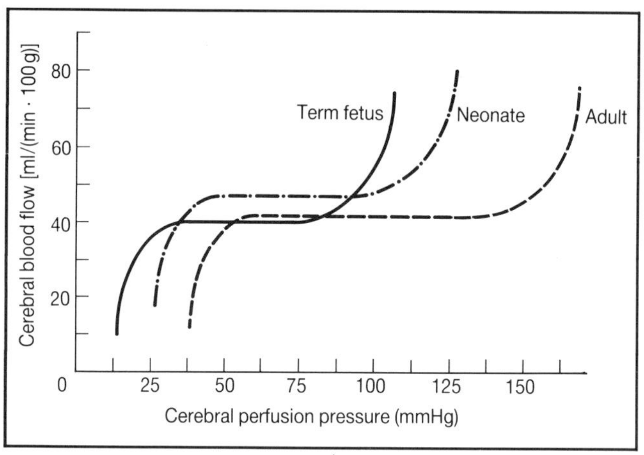

Fig. 10.32. Patterns of autoregulation in the term fetal, neonatal and adult cerebral circulations.

adults (Fig. 10.32). Thus indomethacin may have additional mechanisms of action not mediated by PGs. This tendency to widen the range of effective autoregulation may explain the reduced incidence of *intraventricular hemorrhage (IVH)* associated with cyclooxygenase inhibitors.

PGE_2 is a potent vasodilator in both the piglet and the

fetal baboon. Because plasma PGE_2 concentrations are higher in the baboon fetus than in the mother, and its vasodilator potency is greater in newborns than adults, PGE_2 has been proposed to contribute to the lower cerebrovascular resistance characteristic of fetal life. PGE_1 is also a potent vasodilator of cerebral arteries of the fetal baboon and as is true of PGE_2, sensitivity to PGE_1 appears to diminish with maturity.

During the perinatal period, prostacyclin (PGI_2) reduces tone in cerebral, mesenteric, and pulmonary arteries of both piglets and baboons. $PGF_{2\alpha}$ has also been reported to produce vasodilatation, but only at very low concentrations in the fetal baboon middle cerebral artery. Contractile responses to $PGF_{2\alpha}$ predominate in adult baboons and in pigs of all ages. Thromboxane (Tx) analogs produce vasoconstriction of the cerebral arteries in newborn piglets; the leukotrienes C_4, D_4, and E_4 all promote cerebral vasoconstriction in newborn piglets but their physiological role is not established.

As indicated above, an important feature of prostanoid metabolism is that it mediates and/or modulates the cerebrovascular responses to a wide variety of both physiological and pharmacological stimuli. Opioids, such as **enkephalins and dynorphins**, promote the synthesis and release of vasodilator PGs, which mediate the vasodilator effects of these opioids. Lysine vasopressin also appears to promote the release of vasodilator PGs. Conversely, the contractile responses of piglet cerebral arteries to the free radicals released by hydrogen peroxide appear to involve the synthesis and release of vasoconstrictor prostanoids. However, not all cerebrovascular responses in newborn piglets involve prostanoid release; cerebral vasodilator responses to the amino acids *N*-methyl-D-aspartate (NMDA), glutamate, aspartate, and taurine, for example, all appear independent of PG release.

Cerebral endothelium

The vascular endothelium is one source of vasodilator PGs, particularly PGI_2, in the neonatal cerebral circulation. However, the cerebral endothelium of most species, including humans, is also capable at birth of synthesizing and releasing endothelium derived relaxing factor (EDRF) (see p. 469). EDRF is widely held to be nitric oxide (**NO**) synthesized from L-arginine by the enzyme nitric oxide synthase. NO released by the cerebral endothelium readily diffuses into the adjacent vascular smooth muscle where it activates guanylyl cyclase, elevates vascular levels of cGMP, and precipitates vasodilatation through the actions of cGMP-dependent protein kinase. This pathway appears fully intact at birth in multiple species, including humans, although the magnitude of endothelium-dependent relaxation may be less in neonates than in adults of some species. Cerebral endothelium can also release the peptide **endothelin**, which in the newborn piglet causes vasoconstriction at maximum physiological concentrations. At present, however, the physiological stimuli which promote the release and action of vasoactive endothelial factors from cerebral arteries during the perinatal period remain uncertain. Current candidates include hypoxia, flow-induced shear stress, and stretch of the cerebral arterial wall.

Blood–brain barrier

Aside from its potential influence on cerebrovascular tone, the cerebral endothelium also serves another important function, that of the blood–brain barrier. The tight junctions typical of cerebral endothelium develop early in fetal life, and then undergo active modifications during the late prenatal period in both puppies and lambs. At birth, the cerebral endothelium is slightly more permeable than at maturity; this 'leaky' endothelium allows a higher protein concentration in the cerebrospinal fluid of neonates than in adults, and certain dyes penetrate the brain more easily in fetuses and newborns than in adults. Nevertheless, the blood–brain barrier of newborns is largely impermeable to norepinephrine, angiotensin II, and hydrogen ion, suggesting that the most important aspects of blood–brain barrier function are intact at birth.

Cerebrovascular innervation

In adults, the cerebral arteries are innervated by fibers containing adrenergic, cholinergic, and peptidergic neurotransmitters. For all of these nerve types, there are three general phases of nerve development: (1) the outgrowth of new axons, (2) the development of transmitter synthesis and storage capacity, and (3) the growth and differentiation of nerve varicosities. In general, postsynaptic function, reflecting the presence of appropriately coupled receptors, can be demonstrated before presynaptic elements are fully functional. As for contractility in general, the rate and timing of development of cerebrovascular innervation vary considerably among species and among different neurotransmitter systems.

The neurovascular system best characterized in cerebral arteries during the perinatal period is adrenergic sympathetic innervation. In human fetuses, immature adrenergic nerves with few varicosities can be demonstrated at 19–23 weeks of gestational age, and their density is greatest in the more rostral vessels. In baboons, cerebral arteries contract in response to norepinephrine; the strength of these contractions is greatest in fetuses and diminishes with age. Similarly, cerebral arteries of newborn puppies, piglets, and lambs have all been shown to contract with norepinephrine. In newborn piglets, norepinephrine acts predominantly on α_1-adrenergic receptors in cerebral resistance vessels and on α_2-adrenergic receptors in pial arterioles. In newborn piglets, norepinephrine also stimulates the release of PGE_2, which apparently limits the magnitude of the vasoconstrictor response to norepinephrine. In addition, electrical stimulation of the cerebrovascular sympathetic innervation decreases cerebral blood flow by up to 25 percent in newborn lambs and 15 percent in newborn piglets. In lambs, as in baboons, the responsiveness to norepinephrine is greatest in fetuses and diminishes with age, suggesting that the functional importance of adrenergic cerebrovascular innervation is probably greater during fetal than adult life.

Nerves containing acetylcholine can also be demonstrated in fetal human cerebral arteries between 19 and 23 weeks of gestational age, and as for adrenergic fibers, the fibers generally lack varicosities and are probably functionally immature. In fetal and newborn baboon cerebral arteries, acetylcholine elicits a contractile response that is absent in corresponding arteries from adults. In newborn piglet pial arteries, low concentrations of acetylcholine produce dilation whereas higher concentrations (100 μM) produce vasoconstriction. Interestingly, indomethacin at 5 mg/kg can block pial artery contractile responses to 100 μM acetylcholine, suggesting that vasoconstrictor prostanoids, such as $PGF_{2\alpha}$ and thromboxane A_2, somehow mediate the response.

Although there is some evidence of a serotonergic innervation supplying arteries of the circle of Willis in term human infants, these findings remain controversial and difficult to corroborate. Certainly, serotonin receptors are present in the cerebral arteries of most species at birth, but the pharmacological identity and cross-reactivity of serotonin with these receptors and α-adrenergic receptors in the neonatal cerebral circulation remains uncertain. On the other hand, the presence of a peptidergic innervation supplying human fetal cerebral arteries is more widely accepted. These peptidergic systems supply separate nerves containing neuropeptide Y and vasoactive intestinal polypeptide (VIP) to the major arteries of the circle of Willis and the large pial arteries. In fetal rats, the cerebral arteries are innervated by sensory fibers from the trigeminal ganglion that contain substance P, VIP, cholecystokinin, somatostatin, and calcitonin gene-related peptide. In adults, these peptides are all vasodilators. Their effects on cerebral arteries during the perinatal period, however, remain largely undocumented, as do the physiological stimuli that elicit their release.

Age-related changes in cerebral perfusion and metabolism

In all mammalian species, cerebral perfusion and **cerebral metabolic rate (CMR)** are closely coupled. Although the exact mechanisms responsible for this coupling remain elusive, this matching between flow and metabolism remains a characteristic feature of cerebrovascular regulation, even during the perinatal period. Thus, the key to understanding age-related changes in cerebral blood flow is to focus first on the developmental changes in cerebral metabolic rate. In newborn puppies, the brain is relatively immature at birth, and cerebral metabolic rate is low, as is cerebral perfusion. With postnatal maturation in the puppy, both cerebral metabolic rate and cerebral blood flow rise to reach adult levels. In contrast, the lamb cerebrum is largely mature at birth, the reticular activating system is fully functional, and cerebral blood flow is higher than in adults. The pattern in term human infants is somewhere between these two. At birth, human cerebral blood flow and cerebral metabolic rate are low, and both variables increase steadily through the first 6 years of life, after which cerebral flow and metabolism gradually decline throughout the remainder of life.

Cerebral metabolic rate is not the only factor influencing cerebral perfusion in the neonate. As shown in an extensive series of studies in fetal and newborn lambs, cerebral O_2 delivery is an actively regulated variable (Fig. 10.33).

Cerebral O_2 delivery =
cerebral blood flow × arterial blood O_2 content (CaO_2)

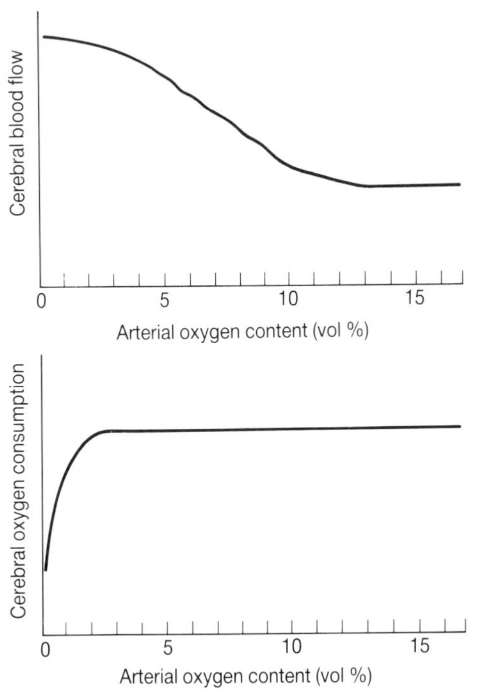

Fig. 10.33. Relationship of arterial blood O_2 content and cerebral blood flow (top panel) and cerebral O_2 consumption (lower panel).

Because the position of the oxyhemoglobin dissociation curve directly determines the amount of O_2 that can be extracted from blood by the tissue (see p. 549), shifts in the hemoglobin P_{50} produce corresponding shifts in the rate of cerebral perfusion; leftward shifts in the oxyhemoglobin dissociation curve decrease the amount of tissue-extractable O_2 and produce an increase in flow. Correspondingly, other maneuvers that alter O_2 carrying capacity, such as hemodilution or carbon monoxide poisoning, also alter the ratio of cerebral perfusion to metabolism. Central to the concept of the regulation of O_2 delivery is the assumption of a feedback mechanism matching tissue O_2 supply and demand. Although the mechanisms mediating this matching remain elusive, the 'O_2 coupling hypothesis' remains of great value in predicting the behavior of cerebral perfusion in response to a wide variety of physiological stimuli.

Other stimuli that influence cerebral perfusion include direct vascular stimuli, such as neurotransmitters or PGs, which act primarily on vascular smooth muscle, and metabolic stimuli, such as catabolic hormones or anesthetics, which act primarily to alter cerebral metabolic rate. For both classes of stimuli, the net effect is determined by how the stimulus affects the cerebral O_2 supply/demand ratio, and how the mechanisms maintaining this coupling compensate. As with most biological control systems, compensation is often not complete, and some 'steady-state error' will remain at equilibrium. Thus, the high carbon dioxide and PGE_2 levels typical of fetal life may contribute to a relative overperfusion of the fetal brain, at least in the ovine species. In human infants, the mechanisms matching tissue O_2 supply and demand appear fully intact at birth.

Cerebrovascular autoregulation

Another feature of cerebrovascular regulation in both neonates and adults is autoregulation, defined as the ability to maintain a constant rate of cerebral perfusion despite changes in cerebral perfusion pressure.

Cerebral perfusion pressure =
arterial blood pressure − cerebrospinal fluid pressure

A key characteristic of autoregulation is the range of perfusion pressures over which autoregulation is effective (Fig. 10.32). In adults, this range extends from a lower limit of approximately 50–60 mmHg (6.6–8.0 kPa) to an upper limit of approximately 140–150 mmHg. In fetuses and neonates, cerebral perfusion pressure is considerably lower than in adults (largely due to a lower mean arterial pressure), and correspondingly, the lower limit of autoregulation extends to lower perfusion pressures of 30–40 mmHg in most species, including human infants. Similarly, the upper limit of autoregulation is also lower in neonates (70–100 mmHg), rendering the neonates of most species, including human infants, more vulnerable than adults to hypertensive transients. In most species, including humans, cerebral autoregulation is fully functional at birth.

One possible mediator of autoregulatory cerebral vasodilatation induced by *hypotension* is tissue **adenosine**. Cerebral adenosine, an excellent vasodilator, increases as cerebral perfusion pressure is lowered. In addition, cerebral adenosine increases as cerebral O_2 supply is decreased, suggesting a possible common mechanism for the coupling of cerebral flow and metabolism, and cerebral autoregulation. However, hypotension also increases the cerebrospinal fluid concentrations of a variety of other compounds including both vasodilator and vasoconstrictor PGs, thromboxane and opioids. At the other end of the autoregulatory range, sympathetic vasoconstriction limits the increases in cerebral perfusion caused by elevated perfusion pressure in newborn piglets, and thus extends the upper limit of cerebral autoregulation. Clearly, cerebral autoregulation is a complex response involving multiple mechanisms, which may explain why it is vulnerable to a wide variety of insults including *metabolic acidosis*, severe *hypoxia* or *asphyxia*, *cerebral ischemia*, and *intracranial hemorrhage*.

Hypercapnic and hypoxic cerebral vasodilatation

One of the oldest known cerebral vasodilators in adults is carbon dioxide. *Hypercapnia* can also increase cerebral perfusion in both newborn and fetal lambs, as well as in newborn and preterm human infants. In general, hypercapnia is a less potent vasodilator in newborns and infants than in adults; the reasons for this difference are unclear. Some of this difference might be due to the possibility that acidosis, in the range which typically accompanies hypercapnia, is a better vasodilator in adult than in newborn cerebral arteries. Alternatively, age-related changes in hematocrit may be involved, as **hematocrit** is inversely proportional to cerebral CO_2 reactivity in newborn baboons. In newborn piglets, vasodilator prostanoids mediate up to 50 percent of the cerebral response to hypercapnia, suggesting that, at least in this species, age-related differences in prostanoid metabolism may contribute to age-related differences in hypercapnic sensitivity. Hypercapnic vasodilatation in newborns apparently does not involve reflex changes in sympathetic discharge or changes in cerebral metabolic rate.

Acute hypoxia also elicits cerebral vasodilatation in neonates of most mammalian species, including rats, piglets, puppies and fetal and newborn lambs. In newborn lambs, the response is greater than in adults, but in newborn puppies it is less, suggesting that the magnitude of response may be related to the extent of cerebral maturation and/or cerebral metabolic rate. Consistent with this view, the brainstem regions of both lambs and puppies, which are generally the most mature of any brain region at birth and have the highest metabolic rates, also exhibit greater responsiveness to hypoxia than do other brain regions.

With the onset of *cerebral hypoxia*, the cerebrovascular response first involves a pronounced vasodilatation, which serves to increase cerebral perfusion and maintain O_2 delivery with little change in the O_2 extraction fraction (O_2 uptake / O_2 delivery) (Fig. 10.33). With increasing hypoxia, the cerebral O_2 extraction fraction begins to increase until maximum O_2 extraction is attained. If hypoxia becomes even more severe, then cerebral O_2 consumption may decrease and anaerobic glycolysis may ensue with attendant lactic acidosis. Thus hypoxic vasodilatation may be viewed as an intrinsic extension of the autoregulatory mechanisms coupling cerebral O_2 supply and demand. As stated above, adenosine is a possible mediator of hypoxic cerebral vasodilatation because acute hypoxia increases cerebral adenosine in adult and newborn rats and pigs. In newborn puppies, however, acute hypoxia also increases vasodilator PGs. Furthermore, hypoxia may also directly affect vascular smooth muscle and endothelium of cerebral arteries. Clearly, hypoxia is a complex stimulus that elicits multiple mechanisms of cerebrovascular response in both neonates and adults.

Cerebral pathophysiology

Hypoxia-ischemia (HI) is a common insult during the perinatal period, in which a number of stimuli are combined. Initially there is hypoxia and hypercapnia (*asphyxia*), which increase cerebral perfusion and, at least in piglets, simultaneously increase adenosine and vasodilator PGs. During prolonged or severe insults, there often is relative hypoperfusion due to redistribution of CBF, or overt ischemia due to hypotension. During *asphyxia*, in all species studied, neonates show a preferential increase in perfusion to the brainstem relative to the telencephalon (cerebral hemispheres); this response may be related to reflex sympathetic cerebral vasoconstriction in the latter regions. This pattern is in marked contrast to adults where increases in CBF are more evenly distributed. This difference may improve neonatal resistance to asphyxia while increasing the risk of survival with hemispheric damage (*hypoxemic-ischemic encephalopathy*). In human newborns, the threshold rate of CBF below which irreversible ischemic damage is certain is lower than in adults and is between 10 and 15 ml/(min·100 g). In lambs cerebrovascular regulatory mechanisms will maintain O_2 delivery until a CaO_2 of below 1 mM is reached. In both newborn lambs and humans, the mechanisms responsible for matching cerebral O_2 supply and demand and of cerebral autoregulation may be reversibly impaired during, and for variable periods after, asphyxia. Thus during a severe HI insult, CBF may become 'pressure passive', i.e. directly related to blood pressure, explaining the critical importance of hypotension in promoting post-asphyxial cerebral damage.

Ischemia is a severe insult that precludes vascular exchange of gases, substrates and wastes. Thus even short-term *cerebral ischemia* is often associated with prolonged post-recovery increases in brain water content, inhibition of protein synthesis, disruption of cellular Ca^{2+} homeostasis, and depressed PG synthetic capacity, in addition to the suppression or death of cerebral neurons associated with asphyxia.

Intraventricular hemorrhage is a common neurological occurrence in most neonatal intensive care units, with a significant incidence of periventricular hemorrhage in infants less than 35 weeks of gestational age. The prevalence of periventricular hemorrhage is inversely related to body weight, with perhaps up to 60 percent of neonates weighing less than 1250 grams ultimately experiencing some degree of hemorrhage. Of particular interest is the tendency for intraventricular hemorrhage to occur predominantly in the germinal matrix region, a finding attributed to the relative immaturity of blood vessels located there. Although multiple factors, including cerebral venous infarction, altered coagulation characteristics, fluctuating blood pressure, acid–base imbalance, and deranged prostanoid metabolism, probably are involved, it is clear that once periventricular blood appears, most normal cerebrovascular regulatory mechanisms are compromised. Perivascular blood attenuates adrenergic vasoconstriction, endothelium-mediated relaxation, hypercapnic vasodilatation, autoregulation, and a host of other responses. Although treatment with phenobarbital can reduce O_2 demand and thereby perhaps stabilize and/or ameliorate the immediate injury, the primary goal for management of periventricular hemorrhage is to attempt to minimize the influences which predispose its occurrence.

Selected reading

Edvinsson L, Owman C, Sjoberg NO. Autonomic nerves, mast cells, and amine receptors in human brain vessels. A histochemical and pharmacological study. *Brain Res* 1976; **115**: 377.

Hayashi S, Park MK, Kuehl TJ. Relaxant and contractile responses to prostaglandins in premature, newborn and adult baboon cerebral arteries. *J Pharmacol Exp Ther* 1985; **233**: 628.

Leffler CW, Busija DW. Prostanoids in cortical subarachnoid cerebrospinal fluid and pial arterial diameter in newborn pigs. *Circ Res* 1985; **57**: 689.

Pearce WJ, Longo LD. Developmental aspects of endothelial function. *Semin Perinatol* 1991; **15**: 40.

Pryds O, Griesen G, Lou H, Friis-Hansen B. Vasoparalysis associated with brain damage in asphyxiated term infants. *J Pediatr* 1990; **117**: 119.

Volpe JJ. Neonatal intraventricular hemorrhage. *N Engl J Med* 1981; **304**: 886.

G2. The Pulmonary Circulation

S J Soifer, J R Fineman and M A Heymann

Morphological development

The morphological development of the pulmonary circulation affects the physiological changes that occur in the perinatal period. In the fetus and newborn, pulmonary arteries (regardless of their size) have a thicker medial smooth muscle coat relative to the external diameter of the artery than do similar size (external diameter) pulmonary arteries in the adult. This greater muscularity accounts, in part, for the higher pulmonary vascular resistance (PVR) and greater pulmonary vascular reactivity in the near-term fetus than in the adult. In the fetus, pulmonary arteries 20–50 μm in external diameter have the thickest medial smooth muscle coat. These are the resistance vessels. After birth and for the first few months of life, the medial smooth muscle coat of the arteries thins. These morphological changes account, in part, for the gradual decrease in PVR and pulmonary vascular reactivity over the first few months of life.

Small pulmonary arteries (20–50 μm in external diameter) can be identified by their relationship to airways (Fig. 10.34). Pre-acinar pulmonary arteries are proximal to, or course with, the terminal bronchioli, while intra-acinar pulmonary arteries course with the respiratory bronchioli and alveolar ducts, or are within the alveolar walls. In the late-gestation fetus, only about 50 percent of the pulmonary arteries associated with respiratory bronchioli are muscularized (either partially or completely). The pulmonary arteries within the alveolar wall are nonmuscularized. The partially and non-muscularized pulmonary arteries contain pericytes and intermediate cells (intermediate in position and structure between pericytes and smooth muscle cells), which are the precursors of smooth muscle cells. With advancing age after birth, these cells differentiate into smooth muscle cells, completely muscularizing the majority of the small pulmonary arteries within alveolar walls in the adult.

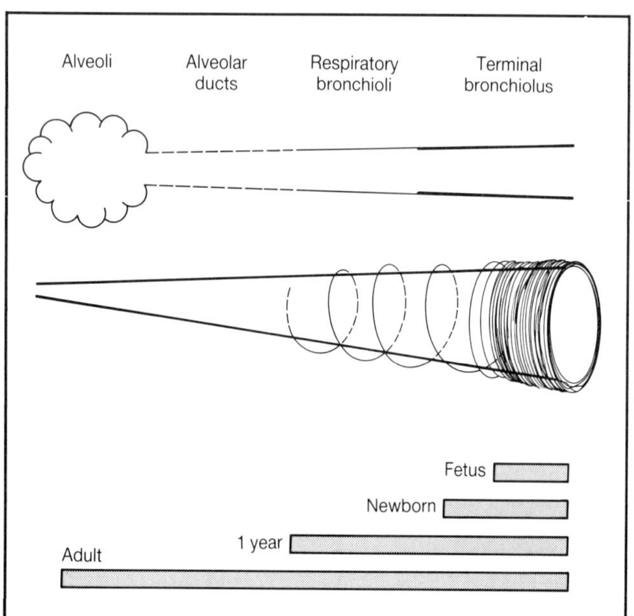

Fig. 10.34. Diagrammatic representation of smooth muscle distribution in normal human pulmonary vessels. (Adapted from Reid LM. *Chest* 1986; **89**: 279, with permission.)

Physiology

Fetal pulmonary circulation

In the fetus, because gas exchange occurs in the placenta, pulmonary blood flow is low, supplying only nutritional requirements for lung growth and performing some metabolic functions. In the mid-gestation fetal lamb (term is approximately 145–150 days), pulmonary blood flow is approximately 3–4 percent of the total combined left and right ventricular outputs of the heart (fetal cardiac output), while in the near-term fetal lamb, pulmonary blood flow is approximately 100 ml/100 g of lung weight per minute, or 8–10 percent of the fetal cardiac output [400–450 ml/(kg·min)]. Fetal pulmonary arterial pressure increases with advancing gestation. At term, mean pulmonary arterial pressure is about 50 mmHg (6.6 kPa), generally exceeding mean descending aortic pressure by 1–2 mmHg.

Determinants of pulmonary vascular resistance

PVR changes throughout gestation and after birth. PVR is related to several factors and can be estimated by applying the **resistance equation** and the **Poiseuille–Hagen relationship**. The resistance equation (the hydraulic equivalent of Ohm's law) states that the resistance to flow between two points along a tube equals the decrease in pressure between the two points divided by the flow. For the pulmonary vascular bed, where R_p = pulmonary vascular resistance and $\dot{Q}_p$ = pulmonary blood flow per min, the decrease in mean pressure is from the pulmonary artery (P_{pa}) to the pulmonary vein (P_{pv}):

$$R_p = \frac{(P_{pa} - P_{pv})}{\dot{Q}_p}$$

Pulmonary vascular resistance increases when pulmonary arterial or pulmonary venous pressure increase. The latter also causes an increase in pulmonary arterial pressure to maintain the driving pressure across the lungs. Similarly, PVR also increases when pulmonary blood flow decreases.

Other factors that affect PVR can be defined by applying a modification of the Poiseuille–Hagen relationship, which describes the resistance (R) to flow of a Newtonian fluid through a system of round, straight glass tubes of constant cross-sectional area:

$$R_p = \frac{8 \cdot l \cdot \eta}{\pi r^4}$$

where l is length of the system of vessels, r is the internal radius of the system of vessels, and η is the viscosity of the fluid. The assumption is that each pulmonary artery is a round, straight glass tube, and that the pulmonary circulation consists of many of these tubes. Changes in **viscosity** or radius affect PVR; increasing the viscosity of blood perfusing the lungs or decreasing the radius or **cross-sectional area** (πr^4) of the pulmonary vascular bed increases PVR. Early in gestation, PVR is much higher than in the newborn or the adult because there are fewer pulmonary arteries in the fetal lung, and therefore a decreased cross-sectional area. Secondary to the growth of new pulmonary arteries and the increase in cross-sectional area of the pulmonary vascular bed, PVR decreases during fetal life. However, near term, PVR is still much higher than after birth.

Differences between physical and biological systems may make these relationships inaccurate. First, blood is not a Newtonian fluid. The viscosity of blood is related to red-cell number, fibrinogen concentration, and red cell deformability. An increased **hematocrit** (secondary to fetal *hypoxemia*, *twin-to-twin blood transfusion* or *maternal-to-fetal blood transfusion*, or *delayed clamping of the umbilical cord*) will increase viscosity. PVR increases logarithmically (not linearly) when the hematocrit increases (Fig. 10.35). Second, blood flow through the pulmonary circulation is pulsatile, not laminar, and the small pulmonary arteries are branched, curved, and tapered, not smooth. In addition, the small pulmonary arteries are in parallel, and the radii of these arteries may differ in different lung zones. Although these factors tend to increase PVR, their actual effects on fetal PVR are minimal.

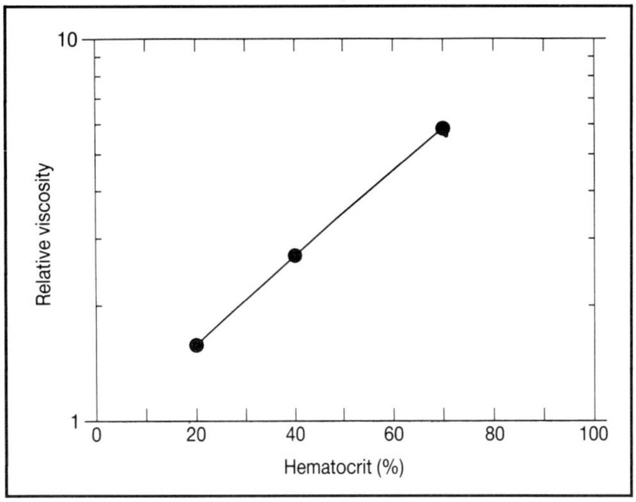

Fig. 10.35. Relationship of relative viscosity (blood viscosity relative to plasma viscosity) and hematocrit at a shear rate likely to be found in the pulmonary circulation.

Regulation of fetal pulmonary vascular resistance

Many factors, including mechanical effects, state of oxygenation, and the production of vasoactive substances, regulate the tone of the fetal pulmonary circulation (Fig. 10.36). In unventilated fetal lungs, fluid filling the alveolar space compresses the small pulmonary arteries, increasing the PVR. In addition, the high PVR is associated with the normally low O_2 tension in pulmonary and systemic arterial blood. In fetal lambs, the pulmonary

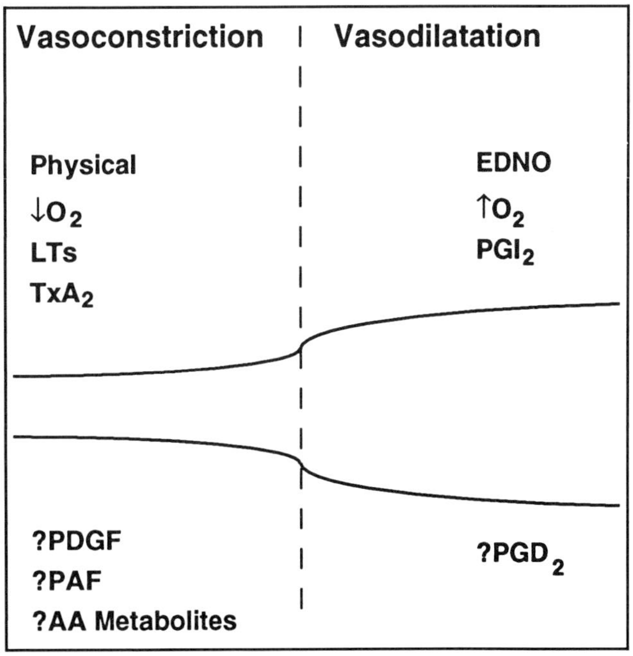

Fig. 10.36. Factors considered to be involved in the control of pulmonary vascular resistance and pulmonary blood flow during fetal life.

arterial blood PO_2 is 17–20 mmHg (2.6 kPa) and the femoral arterial PO_2 is 20–24 mmHg. Reducing PO_2 to similar values in newborn lambs after birth increases PVR. The mechanism of this hypoxia-induced pulmonary vasoconstriction is unknown. Similarly, fetal PVR is increased by decreasing fetal PO_2 either by maternal hypoxia or by compression of the umbilical cord, and is decreased by increasing PO_2 by maternal hyperoxia. Whether the low fetal PO_2 acts directly to constrict pulmonary vascular smooth muscle and increase PVR or indirectly through the release of vasoactive substances is not known. O_2-related changes in PVR are affected by pH; acidemia increases PVR and also accentuates hypoxic vasoconstrictor responses.

Metabolites of arachidonic acid may be actively involved in the control of fetal PVR either directly or as mediators of 'hypoxia-induced' pulmonary vasoconstriction. Leukotrienes (LTs) are synthesized from arachidonic acid by a 5′-lipoxygenase enzyme in pulmonary arterial tissue. LTC_4 and LTD_4 produce pulmonary vasoconstriction in newborn and adult animals. Inhibition of LT synthesis or action prevents hypoxia-induced pulmonary hypertension in older animals, and markedly decreases fetal PVR and increases fetal pulmonary blood flow similarly to ventilation at birth (see below). LTs have been isolated from tracheal fluid of near-term fetal lambs and from lung lavage fluid of newborns with the syndrome of *persistent pulmonary hypertension*. This suggests that LTs may contribute to maintaining the high PVR in the fetus. The pulmonary vasoconstriction produced by LTs is not mediated through secondary production of constrictor prostaglandins (PGs).

Other vasoactive substances may also play a role in maintaining the high PVR in the fetus. Thromboxane A_2, synthesized from arachidonic acid by the cyclooxygenase enzymes, is a vasoconstrictor, as is platelet activating factor. Both produce potent pulmonary vasoconstriction in newborn and adult animals. Several **growth factors**, particularly platelet derived growth factor (PDGF), which are involved in vascular smooth muscle growth and proliferation, also have vasoconstrictor effects. Whether any of these, or other compounds yet to be defined, contribute to maintaining the high PVR in the fetus is unknown.

In addition to the production of vasoconstrictors, the fetal pulmonary circulation actively and continuously produces vasodilating substances that modulate the degree of vasoconstriction under normal conditions and may play a more active role during periods of fetal stress. These substances are mainly endothelial derived and include prostacyclin (**PGI_2**) and endothelial derived relaxing factor (**EDRF**), now known to be nitric oxide (endothelial derived nitric oxide [EDNO]) (see below and also p. 469). In the fetus EDNO production is stimulated both by receptor-mediated mechanisms and by activation of ATP-dependent K^+ channels. The latter pathway is thought to be stimulated by stretch or by increased **shear forces** on the pulmonary vascular endothelium. PGI_2 production by endothelial cells can also be stimulated by increasing shear forces.

Endothelin is a potent vasoconstrictor in adults but produces pulmonary vasodilatation in both the fetal and neonatal lamb. Its role, if any, in normal pulmonary vasoregulation is undefined.

Changes in the pulmonary circulation at birth

After birth, with initiation of ventilation by the lungs, and the subsequent increase in pulmonary and systemic arterial blood O_2 tensions, PVR decreases and pulmonary blood flow increases by 8–10-fold to match systemic blood flow (300–400 ml/min per kg body weight). This large increase in pulmonary blood flow increases pulmonary venous return to the left atrium, increasing left atrial pressure. Then the valve of the foramen ovale closes, preventing any significant atrial right-to-left shunting of blood. In addition, the ductus arteriosus constricts and closes functionally within several hours after birth (see p. 526) effectively separating the pulmonary and systemic circulations. Mean pulmonary arterial pressure decreases, and by 24 hours of age, is approximately 50 percent of mean systemic arterial pressure. Adult values are reached 2–6 weeks after birth.

Regulation of postnatal pulmonary vascular resistance

Many factors cause the decrease in PVR with ventilation and oxygenation at birth (Fig. 10.37). **Physical expansion** or ventilation of the fetal lung without increasing O_2 tension increases fetal pulmonary blood flow and decreases PVR, but not to newborn values. A very small proportion of this decrease relates to replacement of fluid in the alveoli with gas, which allows unkinking of the

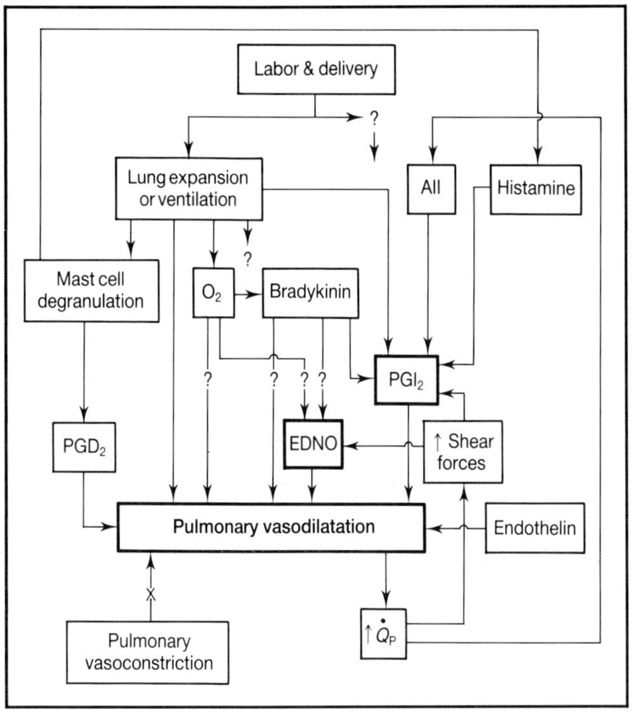

Fig. 10.37. Factors likely to be responsible for the changes of pulmonary vascular resistance and pulmonary blood flow with ventilation and oxygenation at birth.

small pulmonary arteries, and to the changes in alveolar surface tension, which exert a negative dilating pressure on the small pulmonary arteries, maintaining their patency. Physical expansion of the lung releases vasoactive substances such as PGI_2, which increases pulmonary blood flow and decreases PVR in the fetal goat and lamb. PGI_2 is synthesized from arachidonic acid (by cyclo-oxygenase enzymes) in fetal pulmonary arterial endothelial cells. There is also net production of PGI_2 by the lung with the initiation of ventilation at birth. In addition, inhibitors of PG synthesis (such as indomethacin) not only block PGI_2 production, but also attenuate the increase in pulmonary blood flow and decrease in PVR that occur with physical expansion of the fetal lung, although not the changes that occur with oxygenation. Therefore, PGI_2, or perhaps, but less likely, another metabolite of arachidonic acid, plays an important role in the increase in pulmonary blood flow and decrease in PVR that occur in association with the mechanical component (stretch) of ventilation at birth.

Other PGs may also play a role in these circulatory changes. PGE_2, produced in the fetal vasculature and the placenta, not only maintains patency of the ductus arteriosus, but also decreases PVR in fetal lambs and goats. The effects are nonspecific. PGD_2, produced and released by lung mast cells that are located near the small pulmonary arteries, is a selective pulmonary vasodilator in fetal and newborn goats and lambs, and a pulmonary vasoconstrictor in older animals. Because there is mast cell degranulation at birth, PGD_2 may play a role in the postnatal pulmonary circulatory changes.

Ventilation of fetal lungs with air or O_2 to increase O_2 tension increases pulmonary blood flow and decreases PVR to newborn levels. As described above, ventilation of the fetus without **oxygenation** produces partial pulmonary vasodilatation, while ventilation with oxygenation produces complete pulmonary vasodilatation. The increase in alveolar or arterial O_2 tension may decrease PVR either directly by dilating the small pulmonary arteries, or indirectly by stimulating the production of vasodilator substances. **Bradykinin**, a potent pulmonary vasodilator, is produced by the fetal lung during O_2 ventilation and during exposure of pregnant ewes to hyperbaric oxygenation. Bradykinin stimulates PGI_2 production, which would enhance vasodilatation. Increased oxygenation is also a direct stimulus for PGI_2 production, as is **angiotensin II**, which increases markedly in concentration at birth, indicating a complex interaction between various vasodilating stimuli. In addition, bradykinin stimulates (B_1-receptor-mediated) the production of EDRF, specifically endothelium derived nitric oxide (**EDNO**) by endothelial cells. EDNO is synthesized from L-arginine (see p. 469). Once synthesized, EDNO diffuses into vascular smooth muscle cells, stimulates guanylyl cyclase, and increases the concentration of cyclic 3′,5′-guanosine monophosphate (cGMP), which initiates a cascade that results in smooth muscle relaxation and vasodilatation. In fetal lambs, inhibition of EDNO synthesis by N^{ω}-nitro-L-arginine, a competitive inhibitor of L-arginine, increases PVR and attenuates the subsequent increase in pulmonary blood flow and decrease in PVR produced when the same lambs are ventilated with O_2. Therefore, there are at least two components to the decrease in PVR with the initiation of ventilation and oxygenation. First, there is partial pulmonary vasodilatation caused by physical expansion of the lung and the production of prostaglandins (PGI_2 and PGD_2). This probably is independent of fetal oxygenation, and results in a modest increase in pulmonary blood flow and decrease in PVR. Next, there is a further maximal pulmonary vasodilatation associated with fetal oxygenation, which is not necessarily dependent on prostaglandin production. This results in an increase in pulmonary blood flow and decrease in PVR to newborn values. This latter pulmonary vasodilatation is likely caused by the synthesis of EDNO, although the exact stimulus or stimuli for EDNO production are not yet defined. Both components are necessary for the successful transition to extrauterine life. An additional mechanism by which vasodilatation occurs relates to the stimulation by increased shear forces of endothelial cells to produce both EDNO and PGI_2. It is possible that after the initial fall in PVR, due to another mechanism, this particular mechanism acts to maintain pulmonary vasodilatation.

Control of the perinatal pulmonary circulation, therefore, probably reflects a balance between factors producing pulmonary vasoconstriction (low O_2, LTs, and other vasoconstricting substances) and those producing pulmonary vasodilatation (high O_2, PGI_2, EDNO, and other vasodilating substances). The dramatic increase in pulmonary blood flow with the initiation of ventilation and oxygenation at birth reflects a shift from active pulmonary vasoconstriction in the fetus to active pulmonary vasodilatation in the newborn.

Metabolic function

Pulmonary vascular endothelium is capable of producing (e.g. PGI_2, EDNO, bradykinin, angiotensin II) and removing from the circulation (e.g. catecholamines, bradykinin, PGE_2) many different substances. This activity is present in the fetus and changes at the time of transition to air breathing.

Concomitant with the increasing metabolic activity of the fetal lung (particularly increasing antioxidant enzyme and surfactant phospholipid synthesis) in the latter weeks of gestation, resting pulmonary blood flow increases (from about 4 percent of combined ventricular output to about 8 percent). After birth, and associated with the dramatic increase in pulmonary blood flow, pulmonary vascular metabolic capacity also increases markedly, to a large extent due to a significant increase in pulmonary vascular endothelial functional surface area. Angiotensin I conversion to angiotensin II, by the endothelial enzyme angiotensin converting enzyme (ACE), increases and the same enzyme is responsible for the metabolic breakdown of the vasoactive peptide bradykinin. Metabolic removal of PGE_2 also increases, and this is an important component of the transition as PGE_2 is responsible for ductus arteriosus patency (see p. 526).

Failure of pulmonary vascular resistance to decrease at birth

In a number of clinical conditions (e.g. *respiratory distress syndrome*, *meconium aspiration*, or *sepsis*), PVR does not decrease normally at birth, which may result in persistent pulmonary hypertension, right-to-left shunting of blood through the foramen ovale, and/or patent ductus arteriosus and hypoxemia. The *syndrome of persistent pulmonary hypertension of the newborn* accounts for approximately 1 percent of all admissions to newborn intensive care units. Treatment is supportive, consisting of administration of supplemental O_2, mechanical hyperventilation, correction of metabolic abnormalities, infusion of nonspecific vasodilators to lower pulmonary arterial pressure, and infusion of cardiotonic drugs to improve cardiac function. More recently, extracorporeal membrane oxygenation (ECMO) has been used. The clinical course is variable, and the mortality rate is high.

The pathophysiological mechanisms preventing the normal pulmonary vasodilatation and fall in PVR with ventilation and oxygenation at birth are not known. Morphological abnormalities are present, the thickness of the medial smooth muscle coat of the small pulmonary arteries is increased, and this muscle extends to normally nonmuscularized arteries in infants who die with persistent pulmonary hypertension syndrome. The underlying mechanisms (such as alterations in smooth muscle growth-stimulating or growth-inhibiting factors) producing these changes are unknown. These structural changes take time to develop, indicating that prolonged *in utero* events have altered the pulmonary circulation. One such phenomenon that is considered a possible mechanism is chronic partial constriction of the ductus arteriosus. In addition to structural changes there may be functional alterations as well. There may be increased concentrations of or responsiveness to vasoconstricting substances (e.g. LTC_4, LTD_4, and thromboxane A_2) or decreased concentrations of or responsiveness to vasodilating substances (PGI_2, PGD_2, EDNO, and increased O_2 tension). A better understanding of the mechanisms that control PVR in the perinatal period will lead to improved treatment of these infants.

Selected reading

Heymann MA, Soifer SJ. Control of the fetal and neonatal pulmonary circulation. In Weir EK, Reeves JT, eds. *Pulmonary vascular physiology and pathophysiology*. New York: Marcel Dekker, Inc., 1989: 33.

Iwamoto HS, Teitel D, Rudolph AM. Effects of birth-related events on blood flow distribution. *Pediatr Res* 1987; **22**: 634.

Leffler CW, Hessler JR, Green RS. The onset of breathing at birth stimulates pulmonary vascular prostacyclin synthesis. *Pediatr Res* 1984; **18**: 938.

Moore P, Velvis H, Fineman JR, Soifer SJ, Heymann MA. EDRF inhibition attenuates the increase in pulmonary blood flow due to oxygen ventilation in fetal lambs. *J Appl Physiol* 1992; **73**: 2151.

Velvis H, Moore P, Heymann MA. Prostaglandin inhibition prevents the fall in pulmonary vascular resistance due to rhythmic distension of the lungs in fetal lambs. *Pediatr Res* 1991; **30**: 62.

G3. Ductus Arteriosus

R I Clyman

Regulation of ductus arteriosus patency

The ductus arteriosus represents a persistence of the terminal portion of the left pulmonary or sixth branchial arch. More muscular than the elastic pulmonary artery and aorta at either end, the ductus arteriosus also has a looser structure with increased amounts of hyaluronic acid in the muscle media. During fetal life, it serves to divert blood away from the fluid-filled, nonventilating lungs towards the descending aorta and placenta.

Although it was commonly believed that the ductus arteriosus was a relatively passive structure in the fetus, it is now obvious that the relative patency of the ductus arteriosus, even during fetal life, is regulated by both dilating and contracting factors. Evidence that prostaglandins (PGs) participate in maintaining patency of the ductus arteriosus *in utero* is based on their ability to relax the constricted ductus arteriosus and the ability of inhibitors of PG synthesis to constrict the ductus arteriosus both *in vitro* and *in vivo*. What makes the ductus arteriosus unique among blood vessels is its extraordinary sensitivity to the dilating action of PGE_2.

Since the initial studies of Kennedy and Clark in 1942, many investigators have demonstrated that O_2 is responsible for constricting the ductus arteriosus after birth. However, the biochemical basis for the O_2 response has never been fully explained. Recently attention has focused on cytochrome P450-mediated pathways, but no active metabolites have been identified to date. Although neural and hormonal factors (such as catecholamines, acetylcholine, histamine, bradykinin, 5-hydroxytryptamine) produce contractile responses of the ductus arteriosus *in vitro*, and possibly contribute to ductus arteriosus closure under physiological conditions, they do not mediate O_2-induced vessel closure. It is interesting to note that while norepinephrine-containing nerve terminals normally are found throughout the muscle layer of the human fetal ductus arteriosus, ductus arteriosus tissue obtained from children (aged 2 months to 6 years) who had a *patent ductus arteriosus* (PDA) requiring ligation showed no innervation of the media; perhaps this lack of innervation plays a role in persistent patency.

O_2 has a greater constrictor effect on the ductus arteriosus from older than from younger fetuses. Studies in fetal animals indicate that the ability of the ductus arteriosus to achieve maximal contraction is similar in fetuses at 0.7 gestation and in those at full term; therefore, the lesser responsiveness of the ductus arteriosus to O_2 in the moderately immature fetus (greater than 0.7 gestation) is not due to lack of muscular development. The increased contractile response of the mature ductus arteriosus to O_2 is due to a developmental alteration in the sensitivity of the vessel to locally produced PGs: ductus arteriosus smooth muscle from preterm animals is more sensitive to the dilating action of PGE_2 than that from animals near term. On the other hand, the ductus arteriosus from animals less than 0.7 gestation also has decreased muscular development and diminished contractile capacity, in addition to increased sensitivity to dilator PGs. **These factors probably account for the higher incidence of *persistent patent ductus arteriosus* (*PDA*) in preterm newborns.** The exact site of PGE_2 production responsible for ductus arteriosus regulation *in vivo* is currently unclear, but the placenta is one probable source. Isolated rings of ductus arteriosus produce very little PGE_2 at the low ambient O_2 tensions found in the fetus; much more PGE_2 is produced at high

O_2 tensions. Thus it is likely that circulating PGE_2 controls the ductus arteriosus *in utero*. Removal of the placenta and the increased lung circulation after birth reduce circulating PGE_2 concentrations and contribute significantly to ductus arteriosus closure. However, newborn lambs delivered prematurely have decreased pulmonary metabolism of PGE_2, resulting in elevated circulating concentrations. **Thus circulating concentrations of PGE_2 may play a significant role in *PDA* in the premature, but only during the first hours after birth.** On the other hand, after birth, when arterial O_2 tension rises, the ductus arteriosus itself is capable of producing increased quantities of PGE_2. There is some evidence to suggest that PGE_2 production by the ductus arteriosus after delivery may be stimulated by reactive O_2 metabolites. The factors that alter the sensitivity of the ductus arteriosus to locally produced PGE_2 are unknown. Elevated cortisol concentrations in the fetus have been found to decrease the sensitivity of the ductus arteriosus to PGE_2; consistent with these findings, **prenatal administration of glucocorticoids causes a significant reduction in the incidence of *PDA* in premature human infants and animals. The normal increase in endogenous cortisol, which occurs near the end of gestation, probably influences ductus arteriosus development in a manner similar to these experiments, which used exogenously administered steroids.**

In normal, full-term animals, loss of responsiveness to PGE_2 shortly after birth prevents the ductus arteriosus from reopening once it has constricted. Loss of ductus arteriosus responsiveness is directly related to the degree of prior ductus arteriosus constriction. Because luminal blood flow is the major source of ductus arteriosus smooth muscle nutrition, the generalized loss of vessel responsiveness may be due to ischemic damage that occurs when the ductus arteriosus constricts. In contrast to full-term infants, premature infants are more likely to have a ductus arteriosus that continues to dilate in response to PGE_2 after postnatal constriction; consequently, once the ductus arteriosus has closed (either spontaneously or as a result of PG synthesis inhibition by indomethacin administration), it may reopen at a later date, with recurrence of the left-to-right shunt. The incidence of ductus arteriosus reopening is inversely related to birth weight: 33 percent of infants with birth weights <1000 g reopened their ductus arteriosus after initial closure while only 8 percent of infants with birth weights >1500 g reopened their ductus arteriosus. **Premature animals' persistent responsiveness to PGE_2 after ductus arteriosus constriction may account for the high rate of ductus arteriosus reopening observed in preterm infants after successful initial indomethacin-induced closure.** Of those infants whose ductus arteriosus reopens after initial closure, 80 percent apparently remain responsive to indomethacin. The factors that maintain ductus arteriosus responsiveness to PGE_2 in immature animals after postnatal constriction are unknown. Ductus arteriosus smooth muscle cells from premature animals appear to have a lower rate of O_2 consumption than those from animals near term. This might be due to the low circulating concentrations of thyroid hormones in immature fetuses and neonates. If O_2 consumption is less in the preterm ductus arteriosus, then the ductus arteriosus from immature fetuses might be more resistant to ischemic damage during constriction. Consistent with this hypothesis, premature infants with low concentrations of thyroid hormones have an increased incidence of PDA compared with those with normal thyroid hormone concentrations. Conversely, when fetal lambs were infused with triiodothyronine (T_3) *in utero* and subsequently delivered prematurely, there was a generalized loss of ductus arteriosus responsiveness after the ductus arteriosus constricted at birth. The loss of ductus arteriosus responsiveness during postnatal constriction in the T_3-infused premature lambs was similar to that found in full-term lambs. In contrast, the ductus arteriosus in premature control lambs was still responsive to vasoactive agonists after postnatal constriction. Therefore, increases in thyroid hormone concentrations, which occur with advancing gestation, may play a role in preventing ductus arteriosus reopening once it has constricted after birth.

In full-term infants, once the ductus arteriosus constricts, rapid histological changes ultimately lead to obliteration of the vessel's lumen and prevent reopening at a later date. Before birth, there is intimal thickening and fragmentation of the internal elastic lamina with advancing gestation. This intimal thickening appears to be due to extensive constriction and shortening of the ductus arteriosus as well as to migration of smooth muscle cells from the media into the intima, and not due to cellular proliferation. During postnatal closure of the ductus arteriosus, the intima increases in size and forms intimal mounds that partially occlude the lumen. Shortly after birth, cells in the inner part of the media appear to disintegrate. Over the next number of weeks the lumen is obliterated by the increasing size of the intimal mounds, which contain more elastic tissue and increasing amounts of collagen. The muscle fibers of the media ultimately atrophy and are replaced by elastic and connective tissue. Anatomical closure is complete one to several months after birth.

Failure of the normal anatomical remodeling that occurs in full-term neonates also plays a role in late ductus arteriosus reopening. In the preterm infant with a PDA, the vessel is fetal in appearance or has only diminished intimal mounds with an intact subendothelial internal elastic lamina and absence of cytolytic necrosis.

Hemodynamic and pulmonary alterations

The pathophysiological consequences of a PDA depend both on the magnitude of left-to-right shunt through the ductus arteriosus and on cardiac and pulmonary responses to the shunt. There are important differences between immature and mature infants in the heart's ability to handle a volume load (see p. 499). Before term, the myocardium has more water and less contractile mass. Therefore, in the immature fetus the ventricles are less distensible than at term and also generate less force per gram of myocardium (even though they have the same ability to generate force per sarcomere as those in more mature infants). The relative lack of left ventricular distensibility in immature infants is more a function of the ventricle's tissue constituents than of poor muscle function. As a result, left ventricular distension secondary to a large left-to-right PDA shunt may produce a higher left ventricular end-diastolic pressure at smaller ventricular volumes in the immature than in the mature infant. Elevations in left ventricular end-diastolic pressures, which increase pulmonary venous pressures and cause pulmonary congestion, occur with smaller left-to-right shunts in immature than mature infants. In addition several studies have demonstrated that immature infants have less cardiac sympathetic innervation.

Studies in preterm lambs with a patent ductus arteriosus have shown that the lambs are able to increase left ventricular output to maintain 'effective' systemic blood flow, with left-to-right shunts less than 40–50 percent of left ventricular output. With shunts greater than 50 percent of left ventricular output, 'effective' systemic blood flow falls despite an increase in left ventricular output. The increase in left ventricular output is accomplished not by an increase in heart rate, but by an increase in stroke volume. Stroke volume increases primarily as a result of the simultaneous decrease in afterload resistance on the heart and the increase in left ventricular preload. Despite the ability of the left ventricle to increase its output with increasing amounts of ductus arteriosus shunt, blood flow distribution is significantly rearranged. This redistribution of systemic blood flow occurs even with small shunts. Blood flow to the skin, bone, and skeletal muscle is most likely to be affected by left-to-right ductal shunts; the next most likely organs to be affected are the gastrointestinal tract and the kidneys. These organs receive decreased blood flow due to a combination of decreased perfusion pressure (related to a drop in diastolic pressure) and localized vasoconstriction. These organs may experience significant hypoperfusion before there are any signs of left ventricular compromise.

Similarly, in preterm human infants left ventricular output is increased in the presence of a left-to-right ductus arteriosus shunt and falls significantly after closure of the ductus arteriosus. As has been observed in preterm lambs, human preterm infants increase their left ventricular output predominantly by an increase in stroke volume, not by an increase in heart rate. The increase in left ventricular output seen in the presence of PDA does not provide an increase in effective systemic blood flow; femoral blood flow velocity is low prior to closure of the PDA and returns to normal after closure.

Very-low-birth-weight infants with a PDA have been found to have increased flow in the ascending aorta (with increased forearm blood flow) and decreased flow in the descending aorta, with an associated metabolic acidosis. **Such alterations in cardiac output distribution have been implicated in the high incidence of intracranial hemorrhage and necrotizing enterocolitis associated with PDA.** Significant aortic backflow has been observed over large distances in some infants with PDA, consistent with a 'diastolic steal' of blood from the aorta and abdominal organs to the pulmonary artery. The continuous distension of the pulmonary vessels during diastole may be important in the production of pulmonary vascular disease and bronchopulmonary dysplasia.

The decreased ability of the preterm infant to maintain active pulmonary vasoconstriction may be responsible in part for the earlier presentation of a 'large' left-to-right PDA shunt in the most immature infants. Therapeutic maneuvers (e.g. surfactant replacement) that lead to decreased pulmonary vascular resistance can exacerbate responsible for the observed decrease in fetal blood volume during hypoxemia.

The mechanism whereby hypoxemia increases resistance in the umbilical veins is mediated at least in part by catecholamines. Neural reflexes are not likely to be involved because, at least in the human, the umbilical veins have no autonomic innervation. Several vasoactive hormones, including norepinephrine, epinephrine, vasopressin, and angiotensin II, constrict the umbilical vein *in vitro*. However, in fetal lambs receiving these same vasoactive hormones by a constant infusion, resistance in the umbilical veins was increased only by catecholamines (norepinephrine and epinephrine).

Role of hepatic microcirculation and ductus venosus

The other major resistance to umbilical venous return is actually a combined resistance of two alternate pathways, the ductus venosus and liver. As a unit, the ductus venosus and liver are anatomically arranged as circulations in parallel; resistance changes in one may be offset by reciprocal changes in the other so that the combined resistance does not change. In fact, this is seen in response to many types of fetal stress; for example, fetal hypoxemia increases the vascular resistance of the liver. However, this increase is offset by a reciprocal decrease in ductus venosus resistance. Umbilical venous return is thus redistributed so that less umbilical venous blood flows through the liver, and more through the ductus venosus. While neither ductus venosus nor liver is a major regulator of the overall resistance to umbilical venous return, redistribution of blood between these parallel pathways may be an important fetal adaptation to stress.

A sphincter is generally assumed to be present in the ductus venosus at its origin from the portal sinus; it apparently has no resting autonomic nervous constrictor tone because atropine and phentolamine do not alter ductus venosus blood flow. In contrast, norepinephrine or epinephrine increase fetal hepatic vascular resistance by about 50 percent, leading to redistribution of umbilical venous return as described above. Conditions that decrease umbilical–placental blood flow, e.g. umbilical cord compression and fetal hemorrhage, most strikingly increase shunting of umbilical venous return through the ductus venosus.

Like the increased resistance of the umbilical veins during hypoxemia, the increased shunting of umbilical venous return through the ductus venosus may be an important fetal circulatory adaptation during conditions of stress such as hypoxemia, umbilical cord compression, or fetal hemorrhage. Ductus venosus blood flow is derived almost exclusively from umbilical venous return; only 5–10 percent is derived from portal venous return. Therefore, blood passing through the ductus venosus has a high glucose concentration and a high O_2 content. Ductus venosus-derived blood is preferentially distributed to upper body organs, including the brain and heart. During hypoxemia, umbilical cord compression, hemorrhage, and catecholamine infusion, ductus venosus-derived blood flow to the brain and heart increases, in part because of the increase in ductus venosus blood flow. The redistribution of blood flow between the ductus venosus and liver therefore has been postulated to help maintain O_2 and substrate delivery to the most vital organs during fetal stress.

Many studies have documented this increase in ductus venosus blood flow during stress in fetal lambs. However, some species such as the horse, pig, and guinea-pig lack a ductus venosus, which calls into question the role of the ductus venosus as an essential factor to establish preferential distribution of umbilical venous return to the upper body. The late-gestation fetal pig, for example, lacks a ductus venosus but instead has intrahepatic vascular channels over 100 μm in diameter in both lobes of the liver; these allow umbilical venous return to bypass the hepatic sinusoids. Nevertheless, in the fetal pig as in the fetal lamb, upper body arterial O_2 saturation consistently exceeds lower body arterial O_2 saturations during normoxemia and hypoxemia. Moreover, fetal lambs in which a balloon-tip catheter was used to occlude the ductus venosus during both normoxic and hypoxic conditions showed that neither the characteristic patterns of fetal organ blood flows nor O_2 delivery were changed by prolonged occlusion of the ductus venosus. Therefore, as an anatomical shunt, the ductus venosus may not be crucial to the maintenance of inferior vena caval streaming patterns that preferentially distribute umbilical venous return to the upper body.

Because the fetal liver contains 10–15 percent of the total fetal blood volume, alterations in the distribution of umbilical venous return, rather than inferior vena caval streaming patterns, may regulate fetal hepatic and total body blood volume. Because the fetal liver is extremely compliant, small changes in intrahepatic pressure lead to large changes in volume. Increasing the quantity of blood shunted through the ductus venosus would decrease liver volume and increase fetal circulating blood volume. This is supported by the observation that stimuli that decrease fetal intravascular volume, e.g. hemorrhage or umbilical cord compression, cause the most dramatic increases in the proportion of blood shunted away from the liver and through the ductus venosus. This results in a sort of autotransfusion of blood out of the liver and into the circulation. As described above, catecholamines appear to play an integral part in control of this redistribution through their constriction of the hepatic microvasculature.

A role for prostaglandins in the control of the distribution of umbilical venous return between the liver and ductus venosus has been postulated. While the vascular resistance of both ductus venosus and liver increases with indomethacin and decreases with prostaglandin E_1, both are similarly affected so that the relative distribution of blood flow between the two does not change. Therefore, perhaps prostaglandins play a role in maintaining a chronic low resting resistance to umbilical venous return.

It is possible that the umbilical–placental circulation is maximally dilated under normal conditions, including maximal vasodilation of the umbilical veins, ductus venosus, and liver, resulting in minimal resistance to umbilical venous return. This hypothesis was tested with four different vasodilating agents—prostacyclin, adenosine, forskolin, and nitroglycerin—each with a different mechanism of action. Both prostacyclin and adenosine reduced total umbilical–placental blood flow, in part due to systemic hypotension. This decrease in umbilical–placental blood flow was accompanied by an increase in venous resistance with adenosine, but there was no change with prostacyclin. Second, both forskolin and nitroglycerin maintained umbilical–placental blood flow. Forskolin was the only agent to decrease significantly the venous resistance. Therefore, while three of these vasodilators had no direct effect on resistance in the umbilical veins, the response to forskolin indicates at least a small degree of vasodilatory reserve.

Postnatal closure

The ductus venosus closes after birth as the postnatal circulatory pattern is established. While the precise mechanism regulating its closure is not known, several possibilities have been suggested, including loss of a chronic prostaglandin effect, local hypoxemia with loss of the highly oxygenated umbilical venous return, and passive pressure changes with loss of the high volume of blood returning to the portal sinus. There have been anecdotal reports of pharmacological reopening of the ductus venosus with prostaglandin E_1 in a child with total anomalous pulmonary venous return below the diaphragm, and experimentally in fetal lambs. However, there are also reports of prolonged postnatal patency of the ductus venosus in the absence of pharmacological manipulation; therefore, the importance of the findings is not known.

Selected reading

Edelstone DI. Regulation of blood flow through the ductus venosus. *J Dev Physiol* 1980; **2**: 219.

Edelstone DI, Rudolph AM. Preferential streaming of ductus venosus blood to the brain and heart in fetal lambs. *Am J Physiol* 1979; **237**: H724.

Edelstone DI, Rudolph AM, Heymann MA. Effects of hypoxemia and decreasing umbilical blood flow on liver and ductus venosus blood flows in fetal lambs. *Am J Physiol* 1980; **238**: H656.

Paulick RP, Meyers RL, Rudolph CD, Rudolph AM. Venous responses to hypoxemia in the fetal lamb. *J Dev Physiol* 1990; **14**: 81.

Paulick RP, Meyers RL, Rudolph AM. Vascular responses of the umbilical-placental circulation to vasodilators in fetal lambs. *Am J Physiol* 1991; **261**: H9.

Paulick RP, Meyers RL, Rudolph CD, Rudolph AM. Umbilical and hepatic venous responses to circulating vasoconstrictive hormones in fetal lamb. *Am J Physiol* 1991; **260**: H1205.

Silver M, Barnes RJ, Fowden AL, Comline RS. Preferential oxygen supply to the brain and upper body in the fetal pig. *Adv Exp Med Biol* 1988; **222**: 683.

H. CIRCULATORY CHANGES DURING GESTATION

H1. Maternal Cardiovascular Alterations during Pregnancy

R R Magness and C R Rosenfeld

Major changes occur in the maternal circulation during advancing gestation. These include changes in the systemic as well as the uteroplacental vascular beds; the changes in both are interdependent. The 'peripheral or systemic cardiovascular system' is defined collectively to include all vascular beds other than the uteroplacental.

Uteroplacental vascular changes in pregnancy

Changes in the uterine vascular bed during normal gestation must be evaluated with regard to both the uterus as a single unique vascular bed, and its component vascular beds, the endometrium, myometrium, and placenta. Most investigative work has been in the ewe, much of which correlates with human pregnancy when gestational age-adjusted; term pregnancy in the ewe is 145 days.

Total uteroplacental perfusion

Total uterine blood flow rises 20–80-fold above non-pregnant values during the course of normal gestation in women and sheep; even larger increases occur in multifetal gestations. This rise in uteroplacental perfusion accounts for 10–20 percent of cardiac output at term in the sheep, dog, guinea-pig, rhesus monkey, rabbit, and human. Because blood flow to any organ is controlled by relative changes in both vascular resistance and perfusion pressure (i.e. mean arterial blood pressure), it is important to note that this dramatic increase in blood flow occurs while perfusion pressure falls, although slightly (see below). Thus there are substantial decreases in uterine vascular resistance, which can be estimated using the equation:

$$\text{Uterine vascular resistance} = \frac{\text{Mean arterial pressure}}{\text{Uterine blood flow}}$$

During ovine pregnancy, uterine vascular resistance decreases from about 5 mmHg/(min·ml) in nonpregnant ewes to 0.2 mmHg/(min·ml) by 60–100 days and to 0.1 mmHg/(min·ml) by 130–140 days of gestation, providing direct evidence of profound vasodilatation.

The increase in total uterine perfusion may be explained by two phenomena: initially, growth of existing vascular beds and development of the placental vascular bed, and subsequently, vasodilatation of each of these vascular beds. Vascular growth is reflected by an increase in capillary density relative to tissue mass and is seen as an increase in total organ blood flow. Vasodilatation is reflected by total blood flow per gram of tissue. These patterns of change in total uterine weight, uterine blood flow, and blood flow per gram of tissue during ovine pregnancy are illustrated in Fig. 10.39. Total uterine weight is the sum of metabolically active tissues, i.e. endometrium, myometrium, placenta, fetal membranes, and fetus. Prior to about 50 days of gestation (**first trimester**) there are relatively small increases in uterine weight (Fig. 10.39a). Thereafter weight increases rapidly, continuing in a logarithmic manner throughout the remainder of gestation. This increase during the last two trimesters reflects growth and development of not only the uterine tissues and placenta, but also the fetus, and is accompanied by large increases in blood flow (Fig. 10.39b). The pattern of increase in uterine blood flow suggests two periods of rapid change, the first between 40 and 70 days of gestation and the second from 120 days gestation to term (**third trimester**). The first is associated with placentation (as discussed later), and the second with fetal growth. When these changes in blood flow are expressed per gram of tissue (Fig. 10.39c), thereby taking into account both tissue mass and growth as well as blood flow, an inverse pattern is observed, i.e. there are extremely high blood flows in the first 50 days of pregnancy (early implantation/attachment and initiation of placentation), followed by a gradual fall until 90–100 days, after which blood flow remains relatively

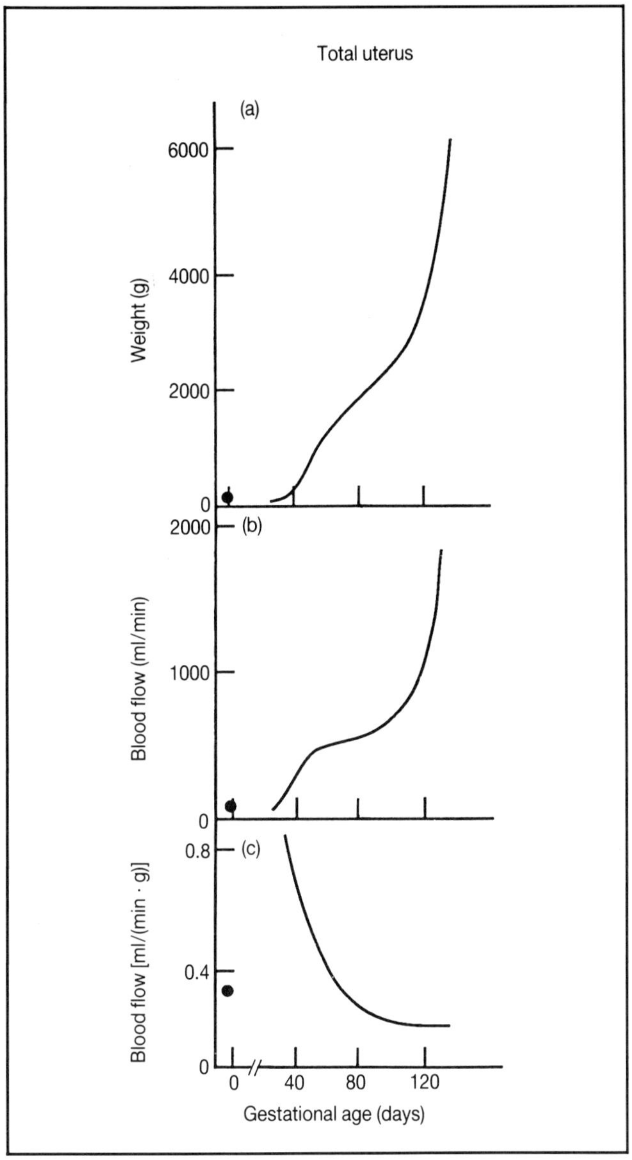

Fig. 10.39. Changes in uterine weight (a), blood flow (b), and blood flow per gram of total uterine weight (c) during ovine gestation. Total uterine weight is defined in the text. ● nonpregnant. (From Rosenfeld CR, Morris FH, *et al. Gynecol Invest* 1974; **5**: 252 with permission of Karger, Basel.)

unchanged. This suggests that during the first two trimesters, the increase in uterine weight is substantially greater than the increase in total uterine blood flow, while thereafter increases in tissue weight and blood flow are proportionate, demonstrating that vasodilatation is occurring.

The high rate of perfusion observed early in gestation may reflect the high metabolic needs of the uterine tissues and early embryo, increased production of steroid hormones (estrogen and progesterone) necessary for the maintenance of pregnancy, or a combination of these factors. Therefore, these blood flow patterns reflect the need for increased uterine O_2 and substrate delivery.

Distribution of uterine blood flow

Changes in distribution of blood flow to individual uterine tissues during ovine pregnancy can be measured with the radiolabeled microsphere technique (Fig. 10.40). In nonpregnant sheep, uterine blood flow is evenly distributed among the endometrium, myometrium, and caruncles (specialized sites for implantation/placentation in the sheep). At 40–50 days of gestation, before placentation is complete, the endometrium receives more than 60 percent of total uterine blood flow, while the remaining blood flow is evenly distributed between myometrium and hypertrophied caruncles (which subsequently become the maternal portion of the placentome). This suggests that significant functional and metabolic alterations occur in the endometrium and the caruncles early in gestation, which may be important in the maintenance of early pregnancy. Between 60 and 80 days of gestation (**second trimester**), when placentation is

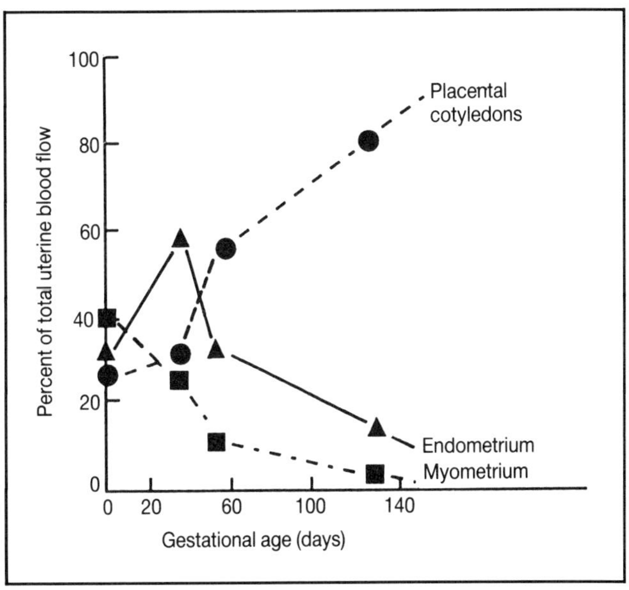

Fig. 10.40. Distribution of uterine blood flow during ovine pregnancy; term = 145 days. (From Rosenfeld CR. *Semin Perinatol* 1984; **8**: 42, with permission of WB Saunders Co.)

being completed, there is a dramatic redistribution of uterine blood flow, and by 80 days placental blood flow accounts for 60 percent, endometrial flow 30 percent, and myometrial flow 10 percent. Thereafter, the proportion to the placentome continues to increase, with commensurate decreases to endometrium and myometrium, until at term, placental blood flow accounts for 80–85 percent, endometrium 10 percent and myometrium 5 percent. This redistribution toward placental blood flow likely reflects the needs of both placental and fetal growth and demonstrates that anatomically and physiologically, the placenta is the key link between the maternal and fetal circulations and that changes in total uterine blood flow late in gestation (Fig. 10.39) primarily reflect alterations in the placental vascular bed.

When the changes in endometrial (Fig. 10.41) and myometrial (Fig. 10.42) blood flow are examined throughout gestation, the patterns are similar for weight and blood flow per gram of tissue, but the magnitudes differ. The phases of blood flow increase likely reflect placental development and the expression of fetal/placental factors, such as estrogen and growth-promoting peptides, which are necessary for the observed increases in tissue blood flow and growth. Because of the disproportionate increase in tissue growth versus blood flow in both the endometrium and myometrium, there are substantial decreases in blood flow per gram of tissue in both tissues as pregnancy progresses until the very end of gestation, when a relatively small increase is seen. The extremely high endometrial blood flow prior to 40–50 days of gestation (Fig. 10.41c), probably affected by embryonic and/or ovarian steroid hormones, most likely reflects the need to perfuse this tissue highly so that placentation and implantation can occur.

Patterns of change in weight and blood flow differ in the placentomes (Fig. 10.43). In the sheep, placental growth begins around 60 days and is complete by 80–90 days of gestation; thereafter, placental weight remains relatively unchanged or even decreases slightly in the last 1–2 weeks of gestation. Similar patterns have been reported for placental DNA content and for morphometric analysis of maternal placental stromal cells. The pattern of change for placental blood flow (Fig. 10.43b) is similar to that observed for the uterus as a whole, i.e. there is a biphasic pattern. When placental growth and blood flow are combined and expressed in terms of blood flow per gram of tissue (Fig. 10.43c), the pattern is different from that observed for the total uterus, endometrium, and myometrium. Rather than a decrease in blood flow with only a minor rise at term, there is a dramatic rise that continues to term. The first increase at 60–90 days (second trimester) represents development and growth of the placental vascular bed; the second rise after 90 days represents vasodilatation of the placental vascular bed because there are no increases in perfusion pressure, placental weight, or in the total numbers of maternal

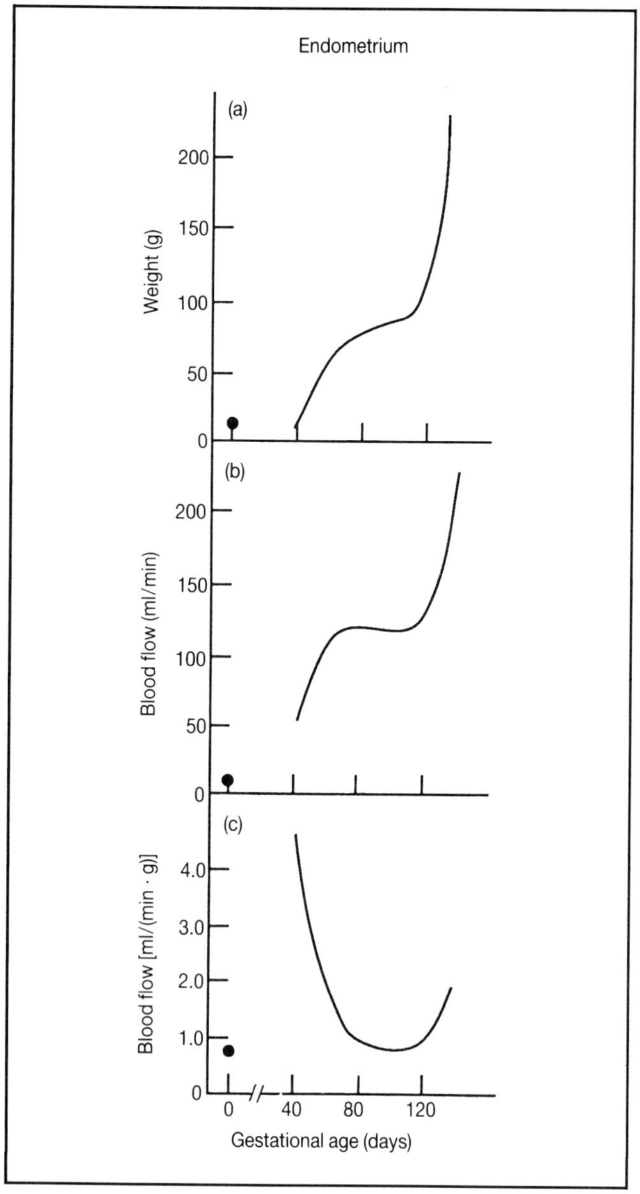

Fig. 10.41. Changes in endometrial weight (a), blood flow (b), and blood flow per gram of endometrium (c) during ovine gestation. ● nonpregnant. (From Rosenfeld CR, Morris FH, *et al. Gynecol Invest* 1974; **5**: 252, with permission of Karger, Basel.)

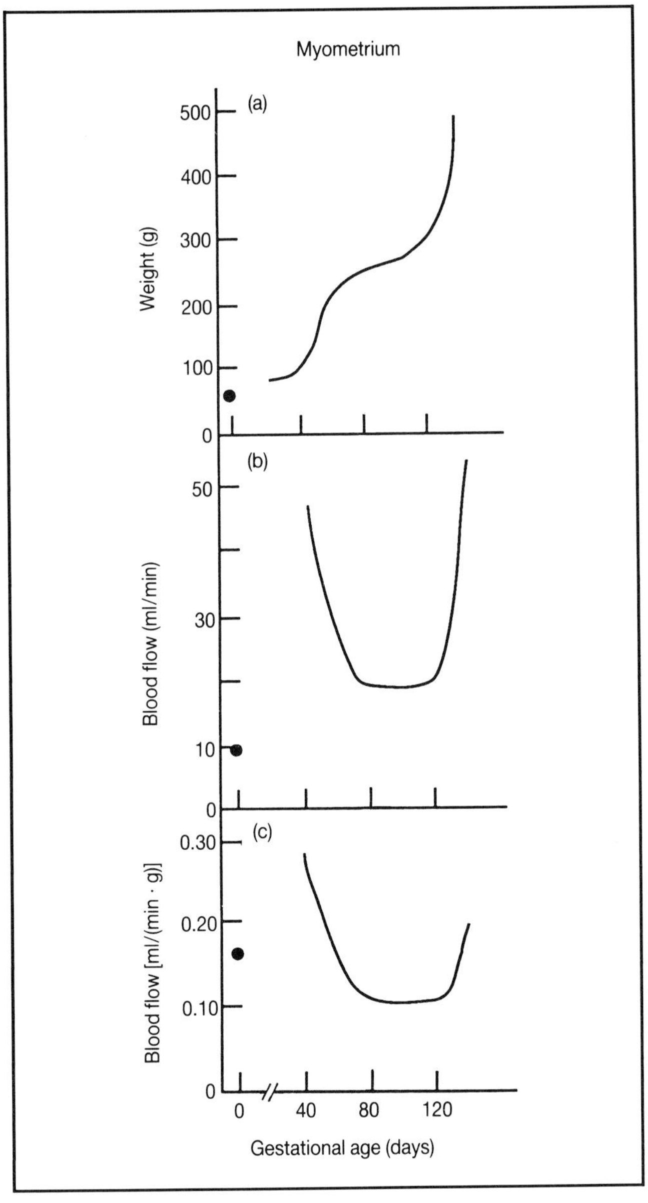

Fig. 10.42. Changes in myometrial weight (a), blood flow (b), and blood flow per gram of myometrium (c) during ovine gestation. ● nonpregnant. (From Rosenfeld CR, Morris FH, *et al.* *Gynecol Invest* 1974; **5**: 252, with permission of Karger, Basel.)

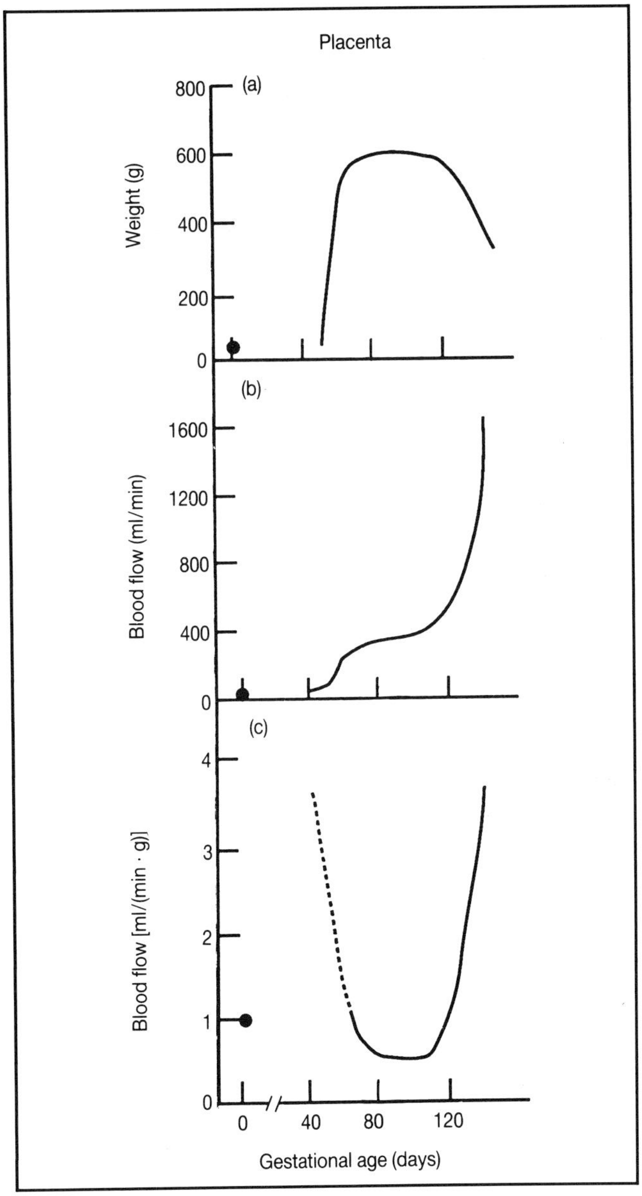

Fig. 10.43. Changes in placental weight (a), blood flow (b), and blood flow per gram of placenta (c). Observations on the nonpregnant animals; ● represent the caruncles or future sites of implantation. (From Rosenfeld CR, Morris FH, *et al.* *Gynecol Invest* 1974; **5**: 252, with permission of Karger, Basel.)

stromal cells so that blood flow/gram increases substantially (Fig. 10.44). Moreover, this placental vasodilatation progresses throughout the remainder of pregnancy. Changes in placental blood flow observed in sheep correspond to patterns reported in women. Although the human and ovine placentas are anatomically different, the overall local and systemic (see below) hemodynamic changes are similar and occur at relatively similar times in gestation.

Peripheral vascular changes in pregnancy

In addition to the dramatic alterations in the utero-placental vascular bed, with advancing gestation there also are numerous changes in the peripheral vascular bed. For example, although there is a relatively minor decrease

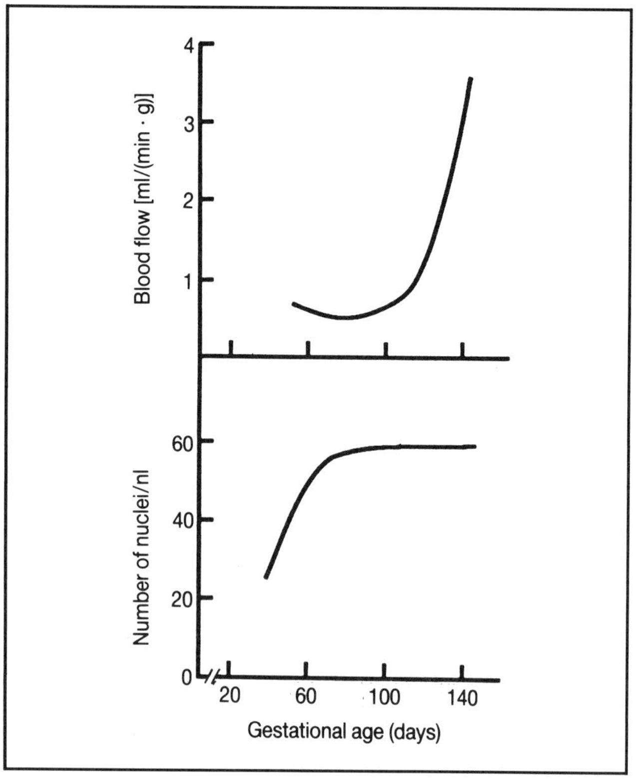

Fig. 10.44. Comparison of maternal placental blood flow per gram of placenta (upper) with the numerical density of nuclei of the maternal placental stroma (lower). (From Teasdale F. *Anat Rec* 1976; **185**: 187. Copyright © 1976. Wiley–Liss. Reprinted by permission of Wiley–Liss, a division of John Wiley and Sons, Inc.)

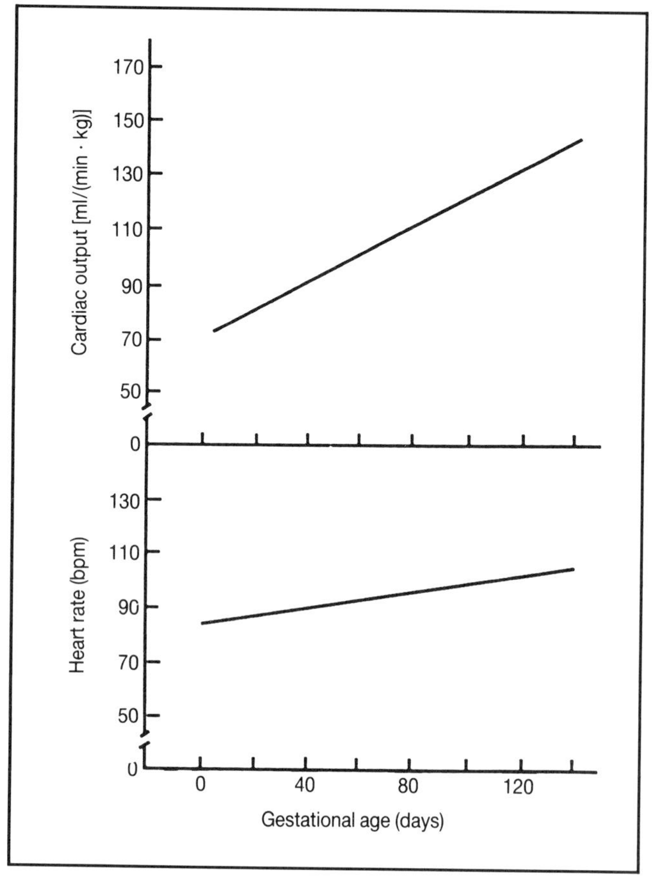

Fig. 10.45. Changes in cardiac output and heart rate during ovine pregnancy. (From Rosenfeld CR. *Am J Physiol* 1977; **232**: H231, with permission.)

in arterial blood pressure, there is a gradual but substantial increase in cardiac output (Fig. 10.45) associated with a similarly substantial fall in peripheral vascular resistance. This clearly demonstrates that pregnancy is a state of both uterine and systemic vasodilatation. Blood volume also increases, and there is relative refractoriness to the pressor effects of infused angiotensin II, α-agonists, and several other vasoconstrictors. Cardiac output is redistributed, primarily reflecting the growth and development of the uteroplacental vascular bed, and later in pregnancy, the growth of the mammary gland vascular bed (Fig. 10.46). Of particular physiological interest, these cardiovascular alterations are temporary, i.e. during the postpartum period, they return to nonpregnant levels within 3–5 weeks.

In normal pregnant women, in the second trimester (12–20 weeks), cardiac output increases approximately 25–40 percent in singleton and 50–60 percent in multifetal pregnancies. It then plateaus and remains unchanged or falls slightly during the third trimester. Definitive information in humans has been elusive because it is difficult to obtain consistent measurements of cardiac output after the second trimester. This is due to the increasing size of the gravid uterus, which often compresses and partially occludes both the vena cava and aorta, causing transient falls in cardiac output as venous return is reduced; e.g. cardiac output may be 22 percent lower in the supine versus the lateral recumbent position. More definitive data have been obtained in sheep in which the uterus does not rest upon the great vessels; cardiac output rises progressively throughout gestation (Fig. 10.45), increasing from nonpregnant values of about 75 ml/(min·kg) to about 150 ml/(min·kg) by the end of gestation. This has been confirmed in several species using different techniques, e.g. dye-dilution, thermal

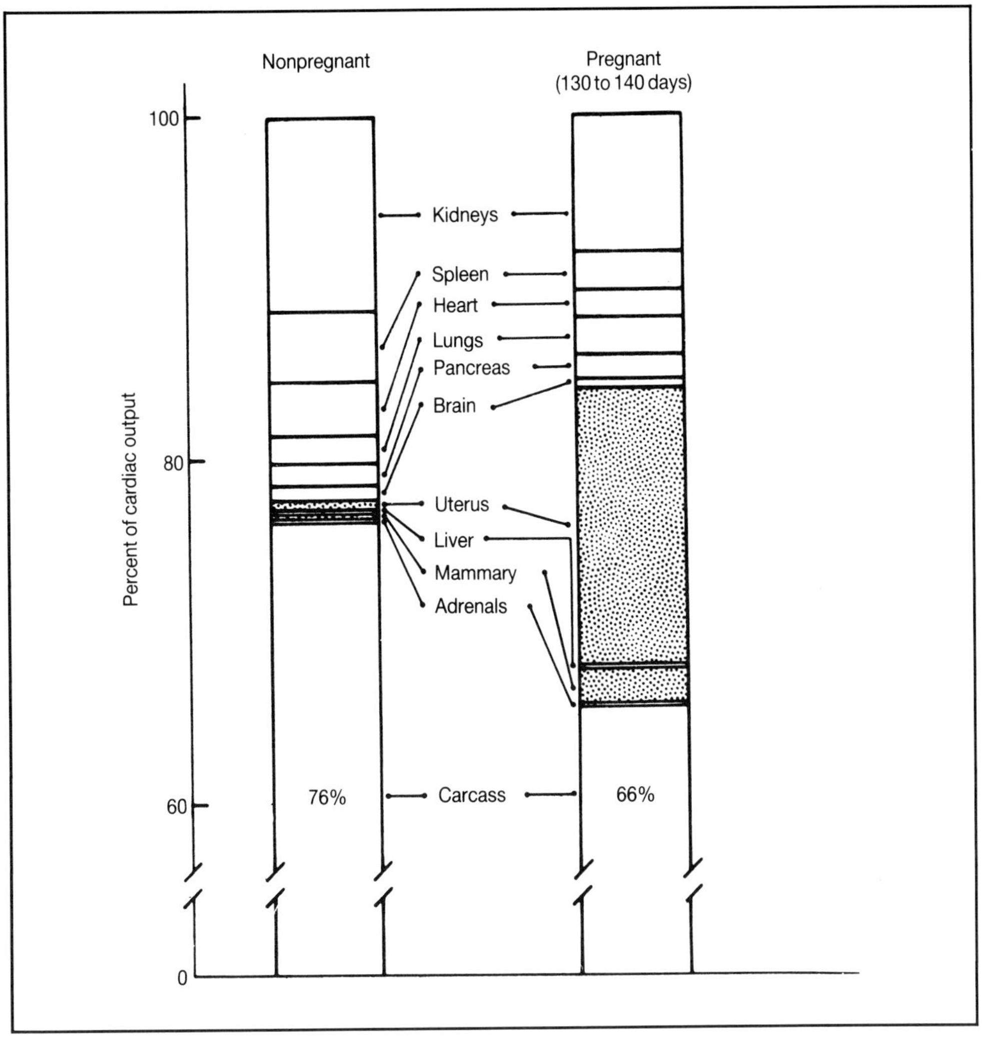

Fig. 10.46. Distribution of cardiac output in nonpregnant and pregnant ewes at 130–140 days of gestation. Stippled areas represent mammary gland and uterine mass. (From Rosenfeld CR. *Am J Physiol* 1977; **232**: H231, with permission.)

dilution, radiolabeled microspheres, and electromagnetic flow transducers.

Because cardiac output is expressed by the equation

$$\text{Cardiac output} = \text{Heart rate} \cdot \text{Stroke volume}$$

it is important to determine which component is responsible for the observed increase. In both humans and sheep, heart rate increases similarly, i.e. 20–30 percent (Fig. 10.45). This rise in heart rate has been attributed both to changes in the autonomic nervous system and to increases in placental steroids; however, their specific roles remain unproven. Because the rise in heart rate is proportionately less than the rise in cardiac output, the increase in cardiac output must also reflect a substantial increase in stroke volume. By echocardiography both left ventricular wall mass and end-diastolic dimensions increase during normal pregnancy. Furthermore, increases in stroke volume are directly proportional to end-diastolic volume, implying little change in myocardial inotropic state during normal singleton pregnancy. However, in multifetal gestations, the additional 20–30 percent rise in cardiac output occurs predominantly by increased inotropic effects as indexed by an increased fractional shortening of the ventricular diameter. Together these changes suggest a decrease in cardiac reserve in normal pregnancy. In addition, the aorta has been noted to be larger and more compliant in pregnant women, which may contribute to the decreased afterload on the heart seen in pregnancy.

The rise in cardiac output in pregnancy also correlates

with an increase in blood volume. This follows from the direct proportionality between stroke volume/end-diastolic volume and blood volume as described by Starling's law of the heart. The magnitude of the increase in blood volume depends on the presence of a singleton or multifetal pregnancy and varies from 30 to 50 percent. In pregnancy there is enhanced erythropoiesis; thus total red blood cell mass also increases; however, the rise in plasma volume exceeds the increase in red cell mass, which explains the development of the *'physiological anemia of pregnancy'*. The following equation defines this relationship:

$$\text{Blood volume} - \text{Plasma volume} = \text{Red blood cell mass}$$

Of particular interest to perinatal clinicians studying *pregnancy-induced hypertension* is the small but significant fall in mean arterial blood pressure early in the second trimester; this transient decrease may not occur in pregnancies complicated by hypertension. In ovine pregnancy, this decrease in mean arterial pressure persists throughout gestation. Nevertheless, the best index of systemic vasodilatation is not blood pressure, but rather peripheral vascular resistance, which takes into consideration changes in both blood pressure and cardiac output during pregnancy, i.e. the increases in systemic flow. Peripheral vascular resistance is calculated by the equation:

$$\text{Peripheral vascular resistance} = \frac{\text{Mean arterial pressure} - \text{Central venous pressure}}{\text{Cardiac output}}$$

Because central venous pressure is generally very low (1–3 mmHg), this calculation can be estimated more easily as: Peripheral vascular resistance = Mean arterial pressure / Cardiac output. Measurements of blood pressure and cardiac output early in pregnancy show substantial decreases in peripheral vascular resistance that begin well **before** the time that the uterine vascular bed enlarges, placentation occurs, or uterine vascular resistance has changed very much. Therefore, these changes reflect peripheral vasodilatation at a time when changes in the uteroplacental vascular bed cannot account for the observed systemic vasodilatation and rise in cardiac output, thereby dispelling the theory that the systemic alterations merely reflect formation of a 'uterine arteriovenous shunt'.

In view of the 40–80 percent fall in peripheral vascular resistance in pregnancy, few have considered why substantial hypotension does not occur during normal pregnancy. If we reverse the above equation to evaluate pressure as the dependent variable, i.e. Mean arterial pressure = Peripheral vascular resistance · Cardiac output, then it can be expected that as resistance falls, the rise in cardiac output will in part maintain blood pressure. Additional data suggest that activation of both the renin–angiotensin system and the sympathetic division of the autonomic nervous system play key roles in maintaining blood pressure in this vasodilated state. However, the role of the integrative reflex functions of these systems on blood pressure control have not been critically evaluated in human pregnancy.

Another critical issue is the distribution of the increased cardiac output, which presently cannot be determined in pregnant humans. In the pregnant ewe, cardiac output increases as much as 3.5 liters/min (100 percent) by term. The greatest increase in organ or tissue blood flow occurred to the uteroplacental vascular bed (Fig. 10.46), increasing from about 0.01 percent of cardiac output in nonpregnant ewes to about 8 percent and 16 percent at 60–100 and 130–140 days of gestation, respectively. Mammary gland blood flow also increased, particularly in the final week of gestation, rising from 0.2 percent in the nonpregnant ewe to 2 percent at term. It is unclear how much of the increase in uteroplacental blood flow late in gestation results in relative systemic 'underfilling', thereby stimulating the further increase in cardiac output and blood volume via activation of the renin–angiotensin–aldosterone system, all of which are increased in pregnancy. When increases in blood flow to the gravid uterus and mammary gland are summed, only 1.5–2.0 liters/min or 40–55 percent of the observed increase in cardiac output are accounted for. Therefore, 45–60 percent of cardiac output is directed towards other systemic tissues and organs. Even though the percentage of cardiac output received by the nonreproductive tissues falls from 76 percent to 66 percent, this actually reflects a 73 percent increase in absolute blood flow to these tissues. Of particular interest, blood flow through the skin, the largest organ in the body, increases nearly 100 percent. Studies in women also have demonstrated rather substantial increases in blood flow through the extremities as pregnancy progressed, supporting the hypothesis that blood flow to the skin may account for a substantial portion of the observed rise in cardiac output; however, this has not been critically evaluated. The percentage of cardiac output to other major organs falls, but there is little or no change in their absolute blood flows, demonstrating that pregnancy is characterized by a redistribution of cardiac output.

Factors controlling uterine and systemic vasculature in pregnancy

Many hypotheses have been proposed regarding which factors are involved in controlling the uteroplacental and systemic vascular changes in normal pregnancy. Suggested factors include estrogen, progesterone, prostaglandins, sympathetic and parasympathetic mediators of the autonomic nervous system, endothelial derived relaxing factor, histamine, growth factors, and even Ca^{2+} channel blockade. No study published to date has established a conclusive **direct cause-and-effect** relationship between any of these substances or pathways and the pregnancy-associated alterations.

Endogenous estrogen production by the fetoplacental unit is increased during gestation. Moreover, uterine and systemic vasodilatation of pregnancy can be mimicked in part by estrogen administration to nonpregnant castrated sheep (Fig. 10.47); these responses are similar to the systemic responses of postmenopausal women treated with conjugated estrogens. In sheep, estrogen increases uterine blood flow, cardiac output, and blood volume while decreasing uterine and systemic vascular resistance. The uterine and systemic vascular beds vasodilate independently in response to estrogen; furthermore, the uterine vascular bed is more responsive to estrogen than the systemic vascular bed. The ovine uteroplacental vascular bed is **not** maximally vasodilated, and has the capacity to vasodilate further after systemic administration of either estradiol-17β or its C_{19}-androgen precursor, dehydroepiandrosterone. Together, these observations suggest that estrogen may be important in modulating and maintaining uteroplacental blood flow during

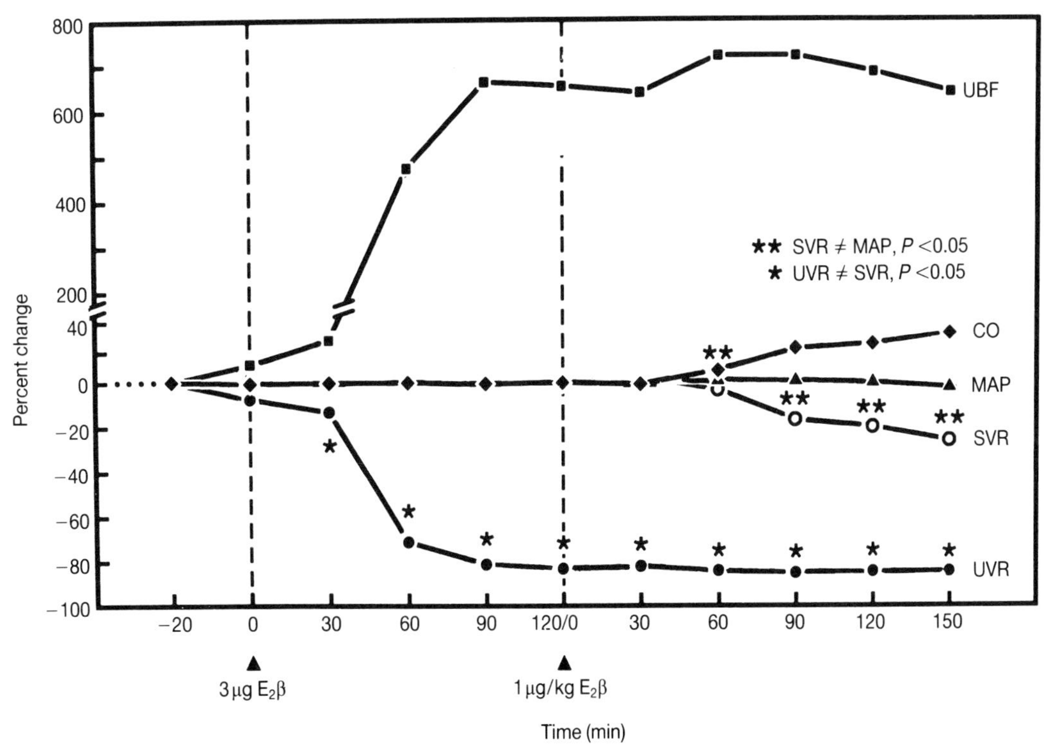

Fig. 10.47. Effects of local and systemic estradiol-17β ($E_2\beta$) on relative responses of uterine blood flow (UBF), cardiac output (CO), mean arterial pressure (MAP), systemic vascular resistance (SVR), and uterine vascular resistance (UVR) in nonpregnant oophorectomized sheep. (From Magness RR, Rosenfeld CR. *Am J Physiol* 1989; **256**: E536, with permission.)

pregnancy; however, cause-and-effect relationships have yet to be established fully.

Suggestions that the increase in prostaglandin production normally seen in pregnancy is necessary for the pregnancy-associated vasodilatation in both the systemic and uteroplacental vascular beds are probably unfounded since a decrease in prostaglandin concentrations of 40–70 percent after systemic and local indomethacin infusion has **no** effect on basal blood flows or other cardiovascular variables. Thus the mechanisms responsible for the systemic vasodilatation seen in pregnancy remain unclear.

Selected reading

Cunningham FG, MacDonald PC, Gant NF. Maternal adaptations to pregnancy. In Patterson L, ed. *Williams obstetrics*. Vol. 18. Norwalk, CT: Appleton & Lange, 1989: 7.

Magness RR. Ovarian secretion and vascular function. In Naftolin F, Sarrel PM, Gutmann JN, DeCherney AH, eds. *Cardiovascular and neurological function and ovarian secretions*. Vol. 80. Norwell, MA: Raven Press, 1990: 93.

Magness RR, Rosenfeld CR. Eicosanoids and the regulation of uteroplacental hemodynamics. In Mitchell MD, ed. *Eicosanoids in reproduction*. Boca Raton, FL: CRC Uniscience Series, CRC Press, 1990: 139.

Magness RR, Rosenfeld CR. Local and systemic estradiol-17β: effects on uterine and systemic vasodilation. *Am J Physiol* 1989; **159**: 252.

Rosenfeld CR, ed. *The uterine circulation*. Vol. 10. Ithaca, NY: Perinatology Press, 1989.

H2. Umbilical–Placental and Uterine Circulations

L Myatt

Development of an adequate and increasing blood flow to both maternal and fetal sides of the placenta is necessary for the increasing nutrient and respiratory demands of the fetus as it develops and grows throughout gestation. In both circulations of the placenta, this is achieved by a combination of remodeling or growth of vessels, the direct influence of vasoactive agents, and by systemic cardiovascular changes.

Umbilical–placental circulation

Anatomy

The human fetal extracorporeal circulation is established by 6 weeks of gestation and adapts to continuous fetal growth and increasing demand throughout gestation so that at term, about 40 percent of fetal cardiac output (combined ventricular output) reaches the umbilical–placental circulation. The umbilical arteries branch from the internal iliac arteries and then run 30–60 cm within the cord without branching. The paired arteries and veins are embedded in a loose connective tissue, Wharton's jelly, consisting of fibroblast-like stellate cells, dispersed in an extracellular matrix. A single layer of amnion cells lines the cord. The three vessels run parallel and are twisted an equal, though highly variable number of times, the twisting protecting the vessels from torsional forces. The vessels have the normal three layers, intima, muscular, and adventitia, each enclosed by a thin connective tissue sheath. Collagen fibers from the adventitia extend between the smooth muscle cells of the muscular layer and also into the Wharton's jelly. The muscle fibers have a defined outer circular and inner layer, which in arteries contains small amounts of elastin and collagen, whereas the vein is richly endowed with connective tissue elements.

Endothelial cells, their basement membrane, and connective tissue constitute the intima. The vein, but not the artery, has an internal elastic lamina. The *in vivo* luminal diameter of the umbilical vein is 6–8 mm, and that of the arteries 3–4 mm. Hoboken's nodules give the cord a segmental appearance. The nodules do not appear to function as valves, though. The umbilical vessels are unusual in that they lack a nerve supply and do not have vasa vasorum, and therefore derive their nutrition by diffusion from the lumen or the amniotic fluid. The umbilical cord is inserted centrally or slightly off-center on the chorionic plate of the placenta. The umbilical arteries each divide into two chorionic arteries, which then divide successively as they move towards the periphery to give first-, second-, third-, and sometimes fourth-order chorionic plate arteries. Each of these terminal umbilical arterial branches then penetrates the chorionic plate to become the stem artery of a cotyledon. Within the cotyledon, the arteries divide to give second, third, and fourth vessels, and finally villous vessels enter the chorionic villi. The previllous arterioles are the major resistance vessels of the placenta. The veins follow the arteries and all drain into the one umbilical vein.

General physiology

Umbilical–placental blood flow increases throughout gestation; however, it decreases as a proportion of fetal cardiac output until at term it is 100–150 ml/(kg·min) (fetal weight) measured by Doppler flow. The flow in the two arteries presumably is equally distributed, but may be unequal in pathological pregnancies. The pressure in the umbilical artery is 40–50 mmHg, and 10 mmHg in the vein. The corresponding blood $P\text{O}_2$ and pH are 25 mmHg (3.3 kPa) and 7.30–7.35 and 45 mmHg and 7.37–7.40 for artery and vein, respectively. To accommodate the increasing flow, resistance in the umbilical–placental circulation normally decreases throughout gestation and can be characterized by an increase in end-diastolic flow velocity relative to peak systolic velocity when umbilical arterial flow velocity waveforms are examined by Doppler ultrasound. Such measurements in the umbilical vessels are indicative of downstream **impedance** in the villous tree. In *pre-eclampsia* and *intrauterine growth retardation (IUGR),* the normal gestational increase in end-diastolic velocity is not seen on ultrasound studies indicating reduced flow. This correlates with a reduced number of vessels and a narrowing of the lumen and thickening of vessel walls in the villous vascular tree, which increases impedance. Blood flow in the umbilical–placental circulation may also be profoundly affected by changes in the fetal cardiovascular system that alter fetal systemic arterial pressure, and hence alter umbilical–placental perfusion pressure.

Regulatory mechanisms

General mechanisms

Changes in blood $P\text{O}_2$, $P\text{CO}_2$, and pH may affect umbilical blood flow. Decreases in $P\text{O}_2$ do not affect umbilical–placental flow in the sheep fetus, whereas flow is increased to the coronary, cerebral, and adrenal circulations. Hypoxemia and acidemia appear to favor the placenta, brain, and heart by redistribution of flow. Very high $P\text{CO}_2$ levels give small decreases in umbilical vascular resistance. Increasing maternal blood pressure in the intervillous space has been suggested to increase fetal–placental vascular resistance and, hence, reduce flow. However, this hypothesis has not been supported. Alterations in the hydrostatic pressure difference across the placenta, e.g. by reducing fetal arterial pressure, is suggested to increase maternal-to-fetal water flow, which would increase fetal venous backflow and cardiac output and restore umbilical pressure and flow. Maternal and fetal flows in the placenta may be matched as are ventilation/perfusion ratios in the lung. This would optimize O_2, nutrient, CO_2, and waste product exchange and requires an agent that easily crosses the placenta and has opposing (vasoconstrictor/vasodilator) effects on either side of the placenta. While prostaglandins (PGs) have been considered as filling this role, conclusive experimental proof is lacking. Indeed, *in vitro* in human placenta, only 6 percent of PGE_2 and $PGF_{2\alpha}$ present in one placental circulation will cross to the other circulation, and the majority of that which crosses ends up as an inactive metabolite. Angiotensin II has also been considered as a possible mediator of perfusion matching. Vascular reactivity and the ability to produce vasoactive agents vary along the length of the umbilical–placental circulation with the umbilical veins responding differently under certain conditions. The villous vascular tree is responsive to vasoactive agents and is the major determinant of resistance in the umbilical–placental circulation, accounting for about 90 percent of the total resistance (umbilical veins account for the remainder). Vasoactive substances (autacoids) affect umbilical blood flow in two ways: (1) by altering perfusion pressure and/or fetal heart rate with no change in umbilical–placental vascular resistance, or (2) by directly altering umbilical–placental vascular resistance. The families of autacoids that may affect umbilical–placental vascular resistance include the renin–angiotensin system, the eicosanoids (arachidonic acid metabolites), catecholamines, and the novel endothelial derived vasoactive factors.

Adrenergic and cholinergic control

In isolated vessels, extremely high concentrations of adrenergic or cholinergic agents are necessary to affect vessel tone, suggesting no or slight physiological effects.

Fetal cholinergic blockade increases umbilical blood flow secondary to increasing systemic pressure and heart rate. β-Adrenergic agonists given to the fetus increase umbilical blood flow and lower vascular resistance, whereas β-antagonists have opposite effects. α-Adrenergic agonists or antagonists do not alter umbilical blood flow. Although circulating catecholamines do not affect arteriolar tone, they do increase umbilical venous tone and almost certainly are responsible for the constriction of those vessels associated with hypoxemia. By increasing umbilical–placental outflow impedance, and thereby distending the veins and recruiting placental exchange area, this may improve gas exchange.

Renin–angiotensin system

Both the umbilical vessels and the villous vascular tree are constricted by angiotensins I and II and also, surprisingly, by angiotensin III, all of which act via the angiotensin II receptor and can be inhibited by receptor antagonists such as saralasin. Angiotensin I acts following its conversion to angiotensin II by angiotensin converting enzyme, which is present in high concentrations in the vascular endothelium. Angiotensin converting enzyme inhibitors should not be used in pregnancy as they cross the placenta and may have detrimental effects on the fetus.

Eicosanoids

Of the eicosanoids, thromboxane A_2 is a potent vasoconstrictor throughout the umbilical–placental circulation. The vasodilator PGs, PGD_2, PGE_1, and PGI_2 (prostacyclin) cannot affect resting tone *in vitro*, suggesting the umbilical–placental circulation is maximally vasodilated. However, all three of these eicosanoids will relax the preconstricted umbilical–placental circulation. The rank order of their potency suggests they all act via a PGI_2 receptor. Increased synthesis of PGI_2 and PGE is found when the umbilical–placental circulation is constricted, for example by angiotensin II, suggesting these eicosanoids act as compensatory vasodilators to attenuate the actions of vasoconstrictors. However, prevention of PG synthesis by cyclooxygenase inhibitors does not affect resting tone, suggesting that PGs are not major determinants of resting tone in the umbilical–placental circulation. The responsiveness of the umbilical–placental circulation to these autacoids appears to be greatest at the placental end of the circulation, i.e. in the villous resistance vessels. Increased synthesis and release of thromboxane and decreased synthesis and release of PGI_2 by maternal and fetal vessels purportedly is characteristic of placental insufficiency syndromes, including *pre-eclampsia* and *IUGR* and may contribute to the altered indices of fetal–placental vascular resistance measured by Doppler ultrasound *in vivo*. Low-dose aspirin therapy (80 mg/day), which selectively inhibits thromboxane synthesis while leaving PGI_2 synthesis relatively unchanged, is reported to increase fetal–placental blood flow and to improve outcome in some patients thought to be at risk of IUGR on the evidence of altered umbilical blood flow velocity waveform indices. The peptidyl leukotrienes C_4, D_4 and E_4 are also vasoconstrictors of the umbilical–placental circulation *in vitro*.

Endothelin and other vasoactive peptides

(see p. 468 for further details)

The endothelins are a family of 21 amino acid peptides (Et-1, 2, and 3) coded for by three separate genes and are potent, long-acting (45–60 minutes) vasoconstrictors. Endothelins usually have greater potency on veins than on arteries. The genes for Et-1 and 3 are expressed in human placenta, and receptors for Et-1 have been characterized in the villous vasculature. Both Et-1 and Et-3 are potent vasoconstrictors of the human fetal–placental circulation *in vitro*. The precursor 39 amino acid peptide big Et-1 is also a vasoconstrictor *in vitro*, but is less potent than Et-1. The action of big Et-1 appears to be indirect following its conversion to Et-1 by a converting enzyme (neutral metalloprotease) in the fetal–placental circulation. Other peptide hormones that are vasoactive in the umbilical–placental circulation include calcitonin gene-related peptide (CGRP), a vasodilator, and vasoactive intestinal peptide (VIP), a vasoconstrictor (see below).

Endothelial derived relaxing factor

(see p. 469 for further details)

The endothelial derived relaxing factor (EDRF) is found in the umbilical–placental circulation. Umbilical cord and chorionic plate vessels appear to produce very little EDRF, but EDRF will relax them if the vessels are preconstricted. One major EDRF appears to be the nitric oxide radical

(NO), which acts via stimulation of cGMP production to cause relaxation. Agents that generate NO will vasodilate the villous vascular tree preconstricted *in vitro* with either thromboxane mimetics, endothelin, bradykinin, serotonin, or angiotensin II. By using competitive substrate inhibitors of the NO synthase enzyme, which forms NO and L-citrulline from the basic amino acid L-arginine, it has been shown that endogenous NO synthesis contributes to maintenance of the low resting tone of the fetal–placental circulation and that it attenuates the actions of vasoconstrictors *in vitro*. The small resistance vessels of the villous vascular tree appear to have a greater capacity to produce EDRF (NO) than the larger umbilical or chorionic plate vessels. In *pre-eclampsia,* the ability of umbilical cord arteries and veins to produce EDRF *in vitro* is significantly reduced compared with vessels from normotensive pregnancies, suggesting that like PGI_2, a deficiency of EDRF synthesis may be associated with increased vascular resistance and reduced flow. Synthesis of NO is greater in arteries than veins and may account for the reduced potency of endothelin in arteries than in veins.

Uteroplacental circulation

Anatomy

Uterine blood flow must increase during pregnancy both to the myometrium and to the decidua and intervillous space of the placenta. The uterine artery arises from the hypogastric or internal iliac artery, descends to the broad ligament and crosses towards the uterus, then divides into the cervicovaginal artery and the ascending uterine artery. The latter vessel runs along the uterus and gives a major branch to the upper portion of the cervix and 8–24 arcuate branches to the uterus. The arcuate arteries are usually paired, traversing the uterus anteriorly and posteriorly within the outer one-third of the myometrium and anastomosing with the vessels from the other side. The radial arteries branch from the arcuates to supply the inner two-thirds of the myometrium and terminate in the spiral arteries, which supply endometrium, decidua, and placenta. The ascending branch of the uterine artery ends as it reaches the Fallopian tube, where it trifurcates to the fundal, tubal, and ovarian branch. The ovarian branch anastomoses with the uterine artery. The spiral arteries supply the endometrium in the nonpregnant uterus and undergo a physiological adaptation to accommodate the increased flow of pregnancy. In the first trimester of pregnancy, extravillous trophoblast migrates in a retrograde manner down the spiral arteries and removes the endothelial and musculoelastic layers of the artery and replaces them with fibrinoid. In the second trimester, the adaptation continues into the myometrial portion of the spiral arteries, the net result being conversion of the tortuous narrow spiral arteries to flaccid, distended vessels with no musculoelastic elements. This implies that the response of these resistance vessels to neural or humoral agents is lost. In *pre-eclampsia* and *IUGR*, the secondary wave of trophoblast invasion is absent and some spiral arteries within the placental bed do not appear to be invaded at all, the net result being an increase in vascular resistance and reduction in flow of up to 50 percent, which can be estimated *in vivo* by Doppler ultrasound measurements in the arcuate arteries. The known uteroplacental pathology associated with these conditions makes it likely that the increased impedance is due to the lack of structural alteration of the spiral arteries rather than an alteration in vascular reactivity.

Physiology

As fetal demands increase, uterine blood flow increases 20–80-fold during pregnancy by virtue of vasodilation and growth of the vascular bed. At term, human uterine blood flow may be up to 800 ml/min or 10–20 percent of cardiac output. The majority of this flow (80 percent) is diverted through the spiral arteries to the intervillous space of the placenta.

Regulatory mechanisms

The vasoactive agents to which the uteroplacental circulation is likely to respond include the same families of autacoids that act on the fetal–placental circulation. The unique features of the uteroplacental circulation include the flaccid distended spiral arteries and the intervillous space that will not respond to neural or humoral agents. Blood flow through these vessels is thus determined by the reactivity of the larger uterine, arcuate, and radial arteries and by systemic cardiovascular changes. What effect the absence of the secondary wave or the total lack of trophoblast invasion of spiral arteries in *pre-eclampsia* or *IUGR* have on uterine vascular reactivity remains to be determined. Overall uterine blood flow has two components, to the myometrium and to the placental intervillous space. Vascular reactivity studies in species such as sheep in which the maternal placenta has a resistance bed obviously bear no relationship to the hemomonochorial human placenta with invaded spiral arteries and an intervillous space with no vascular response elements.

Innervation

The uterus is richly supplied with sympathetic and parasympathetic fibers. There is a reduction in transmitter substances and neural elements in the uterus during pregnancy; this accounts for the reduced response to autonomic agonists in pregnancy. The maximal vasodilation of the uterine circulation makes it difficult to demonstrate vasodilation to local β-adrenergic stimulation. There are very few or no data for autoregulation, i.e. alteration of resistance to maintain constant flow when perfusion is altered, in the human uterine circulation.

Steroid hormones, uterine blood flow, and EDRF

The large increases in estrogen and progesterone synthesis in pregnancy and the correlation with changes in blood flow in pregnancy make the steroid hormones potential candidates for regulating blood flow. Estradiol infusion in nonpregnant animals significantly increases uterine blood flow by a mechanism that is dependent on RNA and protein synthesis with a time delay of 20–30 minutes. Progesterone alone has no effect on uterine blood flow, but will attenuate the estradiol effect. The search for the mediator of this estrogen-induced hyperemia has proven elusive. Recent data suggest that EDRF (NO) may mediate a large proportion of the estrogen-induced increase in uterine blood flow as competitive substrate inhibitors of NO synthesis appear to antagonize the effect in experimental animals. In pregnant animals, NO synthesis inhibitors decrease uterine blood flow, suggesting that NO synthesis is increased in pregnancy, perhaps under estrogenic stimulation. There are at least three isoforms of the NO synthase enzyme. Blood vessels appear to possess both constitutive and inducible forms. The latter form appears to be stimulated by cytokines and inhibited by glucocorticoids, which also inhibit estrogen-induced hyperemia.

Endothelin

Endothelin-1 is also a vasoconstrictor of the uterine circulation in animal models. The contribution of circulating endothelin in humans is unclear as concentrations are below the threshold necessary to activate endothelin receptors. In pre-eclampsia Et-1 concentrations are doubled and yet still do not reach the concentration necessary for receptor activation. Subthreshold concentrations of endothelin may, however, increase the sensitivity of vessels to other vasoconstrictors.

Renin–angiotensin system

The ovine uteroplacental circulation is vasoconstricted by angiotensin II, the responsiveness, however, being less than that of the systemic vasculature. The greater increase in systemic resistance with angiotensin II sometimes indirectly increases uterine blood flow, falsely suggesting that angiotensin II is a uterine vasodilator. Such observations serve to illustrate the interaction between perfusion pressure, vascular resistance, and blood flow in the uterine circulation and the potential dangers of systemic vasodilation of pregnancy. The reduced reactivity of the uteroplacental circulation to angiotensin II, the concentrations of which are increased during pregnancy, has been associated with an increase in PGI_2 production by this vasculature in pregnancy. Of course, increased EDRF synthesis also must now be considered. Blockade of PG synthesis with indomethacin does not affect resting uterine blood flow in late-pregnant sheep, but potentiates the response to angiotensin II, suggesting that as in the fetal–placental circulation, vasodilator PGs attenuate the actions of vasoconstrictors. Indeed, angiotensin II acting via its receptors increases PGI_2 production in isolated uterine vessels.

Eicosanoids

Whole-body and uterine-vessel synthesis of PGI_2 is increased during pregnancy, this perhaps being hormonally regulated, but also possibly arising from increasing flow and/or shear stress over endothelial cells in the vasculature. In *pre-eclampsia* and *IUGR*, there is a generalized deficiency of PGI_2 synthesis relative to thromboxane when compared with normotensive pregnancy, and reactivity to angiotensin II is increased. This deficiency of PGI_2 is associated with the increased vascular resistance of these conditions. This may be more important in the uteroplacental circulation, where PGI_2 plays a greater role in attenuating the action of vasoconstrictors.

Peptide hormones

The presence of unidentified factors that mediate non-adrenergic, noncholinergic nervous control of uterine function has been recognized for a long time. These could include the peptides such as VIP, neuropeptide Y, CGRP, and also radicals such as NO. VIP, a 28 amino acid peptide present in female genital nerves, can give a dose-related increase in myometrial and total uterine blood flow in nonpregnant animals, an effect not mediated via α- or β-adrenergic receptors. Neuropeptide Y, a 36 amino acid peptide with both N- and C-terminal tyrosines and structural homology to other peptides of the pancreatic polypeptide family, is a potent vasoconstrictor in the myometrial circulation *in vitro*. CGRP, a 37 amino acid peptide derived from alternative tissue-specific RNA splicing and transcription of the calcitonin gene, has no structural similarity to calcitonin. CGRP may be distributed in the same nerve fibers as substance P, and CGRP-immunoactive nerve fibers are found adjacent to blood vessels. CGRP is a potent inhibitor of smooth muscle activity.

Calcium channel blockers

An increase in intracellular Ca^{2+} is a common denominator in smooth muscle contraction. A vast array of agents have the ability to block Ca^{2+} influx and have dramatic effects on both vascular and myometrial tissue in the uterus. The Ca^{2+} channel blockers do appear to cross the placenta. In addition to any direct effect on the uteroplacental vasculature, the systemic cardiovascular effects of Ca^{2+} channel blockers will influence uterine perfusion. In pregnant ewes, the dihydropyridine, nifedipine, infused at 10 μg/(kg·min) gives a 22 percent reduction in maternal peripheral resistance, a slight, but significant decrease in maternal arterial pressure, an increase in heart rate, and a 21 percent reduction in uterine blood flow despite no change in uterine vascular resistance. The decrease in uterine blood flow therefore is due to the maternal hypotensive effect. A significant decline in fetal O_2 saturation and a tendency to fetal hypoxia and acidosis is seen. Similar effects are seen in the primate, where transfer of dihydropyridines to the fetus is low, suggesting that changes in fetal oxygenation are secondary to decreases in maternal arterial pressure. The limited number of human studies at present using dihydropyridines as tocolytics show no apparent deleterious effects on neonatal outcome. In human chorionic plate vessels, the dihydropyridines nifedipine and nitrendipine give concentration-dependent inhibition of agonist-induced contractile activity, suggesting that Ca^{2+} channel blockers would increase placental perfusion, although this has not been confirmed *in vivo*.

Smoking, recreational drugs, and exercise

Nicotine from *cigarette smoking* produces a systemic sympathomimetic effect of elevated heart rate and blood pressure. Smoking in pregnancy results in lower-birth-weight babies due either to lower prenatal weight gain in the mother or to direct fetal effects of nicotine or carbon monoxide. In pregnant sheep, nicotine or simulated cigarette smoking do not have an acute effect on uterine blood flow, although constant infusion of nicotine may chronically reduce uterine blood flow. Human intervillous blood flow is reported to decrease acutely about 20 percent by smoking a single cigarette. *Cocaine* stimulates the central nervous system, producing sympathetic stimulation, increased heart rate and blood pressure, and vasoconstriction. An increased incidence of cerebro-vascular accidents and placental abruption is associated with cocaine use. The response to cocaine appears to be heightened during pregnancy in sheep and is somehow related to increased circulating progesterone. Low doses of intravenous cocaine are reported to increase uterine vascular resistance by up to 52 percent in the pregnant sheep. There is no evidence that heroin affects uteroplacental perfusion. Exercise during pregnancy decreased uterine blood flow in animal models in direct relationship to the intensity of exercise, probably by redistribution of cardiac output and increasing catecholamines. Women who exercise vigorously in pregnancy have lighter infants than do sedentary women.

Local anesthetics

Local anesthetics, bupivacaine, lidocaine, and chloroprocaine can decrease uterine blood flow and uterine activity in the pregnant ewe *in vivo*, but only at concentrations exceeding those seen during epidural blocks for labor and delivery. Epidural or spinal anesthesia that results in maternal hypotension can produce a decrease in uterine blood flow and fetal wellbeing as a consequence of decreasing uterine perfusion pressure. In part, these effects may be related to placing the patient in the supine position. Well conducted regional anesthesia without hypotension and supine positioning do not have a detrimental effect on uterine blood flow and fetal well-being. In some studies, an increase in uterine blood flow is seen in patients with epidural analgesia, especially those with pregnancy-induced hypertension, probably by reduction of blood epinephrine and norepinephrine concentrations.

Selected reading

Battaglia FC, Meschia G. *An introduction to fetal physiology*. Orlando: Academic Press, Inc., 1986.

Brinkman CR III. Circulation in the pregnant uterus. In Carsten ME, Miller JD, eds. *Uterine function, molecular and cellular aspects*. New York: Plenum Press, 1990: 519.

Kaufmann P. Basic morphology of the fetal and maternal circuits in the human placenta. In Schneider H, Dancis J, eds. *In vitro perfusion of human placental tissue*. *Contributions to Gynecology and Obstetrics*, Vol. 13. Basel: Karger, 1985: 5.

Magness RR, Rosenfeld CR. Eicosanoids and the regulation of uteroplacental hemodynamics. In Mitchell MD, ed. *Eicosanoids in reproduction*. Boca Raton: CRC Press, 1990: 139.

I. Oxygen Transport

G Lister

Relation between oxygen transport and oxygen consumption

Transport of oxygen (O_2) from the environment to the tissues requires the integration of three organ systems: the lungs, the circulation, and the blood. At rest transport of O_2 to the tissues is in great excess of metabolic rate or O_2 consumption. This buffer between transport and consumption of O_2 permits modest reductions in O_2 transport to be tolerated without any change in O_2 consumption. With stress such as exercise or fever, O_2 consumption increases abruptly, as does O_2 transport. These observations are used as evidence that metabolic rate usually dictates the level of O_2 transport rather than the converse. However, little O_2 is stored in the body. Therefore, severe reductions in O_2 transport or marked increases in metabolic demands can quickly exhaust the usual reserve and cause hypoxia, a mismatch between O_2 supply and demand, unless these organ systems can respond to restore the balance. These integrated responses, which are central adaptations to virtually all forms of cardiorespiratory disturbances, are the focus of this section.

The rate of O_2 transport to the tissues can be quantified as the **systemic O_2 transport** (SOT or $\dot{Q}O_2$), the product of cardiac output or systemic blood flow ($\dot{Q}$) and arterial blood O_2 concentration (CaO_2):

$$\mathrm{SOT} = \dot{Q} \times CaO_2$$

SOT here is expressed in vol of O_2/t, $\dot{Q}$ is in vol blood/t, and CaO_2 is in vol O_2/vol blood. CaO_2 is a function of hemoglobin concentration (Hb), arterial blood hemoglobin O_2 saturation (SaO_2), and arterial blood O_2 pressure or tension (PaO_2) as follows:

$$CaO_2 = (\mathrm{Hb} \times SaO_2 \times 1.34) + (PaO_2 \times 0.003)$$

where Hb is in g/dl blood; SaO_2 is a fraction; PaO_2 is in mmHg; the O_2-carrying capacity of hemoglobin, 1.34, is in ml O_2/g Hb; and 0.003, the solubility of O_2 in blood, is in ml O_2/dl blood per mmHg. These equations demonstrate that O_2 transport may be decreased by reductions in cardiac output (stagnant hypoxia), hemoglobin concentration (anemic hypoxia), or PaO_2 or SaO_2 (hypoxic hypoxia).

The systemic O_2 transport and the rate of O_2 consumption ($\dot{V}O_2$) can be related to each other by rearranging the **Fick equation** for cardiac output:

$$\dot{V}O_2 = \dot{Q}\,(CaO_2 - C\bar{v}O_2)$$

where $C\bar{v}O_2$ is the mixed systemic venous blood O_2 concentration. Multiplying the above equation by CaO_2/CaO_2 and regrouping terms yields:

$$\dot{V}O_2 = \dot{Q} \times CaO_2 \times ([CaO_2 - C\bar{v}O_2]/CaO_2)$$

or

$$\dot{V}O_2 = \mathrm{SOT} \times EO_2$$

where $(CaO_2 - C\bar{v}O_2)/CaO_2$ is the fractional O_2 extraction, EO_2. This equation shows clearly that any decrease in systemic O_2 transport must be attended by a comparable increase in O_2 extraction if O_2 consumption is to be maintained constant. Furthermore, because the fractional O_2 extraction is generally in the range of 0.25–0.30 under normal conditions, this equation also emphasizes the usual abundance of O_2 transport even though O_2 consumption and O_2 transport undergo substantial changes from birth to maturity.

Postnatal changes in O_2 transport and O_2 consumption

O_2 consumption

O_2 consumption per mass in newborns is relatively high compared with adults or fetuses (Fig. 10.48). O_2

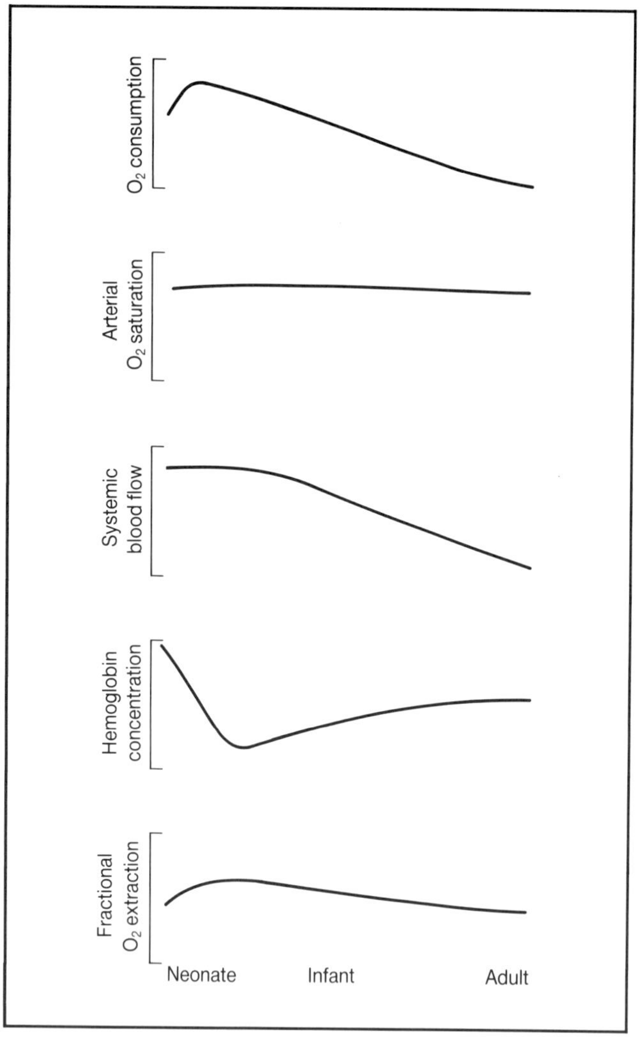

Fig. 10.48. Stylized schema demonstrating postnatal changes in the factors contributing to the changes in O_2 transport. The relationships shown are not precise for humans, but are inferred from data in humans and experimental animals.

consumption increases transiently after birth, then progressively declines to adult values, which are approximately one-half those of the neonate. When O_2 consumption is normalized to body surface area, much of this age-related difference disappears, suggesting that the high newborn rate is in part related to dissipation of heat from a high surface area:mass ratio. In addition, a higher fraction of metabolism is devoted to growth in the newborn than in the more mature subject. These age-related differences are even more accentuated in rapidly growing mammals, such as the premature child. Other factors such as postnatal increases in thyroid hormone (T_3 and T_4) concentrations also contribute to the higher metabolic rate of the neonate.

Some caution must be used when interpreting values of O_2 consumption in infants under widely different conditions. Environmental factors have a marked effect on metabolic rate. For example, O_2 consumption increases by nearly 50 percent when newborns are placed in an environment only 6°C below thermoneutral temperature. Moreover, because activity and sleep state markedly alter O_2 consumption, these need to be specified before comparing data.

Cardiac output

Cardiac output normalized to mass is also much higher in the newborn than in the fetus or in the mature subject. Combined ventricular output of the fetus is about 500 ml/(kg·min), of which 300 ml/(kg·min) contributes to systemic tissues other than the placenta. After birth blood flow from each ventricle is about 400 ml/(kg·min); this decreases progressively to the adult value, which is closer to 80 ml/(kg·min). Because of the high resting cardiac output of the neonate, it has been suggested that there is limited reserve for augmenting blood flow further under conditions of stress. This may be a factor reducing the capacity to respond if O_2 transport must increase suddenly to meet changing metabolic demands. In the mature subject cardiac output can increase by a factor of 3–4 (or as much as much as 6 with training) because stroke volume can increase by a factor of 1.5 and heart rate by 2–4 times. It is doubtful that the infant can sustain such high levels of cardiac output.

Hemoglobin concentration

After birth there is a progressive fall in hemoglobin concentration and hematocrit, with a consequent decrease in O_2-carrying capacity of blood. Hematocrit usually decreases from approximately 55 percent at birth to 33 percent by 2 months and then gradually increases to about 45 percent by adolescence. This decline in hemoglobin concentration is referred to as *'physiological anemia'* because it is unresponsive to transfusion or to hematemic agents and it occurs in healthy infants with no recognized nutritional deficiency. The anemia is accentuated in premature infants and even occurs in chronically hypoxemic infants although the decrease in hemoglobin concentration is less marked than in normal infants. Furthermore, the postnatal anemia occurs in infants with left-to-right shunts and can increase shunting. With the decline in viscosity when hematocrit decreases systemic and pulmonary vascular resistance decrease (roughly in proportion to each other), pulmonary and systemic blood flows increase (also in proportion) in response, and the left-to-right shunt thereby increases. Thus, postnatal changes in hemoglobin concentration may worsen or provoke circulatory failure and not be 'physiological' in the presence of cardiopulmonary pathology.

PaO_2 and *Sa*O_2

Normally, *Sa*O_2 does not change much with postnatal development even though *Pa*O_2 increases from approximately 50–60 mmHg (6.6–8.0 kPa) shortly after birth to approximately 100 mmHg in childhood. Based on changes in *Pa*O_2 breathing 100 percent O_2, the low *Pa*O_2 of the neonate has been attributed to both ventilation/perfusion inequalities and fixed intrapulmonary right-to-left shunting. As a result, healthy newborn infants breathing 100 percent O_2 usually have a *Pa*O_2 of about 300 mmHg, which may represent a right-to-left shunt of approximately 20 percent caused by anatomical shunts (via bronchial and thebesian circulations), atelectasis, and airway closure during expiration. However, owing to the high hemoglobin O_2 affinity (see below) *Sa*O_2 at birth is in the range of 95 percent even with the relatively low *Pa*O_2, and it does not change with postnatal development. Thus, except under unusual circumstances, changes in arterial oxygenation do not contribute to the marked alterations in O_2 transport with postnatal development. Moreover, if hemoglobin concentration or cardiac output are reduced, increases in *Sa*O_2 provide little compensation for the reduced O_2 transport.

O_2 extraction

Simultaneous with the decrease in hemoglobin concentration after birth, there is a progressive rightward shift of the hemoglobin–O_2 dissociation curve (Fig. 10.49). If *Pa*O_2 is normal and mixed systemic venous

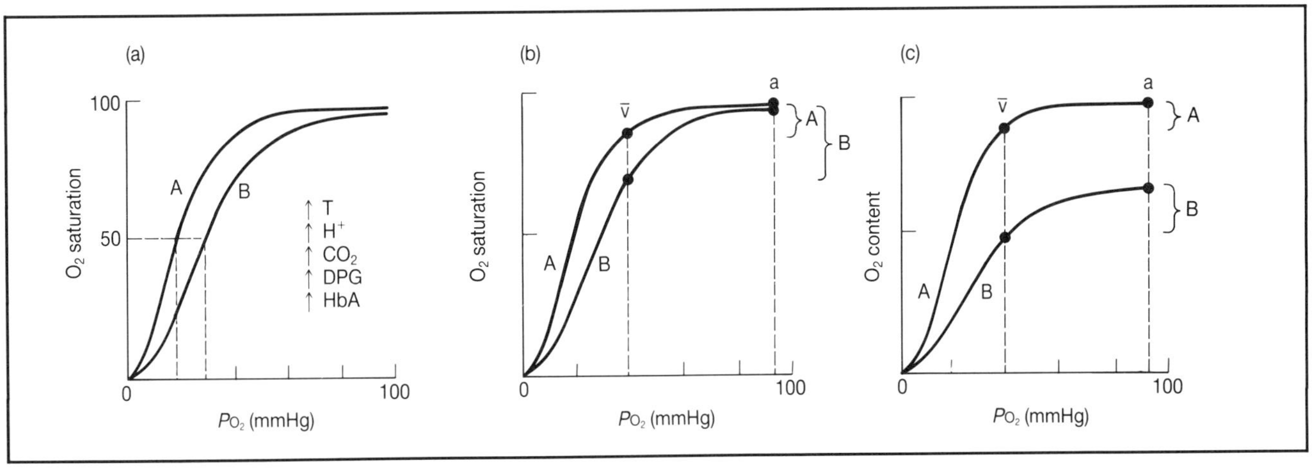

Fig. 10.49. Effect of changes in hemoglobin (Hb) O_2 affinity on O_2 unloading. (a) With increases in temperature (T), serum H^+ concentration, CO_2 concentration, or DPG content in the red cell, the relationship between Hb O_2 saturation and *P*O_2 shifts to the right (curve A to curve B). This shift reduces Hb O_2 affinity and increases P_{50}, the *P*O_2 at 50 percent Hb O_2 saturation. Similarly, when the fraction of adult hemoglobin (HbA) increases during postnatal development, P_{50} also increases because HbA binds to DPG more avidly than does fetal Hb, and this binding to DPG decreases the affinity of Hb for O_2 (see text). Curve A is typical for a newborn, and curve B for an adult. (b) As shown by the brackets, a rightward shift of the dissociation curve (A → B) causes a larger arteriovenous O_2 saturation difference when arterial (a) *P*O_2 and mixed venous ($\bar{v}$) *P*O_2 are normal and fixed. (c) In the presence of postnatal anemia, a rightward shift in the curve permits more O_2 to be unloaded for the same arterial (a) and mixed venous ($\bar{v}$) *P*O_2. When anemia occurs, the relationship between O_2 saturation and *P*O_2 does not fully characterize the effects on O_2 transport; therefore, in this figure O_2 content has replaced O_2 saturation on the Y axis to demonstrate the effect of anemia. Curve A represents the neonate with a low P_{50} (similar to curve A in other panels) and high Hb concentration. Curve B shows the combined effects of an increase in P_{50} and a decrease in Hb concentration. Despite the marked decrease in a total O_2 capacity of blood, curve B permits a larger arteriovenous O_2 content difference, as shown by the brackets.

blood Po_2 ($P\bar{v}o_2$) is constant, this rightward shift would permit progressively more O_2 to be unloaded from oxygenated hemoglobin, increasing arteriovenous blood O_2 content difference, an important mechanism for compensation during postnatal anemia. Thus there is a slight increase in fractional O_2 extraction particularly during the nadir of the anemia. Remarkably, however, **despite large differences in O_2 transport, O_2 consumption, and hemoglobin O_2 affinity during development, there is apparent constancy of $P\bar{v}o_2$,** which is in the range of 39–40 mmHg in normal resting subjects. Therefore, there is reasonable basis for estimates of the capacity to extract O_2 using the position of the O_2 dissociation curve, the hemoglobin concentration, and an assumed $P\bar{v}o_2$.

The postnatal decrease in hemoglobin O_2 affinity (or increase in P_{50}, the Po_2 at which hemoglobin is 50 percent saturated with O_2) is caused by an increase in the proportion of adult relative to fetal hemoglobin and an increase in the concentration of 2,3-diphosphoglycerate (DPG) (or 2,3-bisphosphoglycerate) as follows. There is a gradual decline in fetal hemoglobin from about 77 percent at birth to less than 2 percent by 8 months. DPG, a product of the Rapaport–Leubering shunt present in red cells, decreases the affinity for O_2 (increases P_{50}) through its allosteric interaction with the hemoglobin molecule. Because DPG does not bind to fetal hemoglobin as avidly as it does to adult hemoglobin, hemoglobin O_2 affinity is high immediately after birth (P_{50} approximately 20 mmHg). In contrast, by 8 months P_{50} increases to about 30 mmHg; after adolescence, P_{50} reaches adult values (about 27 mmHg). Therefore, in early infancy when the concentration of fetal hemoglobin is high, change in DPG has little effect on P_{50}, whereas modulation of hemoglobin O_2 affinity is an important compensatory mechanism in the older subject in response to hypoxemia, anemia, or low cardiac output.

Capillary density and surface area also influence O_2 extraction (see below), but no data describe developmental differences in these important factors. Based on observations, when O_2 extraction must increase with acute stress, there seems to be no limitation in the young subject, suggesting that there are no large differences in the microcirculation of newborn and mature subjects.

Physiological O_2-supply dependency

When O_2 transport has been reduced progressively under experimental conditions in which demands are kept relatively constant, the response in whole-body O_2 consumption appears to be biphasic (Fig. 10.50). Initially O_2 consumption is constant and independent of O_2 transport. With further reductions in O_2 transport, O_2 consumption becomes dependent on O_2 transport and declines in proportion, a relationship described as **physiological supply dependency**. Experimental studies comparing the effects of hypoxic hypoxia, anemic hypoxia, and stagnant hypoxia suggest a single, critical O_2 transport above which O_2 consumption is independent of transport. This in turn suggests that resting O_2 consumption is equivalent to metabolic demand, whereas the depressed O_2 consumption (below the critical transport) underestimates true demand. Therefore, when

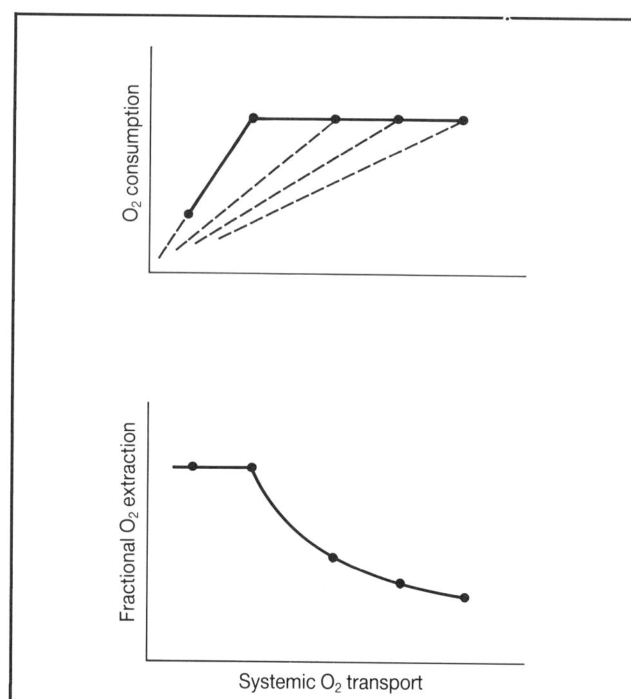

Fig. 10.50. Stylized schema showing the change in O_2 consumption and fractional O_2 extraction as O_2 transport is reduced. Note that O_2 consumption initially remains constant owing to increases in O_2 extraction. O_2 extraction is the instantaneous slope of each point on the top figure, as shown by the dashed lines emanating from the origin. This is typical of the relationships seen in controlled experiments using anesthetized animals during graded reductions in O_2 transport.

O_2 transport is reduced below the critical level, some tissues become hypoxic of necessity. At this point metabolism must be maintained by anaerobiosis or the tissues must decrease metabolic rate, or both. Such a biphasic relationship between O_2 transport and consumption has been demonstrated in intact experimental animals as well as in isolated organs and tissues. Much less evidence is available in intact humans. Although there is no reason to believe that the relationship described in animals is substantially different in humans, this issue has been called into question and is difficult to resolve experimentally in normal subjects.

Effects on metabolic demands

An implicit assumption in studying the effects of changing O_2 transport on O_2 consumption is the maintenance of constant metabolic demands, a condition difficult to ensure in clinical studies. Decreases in O_2 transport may provoke ventilation or cardiac output to increase, raising cardiorespiratory work. Even though this work can be quantified, responding changes in O_2 consumption are not always predictable because the efficiency ([work/*t*]/[energy consumption/*t*]) of these systems can vary widely. When O_2 transport is reduced, other factors increase metabolic demands in a less predictable manner. The release of catecholamines into the circulation or infusion of related drugs with β-adrenergic action can increase O_2 consumption by stimulating thermogenesis. Other drugs may stimulate catecholamines indirectly and produce a similar effect. Finally, if an increase in ventilation (e.g. with hypoxemia) causes alkalemia, this raises whole-body O_2 consumption (as much as 15–20 percent), an effect not related to respiratory work because it occurs with mechanical as well as spontaneous breathing.

On the other hand, some factors decrease metabolic demands when O_2 transport is reduced. For example, if renal blood flow decreases, so does metabolic work of the kidney, because sodium transport (which accounts for 75 percent of renal O_2 consumption at rest) declines. Similarly, metabolic work of the liver, which depends on substrate delivery, decreases if hepatic blood flow is reduced. Thus, for experimental purposes, keeping metabolic demands constant in intact, non-anesthetized subjects as O_2 transport is decreased or increased may be quite difficult.

Matching of flow and metabolism

Fractional O_2 extraction must increase progressively as O_2 transport is reduced if O_2 consumption is to remain constant. The mechanisms by which O_2 extraction increases to maintain O_2 consumption when O_2 transport is disturbed involve regulation of blood flow at both the organ level and in the microcirculation. In general, blood and O_2 flow are distributed to match nutritional demands of the tissue. Such distribution of blood flow occurs both at rest and when metabolic demands are altered. For example, muscle blood flow increases with exercise, and gut blood flow increases following feeding. However, there are important exceptions. Tissues that perform specialized tasks may demand relatively high blood flow. The skin has a high rate of blood flow relative to metabolism because of its importance in heat exchange. The kidney, which is responsible for filtration, also has a very high blood-flow rate relative to its metabolism. Accordingly, both of these organs have relatively low fractional O_2 extractions at rest. The heart and the brain, on the other hand, have low blood-flow rates relative to their metabolic demands and have high fractional extractions at rest. The fractional extraction for the whole body is the flow-weighted average of each organ. When O_2 transport is reduced or metabolic demands are increased, whole-body fractional O_2 extraction is expected to increase in response, as this is a measure of the distribution of O_2 flow relative to demands. Accordingly, in states of limited O_2 supply, a failure of O_2 extraction to increase in response provides strong presumptive evidence of a defect in peripheral O_2 uptake, which could be caused by O_2 consumption–blood flow mismatch (analogous to ventilation/perfusion mismatch in the lung), peripheral arteriovenous shunting, or interference with cellular utilization of O_2.

When O_2 transport is disturbed, overall organ perfusion results from the balance between factors that permit vasodilatation and those that promote vasoconstriction (Fig. 10.51). Three important factors influence organ vascular resistance: the capacity of the organ for autoregulation, the response to neural stimulation, and the response to humoral stimulation. When perfusion pressure to an organ is reduced there can be autoregulation, a simultaneous decrease in vascular resistance that serves to maintain blood flow at its previous level. This vasodilatation and ability to sustain organ perfusion (probably mediated by metabolic feedback) is particularly prominent in the heart, brain,

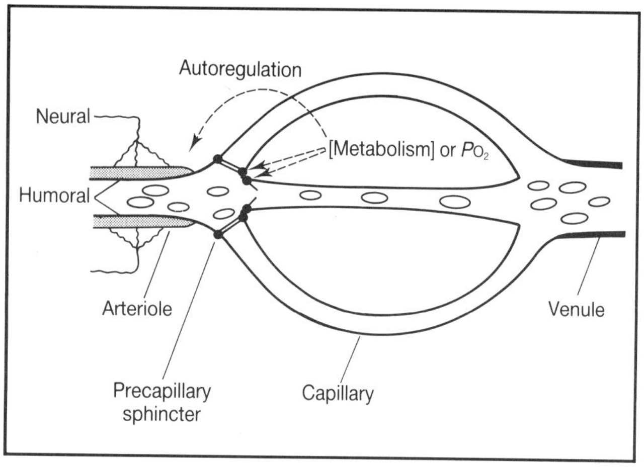

Fig. 10.51. Stylized schema of the microcirculation. This shows that regulation of arterial resistance and flow is governed by neural and humoral factors as well as autoregulation, which is probably regulated by local metabolism. For any given arterial flow, capillaries may be open or closed as regulated by precapillary sphincters, which respond to metabolic factors or local PO_2. Note that the opening of previously closed capillaries reduces distance for diffusion, increases surface area for diffusion, and increases transit time, all of which enhance O_2 extraction.

and kidney, but less important in other organs.

In the intact subject, blood flow is also influenced by an organ's responses to humoral and nervous input that cause vasoconstriction when O_2 transport is limited. Whenever O_2 supply is limited, catecholamines increase, stimulating cardiac contractility and rate and causing peripheral vasoconstriction. In most tissues low cardiac output is accompanied by a local neural release of norepinephrine in response to activation of arterial baroreceptors and cardiopulmonary receptors. In addition, circulating catecholamine concentrations increase in response to chemoreceptor (with anemia and hypoxemia) and baroreceptor (with low cardiac output) activation, which causes the release of epinephrine and norepinephrine from the adrenal medulla. Circulating concentrations of other vasoconstricting hormones also increase. With low cardiac output, renin is released in response to reduced renal blood flow and increased sympathetic stimulation. Renin catalyzes conversion of angiotensinogen to angiotensin I and angiotensin I is hydrolyzed to angiotensin II by angiotensin-converting enzyme. Angiotensin II stimulates the release of aldosterone from the adrenal cortex and vasopressin from the pituitary gland. Vasopressin is also stimulated directly by decreased aortic or atrial pressure. Vasopressin, aldosterone, and angiotensin II are all potent vasoconstrictors. These nervous and humoral responses generally increase regional vascular resistance and divert blood flow away from organs that respond.

Perfusion to a given organ during a reduction in O_2 transport thereby depends on the relative importance of autoregulation, which serves to sustain flow, and the neural and humoral factors, which serve to reduce it. The brain and heart have little sympathetic innervation and are relatively resistant to sympathetic control, whereas the kidney is quite sensitive. Thus, in contrast to the kidney or to other organs that are richly innervated with sympathetic fibers, the brain and heart maintain blood flow during conditions in which O_2 supply is limited. Organs with relatively low resting O_2 extraction (gut, skin, kidney) reduce blood (and O_2) flow relative to demand and increase their fractional extraction as well as that of the whole body when O_2 supply decreases, a response that helps to sustain oxidative metabolism.

Adjustments in the microcirculation

In addition to the alterations in vascular resistance that control organ blood flow, adjustments in the microcirculation enhance O_2 extraction and serve to preserve organ metabolism. These adaptations include the opening of previously closed capillaries and changes in hemoglobin O_2 affinity. Some tissues have precapillary sphincters, which are located at the arterial end of each capillary and maintain the capillary either open or closed. The exact control of these sphincters is not fully understood, although both local metabolic factors and local PO_2 play a role. Whenever the number of perfused capillaries increases, tissues can extract more of the available O_2 via three mechanisms: (1) the increase in capillary density decreases the distance for diffusion between blood and the site of O_2 utilization; (2) the increased number of capillaries increases the lateral surface area for diffusion; and (3) the increase in cross-sectional area of the capillaries reduces the linear velocity of blood and increases transit time for diffusion. These mechanisms permit very high levels of O_2 extraction when O_2 demand is increased or when O_2 supply is curtailed.

In addition to the changes in diffusion as perfusion is altered acutely, H^+ concentration can increase locally, which causes a rightward shift of the O_2 dissociation curve (Fig. 10.49) and permits more unloading of O_2 from hemoglobin (for any given venous blood PO_2, venous O_2 saturation is lower). However, because arterial blood pH is more alkaline than venous blood pH and PaO_2 is on the flat part of the O_2 dissociation curve, O_2 loading usually is not compromised by acidemia. Normally hemoglobin O_2 affinity differs between arterial and venous blood because of the differences in H^+ and CO_2 concentrations in the two circulations. In a state of low O_2 transport this difference is exaggerated, which generally enhances O_2 extraction at the periphery as an acute adaptation. With the marked intraorgan differences in flow relative to metabolism, the shift in the dissociation curve may vary widely.

In addition to this acute shift in hemoglobin O_2 affinity, the O_2 dissociation curve may be affected by changes in the concentration of DPG if the disturbance in O_2 transport is sustained. The concentration of DPG is regulated primarily by the red cell H^+ concentration because the rate-limiting enzyme is pH sensitive. A high pH stimulates DPG synthesis. Because deoxyhemoglobin provides better buffering than oxyhemoglobin and thereby raises red cell pH relative to plasma pH, the low venous O_2 concentration in any form of chronic hypoxia can promote DPG synthesis. However, this adaptive mechanism is less prominent in young infants with fetal hemoglobin, which binds DPG poorly, because synthesis is inhibited by unbound DPG.

Specific disturbances in O_2 transport

Low cardiac output

When cardiac output is reduced abruptly, systemic O_2 transport decreases in parallel because there is little or no change in hemoglobin concentration. Therefore, an increase in O_2 extraction (decrease in $P\bar{v}O_2$) provides the only acute mechanism for sustaining oxidative metabolism. Under some circumstances a reduction in blood flow may even be more disruptive to metabolism than anemia or hypoxemia because it limits the supply of substrates other than O_2 and there may be accumulation of metabolites, which can alter substrate utilization. In experimental animals, cardiac output can be reduced acutely by about 50 percent before there are signs of tissue hypoxia, but this tolerance depends on the hemoglobin concentration; with anemia, the tolerance is less than when the hemoglobin concentration is higher.

When cardiac output is reduced chronically, DPG can increase, which will increase P_{50} and O_2 extraction and restore $P\bar{v}O_2$ towards normal. However, if systemic acidemia persists, this can decrease red cell pH, inhibit DPG synthesis, and interfere with this important hematological adaptation. There is no evidence that a low cardiac output stimulates hemoglobin synthesis even though erythropoietin production is presumably stimulated by low renal venous blood PO_2. It has been suggested that reduced renal blood flow decreases renal O_2 consumption, thereby restoring renal venous blood PO_2 towards normal.

Anemia

When hemoglobin concentration is reduced acutely, cardiac output and O_2 extraction increase. Therefore, O_2 transport does not decrease in proportion to the decline in hemoglobin. In intact animals an isovolemic decrease in hematocrit to the range of 15 percent is tolerated without signs of tissue hypoxia as long as the augmentation of cardiac output can occur. Cardiac output increases with *anemia* because cardiac contractility and heart rate are stimulated by catecholamines and the decrease in blood viscosity reduces vascular resistance. Thus, cardiac output may increase quite significantly at low hematocrit concentrations.

When anemia is sustained, the O_2 dissociation curve shifts to the right, which permits venous O_2 saturation to be quite low and O_2 extraction to be quite high even though $P\bar{v}O_2$ returns towards normal. With anemia there may also be an increase in plasma volume, which helps to increase cardiac output further by increasing stroke volume. Despite these adaptations, the problems of decreased O_2-carrying capacity may be compounded if red cell deformability is abnormal as with *iron deficiency* and *sickle cell disease,* both of which interfere with microcirculatory flow and have been implicated as causes of vascular occlusion and strokes.

Hypoxemia

The response to hypoxemia depends in part on the method used to produce the disturbance. With alveolar hypoxia, O_2 extraction increases and cardiac output

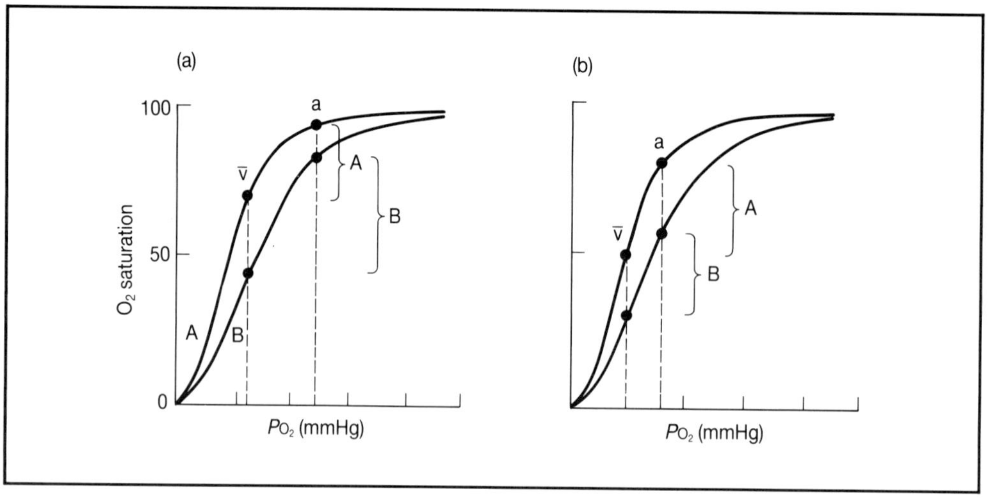

Fig. 10.52. The effect of a shift in the O_2 dissociation curve on O_2 unloading with alveolar hypoxia. The height of the brackets indicates the quantity of O_2 unloaded by hemoglobin. (a) With mild alveolar hypoxia, a shift to the right enhances O_2 unloading while it produces less impairment of O_2 loading. The reason is that the PaO_2 is fixed by the alveolar PO_2, which is on a less steep part of the curve than the mixed venous point ($\bar{v}$). Therefore, the arteriovenous O_2 saturation difference is greater with curve B than curve A. (b) With more severe alveolar hypoxia, both alveolar and arterial PO_2 are very low and both the arterial and mixed venous points are on a steep part of the curve. Hence, in this case the arteriovenous venous O_2 saturation difference is smaller with the right-shifted curve.

increases somewhat, although less so than with a comparable decline in CaO_2 produced by anemia. Part of the contrast relates to the reduced viscosity with anemia and the limitation of systemic blood flow with alveolar hypoxia owing to the increase in pulmonary vascular resistance, which restricts right ventricular output. The concentration of inspired O_2 that is tolerated before there is evidence of tissue hypoxia varies widely with age, species, size, and ambient environment, but in young subjects O_2 consumption usually decreases when inspired O_2 concentration is near 10 percent. However, when neonates are placed in a cool environment (stimulating metabolic demands), even mild alveolar hypoxia can decrease O_2 consumption, which is in contrast to observations in neutral thermal environment.

When hypoxemia is sustained chronically, two important hematological adjustments occur: hemoglobin synthesis increases, and the O_2 dissociation curve shifts. In the presence of hypoxemia from either alveolar hypoxia or from intracardiac shunt, there is an inverse relationship between the hemoglobin concentration and the arterial O_2 saturation, which keeps CaO_2 nearly constant. However, the polycythemia may limit the anticipated augmentation in cardiac output and, when severe, can cause systemic O_2 transport to decrease.

The utility of a change in P_{50} to enhance extraction of O_2 from venous blood depends on the degree to which O_2 loading of arterial blood is affected simultaneously (Fig. 10.52). With anemia or low cardiac output, arterial and pulmonary capillary blood PO_2 are high and O_2 loading occurs on the flat part of the O_2 dissociation curve; thus, there is a large increase in extraction with a rightward shift of the dissociation curve (little decrease in SaO_2 but a marked decrease in $S\bar{v}O_2$). With arterial hypoxemia the effects of the shift in the curve are more complex. If there is alveolar hypoxia, then a rightward shift of the dissociation curve may interfere with O_2 loading; whether a rightward or leftward curve is beneficial depends on the severity of the alveolar hypoxia. In general, rightward shift in the dissociation curve enhances O_2 unloading with mild alveolar hypoxia, and leftward shift enhances unloading with severe alveolar hypoxia. In contrast, with shunt hypoxemia, as occurs with cardiac disease, pulmonary capillary blood PO_2 remains relatively high, and a rightward shift to the dissociation curve interferes minimally with O_2 loading and increases O_2 unloading at the periphery. Accordingly, patients with congenital cardiac disease causing hypoxemia usually have an increase in P_{50} except shortly after birth, whereas the response in subjects with alveolar hypoxia varies.

Metabolic responses

In all subjects the final evidence of impairment of O_2 transport is a disturbance in cellular energy metabolism. When O_2 transport is inadequate, insufficient O_2 is available for oxidative phosphorylation. The electron transport chain slows, the rate of phosphorylation of adenosine diphosphate (ADP) to adenosine triphosphate (ATP) is decreased, and cytochromes remain in the reduced state. There is also an increase in the concentration of adenosine monophosphate (AMP), which is rapidly catabolized to inosine and hypoxanthine during hypoxia. Thus, the state of phosphorylation of the nucleotides, the presence of products of catabolism, and the redox state of one or more of the cytochromes provide inferential information about the state of tissue oxygenation. The tissues of some organs, particularly skeletal muscle, and to some extent brain and heart, can synthesize ATP for brief periods by transferring a high-energy phosphate to ATP. In the presence of the enzyme creatine kinase, creatine phosphate serves as an energy reservoir during hypoxic stress, but such a resource is rapidly depleted.

ADP can also be phosphorylated anaerobically during hypoxia when O_2 supply is reduced, but this is considerably less efficient than aerobic metabolism in terms of moles of ATP per mole glucose. Furthermore, with anaerobic metabolism, lactic acid accumulates in tissues and in venous blood, thereby decreasing serum as well as tissue pH. Each of the metabolic changes has been used as a sign of inadequate tissue oxygenation, although the utility of any one measure depends on experimental conditions and the specific tissue.

More subtle signs of tissue hypoxia are difficult to quantify, but one clear finding in the child with chronic hypoxia is *failure to thrive*. Thus, growth failure of the fetus or the infant is a common consequence of chronic hypoxia, whether produced by hypoxemia, anemia, or limited cardiac output. This finding is strong evidence that adaptation has failed.

Summary

The aim here has been to demonstrate the functioning of a highly integrated system that readily tolerates acute and chronic changes in metabolic demands by adjusting the rate of O_2 transport and extraction. As has been emphasized, disruption in any component of O_2 transport demands quick adaptive changes in other parts of the system. However, any reserve may be exhausted rapidly when such adaptations are disturbed. An infant with cyanotic congenital cardiac disease may maintain sufficient O_2 transport to grow and be active because of an increased cardiac output, increased O_2 extraction, and increased hemoglobin concentration. However, tissue hypoxia may rapidly ensue when cardiac output is compromised, metabolic demands increase, or there is even a mild reduction in hematocrit.

Selected reading

Cain SM. Peripheral oxygen uptake and delivery in health and disease. *Clin Chest Med* 1983; **4**: 139.

Finch CA, Lenfant C. Oxygen transport in man. *N Engl J Med* 1972; **286**: 407.

Lister G, Fahey JT. Oxygen transport. In Chernick V, Mellins RB, eds. *Mechanisms of pediatric respiratory disease: cellular and integrative*. Philadelphia: BC Decker, 1991: 129.

Lister G, Moreau G, Moss M, Talner NS. Effects of alterations of oxygen transport on the neonate. *Semin Perinatol* 1984; **8**: 192.

Schumacker PT, Samsel RW. Oxygen supply and consumption in the adult respiratory distress syndrome. *Clin Chest Med* 1990; **11**: 715.

J. Electrophysiology

G F Van Hare

Impulse formation

Cardiac impulses are formed by cardiac cells that exhibit 'pacemaker activity', or **spontaneous automaticity**. In adults, such cells are found primarily in the sinus and atrioventricular nodes, and to a lesser extent in atrial muscle and the His–Purkinje (distal conducting) system. **Action potentials** recorded from these cells by micro-puncture techniques differ from action potentials recorded from cells in other parts of the heart in several respects (Fig. 10.53). They have a slower rate of rise (phase 0) than action potentials recorded elsewhere, as well as a shorter plateau phase (phase 3). They are known as 'slow-response' potentials, in contrast to 'fast-response' potentials recorded elsewhere. When they are not being overdriven by another source of repetitive stimulation, slow-response cells exhibit a gradual rise in trans-membrane potential during electrical diastole (phase 4) until the threshold potential is reached, giving rise to an action potential. This spontaneous diastolic depolarization is mediated by various ionic mechanisms depending on the location of the cell, and is the origin of normal **pacemaker activity** in the heart.

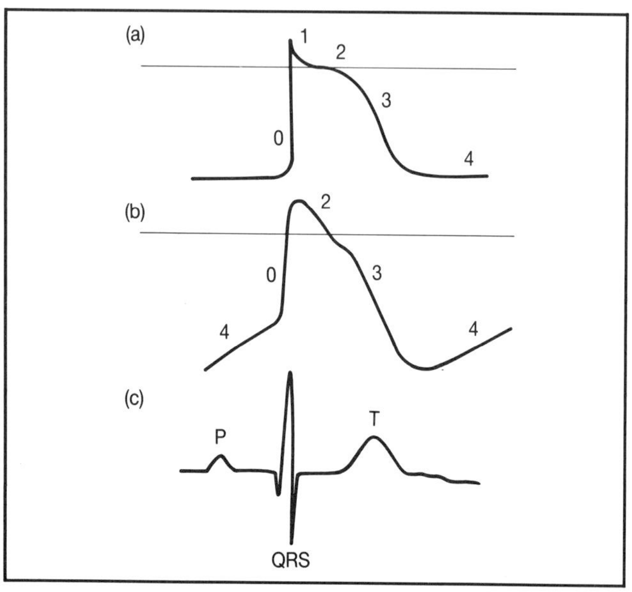

Fig. 10.53. Cardiac action potential. Numbers correspond to the phases of the action potential. (a) Fast-response cells (atrial and ventricular myocardium). (b) Slow-response cells (sinus and atrioventricular nodes). (c) Surface electrocardiogram.

Spontaneous cardiac electrical activity begins very early in embryological development, by 35 hours in the chick embryo. Rhythmic contractions are first observed in the embryonic ventricle, and pacemaker potentials may be recorded in nearly all ventricular cells early in gestation. Very quickly, however, these cells lose their capability for normal automaticity, and the site of cardiac activation shifts to the developing atrium.

The **sinus node** develops quite early as a well demarcated structure at the junction of the right atrium and superior vena cava. This cluster of cardiac cells becomes progressively more compact with further fetal development. It is made up of normal working atrial myocardial cells, a second cell type termed 'typical nodal cells' or 'P cells', and finally 'transitional cells', which are found mainly at the margins of the sinus node. P cells are thought to be primarily responsible for sinus node automaticity, and transitional cells may be important in providing excellent contact with the working atrial myocardium. In addition, the sinus node is well invested with a collagenous matrix that separates cells from one another. While fibrosis of the sinus node has been reported with age, this probably represents loss of sinus node cells rather than the formation of new fibrous tissue.

While sinus node automaticity is mainly responsible for the heart rate, automaticity (at lower rates) may occur in cells lower in the cardiac conduction system, if allowed to 'escape' from overdrive suppression by the sinus node. This may occur in individuals with sinus node disease in response to increased vagal tone or certain drugs, or because of congenital or acquired atrioventricular block (Table 10.3). This escape automaticity is normal and adaptive. In the presence of diseases such as myocarditis or following surgery, abnormal automaticity may develop in any part of the heart, and this abnormal automaticity produces rates that are higher than the escape rates found higher in the conducting system. These sites of abnormal automaticity overdrive other foci.

Impulse propagation

Cardiac muscle cells have the ability to pass electrical impulses to adjacent cells via **gap junctions**, specialized structures that make the cytosol of adjacent cardiac cells electrically continuous. Cardiac muscle is not a syncytium; the cells maintain their cell membranes. However, these specialized cell-to-cell connections allow cardiac muscle to function electrically as a syncytium. An action potential that spreads down one cardiac cell will be passed easily to adjacent cardiac cells, leading to propagation throughout the heart. While cardiac muscle may be viewed as an electrical syncytium, recent evidence suggests this view is overly simplistic. Instead of homogenous conduction in all directions, as one would expect with a syncytial model, in fact propagation is known to be more rapid along the long axis of cardiac cells than along the transverse axis. This property, known as 'anisotropic conduction', reflects greater axial than longitudinal resistivity. Collagenous septa, oriented longitudinally and acting as insulators, may be largely responsible for this difference, along with other factors. These characteristics may lead to discontinuous and heterogeneous conduction, and anisotropic conduction has been hypothesized as an important factor in the genesis of lethal *ventricular arrhythmias*.

Micropuncture studies in fetal and newborn preparations have shown age-related changes in action potential characteristics in several species, including chicks, rats, and canines. There is a gradual increase in negativity of the resting potential from the time the heart beat is first established; in many species, this increase continues into adulthood. The increasing negativity of the resting potential is thought to be due to increasing permeability to K^+ with development, as well as to increasing activity of Na^+-K^+-ATPase.

The velocity of impulse propagation in cardiac muscle depends on a number of factors, including fiber orientation, passive properties of cardiac muscle such as membrane excitability threshold, resistance, and capacitance, and active properties related to the action potential. The most important of these factors is the rate of rise of phase 0 of the action potential, also known as dV/dT or $\dot{V}_{max}$. **Conduction velocity** is directly related to the magnitude of $\dot{V}_{max}$, and factors that affect $\dot{V}_{max}$ also affect conduction velocity.

Table 10.3. Escape rates for intrinsic cardiac pacemaker foci

	0–1 month	1 year	5 years	Adults
Sinus node	90–180	90–150	65–135	60–120
Atrioventricular node	80–90			40–70
Ventricle	30–70			25–50

Phase 0 of the action potential occurs when the transmembrane potential is increased from its resting negative value to its excitability threshold. In fast-response cells, this results in the opening of voltage-sensitive **Na^+ channels** and the rapid entry of positively charged Na^+ ions, and the further increase in the membrane potential toward 0 potential. The Na^+ channel is time dependent and inactivates, allowing other ionic mechanisms eventually to return the membrane potential to its resting potential. Phase 0 corresponds to the QRS complex on the surface electrocardiogram. Phase 1 (early repolarization) occurs due to Na^+ channel inactivation, but also due to a transient outward K^+ current. This is not well seen in slow-response cells. During phase 2 (plateau), membrane conductance is low with respect to all ions, but Na^+-K^+-ATPase and an inward Ca^{2+} current are active. Rapid repolarization occurs during phase 3 and is quite complex. Both time-dependent and voltage-dependent outward K^+ currents are active, and the inward Ca^{2+} current is inactivated, returning the cell to a negative resting potential. In addition, other K^+ channels important in repolarization have been described; they are sensitive to acetylcholine, adenosine triphosphate, and Na^+. The end of phase 3 roughly corresponds to the refractory period of the cell as well as the occurrence of the T wave on the surface electrocardiogram. Finally, in pacemaker cells, phase 4 depolarization occurs. In the sinus node, it is mediated by the inactivation of a repolarizing outward K^+ current, as well as the slow recovery of the inward Ca^{2+} current.

Fast Na^+ channels may be studied using micropuncture techniques, and may be blocked using tetrodotoxin. *Antiarrhythmic agents* with class 1 antiarrhythmic activity, such as procainamide and quinidine, are thought to exert their effects by blocking fast Na^+ channels, therefore slowing the rate of rise of phase 0 and consequently decreasing conduction velocity.

Studies using tetrodotoxin in embryonic chick hearts have shown that these fast Na^+ channels are not present initially. Before they appear, phase 0 of the action potential is mediated by an inward Na^+ current carried by slow-response tetrodotoxin-insensitive Na^+ channels. V_{max} is much lower, and the amplitude of the action potential is lower as well. Tetrodotoxin-sensitive Na^+ channels appear at about 5 days of gestation in the chick heart, and there is a transitional period when both slow and fast Na^+ channels are present. By 8 days of gestation, all Na^+ channels are tetrodotoxin-sensitive. It is not clear whether the same phenomenon exists in other species; tetrodotoxin-insensitive slow Na^+ channels have not been found in canines studied at an early gestational age, nor in human fetuses at 7 weeks.

In slow-response cells like those found in the sinus and atrioventricular node, the upstroke of the action potential, and therefore the velocity of conduction, is much lower than in fast-response cells found elsewhere. Phase 0 of the action potential is not mediated by the opening of fast Na^+ channels, but instead by the slow inward Ca^{2+} current.

In normal sinus rhythm, the **spread of cardiac excitation** proceeds from the sinus node through the atrial muscle to excite both right and left atria (Fig. 10.54). Excitation reaches the atrioventricular node by way of cell-to-cell intra-atrial conduction. Three specialized internodal tracts were once thought to be responsible for conduction directly from sinus to atrioventricular node. However, careful histological studies have failed to find evidence of specialized conduction tissue. The previously described internodal tracts currently are thought instead to be simply preferred routes for intra-atrial conduction, made up of normal atrial myocardial cells.

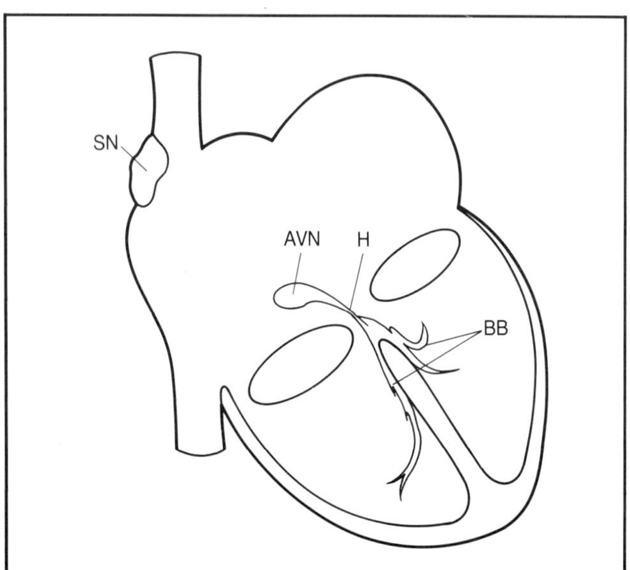

Fig. 10.54. Cardiac conduction system. Abbreviations: AVN, atrioventricular node; BB, bundle branches; H, bundle of His; SN, sinus node.

The **atrioventricular node** is an atrial structure lying at the apex of the triangle of Koch and delineated by three landmarks: the tendon of Todaro (continuous with the eustachian valve), the mouth of the coronary sinus, and the tricuspid valve annulus. The atrioventricular node gives rise to a bundle (**bundle of His**) that penetrates the central fibrous body, then divides to form the left and right bundle branches, made up of Purkinje cells. The atrioventricular node is made up of slow-response cells that are histologically similar to those found in the sinus node. The slower upstroke of the action potential in the atrioventricular node is associated with a lower conduction velocity than elsewhere in the heart, and the atrioventricular node is responsible for introducing a significant delay between atrial and ventricular contraction.

Nodal conduction time is age related. Little is known about conduction time in the node in fetal life. However, **nodal conduction** time may be measured clinically by recording the atrial electrogram at the approaches to the atrioventricular node, and the His electrogram. The 'AH interval' (atrial–His bundle) is a measure of atrioventricular nodal conduction. Normally quite short at birth (20–40 ms), the AH interval increases progressively with age to as long as 200 ms in adulthood. Conduction in the distal conducting system (His bundle and bundle branches) may also be measured by timing the 'HV' interval, i.e. the time from His bundle activation to earliest ventricular activation on the surface electrocardiogram. The HV interval, normally 20 ms at birth, increases to 40–50 ms in adulthood.

In addition to introducing a delay, the atrioventricular node also limits the number of atrial impulses that may conduct to the ventricles. This function is adaptive; arrhythmias such as *atrial flutter* or *atrial fibrillation* occur with atrial rates as high as 500–600 beats per minute. **Refractoriness** in the atrioventricular node limits the resulting ventricular rate. Refractoriness is also age dependent. In late fetal life and in the newborn period, the atrioventricular node may conduct atrial rates as high as 300 beats per minute without block; however, with increasing age, atrioventricular block occurs at progressively slower atrial rates. Atrioventricular node refractoriness is also quite sensitive to autonomic influences.

Regulation of impulse formation and propagation

While both cardiac automaticity and conduction are under autonomic control, various other mechanisms may affect heart rate and conduction velocity. For example, both automaticity and conduction velocity increase with increasing temperature, acidity, and carbon dioxide, and with decreasing O_2.

The adult heart is well invested with nerve fibers, and both the **sympathetic** and **parasympathetic** nervous systems influence cardiac automaticity and conduction. While sympathetic fibers reach the sinus node, atrioventricular node, bundle branches, and atrial and ventricular myocardium, vagal fibers are more limited in distribution, affecting mainly the atrial myocardium and the sinus and atrioventricular nodes. However, innervation of the ventricles by the vagus is limited, and vagal stimulation can lead to mild decreases in ventricular contractility.

Sympathetic fibers, when stimulated, release norepinephrine, which acts on local β-receptors, enhancing the activity of adenylyl cyclase and converting ATP to cyclic AMP, the 'second messenger'. Most norepinephrine is then taken up by the sympathetic terminals to be released again, and a small amount is metabolized. Sympathetic stimulation leads to increased automaticity of both the sinus and atrioventricular nodes, shortening of refractory periods and conduction times through the atrioventricular node, and shortening of refractory periods in both atrial and ventricular myocardium. Fast Na^+ channels do not appear to be regulated by autonomic influences or catecholamines. Calcium channels, on the other hand, are under β-adrenergic control, mediated by a cAMP-dependent protein kinase. Sympathetic stimulation, of course, may have a host of other effects on the circulation, including increased contractility, changes in blood pressure, and effects on the coronary circulation.

Parasympathetic fibers innervating the heart release acetylcholine when stimulated. Cardiac cholinergic receptors are muscarinic in type. Activation of these receptors produces effects that, in general, are the opposite of effects produced by sympathetic stimulation. Therefore, decreases in sinus and atrioventricular node automaticity and increases in atrioventricular node conduction time are demonstrable.

Sympathetic and parasympathetic effects on the heart are age related, and change during fetal and postnatal development. The two opposing influences may develop at different rates during fetal life, but the results of investigations in this area are quite species specific. In sheep, sympathetic effects on the circulation probably appear before parasympathetic effects, but development of both is probably complete by 12 weeks of gestation. In contrast, sympathetic development is not complete at birth in canines, rats, and primates including humans. In these species, heart rate is thought to be primarily under vagal control at the time of birth. Differences in responsiveness to nerve stimulation are not thought to be due to lack of adrenergic or cholinergic receptor activity in the heart. In fact, compared with adults, fetuses appear supersensitive to the effects of infused norepinephrine, isoproterenol, and acetylcholine.

In species that exhibit incomplete sympathetic innervation of the heart at birth, postnatal maturation takes place. Such maturation may be nonuniform and may follow an irregular pattern of progression, as shown by experimental nerve stimulation in puppies. Adrenergic stimulation has been demonstrated to shorten ventricular action potential duration and refractory periods dramatically. Left stellate stimulation, or right stellate removal, is known to lower the threshold for ventricular fibrillation and to prolong the QT interval, and right stellate stimulation, or left stellate removal, raises the threshold. Conceivably, a developmental heterogeneity of sympathetic innervation may create a period of **electrical instability** due to dispersion of refractoriness, when stress and increased sympathetic activity may lead to *ventricular arrhythmias*. Schwartz was the first to propose the idea that autonomic instability could lead to ventricular arrhythmias and subsequently to *SIDS*. There is evidence that abnormalities in the relationship between the QT interval and heart rate changes are detectable in at least some infants who later developed SIDS.

Selected reading

Kralios FA, Millar CK. Functional development of cardiac sympathetic nerves in newborn dogs: evidence for asymmetrical development. *Cardiovasc Res* 1978; **12**: 547.

Mizeres NJ. The anatomy of the autonomic nervous system in the dog. *Am J Anat* 1955; **96**: 285.

Reder RF, Miura DS, Danilo P, Rosen MR. The electrophysiological properties of normal neonatal and adult canine cardiac fibers. *Circ Res* 1981; **48**: 658.

Schwartz PJ. Cardiac sympathetic innervation and the sudden infant death syndrome. *Am J Med* 1976; **6**: 167.

Schwartz PJ, Snebold NG, Brown AM. Effects of unilateral cardiac sympathetic denervation on the ventricular fibrillation threshold. *Am J Cardiol* 1976; **37**: 1034.

Yanowitz F, Preston JB, Abildskov AJ. Functional distribution of right and left stellate innervation to the ventricles. *Circ Res* 1966; **18**: 416.

11 • *Respiratory system*

Editor: Samuel Hawgood

A. STRUCTURE AND FUNCTION

A1. Lung Development

M Post

Embryogenesis

Lung development can be subdivided into five stages: (1) embryonic period—development of major airways; (2) pseudoglandular period—development of airways to terminal bronchioles; (3) canalicular period—development of the acinus and vascularization; (4) terminal sac (saccular) period—subdivision of saccules by secondary crests; and (5) alveolar period—the appearance of alveoli.

Airways and alveoli

Embryonic period

The lung originates from a diverticulum of the ventral wall of the caudal end of the laryngotracheal tube, which divides into two knob-like bronchial buds at 3–4 weeks of gestation. Outgrowth of these buds into the splanchnic mesenchyme produces the left and right primary bronchi. Each primary bronchial bud divides monopodially to give rise to a lateral diverticulum or bud; subsequently, the right lung bud gives origin on its craniodorsal side to a second monopodial diverticulum. Each secondary bronchus is a stem bronchus that will be a lobar bronchus. These stem bronchi are destined to branch and rebranch and, with the surrounding pulmonary mesenchyme, which will provide the elastic tissue, smooth muscles, cartilage, vascular system and other connective tissues, will give origin to the definitive pulmonary lobes that characterize adult lung organization.

Pseudoglandular period

In the pseudoglandular period (6–16 weeks of gestation), the tracheobronchial tree of the fetal lung resembles a system of branching tubules that terminate in exocrine gland-like structures. These tubules are lined by distinct epithelium composed of columnar, or approximately cuboidal, cells and are surrounded by mesenchyme.

Canalicular period

During this period (16–28 weeks of gestation), the gas-exchanging portion of the lung becomes delineated with the appearance of new tubular branches, the respiratory bronchioles. Each respiratory bronchiole terminates in two or three thin-walled dilatations called terminal sacs or primitive alveoli.

Terminal sac period

The terminal sac period (28–36 weeks of gestation) is characterized by further differentiation of the respiratory portion of the lung; respiratory bronchioles rapidly subdivide into an array of thin-walled primitive alveolar ducts and primitive alveoli. The saccules contain both cuboidal and flat types of alveolar epithelial cells, type II and type I epithelial cells, respectively. By the end of the terminal sac period, the organization pattern of the respiratory portion of the lung is complete.

Alveolar period

This period (32 weeks to term and postnatally in humans) is marked by the appearance of the alveoli, lined with extremely thin squamous type I cells. These type I cells become so thin that the underlying capillaries bulge into the space of each terminal sac. By the late fetal period, the lungs are capable of respiration because the alveolar capillary membrane is sufficiently thin to allow gas exchange.

Vasculature

During the first month of gestation, a vascular plexus (originating from the splanchnic plexus) forms within the lung bud, which receives its blood supply both from primitive pulmonary arteries as well as from a pair of branches from the dorsal aorta. Subsequently, numerous paired dorsal intersegmental arteries supply the vascular plexus, but by the end of the fifth week of gestation, as the true pulmonary arteries form and unite with the vascular plexus, the 'primitive' pulmonary arteries become incorporated into the sixth aortic arch and the intersegmental arteries involute. The bronchial arteries develop only after the ninth week of gestation; they supply the bronchi down to a level several generations proximal to the terminal bronchioli.

Differentiation of true intrapulmonary arteries within the vascular plexus occurs at the same time as the airways develop so that by the sixteenth week of gestation, all preacinar branches are present: both the conventional arteries that run alongside the airways and the supernumerary arteries that provide additional blood supply to the alveolar region. After the sixteenth week of gestation the preacinar arteries increase mainly in diameter and length, and the intra-acinar arteries begin to form along the developing acinus (i.e. the primitive alveolar ducts and alveoli).

The pulmonary veins develop from an outgrowth of the left atrium. These structures start as a blind chamber that grows posteriorly to contact the lung buds; it bifurcates, and by the eleventh week of gestation, four separate veins enter the left atrial chamber. The veins within the lung develop at the same time as the arteries so that all preacinar veins are also present halfway through gestation. The conventional veins branch at right angles to the arteries, and there are many supernumerary veins as well. At 20 weeks of gestation, all the veins are nonmuscular, but by 28 weeks, scattered muscle bundles appear.

Tissue interactions

In the embryonic lung, branching of the epithelium is controlled by epithelial–mesenchymal tissue interactions. The mesenchymal component dictates the branching pattern of the epithelium, and the inductive capacity of the mesenchyme is organ- and species-specific. Forces within the epithelial cells themselves alter cell and tissue shape to produce branch points. Extracellular matrix proteins at the epithelial–mesenchymal interface, such as proteoglycans, laminin and collagen, may act as morphogenetic factors controlling the organ- and species-specific pattern of lung branching.

Prenatal growth

As is evident from the preceding section, fetal lung morphogenesis involves major structural changes that are associated with cell proliferation as well as with cell differentiation. The following section summarizes current knowledge of prenatal lung growth.

Physical factors

Increasing evidence suggests that a variety of physical factors influence normal fetal lung growth. These include the amount of amniotic and lung fluid, available space for lung in the thorax, and fetal respiration. How these factors affect lung growth remains to be defined, but the available evidence strongly supports the concept that stretch is an important stimulus for lung growth.

Hormonal factors

Hormones such as glucocorticoids, androgen, thyroid hormone, and insulin affect lung differentiation. Current data, however, suggest that they play no important role in normal fetal lung growth.

Growth factors

Growth factors are a group of small molecular weight (8–40 kDa) polypeptides that regulate the proliferation of cells by inducing DNA synthesis and cell division. Such growth factors have been isolated from a variety of sources including tissue, serum, plasma and conditioned medium from cell cultures. Of the known growth factors, epidermal growth factor (EGF), the somatomedins or insulin-like growth factors (IGFs), and platelet derived growth factor (PDGF) are best defined. Each interacts with target cells through specific cell-surface receptors leading to DNA synthesis. PDGF, EGF, and IGF are present in the fetal lung, and it seems likely that these growth factors mediate the effects of physical factors on cellular proliferation.

Lung cell growth

Lung cell proliferation is confined mainly to morphogenetically active regions, which shift from central to peripheral tubules during development. The rate of proliferation of both epithelial and mesenchymal cells decreases during development, but the decline is unequal. The proportion of dividing cells that are epithelial increases initially during fetal development but declines dramatically near term. The decline in epithelial mitotic activity is associated with an increase in cellular differentiation that occurs in the course of lung morphogenesis. Unlike epithelial cells, the proportion of dividing cells that are mesenchymal decreases in the earlier stages of development, but mesenchymal proliferation increases sharply at the canalicular phase of development because of capillary growth. The capillary formation continues at a rapid rate during late fetal life and, consequently, mesenchymal cells are the predominant dividing cell type near term. The period of alveolarization is accompanied by a phase of rapid cellular proliferation in both epithelial and mesenchymal lung populations. Interstitial fibroblasts proliferate actively early in the period but then slow down, whereas endothelial cell growth is brisk throughout this period. The dividing endothelial and interstitial cells are primarily located in septal crests. Epithelial cell division in this period occurs on septal buds and walls. Both alveolar epithelial cell populations, type II and type I cells, increase during this growth period. However, only alveolar epithelial type II cells proliferate actively, indicating that alveolar type I cells arise from type II cells.

Mesenchymal–epithelial interactions

As mentioned above, the mechanism(s) controlling the ontogenic pattern of lung cell proliferation remains yet to be elucidated. However, it is well known that bronchial epithelial growth is stimulated by bronchial mesenchyme. Embryonic bronchial mesenchyme seems to have the ability to maintain most or all of the epithelial cells at the branching points in the cell cycle, thereby stimulating epithelial budding. The nature of mesenchymal-induced stimulation of epithelial growth is yet unknown.

Differentiation

Epithelium

Type II cells

The commitment of apparently undifferentiated respiratory epithelium to subsequent expression of the type II cell phenotype occurs prior to 13 days of gestation in the fetal rat lung and is dependent upon epithelial–mesenchymal interactions (Fig. 11.1a).

Once the future type II cell is committed to its phenotypic pathway, glycogen deposition precedes lamellar body formation. At the appropriate developmental stage, the synthesis of glycogen in the alveolar epithelium is regulated by corticosteroids, which requires the presence of mesenchyme. Later, the onset of lamellar body formation is associated with glycogen breakdown. Significant quantities of surfactant are not synthesized until close to term. The fine regulation of this quantitative progression in expression of phenotype is under multi-hormonal control, yet local cell and tissue interactions continue to modulate the endocrine signals.

Hormonal factors

A central role in epithelial type II cell maturation is played by endogenous fetal glucocorticoids. They are largely in the inactive form (cortisone), but in the fetal lung fibroblast are 'activated' by reduction at the eleventh carbon to cortisol. Once activated, the glucocorticoid also acts directly within the fibroblast to induce the production of fibroblast-pneumonocyte factor (FPF) (Fig. 11.1c and Fig. 11.2), which in turn acts upon the adjacent type II cell to induce surfactant phospholipid synthesis. The elaboration of FPF in response to glucocorticoid is inhibited in the presence of insulin and androgen. Thyroid hormones increase the responsiveness of fetal type II cells for FPF (Fig. 11.2).

Alveolar type I cells

The alveolar epithelial type I cell is the attenuated alveolar lining cell across which gas exchange takes place. This phenotype appears quite late in development, in keeping with its terminally differentiated state. Its embryonic precursor is the alveolar type II cell. As the appearance of the type I cell occurs at the time that the mesenchyme is regressing and the vascular cells are coming to lie in closer approximation to the alveolar epithelium, it is tempting to speculate that the phenotypic conversion from type II cell to type I cell could be induced by endothelial interactions (or withdrawal of fibroblast interactions).

Vascular cells

The development of blood vessels in the lung (angiogenesis) most likely depends upon a coordinated set of stimulatory and inhibitory signals from a variety of interstitial and blood-borne cell types (see Section 10.A1). The vascular cells themselves contribute. The signals include insulin-like growth factors, interferon-γ, proteins with a high affinity for heparin such as acidic and basic fibroblast growth factors, and the transforming growth factors α and β. The growth and angiogenic factors induce proteolytic activity, which alters basement membrane and other connective tissue proteins. This stimulates not only cell migration and proliferation, but also the elaboration of a different matrix, which may then have an inhibitory or 'stop' action on the proliferating cells and induce proliferation or differentiation of another cell type. Subtle changes in the extracellular protein milieu probably contribute to specialization of vascular cells, and flow patterns ultimately determine whether a vessel is destined to be a capillary, an artery, or a vein. The whole process, while very active in the developing lung, must be held in check after it is completed.

Selected reading

Bernfield M, Banerjee SD, Koda JE, Rapraeger AC. Remodeling of the basement membrane as a mechanism of morphogenetic tissue interaction. In Trelstad RL, ed. *The role of extracellular matrix in development*. New York: Liss, 1984: 545.

Karkinen-Jaakelainen M, Saxen L, Weiss L. *Cell interactions in development.* New York: Academic Press, 1977.

Post M, Van Golde LMG. Metabolic and developmental

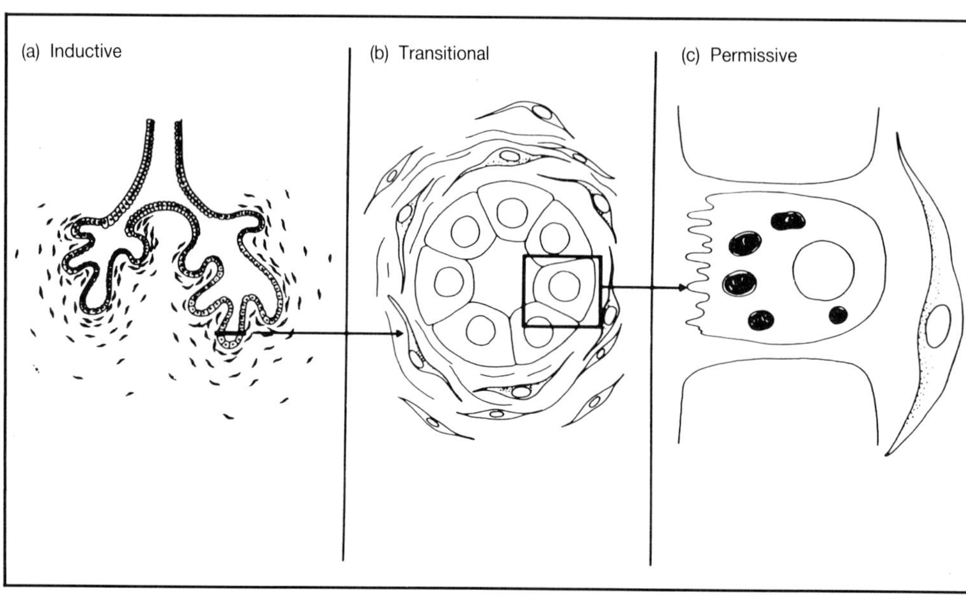

Fig. 11.1. Schematic representation of the time and nature of mesenchymal–epithelial interactions during the organogenesis and differentiation of lung parenchyma. (a) Represents the role of mesenchyme in directing the branching of epithelium and in establishing the future phenotype of the alveolar type II cell. As these involve expression of new gene products, these represent inductive influences. (b) Represents the acquisition of glucocorticoid receptors by mesenchymal cells closest to differentiating epithelium. These influences may involve either new gene expression or quantitative increase in expression of genes, and are termed transitional. (c) Represents the role of fibroblast-derived fibroblast-pneumonocyte factor in enhancing surfactant phospholipid production by the type II cell in anticipation of birth and the need for air breathing. As no new gene products are expressed, but quantitative increases occur, this is termed permissive induction.

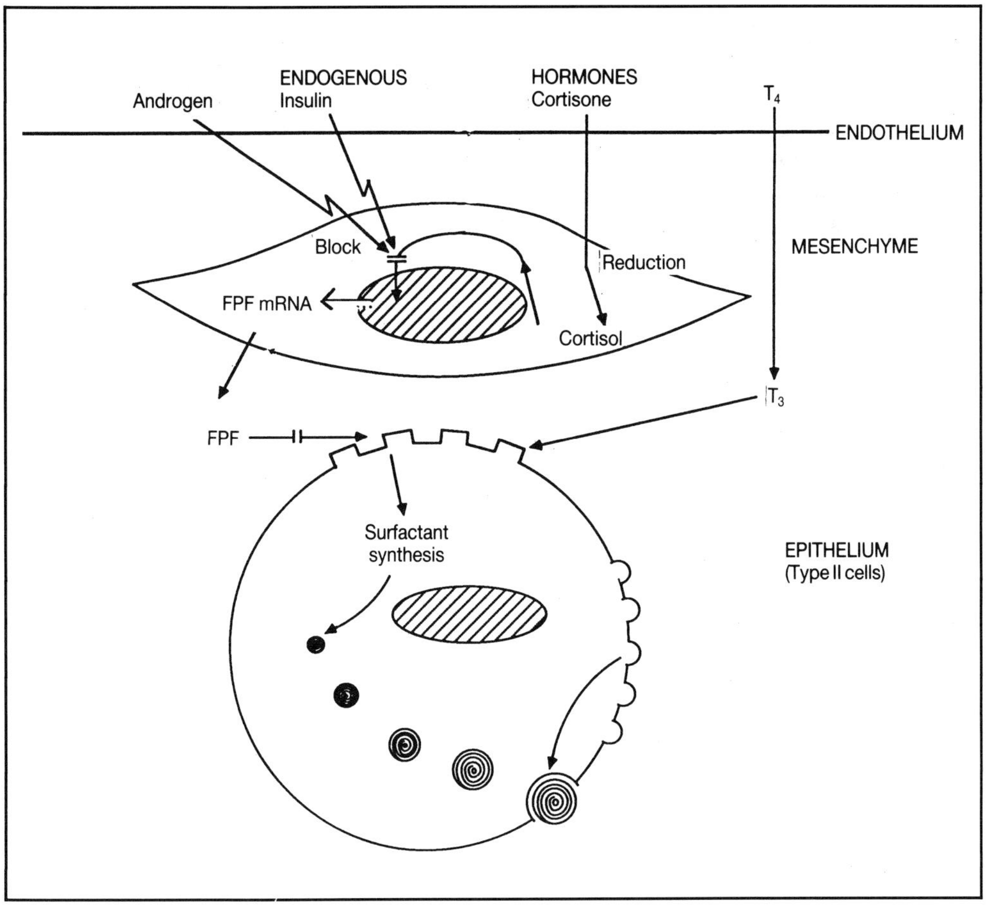

Fig. 11.2. Schematic representation of hormonal influences on epithelial type II cell differentiation. FPF, fibroblast-pneumonocyte factor.

aspects of the pulmonary surfactant system. *Biochim Biophys Acta (Biomembranes Rev)* 1988; **947**: 249.

Reid L. Embryology of the lung. In: DeReuck AVS, Porter R, eds. *Development of the lung*. London: Churchill Ltd, 1967: 109.

A2. Conducting Airways

D L Chapman

The tracheobronchial tree is a continuous system of branching tubes that connect the gas-exchange regions of the lung to ambient air. Although they are continuous, the airways are divided into three major anatomical sections: the cartilaginous airways, including the extrapulmonary airways and the bronchi down to 1 mm in diameter; the membranous bronchioles, comprising the last 4–5 generations of airways leading to the gas-exchange areas of the lung; and the respiratory bronchioles. The conducting airways include the first two sections and make up a large portion of the anatomical dead space. Although the principal function of the conducting airways is to act as a conduit for gas flow, they also have nonrespiratory functions that are important to the lung. The conducting airways humidify, warm, and filter inspired air. They play an important role in defense of the lung against microorganisms, particles, and noxious agents in inspired air. The relatively rigid construction of the conducting airways also provides a supporting framework for the surrounding lung parenchyma.

Airway structure

The conducting airways are organized in three concentric layers: mucosa, submucosa, and adventitia. The mucosa, which lines the airway lumen, is composed of a continuous layer of epithelial cells covered by a thin layer of liquid and mucus. Underlying the epithelium is a basement membrane and lamina propria that separate mucosa from submucosa. The submucosal layer contains glands, smooth muscle, nerves, cartilage, and blood vessels. The outermost layer, the adventitia, is a collection of loose connective tissue that contains nerves, ganglia, and bronchial vessels. The loose connective tissue in this space not only provides a sump for collection of excess liquid from the lung parenchyma, but also contains lymphatics, an important route for clearance of excess liquid from the gas-exchange regions of the lung. The structure of these layers changes as the airways branch out toward the periphery of the lung.

Airway development

Airway development is important in determining the ultimate shape of the mature lung. As the primitive airways grow, a balance between proliferation and migration of epithelial cells as well as specific interactions between the epithelium and the surrounding mesenchyme govern airway branching. Each parent branch gives rise to two smaller daughter branches that differ in length and diameter. This pattern is called irregular dichotomous branching, an important feature of mature airways. After branching, airways become encased in dense mesenchymal tissue that ultimately develops into smooth muscle, connective tissue, and cartilage. Structural development of the airways is complete well before birth. After birth, several terminal generations of airways are lost by development of terminal bronchioles into respiratory bronchioles. This process is complete by about 3 years of age. Thereafter, growth in airway length and diameter continues until growth of the chest cavity stops. In the first years of life, growth in the larger airways may exceed that in the smaller airways.

Airway morphology

Airway morphology in the mature lung is well suited for efficient transport of gas to an expansive gas-exchange surface. The irregular dichotomous branching system results in progressive reduction in length and diameter of the branches as they approach the gas-exchange region. The diameter of a given branch is proportional to the volume of the gas-exchange region that it ventilates. The angles between branches vary according to the diameter of the airway—the smaller the airway, the larger the branch angle. There is considerable heterogeneity in the distance and number of branches required to reach gas-exchange sites. In the mature lung, the total number of divisions between the trachea and the respiratory bronchioles averages about 15 but can vary between 8 and 25. The distance from the carina to the distal bronchioles can vary from 8 to 22 cm.

Functional consequences of airway morphology

Transport of gas in the lung involves bulk movement of gas through the conducting airways and diffusion of gas in the distal lung. The physical characteristics of these two processes differ greatly and place complex requirements on airway structure. Efficient diffusion requires short diffusion distances and large cross-sectional areas. Efficient bulk movement of gas requires increased airway volume in order to decrease air flow resistance. However, increasing airway volume increases wasted ventilation by taking volume away from gas-exchange regions, and increases airway tissue mass.

These opposing requirements are well balanced by the morphological features of conducting airways. As the number of branches increases, the cumulative volume and total cross-sectional area of the airways increases. As the total cross-sectional area of the airways increases, air flow velocity decreases. This decrease in air flow velocity allows for diffusion of gas in terminal respiratory regions. The irregular branching system also enhances bulk flow by minimizing the energy required for gas transport, optimizing air flow that is intermediate between laminar and turbulent, and bringing each point in the gas-exchange region as close as possible to the airway entrance.

Variability in path lengths, airway diameters, and the number of divisions required to reach different gas-exchange areas would be expected to result in higher air flow resistance to more distal gas-exchange sites. Differences in air flow resistances, transit times, and path lengths may contribute to variable time constants and inhomogeneity of ventilation within the lung by mixing inspired air with different amounts of dead-space gas, by altering the location of the interface between bulk flow and diffusion of gas, and by altering the time allowed for diffusion in the distal lung. While longer path lengths and more branch points may lead to higher resistances and longer time constants to distal gas-exchange regions, this is balanced by wider branch angles causing higher resistances in airways to proximal gas-exchange sites. Thus, the balance of structural features that determine air flow in the airways acts to minimize potential differences in ventilation between proximal and distal gas-exchange units.

Structural elements of the airways

(Table 11.1)

Surface epithelium

Cells that line airways and secretory glands are derived from endodermal cells in the primitive foregut. Ciliated and basal cells are seen early in gestation, followed later by secretory cells. Differentiation of the epithelium starts centrally and extends peripherally during development. In the mature lung the mucosal epithelium of the trachea and larger bronchi is a pseudostratified columnar ciliated epithelium. As the airways narrow and branch out toward the lung periphery, the epithelium becomes thinner and more cuboidal. Ciliated cells are the most common cells in the surface epithelium of larger airways; however, they are less numerous in bronchioles. Intermediate cells are relatively undifferentiated cells found submerged within the pseudostratified columnar epithelium. Basal cells form a row of flattened cells along the basement membrane. Brush cells are relatively rare cells located throughout the airways. Goblet cells are mucus-secreting cells seen primarily in the larger airways, and are relatively uncommon in bronchioles under normal conditions. Serous cells are seen in the surface epithelium during fetal life, but are rare after birth. Clara cells are nonciliated cuboidal secretory cells that are common in bronchioles of the mature lung.

The surface epithelium has several important functions. The airway epithelium forms a barrier against foreign material entering the lung tissue and leakage of interstitial liquid into the air spaces. Surface epithelial cells maintain the thin liquid layer that lines airways by transporting ions and water across the epithelial barrier. Secretory epithelial cells provide a variety of substances

Table 11.1. Structural elements of the conducting airways

Structure	Location			Function
	Layer	Cartilaginous airways	Membranous bronchioles	
Surface epithelium				
Ciliated cell	Mucosa	++	+	Clearance, ion transport, barrier
Intermediate cell	Mucosa	+	+	Undifferentiated, ? repair
Basal cell	Mucosa	++	+	Epithelial adhesion
Mucous (goblet) cells	Mucosa	+	+	Secretion
Clara cells	Mucosa	−	++	Barrier, ion transport, secretion, repair and regeneration
Submucosal glands	Submucosa	++	−	Secretion, defense
Smooth muscle	Submucosa	+	+	Control of airway caliber
Neural elements				
Motor nerves	Submucosa, adventitia	+	+	Airway caliber, secretion, ion transport
Sensory nerves	Mucosa, submucosa, adventitia	+	+	Airway caliber, secretion
Neuroepithelial	Mucosa	++	+	Neuroregulatory
Immunological cells	Submucosa	+	+	Defense, airway caliber, secretion, ion transport
Connective tissue				
Cartilage	Submucosa	++	−	Structural support
Elastin and collagen	Submucosa	+	++	Structural support

that contribute to lung defense and clearance mechanisms. Ciliated cells help propel these secretions up the airways. Serous and intermediate cells contribute to repair and regeneration of the epithelium, while basal cells help other epithelial cells adhere to the basement membrane. Clara cells appear to serve regenerative and secretory functions in the bronchioles. Surface epithelial cells also play a regulatory role through interactions with other airway cells.

Submucosal glands

Submucosal glands are acinar structures with tubular ducts opening into the surface epithelium. They first appear in the central airways as clumps of undifferentiated cells, which then migrate into the submucosa. After migration, gland cells differentiate into mucous and serous cells and proliferate to form cystic structures. Ducts form by separation and canalization of cells leading to the surface epithelium. Later in development, primitive glands extend peripherally into the bronchi. Gland formation is largely complete before birth. The glands continue to increase in size and complexity until adolescence and early adulthood. In the mature lung, submucosal glands are seen primarily in the proximal airways. They become smaller and less numerous in more distal airways, and are normally absent in small bronchi and bronchioles.

Submucosal glands aid in lung defense by secreting a complex mixture of mucins and proteins that entraps debris, microorganisms, inflammatory cells, and inhaled foreign particles. The density of glands within the submucosa parallels the deposition of inhaled particles, and increases in chronic inflammatory conditions.

Airway smooth muscle

Smooth muscle cells, elongated contractile cells found in the airway submucosa, are joined by gap junctions and are grouped in muscle bundles. The location and orientation of these bundles in the airway wall varies according to the location in the tracheobronchial tree. In the trachea and larger bronchi, they form bands of muscle that connect the ends of incomplete cartilage rings. Farther down the airway, they form a separate layer of muscle between the surface epithelium and the cartilage. Smooth muscle spirals around smaller airways in a helical fashion.

Smooth muscle begins to develop from dense condensations of mesenchyme around proximal airways, and later develops more peripherally in parallel with developing nerves. Although the amount of smooth muscle in the proximal airways increases substantially after birth, very little increase occurs normally in peripheral airways.

Airway smooth muscle controls air flow within the lung by regulating local air flow resistance through changes in airway caliber. In response to stimulation, the muscles contract slowly, resulting in a gradual increase in tension followed by slow relaxation. The effect of airway smooth muscle contraction depends on the size of the airway. Muscle contraction in the larger cartilaginous airways pulls the ends of the cartilage rings together, diminishing airway caliber. In smaller bronchi, muscle contraction decreases airway diameter and length and increases wall stiffness.

Neural elements

The conducting airways have a generous supply of afferent and efferent nerves as well as receptors that are stimulated by local or humoral substances. These neural elements interact with epithelium, submucosal glands, smooth muscle, and airway vasculature to regulate many airway functions. Development of neural elements in the airways begins early in gestation and continues after birth. Ganglion cells and nerves are seen in the proximal airways early in gestation and extend peripherally along with target structures. Cholinergic nerves are found in airways earlier in gestation than adrenergic nerves. A mature pattern of innervation is achieved by the end of the first year of life.

The airways receive both parasympathetic and sympathetic efferent (motor) nerves. Preganglionic parasympathetic fibers start in the central nervous system, travel to the lung in the vagus nerve, and end in ganglia located around the airway wall. Postganglionic fibers then penetrate into the submucosa to innervate smooth muscle, epithelium, and glands. Parasympathetic innervation is mediated by acetylcholine binding to postsynaptic muscarinic receptors. Preganglionic sympathetic nerves start in the central nervous system and end in the upper thoracic sympathetic ganglia. Postganglionic sympathetic fibers are less numerous than cholinergic fibers. They terminate on glands, airway ganglia, and blood vessels with very little direct input to airway smooth muscle. Despite the sparse sympathetic innervation, adrenergic receptors are found on smooth muscle, glands, epithelial cells, and mast cells, and adrenergic agonists have important effects on these target structures. The physiological agonist for these receptors may be circulating epinephrine released from the adrenal gland.

In addition to the input from the parasympathetic and sympathetic nervous systems, a third system is important in the conducting airways. This system, which does not utilize catecholamines or acetylcholine, has been called the non-adrenergic, non-cholinergic nervous system. Mediators in this system include substance P, neurokinin A, vasoactive intestinal peptide, peptide histidine methionine, calcitonin gene-related peptide, neuropeptide Y, and galanin. These mediators have competing effects on smooth muscle, submucosal glands, and airway vasculature.

Three types of afferent (sensory) nerves are found within the airways. They travel in the vagus nerve and contribute to reflexes that alter bronchial caliber, vascular resistance, and control of breathing. Sensory nerves of the first type, slowly adapting sensory nerves or stretch receptors, are concentrated in the smooth muscle of central airways and decrease in number peripherally. These receptors respond to increases in bronchial wall tension and transpulmonary pressure. Response is diminished in newborns due to higher thresholds of stimulation, lower discharge rates, decreased myelination, and differences in mechanics of the newborn lung. Stimulation of slowly adapting receptors results in laryngeal and bronchial dilatation, increased heart rate, decreased vascular resistance, and apnea during the Hering–Breuer inflation reflex. Sensory nerves of the second type, rapidly adapting nerves or irritant receptors, have nerve endings in the epithelium of the extra-pulmonary airways. They respond to a variety of stimuli including inhaled irritants, inflammatory mediators, prostaglandins, and mechanical deformation of the airways. Response of these receptors is decreased in newborns due to reduced numbers of fibers. Stimulation of these receptors results in reflex bronchoconstriction, cough, increased mucus secretion, and laryngeal constriction. Sensory nerves of the third type, bronchial C-fibers, have nerve endings in the epithelium of the intrapulmonary bronchi. They are very sensitive to chemical stimuli and less sensitive to mechanical stimuli. Stimulation causes reflex bronchoconstriction, mucus secretion, cough, and rapid, shallow breathing. The stimuli and the reflex events caused by sensory nerves overlap; together they play an important regulatory role in cough, control of airway caliber, and airway secretion.

Neuroendocrine cells are granular cells similar to amine precursor uptake and decarboxylation (APUD) cells seen in the gastrointestinal tract. They occur as single cells within the airway epithelium or as clumps (neuro-epithelial bodies) associated with bifurcations in the intrapulmonary airways. They are well positioned to respond to chemical changes in the airway lumen and may serve a sensory function. They also receive external nerve input and may have regulatory effects on lung growth and differentiation, response to hypoxemia, and hypersensitivity immune responses.

Immunological cells

Immunological cells are found predominantly in the larger airways, concentrated where the greatest deposition of inhaled particles and antigens occurs. They include local resident cells such as mast cells, lymphocytes, and macrophages as well as migratory cells derived from the blood. Lymphocytes form lymphoid aggregates, called bronchial-associated lymphoid tissue, that increase during development in response to stimulation by foreign antigen. Mast cells, found predominantly in the submucosa of the proximal airway, release a variety of mediators that cause edema, smooth muscle contraction, and altered function of the epithelium. Resident macrophages within the airspace lumen are phagocytic cells that sequester foreign particles, kill microorganisms, and present digested foreign antigens to other immunological cells.

Connective tissue

Connective tissue elements such as cartilage, elastin, and collagen are important structural components of the airway walls. In the trachea and extrapulmonary bronchi, cartilage forms incomplete rings connected by a muscular membrane. Beyond the mainstem bronchi, rings of airway cartilage are irregularly shaped and helical in configur-ation. Elastin and collagen are present beneath the cartilage in larger airways and become more prominent in small bronchi and bronchioles where cartilage is absent. Elastin is composed of amorphous and microfibrillar components that are closely associated and impart the distinctive springiness to lung tissues. Elastin is most prominent in the parenchyma and contributes to tethering of the airways by lung parenchyma. Loss of parenchymal elastin in *emphysema* results in small airway obstruction. Collagen, a large protein with a complex structure that is found in different forms in the lung, contributes to structural rigidity of airways; excess collagen, as seen in *fibrotic diseases*, decreases compliance of the airway wall.

Control of airway caliber

Airway caliber and resistance to air flow result from a balance of opposing forces produced by the airway structure, elasticity of the airway wall, mechanical interaction between the airway wall and surrounding parenchyma, contraction of airway smooth muscle, fluid balance within the airway wall, and mucus secretion (Fig. 11.3). During inspiration, the pressure gradient across the airway wall (transmural pressure) and traction on the airway by the expanding parenchyma distend the airway. During exhalation, the transmural pressure difference is reversed, and airway distension by the surrounding parenchyma is decreased, resulting in a tendency toward airway collapse.

The degree to which these forces result in dynamic changes in airway caliber is determined by the structural rigidity of the airway wall, the size of the airway, and the elasticity of the airway wall. In the larger airways, cartilage provides structural rigidity to the airway wall that limits these dynamic changes in caliber. Cartilage also limits the reduction in airway caliber that results from smooth muscle contraction. The abnormal shape and laxity of airway cartilage seen in patients with *tracheomalacia* results in excessive dynamic collapse during exhalation. In small bronchi and bronchioles, dynamic changes and contraction of smooth muscle are more directly opposed by traction on the airway wall from surrounding lung parenchyma and the elasticity of the bronchial wall. Smooth muscle contraction has a more direct effect in decreasing airway caliber in the distal airways. The force generated per muscle mass and length is greatest in the peripheral airways. In addition, smaller airways require less increase in wall tension to produce the same percentage decrease in airway caliber. Therefore, equivalent contraction of smooth muscle leads to a greater decrease in airway diameter. All these factors

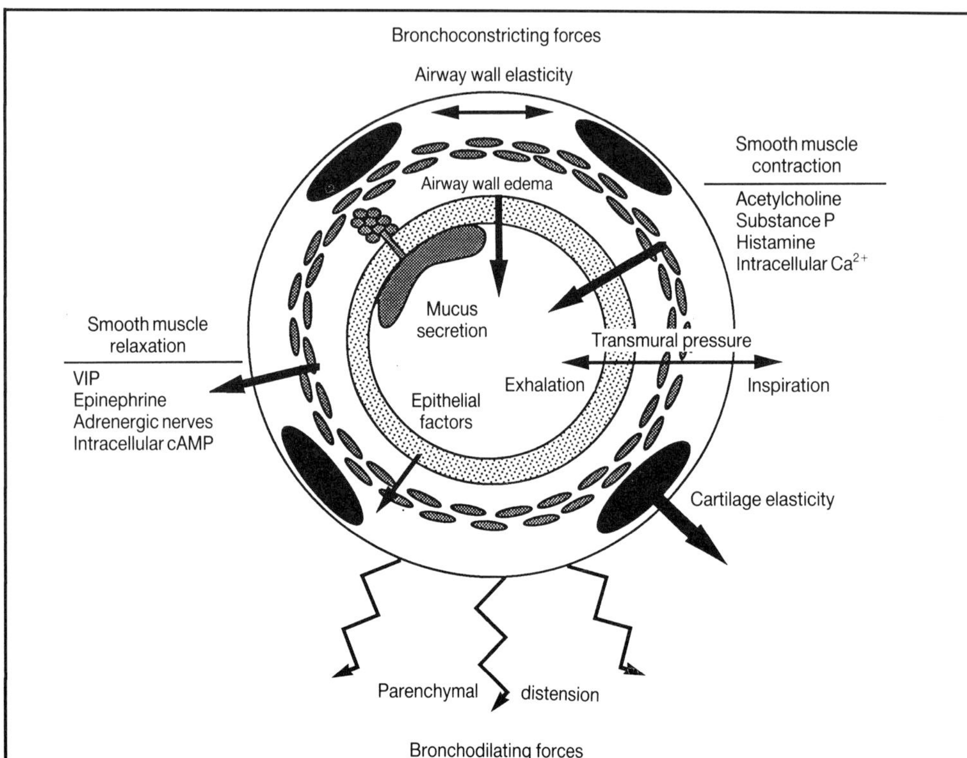

Fig. 11.3. Forces controlling airway caliber. Schematic of an intrapulmonary bronchus demonstrates the forces that determine airway caliber. The caliber of the airway results from the balance of these competing forces.

suggest that control of small airway caliber is more dynamic and sensitive to altered smooth muscle tone than in larger airways. Therefore, smooth muscle contraction within the membranous bronchioles may be important in determining distribution of ventilation to gas-exchange regions.

Contraction of airway smooth muscle is controlled by complex and often competing local interactions between smooth muscle, nerves, epithelium, and inflammatory cells as well as interactions between smooth muscle and neurohumoral input from outside the lung. Smooth muscle tone is determined by the balance of these multiple inputs. Response of smooth muscle to these extracellular stimuli is controlled by a complex biochemical process within the smooth muscle cell. Activation of receptors on the surface of smooth muscle cells stimulates contraction through the production of second messengers that cause phosphorylation of myosin. Phosphorylation causes a conformational change that allows myosin to interact with actin, and resultant hydrolysis of ATP provides the energy needed for shortening of the muscle. The magnitude of the response to receptor stimulation depends on the balance of intracellular enzymes that phosphorylate and dephosphorylate myosin. Thus phosphorylation of myosin is a major regulatory event in the coupling of receptor stimulation to muscle contraction.

Intracellular Ca^{2+} concentration is highly regulated and important to stimulus–contraction coupling. Polyphosphoinositides and their metabolites are important second messengers that increase intracellular Ca^{2+} concentration. Release of intracellular Ca^{2+} results in formation of a Ca^{2+}–calmodulin complex. This complex activates an enzyme that phosphorylates myosin. The Ca^{2+}–calmodulin complex may also regulate enzymes that inactivate myosin. Intracellular concentrations of cAMP have an inhibitory effect on myosin phosphorylation through the activation of a cAMP-dependent kinase. This kinase may decrease the affinity of the myosin phosphorylating enzyme for the Ca^{2+}–calmodulin complex. Alternatively, cAMP may inhibit contraction by causing a decrease in intracellular Ca^{2+} concentration.

The myoneural junction is a major extracellular site for regulating smooth muscle tone. Binding of acetylcholine to muscarinic receptors on the surface of smooth muscle cells stimulates contraction through the release of intracellular Ca^{2+}. Cholinergic nerves participate in bronchoconstricting reflexes that are regulated, at the ganglion, by both local and systemic mediators. Adrenergic input to the smooth muscle is sparse and may not be important in regulating smooth muscle tone under normal conditions. However, when tone is increased, adrenergic input may cause relaxation by inhibition of vagally mediated contraction. Bronchodilation results from stimulation of β-adrenergic receptors that are found with increased density on smooth muscle of the distal airways. Epinephrine can decrease bronchial tone through interaction with these receptors; however, the physiological role of circulating catecholamines in regulating bronchial tone is unclear. Non-adrenergic, non-cholinergic nerves containing vasoactive intestinal peptide and peptide histidine isomethionine are found with greater density in larger airways than peripheral airways and may provide direct inhibitory neural input to airway smooth muscle. These substances cause bronchodilation by stimulating receptors that activate adenylyl cyclase, increasing cAMP levels inside smooth muscle cells. Non-adrenergic, non-cholinergic nerves containing substance P, neurokinin A, and calcitonin gene-related peptide are potent bronchoconstrictors. These neuropeptides are released by local axon reflexes in bronchial C-fiber nerve endings.

Non-neural regulation also plays an important role in regulation of bronchial smooth muscle tone. Resident mast cells found in the submucosa of the airways can be stimulated to release a variety of mediators that cause smooth muscle contraction. Binding of foreign antigen to IgE antibody on the mast cell surface results in release of histamine, eosinophilic chemotactic factor, leukotrienes, and cyclooxygenase products. Release of mediators by mast cells is regulated by cyclic nucleotides, prostaglandins, respiratory heat loss, β-adrenergic agonists, and histamine. The airway epithelium also plays an important role in regulation of airway smooth muscle tone. The integrity of the epithelial barrier affects access of mast cells and sensory nerve endings to foreign antigens and noxious irritants. Epithelial cells release PGE_2 and epithelium derived relaxing factor that act directly on smooth muscle to decrease tone. Epithelial cells also possess neutral endopeptidases that metabolize bronchoconstricting neuropeptides.

Asthma, an important disease in children, is characterized by intermittent and reversible airway obstruction due to bronchial hyperresponsiveness, edema of the airway wall, and excessive mucus secretion. Bronchial hyperresponsiveness may result from an imbalance between endogenous bronchoconstricting and bronchodilating factors. Inflammation appears to play an important role in asthma and airway hyperresponsiveness. Inflammatory cells and their mediators can result in many of the pathological and pathophysiological abnormalities seen in asthmatic patients. How inflammation upsets the normal balance of factors regulating bronchial tone is currently the subject of intense research. Abnormalities in the β-adrenergic receptor have been proposed but probably do not play a major role in the pathogenesis of asthma. Recent evidence suggests imbalances in the non-adrenergic, non-cholinergic nervous system in asthma. Deficiencies in vasoactive intestinal peptide, excesses in bronchoconstricting neuropeptides, and abnormalities in enzymes responsible for degradation of these mediators have been proposed as possible explanations for hyper-responsiveness. Loss of epithelial integrity may play a role in hyperresponsive states associated with epithelial damage through loss of endopeptidase activity, decreased production of smooth muscle relaxing factors, increased exposure of irritant receptors to noxious substances, and increased access of mast cells to foreign antigen. Abnormalities in smooth muscle have also received considerable attention. Increased mass, altered distribution, increased force generation, and increased responsiveness to stimulatory mediators have been proposed to explain the role of smooth muscle in hyperresponsiveness. Morphological features of asthmatic airways are also potential factors in hyperresponsiveness. The thickness of airway walls is increased in asthmatic patients due to smooth muscle hypertrophy and edema. In the presence of thickening, the amount of smooth muscle shortening required to narrow the airway is decreased so that a normal amount of smooth muscle contraction causes increased obstruction. Edema in the airway wall has also been postulated to decrease the tethering of airways by the surrounding lung parenchyma. Thus asthma and bronchial hyperresponsiveness can be considered the final common pathway for any of a variety of abnormalities that upset the normal balance of factors determining airway caliber.

Interaction with the external environment—defense mechanisms

The conducting airways possess a variety of nonspecific and specific mechanisms that contribute to pulmonary defenses. Nonspecific mechanisms include morphological features that result in deposition of inhaled particles and absorption of inhaled gases, airway secretions, ciliary clearance, epithelial barrier function, phagocytic cells, mechanical mechanisms such as cough, and biochemical defenses. Specific mechanisms involve local and systemic, humoral and cellular immunological reactions.

Cleansing of inspired air

The conducting airways remove particles and noxious vapors from inhaled air by deposition of particles along the airway wall and absorption of vapor by the airway epithelium. Factors that govern clearance of inhaled substances may be important in determining airway damage from inhalation injuries and the efficacy of therapeutic aerosols.

Deposition of particles

Deposition of particles along the airway mucosa is determined by the physical characteristics of the particle, air flow properties, and airway anatomy. Particles are deposited by impaction, sedimentation, and diffusion. Deposition of particles by impaction is the result of inertia and is determined by particle mass, air flow velocities, and turbulent flow. It is greatest in the upper airway and proximal large conducting airways. Deposition of particles by sedimentation results from settling of particles by gravity and is determined by the density and size of the particles. Sedimentation occurs primarily in more distal airways where air flow velocity and turbulence are decreased. Deposition of particles by diffusion occurs only with very small particles and in the absence of air flow. Diffusion occurs primarily in the terminal airways and alveoli. Smaller airways, higher respiratory rates, smaller tidal volumes, and increased turbulent flow result in greater impaction of particles. For these reasons, deposition of particles is greater in the proximal airways of children than in adults.

Absorption of vapor

Absorption of vapors by the airway mucosa differs slightly from deposition of particles and is dependent on the physical properties of the gas, gas concentration, tidal volume, and respiratory rate. In general, gases that are highly soluble in water, e.g. sulfur dioxide and ammonia, are readily absorbed by the liquid layer lining the airway and are cleared in the upper and larger conducting airways. Higher concentrations of these gases or deep breathing are required for them to reach the distal lung. In contrast, gases with low solubility in water, e.g. nitrogen dioxide and chlorine, are not readily absorbed by the large airways and are more likely to penetrate deep into the lung.

Mucociliary clearance

Clearance of particles deposited along the airway depends on the production of respiratory secretions by mucosal cells and submucosal glands, the action of cilia on mucus, and the exchange of electrolytes and liquid across the epithelium (Fig. 11.4). Particles that are deposited along the airways are trapped in the mucus or gel layer overlying the mucosa and propelled toward the mouth by cilia. Cilia beat within a liquid or sol layer that contributes to humidification of inspired air and proper hydration of the mucus layer. The volume and composition of this sol layer is maintained by epithelial transport of ions and water. These three processes are regulated by similar mechanisms, constituting a coordinated and integrated system. Abnormalities in any of these processes can result in abnormal airway function and clinical disease.

Airway secretions

Airway mucus is a complex mixture of water, electrolytes, mucins, proteoglycans, and proline-rich proteins produced by secretory cells in the surface epithelium and submucosal glands. The physical

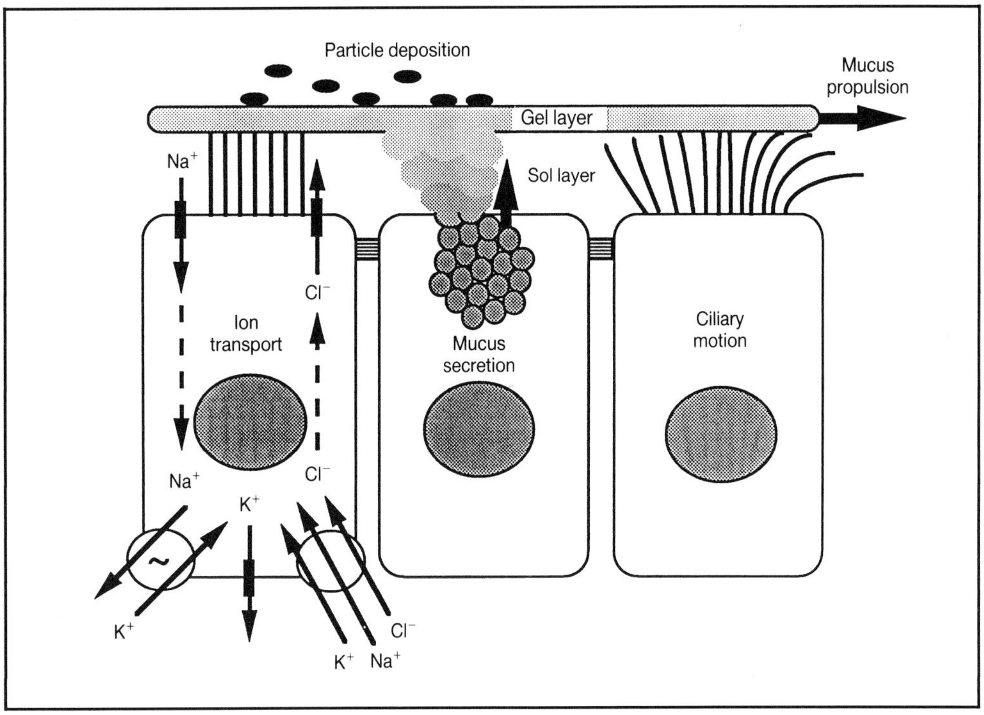

Fig. 11.4. Mucociliary clearance. Schematic shows the major components of normal clearance. Particles deposited along the airway adhere to the gel layer and are propelled up the airways by the action of cilia on mucus. Dense granules of mucus are released by secretory cells and quickly expand as the gel is hydrated by the sol layer. The sol layer is maintained by epithelial ion transport. Cl^- enters surface epithelial cells through a Na^+-K^+-Cl^- cotransporter that is driven by the Na^+ concentration gradient. Cl^- that builds up in the cell exits through apical Cl^- channels. Na^+ moves down its concentration gradient into the cell through apical Na^+ channels and is subsequently removed by the basolateral Na^+-K^+-ATPase. K^+ is recycled across the basolateral membrane in order to maintain the electrical driving force for apical Cl^- movement and to prevent cell swelling.

properties of mucus are largely determined by complex interactions between these elements. Mucins, the major mucoid component of airway secretions, are produced by goblet cells in the surface epithelium and mucous cells in the submucosal glands. Proteoglycans play an important role in hydration of mucins. Proline-rich proteins appear to affect the physical properties of mucus by interaction with mucins. Proteoglycans and proline-rich proteins are secreted by serous cells in submucosal glands. These macromolecules are stored in secretory cells as compact granules that are secreted by exocytosis. After secretion, mucus droplets rapidly swell by absorption of water. Normal hydration appears to be very important in determining the chemical and physical properties of mucus.

In addition to mucus, secretory cells produce a variety of substances that have antimicrobial properties and assist in defense of the lung. Submucous gland serous cells secrete lysozyme, an enzyme that acts on bacterial cell walls and has antimicrobial activity against Gram-positive organisms. Serous cells also secrete lactoferrin, an iron-binding protein with bacteriostatic properties. Epithelial mucous cells secrete peroxidase, which is active against a variety of microorganisms.

The volume and physical properties of respiratory mucus are regulated by neural input, inflammatory mediators, chemical irritants, and mechanical stimulation of the airway mucosa. Cholinergic neural input does not change the physical properties of mucus but increases secretion rate by stimulating both mucous and serous cells. Stimulation of submucosal glands by α-adrenergic input increases the volume of secretions and lowers the viscosity by selectively stimulating serous cells. In contrast, β-adrenergic stimulation has questionable effects on the volume of secretions but increases the viscosity through the relatively selective stimulation of mucous cells. Neuropeptides also act to stimulate mucus secretion. Chemical irritation of the mucosa stimulates goblet cells to increase in number and secretion rate. A variety of humoral and inflammatory mediators including histamine, bradykinin, and arachidonate metabolites can stimulate mucus secretion by both direct and reflex mechanisms.

Cilia

The action of cilia is crucial to normal mucociliary clearance. Cilia beat in waves, and their motion can be divided into three distinct phases. The first, or preparatory stroke phase involves slow backward and clockwise motion of the cilia. At the end of this phase the cilia are extended and pointing upstream. They proceed immediately into the propulsive stroke phase, during which they remain extended and rapidly move forward. After the propulsive phase, the cilia enter a rest phase in which they await the next cycle. Ciliary motion results from mechanical stimulation and is initiated by the preparatory stroke. Waves of ciliary motion, called metachronal waves, can propagate across an area of mucosa by the movement of one cilium mechanically stimulating neighboring cilia. Once the preparatory phase is initiated, the cilia proceed through a complete cycle and return to the resting position. The ciliary beat frequency varies according to the location within the airway, the mechanical load, temperature, and regulatory input. Cilia are more dense and beat more rapidly in the proximal airways than in the distal airways. Cilia also beat faster as the strength of the mechanical stimulus increases. These features of cilia may help prevent excessive accumulation of mucus as it converges on proximal airways from more distal airways. Ciliary beat frequency may also be increased by cholinergic and β-adrenergic stimulation.

Ciliary movement results from interaction between microtubules that are organized in a distinctive longitudinal array within the shaft of the cilia. This organization consists of nine microtubular doublets arranged around a central pair. Doublets are connected to each other by nexin links and to the central pair by radial linkages. One microtubule of each doublet has two dynein arms that contain ATPase. Hydrolysis of ATP by the dynein arms results in sliding of microtubules along each other. Linkages between microtubules direct this sliding so that it results in bending of the ciliary shaft. Defects in this basic structure and the biochemical processes causing ciliary motion have been identified that result in abnormal ciliary motion. This group of primary ciliary dyskinesias result in similar clinical consequences and have been grouped together as the *immotile cilia syndrome*.

Mucus and cilia interactions

Cilia propel mucus with small, claw-like projections that are anchored in the tip of the cilia shaft. These projections allow force to be transmitted from the internal structures that produce ciliary movement to the overlying mucus. The physical properties of mucus are very important to the action of cilia on mucus. The viscosity of mucus tends to decrease in proportion to force that is applied to it, i.e. the harder cilia beat, the less viscous mucus becomes. In addition, the elasticity of mucus allows transmission of applied force; a large sheet of mucus may be moved by acting on only one portion of the sheet. Because the recoil or relaxation time of mucus is relatively slow, ciliary action results in forward propulsion rather than oscillation back and forth as cilia attach and release the mucus sheet. Thus the physical properties of mucus enhance the action of cilia by allowing mucus to help pull itself along the airway.

Ion transport

Epithelial ion transport plays a role in controlling the physical properties of mucus and affects ciliary motion by regulating the volume and composition of the sol layer. Tight intercellular junctions allow epithelial cells to segregate ion-transporting proteins into either the apical or basolateral cell membrane. Segregation of ion-transporting proteins and expenditure of energy to generate ion concentration differences between the inside and outside of the cell allow the epithelium to transport ions across the mucosa. Transepithelial movement of ions generates osmotic differences that draw water back and forth across the epithelium according to the net movement of ions. The airway epithelium can simultaneously secrete Cl^- and absorb Na^+. Secretion of Cl^- into the airway results in liquid production by the airway epithelium. Absorption of Na^+ results in removal of liquid from the airway lumen. Na^+ and Cl^- movement accounts for nearly all the transepithelial ion and water movement. Therefore, the balance of these two ion transport processes regulates the charge, composition, volume, and net production of airway liquid by the airway epithelium.

The importance of the balance between these two ion transport processes to fluid balance across the respiratory epithelium is illustrated by dramatic developmental changes in ion transport. During fetal life the lung is filled with liquid that plays an important role in normal lung development. This liquid is produced by the active secretion of Cl^- and water by the respiratory epithelium. Absorption of Na^+ plays little or no role in fluid balance at this point. In the days immediately preceding birth, the volume of liquid and the rate of liquid secretion slows. During labor, stimulation of Na^+ absorption results in removal of liquid from the lung lumen. This clearance of liquid plays an important role in preparation for air breathing at birth. After birth, Na^+ absorption increases and Cl^- secretion decreases. In the mature airways, Na^+ absorption is the dominant ion-transport process, with Cl^- and bicarbonate moving across the epithelium as counterions.

The importance of a proper balance between secretory and absorptive ion transport processes in the airway epithelium is also illustrated by genetic abnormalities in epithelial ion transport. The mature airway epithelium retains the capacity for Cl^- and water secretion under certain circumstances. Cl^- secretion can be stimulated by a variety of humoral, neural, and inflammatory mediators. These mediators may stimulate Cl^- secretion by increasing intracellular cAMP concentrations. Increased cAMP results in increased intracellular Ca^{2+} concentrations and activation of cAMP-dependent protein kinase which, in turn, activates Cl^- transport pathways within the apical membrane of the epithelial cell. Cl^- secretion can be stimulated by β-adrenergic agonists, prostaglandins, vasoactive intestinal peptide, leukotrienes, adenosine, bradykinin, eosinophil myelin basic protein, and neurokinins. Activation of Cl^- transport by cAMP is abnormal in *cystic fibrosis* patients. This abnormality results in deficient liquid secretion and excessive water absorption by the airway epithelium. This abnormal balance alters the volume of airway liquid and hydration of mucus, resulting in tenacious mucus that obstructs airways in cystic fibrosis patients.

Immunological defenses

Immunological responses in defense of the lung are similar to responses elsewhere in the body and include both humoral and cellular components of the immune system. Immune responses in the conducting airways are largely produced locally and are mediated by immunological cells within the airway. Secretory IgA is the predominate immunoglobulin in airway secretions and assists in viral neutralization, agglutinates microorganisms, and prevents attachment of bacteria to epithelial surfaces. Secretory IgA is derived from local aggregations of lymphoid cells in the submucosa of the large airways. The concentration of IgA decreases toward the periphery of the lung in association with decreases in the size and organization of these lymphoid aggregates. IgG is present in much lower concentrations in the airways. IgE antibody plays an important role in immediate hypersensitivity reactions within the lung. Interferon is produced by macrophages and serves antiviral and immunoregulatory roles within the lung. Complement is normally found in very small amounts in airway secretions but can be increased in inflammatory states, where it serves an immunoregulatory role in controlling vascular permeability and in chemotaxis.

The cellular component of immune responses in the lung involves both local and migratory phagocytic cells and lymphocytes. When circulating leukocytes are activated, they adhere to the vascular endothelium and migrate from the vascular space under the influence of chemotaxins to the site of an immune response. Resident macrophages predominantly serve a local phagocytic role and to a lesser extent an immunoregulatory function. Both local and circulating lymphocytes play a role in the elaboration of immunoglobulin and cell-mediated immunity within the airways. Local T lymphocytes are important to the defense against viruses and have extensive interactions with macrophages that result in the elaboration of lymphokines.

Selected reading

Horsfield K, Cumming G. Morphology of the bronchial tree. *J Appl Physiol* 1968; **24**: 373.

Horsfield K, Cumming G. Functional consequences of airway morphology. *J Appl Physiol* 1968; **24**: 384.

Leff AR. Endogenous regulation of bronchomotor tone. *Am Rev Respir Dis* 1988; **137**: 1198.

Murray JF. Defense mechanisms. In Murray JF, ed. *The normal lung.* Philadelphia: WB Saunders, 1986: 313.

Sleigh MA, Blake JR, Liron N. The propulsion of mucus by cilia. *Am Rev Respir Dis* 1988; **137**: 726.

Weibel ER. Lung cell biology. In Fishman AP, Fisher AB, eds. *Handbook of physiology, Section 3: The respiratory system, Vol. 1, Circulation and non-respiratory functions*. Bethesda, MD: American Physiological Society, 1985: 47.

Widdicombe JH. Ion transport by airway epithelia. In Crystal RG, West JB, eds. *The lung: scientific foundations*. New York: Raven Press, 1991: 263.

A3. The Alveolar Region

S Hawgood

Organization of the alveolar region

The alveolar region of the lung lies distal to the smallest of the conducting airways, the respiratory bronchiole. The primary function of the alveolar region is the exchange of O_2 and CO_2 between the inspired air and the blood. The alveolus is the basic anatomical unit of gas exchange; the human lung contains about 500 million alveoli. The average alveolar diameter in the human lung is approximately 200 μm; at birth, alveolar diameter is about 50–100 μm. When the adult lung is 60 percent inflated, the alveolar surface area available for gas exchange is approximately 140 m^2. Thousands of individual, cup-shaped alveoli, separated by septa and interconnected by alveolar ducts, make up a respiratory acinus. The acinus constitutes the basic unit of ventilation in the lung. Each acinus is connected to a single respiratory bronchiole. The basic perfusion unit, the capillary bed between each pulmonary arteriole and the corresponding pulmonary venule, is less easy to define anatomically but clearly extends over several alveoli because paired arterioles and venules are separated by 0.5–1.0 mm. The pulmonary microvasculature has a large capillary surface area that almost matches the alveolar surface area available for gas exchange. The total estimated volume of the pulmonary microcirculation is approximately 200 ml.

Alveolar structure

The structure of the alveolar region promotes efficient gas exchange between alveolar gases and blood in the microvasculature by keeping the tissue space between the two to a minimum. Adjacent alveoli share a very thin common wall, or alveolar septum, only 5–8 μm thick. Over most of their length the septa are covered by the very attenuated cytoplasmic extensions of specialized epithelial cells (type I cells), which rest on a basement membrane shared with the underlying endothelial cells of the pulmonary capillary in the septum. Through more than half of the enormous gas-exchange area in the lung, there is little to no interstitial space. This fragile architecture creates special problems of maintaining structural stability while allowing for the distensibility necessary during ventilation. As the luminal surface of the alveolar epithelium is lined by a thin, but continuous liquid layer, surface forces also potentially compromise alveolar structural stability.

The alveolar region of the lung is supported, in part, by a system of interstitial fibers, collagen and elastin, that follow the branching of the airways and run through the alveolar ducts to connect with the strands of connective tissue that support the alveolar septa. Additional mechanical support is provided by a fibrous network that extends in from the visceral pleura along the interlobular septa. These three fibrous systems are interconnected and between them provide a supportive scaffolding for the alveolar region. Fibroblasts and other cells are found in the proximity of the fibrous bundles in the interstitial space. The surface forces present in the liquid layer that lines the alveolar epithelium are reduced to low levels by a unique surfactant secreted by a second, specialized epithelial cell of the alveolar lining, the type II cell. Absence or dysfunction of this surfactant leads to volume loss in the gas-exchange region and respiratory failure. These basic elements of the alveolar region will be discussed in greater detail below.

Alveolar epithelium

Because the alveolar region has such an enormous surface area and a generally thin interstitial space, the epithelial cells lining the alveolus constitute more than 20 percent of the total number of cells in the lung. The alveolar epithelium consists of just two cell types, known as type I and type II cells. Each human alveolus is lined by approximately 40 type I cells and 70 type II cells. The specialized design of the alveolar epithelium creates a tight barrier between the interstitial space and the alveolar lumen. This barrier regulates the accumulation and composition of fluid in the alveolus while imposing a minimal resistance to respiratory gas diffusion. The alveolar epithelium, particularly the type II cell, secretes many biologically active substances, including pulmonary surfactant, into the alveolar lumen. Other major cells of the alveolar region, including interstitial fibroblasts and endothelial cells, are discussed in other parts of this section.

Type I cells

Type I cells cover about 95 percent of the alveolar surface area. Type I cells are very large and extremely thin cells with complex branched cytoplasmic extensions. A single type I cell covers an area of approximately 5000 μm^2, but its average thickness over most of this enormous area is only 0.2 µm. This extreme cytoplasmic attenuation presumably facilitates gas exchange by limiting the total tissue space across which gas exchange must occur to less than 0.5 µm in much of the alveolar region. No functions other than this important barrier role have been ascribed to the type I cell. The cells have relatively few mitochondria and a small endoplasmic reticulum and Golgi apparatus, suggesting limited metabolic capacity; however, because of difficulties in isolation and culture, type I cells have not been directly studied *in vitro*. Type I cells do contain a relatively large number of pinocytic vesicles and therefore may have an important role in the bidirectional traffic of small solutes and proteins between the alveolar lining liquid and the interstitial space.

The basement membrane beneath the type I cell appears to be fused or intermingled with the basement membrane of the closely apposed capillary endothelial cell. Along much of the alveolar septum there is almost no discernible interstitial space between type I cells and the underlying capillaries. The contact between type I cells and other type I or type II cells is formed by tight junctions, making the alveolar epithelium a relatively tight or impermeable barrier for solutes and proteins in the interstitial space. Type I cells appear in the fetal lung in the early third trimester. Whether type I cells differentiate directly from the progenitor columnar epithelium or trans-differentiate from type II cells is uncertain. Type I cells are acutely susceptible to a wide variety of lung injury including injury caused by oxidants, barotrauma, and infection. Injured type I cells readily detach from the basement membrane. In the adult lung, epithelial integrity apparently is restored after injury by division and subsequent trans-differentiation of type II cells. Adult type I cells are thought to be terminally differentiated and to lack the capacity for mitosis. The signals regulating the mitogenic responsiveness and differentiated state of alveolar epithelial cells are unknown, but may include soluble factors secreted by mesenchymal cells and alveolar macrophages as well as molecules in the extracellular matrix.

Type II cells

The relatively small, cuboidal type II cells are approximately twice as abundant as type I cells but cover only about 5–10 percent of the alveolar surface area. Type II cells are frequently, but not exclusively situated in the corners of the alveoli. Ultrastructurally, type II cells are distinguished by numerous short microvilli on the luminal surface and unique secretion granules known as lamellar bodies. The lamellar bodies store surfactant and other molecules including lysosomal enzymes. Type II cells each contain about 150 lamellar bodies. Type II cells contribute to the barrier functions of the alveolar epithelium by forming tight junctions with neighboring type I cells. Type II cells have the additional known functions of synthesizing, storing, secreting, and clearing surfactant, actively transporting solutes and possibly proteins between the alveolar and interstitial spaces, and acting as progenitor cells for alveolar epithelial repopulation after injury. Type II cells also appear to synthesize and secrete many other bioactive molecules such as components of the complement cascade, coagulation factors, lysozyme, lysosomal enzymes, growth factors, and cytokines. The biological role of most of these products in the alveolar space is unknown.

Morphologically recognizable type II cells appear in the human fetal lung early in the third trimester of pregnancy. In culture, morphological maturation of the columnar epithelium lining the developing air spaces can be synchronized and induced by a number of factors, including cAMP, prostaglandins, and glucocorticoids, but the precise sequence of signals regulating type II cell differentiation *in vivo* is unknown.

Surfactant

Surface forces and lung mechanics

The presence of the large air–liquid interface in the alveolus (approximately 140 m^2 in the adult lung) leads to a tension in the interface or a surface force that promotes retraction of the interface (*lung collapse*) and accumulation of fluid in the alveolar lumen (*pulmonary edema*). Pulmonary surfactant accumulates at the alveolar air–liquid interface and reduces the tension in the interface. Surfactant therefore stabilizes the alveolus against collapse, or *atelectasis,* on expiration (helps maintain **residual volume**), promotes expansion on inspiration (reduces **compliance** and **work of breathing**), and helps to keep the alveolar space relatively dry. A surfactant-deficient lung has a reduced lung volume and is stiff or has a decreased compliance. If the alveolus is considered as a spherical structure the relationships between alveolar size (r), surface tension (σ) and trans-surface or transpulmonary pressure (P) can be modeled using the law of Laplace for thin-walled spheres

$$P = 2\sigma/r$$

If the surface tension (σ) is high (70 dynes/cm, as in the absence of any surfactant) a trans-surface pressure (P) of approximately 28 cmH_2O would be required to maintain a radius (r) of 50 μm. Simplistically, a similar calculation in the context of the lung infers that a **positive end-expiratory pressure (PEEP)** of 28 cmH_2O would be required to maintain a reasonable **functional residual volume (FRC)** in the absence of any surfactant. Surfactant lowers the surface tension to very low values by accumulating at the air–liquid interface. The transpulmonary pressure required to maintain FRC in the normal lung is therefore very low. The complex geometry of the alveolar region is clearly not adequately modeled as a simple collection of non-interacting, thin-walled spheres. The Laplace law cannot therefore be strictly applied, but it does serve to highlight the importance of surface forces to volume stability.

Surfactant composition

Pulmonary surfactant is predominantly lipid consisting of approximately 45 percent dipalmitoylphosphatidyl-choline (DPPC), 25 percent unsaturated phosphatidyl-cholines, 15 percent phosphatidylglycerol, and lesser amounts of several other lipids. DPPC is the component that accumulates at the air–liquid interface and reduces surface tension. At least three specific apolipoproteins are associated with surfactant. SP-A is a large complex, oligomeric, collagen-like lectin that binds to surfactant lipids and modifies their structure and surface properties. SP-A also may have roles in regulating the alveolar surfactant pool size and possibly immunoregulatory functions in the alveolus. SP-B is a smaller (79 amino acids), hydrophobic, cationic protein with a detergent-like effect on lipid membranes that probably destabilizes surfactant so that it can spread rapidly at the air–liquid interface. SP-C is a very small (35 amino acids), covalently palmitoylated, hydrophobic protein that has similar, but not identical properties to SP-B. All three surfactant apolipoproteins likely act as a cooperative unit to facilitate the delivery of DPPC from the type II cell to the air–liquid interface. The proteins may also have other roles related to the clearance of used surfactant from the alveolar space.

Surfactant metabolism

Surfactant is synthesized in type II epithelial cells. The phospholipids and apolipoproteins are synthesized from blood-borne precursors in the endoplasmic reticulum and are transported through the Golgi apparatus to the lamellar body. These organelles are the intracellular storage site for surfactant. Roughly half the total pool of lung surfactant is stored in lamellar bodies, and half is in the alveolar lumen. Lamellar bodies are released from the type II cell in a regulated manner in response to a number of pharmacological stimuli including β-agonists. Circulating catecholamines may therefore play a role in the secretion of surfactant. Expansion of the lung towards total lung capacity and the hyperventilation of exercise also stimulate surfactant release. Periodic sighs therefore may be an important mechanism to maintain adequate alveolar surfactant levels. Conversely, prolonged ventilation at a fixed tidal volume without intermittent sighs may lead to a deficiency of surfactant in the alveolar lumen with a loss of compliance and *atelectasis*. Approximately 10 percent of the intracellular surfactant pool is secreted into the alveolar space each hour at rest. The secretion rate can increase fourfold during exercise.

The lamellar body contents are secreted into the alveolar lining liquid and transform into an unusual morphological form called tubular myelin. This form of surfactant, containing the apolipoproteins and lipids, appears to be specialized for the transport of phospholipids, particularly DPPC, to the interface. At the air–liquid interface, DPPC forms a surface layer and surface tension falls. Like all phospholipids, DPPC is an amphipathic molecule with a polar head group (choline) and apolar tails (palmitate). This amphipathicity allows DPPC to accumulate in the surface layer. Additionally, the straight acyl chains of DPPC and the high melting point of this lipid allow it to pack very tightly in the surface film, exclude water, and therefore reduce surface tension to very low values. With ventilation some DPPC is lost from the surface layer and must be replaced by new material. Therefore, a continuous and balanced cycle of surfactant secretion and clearance occurs in the alveolus. The pathways of clearance are not well understood but include active reuptake into type II cells (conservation and reuse of surfactant) and clearance by alveolar macrophages (degradation of surfactant). The total amount of surfactant in the alveolar space at rest is about 10 mg phospholipid/kg body weight but only about half this amount is actually in the surface layer. The concentration of surfactant in the alveolar space is more difficult to establish, but is probably about 15 mg/ml.

Surfactant ontogeny

Active synthesis of surfactant components begins early in the third trimester of fetal life. Adult pool sizes are not attained until 35–36 weeks in most fetuses but noticeable disease from *surfactant deficiency* is rare after 34–35 weeks. At term about 10 percent of the normal alveolar luminal surfactant pool is present in lung liquid, which fills the fetal alveoli. A dramatic burst of secretion occurs with lung inflation at birth. A normal pool of alveolar surfactant is established within hours of birth.

The regulation of surfactant synthesis during fetal life is complicated. Several hormones, cytokines, and growth factors interact to bring about the orderly maturation of the surfactant system. **Glucocorticoids** contribute to the normal maturation of the surfactant system and can be used to prematurely stimulate surfactant production from very early in fetal life. Glucocorticoids also stimulate morphological maturation of the alveolar epithelium and pulmonary interstitium. Other hormones, including thyroxine and prolactin, and growth factors such as epidermal growth factor may act synergistically with glucocorticoids in the induction of surfactant synthesis. *In vitro* insulin and transforming growth factor β down-regulate the expression of some of the surfactant apolipoprotein genes, but the biological significance of these findings has not been clarified. Maturation of the surfactant system in male fetuses is delayed by 1–2 weeks relative to female fetuses. This has been attributed to the higher circulating levels of androgens in the male fetus.

Surfactant deficiency—respiratory distress syndrome (RDS)

A relationship between surfactant deficiency or dysfunction and acute respiratory failure has been clearly established. Infants born before the surfactant system has fully matured develop RDS manifested by widespread atelectasis, poor lung compliance, intrapulmonary shunts and pulmonary edema. Following the logic of the Laplace relationship, treatment is directed towards restoring lung volume by the application of positive end-expiratory pressure. Infants breathing spontaneously try to achieve the same result by expiring through a partially closed glottis. This pattern of breathing often is accompanied by a characteristic expiratory grunt.

Therapeutic surfactant can also be administered by the trachea. The formulations of the *exogenous surfactants* vary, but all contain high concentrations of DPPC and an agent included to promote spreading of the DPPC at the air–water interface. Exogenous surfactant therapy approximately halves the mortality from RDS. In several diseases where acute respiratory failure with stiff lungs and low lung volumes is a final common end point (*adult respiratory distress syndrome* or *ARDS*), surfactant may be present in normal amounts but be inactivated by the presence of soluble inhibitory agents present in the edema fluid in the alveolar space. The specific pathway of inhibition is unclear, but the surfactant dysfunction that results undoubtedly contributes to the morbidity of these conditions. The role of surfactant therapy in ARDS has not been clarified.

Alveolar fluid balance

The enormous capillary surface area of the pulmonary microvasculature allows for a large solute, protein and fluid flux between the vascular space and the interstitium. A number of physical forces, classically described by the Starling law of capillary fluid exchange, determine the flux of fluid between these compartments. The lymphatics of the pulmonary interstitium control fluid accumulation in the interstitial space and the relatively tight epithelial barrier limits alveolar flooding and frank *pulmonary edema*. In the normal lung the alveolar epithelium is covered with a thin but continuous fluid layer. The volume and ionic composition of this alveolar lining fluid appears to be primarily regulated by active epithelial processes including ion pumps and transcytotic vesicular pathways.

Capillary fluid exchange

Transcapillary fluid movement in the pulmonary microcirculation is discussed in Section 11A4.

Epithelial barrier

Fluid and protein entering the interstitial space generally does not spill over into the alveolar lumen. This is because under normal circumstances, the alveolar epithelium forms a tight barrier restricting passive fluid, solute, and protein movement. Alveolar epithelial cells are linked by morphologically recognizable tight junctions. Some passive diffusion of water and small solutes occurs across the normal epithelial barrier, but the actual anatomical sites (paracellular or transcellular) through which this flux occurs are not known. Epithelial injury, hyperventilation, and surfactant deficiency increase epithelial permeability.

Active epithelial transport processes appear to be very important in maintaining a dry alveolar lumen. Type I and type II cells have vesicular pathways that may contribute to the selective bidirectional movement of proteins, including albumin and immunoglobulins, between the interstitial space and alveolar lumen. The alveolar epithelium also has active ion transport potential. In the fetal lung the predominant process is thought to be cAMP-dependent Cl^- secretion by the epithelium lining the developing potential air spaces. The actual pump and its location have not been identified. The mature alveolar epithelium actively transports sodium from the luminal to interstitial spaces. This transport is regulated by cAMP and β-agonists *in vitro* and *in vivo*. In the mature epithelium, active Na^+ resorption followed by passive Cl^- and H_2O resorption likely is primarily responsible for keeping the normal alveolar space relatively dry and for clearing fluid that accumulates during *pulmonary edema*. The factors that control the transition from a predominantly Cl^--secreting state before birth to a Na^+-resorbing state after birth are not fully defined, but circulating hormones including catecholamines and vasopressin are thought to play a major role. Although all cells can be expected to express ion pumps on their surface, pulmonary type II epithelial cells appear to be particularly rich in basolateral Na^+-K^+-ATPase and may therefore play a primary role in regulating alveolar liquid homeostasis.

Alveolar liquid lining layer

The alveolus in the mature lung is not completely dry. The epithelial layer is lined by a thin, but probably continuous layer of fluid. The interface between this fluid layer and the respiratory gases imposes the special surface forces problem for the volume stability of the lung. The volume of the liquid layer is difficult to assess but is probably in the order of 35–70 ml in the adult human lung. The average depth of this layer, sometimes referred to as the alveolar subphase or hypophase, is about 1 μm, but in large areas over the type I cells the subphase is very thin, covering little more than the cell's glycocalyx. The alveolar subphase (pH 6.9) is more acidic than plasma (pH 7.4). In the fetal lung, the free Ca^{2+} concentration of the lung liquid is 0.5 mM. The subphase Ca^{2+} concentration rises after birth and rapidly reaches a level (2 mM) similar to the plasma concentration. The importance of these values and their changes with birth is unknown, but Ca^{2+} may regulate certain important aspects of surfactant function such as the rate of surface layer formation. Major derangements in alveolar subphase protein and ion concentration, as may occur in states of pulmonary edema, could interfere with surfactant function.

Pulmonary edema

The normal lung does not become edematous, even though fluid filtration increases, until pressure in the microvasculature rises to very high levels. As fluid filtration increases, compensatory decreases in interstitial oncotic pressure and increases in interstitial pressure slow the rate of fluid filtration (see Starling equation in Section 11A4). The flow through the pulmonary lymphatics can also increase dramatically, limiting accumulation of fluid in the interstitium. In the injured lung, the fluid filtration rate increases at much lower microvascular pressures. Eventually with a sufficiently high rate of fluid filtration, the capacitance of the interstitial space is exceeded; alveolar flooding occurs when the interstitial volume has increased by approximately 50 percent. Epithelial injury from barotrauma, oxidant injury, surfactant deficiency, infection, etc. allows earlier alveolar flooding. Gas exchange deteriorates markedly with alveolar flooding.

The mechanisms involved in the clearance of liquid and protein from the alveolar space after alveolar flooding are not fully understood. Active Na^+ resorption with passive water resorption by the alveolar epithelium, particularly the type II cells, is probably a central mechanism of edema clearance. In diseases with a major component of epithelial injury and permeability edema (high protein concentration in the edema fluid), the subphase protein concentration may rise to very high levels as the water is cleared from the alveolar lumen. The mechanisms of protein clearance from the alveolar space during the recovery phase of pulmonary edema are not known, but probably include alveolar macrophage phagocytosis and degradation and asymmetric epithelial transcytosis.

Immune effector cells in the alveolus

In the normal lung the major immune effector cells in the alveolar region are alveolar macrophages and T lymphocytes. Macrophages are by far the most numerous, but both cell types are found scattered through the alveolar interstitium and in the alveolar space. The functional characteristics of the cells in the interstitium of the lung appear to be similar to those of the luminal cells. In lavage fluid from the distal lung, 80–85 percent of the cells are alveolar macrophages and 10–15 percent are activated or memory T lymphocytes. Less than 5 percent of the cells in normal lavage fluid are neutrophils or eosinophils, but the number of these cells can increase dramatically in disease states. A variety of other alveolar cells can act as antigen-presenting accessory immune cells, including cells of the dendritic lineage, which are scattered throughout the alveolar interstitium. The responses of all these alveolar immune effector cells to foreign antigens, particulates, and pathogens are similar to the responses of immune cells elsewhere in the body. The details of the general immune response are described in detail elsewhere (Chapter 13); only the rather specialized alveolar macrophage will be briefly discussed here.

Alveolar macrophages

Fetal lung liquid is virtually acellular. The number of alveolar macrophages increases steadily after birth. The average adult alveolus contains 10–50 macrophages closely associated with the alveolar epithelium in the subphase fluid. Both tissue macrophages and intravascular macrophages are also found in the alveolar region. Alveolar macrophages are predominantly derived from blood monocytes and are quite long-lived in the alveolus. Alveolar macrophages also have some limited potential to proliferate in the alveolar space. Alveolar macrophages are multifunctional cells with beneficial roles in antigen presentation to T lymphocytes, phagocytosis of particulates and microorganisms, recruitment and functional regulation of other immune cells, and stimulation of repair processes in the injured alveolus. A broad array of receptors, including receptors for complement components and immunoglobulins, have been localized to the surface of the alveolar macrophage. Subpopulations of alveolar macrophages with possibly different functions have been described. The ability of the alveolar macrophage to produce and secrete many bioactive compounds including prostanoids, cytokines, growth factors, proteases, and other enzymes has led to the belief that products of the alveolar macrophage may also play harmful roles in many diseases.

Selected reading

Avery ME, Mead J. Surface properties in relation to atelectasis and hyaline membrane disease. *Am J Dis Child* 1959; **97**: 517.

Clements JA, Hustead RF, Johnson RP, Gribetz I. Pulmonary surface tension and alveolar stability. *J Appl Physiol* 1961; **16**: 444.

Fels A, Cohn Z. The alveolar macrophage. *J Appl Physiol* 1986; **60**: 353.

Taylor AE, Barnard JW, Barman SC, Adkins WK. Fluid balance. In Crystal RG, West JB, eds. *The lung: scientific foundations*. Vol. I. New York: Raven Press Ltd, 1991: 1147.

Weibel ER. Morphological basis of alveolar-capillary gas exchange. *Physiol Rev* 1973; **53**: 419.

A4. The Pulmonary Vasculature

D P Carlton

The pulmonary vasculature plays a central role in normal and abnormal lung function. A critical and obvious role of the pulmonary vasculature is to provide a conduit through the lungs for the oxygenation of systemic venous blood. While providing this pathway is essential, the pulmonary vasculature is not simply a system of inert tubes. It regulates its own blood flow and distribution and is intimately involved with multiple circulating components in the blood.

Integrative physiology

The pulmonary circulation serves the indispensable function of delivering deoxygenated blood to the distal air spaces where O_2 and CO_2 are exchanged.

Blood volume

The fetal lungs contain relatively less blood than they do postnatally. After birth, the blood volume of the lung increases approximately 40 percent. If estimates for adults are applicable to children, then approximately 10–15 percent of the total blood volume is contained in the lungs. Because of this, the lungs can act as a reservoir of volume for the maintenance of cardiac output; this reservoir may be needed during postural changes.

Blood flow

Developmental considerations

In the fetus only about 8 percent of the combined ventricular output of the heart traverses the pulmonary circulation, a result of the high pulmonary vascular resistance, which shunts blood from the pulmonary artery to the descending aorta through the ductus arteriosus. Within the first day after birth, pulmonary arterial pressure, which is slightly greater than aortic pressure in the fetus, falls to roughly 50 percent of the *in utero* value while systemic arterial pressure remains relatively constant. The regulation of this fall in pulmonary vascular resistance, and vasomotor tone in general, are discussed in Section 10G2.

Effect of gravity

Because the postnatal pulmonary circulation is a low-pressure circuit that is influenced by alveolar and interstitial pressure, the distribution of blood within the lungs is not uniform; rather, blood flow depends on the interplay of lung position and gravity.

By convention, physiologists divide the lung into several different zones; blood flow through each is determined by the interrelationship of pulmonary arterial pressure, alveolar pressure, and pulmonary venous pressure. Zone 1 is the uppermost section of lung, and the remaining zones follow one below the other. Furthermore, physiologists label vessels in the lung as either alveolar or extra-alveolar. The alveolar vessels are subject to the pressure in the alveolar space and are compressed by lung inflation, while extra-alveolar vessels are not affected by alveolar pressure and expand with lung inflation. The concepts of lung zones and alveolar and extra-alveolar vessels are functional, and not anatomically based. They are most useful in terms of understanding and explaining the results of experimental manipulations of the lung.

Zone 1 is that area of the lung in which alveolar pressure is greater than pulmonary arterial and pulmonary venous pressures and there is no blood flow through alveolar vessels because alveolar pressure exceeds pulmonary arterial pressure; alveolar pressure acts, in effect, as a clamp on the alveolar vessels in this zone. Blood flow does occur in extra-alveolar vessels in zone 1. In an upright patient, zone 1 comprises the area of the lung near the apices.

In **zone 2**, which begins just below zone 1, pulmonary arterial pressure now exceeds alveolar pressure, but alveolar pressure still exceeds pulmonary venous pressure. Blood flow in zone 2 increases with distance down zone 2 because pulmonary arterial pressure increases with distance down zone 2.

Zone 3 begins at the point where alveolar pressure equals pulmonary venous pressure. In zone 3, resistance to blood flow is determined by the difference between pulmonary arterial and pulmonary venous pressures but measured blood flow increases with distance down zone 3 just as in zone 2. This is rather unexpected because the difference in driving pressure for fluid movement (the difference between pulmonary arterial and pulmonary venous pressures) remains constant in zone 3. The increase in observed blood flow is thought to be secondary to vessel recruitment and anatomical changes resulting in vessel distension.

The most dependent area of the lung is sometimes referred to as **zone 4**. Determinants of blood flow are more complicated in this zone and, as a result, blood flow is influenced to a greater extent by flow in vessels other than those in close approximation to alveoli. Blood flow often decreases with distance down zone 4 as blood vessels are compressed by gravity.

Sites of vascular resistance

In the pulmonary circulation, the total cross-sectional area in the pulmonary vasculature decreases as vessels branch distally. Direct microvascular pressure measurements have shown that as a result of this, the pressure drop across the microcirculation is substantial. This contrasts with the situation in the systemic circulation, where the greatest site of resistance is in the small arterioles, upstream from the microcirculation.

Effect of vascular pressure and lung volume

The pulmonary circulation can accommodate substantial changes in blood volume and flow. For instance, an increase in pulmonary arterial pressure or left atrial pressure decreases pulmonary vascular resistance due to vascular distension and vessel recruitment. Likewise, an increase in pulmonary blood volume also causes vascular distension and recruitment and results in a decrease in pulmonary vascular resistance. Thus, during exercise, even though cardiac output may increase substantially, pulmonary arterial pressure does not rise dramatically because pulmonary vascular resistance decreases.

When the lung is at functional residual capacity (FRC), pulmonary vascular resistance is lowest. An increase in lung expansion or a forced expiration at the end of a tidal breath, which lowers lung volume below FRC, will elevate pulmonary vascular resistance.

Although commonly believed, the concept that interstitial pulmonary edema *per se* increases pulmonary vascular resistance (by 'filling up' the interstitial space) is not supported by experimental evidence at present. There is evidence, however, that alveolar edema results in a local increase in pulmonary vascular resistance secondary to vasoconstriction. This results in redistribution of blood flow to areas of the lung with well ventilated alveoli.

Liquid and solute transport

The pulmonary vasculature is the first barrier to liquid and solute movement into the parenchyma of the lung, and as such is the first line of defense against excessive fluid accumulation, pulmonary edema, in the lung. Although edema in peripheral tissues is cosmetically unappealing, edema in the lungs can be life-threatening. Conditions that increase the rate of transport of liquid into the lungs are common, but fortunately, the pathways for liquid removal can accommodate excess fluid under most circumstances. Pulmonary edema results when the mechanisms for liquid removal are overwhelmed.

Water probably crosses the endothelial barrier directly through the endothelial cell or through interendothelial cell junctions. Macromolecules probably cross the endothelial barrier through interendothelial cell junctions, which do not restrict small particles but do restrict large proteins. There is some evidence for vesicular transport across the endothelial cell itself, but how much this type of solute transport contributes to overall liquid and protein movement is unclear at this point.

In general, fluid transport across a semipermeable membrane can be described conceptually by the Starling equation:

$$Q = Kf[(P_{\mathrm{mv}} - P_{\mathrm{pmv}}) - \sigma(\pi_{\mathrm{mv}} - \pi_{\mathrm{pmv}})],$$

where Q is the net liquid flow across the membrane, Kf represents the conductance of the membrane, P is the hydrostatic pressure term, σ represents the reflection coefficient, and π represents the protein osmotic pressure; the subscripts mv and pmv represent the microvascular and perimicrovascular sites of measurement, respectively. The major portion of the fluid exchange occurs in the vicinity of the alveolar walls in the small vessels, collectively termed the microvasculature.

Permeability

The conductance of the vascular barrier, Kf, is a function of both the permeability to water and the surface area available for fluid exchange. From the above equation, if permeability increases, Kf would increase, resulting in more fluid transport across the pulmonary vasculature. Likewise, if the surface area for fluid exchange increases, Kf would increase, and fluid flow across the endothelial barrier would increase.

The other term in the equation that affects permeability is σ, the osmotic reflection coefficient. The reflection coefficient indicates how resistant a barrier is to solute movement. In the limiting case, an impermeant molecule would have a reflection coefficient of one and a molecule with no restriction to movement, such as serum electrolytes, would have a value of zero. σ represents the sum of the permeability characteristics for all the plasma proteins. As a practical matter, any condition that increases the water conductance of the barrier also increases the protein permeability and results in an increase in Kf and a decrease in σ.

The *adult respiratory distress syndrome* affects not only adults but many pediatric patients as well. The pulmonary endothelium is more permeable than normal (Kf is increased and σ is decreased), which results in an exaggerated filtration of fluid across the vascular barrier and resultant pulmonary edema. In the *respiratory distress syndrome* that occurs in premature infants secondary to surfactant deficiency, the pulmonary endothelium is also abnormally permeable.

Vascular and osmotic pressure

From the Starling relationship, it is clear that a rise in microvascular hydrostatic pressure will increase fluid filtration. The difference between the microvascular and perimicrovasular pressures actually determines whether a change in hydrostatic pressure will change fluid transport. For the most part, however, increases in microvascular pressure are not accompanied by equivalent increases in interstitial pressure; therefore, excess fluid is filtered across the circulation.

Likewise, the protein osmotic pressure terms must be considered together. That is, the difference between the microvascular and perivascular protein osmotic pressures determines the effect on fluid filtration.

Equilibration between protein concentrations in the intravascular and interstitial spaces of the lung is more rapid than is generally appreciated. In normal lungs, for instance, the albumin concentration in interstitial fluid is approximately 80–90 percent that of plasma. It rapidly reaches a new equilibrium when plasma albumin concentration changes. In conditions where the permeability of the endothelial barrier is compromised, the concentration of albumin in the interstitium is even closer to that of plasma. Infusions of albumin to increase plasma oncotic pressure in patients with increased vascular permeability are unlikely to result in any substantial benefit to the patient as the albumin will equilibrate rapidly between the plasma and interstitium. In fact, such an infusion might increase pulmonary vascular pressures and enhance fluid filtration into the lung.

Endothelial cell biology

Metabolic functions

The pulmonary endothelium is not an inert cell lining, but rather is metabolically active and sensitive to a number of agents that come in contact with its surface. After birth the entire cardiac output passes through the pulmonary circulation; therefore, the lung is in a unique position to respond to mediators present in the circulation.

Prostaglandins

Prostaglandins are a class of arachidonic acid metabolites made by virtually all cell types (see p. 103). Pulmonary endothelium is no exception and makes predominantly PGI_2 which has potent effects on vasomotor tone (see Section 10G2). PGI_2 is not metabolized in the lung. In contrast, PGE_2, PGE_1, and $PGF_{2\alpha}$ are all inactivated in the lung. PGE_2 inactivation is gestationally dependent in the perinatal period with less circulating PGE_2 being cleared in a single passage through lungs from immature fetuses. Pulmonary inactivation of circulating PGE_2 is important in functional closure of the ductus arteriosus at birth.

Endothelial derived relaxing factor (EDRF)

Now considered to be nitric oxide (NO) and more recently termed endothelial derived nitric oxide (EDNO), this substance is released in response to various stimuli. It too plays a major role in pulmonary vasoregulation (see Section 10G2).

Inactivation of biogenic amines

Catecholamines, histamine, and serotonin are potent vasogenic bioamines. The pulmonary circulation plays a major role in the inactivation of two of these substances, serotonin and norepinephrine. The pulmonary circulation plays little or no role in the inactivation of epinephrine, dopamine, or histamine.

Serotonin

Serotonin (5-hydroxytryptamine), a potent vasoconstrictor, is found in a variety of tissues. The pulmonary endothelium contains a specific uptake mechanism for the removal of serotonin. This extraction process is carrier mediated, driven by the Na^+ gradient produced by Na^+-K^+-ATPase and it is saturable and temperature dependent. Once inside the cell, serotonin is metabolized by a monoamine oxidase. The uptake system is quite efficient, clearing over 90 percent of plasma serotonin during a single pass through the lung. It is inhibited by cocaine and tricyclic antidepressants.

Norepinephrine

Norepinephrine is also a potent vasoconstrictor. Like serotonin, norepinephrine is taken up and inactivated by the pulmonary endothelium; 25–50 percent of circulating norepinephrine is cleared during a single pass through the lungs.

The uptake of norepinephrine by endothelial cells is biochemically similar to the uptake of serotonin, although the carriers responsible for transport are distinct. Once inside the cell, norepinephrine is metabolized by either a monoamine oxidase or catechol-*O*-methyltransferase. Uptake inhibitors are similar to those for serotonin.

Vasoactive peptides

Bradykinin

Bradykinin is a 9 amino acid peptide formed in plasma by the kininogen–kinin system. It is a potent hypotensive substance and it is inactivated by angiotensin-converting enzyme, an endothelial cell-surface dipeptidylcarboxypeptidase. Roughly 80 percent of the circulating bradykinin is removed during one pass through the lungs.

Angiotensin I

Angiotensin I is a 10 amino acid peptide formed in plasma from angiotensinogen. As angiotensin I passes through the lungs, it is converted by the angiotensin-converting enzyme noted above to angiotensin II, an 8 amino acid peptide that causes hypertension. Although other endothelial cells possess angiotensin-converting enzyme activity, the lung is the most important site for converting angiotensin I to angiotensin II. Angiotensin II is not metabolized by the lung, but is metabolized by other vascular beds.

Pulmonary circulation and hemostasis

The pulmonary endothelium, like other endothelial beds, normally maintains a non-thrombogenic surface. However, a number of lung diseases are associated with disordered hemostasis in the pulmonary circulation. Often it is unclear whether the abnormal hemostasis causes or aggravates the lung disorder or whether it is secondary to a primary endothelial cell abnormality.

Anticoagulant characteristics

Prostaglandins

PGI_2 is not only a potent vasodilator but also inhibits platelet aggregation. This is pertinent because platelet aggregation occurs early in response to vascular injury. Platelet aggregation promotes conversion of prothrombin to thrombin, and aggregating platelets release thromboxane A_2, a powerful vasoconstrictor. PGI_2 released by endothelial cells serves to counteract these responses.

Endothelial derived nitric oxide (EDNO)

EDNO, much as PGI_2, is not only a potent vasodilator but also inhibits platelet aggregation.

Heparan sulfate

In addition to PGI_2 and EDNO formation, endothelial cells also express cell-surface-associated molecules involved in anticoagulation. One such molecule is heparan sulfate, a proteoglycan that has heparin-like characteristics. Heparin, and similarly heparan sulfate on the cell surface, acts as an anticoagulant because it binds to circulating antithrombin III, which inactivates thrombin at an accelerated rate. In addition to inactivating thrombin, antithrombin III also inactivates factors IXa, Xa, XIa, and XIIa. Antithrombin III acts by blocking a serine residue necessary for coagulant enzyme activity. If endothelial cells are damaged in such a manner as to block or destroy the heparan sulfate molecules on the cell surface, their antithrombin III-mediated anticoagulant property is lost.

Thrombomodulin

Endothelial cells express a thrombin-binding protein called thrombomodulin. This protein avidly binds thrombin to form a complex that dramatically enhances thrombin-catalyzed activation of protein C. The endothelial cell provides a surface for activated protein C to interact with protein S, a circulating glycoprotein. When the activated protein C–protein S complex is formed, activated protein C blocks the function of factors Va and VIIIa, inhibiting the coagulation process.

There is also evidence that after thrombin binds to thrombomodulin, this ligand–receptor complex is internalized. This process would promote anticoagulation because thrombin bound to thrombomodulin can still convert fibrinogen to fibrin under the appropriate conditions.

Procoagulant characteristics

The major procoagulant property of endothelial cells is the cell-surface expression of tissue factor, a glycoprotein with a molecular weight of 40–50 kDa. Tissue factor acts as a cofactor with factor VII to enhance the activation of factors IX and X. Normal endothelium does not express tissue factor, but certain molecules known to be associated with pulmonary vascular injury are stimulants for tissue factor expression by endothelial cells. These include thrombin, endotoxin, interleukin-1, and tumor necrosis factor.

Fibrinolysis

The endothelium plays a balancing act in fibrinolysis, producing molecules that promote and inhibit clot lysis. Like every other aspect of the coagulation cascade, regulated production of these factors is the critical element.

Endothelial cells produce two plasminogen activators, urokinase plasminogen activator (uPA) and tissue plasminogen activator (tPA). tPA binds to fibrin and plasminogen, forming a complex that accelerates the formation of plasmin from plasminogen. Plasmin then cleaves fibrin and fibrinogen to begin clot lysis.

Endothelial cells also produce plasminogen activator inhibitor. This molecule inhibits both tPA and uPA. Thus the endothelial cell participates intimately in the regulation of clot formation and dissolution. Factors like endotoxin and tumor necrosis factor disturb this balance and promote endothelial procoagulant activity.

Non-hemostatic effects

Some of the molecules formed during hemostasis have additional effects on the pulmonary vasculature. For instance, thrombin is a crucial clotting enzyme, but also appears to increase pulmonary vascular permeability, pulmonary vascular resistance, and pulmonary arterial pressure. Thrombin also causes neutrophils to adhere and accumulate in the lung and stimulates platelet aggregation and adherence of platelets to endothelial cells. Heparan sulfate proteoglycan produced by endothelial cells also acts as a growth inhibitor for pulmonary vascular smooth muscle.

Neutrophil–endothelial cell interaction

Although the interaction of endothelial cells and circulating neutrophils is absolutely required for normal host defense, when this interaction occurs in an unregulated fashion, neutrophils can initiate or enhance vascular and tissue damage. A number of studies imply that neutrophils play a role in lung injury and the subsequent development of pulmonary edema.

The requisite step in neutrophil migration into the interstitium is adhesion to the vascular wall. This adhesion is modulated by neutrophil-dependent and endothelial cell-dependent mechanisms.

Neutrophil-dependent adhesion

Two general classes of adhesion molecules, present on neutrophils, mediate their binding to endothelial cells, the β_2-integrins and L-selectin.

β_2-integrins

The three β_2-integrins are more commonly recognized by their 'CD' classifications: CD11a-CD18, CD11b-CD18, and CD11c-CD18. All three integrins are normally present on the neutrophil plasma membrane.

A number of diverse agonists induce neutrophil-dependent, integrin-mediated adhesion to endothelial cells, including f-Met-Leu-Phe, fragments of complement activation, platelet-activating factor, and leukotriene B_4. Adhesion appears to be dependent on a conformational change in the β_2-integrins present on the surface to the time of stimulation. Although new β_2-integrins are translocated to the cell surface after agonist stimulation, neutrophil adhesion still occurs, even if new integrins are not expressed on the cell surface.

The β_2-integrins bind to the intercellular adhesion molecules 1 and 2 (ICAM-1, ICAM-2) on the endothelial surface. The β_2-integrins may also bind to other uncharacterized molecules.

L-selectin

L-selectin (also known as LAM-1 and MEL-14) is one of three molecules in the selectin family, the others being E-selectin and P-selectin. L-selectin is the only one, however, known to be present on neutrophils. The adhesion molecule on endothelial cells to which L-selectin binds is uncertain at this time.

The binding characteristics of neutrophil adhesion to endothelial cells mediated by L-selectin have not been explored as extensively as those of the β_2-integrins. It is interesting that under certain conditions there may be a cooperation between L-selectin and β_2-integrins since reagents that interfere with either β_2-integrins or L-selectin inhibit neutrophil adhesion to cytokine-stimulated endothelial cells.

Endothelial cell-dependent adhesion

Platelet-activating factor (PAF)

Platelet-activating factor is a well characterized phospholipid that is rapidly synthesized in endothelial cells in response to a number of agonists including leukotriene C_4, histamine, and thrombin. PAF is expressed on the cell surface after it is synthesized, and is not released. PAF binds to a receptor on the neutrophil surface, a process that results in an increase in neutrophil adhesiveness, further anchoring the neutrophil to the endothelial cell. The enhanced neutrophil binding triggered by PAF is mediated by the β_2-integrins CD11a-CD18 and CD11b-CD18. PAF can also prime the neutrophil to respond in an exaggerated fashion to chemotactic factors.

Interleukin-8 (IL-8)

Another molecule, IL-8, is synthesized by endothelial cells and participates in neutrophil binding and subsequent neutrophil migration. After endothelial cells are stimulated by tumor necrosis factor (TNF), interleukin-1 (IL-1), or lipopolysaccharide (LPS), transcription of IL-8 mRNA begins, ultimately resulting in maximal IL-8 expression 4–24 hours later. IL-8 is secreted by the endothelial cell and exerts its effect by binding to a receptor on the neutrophil. In response to IL-8 stimulation, neutrophil adhesion is mediated through the β_2-integrin complex.

P-selectin

When endothelial cells are activated by histamine or thrombin, P-selectin moves rapidly from storage granules in the endothelial cell to the plasma membrane. Cell-associated P-selectin binds a receptor on the neutrophil surface that is distinct from the β_2-integrin family. The time course for expression of P-selectin activity is similar to expression of PAF activity. Thus, P-selectin may initially bind the neutrophil, allowing PAF to activate the neutrophil. This would result in enhanced neutrophil adhesion secondary to β_2-integrin binding and enhanced responsiveness to chemotactic factors. The receptor for P-selectin on the neutrophil is unknown.

E-selectin

E-selectin (also known as endothelial-leukocyte adhesion molecule 1, or ELAM-1) is a molecule expressed and retained on the endothelial cell plasma membrane in response to stimulation with TNF, IL-1, or LPS. Expression requires protein synthesis and is maximal at 4–8 hours. β_2-integrins are not required for E-selectin-mediated neutrophil binding, nor is neutrophil activation required. The receptor on the neutrophil for E-selectin is unknown.

Mediators of neutrophil-induced damage

There is abundant evidence that oxidants released from stimulated neutrophils are responsible in part for damage caused by these cells. Antioxidants like superoxide dismutase and catalase ameliorate neutrophil-mediated damage *in vivo* and *in vitro*. Likewise, reduced amounts of natural antioxidants like glutathione increase the susceptibility of endothelial cells to neutrophil-mediated damage. The exact mechanism of oxidant injury is unclear, but oxidants may oxidize cell phospholipids and thereby alter membrane function. Oxidants may also inactivate naturally occurring antiproteases.

Neutrophils also cause damage by releasing proteases in response to activation. These proteases may then disturb endothelial cell-matrix attachments and they may alter molecules expressed on the endothelial cell surface such as heparan sulfate.

Selected reading

Carlos TM, Harlan JM. Membrane proteins involved in phagocyte adherence to endothelium. *Immunol Rev* 1990; **114**: 5.

Fishman AP. Pulmonary circulation. In Fishman AP, Fisher AB, eds. *Handbook of physiology*. Vol. I, Sect. 3. Baltimore: Waverly Press, 1985: 93.

Staub NC. Pulmonary edema. *Physiol Rev* 1974; **54**: 678.

Stern DM, Kaiser E, Nawroth PP. Regulation of the coagulation system by vascular endothelial cells. *Haemostasis* 1988; **18**: 202.

A5. The Pulmonary Interstitium

D P Carlton

Anatomically, the pulmonary interstitium is considered to encompass the area between the alveolar epithelium and capillary endothelium. This space is contiguous with the loose connective tissue that surrounds the airways and larger blood vessels; thus this entire region is in series. The interstitium contains a number of different cells and molecules necessary for maintenance of normal lung function, and is also the area through which water and solutes travel after they have filtered across the vascular endothelium or have been reabsorbed from the alveolar air space.

Structural design

The interstitial area throughout the lung contains an organized connective tissue framework that gives the lung its characteristic shape. The elements of this framework are predominantly collagen and elastin. The framework is divided into three components. First, the peripheral fiber system begins in the interstitium of the visceral pleura. These fibers surround the lung in the pleural interstitium and also travel centrally, subdividing the lung into segments as they move towards the hilum. The second component, the central fiber system, begins at the hilum and moves peripherally, surrounding and supporting airways and vessels. The third component, the septal fiber system, is composed of small connective tissue fibers that provide support for the alveoli. This design gives the lung its strength and its elastic characteristics.

Liquid movement

The fibrous network of the interstitium permits efficient liquid movement away from the alveoli to a more central location, thus minimizing interference with gas exchange. Normally, fluid is removed by lymphatics as it moves out of the alveolar septal area, and the volume of lymphatic drainage is considered to be equal to transvascular fluid filtration. There is always a net movement of liquid from the circulation into the interstitial space. The lymphatics do not begin in the alveolar septal area, but rather in the peribronchovascular space around terminal airways and vessels. Lymphatics are lined by continuous endothelium and contain numerous valves, similar in function to those in the systemic veins, which results in unidirectional lymphatic flow centrally. Smooth muscle cells that surround larger lymphatic vessels are responsible for the pulsatile movement of lymph towards the hilum. The lymph eventually drains into regional lymph nodes, and ultimately the systemic circulation.

The alveolar septal connective tissue space is in series with the peribronchovascular space, the loose connective tissue that surrounds the larger airways and blood vessels. When abnormal amounts of fluid are filtered from the circulation and overwhelm the lymphatic system, this excess fluid moves to fill the peribronchovascular space. Again this minimizes the volume of liquid filling the alveolar septal space. The driving force for this movement is an increasingly negative pressure gradient from periphery to hilum.

Extracellular matrix

Together, collagen and elastin in the interstitium are estimated to comprise most of the total protein in the lung, well over 95 percent of the connective tissue, and 15–20 percent of dry lung weight. Of the two, collagen is the most abundant. Together they give the lung its structural integrity, expansive limit, and elastic recoil.

Collagen

Collagen collectively consists of at least 13 different proteins. Their chemical properties give them great tensile strength. Type I and III collagen are the most abundant forms found in the lung, accounting for over 75 percent of the connective tissue. All collagen molecules share relatively unique amino acid sequences of repeating trimers containing glycine. In addition to the large amount of glycine, proline and hydroxyproline are also abundant. The latter is an uncommon amino acid and, in fact, is often used as a marker of collagen as virtually no other protein contains hydroxyproline. The other unique molecular characteristic of collagen is that it is composed of three subunits that form a triple helix. Depending on the collagen type, the subunits may be the same or different.

Collagen synthesis is not restricted to one cell type in the lung, but there appear to be a limited number of types of collagen manufactured. Although fibroblasts, epithelial cells, and endothelial cells can synthesize collagen, the fibroblast is considered to be the model cell for collagen production. Collagen is initially translated as procollagen. While still inside the cell, the appropriate proline, and sometimes lysine, residues are hydroxylated. Three individual procollagen subunits then associate and form a more mature procollagen, which then undergoes helix formation. Before secretion, the hydroxylysine residues are glycosylated. The extra peptides present on the procollagen molecules are thought to have several functions, one of which is to keep the collagen precursor soluble in the cell until secretion. After secretion, C- and N-terminal regions of the procollagen subunits are cleaved to form mature collagen. Mature collagen is known to bind to fibronectin and to certain cells, but the biological significance of these findings is unclear. Collagen synthesized in response to injury is predominantly type I. This is a result of enhanced fibroblast production and an overall increase in fibroblast number.

Collagens are degraded by metalloproteinases referred to as collagenases, but what role collagenases play in the turnover of lung collagen is unclear. Neutrophils, macrophages, and fibroblasts each secrete collagenases, but their specificity for a particular collagen type is different. A number of cells, including fibroblasts, macrophages, and neutrophils, produce enzymes capable of destroying collagen, which is undoubtedly important in lung diseases where destruction of the delicate interstitial elements occurs.

Elastin

Elastin is the other major component of the connective tissue in the lung. Although not as prominent as collagen, it is extremely important, giving the lung its 'elastic' quality. Although elastin can be found relatively early in gestation, the majority of elastin production takes place during the latter part of gestation, temporally associated with alveolarization; after this portion of lung development is complete, new elastin formation is minimal.

Elastin is first secreted in a soluble form, tropoelastin. Tropoelastin then associates with microfibrils, after which lysyl oxidase links tropoelastin molecules together to form mature elastin; chemically, mature elastin is quite insoluble. A variety of cells, including smooth muscle cells, endothelial cells, myofibroblasts, and some types of fibroblasts, are believed to be capable of producing elastin. The normal turnover rate for elastin is extraordinarily slow. Mature elastin that does turn over is degraded by elastases. These enzymes are promiscuous and degrade not only elastin but also proteoglycans, collagen, and fibronectin. The normal site in the lung for elastase production is unknown.

Fibronectins

The role of fibronectins in the extracellular matrix of the lung is unclear. They are large glycoproteins with molecular weights of approximately 500 kDa and at least 20 isoforms have been identified. Although plasma fibronectin is produced by hepatocytes, a 'cellular' fibronectin produced locally by lung cells is considered important in normal lung development. Pulmonary endothelial cells, epithelial cells, fibroblasts, alveolar macrophages, and smooth muscle cells all are capable of producing fibronectin *in vitro*. Although at this time it is uncertain whether fibronectin detected in the lung is derived from plasma or is produced in the lung, the balance weighs in favor of plasma deposition.

Fibronectins contain an RGD (Arg-Aly-Asp) sequence that acts as a binding site for lung fibroblasts, which possess a fibronectin receptor complex. Fibronectin–fibroblast interactions allow the fibroblasts to migrate and spread. Other cell types, including endothelial and epithelial cells, also bind to fibronectin, but whether this binding is mediated in the same fashion as fibroblasts is unclear.

The role of fibronectin in lung development is deduced from experiments showing increased fibronectin content associated with cell differentiation. This role for fibronectin in a general biological sense is strengthened because of similar associations in other organs during development. Furthermore, experiments with antibodies that interfere with fibronectin–fibronectin receptor binding *in vitro* disturb normal lung development.

Although normal adult lungs have very little cellular fibronectin, injured lungs show a dramatic increase in cellular fibronectin production. The importance of this finding is unknown, but probably reflects the role of fibronectin in cell migration.

Basement membrane

Basement membranes consist of molecules assembled together to form a matrix that supports and surrounds the endothelium and epithelium. Basement membranes are also associated with smooth muscle cells and nerves. The basement membrane serves as a somewhat selective barrier for macromolecules and inhibits cell movement, unless the cells possess specific proteases that dissolve the matrix (e.g. inflammatory cells).

Collagen

Type IV collagen is a major constituent of basement membranes. It is similar in basic constitution to other collagens and has a molecular weight of approximately 500 kDa. The COOH-terminal globular domains are joined together, which allows the NH_2-terminal ends from four collagen molecules to interact. This interaction results in a lattice or meshwork of collagen.

Laminin

Laminin, another major component of basement membranes, is a large glycoprotein with a molecular weight of around 850 kDa. Fully assembled, laminin exists as a four-armed 'cross'-like structure composed of three distinct chains. Laminin is not one molecule but, like fibronectin, exists as several different isoforms. Also like fibronectin, laminin has several sites of attachment that permit binding of cells and other constituents of the extracellular matrix. Laminin probably plays a role in cell migration.

Entactin

Entactin, also known as nidogen, is a glycoprotein of molecular weight 150 kDa. It apparently exists in basement membrane only, and is closely associated with laminin. The entactin molecule has binding sites for type IV collagen; therefore, entactin may serve to link laminin and collagen.

Heparan sulfate proteoglycans

These molecules are proteins bound to heparan sulfate chains. Because of their negative charge, they may serve to restrict movement of negatively charged molecules. There are a number of different heparan sulfate proteoglycans. Some are known to bind laminin, type IV collagen, and fibronectin.

Interstitial cells

Fibroblasts

These cells constitute the major cell type of the lung interstitium. Although sometimes presented as distinctly different cells, fibroblasts, myofibroblasts, and pericytes probably represent different forms of a similar cell type.

Fibroblasts contain many mitochondria, a large amount of endoplasmic reticulum, and an obvious Golgi complex. These findings are consistent with the synthetic capabilities of the fibroblast to produce collagen, fibronectin, and proteoglycans. Fibroblasts possess cell-surface receptors capable of binding a number of interstitial elements including fibronectin, laminin, and collagen. The fibroblast–connective tissue interactions may serve to arrange the interstitial components during development and repair.

Pericytes

Pericytes are associated with the capillaries in the alveolar system. They are partially surrounded by a basement membrane, and cytoplasmic extensions are often found in direct contact with the endothelial cells. Their function is uncertain but they are considered by some to be smooth muscle cell precursors.

Myofibroblasts

Myofibroblasts are present in the alveolar septum. They possess contractile characteristics, but their biological significance is unknown. They are abundant, perhaps constituting 40 percent of the volume of the interstitial space.

Certain diseases resulting in *pulmonary fibrosis* are associated with alterations in fibroblasts and extracellular matrix. For instance, bleomycin induces pulmonary fibrosis and is associated with diminished fibroblast growth, but it enhances collagen production.

Selected reading

Foster JA, Curtiss SW. The regulation of lung elastin synthesis. *Am J Physiol* 1990; **259**: L13.

Goldstein RH. Control of type I collagen formation in the lung. *Am J Physiol* 1991; **261**: L29.
McDonald JA. Extracellular matrix assembly. *Annu Rev Cell Biol* 1988; **4**: 183.
Yurchenco PD, Schittny JC. Molecular architecture of basement membranes. *FASEB J* 1990; **4**: 1577.

A6. Lung Injury

J R Wispé

Aerobic organisms are continually exposed to the risk of oxidant injury caused by partially reduced, reactive oxygen metabolites (ROM). Reactive oxygen metabolites can cause injury by reacting with cellular proteins, lipids, and nucleic acids. To protect against oxidant injury, aerobic cells evolved a multilayered, interdependent antioxidant system that includes enzymatic and non-enzymatic components. This antioxidant system exists in the mature lung of all air-breathing organisms. In human diseases, an imbalance between oxidants and antioxidants is involved in the pathogenesis of diverse pulmonary and non-pulmonary disorders. This section characterizes the nature and source of reactive oxygen metabolites and describes the function of key antioxidant compounds.

Pulmonary oxidant injury

An imbalance between pulmonary oxidants and antioxidants may arise under several circumstances. Increased production of oxidants is a common factor in lung injury. Oxidants arise from three major sources in the lungs: (1) normal cellular processes may produce increased amounts of ROM, especially during exposure to hyperoxia (for example, hyperoxia increases mitochondrial production of ROM); (2) activated inflammatory cells, neutrophils and macrophages, generate ROM intracellularly that can be released; and (3) metabolism of xenobiotics frequently generates reactive metabolites. Ozone is metabolized in the airway to reactive oxygen and lipid peroxide compounds. Compounds in tobacco smoke are also used by lung cells to produce reactive metabolites. Reactive oxygen species include the partially reduced oxygen metabolites superoxide anion (O_2^-), hydrogen peroxide (H_2O_2), hydroxyl radical ($OH^\bullet$), and singlet oxygen (O^-) (see p. 108). The initial reaction of oxygen radicals with cellular constituents can also generate a secondary cascade of lipid and protein 'radicals' that further propagate oxidant injury. One should recognize three key features of oxidant injury. First, oxidants are produced at specific subcellular sites, which vary depending on the oxidant stress. Second, because of their reactivity, ROM are diffusion-limited and oxidant injury tends to occur near the site of ROM production. For example, during hyperoxia mitochondrial production of ROM increases, and mitochondrial injury is an important component of oxygen injury. Hydrogen peroxide, which crosses cellular and subcellular membranes, may be an exception to this. Third, because of the specificity of ROM production and injury, protective antioxidants must be located either at the site of ROM production or at the oxidant target. Therefore, increased mitochondrial antioxidants would be expected to protect mitochondria from locally produced ROM during hyperoxia, while an increase in extracellular or cytoplasmic antioxidants might not.

Pulmonary antioxidant enzymes

The cascade of oxidizing radicals requires a matched system of substrate-specific antioxidant enzymes. Superoxide anion (O_2^-), the initial radical formed by one electron reduction of molecular oxygen, is eliminated by the superoxide dismutases (SOD). Eukaryotic organisms contain at least three SODs—a cytosolic CuZn-SOD, a mitochondrial Mn-SOD, and an extracellular SOD. All three SODs efficiently catalyze the reaction:

$$2O_2^- + 2H^+ \rightarrow H_2O_2 + O_2$$

Eukaryotic cells are well protected against H_2O_2 by catalase and glutathione peroxidase, which eliminate H_2O_2. The subcellular distributions of catalase and glutathione peroxidase are different; catalase is present in peroxisomes, and glutathione peroxidase in cytosol and in the mitochondria. Their affinity for H_2O_2 also differs; glutathione peroxidase: $K_m = 10^{-6}$ M; catalase: $K_m = 10^{-3}$ M. Although glutathione peroxidase has a greater affinity for H_2O_2, it has a smaller capacity than catalase. Glutathione peroxidase may, therefore, be important at times of low H_2O_2 production, with catalase assuming greater importance during times of high H_2O_2 production. It is imperative that the cell eliminate both O_2^- and H_2O_2. Through the Haber–Weiss reaction, O_2^- and H_2O_2 react together, in the presence of iron, to produce hydroxyl radical ($OH^\bullet$), an extraordinarily reactive metabolite capable of oxidizing any cellular constituent:

$$\text{(i)}\ Fe^{3+} + O_2^- \rightarrow Fe^{2+} + O_2$$

$$\text{(ii)}\ Fe^{2+} + H_2O_2 \rightarrow Fe^{3+} + OH^\bullet + OH^-$$

Eukaryotic cells have no specific enzymatic protection against $OH^\bullet$, other than 'suicide' reactions in which sulfhydryl groups or unsaturated fatty acids react nonspecifically with $OH^\bullet$. These reactions irreversibly oxidize the SH or lipids and frequently produce other reactive compounds.

Inherent in the eukaryotic cellular antioxidant system is the interdependence of the components. Augmentation of one antioxidant, without commensurate changes in other components, may not be beneficial. When SOD is increased in single-cell organisms, and in some mammalian cells in culture, oxidant cytotoxicity is increased. Presumably, the increased toxicity results from an inability to cope with the increased H_2O_2 that is generated by the SOD.

Non-enzymatic antioxidants

Several important antioxidants are non-enzymatic. Vitamin E (more precisely α-tocopherol) is a membrane antioxidant that detoxifies oxygen and lipid radicals to protect membrane fatty acids. When there is *vitamin E deficiency,* membrane polyunsaturated fatty acids are more sensitive to reactive species that are formed in normal metabolism, and to any oxidative stress (hyperoxia, radiation, ozone, oxidant drugs). Peroxidation of membrane polyunsaturated fatty acids (PUFA) changes the physical and functional characteristics of the membrane.

Although not strictly an antioxidant, glutathione (GSH), a peptide thiol, is an important component of the antioxidant system. GSH is a required cofactor in detoxification pathways of xenobiotics, is used by glutathione peroxidase in metabolism of H_2O_2 and lipid peroxides, and is necessary for regeneration of several antioxidants including ascorbate and α-tocopherol. When cellular GSH is insufficient, eukaryotic cells are more sensitive to reactive species generated during normal metabolism, and to exogenous oxidant stress. Manifestations of GSH deficiency are diverse, but include profound mitochondrial damage, presumably due to oxidant damage by mitochondrially produced ROM.

Vitamin A (retinoic acid) is often classified as an antioxidant. Although vitamin A may have antioxidant properties, it is more important as a regulator of cell growth and differentiation. Repair and regeneration of damaged epithelia requires adequate vitamin A. *Vitamin A deficiency* is associated with dysplastic epithelial changes that are reminiscent of the chronic lung changes that develop after pulmonary oxygen injury. There is strong evidence that inadequate vitamin A worsens the chronic lung sequelae that result from *neonatal pulmonary oxygen injury*.

Developmental aspects of pulmonary antioxidants

The developmental patterns of antioxidants have an important impact on *neonatal pulmonary oxygen injury*. The ontogeny of the pulmonary antioxidants mirrors the development of the surfactant system; maturation of the surfactant and antioxidant systems is part of a generalized preparation of the lung for birth. Lung antioxidant enzyme activities are low until immediately prior to term, when they are strongly induced. Activities peak in the immediate postnatal period and then decline to normal adult levels. The genetic and cellular mechanisms involved in regulation of lung antioxidant activities involve complex interactions between hormones, growth factors, and local substances. Less is known about the ontogeny of non-enzymatic lung antioxidants. Several are nutritionally regulated, and vitamin E and A levels in the lung require adequate liver stores. For most nutritional factors, lung levels are low throughout gestation, and normal postnatal increases require adequate enteral intake.

The preterm infant is ill prepared for an increase in oxidant stress because of low enzymatic and non-enzymatic antioxidant capabilities. Many preterm infants require supplemental oxygen because of pulmonary immaturity. The combination of increased oxidant stress and low antioxidants places important biological components at risk of oxidant damage. Although life-saving, hyperoxia causes significant morbidities that are mediated by reactive oxidant metabolites.

Lung proteases and antiproteases

The human lung is normally protected from proteases capable of attacking the extracellular matrix by a group of proteins, the antiproteases. The extracellular antiproteases in lung include α_1-antitrypsin (α_1AT), secretory leukoprotease inhibitor (SLPI), α_1-antichymotrypsin (α_1ACT), tissue inhibitor of metalloproteases (TIMP) and α_2-macroglobulin (α_2M). Antiproteases functionally inactivate proteases by specific binding, usually at the active proteolytic site. The binding is either irreversible or slowly reversible. Thus, the antiproteases act as a 'substrate' with a greater affinity for the protease than other substrates. The kinetics of protease inhibition involve both the time of inhibition (association rate constant) and the concentration of antiprotease required for inhibition (equilibrium constant), again emphasizing the concept of balance between protease and antiprotease. None of the lung antiproteases is protease specific; however, most are class specific. For example, α_1AT and SLPI inhibit all serine proteases, while TIMP inhibits metalloproteases.

α_1AT, the most abundant pulmonary extracellular antiprotease, provides most of the protection against neutrophil elastase in the lower respiratory tract. The major site of α_1AT production is liver hepatocytes, although other cells make small amounts. Pulmonary levels of α_1AT are ultimately controlled by hepatocyte synthesis and secretion. The critical importance of α_1AT is demonstrated by the genetic condition *α_1-antitrypsin deficiency*. In these patients, plasma α_1AT levels are less than 35 percent of normal, and the patients develop severe emphysema in young adulthood. Relative α_1AT deficiency probably is involved in other conditions. Merritt and co-workers reported that airway α_1AT was inactive in premature infants who later developed bronchopulmonary dysplasia.

Serum leukoprotease inhibitor, a serine antiprotease, is produced in the lung by mucosal cells in large and small airways. In distal respiratory tract, SLPI is made in nonciliated (Clara) epithelial cells. The major role of SLPI appears to be to protect the upper respiratory tract from neutrophil elastase. TIMP is a specific inhibitor of metalloproteases, such as collagenase, gelatinase, and the stromolysins. TIMP is produced within the lung by fibroblasts and alveolar macrophages. Although the exact role of TIMP in the lung is unclear, TIMP was recently reported to be specifically induced by pulmonary oxygen injury, perhaps as an adaptive-protective response.

Proteases and lung injury

The balance between proteases and antiproteases appears to be heavily weighted towards excess antiprotease protection in the healthy lung. Disturbance of this balance, with unlimited proteolysis, results in damage to and loss of the extracellular matrix. Without the support of their underlying connective tissue, alveoli are lost, resulting clinically in *emphysema*. Extensive work with animal models has demonstrated that administration of exogenous proteases, or stimulation of endogenous proteases, causes lung injury. Imbalance between proteases and antiproteases can occur as a primary pathophysiology in human lung; the best evidence for this mechanism is α_1AT deficiency, *cigarette smoke toxicity*, and *idiopathic pulmonary fibrosis*. More commonly, increased proteolytic injury occurs subsequent to *lung inflammation* with release of proteolytic enzymes from neutrophils and alveolar macrophages. The influx of inflammatory cells can occur in response to a variety of stimuli, including infection, acute lung injury, or complement activation. The acutely injured lung produces many substances that are chemotactic for neutrophils. These activated inflammatory cells release proteases and reactive oxygen species that cause further lung injury. Reactive oxygen species may also oxidize the active site of α_1AT, rendering it inactive, further tipping the balance towards proteolysis and lung injury. Because pulmonary inflammation is an almost universal response to lung injury, the major role of proteolysis in human lung disease may be to amplify and prolong acute lung injuries incited by diverse causes. In the future, it may be possible to augment the antiprotease defenses of the lower airway in order to prevent proteolytic injury.

Selected reading

Crystal RG, West JB, eds. *The lung, scientific foundations*. Vol. 2. New York: Raven Press, 1991; chapters 7.1, p. 1763, 7.2, p. 1803.

Fridovich I. Antioxidant defenses in the lung. *Annu Rev Physiol* 1986; **48**: 693.

Halliwell B, Gutteridge JMC. Oxygen toxicity, oxygen radicals, transition metals and disease. *Biochem J* 1984; **219**: 1.

Hubbard RC, Ogushi F, Fells GA, *et al*. Oxidants spontaneously released by alveolar macrophages of cigarette smokers can inactivate the active site of α_1-antitrypsin, rendering it ineffective as an inhibitor of neutrophil elastase. *J Clin Invest* 1987; **80**: 1289.

Merritt AT, Cochrane CG, Holcomb K, *et al*. Elastase and α_1-proteinase inhibitor activity in tracheal aspirates during respiratory distress syndrome. *J Clin Invest* 1983; **72**: 656.

Wispé JR, Roberts RJ. Molecular basis of pulmonary oxygen toxicity. *Clin Perinatol* 1987; **14**: 651.

B. Control of Breathing

B1. Neural Regulation of Respiration

B M Johnston and H Lagercrantz

The respiratory system functions to ventilate the lungs with air to allow the absorption of O_2 and removal of CO_2 according to the thermometabolic needs of the body. However, it is also involved in a number of behavioral reactions such as fright, locomotion and exercise and is of fundamental importance for oral communication. The ventilatory apparatus, consisting of the lungs and the chest wall, is activated by the respiratory muscles, which increase and decrease thoracic cavity size. During inspiration, contractions of the diaphragm and external intercostal muscles expand the chest and inflate the lungs. Respiratory motor activity is transmitted to the diaphragm via the phrenic nerve and along spinal nerves to the intercostal and abdominal muscles. The laryngeal muscles of the upper airway are innervated by a branch of the vagus nerve and the tongue (genioglossus) and pharyngeal muscles, also important respiratory muscles, are innervated by the XIIth and IXth cranial nerves respectively. Spontaneous respiration occurs as a result of the rhythmic and coordinated discharge of the motor neurons innervating the respiratory muscles. Motor neuron discharge originates in the caudal part of the brainstem. Ventilation ceases if the medulla is separated from the spinal cord above the origin of the phrenic nerves, but transection of the brainstem above the medulla at the pontine-medullary junction does not prevent rhythmic respiration even though breathing becomes irregular.

Respiration is controlled by two separate neural mechanisms, one voluntary , the other automatic (Fig. 11.5). Voluntary control, e.g. modulation of respiration during vocalization and cessation of respiration during voluntary breath holding, results from cerebral cortical

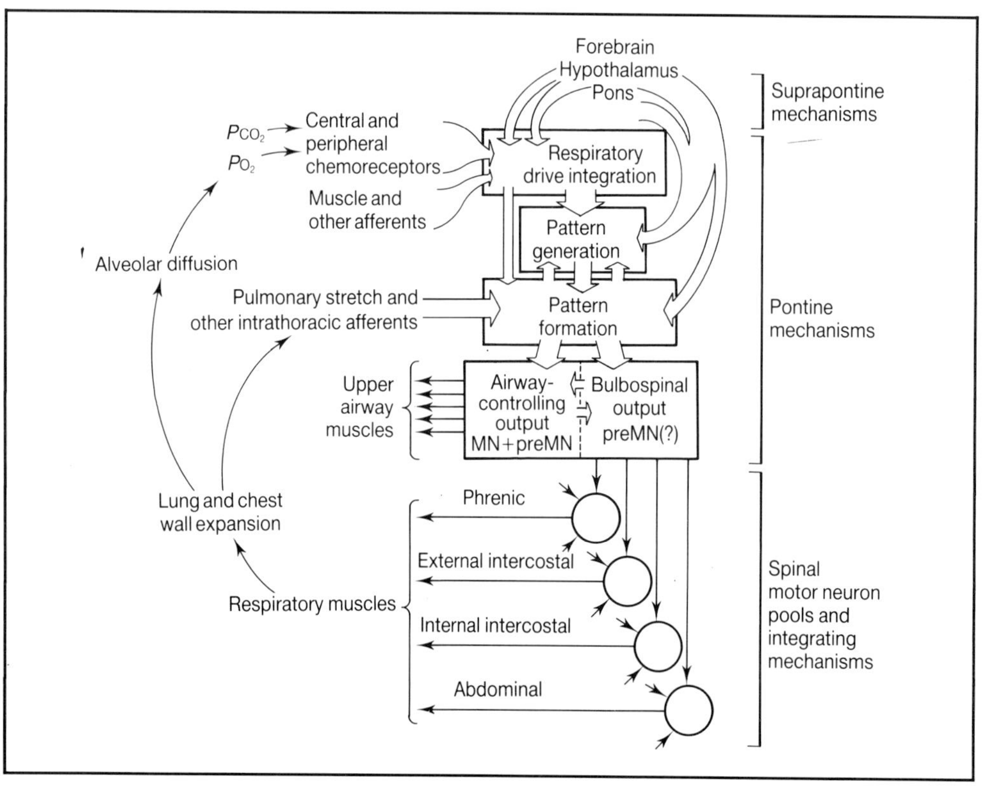

Fig. 11.5. Organization of the neural control of breathing. Emphasis is placed on the mechanisms for respiratory drive integration, respiratory pattern generation and formation and their influences on the two main output systems which control the upper airway and respiratory muscles. (From Euler CV. Breathing behaviour. In Euler CV, Lagercrantz H, eds. *Neurobiology of the control of breathing*. New York: Raven Press, 1987: 4. Reproduced with permission of Raven Press.)

activity activating respiratory motor neurons directly via the corticospinal tracts. Automatic respiration is controlled by a central pattern generator which spontaneously generates a characteristic pattern, even in the absence of extrinsic reflexes or feedback loops, provided there is sufficient tonic drive input. However, optimal control is achieved by integration of a number of reflexes as well as by feed-forward and feedback control mechanisms (Fig. 11.5). The respiratory control system can be considered as a neural oscillator with multiple inputs including non-sensory (cortex, hypothalamus, reticular formation), respiratory (chemoreceptor and mechanoreceptor) and non-respiratory (muscular, mechanoreceptor, pain, thermal and baroreceptor) feedback inputs.

There is some controversy regarding the existence of a circumscribed 'vital center' where respiratory rhythmicity is generated. There is no conclusive evidence that any pacemaker cells are involved in the generation of breathing in mammals. However, in isolated neonatal rat brain, spontaneously firing units are present in the rostral ventrolateral medulla.

Organization of central respiratory neurons

Medullary respiratory neurons are of two types: inspiratory (I neurons) which discharge during inspiration and expiratory (E neurons) which discharge during expiration. During quiet breathing, expiration is passive and E neurons are active only when ventilation is increased. Medullary respiratory neurons are grouped into two main areas. The predominantly inspiratory **dorsal respiratory group** (DRG) is located dorsally in the nucleus tractus solitarius (NTS) near the exit of the IXth cranial nerve. The **ventral respiratory group** contains both inspiratory and expiratory neurons and extends rostrally from the first cervical spinal segment to the caudal border of the pons in the retroambiguous, para-ambiguous and retrofacial nuclei. The exact anatomical and functional organization of the medullary respiratory neurons is the subject of active research.

Groups of respiratory-related neurons have also been described in the pons, but unlike the medullary respiratory neurons the majority of pontine neurons show phase spanning activity across both inspiration and expiration with peak firing frequency at either the I–E or E–I transition. It is believed that these pontine neurons influence the switching between inspiration and expiration. Two rostral areas in the pons (the medial parabrachial and Köllike–Fuse nuclei) intermittently inhibit tonically discharging neurons in the caudal, so-called, medullary apneustic center. Vagal afferents are also important for the transition from inspiration to expiration (see below). Transection of the pons between the rostral and caudal respiratory groups or vagotomy result in deep and sustained inspirations lasting tens of seconds. This arrest of respiration in inspiration is known as apneusis.

The mechanism causing switching between inspiration and expiration is still unresolved. Respiratory oscillations may result from direct reciprocal inhibition of interconnected networks of inspiratory and expiratory neurons. Alternatively, generation of inspiratory activity may be the primary event, and respiratory rhythmicity may result from recurring inhibition of inspiratory activity. Thus the generation of increasing respiratory drive by a group of neurons influenced by chemoreceptor input leads to excitation of a second group of neurons, which also receive vagal afferent input from the lungs. Reaching a threshold triggers a third neuronal group, which receives input from the pons, and inspiration is turned off.

Suprapontine drive

The forebrain drive usually overrides the metabolic or autonomic control of breathing in awake adults. Respiration during wakefulness, therefore, is fairly irregular and easily can be modulated by sensory inputs. This probably also applies to infants; for example, during sucking, breathing is intermittently interrupted to the point that blood gases can become deranged.

The hypothalamus and other higher centers have afferent connections to the central respiratory neurons, and thermal, painful and emotional stimuli can all affect respiration (Fig. 11.6). Respiratory drive is greater during wakefulness than during sleep, due to tonic excitation by the reticular system, which is involved in the maintenance of central nervous system arousal. In addition, sensitivity to hypercapnia and hypoxia is lower during sleep than during wakefulness. Nevertheless, during quiet sleep, maintenance of respiratory rhythm is critically dependent on chemical and vagal afferents. Withdrawal of all these afferent inputs leads to apnea

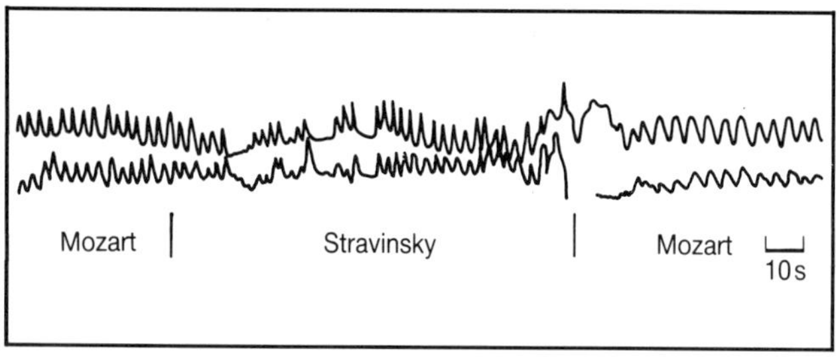

Fig. 11.6. An example of the influence of forebrain drive on the respiratory pattern (recorded by induction plethysmography) in a healthy newborn infant. During the playing of a Mozart serenade breathing was regular; during the playing of 'The Firebird' by Stravinsky, breathing became very irregular but returned to a slower, regular pattern on the reintroduction of music by Mozart. (Lagercrantz, unpublished.)

during this sleep state, whereas in wakefulness and in active sleep, respiratory rhythm is maintained due to reticular activation.

Chemical regulation of breathing

Respiratory depth and rate are regulated by chemical mechanisms which monitor Po_2 and Pco_2 and adjust ventilation so that blood gases and pH are kept within normal limits. Rises in $Paco_2$ or a fall in Pao_2 increase inspiratory activity and stimulate ventilation to facilitate excretion of CO_2 and absorption of O_2. Conversely, blood gas changes in the opposite direction have a depressive effect. These effects on respiration are mediated by **chemoreceptors** responsive to changes in respiratory gases or hydrogen ion concentration. Arterial and alveolar CO_2 tensions are regulated more precisely than O_2 levels.

Inputs from central chemoreceptors; CO_2 drive (see p. 615)

The linear ventilatory response to 7–8 percent inhaled CO_2 is mediated predominantly by central chemoreceptors located on the ventral surface of the medulla. However, the peripheral chemoreceptors are also CO_2 responsive and account for 10–20 percent of ventilatory stimulation. There remains some controversy regarding the exact location of the central chemoreceptors; the areas most likely involved (the rostral Mitchell area, the caudal Loeschcke area and the intermediate non-sensitive Schläfke area where the afferents enter the brainstem) are not located within either the dorsal or ventral respiratory groups and are believed to be distinct from the respiratory neurons.

The central chemoreceptors respond to changes in $Paco_2$ via changes in interstitial fluid, and possibly cerebrospinal fluid (CSF), but the final stimulus may be an increase in H^+ concentration within the chemoreceptor cells. Although H^+ and HCO_3^- penetrate the blood–brain and CSF barriers slowly, CO_2 is readily transferred and is promptly hydrated. The H_2CO_3 dissociates so that the local H^+ rises. Normally H^+ concentration in brain interstitial fluid parallels changes in $Paco_2$, although because CSF bicarbonate concentrations change slowly, this may not be true in conditions of metabolic acidosis or alkalosis or following rapid changes in altitude.

Inputs from peripheral chemoreceptors; hypoxemic drive
(see p. 612)

A fall in Pao_2 results in a hyperventilatory response which is mediated by peripheral chemoreceptors located in the carotid and aortic bodies. The carotid bodies are innervated by a branch of the IXth nerve and are situated at the junction of the internal and common carotid arteries. The aortic chemoreceptors, situated in the aortic arch, are innervated by the vagus nerve. The peripheral chemoreceptors project afferents to the NTS in the medulla. Afferent discharge increases when Pao_2 falls and is silenced by inhalation of 100 percent O_2. Removal or denervation of the carotid bodies has little effect on resting ventilation but results in loss of the respiratory stimulatory response to hypoxia and a diminished response to hypercapnia.

Pattern formation

Infants, particularly premature infants, are highly dependent on vagal afferent input from the lung to the brainstem to maintain lung volumes and promote inflation. Abolition of this receptor feedback, either by bypassing the larynx or by vagotomy, results in disruption of normal inspiratory activity.

Pulmonary mechanoreceptors

Inflation of the lungs inhibits inspiratory discharge by a reflex mechanism known as the **Hering–Breuer inflation reflex**. The reflex is more pronounced in anesthetized animals than in adult man. Lung stretch receptors, whose afferents run in the vagus nerve to the NTS, are stimulated by lung inflation and this terminates inspiration and promotes expiration. Larger volume changes are required to halt inspiration early in inspiration than later in inspiration. A further reflex, the Hering–Breuer deflation reflex, involves stimulation of J(juxtacapillary)-receptors located in lung interstitium near alveolar capillaries. Innervated by unmyelinated vagal fibers, J-receptors are stimulated by pulmonary edema and chemicals such as histamine. The response results in laryngeal closure and apnea followed by rapid, shallow breathing.

In contrast to the slowly adapting pulmonary stretch receptors, other vagally innervated pulmonary receptors, the irritant receptors, are rapidly adapting. They can be stimulated both chemically (e.g. by noxious gases, histamine, bradykinin, antigens) and mechanically (e.g. by particulate matter or increases in airflow [Head paradoxical inflation reflex]). The receptors are spread throughout the epithelial cells of the trachea, bronchi and lungs. Stimulation of these receptors augments inspiratory activity, but can also constrict the airway and cause coughing or rapid, shallow breathing. Irritant receptor stimulation may also initiate augmented breaths or sighs that occur periodically during normal breathing and that maintain lung expansion. Irritant receptor stimulation by histamine and other substances released in response to allergens may increase ventilation during *asthma* attacks by augmenting inspiration. Rapid, forceful inspiration, as may occur with mechanical ventilation, particularly in infants, may also augment inspiration and promote lung inflation.

Proprioceptor afferents

Afferents from chest wall proprioceptors convey information about chest wall movement and forces exerted by respiratory muscles. This can help coordinate breathing during speech or postural changes and may also assist ribcage stabilization when breathing is impeded by increased airway resistance or decreased lung compliance. Joint and tendon afferents also stimulate the respiratory centers and may increase ventilation during exercise.

Selected reading

Bryan AC, Bowes G, Maloney JE. Control of breathing in the fetus and newborn. In Cherniack NS, Widdicombe JG, eds. *Handbook of physiology. Section 2: The respiratory system*. Vol. II. Bethesda, MD: American Physiological Society, 1986: 621.

Cohen MI. Neurogenesis of respiratory rhythm in the mammal. *Physiol Rev* 1979; **59**: 1105.

Lagercrantz H, Milerad J, Walker D. Control of breathing in the neonate. In Crystal RG, West JB, *et al*. *The lung*. New York: Raven Press Ltd, 1991: 1711.

Phillipson EA, Bowes G. Control of breathing during sleep. In Cherniack NS, Widdicombe JG, eds. *Handbook of physiology. Section 2: The respiratory system*. Bethesda, MD: American Physiological Society 1986: 649.

von Euler C. On the central pattern generator for the basic breathing rhythmicity. *J Appl Physiol* 1983; **55**: 1647.

B2. Respiratory Muscles

W E Cameron

Function of respiratory muscles

The muscles of respiration are characterized by phasic activity during the respiratory cycle. Although the external intercostal muscles are active, the diaphragm is predominant in controlling inspiration. During quiet breathing, the diaphragm generates the negative intrathoracic pressure that creates airflow into the lungs. The expiratory phase during quiet breathing is a passive event requiring no muscular contraction. Expiratory muscles (internal intercostal and abdominal) do become active during loaded breathing as occurs in some disease states. The accessory muscles (scalene and sternomastoid) are recruited during strenuous exercise. Because of its dominant role in all levels of respiratory effort, the diaphragm has been the focus of most investigations of respiratory muscles.

Biomechanics of respiration

The vertical dimension of the thoracic cavity is increased by the descent of the dome of the diaphragm and the transverse diameter is increased by lifting and expanding the lower margins of the rib cage. The diaphragm comprises a type of a skeletal muscle with an optimal length at which maximal contractile force is generated. This length corresponds to the maximal overlap of crossbridges between the actin and myosin filaments in the muscle fiber. Equivalent to an appendicular muscle having a particular joint angle that corresponds to this optimum for force production, the diaphragm has a particular lung volume at which it can generate maximum negative intrathoracic pressure.

In the adult, a rigid rib cage provides a stable origin for the diaphragm to pull against as its dome descends. However, the rib cage of the newborn, and even more particularly the preterm infant, is very compliant and the diaphragm must contract initially to draw in the edges of the rib cage and then contract still further to initiate air movement into the lungs. Because of this mechanical disadvantage in the newborn, the diaphragm must perform more work over a broader range of lengths than is required in the adult. The contraction of the intercostal muscles does provide some stiffness to the chest wall in the newborn but this contribution is less in preterm infants and is lost when these muscles become atonic during the frequent epochs of rapid eye movement (REM) sleep. Therefore, the greatest demand on the performance of the diaphragm occurs during the newborn period. The diaphragm of the full-term infant can defend its ventilation under normal conditions and most respiratory challenges (e.g. hypoxia, hypercapnia). However, the preterm infant is more susceptible to diaphragmatic failure when faced with more serious challenges (e.g. decreased lung compliance).

Biochemistry of respiratory muscles

The biochemical composition of a muscle fiber is correlated to its contractile properties. At a cellular level, muscle fibers are endowed with a variety of metabolic enzymes that underscore their dependence on oxidative and/or glycolytic pathways. Muscle fibers rich in enzymes of the Krebs cycle are resistant to fatigue while muscle fibers possessing enzymes of glycolysis fatigue more rapidly. In those muscles having a large proportion of oxidative muscle fibers, there is a high density of capillaries to supply required oxygen. At the level of the contractile proteins, different subspecies of the myosin heavy chain (MHC) molecule have been correlated with the speed of contraction. In general, muscle fibers possessing fast MHC are more dependent on glycolysis and are more prone to fatigue than fibers possessing slow MHC which utilizes more oxidative pathways. There also is a hybrid of these two classes of muscle fibers. One group of muscle fibers contains a unique isoform of the fast MHC and a high concentration of both oxidative and glycolytic enzymes. These fibers exhibit fatigue properties that are intermediate to the two other muscle fiber types. The adult mammalian diaphragm comprises all three fiber types.

In both preterm and full-term infants, the concentration of oxidative enzymes is relatively high and uniform among all muscle fibers of the diaphragm. This endows these muscles with relatively high resistance to fatigue. In the adult, but not in early postnatal life, there is a strong correlation between the concentration of oxidative enzymes and the fatigue resistance of the muscle fibers. With maturation, the concentration of oxidative enzymes in some muscle fibers tends to increase while the diaphragm as a whole is becoming more susceptible to fatigue.

In the newborn, respiratory muscles are found to express two developmental forms of MHC that are not found in the adult. Both embryonic and neonatal isoforms are present at birth, with the embryonic the first to disappear. The process of muscle maturation can be altered by a variety of factors. Perinatal undernutrition retards the maturation of respiratory muscles by delaying the disappearance of the neonatal isoform. During development, the embryonic MHC coexists in some developing muscle fibers with the adult slow MHC. The ultimate expression of this slow adult isoform depends upon the neural activity pattern imposed on the muscle fibers. Without appropriate activity, as occurs in denervation, these muscle fibers will continue to coexpress both isoforms of MHC and will not attain adult contractile properties.

Contractile properties of the diaphragm

Shortly after its formation in mid-gestation, the diaphragm begins to contract at irregular intervals. These contractions become more regular with further development. The first muscle fibers to differentiate contain adult slow MHC along with developmental isoforms. Each of these primary myofibers then becomes surrounded by a cluster of second generation myofibers that contain fast MHC and there is then a majority of muscle fibers expressing the fast isoform. With maturation, the proportion of muscle fibers expressing slow MHC increases, presumably by conversion of some fast secondary myofibers. Contrary to what might be expected, the newborn diaphragm and intercostal muscles contract slower at birth than they will in the adult. This contradiction is because the contractile speed during the early postnatal period is dominated by the properties of the slow contracting embryonic and neonatal MHC that coexists with adult MHC and is not due to the properties of the adult isoforms. As a result of this slower contraction speed, the muscle twitches of developing respiratory muscle fuse into a smooth tetanus at a lower firing rate than that found in the adult. In summary, the contractile properties of the various muscle fibers at birth are relatively homogeneous and the broad range of contractile speeds characteristic of the adult only emerges as development continues.

Development of respiratory motor units

The motor unit is the functional subunit of muscle and consists of the α-motoneuron and all the skeletal muscle fibers that it innervates. In the adult diaphragm, each motoneuron innervates several hundred muscle fibers and each muscle fiber receives input from only a single motoneuron. However, during early development, each muscle fiber is contacted by more than one neuron. Over the course of the first few weeks of postnatal life, this multiple or polyneuronal innervation is eliminated. With elimination of polyneuronal innervation, more than one-half of the phrenic motoneurons develop a leakier membrane (lower input resistance). Up to this time, the newborn utilizes the vast majority of its phrenic motoneurons to generate each inspiration. After this time, these leakier cells are no longer activated during each breath but form a reserve of quiescent diaphragmatic motor units that can be recruited when larger forces are necessary as in a sigh or a sniff. Coincident with these cells becoming inactive, more muscle fibers that generate larger forces and are more easily fatigued appear in the diaphragm. This progression provides the newborn with the ability to sustain moderately strong contractions of the diaphragm without fatigue while later in development, the diaphragm can generate much larger forces but has become more susceptible to muscular fatigue.

There are two mechanisms available to increase the force generated by a muscle: increase in firing rate of the active motoneurons and/or recruitment of previously inactive motor units. In the newborn, an increase in diaphragmatic force must be achieved mainly by modulation of the discharge frequency of the active phrenic motoneurons because there are very few inactive units. Older animals can employ both recruitment and frequency modulation to achieve the large forces that may be important to adequately defend the patency of upper airways.

Respiratory muscle fatigue

There are several possible sites of muscle fatigue. First, there could be a decreased central drive to the respiratory motoneurons (central fatigue). Second, there could be transmission failure at the neuromuscular junction. Finally, there could be failure of the excitation–contraction coupling mechanism. In most instances, the contribution of neuromuscular failure is minimal. However, in the neonate, there is evidence for both central and contractile fatigue of the diaphragm. During a respiratory challenge, the central drive will increase to a point to compensate for decreasing diaphragmatic contraction. Beyond this point, some yet unknown central mechanism prevents any further increase in the drive to the diaphragm and instead, recruits the accessory muscles, driving them in some instances to complete exhaustion. This safety mechanism that limits the excitatory drive to the diaphragm must insure that this muscle will continue to perform in some capacity even in the face of prolonged respiratory loads.

The diaphragm is more prone to fatigue when it must perform more mechanical work. The compliance of both the rib cage and the lung parenchyma influence the amount of work that the diaphragm must perform to defend ventilation. One serious challenge occurs in the premature infant with lung disease (decreased compliance) where there is severe distortion of the rib cage. The diaphragm must compensate not only for the compliant rib cage but also for the increased resistive load of the disease state. The increased diaphragmatic work required to maintain ventilation in the premature infant can account for as much as 10 percent of basal metabolic rate.

As indicated above, there is a strong correlation between activity of the motoneuron and the properties of the muscles fibers. A complication can arise when premature or term infants are artificially ventilated. Even with assisted ventilation, the activation of respiratory muscle by the central nervous system is dramatically altered and the muscles can undergo disuse atrophy (including a decreased resistance to fatigue). Unfortunately to date, the weaning of an infant from a ventilator remains an art and not a procedure dictated by scientific understanding.

The most prominent symptoms of inspiratory muscle fatigue are dyspnea and respiratory distress. Clinical features, in order of appearance, are tachypnea, decreased tidal volume, paradoxical inward movement of the abdomen during inspiration, and alternation between abdominal and thoracic breathing. CO_2 retention is a late manifestation. In infants, apnea quickly follows.

Power spectrum analysis of the electromyogram shows that with the onset of fatigue there is a redistribution of power in the EMG signal away from high frequencies toward lower frequencies, possibly because the conduction velocity of muscle depolarization is retarded.

In respiratory diseases with hyperinflation, such as *cystic fibrosis* or *asthma*, the diaphragm is passively shortened, inspiratory muscle force is reduced and inspiratory muscle fatigue should be anticipated. Numerous metabolic factors, including hypoxemia and acidosis, combine to further compromise the performance of the inspiratory muscles. Impaired nutritional status and other destructive processes alter muscle membrane function and damage the contractile machinery of the muscle fibers. Inspiratory muscle fatigue is also associated with *acute upper airway obstruction*, *chest wall disorders* (e.g. *scoliosis*), and neuromuscular conditions (e.g. *Duchenne muscular dystrophy*). With chronic diseases specific training techniques can increase inspiratory muscle strength and endurance.

Selected reading

Monteau R, Hilaire G. Spinal respiratory motoneurons. *Prog Neurobiol* 1991; **37**: 83.

Muller N, Volgyes G, Bryan MH, Bryan AC. The consequences of diaphragmatic muscle fatigue in the newborn infant. *J Pediatr* 1979; **95**: 793.

Rochester DF. Fatigue of the diaphragm. In Fishman AP, ed. *Update: pulmonary diseases and disorders*. New York: McGraw-Hill, 1982.

Sieck GC, Fournier M. Developmental aspects of diaphragm muscle cells: structural and functional organization. In Haddad GG, Farber JP, eds. *Developmental neurobiology of breathing*. Vol. 53. New York: Marcel Dekker, 1991: 375.

Vrbova G, Navarrete R, Lowrie M. Matching of muscle properties and motoneurone firing patterns during early stages of development. *J Exp Biol* 1985; **115**: 113.

B3. Perinatal Development of Central Respiratory Control

B M Johnston

Fetus

Spontaneous rhythmic activity of the diaphragm and other respiratory muscles occurs from early in gestation in human and other mammalian fetuses. Rapid and irregular bursts of diaphragmatic activity generate negative tracheal pressure fluctuations of 2–6 mmHg (0.3–0.8 kPa). The diaphragmatic electromyogram (EMG) correlates with phrenic nerve activity and firing of medullary inspiratory motoneurons, indicating that movement of the respiratory muscles represents respiratory center output. These diaphragmatic movements, termed fetal breathing movements, serve no respiratory function as gas exchange takes place through the placenta. Teleologically, prenatal respiratory practice is presumed necessary for the development of the respiratory musculature and organization of the central processes controlling respiration after birth. Also fetal breathing movements are essential for normal lung growth and development.

Regulation of fetal breathing movements

Effect of sleep state

Breathing activity before birth is unique in that it is not continuous. With advancing gestation fetal breathing movements become progressively more episodic as prolonged periods of apnea alternate with epochs of fetal breathing movements. In fetal sheep, from the beginning of the third trimester onwards, the development of apneic periods is associated with differentiation of the electrocorticogram (ECoG) into periods of low voltage (LV) and high voltage (HV) activity which correspond to rapid eye movement (REM) sleep and nonREM sleep postnatally (see p. 250). Fetal breathing movements occur only during low voltage ECoG activity but do not necessarily occupy the entire period of low voltage activity; episodes of fetal breathing movements (FBM) therefore may last from a few minutes to an hour.

ECoG	LV	HV
REM	+	–
FBM	+	–

By late gestation fetal breathing movements are present for only about 40 percent of the time in sheep (Fig. 11.7) and 25–30 percent in humans, as identified by ultrasonography. While the definition of state is less certain (see p. 250), in the human fetus, fetal breathing movements are also behavioral state related. During periods of high voltage ECoG activity, which alternate with low voltage activity, fetal sheep are apneic apart from occasional isolated deep gasp-like activity. Such gasps are a normal feature of high voltage activity and are not associated with asphyxia. However, during periods of acute fetal distress, asphyxia may cause gasping which can result in *meconium aspiration*.

In adult physiology the classical view is that continuous respiration is generated by spontaneous rhythmic discharge of inspiratory and expiratory neurons of the medullary respiratory centers. Pontine influences and

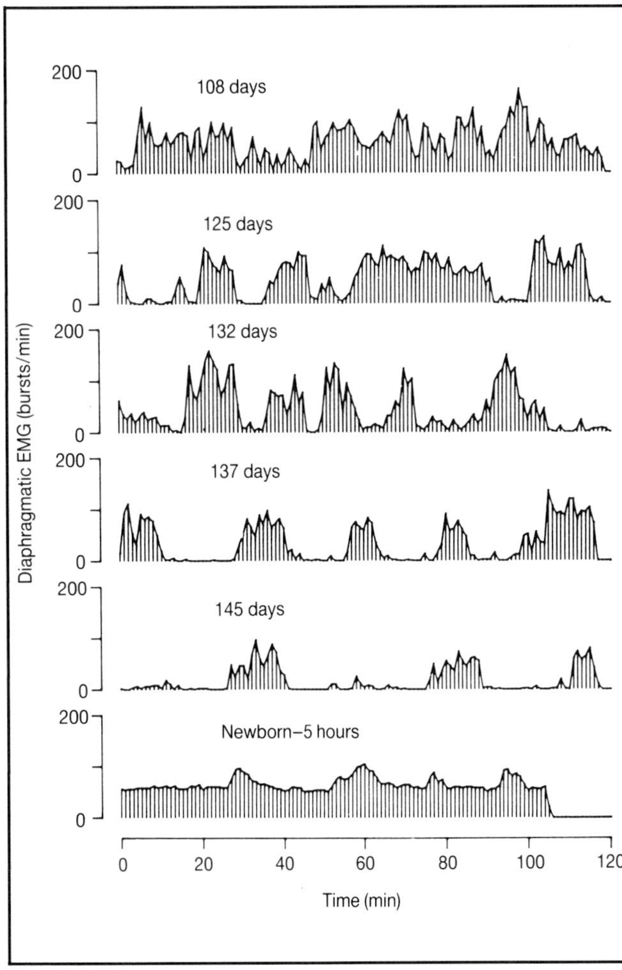

Fig. 11.7. Analysis of diaphragmatic EMG of a fetus at five gestational ages (108–145 days) and as a 5-hours-old newborn. Each graph displays time in minutes on abscissa and diaphragmatic EMG activity in bursts/min on ordinate. (Reproduced with permission from Bowes G *et al*. *J. Appl Physiol* 1981; **50**: 693–700).

afferent inputs (chemoreflex, mechanoreflex and thermal) were thought only to modify the intrinsic rhythm, but recently the profound influence of sleep state on respiratory control has been recognized. During slow wave (quiet) sleep chemical and peripheral afferents are critical in maintaining respiratory rhythm. In contrast in REM sleep there is relative insensitivity to metabolic stimuli (e.g. hypoxia, hypercapnia) and breathing is driven by intrinsic central nervous system activity associated with reticular and cortical activation.

Recognition of the importance of sleep state in control of respiration in adults led to the theory that the apnea associated with high voltage ECoG activity in the fetus resulted from lack of afferent input, but this is not fully resolved. While bilateral vagotomy has no effect on the episodic nature or character of fetal breathing movements, pulmonary stretch receptors are functional well before birth in fetal lambs. Evidence of a role for carotid chemoreceptors in the normal regulation of fetal breathing movements is conflicting. There is a powerful inhibitory mechanism operating during high voltage ECoG activity which overrides any stimulatory effects from peripheral or chemical afferents. Brainstem transection at the midbrain/pontine junction in fetal sheep results in dissociation of fetal breathing movements from the low voltage activity ECoG and progressive emergence of almost continuous fetal breathing movements after 10–12 days. An area in the rostral lateral pons is believed to be involved in this central inhibitory process.

Chemical regulation of fetal breathing movements

Hypoxia

In addition to the inhibition of fetal breathing movements associated with high voltage ECoG activity, the fetus exhibits a unique response to acute hypoxia which causes a rapid suppression of fetal breathing movements. This is interpreted teleologically as a protective mechanism to reduce fetal O_2 consumption. The ensuing apnea occurs independently of electrocortical state although hypoxia also increases the proportion of high voltage activity; in contrast to the adult, there is no evidence of arousal. The fetal response contrasts with the adult where hypoxia causes arousal and stimulates respiration via peripheral chemoreceptors. Originally attributed to direct depression of the medullary respiratory centers or nonfunctional carotid chemoreceptors, the depressive effect of hypoxia on fetal breathing movements is now known to result from a central inhibitory mechanism. Upper pontine brainstem transections, which abolish the depressive response and cause fetal breathing movements to be stimulated by hypoxia, point to an inhibitory influence arising in or above the upper pons; the region appears to be the Köllike–Fuse and lateral parabrachial nuclei but is located more lateral than the 'pneumotaxic' center which is classically considered to encompass the medial parabrachial nuclei. The neuropharmacology of the hypoxic inhibitory pathways is not well defined, but there is evidence for involvement of adenosine or an α_2-adrenergic mechanism.

Hypercapnia

Central chemoreceptors, located on the ventral surface of the medulla, and which mediate the hyperventilation produced by increases in arterial blood $P\text{CO}_2$ ($P\text{aCO}_2$) in the adult, are certainly functional in fetal life. Fetal hypercapnia, induced by maternal inhalation of 4–6 percent CO_2 in air, increases the incidence of fetal breathing movements to around 70 percent of the time; breathing becomes more regular with increased depth and inspiratory slope. Hypercapnia also increases time spent in low voltage ECoG activity to around 80 percent. However, the fetal response to hypercapnia is unique in that these stimulatory effects occur only during low voltage ECoG activity. Once the ECoG shows high voltage activity, fetal breathing movements cease immediately and the normal apnea associated with high voltage ECoG activity dominates. Even inspired concentrations of CO_2 as high as 10 percent will not induce fetal breathing movements during high voltage ECoG activity.

Acidemia

Fetal responses to metabolic acidemia are not entirely resolved. Lactic acid infusion decreases the incidence of fetal breathing movements, whereas HCl or NH_4Cl stimulate fetal breathing movements, with a delay of several hours perhaps due to slow penetration of H^+ ions to medullary chemoreceptors. Direct stimulation of central chemoreceptors by ventriculocisternal perfusion of artificial CSF low in HCO_3^- increases the depth and incidence of fetal breathing movements. Although fetal breathing movements can occur intermittently during high voltage ECoG activity with low HCO_3^- perfusion, the effect is not persistent.

Lateral pontine lesions which abolish fetal inhibitory responses to hypoxia also stimulate fetal breathing movements continuously through both high and low voltage ECoG activity under conditions of hypercapnia or acidemia. However, because lateral pontine lesions do not themselves produce continuous fetal breathing movements when blood gases and pH are normal, and because raising H^+ and/or CO_2 does not induce fetal breathing movements during high voltage ECoG activity in brainstem-intact fetuses, it is now believed that the lengthening periods of apnea seen with the development of high voltage ECoG activity late in gestation result from two processes. The first is the brainstem inhibitory mechanism involving the lateral pons and the second is a raised threshold for chemosensitivity. Because fetal breathing movements are not stimulated by the normal resting fetal $Paco_2$ which is about 15 mmHg higher than that of the mother, it is possible that central chemoreceptors reset after birth as do peripheral chemoreceptors (see p. 610).

Pharmacological agents affecting fetal breathing movements

Many attempts have been made to define the neurochemical basis of the episodic nature of fetal breathing movements but this is not resolved. Several neurotransmitter agonists stimulate fetal breathing movements during low voltage ECoG activity but have no effect in high voltage ECoG activity. Other agents inhibit fetal breathing movements but administration of appropriate antagonists does not result in continuous fetal breathing movements. Table 11.2 summarizes some of the agents and stimuli known either to stimulate or to inhibit fetal breathing movements. Of these, most strongly implicated in inhibition of fetal breathing movements during high voltage ECoG activity is prostaglandin $(PG)E_2$, particularly since the PG synthesis inhibitors indomethacin and meclofenamate stimulate prolonged periods of fetal breathing movements during both high and low voltage ECoG activity. In addition to the pharmacological agents listed, other factors influencing fetal breathing movements are maternal food intake or glucose administration which increase the rate and incidence of fetal breathing movements, though not during high voltage ECoG activity, and the onset of labor which is associated with a marked reduction in fetal breathing movements, possibly due to increased PG concentrations.

Table 11.2. Pharmacological and other stimuli affecting fetal breathing movements

Stimulus	Effect
High voltage ECoG	↓
Fetal hypoxia (fetal distress)	↓
Labor	↓
Prostaglandins (PGE_1, PGE_2)	↓
Starvation (hypoglycemia)	↓
Barbiturates	↓
Ethanol	↓
Diazepam	↓
Meperidine (pethidine, Demerol)	↓
Adenosine	↓
Norepinephrine	↓
ACTH	↓
Clonidine	↓
Low voltage ECoG	↑
Hypercapnia (only during low voltage)	↑
Glucose	↑
Prostaglandin synthetase inhibitors (indomethacin)	↑
Isoproterenol	↑
Epinephrine	↑
Morphine	↑
Theophylline/caffeine	↑
Thyrotropin releasing hormone	↑
Corticotropin releasing factor	↑

Neonate

Although breathing movements are present in the fetus, at birth there is a fundamental change in their purpose. With removal of the placenta, continuous rhythmic respiratory movements are critical for insuring adequate ventilation and gas exchange, essential to the metabolic needs of independent life. Respiratory control after birth is multifactorial, with many influences such as airway mechanoreflexes, chemoreflexes, thermal balance and behavioral state all acting to determine effective respiratory control rather than merely modify it. Furthermore, the relative importance of the various influences in sustaining effective respiration changes with development and in the immediate neonatal period, thermal and metabolic influences represent a more important drive to respiration than chemoreceptor inputs which become dominant later in postnatal development (Fig. 11.8).

Brainstem (bulbopontine) rhythm generation

The bulbopontine respiratory control system is functional from an early fetal stage, but the brainstem

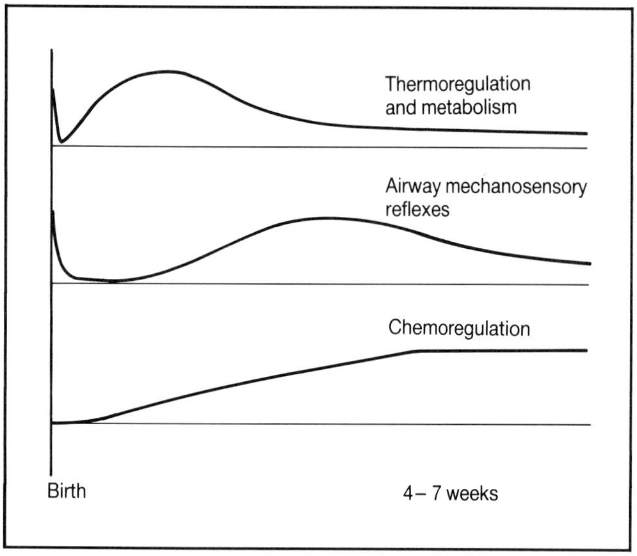

Fig. 11.8. Diagrammatic representation of the phases of postnatal respiratory control. (Reproduced with permission from Johnson P. In: *Respiratory control and lung development in the fetus and newborn*. Ithaca NY: Perinatology Press, 1986: 384).

neural network and its connections are still immature at birth, synaptogenesis is incomplete, the dendritic network is sparse and since myelinization is incomplete, nerve cell conduction is slower. Considerable maturation occurs postnatally. Myelinization continues, dendritic pathways become more organized as arborization progresses and synapse formation is completed. The effect of behavioral state on respiratory rhythm is particularly important in the neonate because of the large amount of time spent asleep. Wakefulness occupies only a small proportion of time, but because cortical and forebrain influences usually override metabolic or autonomic control, respiration is irregular during wakefulness and activities such as crying and feeding affect the pattern. At 30 weeks of gestation REM sleep occupies about 90 percent of the time in preterm neonates but by term this has fallen to 50 percent. Breathing is irregular during REM sleep, sustained more by intrinsic activity of the reticular formation than by afferent inputs, to which sensitivity is generally reduced. Overall minute ventilation is a little higher during REM sleep, though there are marked fluctuations. Clearly defined quiet sleep does not develop before 32 weeks of gestation and does not display all of the characteristics of adult non-REM sleep until late in the first year of postnatal life. Breathing is slower and more regular than in REM and tidal volume is slightly increased.

Metabolic and thermal influences

At birth emergence into the cooler extrauterine environment is a major stimulus to breathing (probably by hypothalamic mechanisms) and to maintain continuous breathing there must be a negative thermal gradient between skin and core temperatures. Recent studies have highlighted the importance of changes in thermoregulation, close to the thermoneutral range, in controlling respiratory pattern and rate after birth. In newborn lambs the thermoneutral zone is narrow and the high metabolic rate necessary to achieve thermoregulation is a major drive to respiratory rhythmicity. In humans, the incidence of *apnea of prematurity* increases with elevated environmental temperatures. Upper airway bypass, with consequent loss of laryngeal braking, causes significant respiratory dysrhythmia after 14 days of age; however, it has little effect on respiratory rate or pattern during the first week of life because the metabolic influences are a sufficient stimulus to respiration. With increasing postnatal age thermal efficiency improves, the thermoneutral zone widens and metabolic rate and O_2 consumption fall. Along with the decrease in metabolic rate, respiratory frequencies are reduced and lung volume is no longer maintained by high respiratory rates. Instead vagal stimuli become more important in sustaining rhythmicity.

Vagal reflexes

Stretch receptors

Afferent influences carried via the vagus nerve from stretch receptors in the airways, lung parenchyma and chest wall are major determinants of respiratory depth and timing in the newborn. Lung inflation increases the discharge rate of stretch receptors and terminates inspiration. This reflex, known as the Hering–Breuer inflation reflex, is markedly more pronounced in newborn than adult humans, peaking at 38 weeks of gestation in the preterm infant and declining post-term. The reflex predominates during quiet sleep and is diminished or abolished during active sleep. Clinically the reflex is important because preterm babies with *respiratory distress syndrome* who 'fight' the ventilator may develop *pneumothorax* as a result of active expiration. Vagal reflexes are important in the maintenance of lung volume, especially in the premature infant. In lambs expiratory laryngeal braking, or glottic closure, becomes more prominent in the post-neonatal period, particularly in quiet sleep. This mechanism imposes expiratory pressures on the lung stretch receptors and because of the Hering–Breuer reflex influences respiratory cycle timing and maintains lung volume.

The paradoxical reflex of Head is another vagal reflex which predominates neonatally. Rapid and forceful inspiration acts to augment inspiration further and this reflex may be important when hand ventilating neonates during resuscitation.

Irritant receptors

In full-term infants, as in adults, the airways are extremely sensitive to mechanical irritation and airway stimulation produces bronchial constriction, coughing, hyperventilation and arousal; however, the preterm infant rarely coughs during tracheal intubation or suctioning and below 35 weeks of gestation respiratory slowing or apnea is frequently the only response. This may be due to incomplete vagal myelinization before term or to decreased vagal reflex sensitivity in active sleep which is the predominant state of the preterm.

Chemical regulation of respiration

Hypoxia

Respiratory responses of the neonate to acute hypoxia are biphasic. The initial hyperventilation is not sustained and within 5 minutes ventilation falls towards or below control. There are some species differences in magnitude and duration of the initial increase in ventilation and also in the degree of the so-called 'ventilatory depression' which characterizes the second phase of the response. This is most marked in preterm infants and can lead to apnea. In human infants reduced minute ventilation occurs primarily because of a fall in respiratory frequency, but in some species tidal volume is also reduced. Because $P\text{aCO}_2$ usually remains below control despite reduced minute ventilation, there is controversy as to whether this second phase should be termed 'ventilatory depression'. In human infants, where ventilation falls below control levels, this depressive response pattern is seen during the first week after birth in term infants and for 3–4 weeks in preterm infants.

Species differences in the effect of sleep state on ventilatory responses to hypoxia are apparently related to the effect of sleep state on the ribcage. Human infants and puppies have a similar response in REM and nonREM sleep, but in lambs and calves, where there is a loss of intercostal muscle tone in REM sleep, the ventilatory response is attenuated.

The mechanisms underlying the secondary fall in ventilation are not fully resolved. It is not due to peripheral chemoreceptor failure since carotid afferent discharge is maintained at high rates throughout hypoxia. Peripheral mechanisms including mechanical effects have been proposed but the response is unlikely to be due to respiratory muscle fatigue. In newborn rabbits a central inhibitory mechanism, similar to that in the fetus, may be involved because decerebration at the midbrain/pontine junction reverses the fall in ventilation. The neurochemical basis of the hypoxic depression is not defined with certainty, but adenosine and endogenous opiates have both been implicated. Theophylline prevents the secondary fall in ventilation in piglets, prevents the hypoxic ventilatory depression in rabbit pups and is widely used in the treatment of *apnea of prematurity*. However, these effects may be due to a nonspecific excitation of central nervous system neurons.

Hypercapnia

The CO_2 drive is very weak in the fetus but after birth there is an immediate shift of CO_2 sensitivity to a lower threshold, possibly caused by cooling. The resistance to CO_2 stimulation during quiet sleep disappears and hypercapnia stimulates ventilation in all behavioral states. The slope of the ventilatory response in term infants is similar to the adult, although the lower resting $P\text{aCO}_2$ in infants shifts the curve to the left. Preterm infants show a decreased sensitivity to CO_2; the sensitivity increases with advancing gestational age and postnatal growth. However, it is uncertain whether the increased response is due to a true change in neural sensitivity or improved mechanical efficiency of the thorax.

Whether or not a deficient CO_2 response explains apnea of prematurity is somewhat controversial, although there are reports of lower CO_2 sensitivity in preterm infants with apnea. It is also possible that in the neonate the CO_2 response is attenuated by hypoxia rather than being potentiated as in the adult.

Selected reading

Henderson-Smart DJ, Cohen GL. Regulation of breathing and apnea in the newborn infant. In Johnston BM, Gluckman PD, eds. *Respiratory control and lung development in the fetus and newborn*. New York: Perinatology Press, 1986: 397.

Johnson P. Non-chemical factors in postnatal respiratory control. In Johnston BM, Gluckman PD, eds. *Respiratory control and lung development in the fetus and newborn*. New York: Perinatology Press, 1986: 377.

Johnston BM. Brainstem inhibitory mechanisms in the control of fetal breathing movements. In Hanson MA, ed. *The fetal and neonatal brainstem*. Cambridge: Cambridge University Press, 1991: 21.

B4. Perinatal Control of Breathing by Peripheral Chemoreceptors

M A Hanson

Fetus

Under normal circumstances the peripheral chemoreceptors (carotid and aortic bodies) probably play no role in regulating the incidence of fetal breathing movements either during normoxia or hypoxemia. This is not due to chemoreceptor immaturity as in the last third of gestation they are spontaneously active and respond to a fall in arterial blood PO_2 (PaO_2) or pH or to a rise in PCO_2. Peripheral chemoreceptors are involved in vital circulatory reflexes, operating to redistribute combined ventricular output to certain organs and to minimize O_2 consumption during acute episodes of hypoxemia. Central nervous control mechanisms operate to preserve cardiovascular chemoreflexes while the respiratory chemoreflexes are suspended or inhibited.

Birth

Peripheral chemoreceptors and changes in arterial blood gas tensions and pH are not necessary for establishing continuous breathing in the first few minutes after birth, as this occurs even when the vagus and carotid sinus nerves are cut (peripheral chemodenervation). However, elevation of arterial blood PCO_2 ($PaCO_2$) reduces the time before breathing becomes continuous after birth. This CO_2 sensitivity is likely to be conveyed by both peripheral and central (medullary) chemoreceptors. Hypoxemia does not potentiate the responses, as would be expected if the peripheral chemoreflexes acted purely as in the adult, but inhibits breathing, since the central nervous inhibitory processes operating in fetal life can still be evoked. There also are other factors, e.g. change in environmental temperature and the increase in metabolism, which operate to affect the gain of chemoreflexes in the neonate.

Stimulus to the chemoreceptors

Despite their tiny size, the carotid bodies receive the highest blood flow per unit weight of any organ in the body. Although arteriovenous anastomoses exist, a high proportion of the blood reaches chemoreceptor tissue. O_2 consumption of the organ is very small in relation to O_2 supply and therefore tissue PO_2 near the chemoreceptor cells is little different from arterial PO_2. Thus carotid chemoreceptor responses depend on PaO_2 rather than O_2 content. Whether the aortic chemoreceptors (located in the walls of several thoracic great arteries and the aortic arch) similarly receive such a high blood flow is not known, but they also respond to PaO_2 rather than to O_2 content.

As CO_2 is much more readily diffusible than O_2, there is an insignificant PCO_2 gradient between chemoreceptor tissue and blood. Chemoreceptor responses are therefore described in terms of PaO_2 and $PaCO_2$ (Fig. 11.9). Responses to changes in PCO_2 are more rapid than to changes in PO_2, and depend on the hydration of CO_2 by intracellular carbonic anhydrase. Thus the response is mediated by changes in intracellular pH. The stimuli of increased PCO_2 and reduced PO_2 interact, such that asphyxia is a very potent stimulus to chemoreceptors. This suggests a common (but unknown) intracellular transduction mechanism for the two stimuli that may

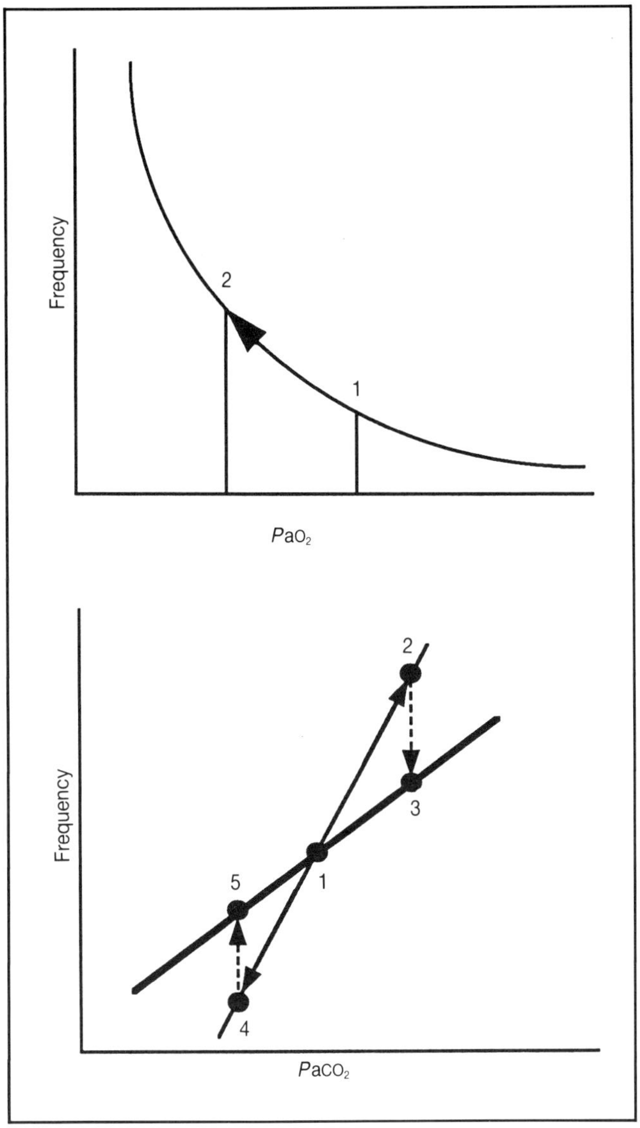

Fig. 11. Effects on frequency of arterial chemoreceptor discharge of changes in arterial blood P_{O_2} (top) or P_{CO_2} (bottom). The steady-state response to hypoxia is hyperbolic. The dynamic response to rapid changes in P_{O_2}, e.g. from point 1 to point 2, follows the steady-state line, i.e. there is no adaptation. As seen in the lower graph, increasing P_{CO_2} rapidly elevates discharge along a dynamic response line from point 1 to point 2, but discharge then adapts down to point 3 on the steady-state line. Conversely, rapid reduction of P_{CO_2} reduces discharge along a line from point 1 to point 4 but discharge then adapts up to point 5.

involve the effects of P_{O_2} and pH changes on membrane channels and mitochondrial processes determining intracellular Ca^{2+}. Increases in plasma K^+ as occur during muscular exercise or hyperkalemia are also potent stimuli. The sensory transmitters involved in carotid body chemoreception are not unequivocally established, but excitatory amino acids and substance P seem to be likely candidates. Dopamine, found in high concentration in the glomus cells, might act as a modulator.

P_{O_2} changes at birth and chemoreceptor resetting

Pa_{O_2} rises sharply from a fetal value of about 25 mmHg (3.3 kPa) to over 60 mmHg (8 kPa) once air breathing starts. This P_{O_2} is well above the range over which the chemoreceptors have been active in fetal life, and silences them. The range of chemoreceptor sensitivity to P_{O_2} then shifts over the first few days of postnatal life, so that it comes to occupy its 'adult' position (Fig. 11.10). After complete resetting, the arterial chemoreceptors are spontaneously active at a Pa_{O_2} of about 90–100 mmHg and increase their discharge if Pa_{O_2} falls below this value. Unlike the linear response to hypercapnia, the relationship between Pa_{O_2} and ventilation is hyperbolic. The resetting increases the gain of respiratory chemoreflex responses to changes in P_{O_2}. This is seen both in the magnitude of stimulation of ventilation in response to small reductions in Pa_{O_2} and in the fall in ventilation in response to

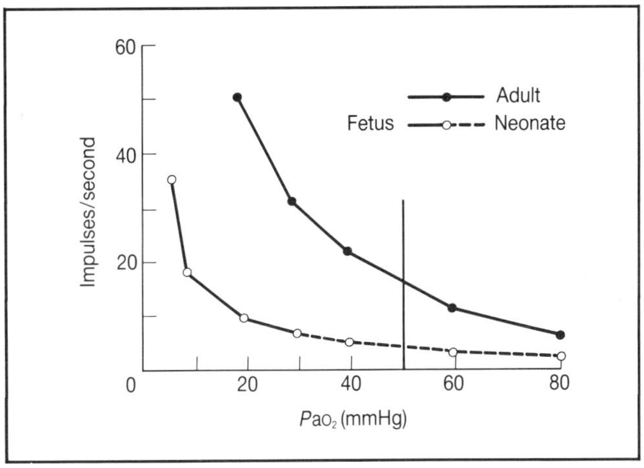

Fig. 11.10. Arterial chemoreceptor response curves to changing arterial blood P_{O_2} in sheep. The fetal curve (open symbols, continuous line) lies to the left of the adult curve (solid symbols, continuous line). In the neonate (open symbols, interrupted line) the P_{O_2} has risen well above the fetal range and discharge is quiescent. Resetting then shifts the response curve up and to the right to its adult position. At any P_{O_2} (e.g. 50 mmHg shown by vertical line) both mean discharge and slope of the response line to changes in P_{O_2} are greater.

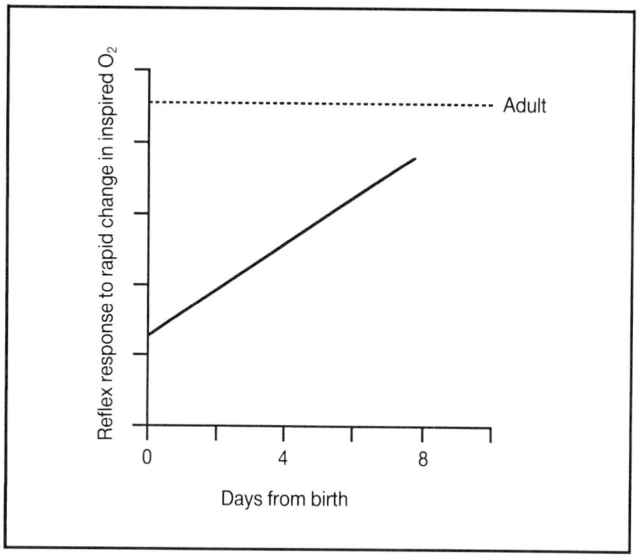

Fig. 11.11. Maturation of the respiratory chemoreflex response to rapid changes in Po_2 (tested either by lowering or raising inspired O_2) in early neonatal life.

artificially raising PaO$_2$, both of which are larger in infants at 1 week of age than on the day of birth (Fig. 11.11). As chemoreceptor stimulation increases ventilation and makes breathing more regular, weak chemoreflexes may play a role in *apnea of prematurity*.

Mechanism of resetting

Since the biochemical mechanisms enabling the adult carotid body to respond to changes in Po_2 at a mean PaO$_2$ near 100 mmHg are unknown, it is not surprising that the mechanism whereby sensitivity to changes in Po_2 resets postnatally has not been identified. This resetting occurs for both carotid and aortic chemoreceptors. The process appears to be Po_2 dependent because elevating PaO$_2$ in the fetus *in utero* initiates the resetting process even before birth. Resetting does not involve changes in blood flow to the carotid body. In the newborn, relatively high levels of dopamine are present in the carotid body in the first few hours after birth and this may modulate sensitivity; however, dopamine turnover is also high. Changes in catecholamine turnover occur over a similar time course to that of chemoreceptor resetting.

Pathological changes in chemoreceptor function

Chronic hypoxemia

Since the normal resetting process depends on the rise in PaO$_2$ at birth, limiting this increase reduces the extent of resetting. Infants born at high altitude and animals reared in 15 percent O_2 have a blunted chemoreflex response to hypoxia. Chronic hypoxemia due to *bronchopulmonary dysplasia* or repeated acute hypoxemia from *recurrent apnea* have similar effects. The blunting seems to be in part at the carotid body but, as for resetting itself, the precise mechanism is not known. The carotid body hypertrophies by an unknown mechanism in high altitude natives and adults suffering from chronic hypoxemia.

Sudden infant death syndrome (SIDS)

Poor chemoreflexes have been reported in some groups of infants at high risk for *sudden infant death*, i.e. those with *recurrent apnea* or *bronchopulmonary dysplasia*. This may represent a genetic or environmental difference or could be a pathophysiological change resulting from hypoxemia. There have been reports that the carotid body dopamine levels of some SIDS victims are higher than those of infants dying of other causes. This is not consistent, and its significance is unknown.

Other effects of peripheral chemoreceptors

The reflex effects of increased peripheral chemoreceptor discharge on respiration are the best known, but chemoreflexes also exert powerful effects on other systems. The reflexes are integrated into an overall response. The other most important components of this response are:

1. Cardiovascular, producing vasoconstriction, a rise in systemic arterial blood pressure and a change in heart rate. If ventilation does not increase, there is bradycardia but if breathing is spontaneous, the increase in ventilation produces an overriding tachycardia. These components of the response are

similar to aspects of the diving reflex seen in adult animals, especially in species such as seals.
2. Behavioral, producing arousal from sleep. The threshold for arousal is less in quiet than active sleep.
3. Maintaining upper airway patency. Chemoreceptor afferents project to the hypoglossal motorneurons, affecting rhythmic contraction of muscles which maintain a patent airway, e.g. the genioglossus. Contraction of this muscle protrudes the tongue, and its activity in inspiration prevents obstruction produced by relapse of the tongue. Cessation of genioglossus activity is important in *obstructive apnea.*
4. Metabolic, inhibiting thermoregulation from shivering and possibly also from brown adipose tissue.
5. Endocrine, causing release of a range of hormones, e.g. arginine vasopressin, epinephrine, ACTH and cortisol.

Endocrine effects on chemoreceptors

Adenosine, released from neurons in response to hypoxemia, and acting centrally, may produce respiratory depression. However, adenosine stimulates arterial chemoreceptors and this may, at least partially, offset the central depression.

Prostaglandin E_2 also inhibits breathing in both the fetus and newborn, partially via a central mechanism but also by reducing chemoreceptor discharge in the newborn.

Effects of anesthetics and drugs on chemoreceptors

Inhalation anesthetics, such as halothane, depress resting chemoreceptor discharge in animals (Fig. 11.12). This effect is independent of the accompanying hypotension, which would be expected to increase chemoreceptor discharge. Halothane also impairs the reflex ventilatory response to hypoxemia, and its effects may be long-lasting (at least several hours). It has been implicated in respiratory failure after general anesthesia, especially in preterm babies.

Metabolic inhibitors, such as cyanide, stimulate chemoreceptors, mimicking hypoxia at the carotid body. Doxapram and almitrine are stimulants of chemoreceptors which may also act at the hypoxia-sensing mechanism. The former has been used clinically as a respiratory stimulant in the neonate.

Selected reading

Biscoe TJ, Duchen MR. Cellular basis of transduction in carotid chemoreceptors. *Annu Rev Physiol* 1990; **2**: 271.

Fidone SJ, Gonzalez C. Initiation and control of chemoreceptor activity in the carotid body. In Fishman AP, ed. *Handbook of physiology: Section 3. The*

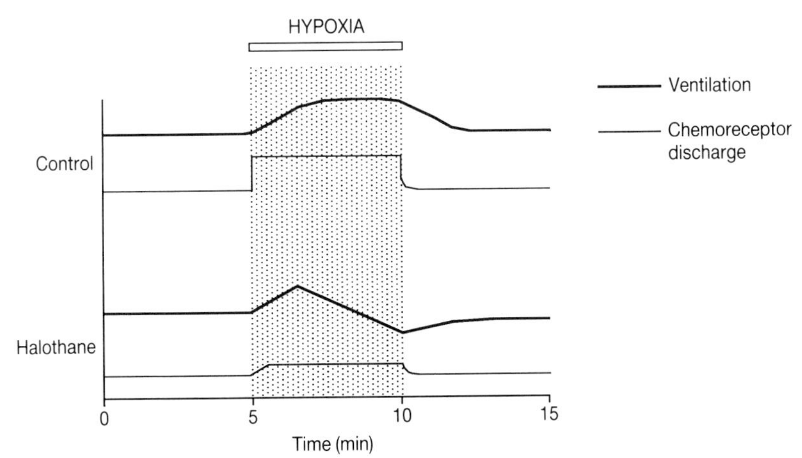

Fig. 11.12. Effects of inspired halothane (0.5–1.0 percent) on the ventilatory and carotid chemoreceptor responses to a brief period of hypoxia. Chemoreceptor discharge in normoxia and in hypoxia is reduced by halothane. With halothane, stimulation of ventilation during hypoxia is not maintained.

respiratory system. Vol. 2, Part 1. Bethesda, MD: American Physiological Society, 1986: 247.

Hanson MA. Peripheral chemoreceptor function before and after birth. In Johnston BM, Gluckman PD, eds. *Respiratory control and lung development in the fetus and newborn*. New York: Perinatology Press, 1986: 311.

Hanson MA, Eden GJ, Nijhuis JG, Moore PJ. Peripheral chemoreceptors and other O_2 sensors in the fetus and newborn. In Lahiri S, Forster RE, Davies RO, Pack AI, eds. *Chemoreceptors and reflexes in breathing*. New York: Oxford University Press, 1989: 113.

Kumar P, Hanson MA. Postnatal resetting of the hypoxic sensitivity of aortic chemoreceptors in the lamb. In Eyzaguirre C, Fidone SJ, Fitzgerald RS, Lahiri S, McDonald DM, eds. *Arterial chemoreceptors*. Berlin: Springer-Verlag, 1990: 279.

B5. Respiratory Control during the Transition at Birth

S L Adamson

The first postnatal breath is taken either during or within seconds of delivery. Within minutes, a regular breathing rhythm is established which remains virtually continuous for life. One or more of the many potential respiratory stimuli associated with birth cause the rapid onset of breaths vigorous enough to initiate lung aeration, and the transition from an intermittent to a continuous breathing pattern.

Transition to lung gas exchange

As labor approaches, the incidence of fetal breathing movements decreases. Lung liquid is produced at a gradually decreasing rate and, during labor, absorption of lung liquid begins, possibly related to increased epinephrine or vasopressin concentrations. The first breath causes air to enter the lungs where it mixes with lung liquid to create a foam. Initially, breathing is highly irregular and very deep breaths are often observed. After several minutes, continuous breathing becomes established, lung liquid is absorbed from the alveoli into the perivascular spaces, and the foam is gradually replaced with air. Clearance of lung liquid from the pulmonary perivascular spaces continues until several hours after birth. Abnormally slow resorption of fetal lung fluid may cause *transient tachypnea of the newborn*, which normally resolves with supportive treatment within 24 hours.

Role of arterial blood $P\text{O}_2$, $P\text{CO}_2$ and pH

The primary function of the postnatal respiratory control system is to maintain arterial blood gas tensions within normal limits based on feedback received from peripheral and central chemoreceptors. Although long speculated to be crucial in the stimulation of breathing at birth, it now appears that changes in arterial blood gas tensions and pH are not the primary stimuli for the onset of continuous air breathing.

Serial measurements in humans indicate a modest impairment of gas exchange during the first 20 seconds after birth and several breaths are required to reverse this. By 1 minute of age, arterial blood $P\text{O}_2$ ($P\text{aO}_2$) and O_2 saturation levels are similar to normal fetal values. Over the next 30 minutes $P\text{aO}_2$ rises and $P\text{aCO}_2$ declines to reach fairly stable levels (approximately 60 mmHg and 35 mmHg; 8.0 and 4.7 kPa respectively). Arterial blood pH decreases transiently after birth (to pH $\approx$ 7.2) but this mild acidosis is largely resolved within 30–60 minutes.

The initial small decrease in $P\text{aO}_2$ is not responsible for stimulating the first breath; decreases in $P\text{aO}_2$ inhibit rather than stimulate respiratory activity in fetal sheep. Similarly, over the short term, experimentally induced metabolic acidosis in fetal and newborn sheep (and by inference, transient metabolic acidosis in the first hour) does not contribute to respiratory stimulation. $P\text{aCO}_2$ increases transiently after birth; however, hypercapnia alone cannot account for the dramatic change in breathing pattern after birth. Hypercapnia does not cause fetal breathing to become continuous in all sleep states (see p. 605), and does not stimulate deep, vigorous breathing efforts similar to those seen immediately after birth.

Once breathing is initiated, $P\text{aO}_2$ increases. Whether this rise feeds back to further stimulate breathing is not known. Large increases in $P\text{aO}_2$ can stimulate continuous breathing in fetal sheep near term but more physiological increases in $P\text{aO}_2$ (i.e. to normal newborn levels of 50–60 mmHg) do not.

Role of central and peripheral chemoreceptors (see pp. 606 and 610)

Transient impairment of gas exchange after birth causes $Pa{O_2}$ and pH to fall, and $Pa{CO_2}$ to rise. Hypercapnia stimulates breathing via central chemoreceptors and might accomplish this in the newborn. Changes in $Pa{CO_2}$ and $Pa{O_2}$ should be detected by peripheral chemoreceptors but their afferent input may remain ineffective in changing respiratory drive, as in fetuses. Once gas exchange is established $Pa{O_2}$ rises to levels that silence peripheral chemoreceptors so any possible role they may play in stimulating breathing would quickly end. In practice, peripheral chemodenervation in fetal sheep has no effect on breathing initiation so peripheral chemoreceptors appear to play little, if any, role in this process.

Asphyxia and gasping

Cessation of placental gas exchange before the onset of lung aeration causes a rapid fall in $Pa{O_2}$ (within 90–120 seconds) because of very limited fetal O_2 stores. Normally a marked fall in $Pa{O_2}$ at birth is prevented by rapid initiation of lung gas exchange. However, if this fails, hypoxemia develops which inhibits regular breathing. When $Pa{O_2}$ falls to $\leqslant 5$ mmHg 'gasping' is stimulated. Gasps are generated by a discrete region of the medulla and are distinguishable from breaths by their steep inspiratory slopes, higher amplitude, and long expiratory phase. Continuous breathing will occur only if gasping or *resuscitation* successfully raises arterial oxygenation above the apneic threshold.

Role of sensory input at birth

Birth is associated with massive tactile and probably painful stimulation. Once delivered, the baby is exposed to cutaneous cooling in room air, an effect which will be exaggerated by evaporative heat losses. There are also large changes in tactile, visual, and auditory stimulation due to the change in physical environment and to obstetrical or maternal interventions. Cutaneous cooling is particularly effective in stimulating the onset of continuous breathing (see p. 607) and even mild tactile stimulation increases respiratory drive sufficiently to reduce the incidence of *apnea* in premature human newborns. Sciatic nerve stimulation (which would stimulate fibers from pain, temperature, and touch receptors) and cutaneous cooling can initiate respiratory responses within seconds in fetal sheep, so the time course of the response is appropriate to explain the rapid stimulation of breathing at birth. The transition from the 'weightless' fetal condition to gravitational forces might also be of importance in sustaining breathing in the neonate as vestibular stimulation, such as by rocking, is an effective method of preventing apnea of prematurity.

Behavioral arousal

Human newborns awake within seconds of birth and remain awake and alert, with frequent bursts of motor activity for 30 minutes or more. Crying frequently occurs, which generates large intrathoracic pressure changes and which may assist in establishment of lung gas volume. Coughing and sneezing may help clear the upper airways. The ventilatory response to hypoxia and hypercapnia in adults is enhanced in the awake state. Thus, arousal at birth may increase respiratory drive as well as promote the rapid onset of lung gas exchange.

Role of the endocrine system

The fetus is relatively unresponsive to stimuli which would provoke prompt arousal in postnatal animals, and the respiratory system is relatively unresponsive to peripheral chemoreceptor stimulation and to stimulation by hypercapnia (in that hypercapnia fails to cause continuous breathing movements). Thus, it is possible that at birth a source of inhibition of respiration and arousal is removed. Possibly this is mediated by changes in endocrine environment.

Marked changes in concentrations of many hormones occur at birth. Placental hormones, such as progesterone and prostaglandin (PG) E_2 decrease due to the loss of an important site of production. In contrast, other hormones such as vasopressin, angiotensin II, norepinephrine and epinephrine show large and transient increases. Many of these hormonal changes elicit other primary adaptations to birth such as lung fluid resorption, arousal, or cardiovascular changes and may have only an indirect impact on the control of breathing. However, removing the placenta from the circulation stimulates breathing and resuming placental blood flow inhibits breathing in fetal sheep by a mechanism unrelated to changes in arterial blood gas tensions or pH. Possibly, this is mediated by a change in circulating concentration(s) of a respiratory inhibitor(s) of placental origin.

PGE_2 and adenosine, respiratory inhibitors in the perinatal period, are produced by the placenta, and are present in the fetal circulation in higher concentrations than in postnatal animals. A notable effect of reducing fetal plasma PG concentrations with PG synthesis inhibitors (e.g. indomethacin) is that continuous breathing is evoked without disrupting normal sleep state patterns. PG synthesis inhibitors induce fetal breathing in all sleep states, a change in breathing pattern similar to that which occurs at birth. After birth, it takes some time for PGE_2 and adenosine concentrations to fall. Therefore, other factors are likely responsible for stimulating the very rapid increase in respiratory activity which occurs within seconds or minutes after birth. The role of these substances, as well as other neuroactive agents such as endorphins, in the transition in respiratory control at birth are subjects of continuing study.

Role of the cardiovascular system

Lung ventilation will not effectively accomplish gas exchange unless pulmonary blood flow increases dramatically from fetal levels. Lung aeration and oxygenation cause a tenfold increase in pulmonary blood flow to occur within 15 minutes of birth. Could the increase in pulmonary blood flow feed back and affect breathing? Increasing pulmonary blood flow by sevenfold increases lung ventilation approximately twofold in adult dogs, and this effect can be abolished by vagotomy. Since a change in pulmonary blood flow of this magnitude occurs within minutes of birth, this mechanism could promote the onset of continuous lung ventilation. However, fetal sheep vagotomized either before or at birth initiate breathing with a time course similar to intact newborns which suggests that this mechanism is not essential for the transition to continuous breathing although it could still be a contributing factor.

Summary

The initiation of lung ventilation at birth is caused by a combination of factors which act together to stimulate respiratory drive and to reduce respiratory inhibition (Fig. 11.13). Evidence suggests that sensory stimuli associated with birth and delivery are of central importance in promoting the very rapid onset of postnatal breathing. Any increase in $P\text{CO}_2$ or decrease in pH which occurs may further promote this process by stimulating the central chemoreceptors but these stimuli alone would be ineffective. If the rapid initiation of lung gas exchange fails, then the gasping reflex may provide a physiological backup mechanism for the establishment of lung aeration. Breathing will probably be stimulated only transiently by

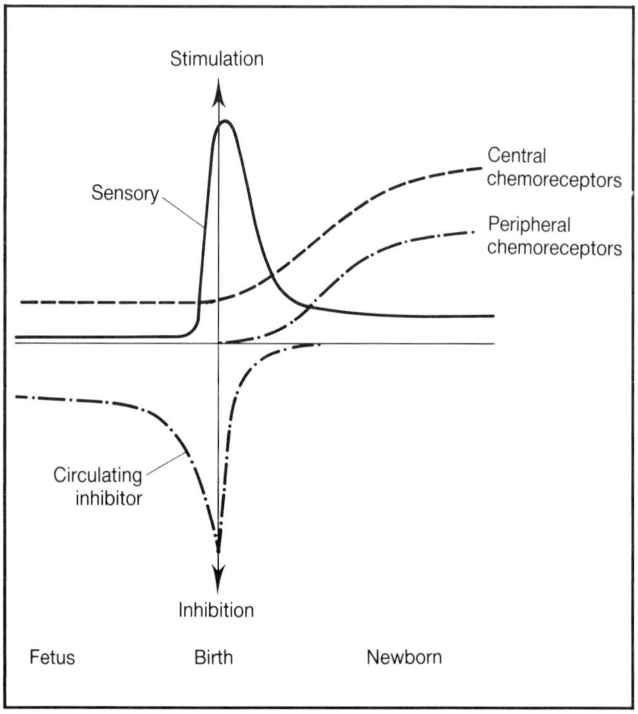

Fig. 11.13. Model of factors regulating breathing in the perinatal period. Central chemoreceptors influence respiration throughout the perinatal period whereas peripheral chemoreceptors gradually become effective during the first few days of postnatal life. Sensory stimulation (e.g. thermal, tactile, visual, auditory) acts as a powerful nonspecific respiratory stimulus during labor and for several hours after birth. During this time newborns are in the awake state. Circulating respiratory inhibitor(s) suppress fetal respiratory activity and the degree of suppression increases during labor. After birth, the inhibitor is rapidly removed from the circulation. Not shown is the sleep state-dependent stimulation of breathing which occurs in rapid eye movement sleep both before and after birth.

arousal and by sensory changes at birth. The newborn will eventually go to sleep, and either will adapt to the sensory stimuli or the stimuli may wane with time. Thus, a more sustained respiratory stimulus is required to explain the maintenance of continuous breathing. This is particularly evident 24 hours after birth when $Pa\text{O}_2$ and pH become higher, and $Pa\text{CO}_2$ becomes lower than during fetal life. Experimental evidence indicates that removal of the placenta from the circulation causes a gradually increasing stimulation of breathing, as well as increasing the respiratory response to CO_2 stimulation. This may be caused by the withdrawal from the circulation of a placentally produced respiratory inhibitor.

Selected reading

Adamson SL. Initiation of lung ventilation at birth. *Fetal Med Rev* 1991; **3**: 133.

Jansen AH, Chernick V. Onset of breathing and control of respiration. *Semin Perinatol* 1988; **12**: 104.

Karlberg P, Wennergren G. Respiratory control during onset of breathing. In *Cardiovascular and respiratory physiology in the fetus and neonate*. Colloque INSERM Vol. 133. Paris: John Libbey Eurotext, 1986: 131.

B6. Control of Upper Airway Patency

J Milerad and S L Davis

The upper airway between the choanae and larynx is unsupported by skeleton or cartilage and tends to be closed in the absence of muscle action. The muscles that provide tension to the upper airway walls include those that are tonically active (e.g. tensor palatini) and those that, in addition, increase their action phasically during inspiration (e.g. alae nasi, genioglossus). The level of activity in these upper airway maintaining muscles is influenced by central ventilatory drive so that their action is diminished when ventilatory drive is decreased (e.g. during sleep). During inspiration there is a sequential activation of the alae nasi, the genioglossus muscle and the vocal cords before the diaphragm contracts. The ability to synchronize the air pumping and upper airway activity is related to gestational age and the high incidence of respiratory arrhythmias in preterm infants may in part be related to a lack of coordination.

Upper airway maintaining muscles are also influenced by reflex mechanisms arising in the upper airway and chest (e.g. reflexes activated by stretch, inflation and air flow) and by peripheral and central chemoreceptor stimulation (e.g. hypoxia and hypercapnia). However, the inspiratory activity of the upper airway is not uniformly increased by chemosensory stimulation. The CO_2 threshold is higher for the genioglossus compared to the alae nasi and the diaphragm, which may affect airway patency during hypercapnia. Whether this is related to differential output from the central chemosensory area or can be attributed to differential stimulation of airway CO_2 receptors is not clear. In general CO_2 stimulation stabilizes the chest wall and increases activity in the laryngeal dilators; CO_2 breathing has been used therapeutically in *severe obstructive apnea.*

There is some evidence that the mechanics of the collapsible human upper airway are best modeled by a Starling resistor. In this model, when the tension in the upper airway wall is greater than the potentially collapsing negative pressures generated in the airway by action of inspiratory muscles (Fig. 11.14a) air flow is dependent on the pressure drop between the nares (atmospheric pressure) and the thorax, and on upper airway resistance. When tension in the upper airway wall is inadequate to maintain patency during inspiration (Fig. 11.14b), the upper airway tends to collapse and a situation of air flow limitation is created where air flow is driven by the pressure difference between the nares (atmospheric pressure) and the level of negative pressure in the collapsible portion of the airway at which it collapses, the critical pressure. When upper airway muscles fail to maintain airway patency at atmospheric pressure (Fig. 11.14c) the airway is closed and there is no air flow.

In newborns the anatomical relation between the tongue, soft palate and posterior pharyngeal wall favors nasal breathing. This breathing route also offers the lowest airway resistance. The air flow in the nasal cavity contributes to the timing between inspiration and upper airway activity through sensory information from the nasopharyngeal pathway. The normal pattern is disrupted when this input is abolished, either by diverting air flow through a tracheostomy or by topical anesthesia, and in experimental animals has led to asphyxia and even death. Therefore it is important to relieve airway obstruction in infants with conditions such as *cleft palate*.

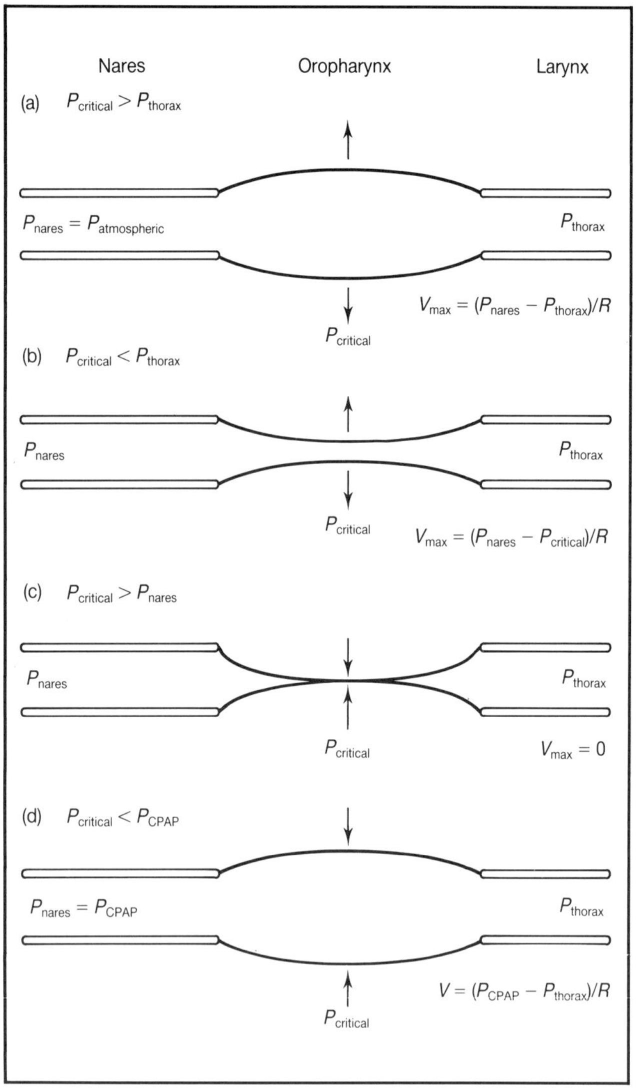

Fig. 11.14. Schematic representation of pressure–flow relationships in the collapsible segment of the upper airway based on the Starling resistor model: (a) the normal airway, (b) the airway with air flow limitation, (c) the airway at the point of collapse, (d) the airway during CPAP therapy. P_{nares}, pressure in airway above collapsible segment; $P_{critical}$, pressure in collapsible segment at which it collapses; P_{thorax}, pressure in airway below the collapsible segment; R, airway resistance; V_{max}, maximum flow.

Upper airway (laryngeal) reflexes

Upper airway reflexes serve not only to modulate respiratory timing, but also to prevent entry of foreign matter into the lower airways. The upper laryngeal mucosa contains receptors sensitive to mechanical as well as chemical and thermal stimuli. The excitation of laryngeal chemoreceptors with liquid induces apnea, active upper airway constriction and repeated swallowing as a protective reflex against aspiration of foreign matter, e.g. *gastroesophageal reflux*. The laryngeal reflex is exaggerated in immature animals and is enhanced by hypoxia. It is especially active in preterm infants in whom it can be elicited not only by hypotonic solutions but also by normal saline. In addition to the changes in ventilation the laryngeal chemostimulation has prominent autonomic effects and induces bradycardia, peripheral vasoconstriction and redistribution of blood flow. The apneic and bradycardic components can be reinforced powerfully by hyperthermia and hypoxia, a finding of potential significance with regard to life-threatening *apnea of infancy* and *sudden infant death syndrome (SIDS).*

Selected reading

Bryan AC, Bowes G, Maloney JE. Control of breathing in the fetus and newborn. In Cherniack NS, Widdicombe JG, eds. *Handbook of physiology. Section 2: The respiratory system.* Vol. II. Bethesda, MD: American Physiological Society, 1986: 621.

Lagercrantz H, Milerad J, Walker D. Control of breathing in the neonate. In Crystal RG, West JB, *et al. The lung.* New York: Raven Press Ltd, 1991: 1711.

B7. Apnea

S L Davis

Mechanisms

Two basic mechanisms may contribute to the interruption of effective breathing in clinically significant apnea. In *central apnea,* neural drive is interrupted to inspiratory muscles, including the diaphragm, intercostal, and upper airway-maintaining muscles. In *obstructive apnea,* diaphragm contraction fails to result in movement of air in the upper airway because of upper airway closure. The action of muscles during inspiration can be measured using the surface-recorded diaphragmatic electromyogram or by intrathoracic pressure monitoring (e.g.

with an esophageal balloon), and can be detected by monitoring abdominal or chest wall movement (e.g. with strain gauge, electrical impedance, or electrical inductance techniques). Air flow can be measured with a flow meter (e.g. pneumotachometer) attached to a facial or nasal mask, or detected by monitoring air temperature at the nares (e.g. with a thermistor), $P\text{CO}_2$ at the nares, or sounds of air movement in the upper airway with a microphone.

Brief (less than 15 seconds) central pauses in breathing are common during both waking and sleep and are unrelated to age. In waking they are related to volitional activity (e.g. speech); in rapid eye movement (REM) sleep they are associated with REM motor activity; in nonREM sleep they characteristically follow augmented breaths (sighs). Many movements involving the trunk and upper limbs are accompanied by splinting of the thorax by contraction of expiratory intercostal and abdominal muscles and with active closure of the glottis (Valsalva maneuver). Such movement-related breathing pauses can be recognized by the re-initiation of respiratory air flow in expiration.

In *cyanotic breath-holding spells,* some children, when frustrated or angry, actively expire without glottic closure so that lung volume is reduced below functional residual capacity. The rapid fall in O_2 saturation recorded during these attacks is attributed to alveolar collapse and pulmonary arterial–venous shunting. Rapid desaturation frequently results in loss of consciousness, which is characteristically brief as relaxation of expiratory muscles terminates the apnea. These spells can occur as early as 2–3 months of age, but are most common between 6 months and 4 years.

Hypoventilation and central apnea resulting from depression in central ventilatory drive occurs in *diffuse encephalopathies with reduced level of consciousness,* with *focal brainstem lesions,* and from the action of depressant drugs (e.g. barbiturates, benzodiazepines, narcotics, ethanol). Immaturity increases susceptibility to central ventilatory depression so that preterm infants may manifest recurrent central apnea with *sepsis, hyperthermia,* or *hypoxia*. Depression of central ventilatory drive usually results in reduced tidal volume and, by reduced phasic drive to upper airway-maintaining muscles, upper airway collapse. The distinction between central and obstructive apnea therefore is not always clear. A progressive decrease in respiratory drive may result initially in reduced tidal volume (*hypoventilation*), followed by flow-limited breathing (*obstructive hypopnea*), upper airway closure (*obstructive apnea*), then *central apnea*. On the other hand, *primary central apnea* is often accompanied by airway closure, signaled by a failure of the pressure changes in the airway with each heart beat to be transmitted to the nares. Persistence of airway closure when breathing recommences may be a result of the added load on airway-dilating muscles created by surface tension forces.

Clinical syndromes

Apnea of prematurity

Physiological respiratory pauses are not associated with bradycardia or significant O_2 desaturation. However, preterm infants frequently experience recurrent 15–20 second pauses in respiration, sometime accompanied by bradycardia and O_2 desaturation. This defines *apnea of prematurity* which is associated with immaturity of central ventilatory control. The incidence and severity is inversely related to conceptual age and as defined above most infants under 32 weeks of gestation have apnea. Although generally not related to pulmonary or central nervous system pathology, recurrent apnea in these infants may be the first sign of septicemia, hypoglycemia, hydrocephalus or intraventricular hemorrhage.

Apnea of prematurity can be central, obstructive, or mixed in character with obstructive and mixed apnea occurring particularly in the first several days after birth. Oscillations in central respiratory drive and upper airway collapse appear to be important causes, although *laryngeal reflex apnea* and *cyanotic breath-holding spells* may play a minor role. One aspect of immaturity that contributes to upper airway dysfunction in apnea of prematurity is incomplete synchronization of the upper airway muscles and diaphragm. In adults, airway muscles that are phasically active in inspiration begin to contract immediately before the onset of diaphragmatic contraction. In contrast, in ovine fetuses *in utero*, synchronization of the upper airway-dilating muscles and diaphragm is absent. Failure of an upper airway muscle (genioglossus) to activate in response to nasal occlusion in some preterm infants with recurrent *obstructive apnea* supports the notion that the control of upper airway maintaining muscles is immature in them. A primary role for upper airway dysfunction in this disorder is underlined by the effectiveness of low levels of continuous positive airway pressure (CPAP) in its management. CPAP appears to act by mechanically splinting the upper airway, assisting muscles that provide tension to the airway walls. In the Starling resistor model of the upper airway described earlier (p. 618), when airway-maintaining muscles fail to counter effectively the negative airway pressures generated during inspiration, air flow is maintained by the pressure difference between the airway inlet (the nares), which is held at 2–10 cmH_2O by CPAP, and the pressure at which the airway walls collapse (Fig. 11.14d).

Although controversial, providing there is no associated underlying pathology, e.g. septicemia (see above), central and mixed apnea of prematurity have been regarded by some as 'physiological' phenomena because the fetus of equivalent maturity only breathes episodically. This is proposed despite major differences between the fetus and newborn: the discontinuity of fetal breathing is state related whereas this is not so in the newborn and further, periodic breathing related to oscillations in respiratory control systems is prominent in the newborn and is not evident in the fetus. Immaturity of neuronal networks and slow neural conduction certainly may contribute to the instability of respiratory control feedback mechanisms that result in periodic fluctuations in central respiratory drive. However, respiratory rhythm generation and central respiratory drive are not deficient. It is likely that there are residual fetal inhibitory mechanisms, which may be activated when an infant is placed in an 'intrauterine-like' environment (e.g. sensory deprivation, increased environmental temperature, hypoxemia). Sensory stimulation as might occur with gentle cutaneous stimulation or gentle rocking (as on a water bed) may decrease or inhibit apneic episodes. Apnea is more common when incubator or skin temperatures approximate or are higher than core temperature. During hypoxemia, where $Pa\text{O}_2$ is lowered towards fetal levels, if a 'critical' level is reached apnea may occur. This could be due to neurochemical stimulation (e.g. adenosine, dopamine) or to stimulation of a suprapontine region, possibly the Köllike–Fuse region (see p. 599) which depresses breathing. Correction of hypoxemia by appropriate low concentration O_2 therapy may attenuate or abolish this mechanism of apnea.

Xanthine derivatives, such as theophylline and caffeine, are often effective in the management of apnea of prematurity. Their exact mechanism of action is unknown but they may antagonize endogenous adenosine which both depresses respiration and slows the release of excitatory amino acids; the latter increase neuronal discharge and may thereby increase the forebrain respiratory drive. It also is possible that the xanthines actively stimulate the release of these excitatory amino acids.

Congenital central hypoventilation syndrome (Ondine curse)

In this disorder, central ventilatory drive declines progressively at the onset of sleep to the point that breathing efforts may cease altogether at the onset of stage 2 nonREM sleep. When severe, newborn infants may become apneic at the onset of quiet sleep on the first day of life. More frequently the disorder presents during the first days or weeks of life as hypoventilation during quiet sleep with cyanosis and apnea terminated by spontaneous or forced arousal. The failure of central ventilatory drive during nonREM sleep appears to result from a selective disorder in the system regulating the feedback of peripheral and central chemoreceptors to the respiratory center in the brainstem; therefore, both hypoxia and hypercapnia fail to stimulate breathing.

Apparent life-threatening events (ALTEs)

Infants who experience isolated or recurrent events manifested by apnea, pallor or cyanosis, and hypotonia, especially if there is failure to arouse from sleep briskly and to recover without breathing assistance by the caretaker, have a substantially increased risk of *SIDS*. Hence, managing infants who experience such unexplained *ALTEs* on monitors which detect breathing movements, and in some cases the heart beat, is now customary. However, the routine use of these monitors has not apparently altered the incidence of SIDS. Polygraphic studies in infants who presented with an ALTE have shown a significant increase in the incidence of subsequent SIDS in infants in whom prolonged (more than 14 seconds) obstructive apnea was documented. Infants with well recognized anomalies involving the upper airway (e.g. *Pierre Robin syndrome*), who often show signs of increased upper airway resistance such as inspiratory chest and lateral neck indrawing, may experience severe apnea or even sudden death during sleep. Lesser degrees of anatomical upper airway narrowing may be found in infants with a small lower jaw; this craniofacial appearance occurs in families of infants with ALTEs and is also associated with *obstructive sleep apnea syndrome* in adulthood. A possible role of upper airway dysfunction in determining the timing of SIDS, which reaches peak incidence at 6–12 weeks of age, is suggested by the finding that oropharyngeal airway dimensions, measured radiographically, are smaller during inspiration at 6 weeks than in the newborn period. Fundamental differences distinguish infants under 6 months with upper airway dysfunction from older individuals with obstructive sleep apnea syndrome (described below). Infants do not snore because the redundant upper airway tissues that vibrate to create snoring are not yet formed. Many infants with increased upper airway resistance from anatomical anomalies (e.g. *large alar flaps, choanal stenosis, small jaw, large tongue*) may experience flow-limited breathing (Fig. 11.14b) because of increased inspiratory effort generated to maintain tidal volume, but generally are able to resist upper airway collapse during waking and sleep. Maturation of processes controlling the regulation of breathing in quiet sleep, which evolves into mature adult nonREM sleep between birth and 6 months of age, with an increased propensity to deeper stages of sleep during the night after 6 weeks, may contribute to decreasing upper airway collapse during sleep following the first months of life.

Obstructive sleep apnea syndrome

Sleep-related upper airway dysfunction can occur even in infants as young as 6 months; however, it is overwhelmingly a disorder of obese, middle-aged men. In childhood, it frequently results from airway compromise by *enlarged tonsils and adenoids,* and less frequently is associated with an enlarged tongue (e.g. *Down syndrome, lipid storage disorders*). *Snoring* and *obstructive sleep apnea* form a continuum of severity. They are both exacerbated by conditions that depress ventilatory drive during sleep (e.g. sleep loss or fragmentation, depressant drugs and ethanol) and by conditions that cause airway mucosal swelling (e.g. *infection* or *trauma*).

Obstructive sleep apnea involves a recurring cycle of sleep onset with apnea, followed by arousal and re-initiation of effective breathing, followed by sleep onset and apnea, etc. The duration of apnea and level of O_2 desaturation before arousal in each cycle are both measures of severity. Increased upper airway resistance may be present during waking. Tidal volume decreases progressively as the subject becomes drowsy and enters stage 2 sleep. Because severe sleep debt is common, sleep onset may progress rapidly to deeper stages and even to REM sleep. As tidal volume declines with deepening sleep state, the tension of muscles maintaining the upper airway also declines. When the critical airway pressure, i.e. the maximum negative airway pressure at which airway patency can be maintained, rises above peak inspiratory intrathoracic pressure (Fig. 11.14b), air flow is limited and vibration of airway soft tissues (snoring) results. When the critical airway pressure falls further (Fig. 11.14c), i.e. airway muscles cannot maintain airway patency even at atmospheric pressure, the airway collapses. The site of collapse varies, but usually occurs between the level of the soft palate and the base of the tongue. The inability of the upper airway-dilating muscles to maintain airway patency results from a combination of decreased ventilatory drive during sleep and mechanical load placed on these muscles by pathological changes in the airway walls that alter airway shape, dimensions, and compliance (e.g. *lymphoid hyperplasia* or *fat deposition*). Following initial airway collapse, inspiratory efforts against the closed airway may continue to decline until failure of ventilation causes sufficient hypoxia to stimulate peripheral chemoreceptors. Hypoxic drive then results in increased inspiratory efforts. The resulting increase in the level of negative intrathoracic pressure generated by inspiratory efforts can be substantial and can have an important effect on venous return. In the fully developed syndrome, hypoxia and the subsequent increase in inspiratory drive both fail to result in airway reopening or to cause arousal. Arousal with simultaneous recovery of airway patency is triggered by a critical level of intrathoracic pressure. The cycle of sleep onset, airway collapse, and arousal repeats every 20–120 seconds, resulting in a marked fragmentation of sleep and disruption of sleep architecture. Complete airway collapse is not necessary for the significant consequences that result from sleep-related upper airway dysfunction. Severe air flow limitation, *obstructive hypopnia,* with *snoring* may also cause intermittent hypoxia, cardiovascular mechanical changes, and sleep disruption.

Sleep disturbance may result in irritability, hyperactivity, and short attention span as well as poor appetite and failure to thrive. In adults, daytime sleepiness, headaches, and depressed mood are prominent, and sudden death has been reported.

Effective management involves reversal of the anatomical airway abnormality (e.g. tonsillectomy and adenoidectomy, weight loss) or avoidance of factors that depress ventilation during sleep (drugs, ethanol, sleep loss). Where these therapeutic modalities are not appropriate or feasible, nocturnal nasal CPAP is frequently effective; however, tracheostomy may be necessary.

Selected reading

Guilleminault C, Heldt G, Powell N, Riley R. Small upper airway in near-miss sudden infant death syndrome infants and their families. *Lancet* 1986; **i**: 402.

Kahn A, Blum D, Rebuffat E, *et al*. Polysomnographic studies of infants who subsequently died of sudden infant death syndrome. *Pediatrics* 1988; **82**: 721.

Poets CF, Stebbens VA, Southall DP. Arterial oxygen saturation and breathing movements during the first year of life. *J Dev Physiol* 1991; **15**: 341.

Smith P, Wise RA, Gold AV, *et al*. Upper airway pressure-flow relationships in obstructive sleep apnea. *J Appl Physiol* 1988; **64**: 789.

Southall DP, Croft CB, Stebbens VA, *et al*. Detection of sleep associated dysfunctional pharyngeal obstruction in infants. *Eur J Pediatr* 1989; **148**: 353.

C. Mechanics of Breathing

J J Pérez Fontán

As aquatic animals adapted to life on land, their gas-exchange systems needed to maintain a large contact surface with air without losing large amounts of water to evaporation. Therefore, the lungs of most terrestrial species evolved as invaginated structures. An invaginated lung, however, required a mechanism to force air in and out of the gas-exchanging spaces. In mammals and other higher vertebrates, this mechanism resembles a bellows pump, in which a group of respiratory muscles apply force on the passive elements of the chest wall (rib cage and abdomen) to inflate and deflate the lungs. The function of the pump is regulated by a complex network of sensors, which relay both mechanical information from the pump's components and chemical information from arterial blood to a control center in the brainstem. Despite the relative simplicity of the pump and the obvious complexity of the regulatory network, the respiratory system is more vulnerable to mechanical than to control dysfunctions. In fact, the increase in energy demand imposed by various types of mechanical breakdown usually causes most of the signs and symptoms of respiratory disease and ultimately leads to respiratory failure.

From a mechanical point of view, the function of the respiratory system is best analyzed in terms of work and energy. Above, we compared the mammalian respiratory system to a bellows pump. Basic physics indicates that the amount of work (ΔW) done by such a pump in order to produce a certain volume change (V_0 to V_1) with a pressure change P can be computed as (equation 1):

$$\Delta W = \int_{V_0}^{V_1} P \, \mathrm{d}V$$

For the respiratory system, the total amount of work done by the respiratory muscles during a single breath depends on the mechanical characteristics of the lungs and chest wall (which define the magnitude of P) and on the needs for gas exchange (which define the limits of the volume change, V_1–V_0).

Work alone, however, is not a direct measure of the energy that the muscles must extract from the metabolic fuels provided by the circulation. The reason is that the respiratory muscles transform energy (ΔQ) into work with variable efficiency (ε) (equation 2):

$$\Delta Q = \Delta W / \varepsilon$$

In this regard, energy and work can be envisioned as if on a see-saw on a sliding fulcrum, the position of which is defined by the efficiency of the system. Excluding extreme conditions (e.g. circulatory shock), the circulation provides the respiratory muscles with abundant substrates, and small increases in work or decreases in efficiency caused by mild, or even moderate, mechanical derangements can be compensated by extracting more energy from these substrates and by processing this energy into contractile force. With more severe derangements, however, substrates either may not be available or, more commonly, may not be processed fast enough into work by the muscles' metabolic and contractile apparatus. If so, the balance is tipped beyond the limits of compensation, leading to the gas-exchange abnormalities that characterize *respiratory failure*. We will discuss separately how respiratory work and efficiency are determined in both health and disease, paying particular attention to the unique characteristics of the developing respiratory system.

Determinants of volume–pressure work

As shown by equation 1, the volume–pressure relationships of the respiratory system are the only determinants of how much work the respiratory muscles must do during breathing. These relationships summarize the mechanical behaviors of the lungs and the chest wall. Because lungs and chest wall are linked by a non-compressible boundary (the pleural space), their volumes cannot change independently of each other or of the respiratory system as a whole, and therefore (equation 3):

$$\Delta V_L = \Delta V_W = \Delta V_{RS}$$

where ΔV_L, ΔV_W, and ΔV_{RS} represent the volume changes that the lungs, chest wall, and respiratory system, respectively, undergo during breathing.

In contrast, the pressures that the respiratory muscles need to generate in order to inflate the lungs (P_L), chest wall (P_W), and respiratory system (P_{RS}) depend on the pressure difference across each component, and consequently they are all different (equations 4–6):

$$P_L = P_{ao} - P_{pl}$$
$$P_W = P_{pl} - P_B$$
$$P_{RS} = P_{ao} - \mathrm{P_B}$$

where P_{ao} is the pressure at the airway opening (the nares or the mouth, during normal breathing), P_{pl} is the representative pressure in the pleural space, and P_B is atmospheric pressure. These equations can be easily reworked into the following expression (equation 7):

$$P_{RS} = P_L + P_W$$

which indicates that, at any time during breathing, the total pressure needed to produce a certain volume change in the respiratory system is equal to the sum of the pressures needed to produce the same change individually in the lungs and the chest wall.

Pressures acting on the respiratory system

To move both air and respiratory tissues during breathing, the respiratory muscles must overcome several types of forces, which when applied on tissue surfaces, are translated into pressures. Depending on whether the energy consumed in the effort leaves the system as heat or simply remains stored to be recovered later, the pressures acting on the respiratory system can be classified into non-dissipative and dissipative. **Non-dissipative** pressures include elastic or volume-dependent pressures that arise from the tendency of the lung and chest wall to recover their original shape upon deformation, inertial or acceleration-dependent pressures produced by the changes in velocity experienced by gas and tissues during breathing movements, and gravitational or mass-dependent pressures related to the mere weight of the tissues. **Dissipative** pressures, on the other hand, are commonly grouped together as resistive pressures, and include flow-dependent pressures generated primarily by the friction of the gas against the airway walls, and viscoelastic or time-dependent pressures created by the molecular movements that occur in the tissues and in the gas–liquid interface as the respiratory system changes volume.

Non-dissipative pressures

Inertial and gravitational pressures are small during normal breathing in children and can be neglected. Elastic pressures, in contrast, can be quite large. Their magnitude depends on the volume of the respiratory system, somewhat as the tension developed by a rubber band depends on the extent to which it is stretched. Elastic pressures are best characterized when there are no other pressures operating in the respiratory system. For this to happen, respiratory system volume must be maintained constant for at least a few seconds (e.g. by breath holding at a given level). Under such circumstances, gas ceases to flow in the airways, and pressures at the airway opening and in the alveoli (P_A) become the same. Equations 4–6 can then be rewritten (equations 8–10):

$$P_{L,el} = P_A - P_{pl}$$
$$P_{W,el} = P_{pl} - P_B$$
$$P_{RS,el} = P_A - P_B$$

where $P_{L,el}$, $P_{W,el}$, and $P_{RS,el}$ represent the elastic pressures generated by the lungs, the chest wall, and the whole respiratory system, respectively.

The relationships between volume changes and elastic pressures in the respiratory system and its components are quite complex. Graphically, their shape can be described by a sigmoid curve: volume increases much less for a given pressure change at low and high volumes than at intermediate volumes, when the volume–pressure relationship is steeper (Fig. 11.15). From a mathematical point of view, the description is more difficult. Like any other continuous function, each volume-pressure relationship has a well specified slope at each volume ($\Delta V/\Delta P$). This slope defines the **compliance** of the lungs, chest wall, or respiratory system for that volume depending on whether $\Delta P_{L,el}$, $\Delta P_{W,el}$, or $\Delta P_{RS,el}$ is substituted for ΔP. Unfortunately, no single slope or compliance can accurately describe the totality of the volume–pressure relationship. Only for the intermediate range of volumes is the relationship relatively linear, and $\Delta V/\Delta P$ can be considered constant.

If we rearranged equations 8–10 in a way similar to equation 7, we would find that, just like the total pressure, the elastic pressure developed by the respiratory system is the sum of the elastic pressures developed by the lungs and the chest wall. A graphic analysis demonstrates how this additive interaction of the lungs and the chest wall shapes the volume–pressure behavior of the entire respiratory system (Fig. 11.16). For instance, at the points at which the volume–pressure curves intersect the volume axis, the respiratory system and each of its components (lungs and chest wall) are at their respective **relaxation volumes** (i.e. the volumes at which the elastic elements generate no recoil). Lungs and chest wall have different relaxation volumes. The relaxation

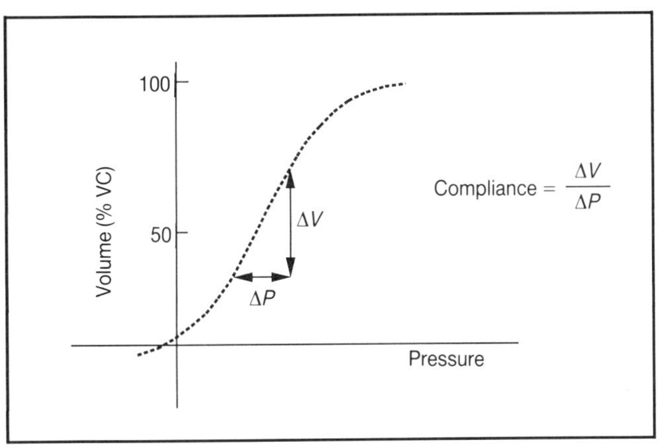

Fig. 11.15. Idealized relationship between volume and elastic pressure in the lungs. Volume is represented as a proportion of the vital capacity of the lungs (VC, the maximal volume that can be inhaled after a complete exhalation). The relationship is relatively flat at high and low lung volumes and steeper at intermediate volumes, where breathing normally takes place. At these intermediate volumes, the slope is relatively constant, and the relationship can be described with a single compliance.

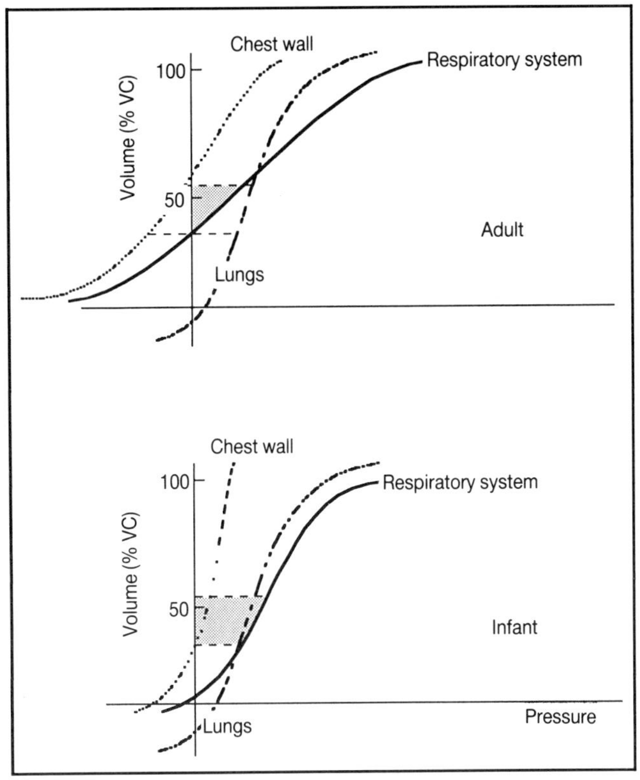

Fig. 11.16. Elastic volume–pressure relationships of the lungs, chest wall, and respiratory system for the range of vital capacity (VC) in an adult and in an infant. These relationships show that the pressure needed to inflate the respiratory system to any given volume is the sum of the pressures that would be needed to inflate the lungs and the chest wall individually to the same volume. The intersection of each relationship with the ordinate represents the relaxation volume of each component. The volume–pressure relationships of the lungs are similar in the adult and in the infant; the volume–pressure relationship of the chest wall, however, is much steeper in the infant, causing both the relaxation volumes of the chest wall and the respiratory system to be lower as well. The stippled area represents the elastic work done by the respiratory muscles for a typical tidal volume. Note that this work tends to be greater in the infant because, at normal breathing volumes, the recoil of the chest wall does not contribute to inflating the lungs as it does in the adult.

volume of the lungs is rather small; if allowed to collapse freely, the lungs would end up containing a gas volume smaller than the normal **residual volume** (the gas volume of the lungs after a forced expiration). The relaxation volume of the chest wall, on the other hand, is considerably larger; in the adult, it exceeds 50 percent of the **vital capacity** (the gas volume of the lungs after a maximal inspiratory effort). The discrepancy between the relaxation volumes of the lungs and the chest wall has three important mechanical consequences. First, it causes the relaxation volume of the respiratory system to occupy a position intermediate between those of the lungs and the chest wall; beyond the newborn period, the relaxation volume of the respiratory system coincides with the **functional residual capacity** of the lungs (the gas volume of the lungs at the end of a tidal breath). Second, the opposing recoils of the lungs and chest wall create a negative pressure in the pleural space at the end of a normal breath. This negative pressure attaches the lungs to the chest wall and promotes venous return into the heart. Finally, for at least a portion of the volume range, the passive outward recoil of the chest wall contributes to the work of expanding the lungs, thereby reducing the energetic demands on the respiratory muscles (Fig. 11.16).

The elastic recoil generated per unit of lung volume is relatively constant during development. In contrast, the recoil of the chest wall increases substantially after the perinatal period, when a high chest-wall compliance is essential to facilitate passage through the birth canal. As a result of this high chest-wall compliance, the inward recoil of the newborn's lungs is partially unopposed, and the relaxation volume of the respiratory system is proportionally smaller than that of the adult (Fig. 11.16). Because a small lung volume represents a disadvantage in terms of both alveolar stability and oxygenation, newborns of most mammalian species have developed strategies to maintain the functional residual capacity of their lungs above the relaxation volume of their respiratory system. These strategies combine mechanisms directed at prolonging expiratory flow (such as sustaining the tonic activity of the inspiratory muscles during expiration or contracting the adductor muscles of the larynx) with a relatively high breathing rate, which reduces the time available for expiration. The resultant dependence of lung volume on neural control renders the functional residual capacity of newborn and small infants' lungs very vulnerable to changes in muscle coordination and tone. Concurrent decreases in intercostal and upper airway muscle tone during rapid eye movement (REM) sleep, for example, prevent expiratory flow prolongation and may decrease lung volume substantially, particularly in the premature infant. Likewise, muscle weakness, deep sedation, and central nervous system depression all can reduce the functional residual capacity of the lungs, increasing the work of breathing and impairing gas exchange.

Dissipative pressures

A pressure is characterized as dissipative when the energy that is used to overcome it leaves the system (usually as heat) and cannot be used again. In the respiratory system, most dissipative energy losses are produced by the friction of the gas against the internal surface of the airways. A measurable amount of energy, however, is also permanently invested in rearranging molecules in both the tissues and the gas–liquid interface. If this energy is primarily dependent on time then the dissipative pressures are known as viscoelastic. If, on the other hand, the energy used for the molecular rearrangements varies depending on the direction of the breathing movements, then the dissipative pressures are known as plastoelastic (certain materials, like pulmonary surfactant, exhibit high plastoelasticity). Regardless of whether the final pathway is frictional, viscoelastic, or plastoelastic, the energy dissipated during inspiration can no longer contribute to work performed during expiration. Thus, whenever present, dissipative forces cause the volume–pressure behavior of the respiratory system to vary depending on the inspiratory or expiratory direction of the volume changes, a property known as **hysteresis**.

Hysteresis is responsible for the formation of loops when the volume–pressure relationships of the respiratory system are plotted during breathing (Fig. 11.17). In such graphic representation, the dissipative pressures can be identified at any volume as the distance

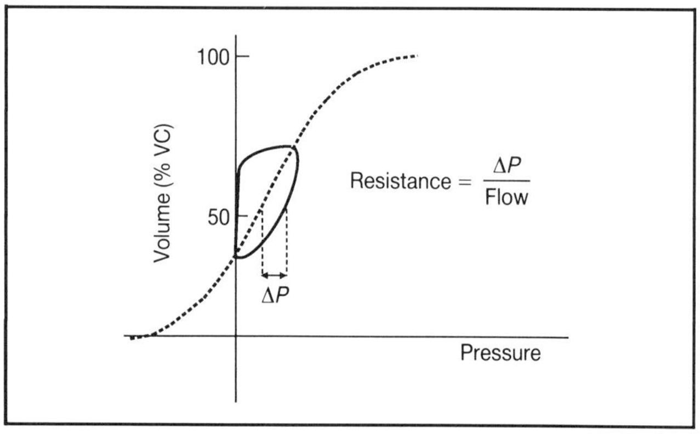

Fig. 11.17. Dynamic volume–pressure relationship showing hysteresis (loop) caused by dissipative energy losses. The magnitude of the dissipative pressure losses can be estimated at any point as the distance between the hysteretic loop and the elastic volume–pressure relationship (ΔP). The resistance of the respiratory system is usually calculated by dividing the dissipative pressure losses calculated in this fashion by the gas flow.

between the point in the loop and the point that the elastic volume–pressure relationship would occupy at a similar volume (ΔP in Fig. 11.17). In the same representation, the area enclosed by the loop provides a measure of the total amount of work done against dissipative pressures (Fig. 11.18). Under normal circumstances, however, only the inspiratory portion of this work is performed by the respiratory muscles. The dissipative work done during expiration is performed at the expense of the energy accumulated in the elastic elements of the lungs and the chest wall during inspiration.

Similar to the elastic pressures, the dissipative pressures in the respiratory system cannot be predicted with a simple mathematical expression. Viscoelastic and plastoelastic pressures, for instance, are complex, nonlinear functions of gas flow, respiratory system volume, and time. In contrast, frictional pressures are generally considered to relate linearly to gas flow in the airways ($\dot{V}$). Based on this consideration and the fact that friction causes the difference between the pressure at the airway opening (P_{ao}) and at the alveoli (P_A), we can write equation 11:

$$P_{ao} - P_A = R_{aw} \dot{V}$$

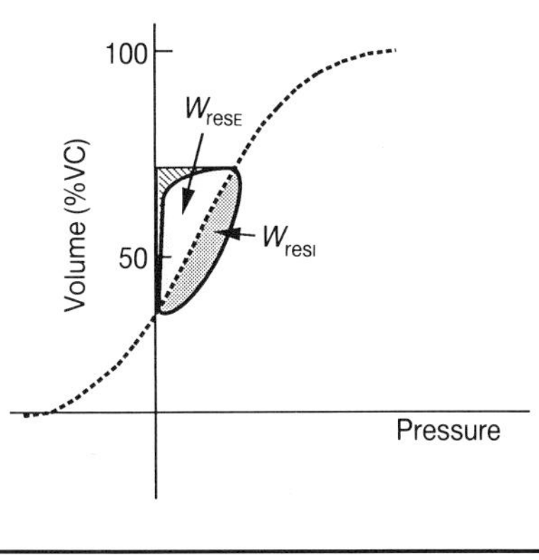

Fig. 11.18. Graphic representation of the work performed during a typical tidal breath. The area enclosed by the loop is a measure of the work done against dissipative forces. Only the inspiratory portion of this work (W_{resI}, stippling), however, needs to be performed by the respiratory muscles; the expiratory portion of the dissipative work (W_{resE}, no stippling) is done by the energy accumulated in the elastic elements of the system during inspiration. A small portion of this elastic energy is used to overcome the tone left in the inspiratory muscles during expiration (cross-hatched area).

where the constant R_{aw} represents the flow resistance of the airways. However, even this formulation is an over-simplification: volume-dependent variations in airway caliber as well as turbulence and other flow perturbations common at points of airway narrowing and bifurcations cause substantial departures from flow–pressure linearity that cannot be accounted for by a constant R_{aw}.

Airway dynamics

An understanding of the relationship between airway caliber and lung volume is essential for the recognition and diagnosis of *airway obstruction*. Central to this understanding is the idea that the airways are elastic tubes, the caliber of which is determined by the coupling of airway wall compliance and airway transmural pressure. Airway wall compliance determines both the distensibility and collapsibility of the airways; it depends on the state of health and maturity of the airway tissue and is modulated by the airway smooth muscle tone. Airway transmural pressure, defined as the difference between the pressures of the gas column inside the airway and the tissue outside the airway, varies during the breathing cycle in a fashion that depends on whether the airway is extra- or intrathoracic.

Extrathoracic airways (nose, pharynx, larynx, and trachea to the thoracic inlet) are exposed to atmospheric pressure on the outside. Because the pressure inside is subatmospheric during inspiration and supra-atmospheric during expiration, the transmural pressure of these airways is always negative (promoting airway collapse) during inspiration and always positive (promoting airway distension) during expiration. The outside surface of the intrathoracic airways (trachea and bronchi) is exposed to a pressure similar to pleural pressure (independent of whether they are embedded in the lung tissue or the mediastinum). Because inspiratory flow requires the pressure inside the airways to be greater than alveolar pressure, and alveolar pressure must in turn be greater than pleural pressure (the difference being equivalent to the elastic recoil of the lungs—$P_{L,el}$ in equation 8), the transmural pressure of the intrathoracic airways becomes increasingly positive (causing the airways to become distended) during inspiration. Expiratory flow, in contrast, requires the pressure inside the airways to be lower than alveolar pressure. Whether the pressure at a specific point inside an airway (P_{aw}) is higher or lower than the outside pleural pressure (P_{pl}), however, depends on the balance between the frictional pressure losses that occur upstream from the airway ($P_A - P_{aw}$) and the elastic recoil of the lungs ($P_{L,el}$). If, at a certain point, friction causes ($P_A - P_{aw}$) > $P_{L,el}$, then it follows that (equation 12):

$$P_A - P_{L,el} > P_{aw}$$

or, from equation 8 (equation 13):

$$P_{pl} > P_{aw}$$

which means that from this critical point all the way to the thoracic inlet, the transmural pressure is negative and the airway tends to collapse. Obviously, diseases that increase the frictional resistance of the airways (e.g. *asthma*) or decrease the elastic recoil of the lungs (e.g. *emphysema*) will move the critical point closer to the alveoli, causing airway collapse and further increasing airway resistance during expiration.

Depending on the airway wall compliance and caliber, airway collapse during expiration can lead to **flow limitation**, a situation in which expiratory gas flow remains constant even if the subject makes a maximal effort to raise alveolar pressure. Flow limitation can be caused by both the increase in frictional pressure losses (viscous flow limitation) and the formation of areas of critical velocity above which pressure disturbances cannot travel upstream (wave-speed flow limitation) as airway flow increases. Regardless of which of these two mechanisms is operative, the flow rate at which flow limitation occurs at a given lung volume depends only on the caliber and collapsibility of the airways and is highly reproducible. Determinations of maximal expiratory flow during respiratory function testing take advantage of this reproducibility to assess and follow the functional state of the intrathoracic airways over time or in response to therapeutic interventions.

Airway obstruction

Airway obstruction exaggerates the normal changes of the airway caliber during breathing (Fig. 11.19). When

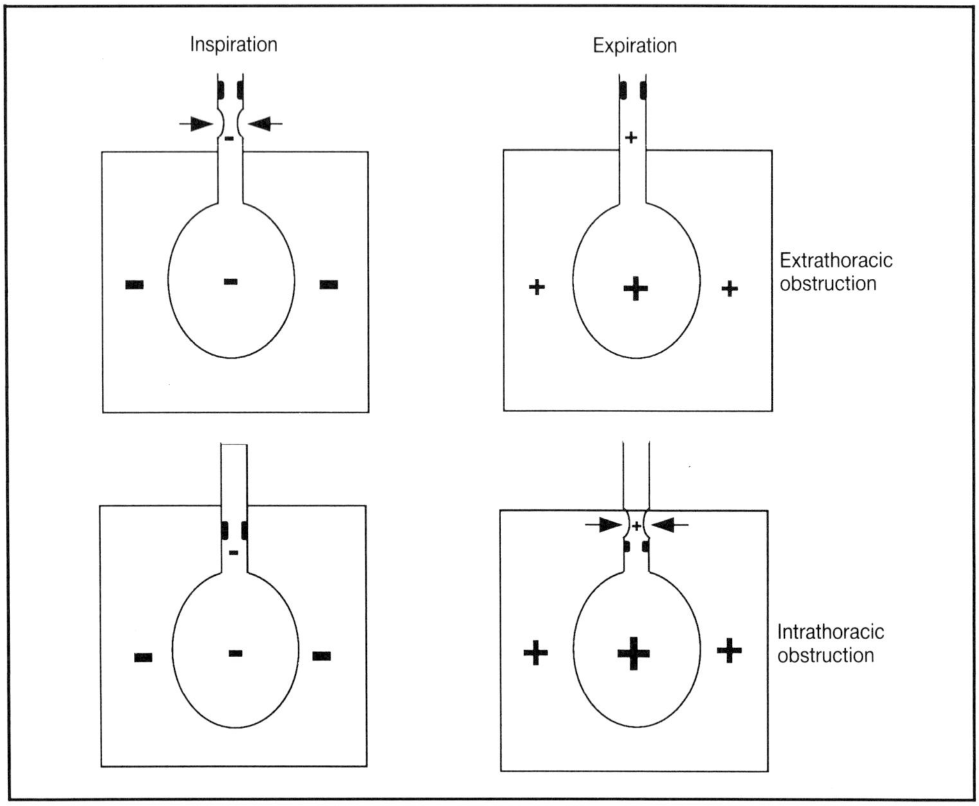

Fig. 11.19. Effects of airway obstruction on airway caliber during inspiration and expiration. Extrathoracic obstruction is exacerbated during inspiration because the highly negative pressure inside the airways is unopposed by the atmospheric pressure outside, causing the airway to collapse (arrows). Intrathoracic obstruction, in contrast, worsens during expiration because, as gas starts to flow towards the mouth, the pressure outside the airways (which is similar to pleural pressure) rapidly exceeds the pressure inside, causing the airways downstream from the obstruction point to collapse (arrows). (From Pérez Fontán JJ, Lister G. In Touloukian RJ, ed. *Pediatric trauma*. 2nd Edition. Saint Louis: Mosby-Year Book Inc., 1990: 46, with permission.)

the obstruction is extrathoracic (e.g. *croup*), the pressure inside the airway segment downstream from the narrow point must become more negative during inspiration in order to overcome the increased frictional resistance of the narrowing. The segment therefore tends to collapse, producing both an inspiratory exacerbation of the obstruction and a characteristic turbulent noise (inspiratory stridor). The obstruction is somewhat relieved during expiration, as the pressure inside the airways must become more positive, again to overcome the narrowing's increased resistance. When the obstruction is intrathoracic (e.g. *asthma* or *tracheobronchomalacia*), very negative pleural pressures tend to dilate the airways during inspiration. During expiration, however, increased frictional pressure losses create a marked pressure gradient from the alveoli toward the airway opening. As a result, the pressure inside the airways is rapidly exceeded by pleural pressure as the lungs deflate, causing an expiratory exacerbation of the obstruction and a distinctive mid- to end-expiratory wheeze on auscultation.

Restrictive and obstructive respiratory disease

The total amount of work that the respiratory muscles must do during breathing is the sum of the work done to overcome the non-dissipative and dissipative pressures. Depending on which of these two work components predominates, the mechanical dysfunctions of the respiratory system can be classified as restrictive or obstructive.

Restrictive disease is caused by processes that increase the elastic recoil of the lungs (e.g. *pulmonary edema, respiratory distress syndrome of the newborn*) or the chest wall (e.g. *abdominal distension, scoliosis*). The increased recoil has two major consequences. First, it increases the amount of work that the respiratory muscles must do during inspiration (expiration continues to be passive). In addition, by lowering the relaxation volume of the respiratory system, the increased recoil also decreases the functional residual capacity of the lungs, promoting alveolar collapse and increased venous admixture. In an attempt to counteract the effects of restrictive disease on lung volume, infants and children often close their glottis toward the end of expiration, generating a grunt, which is a helpful diagnostic sign. Positive end-expiratory pressure and continuous airway pressure are therapeutic modalities both directed at preserving alveolar stability.

The small caliber and high compliance of the developing airways renders them particularly vulnerable to obstruction. During normal breathing, small airways represent no particular disadvantage for the child because gas flows are low and dissipative pressure losses also remain small. When obstruction occurs, however, frictional pressure losses increase exponentially with the reduction in airway diameter, an increase that is compounded by the tendency of flow to develop into turbulent patterns in low-caliber tubes. Consequently, the same degree of obstruction has much more dire consequences in the small infant and child than in the adult.

Determinants of breathing efficiency

In a thermodynamic system, efficiency can be defined as the proportion of free energy that is transformed into external work. In the case of the respiratory system (equation 14):

$$\varepsilon = \frac{\text{Work/Time}}{\text{Respiratory Muscle Energy Consumption}}$$

The numerator of this expression represents the amount of volume–pressure work done by the respiratory muscles to inflate the lungs per unit of time (in physical terms, the power of the respiratory system), which depends on the mechanical behavior of the lungs and chest wall, the range of the tidal volume, and the breathing frequency. The denominator includes not only the energy consumed by the muscles to do volume–pressure work, but also the energy applied to perform isometric and postural tasks (which involve no change in volume, and therefore are not proper work) and that wasted in distorting the rib cage (which is proper work, but does not contribute to lung inflation).

Considered in these terms, the respiratory system is an extremely inefficient machine. Efficiency values as low as 8–25 percent occur in adult humans at rest; even lower ones in healthy premature infants (4 percent) and in patients with respiratory disease (1–3 percent). Because of these low starting values, very small changes in efficiency have a large effect on the energy required for breathing. A clear understanding of the factors that influence respiratory system efficiency is important for both the diagnosis and the treatment of most breathing disturbances. Among these factors are breathing pattern, diaphragmatic configuration, chest wall distortion, and the contractile state of the respiratory muscles.

Breathing pattern

The amount of work that the respiratory muscles must do to generate a given alveolar ventilation (and thus maintain a certain $Pa\text{CO}_2$) depends on the breathing pattern (Fig. 11.20). Each individual has a well defined optimal breathing frequency, above and below which the work of breathing increases hyperbolically. This theoretical frequency is linked to the volume–pressure relationships of the respiratory system; it increases when the elastic recoil of the lungs or the chest wall increases (e.g. with *pulmonary edema*) and decreases when the dissipative pressures of the respiratory system increase (e.g. with *airway obstruction*). In practice, most subjects, including those with respiratory mechanical disturbances, adopt breathing frequencies that approach their predicted optimal frequency. As a result, one can usually categorize respiratory disease as primarily restrictive or obstructive depending on whether the patient breathes rapidly or slowly. However, the breathing pattern is regulated through neural pathways that respond more to mechanical and irritant stimuli from the respiratory system or to cortical influences than to energetic convenience. Therefore, it is not uncommon for children with respiratory disease to breathe transiently at frequencies that depart substantially from the optimal frequency. In this manner, airway irritation, stretch receptor stimulation, crying, and agitation can reduce the energetic efficiency of the respiratory system and precipitate respiratory failure.

Diaphragmatic length and configuration

Just like any other muscle, the diaphragm develops its maximal contractile force at a certain optimal length (see p. 602), which happens to be attained when the lungs approximate their functional residual capacity. At this volume, the diaphragm is configured as a dome-capped cylinder, an arrangement that has several advantages. First, a cylindrical shape allows a much greater volume displacement for a given fiber shortening than a simple dome shape. Second, as the sides of the cylinder shorten during inspiration, making the dome descend toward the abdomen in a piston-like motion, the area of contact between the internal surface of the rib cage and the lungs increases. This increase provides a way to accommodate

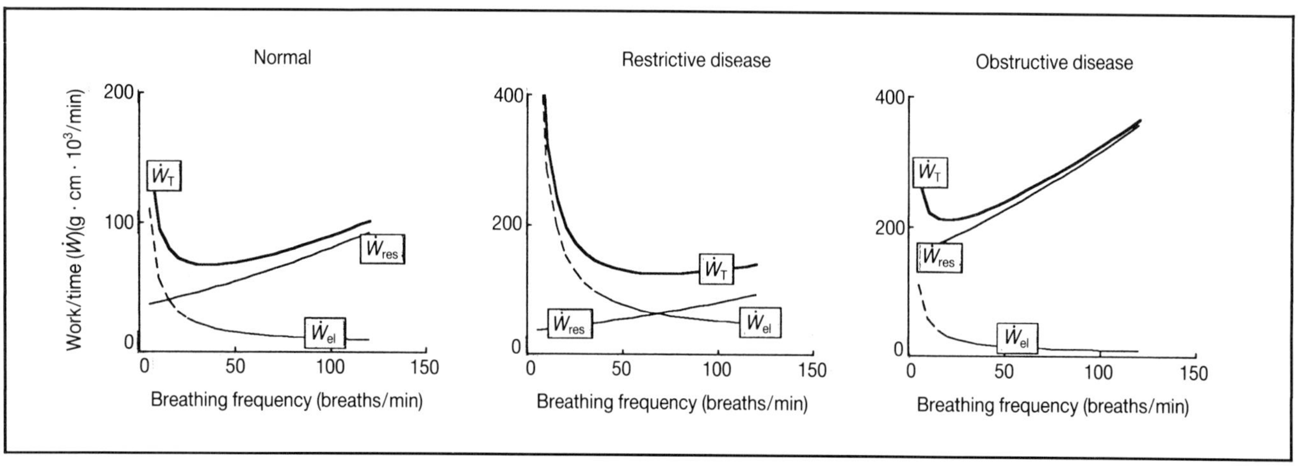

Fig. 11.20. Calculated effect of breathing frequency on the energy expended per unit of time (breathing power, $\dot{W}$) to overcome elastic forces ($\dot{W}_{el}$), resistive forces ($\dot{W}_{res}$), and their sum ($\dot{W}_T$) in a normal infant and in two infants with respiratory disease, one restrictive and the other obstructive. Calculations are based on assumptions that minute alveolar ventilation is constant, breathing pattern is sinusoidal, and volume and flow–pressure relationships are linear. Elastic and resistive power decrease and increase with frequency, respectively. As a result, total power follows a bimodal course, decreasing at low frequencies and increasing at high frequencies. The point at which total power reaches a minimum is the optimal frequency in terms of energy expenditure. The figure shows that the predominance of elastic and resistive power shifts this optimal frequency to higher frequencies in restrictive disease and to lower frequencies in obstructive disease. Note different scales used to accommodate the increase in breathing power caused by restrictive and obstructive disease.

without distortion the inevitable increase in lung surface that occurs as the lungs expand. Finally, for most of the tidal volume range, the sides of the diaphragmatic cylinder are apposed to the internal surface of the rib cage. By transmitting to the ribs and the sternum the increase in intra-abdominal pressure that occurs as the diaphragm descends into the abdomen, this area of apposition establishes a mechanical link between the abdomen and the rib cage, helping to stabilize the chest wall and facilitating inspiration.

The developing diaphragm may lack some of these advantages. Particularly in the newborn and small infant, the lower portion of the rib cage has proportionally wider diameters than in the adult. As a result, the muscle's insertions are spread out, and the sides of the diaphragmatic cylinder are short (Fig. 11.21). Under such conditions, fiber contraction can only increase the radius of the dome; therefore, the volume displaced (and the work done) by a given fiber shortening (or for a certain energy expenditure) is limited. In addition, the shortness of the area of apposition lessens the stabilizing and inspiratory effects of intra-abdominal pressure, further reducing the work/energy ratio and the efficiency of the respiratory system.

Chest-wall distortion

Until this point, we have assumed that every portion of the chest wall undergoes a similar displacement during breathing, regardless of its location. In reality, not only can different portions of the rib cage and abdomen change volume independently of each other, but they often do it in opposite directions.

Chest-wall distortion is primarily the consequence of regional variations in chest-wall compliance. In the case of the rib cage, areas without bony support (intercostal, suprasternal, and subcostal spaces) are particularly prone to move inward as pleural pressure decreases during inspiration. When pleural pressure becomes very negative to overcome an increased elastic recoil or an airway obstruction, this inward movement of the rib cage becomes more pronounced, causing visible **retractions**.

The chest walls of newborns and infants are very susceptible to distortion. As discussed above, the limited ossification of ribs and sternum increases markedly the passive compliance of the rib cage during early life. In addition, the developing intercostal muscles, the main function of which is to stabilize the chest by contracting simultaneously with the diaphragm, appear to have decreased tone, especially during REM sleep. Finally, the lack of a substantial area of apposition between the

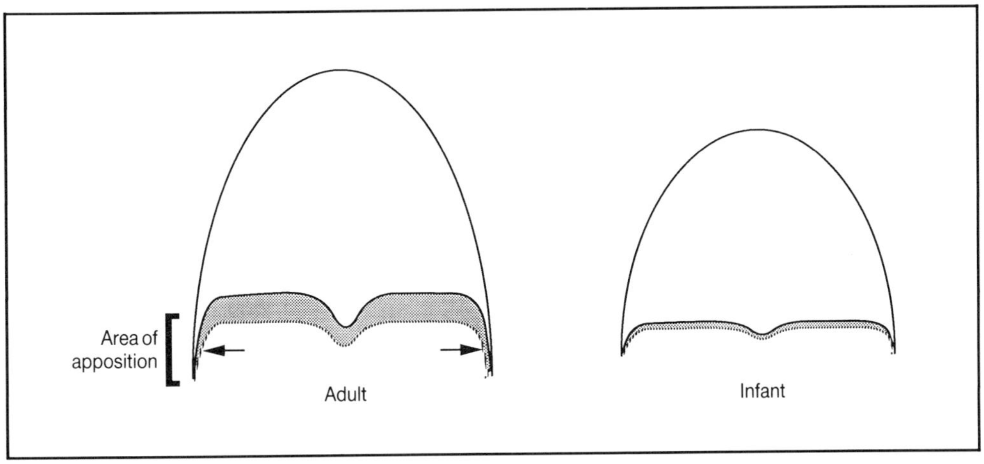

Fig. 11.21. Diagrams of the configuration of the diaphragm in the adult and the infant. In the adult, the diaphragm has the shape of a cylinder with a dome cap. The sides of the cylinder adhere to the internal surface of the rib cage, forming an area of apposition that is used by intra-abdominal pressure to push the ribs and the sternum during inspiration. In the infant, the diaphragmatic insertions are more spread out and both the sides of the cylinder and the area of apposition are smaller. As a result, the volume displaced by the muscle's contraction (stippling) is smaller, and the abdomen and rib cage are linked in a less efficient manner.

diaphragm and the rib cage eliminates the additional stabilizing effect of intra-abdominal pressure on the lower ribs and subcostal area at these ages.

Chest-wall distortion can be quantified as a change in volume caused by a change in pressure. Therefore, it represents a form of work and has a measurable energy cost. Unfortunately, the work done to produce the distortion is not applied to lung inflation, and therefore distortion can be considered a source of inefficiency. This point of view is well illustrated by a simple analysis of the work done by the diaphragm in the presence of rib cage retractions (Fig. 11.22). Regardless of whether such retractions are present or not, the tidal volume of the lungs (ΔV_L) has to be equivalent to the sum of the volume changes undergone by the rib cage (ΔV_{rc}) and abdomen (ΔV_{ab}) (equation 15):

$$\Delta V_L = \Delta V_{rc} + \Delta V_{ab}$$

Consequently, decreases in ΔV_{rc} caused by rib cage retractions during inspiration must be accompanied by a commensurate increase in ΔV_{ab}, if ΔV_L is to remain constant. In extreme cases, ΔV_{ab} can in fact be greater than ΔV_L if ΔV_{rc} becomes negative. Because ΔV_{ab} approximates the volume displaced by the diaphragm, the work performed by the muscle is increased markedly by rib cage distortion without a parallel change in the work done on the lungs. The resultant energy waste may contribute to the poor weight gain and easy diaphragmatic fatigability of small infants suffering from respiratory distress.

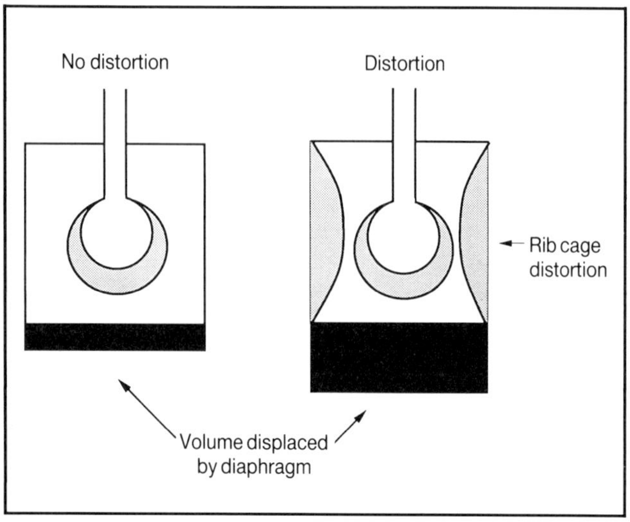

Fig. 11.22. Schematic representation of the effects of rib cage retractions on the volume displaced by the diaphragm during inspiration. During a non-distorted inflation, both rib cage and abdomen expand. During a distorted inflation, however, the diaphragm must increase its volume displacement (and therefore do more work) to offset the inward movement of the rib cage and maintain the tidal volume of the lungs constant. (From Pérez Fontán JJ. Mechanical dysfunction of the respiratory system. In Fuhrman BP, Zimmerman JJ, eds. *Pediatric critical care*. Saint Louis: Mosby-Year Book Inc., 1992: 399, with permission.)

Contractile state of the respiratory muscles (see p. 603)

Muscle fatigue (the decrease in contractile force that follows excessive muscle activity) appears to increase the energy needed by respiratory muscles to perform a certain amount of work on the lungs, thereby reducing their efficiency. Metabolic disturbances and simple malnutrition may have similar effects.

Summary

As the previous discussion establishes, the developing respiratory system has some mechanical disadvantages. The reader, however, should not be left with the impression that infants and children are constantly on the brink of respiratory failure. On the contrary, they have a remarkable capability to compensate for most mechanical disturbances. This capability is based on the maintenance of a large functional reserve. Recognizing when this reserve becomes threatened is perhaps the most important point in the rational management of children with respiratory disease.

Selected reading

Mead J. Mechanical properties of the lungs. *Physiol Rev* 1961; **41**: 281.

Mortola JP. Dynamics of breathing in newborn mammals. *Physiol Rev* 1987; **67**: 187.

Roussos C, Campbell EJM. Respiratory muscle energetics. In Macklem PT, Mead J, eds. *Handbook of physiology: The respiratory system*. Vol. III, Part 2. Bethesda MD: American Physiological Society, 1986: 481.

12 ◆ *Blood*

Editors: Charles A J Wardrop and B M Holland

A. Leukopoiesis and the Lymphoid System

K R Schibler and R D Christensen

Hematopoiesis

Each of the cellular elements of blood has a finite life span, and consequently must be continually replaced. The collective process by which new blood cells are generated is termed hematopoiesis. In the 'steady state', hematopoiesis proceeds at a relatively fixed pace, constantly maintaining the circulating concentration of each cell type within remarkably narrow limits. Despite this usual stability, the hematopoietic system is highly responsive, with the capacity to markedly up-regulate production of any of the various cell types on demand.

The processes regulating hematopoiesis are necessarily complex. This intricacy is needed not only to maintain equilibrium between cellular production and utilization and to assure the necessary responsiveness to rapidly changing demands for cells, but also to accommodate the unique life spans of the various cellular elements. For instance, in adults erythrocytes circulate for about 120 days, platelets for about 10 days, and neutrophils only for hours (steady-state $t_{1/2}$ = 6.5 hours). Empirically, independent mechanisms would be needed to regulate the production of each variety of blood cell. Indeed, a large and constantly increasing list of hematopoietic growth factors can now be assembled, each with a unique set of actions on clonal development of the various mature blood cell types from hematopoietic progenitors.

Hematopoietic progenitor cells

A schematized hierarchy of the hematopoietic progenitors is shown in Fig. 12.1. Although the progenitors can be categorized as existing at the various developmental stages shown, progress from pluripotent progenitors to mature hemic cells undoubtedly occurs as a continuous process, proceeding through numerous intermediate stages.

Bradley and Metcalf first established the existence of pluripotent, self-renewing, hematopoietic stem cells by showing that transfusing irradiated mice with marrow cells obtained from normal mice would repopulate their entire hematopoietic system. Subsequently, the capacity to culture hematopoietic progenitors in semisolid media, beginning with the work of Pluznick and Sachs, permitted the categorization, functional analysis, and definition of growth factor requirements of the various hematopoietic progenitors.

Progenitor cells that develop into clones containing neutrophils, macrophages, erythrocytes, and megakaryocytes (and sometimes eosinophils and mast cells) are termed CFU-GEMM (colony-forming unit–granulocyte, erythrocyte, macrophage, megakaryocyte). These progenitor cells are categorized as 'primitive' on the basis of their pluripotentiality. They appear to have a limited capacity for self-renewal, however, and therefore are not true 'stem cells'. In contrast to pluripotent progenitors, committed progenitors are those that give rise to colonies containing cells of only one (or sometimes two) types. Examples include BFU-E (burst-forming unit–erythrocyte), CFU-E, CFU-GM, CFU-Eo, CFU-Baso, and CFU-Meg.

The more primitive variety of erythroid progenitors, BFU-E, appears to be derived from pluripotent progenitors. BFU-E subsequently differentiate into clones of mature erythroid progenitors, CFU-E (colony-forming unit–erythrocyte). Subsequently, under the influence of erythropoietin, CFU-E generate clones of normoblasts. Although BFU-E and CFU-E appear to be two stages in a continuum, they differ in important ways. For instance, BFU-E require factors with 'burst promoting' activity (detailed in the next section) in order to develop into CFU-E, while CFU-E do not require such factors to differentiate into clones of normoblasts. BFU-E are found in the blood as well as in the bone marrow, but CFU-E are scarce in blood. (Fetal blood is an exception, particularly blood of extremely preterm infants, which is rich in CFU-E.) Other differences between BFU-E and CFU-E include the large number of normoblasts per mature BFU-E colony (often as many as 10 000 normoblasts/colony) versus the small number per CFU-E colony (64 to 200–300). Another difference is the length of time required in culture to produce a mature clone of normoblasts from BFU-E (14 days) versus CFU-E (7 days). Of note, both

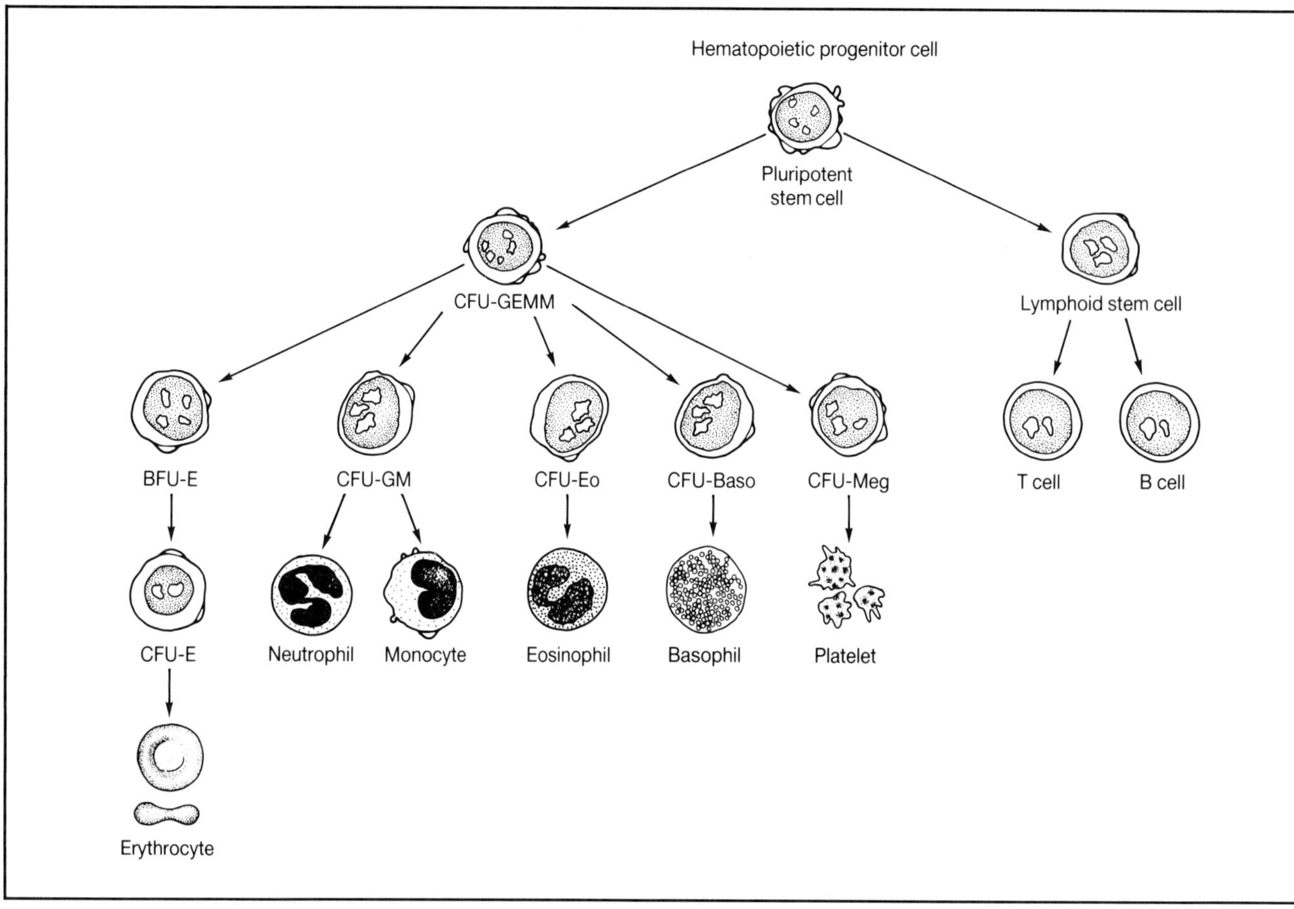

Fig. 12.1. Pluripotent hematopoietic progenitors (see text) differentiate into either myeloid multipotent progenitors (CFU-GEMM) or lymphoid multipotent progenitors that further clonally differentiate into mature hematopoietic cells. Stages of intermediate progenitors are recognized by the colonies formed from them *in vitro*, as well as their unique sensitivities to recombinant hematopoietic growth factors.

BFU-E and CFU-E of fetal origin mature into clones of normoblasts in culture more rapidly than do those of adult origin.

Granulocyte-macrophage progenitors (CFU-GM) also appear to be differentiated from pluripotent progenitors, having been restricted in their capacity to produce only granulocytes and macrophages. CFU-GM can differentiate further into cells capable of generating clones of macrophages only (CFU-M) or neutrophils only (CFU-G).

Progenitors with features that are intermediate between those shown in Fig. 12.1 are identified frequently. For instance, colonies are seen that contain neutrophils, macrophages, and normoblasts, but no megakaryocytes. Others contain neutrophils and normoblasts. Any colony that contains a mixture of normoblasts with another variety of cells is referred to as a MIX colony, and thus, derived from a progenitor termed CFU-MIX. Such a progenitor might be thought of as intermediate between a CFU-GEMM and a committed progenitor.

The proliferative state of hematopoietic progenitors can be categorized as either quiescent (in the G_0 phase of the cell cycle) or as actively cycling. Further categorization of cycling cells can be accomplished by assessing, during a 'flash label' (a 20-minute exposure to tritiated thymidine of high specific activity), the proportion of progenitors that are in 'S' phase. The proliferative state, as well as clonogenic maturation, of hematopoietic progenitors appears to be regulated by hematopoietic growth factors.

Pluripotent progenitors (CFU-GEMM and CFU-MIX) obtained from the bone marrow of healthy adults are generally relatively quiescent. In contrast, at least 10–30 percent of the committed progenitors (such as CFU-E and CFU-GM) are generally in 'S' phase. On this basis it has been proposed that 'steady-state' demands are met by the committed progenitors. During a period of increased demand for cells, a greater percentage of committed progenitors will usually be found to be in 'S' phase, and pluripotent progenitors might also be found to be cycling. For instance, during bacterial infection, cycling of CFU-MIX as well as CFU-GM increases, and following acute blood loss, cycling of BFU-E as well as CFU-E increases.

Unlike the situation in adult marrow, pluripotent progenitors in fetal blood and marrow (and in animals, progenitors in the liver and spleen as well) are actively cycling. For instance, generally less than 5 percent of CFU-MIX cultured from adult bone marrow are in 'S' phase, versus 20–30 percent from fetal blood or marrow. Similarly, as many as 40–60 percent of CFU-GM from fetal blood or marrow are generally in 'S' phase, versus 10–30 percent from adult marrow. This high rate of progenitor cell cycling is consistent with the rapid myeloid (and somatic) growth of the fetus. Rapid cycling of CFU-GM in the noninfected fetus has been interpreted as a potential limitation in capacity to further up-regulate neutrophil production during an infectious challenge. Indeed, in infected newborn rats the percentage of CFU-GM in 'S phase' does not appear to increase substantially from the already high baseline rate. Whether human neonates have a similar limitation is not known. An argument against a limitation as severe as that observed in neonatal rats is that the baseline CFU-GM cycling rate in noninfected human neonates, although high, is not maximal.

Hematopoietic growth factors

Recent advances in molecular biology have permitted the production, purification, and characterization of factors that support hematopoiesis *in vitro*. Experiments using such factors have permitted a more sophisticated scrutiny of hematopoietic regulation. Moreover, production of relatively large amounts of these factors has permitted clinical trials in which their *in vivo* actions have been assessed.

Table 12.1 lists the factors known to influence hematopoietic growth and differentiation, their molecular mass, chromosomal location, and the principal varieties of cells that they influence.

Table 12.1. Hematopoietic growth factors

Factor	Molecular mass (kDa)	Chromosomal location	Target cell
Interleukin-1 (IL)	17	(beta) 2q13–21	Hepatocyte, endothelial cell
		(alpha) 2q13	Osteoclast, neutrophil, macrophage, TH2 lymphocyte
Interleukin-2	15.5	4q26–27	T lymphocyte, cytotoxic lymph
Interleukin-3	15–30	5q23–31	CFU-GEMM, CFU-MIX, CFU-MEG, CFU-GM, BFU-E, cytotoxic lymph, macrophage
Interleukin-4	16–20	5q31	T lymphocyte, B lymphocyte
Interleukin-5	46 (Dimer)	5q31	CFU-Eo, B lymphocyte
Interleukin-6	19–21	7p15	CFU-GEMM, CFU-MIX, B lymphocyte, T lymphocyte, fetal CFU-GM, fetal BFU-E, macrophage, hepatocyte, neural cell
Interleukin-7	25	8q12–13	B lymphocyte
Interleukin-8	8–10	4	Neutrophil, endothelial cell, T lymphocyte
Interleukin-9	16	5q31–32	BFU-E, CFU-GEMM, CFU-MIX, fetal CFU-GM
Interleukin-10	35–40	—	B and T lymphocyte, mast cell
Interleukin-11	20	19q13.3–13.4	CFU-GEMM, CFU-MIX, fetal BFU-E
Interleukin-12	70–75 (Dimer)	—	T lymphocyte
GM-CSF	18–30	5q23–31	CFU-GM, CFU-MIX, BFU-E, CFU-GEMM, macrophage, neutrophil
G-CSF	20	17q11.2–21	CFU-G, neutrophil, CFU-GM, CFU-MIX,CFU-GEMM, BFU-E?
M-CSF	70–90 (Dimer)	5q33.1	CFU-M, CFU-GM, macrophage, uterine epithelium? placenta?
Stem cell factor	28–35	12q4.3–12	All hematopoietic progenitors
Erythropoietin	34–39	7q11–22	CFU-E, mature BFU-E, fetal BFU-E

Cell-surface receptors for hematopoietic growth factors

All of the hematopoietic growth factors appear to interact with target cells by way of specific cell-surface receptors. Although not all have been identified, the receptors appear, in general, to be members of the superfamily of receptors that couple to guanine nucleotide binding proteins (G-proteins). Little information is available to date concerning the signal transduction mechanisms resulting from interaction of hematopoietic growth factors with their receptors. Certain inherited and acquired disorders of hematopoiesis likely will be identified eventually as due to defects in hematopoietic growth factor receptors or the subsequent signal transduction mechanisms.

Clinical aspects

Human and animal studies indicate that, compared with adults, neonates have an increased susceptibility to acquiring certain infections and, when infected, have an increased likelihood of developing a severe resultant illness. This susceptibility is considerably more marked in neonates delivered prematurely. Multiple factors appear to contribute to this reduced host defense status of neonates; including hyporesponsiveness of B cells, T cells, and granulocytes, and reduced quantities of granulocytes and their progenitors per kg of body weight. Specific defects include delayed maturation of B cells into antibody-producing cells, deficient stimulation of T-cell maturation, and delayed induction of hematopoietic progenitor cell cycling.

Actions of several hematopoietic growth factors, including G-CSF, GM-CSF, IL-6, and IL-8, closely parallel these areas of diminished host defense. For example, the actions of G-CSF include stimulation of myeloid progenitor cycling, clonal development of neutrophils, and enhancement of neutrophil functions such as phagocytosis, superoxide production, and bactericidal activity. Similarly, IL-6 acts to induce antigen-specific antibody production, T-cell maturation, and hematopoietic progenitor cell cycling. Thus, one possible mechanism accounting for a number of the host defense defects in neonates is defective production or action of certain of the hematopoietic growth factors.

Generation of hematopoietic growth factors by the fetus and neonate

Studies of explanted human fetal cells support the hypothesis that preterm neonates produce certain hematopoietic growth factors poorly. Normal term newborns exhibit diminished production of interferon-γ by leukocytes, decreased GM-CSF production by mononuclear cells, diminished IL-6 production, and decreased IL-6 gene transcription, by explanted monocytes. Preterm neonates exhibit much more severe decreases in IL-6 production by monocytes. To date, studies of hematopoietic growth factor production *in vivo*, during bacterial infection, are incomplete, but such studies will be needed to determine the clinical significance of the *in vitro* observations.

In order to interpret the significance of the reduced production of certain hematopoietic growth factors by preterm neonates, information must be obtained regarding the actions of such factors on fetal and neonatal target cells. For instance, reduced production of G-CSF by fetal marrow stroma during bacterial infection might be completely counterbalanced by a heightened responsiveness of fetal CFU-G to the actions of G-CSF. If diminished production of certain hematopoietic growth factors by fetal cells is a clinically relevant limitation, the mechanism that results in this limitation will also be an important topic for investigation. Such a mechanism might include either 'programming' of otherwise fully functional fetal cells by extrinsic factors to produce certain products efficiently and others poorly, or a 'developmental defect', such that fetal cells lack a specific capacity to respond to an inflammatory agonist. Potential examples of this include a reduced density of cell-surface receptors capable of interacting with a particular ligand critical to hematopoietic growth factor generation, reduced signal transduction specific for that ligand, a limitation relating to specific gene transcription for that growth factor, diminished message stability, and diminished stability of that protein. Understanding the biology responsible for the diminution in production of certain hematopoietic growth factors by fetal cells is a critical step toward the clinical testing of cytokine-based therapy for infected neonatal subjects.

Neutrophil production in the fetus and neonate

During bacterial sepsis, newborn mice, rats, dogs, and humans are much more susceptible than adults to developing neutropenia, exhaustion of the marrow neutrophil reserves, and death. The basis for this susceptibility appears to include: (1) lack of rapid up-regulation of neutrophil production during infection, (2) a small neutrophil storage pool/kg body weight, and (3) specific defects in neutrophil function, permitting greater bacterial growth and, subsequently, the requirement for more neutrophils than would be needed if the infection was sterilized rapidly.

Whether the development of neutropenia and marrow neutrophil reserve exhaustion could be prevented or treated by administration of hematopoietic growth factors is not known. In part, this depends on such factors as the extent to which neutrophil production can be further increased in infected neonates, the sensitivity of hematopoietic progenitors from infected neonates to recombinant hematopoietic growth factors, and the likelihood of adverse reactions to administration of cytokines. Indeed, studies aimed at assessing the benefits versus risks of administration of recombinant hematopoietic growth factors to infected infants should probably await a better definition of precisely which hematopoietic growth factors are produced poorly by infected preterm neonates. Also, the actions of those specific recombinant growth factors on target cells of neonates should probably be assessed *in vitro* before such trials begin.

Neutrophil function in the fetus and neonate

Among the many explanations for the unique susceptibility of neonates to overwhelming infection are biochemical, structural, and functional abnormalities of neutrophils. Developmental defects in signal transduction, cell-surface receptor up-regulation and mobility, cytoskeletal rigidity, microfilament contraction, O_2 metabolism, and intracellular antioxidant generation have all been described.

The lymphoid system

The goals of lymphopoiesis are to produce cells that possess the capacity to: (1) distinguish between foreign and self antigens, (2) facilitate elimination of antigens determined to be foreign, and (3) maintain a memory of previous foreign antigen exposures. To accomplish these tasks, lymphoid development proceeds along two pathways, culminating in the formation of B lymphocytes involved in antibody-mediated immunity, and T lymphocytes responsible predominantly for cell-mediated immunity.

T lymphocytes

Ontogeny

Differentiation of T-cell precursors into functional T lymphocytes involves interaction between non-lymphoid and lymphoid elements of the thymus. The thymus develops relatively early in humans. Morphologically, the primitive thymic rudiment formed from the ectoderm of the third branchial cleft and the endoderm of the third branchial pouch is evident at approximately 4 weeks of gestation. These structures move caudally, and at week 8 fuse in the midline. Distinct cortical and medullary regions are identified at 14 weeks, and by 16 weeks Hassall bodies are present and the thymus assumes the histological configuration seen postnatally.

Before week 7, T-cell precursors, identified by monoclonal antibodies to early T-cell markers CD7 and CD45, are present in the yolk sac, neck, upper thorax, and liver. Between 7 and 8.5 weeks of gestation they migrate to the thymic rudiment, an event that appears to be regulated by chemotactic factors elaborated from the thymic epithelium. These cells colonizing the thymus differentiate into T-cell colonies expressing markers of T-cell lineage (CD2, CD4, CD8, and WT31) if cultured *in vitro* with T-cell conditioned medium and interleukin-2 (IL-2). They retain capacity to differentiate into cells of myeloid lineage, however, if provided an appropriate environment.

Lymphoid cells from the thymus at 8.5 weeks react with antibodies to CD2 (sheep erythrocyte rosette receptor). Arrest of T-lymphocyte maturation at this stage is identified in some cases of *severe combined immunodeficiency disease*. At 8.5 weeks thymocytes fail to react with monoclonal antibodies directed against CD3, CD5, CD4, CD8, and A1G3-p80; however, at 10 weeks these antigens are present. Thus, between 8.5 and 10 weeks gestation thymocytes develop from stage I ($CD7^+$, $CD2^+$) to stage II ($CD4^+$, $CD8^+$, and $CD3^+$).

Generation of diversity

During maturation, T cells are programmed to recognize antigenic determinants in the context of the self-major histocompatibility (MHC) antigens. T lymphocytes of the CD4 population recognize antigens in conjunction with MHC class II molecules, while CD8 T cells recognize antigens in conjunction with MHC class I molecules. To acquire these capacities, prothymocytes migrate to the thymus and undergo rapid division and rearrangement in the T-cell receptor gene. There are two sets of the receptor gene, γδ and αβ, which encode different receptors. Each gene comprises multiple components that rearrange; these are designated as diversity (D) sequences, variable (V) sequences, joining (J) sequences, and constant (C) sequences of DNA. Successful rearrangement of genes encoding γδ stops rearrangement of αβ genes. Likewise, αβ rearrangement precludes further γδ rearrangement. The tremendous diversity of T-cell receptors is generated through rearrangement and joining of these gene elements. The most common T-cell receptor lineage is the αβ heterodimer pair. Following successful rearrangement of these genes, thymocytes stop proliferating.

Peripheral T-cell maturation and proliferation is influenced by exposure to antigens and soluble factors. Exogenous antigen encountered by antigen-presenting cells is processed and presented to T cells expressing the appropriate MHC determinants. The signal thereby delivered induces interleukin-2 (IL-2) secretion by T cells, which initiates a cascade of events leading to proliferation. A second signal initiating activation of T cells is interleukin-1.

Recognition of a foreign antigen by accessory cells such as macrophages initiates the following chain of events culminating in T-cell activation. The macrophage processes the antigen and re-expresses this modified antigen on its surface. Additionally, the macrophage secretes IL-1 in response to the antigenic stimulus. The T cells recognize the foreign antigen in the context of their appropriate MHC antigen.

Soluble factors influencing T-cell function include the interleukins and interferons. Interleukin-1, which is produced by monocytes and thymic epithelial cells, has varied effects on T cells, B cells, monocytes, neutrophils, fibroblasts, and a host of other cells. Its chief effect on T cells is to induce IL-2 production. IL-2, also called T-cell growth factor, induces proliferation and maturation of T cells, B cells, and natural killer (NK) cells. The interferons are a group of glycoproteins produced in response to viral infection and by other immune stimulatory events. Three classes of interferons have been characterized. Interferon-α and interferon-β are produced by leukocytes and by fibroblasts in response to viral infection. Interferon-γ is synthesized by T cells in response to antigenic stimulation. Interferons induce a number of cell membrane effects including augmentation of MHC I and II expression, and up-regulation of IgG receptors. Interferons stimulate increased macrophage cytotoxicity, increase cytotoxic activity of NK cells, and increase the reactivity of cytotoxic T cells. Paradoxical effects of interferon have been reported with respect to its effect on lymphocyte proliferation and immunoglobulin production.

Alterations in T-cell function

Congenital T-cell defects are relatively rare, e.g. *DiGeorge syndrome (congenital thymic aplasia)*. More commonly, T-cell defects are combined with defects in humoral immunity. This category includes *severe combined immunodeficiency (SCID)*, *Wiskott–Aldrich syndrome*, *ataxia-telangiectasia*, and *adenosine deaminase deficiency*. These diseases generally become clinically apparent during infancy due to repeated infections with a wide variety of microorganisms.

Acquired abnormalities in T-cell function are relatively common, occurring in conjunction with *viral infections*, *malignancy*, *immunosuppressive drug administration*, *renal failure*, *autoimmune diseases*, *human immunodeficiency virus (HIV) infection*, and *malnutrition*. Transient T-cell dysfunction often accompanies infections such as *measles*, *rubella*, and *mycoplasma*. Quantitative and functional abnormalities in the suppressor T-cell population are observed in a variety of autoimmune disorders.

Infection with HIV causes profound derangements in T-cell-associated immunity. Marked reduction in CD4 (helper/inducer) T-cell numbers and in T-cell function render these patients susceptible to a variety of microorganisms and to malignancy.

T-cell function in the fetus and neonate

Mitogen-responsive T cells are identifiable in the peripheral blood and spleen by week 12 of gestation and increase in number until approximately 20 weeks, at which time they approach numbers seen at term. While the proportion of T cells in the blood at term has been reported to be low in some studies and normal in others, their absolute numbers generally exceed adult levels due to a relative lymphocytosis. Response to the mitogens phytohemmagglutinin and concanavalin A is diminished in very-low-birth-weight infants, but is normal or increased in term infants.

While T-cell numbers and mitogen sensitivity are relatively normal in term neonates, a number of functions are deficient, including cytotoxic effector functions of T cells and NK cells, lymphokine production, and regulation of B-cell function. T-cell-mediated cytotoxicity requires sensitization followed by cell lysis. Cell-mediated lympholysis has been detected as early as 18 weeks of gestation. However, in term infants it is only 50 percent of adult levels. Similarly, NK cell function has been demonstrated early in gestation (9 weeks); however, NK activity and cell numbers are decreased at birth.

Production of some lymphokines by fetal and neonatal T cells appears to be normal, while others are diminished. Normal production of IL-2 and IL-2 receptor have been reported, but production of other lymphokines is defective. Among these are interferon-γ, lymphocyte-derived chemotactic factor, and macrophage-activating factor.

Immunoregulatory functions of neonatal T cells have been studied, particularly with regard to interaction with B cells. The impaired capacity of human newborns to produce specific immunoglobulins despite normal numbers of B cells in peripheral lymphoid organs and in the blood is at least in part due to interaction between T cells and B cells. Experiments in which neonatal T cells were cultured with adult B cells demonstrated suppression of B-cell proliferation and immunoglobulin secretion. Conversely, when adult T cells were co-incubated with neonatal B cells, they were transformed into plasma cells capable of producing immunoglobulins including IgA and IgG, although at lesser quantities than similar studies involving adult B cells. Although a number of investigators have identified increased suppressor activity in neonatal cord blood, controversy remains as to the cellular or humoral nature of this suppression.

B lymphocytes

Ontogeny

Pluripotent stem cells in the fetal liver and bone marrow give rise to pre-B cells identified by intracytoplasmic IgM. These B-cell precursors appear first in the fetal liver at 8 weeks of gestation. By 10 weeks of gestation IgM surface receptors are detectable. Between 10 and 12 weeks, clones of immature B cells segregate, which develop isotype specificity (i.e. IgE, IgG, IgM, etc.). By 15–18 weeks the absolute number and proportion of B cells expressing each of the different immunoglobulin isotypes reaches adult numbers; however, immunoglobulin secretion remains limited.

Generation of diversity

The molecular basis for generation of antibody diversity results from extensive rearrangement of genetic information encoding heavy-chain variable (V_H), diversity (D_H), and joining (J_H) regions and light-chain variable (V_L) and joining (J_L) regions. Heavy-chain variable and constant genes are located on chromosome 14 in humans. Genes encoding κ light chains are located on chromosome 2, and those encoding λ light chains are on chromosome 22. There are approximately 1000 heavy-chain variable regions, 20 diversity regions, and 6 joining segments. Heavy-chain diversity generated by DNA excision and splicing of these elements would account for one million antigenic determinants. Light-chain diversity occurring in a similar manner also accounts for about one million combinations. Thus, combinatorial joining of heavy- and light-chain products of these genetic rearrangements forms a repertoire of complete immunoglobulin molecules capable of recognizing approximately one billion antigenic specificities. Somatic mutations occurring during the rearrangement of these elements further expand this array of antibody determinants.

B-cell development

During the pre-B-cell stage, DNA rearrangements, joining of $V_HD_HJ_H$ elements, occur culminating in assembly of a complete heavy-chain variable gene, termed the mu gene. Expression of this gene produces mu chains evident in the cytoplasm of pre-B cells. The absence of light-chain production at this stage precludes formation of complete Ig molecules. The next stage of maturation, the early B cell, is marked by assembly and expression of light-chain genes. The mu and light chains are assembled into complete IgM molecules, which are expressed on the cell surface. The final stage of B-cell maturation is distinguished by secretion of immunoglobulin molecules. Interaction with T cells and exposure to antigens are integral in maturation of B cells into activated B cells or plasma cells. This transition requires RNA splicing to express secretory exons preferentially. Switching of heavy-chain isotypes, regulated by the T cell, also occurs at this stage of development.

Antibody response

Following initial exposure to an antigen there is a 10–14-day delay before appearance of specific antibody in the circulation. During this primary response to an antigen, the predominant immunoglobulin class is IgM. Upon subsequent exposure to the same antigen, an antibody response of far greater magnitude and consisting predominantly of IgG isotype occurs within 4 days. This secondary response is initiated by binding of the foreign antigen to long-lived memory B cells expressing specific antigen receptors on their surface.

The antibody response is a regulated process involving interaction between macrophages, T cells, and B cells. During the initial phase of this response the antigen is contacted by cells of the monocyte/macrophage system within the spleen and lymph nodes. The antigen is processed by these antigen-presenting cells and displayed on the cell surface in conjunction with MHC antigens to facilitate recognition by T cells. The requirement for a dual signal, antigen plus MHC determinants, is required for T-cell interaction, but not B-cell interaction with an antigen. The second phase (proliferative phase) of the antibody response involves both cellular interaction and response to lymphokines. Direct interaction between T cells and B cells enables the B cell: (1) to differentiate into an antibody-producing plasma cell, (2) to become a long-term memory B cell, or (3) to proliferate, forming clones of antigen-sensitive cells. In addition to direct cellular interactions, B cells are influenced by exposure to lymphokines elaborated by T cells. Activated T cells release interleukin-4 (IL-4), which induces proliferation of antigen-specific B cells and up-regulates the expression of IL-6 receptors on B cells. In addition, T cells secrete interleukin-6 (IL-6), which induces B cells to differentiate into antibody-producing plasma cells. The final stage of the antibody response involves production and secretion of specific antibodies.

Developmental aspects of B-cell function

Immunoglobulin synthesis by the fetus is limited, constituting primarily IgM. The fetus acquires circulating levels of maternal IgG through placental transport. This transplacental acquisition begins at approximately 12 weeks. Maternal IgG renders the infant relatively protected from many viral and bacterial diseases during the first 4–6 months of postnatal life. Infants born prematurely, however, particularly those delivered before 30 weeks of gestation, generally do not receive sufficient quantities of maternal IgG to provide the same level of protection.

Following birth, serum concentrations of IgG fall gradually, due to catabolism of maternal IgG, to 300–500 mg/dl by 4 months of age. This *physiological hypogammaglobulinemia* is more protracted in infants born prematurely. Significant IgG production generally begins at 4 months of age and increases gradually over the first 10 years of life. By 1 year of age the infant's serum IgG concentrations are approximately 60 percent of adult levels.

The capacity for IgM production is intact *in utero*. In fact, during congenital infection the fetus produces IgM usually exceeding 20 mg/dl. After birth, production of IgM precedes that of IgG. The majority of antibodies to enteric Gram-negative bacteria are of IgM isotype, and production of IgM accelerates during the first week of life as colonization of the gastrointestinal tract occurs. IgM synthesis reaches 80 percent of adult levels by 1 year of age. IgA, IgD, and IgE are not transplacentally acquired. Synthesis of these immunoglobulins increases slowly, approaching adult levels by about 15 years of age.

Selected reading

Cairo MS. Neonatal neutrophil host defense. *Am J Dis Child* 1989; **143**: 40.
Christensen RD. Hematopoiesis in the fetus and neonate. *Pediatr Res* 1989; **26**: 531.

Hill HR. Biochemical, structural, and functional abnormalities of polymorphonuclear leukocytes in the neonate. *Pediatr Res* 1987; **22**: 375.

Lobach DF, Haynes BF. Ontogeny of the human thymus during fetal development. *J Clin Immunol* 1987; **7**: 81.

Nathan DG. Regulation of hematopoiesis. *Pediatr Res* 1990; **27**: 423.

Schwartz RH. Acquisition of immunologic self-tolerance. *Cell* 1989; **57**: 1073.

Sieff CA. Hematopoietic growth factors. *J Clin Invest* 1987; **79**: 1549.

B. Red Cell Physiology

C A J Wardrop, B M Holland and J G Jones

Oxygen transport

O_2 is transported as a complex with hemoglobin (Hb), which is contained within a flexible red blood cell—the erythrocyte. Adequate production of healthy erythrocytes is essential for proper tissue oxygenation as these cells determine the concentration of hemoglobin, control hemoglobin–O_2 affinity, and contribute to both blood volume and viscosity.

Erythropoiesis

Erythrocytes develop from pluripotent stem cells, which are capable of both replication and differentiation to a wide spectrum of blood cells including red cells, granulocytes, monocytes, and megakaryocytes/platelets (see Fig. 12.1). The earliest recognizable red blood cell is the normoblast, which matures, without further replication, to a reticulocyte, and finally becomes an erythrocyte. The normoblast is preceded by other cell lines that, although committed to becoming red cells, are still capable of replication. These are represented *ex vivo* by the burst-forming unit–erythrocyte (BFU-E) and colony-forming unit–erythrocyte (CFU-E). *In utero*, erythropoiesis begins in the yolk sac, but this function migrates to the liver at about 6 weeks and ultimately to the bone marrow at about 20 weeks of gestation. Blood serves as the intermediary medium for this transfer, and blood from premature neonates still contains measurable numbers of hemopoietic progenitor cells (Table 12.2).

Erythropoietin

The maturation of these red cell precursors, in neonates and adults, is controlled by the hormone erythropoietin (EPO), which binds to specific receptor sites in the membrane. If the receptor sites are not complexed with EPO, then the progenitor cells do not survive. In general the responsiveness to EPO is inversely related to the ability of the progenitor cells to replicate. Hence BFU-E are very proliferative cells but are not very responsive to EPO, while in contrast, CFU-E are less able to replicate but are entirely dependent on EPO for further maturation to normoblasts. EPO, a glycoprotein containing about 30 percent carbohydrate, is produced in fetal liver but largely in adult kidney, although adults retain some potential for hepatic synthesis. EPO synthesis is regulated by blood PO_2, and the sensor, in adults, is believed to be a heme protein synthesized largely, but not exclusively, in the kidney. Like hemoglobin, this protein is thought to be an allosteric molecule that exists in two separate conformations, corresponding to oxygenated and deoxygenated forms, the latter postulated to stimulate EPO synthesis. EPO concentrations peak about 24 hours following acute blood loss. The kinetics of EPO synthesis are insensitive to the degree of hypoxia, suggesting that the sensor 'flips' from low to high saturation with O_2 over a narrow range

Table 12.2. Numbers of stem cells in cord blood from preterm and term infants

	CFU-GM		CFU-E	
Gestational age (weeks)	per 10^5 LDNAs	per ml	per 10^5 LDNAs	per ml
25–31	175	10 000	4 200	21 000
32–36	75	4 000	100	6 500
38–41	35	3 000	125	11 000

LDNAs, low-density non-adherent cells.
Adapted from Clapp DW, Baley JE, Gerson SL. Gestational age-dependent changes in circulating hematopoietic stem cells in newborn infants. *J Lab Clin Med* 1989; **113**: 422, with permission.

of concentration of the gas. This behavior is entirely consistent with the view that the sensor is an allosteric protein with a sigmoidal binding curve for O_2. The deoxygenated form of the sensor is believed to enhance EPO synthesis by stimulating the EPO gene, and it may also stabilize the resulting messenger RNA. The consequence of this sensitive control is an inverse relationship between hematocrit and the **mean** plasma concentration of EPO (Table 12.3), but there can be a 10-fold difference in measured EPO at any hematocrit. This individual variability stems from the complex relationships between plasma $P\text{O}_2$ and a variety of interrelated physiological processes. Hence, in addition to red cell numbers, the tissue $P\text{O}_2$ depends on other factors such as cardiopulmonary function, blood volume, hemoglobin concentration, hemoglobin–O_2 affinity, and O_2 consumption. In response to anemic hypoxia, cardiac output is increased, and there are compensatory changes in hemoglobin–O_2 affinity and inter-organ distribution of blood (see below). Each of these physiological functions has a separate O_2 sensor with its own unique response time. Although these different control mechanisms are interrelated, it is not surprising that there is considerable individual variation in the relationship between EPO concentration and hematocrit, which is just one hematological variable measured at a single moment in time.

Table 12.3. Erythropoietin concentrations and hematocrit

Hematocrit	EPO concentration (mU/ml)
45	10–20
30–45	20–200
20–30	200–2 000
Transfusion-dependent	2 000–20 000

Adapted from Erslev AJ. *Semin Hematol* 1991; **28**: 2, with permission.

The EPO gene has been isolated, copied, cloned, and expressed in a biologically active form in Chinese hamster ovarian cells. This recombinant human EPO has been used therapeutically, at doses of 50–150 U/kg three times per week, with spectacular success as replacement therapy in patients with *anemia associated with renal failure*. Larger doses of 600 U/kg three times per week have been used to facilitate therapeutic venesection in *iron overload* and to provide blood for later *autologous transfusion*. Such pharmacological doses can also promote red cell production in patients with mild to severe *anemia,* but the response is variable and the proper dosage requires further investigation.

EPO after term and preterm birth

The increase in plasma $P\text{O}_2$ after birth switches off EPO production and concentrations decline, with a half-life of about 4 hours. In term infants, red blood cell numbers then decline, more gradually, from a mean count of 5.4×10^{12}/liter of blood at birth to a nadir of 3.4×10^{12}/liter at 7 weeks, rising again to 3.7×10^{12}/liter at 12 weeks; this is then maintained by renewed and balanced EPO synthesis. The timing of these maturational processes is not affected by preterm delivery. Anemia, associated with low EPO, is seen in children with *renal failure* and in *preterm infants*. The former reflects failure of synthesis due to renal damage and can be treated with recombinant EPO. The *anemia of the preterm infant* represents 'immaturity' of the hormonal response, but evidence is growing that this may also respond to higher pharmacological doses of EPO. In this context, it is pertinent to note that an infant growing from 1 kg to 3 kg requires, at least, a further 90 ml of red blood cells, and this degree of synthesis demands adequate nutritional and hematinic support.

Hemoglobin and O_2 transport

Genetics of hemoglobin synthesis

The decline in hemoglobin concentration after birth is accompanied by a change in the type of circulating hemoglobin. During human development, six genetic variants of hemoglobin are produced. Each complete protein is a tetramer made from two pairs of identical dimers, and each dimer contains one α-like subunit (ζ OR α) combined with one β-like subunit (ε OR γ OR β OR δ). α-Like globins are coded by genes on chromosome 16, while β-like globins are coded by genes on chromosome 11. Adult hemoglobin (HbA) is composed of two α-β dimers with a minor form (HbA_2, < 5 percent of total circulating hemoglobin) containing ε globins in place of β. The major fetal form of hemoglobin (HbF) is composed of two α-γ dimers and is first produced at about 6 weeks of gestation; prior to that, three separate embryonic proteins are produced from dimers of ζ-ε (hemoglobin Gower 1), ζ-γ (hemoglobin Portland), or α-ε (hemoglobin Gower 2). HbF is itself heterogeneous with 75 percent of the γ globin (G-γ) having glycine in position 136, while the remainder (A-γ) contain alanine in this position. In functional terms, both forms of HbF are identical and are usually considered as one. The switching from HbF to HbA synthesis begins *in utero* at 34 weeks of gestation and proceeds with a half-life of about 6 weeks. This is not altered by preterm delivery but can be delayed by *maternal hypoxia* or by *diabetes* and in infants who are *small for gestational age*. In term infants at birth, 60 percent of hemoglobin is HbF; this declines to below 1 percent over the first year of life. The switching from HbF to HbA synthesis changes the affinity of the hemoglobin for O_2 with important consequences in terms of O_2 delivery. An understanding of these changes in O_2 affinity requires a brief description of the quaternary molecular structure of human hemoglobin.

Structure and function of hemoglobin

All hemoglobins exist in two different quaternary structures (tense or T-state and relaxed or R-state) that are linked by a reversible equilibrium. The R-state has an affinity for O_2 100-fold higher than that of the T-state and, in the absence of O_2, the ratio of T/R is 1×10^5. Thus, as O_2 binds to hemoglobin, the equilibrium shifts to give a higher concentration of the high affinity R-state, and this accounts for the sigmoidal hemoglobin–O_2 binding curve. The affinity of hemoglobin for O_2 can be modified by altering the equilibrium between the T and R states of the protein. Compounds that inhibit O_2 binding will bind to the T-state, and there are three important physiological inhibitors. H^+ ions and CO_2 are important extra-erythrocytic modulators of binding, and both decrease O_2 affinity when blood moves from the lungs to the tissues, thereby enhancing O_2 release. A more long-term modulator of hemoglobin–O_2 affinity is provided by the intra-erythrocytic metabolite 2,3-bisphosphoglycerate (BPG) (2,3-diphosphoglycerate, 2,3DPG). Hypoxic or anemic *hypoxia* is often compensated for by an increase in BPG with a resulting decrease in hemoglobin–O_2 affinity. In contrast, a decrease in plasma pH decreases the rate of BPG production and increases the affinity of hemoglobin for O_2. This effect is seen in *diabetic keto-acidosis* or in bank blood stored at low pH. Fetal blood has a higher affinity for O_2 than adult blood, again related to the physiological function of BPG. HbF has a lower affinity for BPG than HbA and hence, at a given concentration of BPG, a higher affinity for O_2. The O_2 tension required to half saturate blood (P_{50}) at pH 7.4 and $P\text{CO}_2$ of 40 mmHg (5.33 kPa) is 27 mmHg in adults and 20 mmHg in preterm infants with 90 percent HbF. These various differences in hemoglobin O_2 affinity are generally too small to affect O_2 loading in the lungs but make a significant contribution to O_2 release in the tissues.

Available O_2

The predicted physiological consequence of simultaneous changes in hemoglobin concentration and O_2 affinity, is provided by the derived 'available O_2' (AO). It is the calculated difference in O_2 content of blood at arterial $P\text{O}_2$ and at an assumed mixed venous $P\text{O}_2$ of 20 mmHg and represents the amount of O_2 that can be extracted from blood before the need arises for an increase in cardiac output. Available O_2 can be calculated from the measured O_2 affinity of the blood or, for untransfused preterm infants up to 10 weeks of postnatal age, can be estimated from the total post-conceptual age:

$$\text{AO (ml/g Hb)} = 0.54 + 0.005 \times \text{age (weeks)}$$

This predicts age-dependent increases in the available O_2 reflecting the decreasing affinity of hemoglobin for O_2, which compensates for the decline in circulating hemoglobin in term infants. The compensatory value of a decrease in O_2 affinity in *anemia* is often illustrated with another calculation analogous to, but different from, available O_2. This is the O_2 release capacity, which uses an assumed mixed venous $P\text{O}_2$ of 40 mmHg, chosen to reflect *in vivo* conditions at rest rather than in a period of high O_2 demand. This difference appears trivial but is highly significant; changes in P_{50} that restore O_2 release capacity to normal, after preterm delivery, may leave the available O_2 suboptimal. In these circumstances, the infant will not cope with O_2 demands above those required at or near to resting conditions. Symptoms of anemic hypoxia can arise in preterm infants born at less than 30 weeks of gestation when the nadir of hemoglobin occurs before there is significant switching to HbA synthesis, and this tips the balance to clinical signs of anemia. This is likely to occur when the available O_2 drops to 6.0 ml/dl of blood. In healthy adults the normal available O_2 is 12.2 ml/dl. Similar problems will be relevant in older infants with abnormal hemoglobin or with metabolic disturbances that alter the hemoglobin–O_2 affinity. An abnormal, high-affinity hemoglobin will result in chronic hypoxia, which may stimulate EPO synthesis and an elevated production of red cells. The resulting *polycythemia* will be associated with abnormal blood flow due to the increase in blood viscosity (see below).

Blood volume and O_2 transport

In addition to the concentration of hemoglobin, the total volume of circulating red cells (RCV) is also an important hematological variable that influences tissue oxygenation. When considering blood volume variables, it is useful to consider hemoglobin concentration as the proportion of blood occupied by the red blood cells, which for a sample of peripheral blood, is defined as hematocrit (Hct). The relationship between Hct and hemoglobin concentration will, of course, vary with the amount of hemoglobin contained within each cell, the mean corpuscular hemoglobin (MCH). The whole body hematocrit (HctB) is defined by the equation (1):

$$\text{HctB} = \frac{\text{RCV}}{(\text{RCV} + \text{PV})}$$

where RCV is the total volume of circulating red cells, PV is the volume of plasma within which these cells are circulating, and the sum of RCV and PV is blood volume (BV). In neonates and adults, a plot of peripheral Hct versus RCV is hyperbolic with a large degree of individual scatter attributed to inequality in maintenance of plasma volume between individuals. Importantly, there is little evidence of compensatory changes in PV to maintain circulating BV at low RCV. The corollary to this is a linear relationship between BV and RCV, and a low RCV is likely to be associated with oligovolemia as well as anemia (Fig. 12.2). This reduction in blood volume decreases venous compliance and capacity, which occurs unevenly, leading to redistribution of blood flow through organs such as the heart and brain to protect them from O_2 deprivation. This circulatory adaptation delays major physiological responses, such as an increase in cardiac output at rest, until anemia becomes severe. Theory predicts a biological response will occur when RCV in neonates falls to about 15–20 ml/kg. The biological responses could be normal physiological compensatory mechanisms as well as signals of the need for clinical intervention in

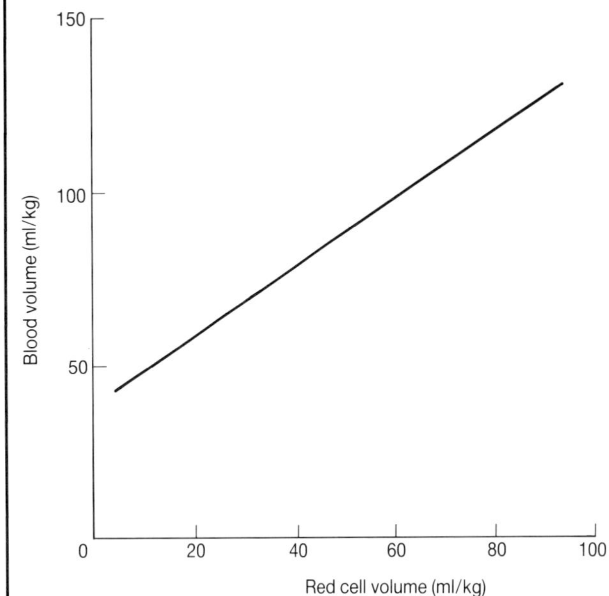

Fig. 12.2. Relationship between red cell volume and blood volume. (From Jones JG, Holland BM, Hudson IR, Wardrop CA. *Br J Haematol* 1990; **76**: 288, with permission.)

severely affected individuals. Clinical data from preterm neonates support these conclusions and identify 25 ml/kg as the critical RCV below which cardiac output at rest and the level of clinical attention increases (Fig. 12.3). From the early stages of anemia, however, a more immediate, but equally undesirable result of uneven redistribution of blood in oligovolemia is chronic underperfusion and possible hypoxia in some tissues. The liver and bowel are particularly vulnerable to decreasing blood O_2 content, and the bowel is a major source of lactic acid in endotoxic shock. It is therefore important to address problems associated with reduced RCV early before the situation is serious enough to invoke an increase in cardiac output at rest. The increased cardiac output, which is stimulated by, and correlated with, a low RCV is not related to hematocrit alone but is correlated with both Hct and BV as independent predictors. The hematocrit predicts O_2-carrying capacity of the blood, and BV is a measure of the effective proportion of the total tissue vasculature that is perfused. RCV has been used in some investigations as the single measurement reflecting both of these important variables and has been considered the logical target and monitor in red cell transfusion regimens. However, the

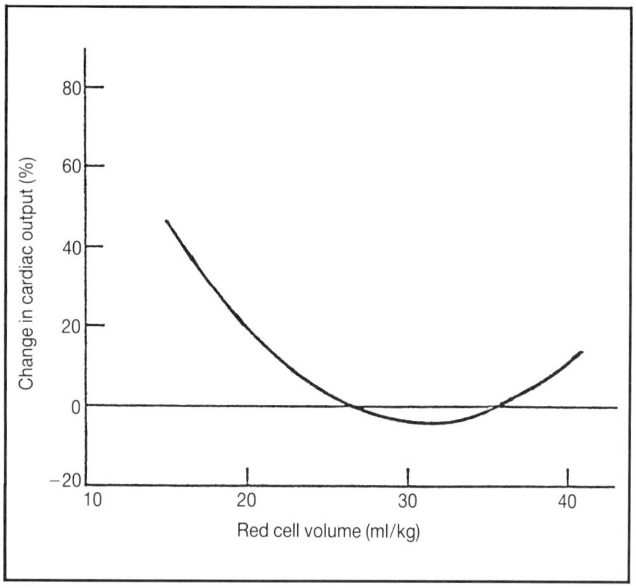

Fig. 12.3. Association between red cell volume and changes in cardiac output after altering red cell volume with blood transfusion in preterm neonates. (From Hudson I, Cooke A, Holland B, *et al. Arch Dis Child* 1990; **65**: 672, with permission.)

best hematological guide to possible tissue hypoxia is a combination of Hct and BV, and methods for measuring BV are becoming increasingly important. Apart from indirect methods such as hydrostatic pressure in major blood vessels, there are two ways of obtaining this measurement:

1. Independent measures of RCV and PV; or
2. From equation (1) using measured Hct and **either** RCV **or** PV.

Measurement of red cell volume

In general, measurements of RCV depend on labeling autologous cells with radioisotopes or biotin and measuring the degree of dilution after retransfusion of the labeled cells into the original donor. Radioisotopes are invasive, and biotin involves lengthy and labor-intensive procedures. Neonatologists, however, often transfuse neonates with adult red cells as part of clinical therapy, and the administered cells are diluted with those of the infant receiving the transfusion. In these circumstances, dilution of autologous HbF by donor HbA forms the basis of a simple, rapid, and proven graphical method for RCV measurement. It does, however, become less sensitive with multiple transfusions as the proportion of HbA in the circulation increases.

RCV measurement is also relevant in the clinical management of *polycythemia,* presently recognized as an elevated Hct or hemoglobin concentration. The distinction between true erythrocytosis and contracted PV, an essential part of hematological diagnosis in adults, is less appreciated in infants. In these patients, the estimation of RCV must depend on more traditional dilution techniques, and the biotin method, proven effective in neonates as well as adults, may be a possibility in an environment with the appropriate trained staff and technology. The need is growing for easier methods of RCV estimation.

Measurement of plasma volume

PV, the volume of fluid within which the red cells are distributed, is estimated in practice as the volume of distribution of macromolecules believed to be confined to the vascular space. The usual molecule is albumin, labeled with a suitable radioactive isotope or chromophoric dye. The volume of distribution of albumin is probably greater than that of the larger erythrocyte; this difference is likely to be exaggerated in sick infants with compromised capillary permeability. This method of estimating plasma volume is therefore unsatisfactory, and an alternative is required. In neonatology, the immunoglobulin IgM is emerging as a useful molecule in this context as it is reduced or absent from neonatal blood and is administered clinically during plasma transfusion. In these circumstances, the volume of distribution of IgM is easily calculated and has been used as a measure of PV. From studies of neonatal blood, it is now clear that the volume of distribution of red blood cells is closer to that of IgM than to that of albumin.

Measurement of blood volume

The use of equation (1) for estimating BV from Hct and either RCV or PV has been questioned because of the reported variable relationship between measured peripheral Hct and whole-body hematocrit (HctB). The ratio HctB/Hct varies from 0.75 to 0.97 in neonates for two possible reasons. First, the distribution of flowing blood cells and plasma in the vasculature depends on the diameter of the vessel, and Hct is a variable, site-specific variable. Second, HctB is calculated from independent measures of RCV and PV, and the latter is accepted as the volume of distribution of labeled albumin. The use of RCV to calculate PV from equation (1) would be subject to the first of these errors, but not the second. Conversely, the use of PV, as measured above, to calculate RCV would be subject to both errors. Equating the volume of distribution of albumin with that of red cells therefore seems particularly undesirable as variations, which are irrelevant to tissue oxygenation, will affect the calculation of RCV from equation (1). For the present, and provided care is taken to standardize the drawing of blood samples, to estimate BV from the peripheral Hct and RCV should be acceptable. The BV, calculated in this way, and the peripheral Hct are the primary determinants of whole-body tissue oxygenation.

Blood viscosity

The oxygenation of tissues also depends on blood flow, which is sensitive to changes in blood viscosity that effect vascular resistance to flow (see p. 520). Hyperviscosity has been reported in about 5 percent of infants at birth, and 2 percent of those may present with clinical problems. The viscosity of blood is determined by plasma viscosity, the number of red cells, and the rheological properties and aggregability of those cells. Except in extreme leukocytosis, the white cells do not influence blood viscosity but have profound effects on flow through the microcirculation. Plasma viscosity reflects the concentration of high molecular weight proteins such as fibrinogen. The concentration of fibrinogen increases from about 25 g/l in term infants to about 35 g/l in adults with a concomitant increase in plasma viscosity from 1.25 mPa to 1.46 mPa. The viscosity of blood at a high shear rate is typically 10-fold higher than that of plasma due to the red blood cells. This difference is exaggerated at low shear rate due to the aggregation of the red cells. The viscosity of blood is therefore very sensitive to Hct but, at any Hct, is lower in neonates than adults due to the lower concentration of plasma fibrinogen and the larger size of the red cells.

In terms of O_2 delivery there is a delicate balance between blood O_2 content and blood flow. An increase in Hct increases the first but decreases the second due to changes in blood viscosity and thereby vascular resistance. Calculation and experimental measurements show that the optimum Hct for O_2 delivery is about 40 percent in adults (RCV = 30 ml/kg) but about 50 percent in term neonates (RCV = 45 ml/kg). This difference reflects the larger size of neonatal red cells. An increase in Hct above the optimum therefore will not necessarily benefit tissues as it will be offset by an increase in blood viscosity. There is evidence that normovolemic reduction in hematocrit improves muscle oxygenation in dogs, and conversely, increases in hematocrit can reduce pulmonary blood flow in children with *high flow congenital heart disease* (e.g. *VSD*). It is therefore common, in clinical transfusion practice, to aim for a hemoglobin concentration below that found in healthy subjects. This practical interpretation of the data may be mistaken; a chronic anemia in neonates, children, and adults is hypovolemic and probably associated with hypoperfusion of some tissues in order to protect others. Hence a Hct below the normal value will not correct the oligovolemia, will leave an impaired **total** tissue oxygenation, and is the wrong target in blood transfusion therapy.

Selected reading

Christensen RD. Hematopoiesis in the fetus and neonate. *Pediatr Res* 1989; **26**: 531.

Jones JG, Holland BM, Hudson IRB, Wardrop CAJ. Total circulating red cells versus haematocrit as the primary descriptor of O_2 transport by the blood. *Br J Haematol* 1991; **76**: 288.

Jones JG, Holland BM, Wardrop CAJ. Disorders of red cells 3: red cells and O_2 transport. In Lilleyman JS, Hann IM, eds. *Paediatric haematology*. 2nd ed. Edinburgh: Churchill Livingstone, in press.

Lipton JM, Nathan DG. The anatomy and physiology of hematopoiesis. In Nathan DG, Oski F, eds. *Hematology in infancy and childhood*. Vol. I. Philadelphia: WB Saunders, 1987: 128.

Wardrop CAJ, Jones JG, Holland BM. Detection, correction and ultimate prevention of anaemias in the preterm infant. *Transfusion Sci* 1991; **12**: 257.

C. Hemostasis

M Andrew

Children may develop hemorrhagic or thrombotic complications secondary to either inherited or acquired disorders of hemostasis. The diagnostic and therapeutic approach to pediatric patients is usually extrapolated from adult information because many hemostatic problems, particularly thrombotic complications, are rare in pediatrics. The use of adult guidelines in children is not optimal for several reasons. First, the epidemiology of many hemostatic problems is distinctly different. Second, several unique physiological forms of hemostasis are present during the first months and years of life. Indeed, hemostasis is a dynamic continuum of gradually maturing systems. The very low incidence of thrombotic complications during childhood, secondary to either inherited or acquired disorders, raises the intriguing possibility that the hemostatic systems in the young have advantages over those in adults. Finally, the interaction of anticoagulants and thrombolytic agents with the hemostatic systems differs significantly in childhood. Optimal management of children with hemostatic problems depends upon a thorough understanding of developmental hemostasis.

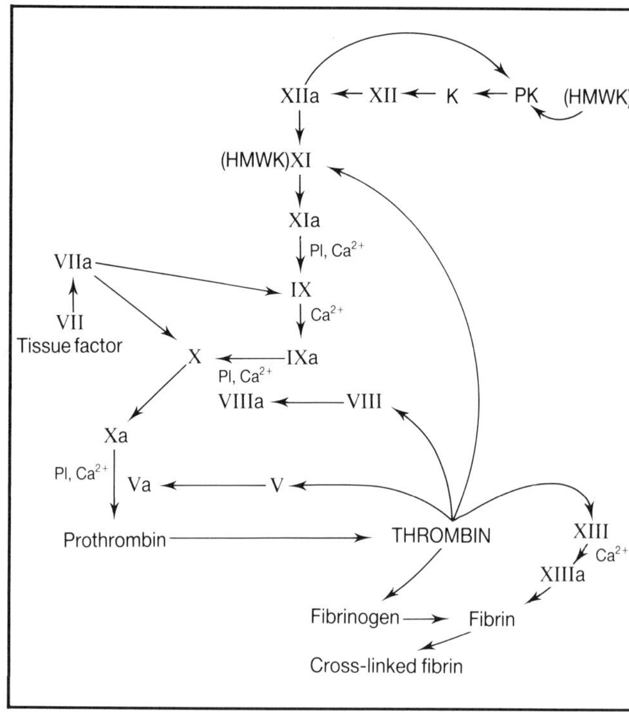

Fig. 12.4. The generation of thrombin from prothrombin can be considered a central event in blood coagulation. HMWK, High molecular weight kininogen; PK, prekallikrein; K, kallikrein; Pl, phospholipid.

Coagulation

Thrombin generation: general

Thrombin generation is a complicated process that involves the interaction of many coagulation proteins. All components of coagulation are present from early fetal life. Just as for adults, blood is maintained in a fluid phase, and in response to damage to the vessel wall, platelets, plasma coagulation proteins, and the damaged vessel contribute to the formation of a hemostatic plug. Fig. 12.4 shows a schematic outline of blood coagulation. Although blood coagulation theoretically can be initiated by the contact system or by exposure of blood to tissue factor, the latter is the physiologically important activation pathway. The binding of factor VII to tissue factor initiates coagulation by factor VIIa catalysis of both factor X and factor IX. Activation of the contact system (factors XII, XI, prekallikrein [PK], high molecular weight kininogen [HMWK]) results in the generation of factor XIa. Factors XIa and VIIa both cleave factor IX to factor IXa. Factor IXa (enzyme) in the presence of factor VIIIa (cofactor), factor X (substrate), Ca^{2+}, and a phospholipid surface forms one of two tannase complexes. Factor VIIa proteolytic activation of factor X (substrate) in the presence of tissue factor, Ca^{2+}, and a phospholipid surface forms the second tannase complex. The final common pathway of coagulation is the formation of the prothrombinase complex, which consists of factor Va (cofactor), factor Xa (enzyme), prothrombin (substrate), Ca^{2+}, and a phospholipid surface. The final product of the prothrombinase complex is the key enzyme in coagulation, thrombin. Thrombin is a serine protease with many coagulant functions. It cleaves fibrinopeptide A and B from fibrinogen, resulting in fibrin formation; it activates factors VIII and V, thereby enhancing its own generation; it activates factor XI directly, bypassing the other contact factors; it activates factor XIII, promoting fibrin crosslinking; and it activates platelets.

An overall assessment of the coagulation system can be made with two general screening tests, the prothrombin time (PT) and the activated partial thromboplastin time (APTT). The PT measures thrombin generation following activation of factor X by factor VIIa, and the APTT measures thrombin generation following activation of the contact system. Plasma concentrations of individual coagulation proteins can also be measured directly with functional or immunological assays. These assays provide an important means of assessing the coagulation system; however, they do not determine whether the coagulation system was activated *in vivo*. Sensitive laboratory tests that reflect *in vivo* generation of thrombin are now available. These include measurement of a fragment formed following proteolytic cleavage of prothrombin, fragment F1.2; a peptide released by thrombin cleavage of fibrinogen, fibrinopeptide A; the remaining portion of the fibrinogen molecule called fibrin monomer, and thrombin complexed to its natural inhibitor, antithrombin III, thrombin–antithrombin III complexes (TATs). Together these tests provide an effective means to evaluate hemostasis under physiological and pathological conditions.

Table 12.4. Mean values from full-term and premature infants on the first day after delivery

	Full-term	Preterm
Fibrinogen (g/l)	2.9[a]	2.4[a, b]
II	0.5	0.5
V	0.7	0.9[a, b]
VII	0.7	0.7
VIII	1.0[a]	1.1[a]
vWF	1.5	1.4
IX	0.5	0.4[b]
X	0.4	0.4
XI	0.4	0.3[b]
XII	0.5	0.4[b]
PK	0.4	0.3
HMWK	0.5	0.5
XIII_a	0.8	0.7
XIII_b	0.8	0.8
ATIII	0.6	0.4[b]
α_2M	1.4	1.1[b]
C_1E-INH	0.7	0.7
α_1AT	0.9[a]	0.9[a]
HCII	0.4	0.3[b]
Protein C	0.4	0.3[b]
Protein S	0.4	0.3[b]

VIII, Factor VIII procoagulant; vWF, von Willebrand factor; PK, prekallikrein; HMWK, high molecular weight kininogen; ATIII, antithrombin III; α_2M, α_2-macroglobulin; C_1E-INH, C_1-esterase inhibitor; α_1AT, α_1-antitrypsin; HCII, heparin cofactor II.
All factors, except fibrinogen, units per milliliter (U/ml).
[a] Values indistinguishable from the adult.
[b] Values different from the full-term infant.

Thrombin generation: infancy and childhood

Thrombin generation is critical to physiological hemostasis and the prevention of bleeding. Clinically, infants and children are not at greater risk of bleeding than adults. Therefore, the ability of their systems to generate thrombin must be considered physiological, even if it differs significantly from the adult system. Components of the coagulation system do not cross the placenta from mothers to fetuses; rather, they are synthesized by fetuses, initially appearing by approximately 10 weeks gestational age. Samples obtained at fetoscopy provide the best assessment of the fetal coagulation system for the first weeks of gestational age and for the very premature infant (Table 12.4). Study of hemostasis following birth and during infancy and early childhood has been hindered by problems in obtaining adequate samples from healthy infants, by greater variability in plasma concentrations of coagulation proteins, and by the need for microassays to measure coagulation proteins on small volumes of plasma. Normal ranges for the coagulant proteins were generated from premature (30–36 weeks gestational age) and full-term infants at several times during the first 6 months of postnatal life, from healthy children evenly distributed throughout childhood, and from healthy adults. Figures 12.5, 12.6, and 12.7 summarize data for the vitamin K-dependent factors (Fig. 12.5: factors II, VII, IX, X), the contact factors (Fig. 12.6: factors XII, XI, PK, HMWK), and other coagulants (Fig. 12.7: factors V, VIII, XIII, and vWF) throughout infancy and childhood.

A notable feature of coagulation during infancy is that plasma concentrations of coagulation proteins are not all similarly different from adult values. For example, plasma concentrations of the four vitamin K-dependent proteins

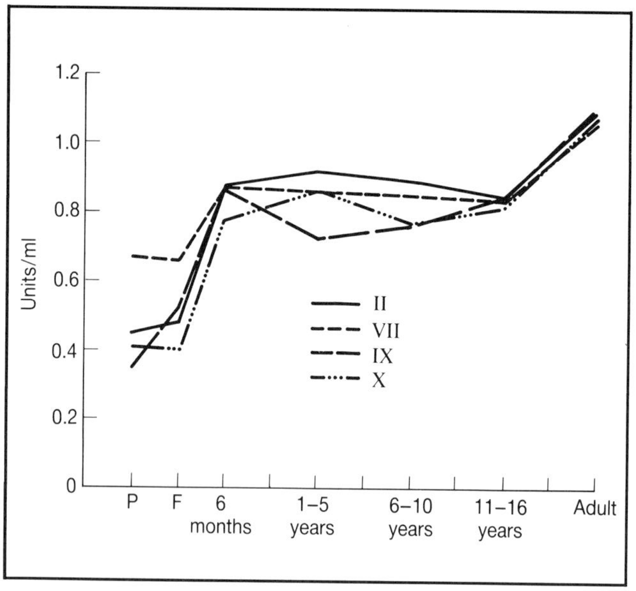

Fig. 12.5. Plasma concentrations of vitamin K-dependent factors (II, VII, IX, X) in healthy premature infants on day 1 of life (P), in healthy term infants on day 1 (F) and at 6 months of life, during childhood (ages 1–5, 6–10, 11–16 years), and in adults.

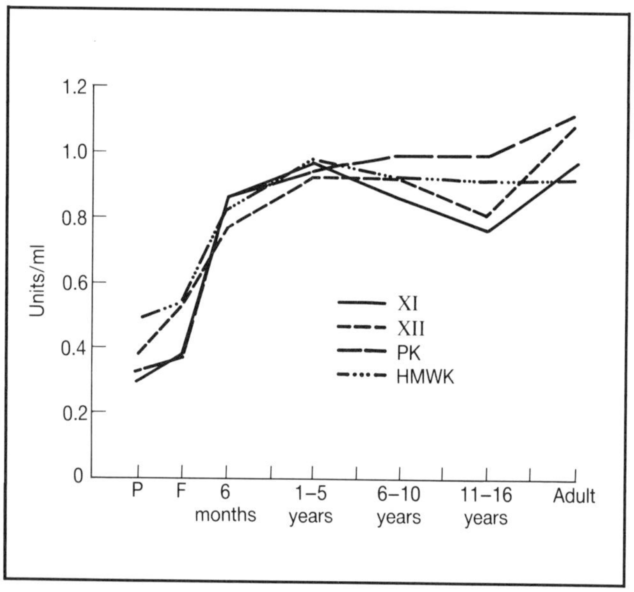

Fig. 12.6. Plasma concentrations of contact factors (XII, XI, prekallikrein [PK], and high molecular weight kininogen [HMWK]) in healthy premature infants on day 1 of life (P), in healthy term infants on day 1 (F) and at 6 months of life, during childhood (ages 1–5, 6–10, 11–16 years), and in adults.

and the four contact factors at birth are approximately 50 percent of adult values (Table 12.4, Figs 12.5, 12.6). In contrast, plasma concentrations of fibrinogen and factors VIII, vWF, and V are not decreased at birth (Table 12.4)

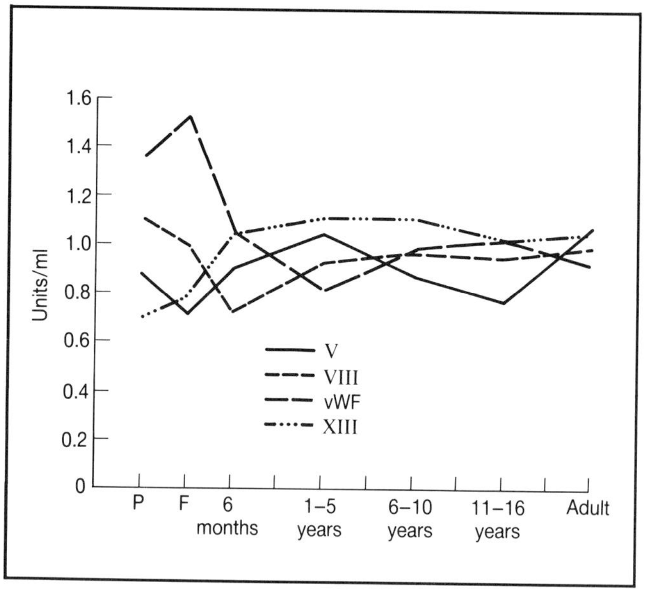

Fig. 12.7. Plasma concentrations of factors V, VIII, vWF, and XIII in healthy premature infants on day 1 of life (P), in healthy term infants on day 1 (F) and at 6 months of life, during childhood (ages 1–5, 6–10, 11–16 years), and in adults.

nor during early childhood (Fig. 12.7). The first clue that these physiological differences affect thrombin generation is the presence of prolonged PTs and APTTs during infancy (Table 12.4). More recently, thrombin generation in newborn plasma has been quantitated with a sensitive chromogenic assay, and is both delayed and decreased compared with adult plasma (Fig. 12.8). The degree of impairment is similar to that in plasma from adults receiving therapeutic amounts of Coumadin or heparin. The amount of thrombin generated is directly proportional to the plasma prothrombin concentration, while the rate at which thrombin is generated depends upon the concentration of all procoagulants. Once generated, thrombin cleaves fibrinopeptides A and B from fibrinogen, resulting in fibrin formation. During childhood, fibrinogen is present with plasma concentrations similar to adults. However, in newborns fibrinogen is characterized by greater sialic acid content than adult fibrinogen. The thrombin clotting time (TCT), if performed without Ca^{2+} in the system, is prolonged in newborns, reflecting the 'fetal' fibrinogen. If the sialic acid is removed, 'fetal' fibrinogen appears indistinguishable from adult fibrinogen. The physiological significance of 'fetal' fibrinogen is unknown. Factor XIII concentrations are similar to adult values, and 'fetal' fibrinogen cross-links normally.

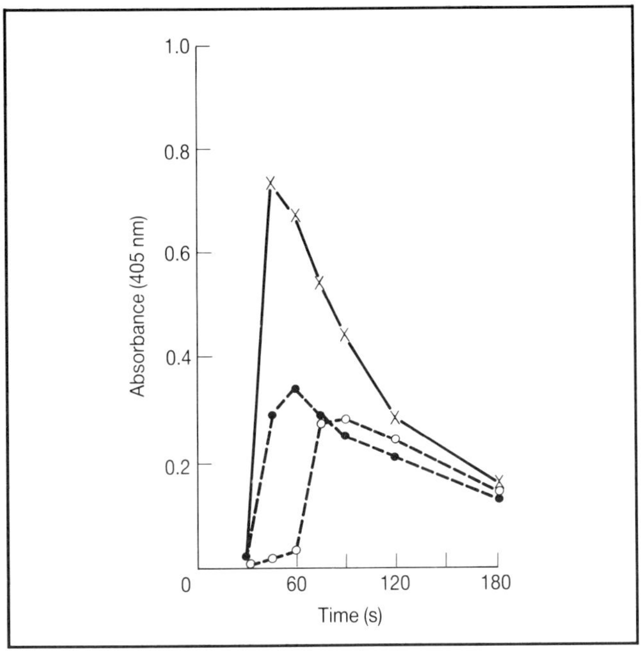

Fig. 12.8. Thrombin generation following activation in the APTT system in plasma from adults (×), from full-term infants on day 1 of life (●), and from premature infants on day 1 of life (○). The amount of thrombin generated was determined by its ability to cleave a chromogenic substrate, resulting in a change in the absorbance reading at 405 nm.

Patients with *inherited disorders of hemostasis* frequently present first with bleeding complications during infancy or early childhood. The physiological status of the coagulation system during childhood directly affects the diagnosis and treatment of inherited coagulopathies. For example, in newborns the physiological lower limit of normal for plasma concentrations of some coagulation proteins overlaps with pathological values as defined in the adult coagulation system (Table 12.4). In contrast to children and adults, the most common congenital coagulation defects to present clinically in newborns are the *hemophilias*. Severe (< 0.01 units/ml) and moderate (0.01–0.05 units/ml) forms of both hemophilia A (factor VIII deficiency) and hemophilia B (factor IX deficiency) can be diagnosed at the time of birth because physiological and pathological concentrations do not overlap (Table 12.4). However, mild forms of hemophilia B may overlap with the lower physiological limit of normal for infants (0.15 units/ml). Correctly identifying patients with potentially significant problems from hemophilia C (factor XI deficiency) can be difficult because the lower limit of normal for factor XI at birth is 0.05 units/ml (Table 12.4). Whether a combination of physiological and congenital factor XI deficiency would result uniformly in plasma concentrations less than 0.05 units/ml for all affected infants is unknown. *von Willebrand disease* (vWD), the most common inherited bleeding defect in adults, cannot be diagnosed in newborns by assays reflecting vWF activity or protein concentrations. There are rare forms of vWD, usually homozygous forms associated with marked decreases of both vWF and factor VIII, that can present with bleeding in newborns, and can be identified by specific assays of factor VIII and vWF. Other clinically significant coagulation protein deficiencies that may be difficult to diagnose in infancy include homozygous deficiencies of factors II and X (Table 12.4).

Infants may also develop the same acquired coagulation problems as adults. The most common *acquired coagulopathies* include *disseminated intravascular coagulation (DIC)*, *vitamin K deficiency*, and *liver failure*. Adult guidelines for diagnosing these acquired coagulation disorders are not appropriate for infants. For example, DIC is characterized in part by activation of the coagulation system with the generation of thrombin and consumption of many coagulation factors and inhibitors. Activation of coagulation also occurs as part of the physiological process of birth, resulting in increased plasma concentrations of fibrinopeptide A, as well as thrombin–antithrombin III complexes in cord blood. Clearly, healthy newborn infants do not have DIC, yet the values of some coagulation laboratory tests would be compatible with that diagnosis in adults. Similarly, vitamin K deficiency in adults can be diagnosed when plasma concentrations of the four vitamin K-dependent coagulant proteins are low (< 0.50 units/ml) and plasma concentrations of factors V and VIII are normal (0.50–1.50 units/ml). The latter pattern represents the physiological form of the newborn coagulation system and not vitamin K deficiency (Table 12.4).

By 6 months of age, the coagulation system has evolved to one with many similarities to the adult. At the same time, the coagulation system of 6-month-old infants still differs significantly from that of adults in several important ways (Figs 12.5, 12.6). Plasma concentrations of vitamin K-dependent factors and contact factors are 10–20 percent lower than adult values, and the lower boundaries of normal are also decreased compared with adults. The physiological significance of these differences is still unknown and will not likely alter the correct identification of patients with inherited or acquired deficiencies of coagulation proteins. However, some of the subtle differences in plasma concentrations of certain coagulation proteins may contribute to observed differences in the risk of *thromboembolic disease* during childhood. Prospective studies in adults have shown a significant positive relationship between plasma factor VII concentrations and the occurrence of *ischemic cardiovascular events*.

In addition, plasma concentrations of prothrombin are directly related to the amounts of thrombin generated. Whether lower plasma concentrations of factors VII and prothrombin during childhood are in part responsible for the lower risk of thrombotic complications is plausible, but remains to be proven.

Thrombin regulation: general

Thrombin generation and activity are regulated by plasma inhibitors, endothelial cells, and fibrin. The direct plasma inhibitors of thrombin include antithrombin III (ATIII), α_2-macroglobulin (α_2M), and heparin cofactor II (HCII). ATIII is an important inhibitor of several serine proteases in coagulation, thereby controlling both the generation of thrombin and thrombin activities. ATIII belongs to the serine proteinase inhibitor family (serpins). It inactivates thrombin by forming a 1:1 covalent bond with the active site of thrombin. ATIII-mediated inhibition of thrombin is potentiated by certain glycosaminoglycans, most importantly heparan sulfate and heparin. *In vivo*, endothelial cell-surface-associated heparan sulfate provides an important mechanism for potentiating ATIII-mediated inhibition of thrombin. Therapeutically, heparin and its derivatives are the most commonly used anticoagulants for the prevention and initial treatment of deep venous thrombosis. α_2M, like ATIII, is an inhibitor that binds to several serine proteases involved in blood coagulation. When α_2M binds to thrombin, it inhibits the ability of thrombin to cleave fibrinogen but not small molecules such as chromogenic substrates. α_2M is not as important an inhibitor of thrombin as ATIII in adults, and its inhibition of thrombin is not enhanced by glycosaminoglycans. HCII is a specific inhibitor of thrombin that, like ATIII, forms a 1:1 covalent bond with thrombin, completely neutralizing its enzymatic activity. In addition, HCII inhibition of thrombin can be potentiated by a glycosaminoglycan, dermatan sulfate. In adults, HCII inhibits only small amounts of thrombin compared with ATIII. Dermatan sulfate is present on endothelial cell surfaces as well as several other locations. Dermatan sulfate has only recently been available for clinical testing. It is an effective and safe anticoagulant in animal models of thrombosis and in initial studies in humans.

Thrombin also functions indirectly as an inhibitor of coagulation by binding to the endothelial cell receptor, thrombomodulin. Thrombin bound to thrombomodulin can no longer cleave fibrinogen or factors V and VIII. However, it can then activate protein C to its activated form (APC). APC, a vitamin K-dependent serine protease, enzymatically inactivates factors Va and VIIIa by limited proteolytic cleavage. The enzymatic activity of APC is enhanced by another vitamin K-dependent protein, protein S. Protein S circulates in blood in two forms, a free active form and a bound (C4B) inactive form. APC is inhibited by at least two plasma inhibitors, protein C inhibitor (PCI) and α_1-antitrypsin inhibitor. Another mechanism by which thrombin coagulant activity is controlled is the fibrin clot itself. In pathological conditions when a fibrin clot is formed, thrombin binds to fibrin and is relatively protected from inactivation by plasma antiproteases. However, thrombin can still cleave fibrinogen to fibrin, resulting in propagation of the fibrin clot.

Thrombin regulation: infancy and childhood

During infancy and childhood, thrombin is regulated by the same basic mechanisms as in adults. However, several important physiological differences provide at least a partial explanation for the lower incidence of *thrombotic complications* in children than in adults. First, during the first weeks of life plasma concentrations of ATIII and HCII are approximately 50 percent of adult values (Table 12.4, Fig. 12.9). In contrast, plasma concentrations of α_2M are significantly higher than in adults. Low physiological plasma concentrations of ATIII and HCII result in a slower rate of thrombin inhibition in healthy infants than in adults (Fig. 12.10). However, the magnitude of difference in thrombin inhibition between newborns and adults is reduced by the high plasma α_2M concentrations. Significantly more thrombin is inhibited by α_2M than by ATIII in newborn plasma, reflecting the high plasma α_2M

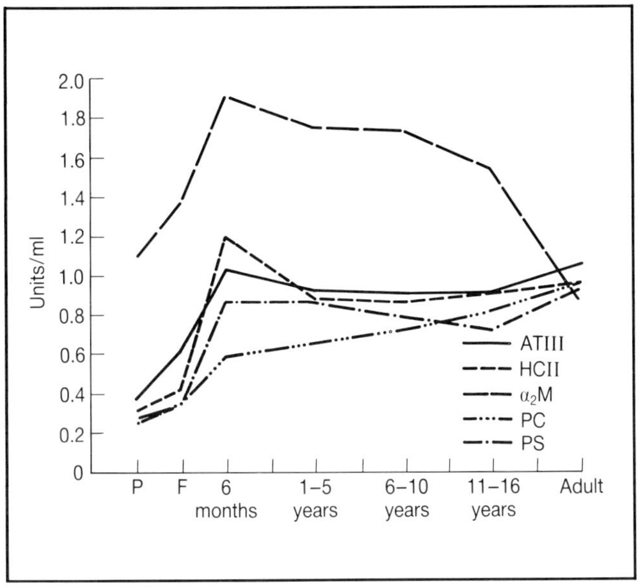

Fig. 12.9. Plasma concentrations of inhibitors antithrombin III (ATIII), protein C, protein S, heparin cofactor II (HCII) and α_2-macroglobulin (α_2M) in healthy premature infants on day 1 of life (P), in healthy term infants on day 1 (F) and at 6 months of life, during childhood (ages 1–5, 6–10, 11–16 years), and in adults.

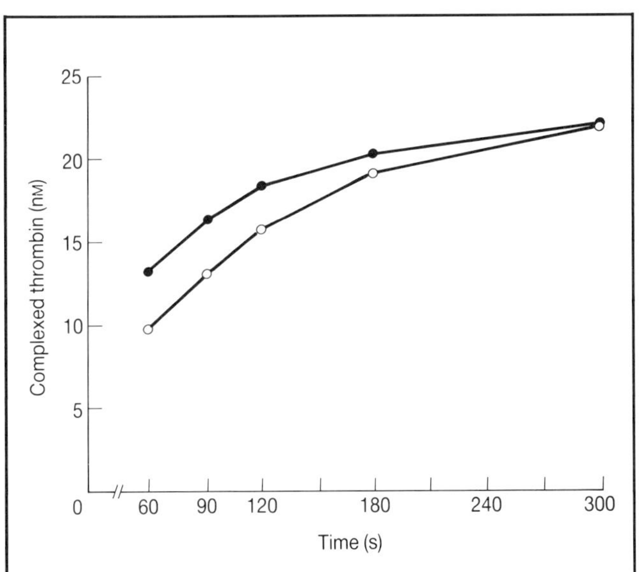

Fig. 12.10. Inhibition of ^{125}I-thrombin (25 nM) in adult (●—●), and neonatal (○—○) plasma is dependent on incubation time and differs between the two age groups.

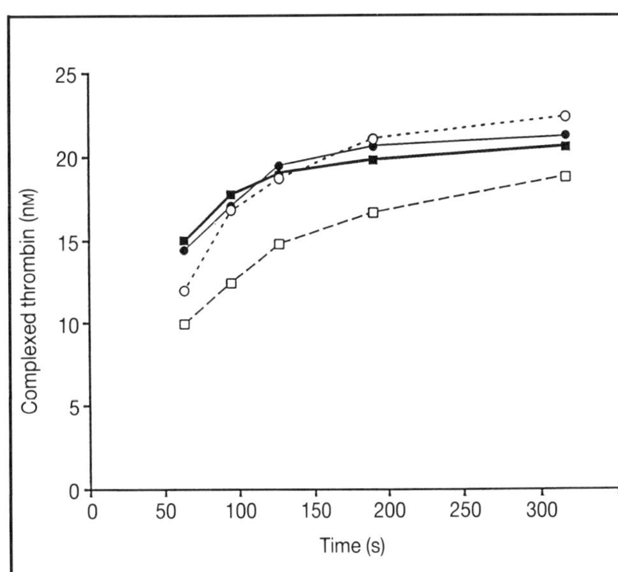

Fig. 12.11. The amount of ^{125}I-thrombin complexed to inhibitors over time in antithrombin III (ATIII) deficient children (○—○), healthy children (●—●), ATIII-deficient adults (□—□), and healthy adults (■—■). ATIII-deficient children inhibited ^{125}I-thrombin as well as healthy children and adults. In contrast, ATIII-deficient adults inhibited ^{125}I-thrombin at a significantly slower rate than the other groups.

concentrations. There is some evidence that increased binding to α_2M also occurs *in vivo* in newborns.

Plasma α_2M concentrations remain increased throughout childhood and do not reach adult values until the third decade of life. The persistently increased plasma α_2M concentrations result in greater inhibition of thrombin by α_2M throughout childhood. It seems likely that increased plasma α_2M concentrations provide additional protection from thrombotic events in healthy children. Patients with congenital ATIII deficiency, an autosomal-dominant disorder that accounts for a small proportion of patients with *venous thrombosis*, usually have plasma ATIII concentrations that are 40–60 percent of physiological adult values, suggesting that protective mechanisms are in place. The first thromboembolic events rarely occur during childhood and coincide with the decline of plasma α_2M concentrations to adult levels. A recent study showed that plasma from ATIII-deficient children inhibited thrombin as effectively as healthy children and adults and that this ability to inhibit thrombin effectively was due to increased binding of thrombin by α_2M. In contrast, thrombin was inhibited more slowly in plasmas from ATIII-deficient adults than in either ATIII-deficient children or healthy children and adults (Fig. 12.11).

Thrombin inhibition by HCII is also increased in newborn plasma. This does not reflect the decreased plasma concentrations of HCII in newborns (Table 12.4,

Fig. 12.9), but rather a circulating glycosaminoglycan that catalyzes thrombin inhibition by the natural inhibitor HCII. This fetal anticoagulant circulates as a proteoglycan (0.3 μg/ml), with a molecular weight of approximately 150 kDa; it is also present in plasma from pregnant women. The fetal anticoagulant has properties similar to dermatan sulfate (DSPG), not heparan sulfate, and is likely released from the placenta. DSPG disappears from maternal blood within days of delivery. The length of time that the DSPG remains in newborn blood is not known, except that it is still present during the first week of life in sick premature infants with respiratory distress syndrome.

The generation of thrombin is also controlled by several other inhibitors of coagulation that inhibit other serine proteases involved in coagulation. α_1-Antitrypsin and C_1-esterase inhibitor regulate the contact phase of coagulation and have similar or increased plasma concentrations when compared with adult values. In contrast, plasma concentrations of the vitamin K-dependent inhibitors protein C and protein S are significantly lower in newborns than in adults (Table 12.4, Fig. 12.9). Protein S circulates completely in the free, active form in newborns because C4B-binding protein is absent in newborn plasma. This likely compensates for the low plasma concentrations of total protein S. Recently, adult and fetal protein C were purified and the compositions compared. Protein C from cord plasma was identical to adult protein C, except that there was a twofold increase in cord single-chain protein C. The investigators suggested that the processing of fetal protein C may be developmentally influenced. Cord plasma protein C appears to have normal functional activity. The lower limits of normal for protein C and protein S, which remain low throughout early childhood, are important to consider when assessing children for inherited deficiencies of these inhibitors. The physiological lower limit for protein C is 0.40 units/ml until 10 years of age, and 0.55 units/ml until the third decade of life (Fig. 12.9). Similarly, the physiological lower limit for total protein S is 0.41–0.54 units/ml, and approximately 0.20 units/ml for free protein S in early childhood.

Thrombin regulation: mechanisms

Potential mechanisms responsible for differences in plasma concentrations of coagulation components are: decreased synthesis, increased clearance or consumption, and presence of proteins with decreased activity. RNA levels have been measured for factors VII, VIII, IX, and X, fibrinogen, ATIII, and protein C in hepatocytes from 5–10-week-old human embryos and fetuses, and from adults. The embryonic–fetal transcripts and adult mRNAs were similar in size, and the nucleotide sequences of factor IX and X mRNA were identical. However, the expression of RNA was variable, with adult levels for some coagulation proteins and decreased expression for others. Similar concentrations of prothrombin mRNA are found in newborn and adult rabbit livers; one study has reported lower prothrombin mRNA concentrations in sheep. At least some coagulation proteins are cleared more rapidly in newborns than adults. The half-life of fibrinogen is significantly shorter in newborn animals and in infants with respiratory distress syndrome than in corresponding adults. The half-life of ATIII is shorter in infants requiring an exchange transfusion for hyperbilirubinemia than in healthy adults. Reasons for the faster clearance of these proteins in newborns are incompletely understood, but may in part be due to an increased basal metabolic rate in newborns. Activation of coagulation, as discussed earlier, does occur but does not provide an explanation for low concentrations of coagulation proteins in newborns. Similarly, there is no evidence that fetal proteins are significantly affecting functional measurements of coagulation proteins and thereby contributing to low plasma concentrations of the proteins involved.

In summary, healthy infants and children rarely develop thrombotic complications, strongly suggesting that protective mechanisms are in place. Superficially, the physiologically low plasma concentrations of ATIII and HCII in newborns would suggest that this population is at greater risk for thrombotic complications. However, newborns compensate for low plasma concentrations of ATIII and HCII through several novel mechanisms that all enhance thrombin regulation. These include: generation of smaller amounts of thrombin than adults, reflecting low plasma concentrations of certain coagulation proteins, particularly prothrombin; enhanced thrombin inhibition by α_2M, reflecting increased plasma concentrations of α_2M; enhanced thrombin inhibition by HCII, reflecting the presence of DSPG; and the presence of protein S in the free functional form. Some of these mechanisms persist into early childhood.

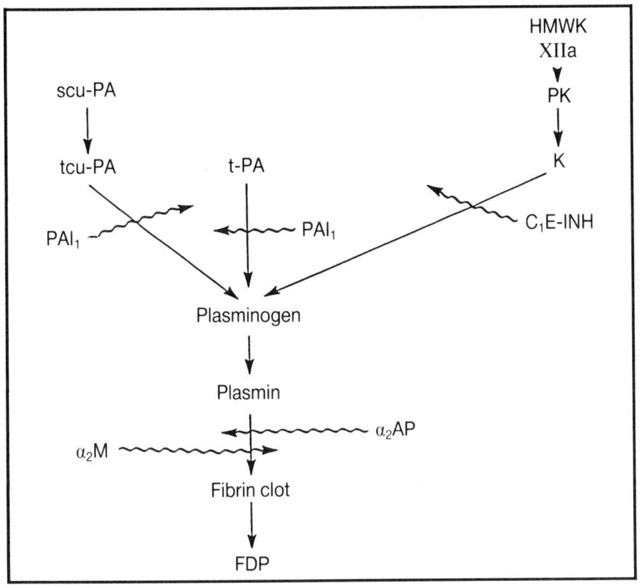

Fig. 12.12. A schematic of the normal fibrinolytic system. Inhibitors are indicated by a ～～～. scu-PA, single-chain urokinase plasminogen activator, tcu-PA, two-chain urokinase plasminogen activator; PAI_1, plasminogen activator inhibitor; t-PA, tissue plasminogen activator; HMWK, high molecular weight kininogen; PK, prekallikrein; K, kallikrein; C_1E-INH, C_1-esterase inhibitor; α_2M, α_2-macroglobulin; α_2AP, α_2-antiplasmin; FDP, fibrin degradation products.

Fibrinolysis

Plasmin regulation: general

Once a fibrin clot has formed *in vivo*, it is modified by the fibrinolytic system (Fig. 12.12). Analogous to thrombin, plasmin is the critical enzyme in fibrinolysis. Plasminogen circulates in two forms, one with an NH_2-terminal glutamic acid residue (glu-plasminogen) and a second form with NH_2-terminal lysine, valine, or methionine residues (lys-plasminogen). Glu-plasminogen can be converted to lys-plasminogen by limited proteolytic degradation. Lys-plasminogen has both a higher affinity for fibrin and increased fibrinolytic activity than glu-plasminogen. Both forms of plasminogen bind to fibrin through specific lysine-binding sites that also mediate the interaction of plasminogen with its inhibitor, α_2-antiplasmin (α_2AP). Plasminogen is converted to its enzymatically active form, plasmin, by several activators. Tissue plasminogen activator (t-PA) is the most important physiological activator of plasminogen. t-PA is a serine protease that also binds to fibrin through lysine-binding sites. t-PA is a relatively poor enzyme in the absence of fibrin; however, fibrin greatly enhances the rate of plasminogen activation by t-PA. Urokinase (u-PA) is a second physiological activator of plasminogen. Single-chain urokinase (scu-PA) has relatively low thrombolytic activity until it is activated to its two-chain form (scu-PA) by limited cleavage by plasmin or kallikrein. Plasminogen is also activated by components of the contact system; however, this does not appear to be of physiological importance. The plasmin molecule is a two-chain, trypsin-like serine proteinase. Once formed on the fibrin clot, plasmin cleaves fibrin in sequential steps, resulting in fibrin degradation products. When bound to the fibrin surface, plasmin is relatively protected from inhibition by its major inhibitor α_2AP. α_2AP belongs to the serpin family of inhibitors and binds to the active site of plasmin, forming a 1:1 stoichiometric complex that has no further activity against fibrin. α_2M is a less important inhibitor of plasmin than α_2AP in adults. Plasmin bound to α_2M retains some fibrinolytic activity. The fibrinolytic system is also regulated by inhibitors of t-PA and u-PA. Three plasminogen activator inhibitors have been described, PAI_1, PAI_2, and PAI_3. PAI_1 is the major inhibitor of t-PA and tcu-PA in adults. PAI_2 is present in plasma during pregnancy and is produced by the placenta. PAI_2 is likely the physiological mechanism by which fibrinolysis is suppressed during pregnancy. Recently PAI_3 was shown to be identical to the protein C inhibitor.

Plasmin regulation: infancy and childhood

During infancy and childhood, plasmin is generated and inhibited in a similar fashion as for adults. However, as with thrombin regulation, there are important differences when compared with the adult fibrinolytic system (Fig. 12.12). First, plasma concentrations of fibrinolytic proteins differ significantly in newborns from adults (Table 12.5). In newborns, plasminogen concentrations are only 50 percent of adult values, α_2AP concentrations are 80 percent of adult values, and plasma PAI_1 and t-PA concentrations are significantly increased. The increased plasma t-PA and PAI_1 concentrations in newborns on day 1 of life are in marked contrast to values from cord blood, in which concentrations of these two proteins are significantly lower than in adults. PAI_2 concentrations are low in cord blood and have not been measured in

Table 12.5. Fibrinolytic system values (mean) on day one for full-term and preterm infants

	Full-term	Preterm
Plasminogen (U/ml)	2.0	1.7[b]
TPA (ng/ml)	9.6	8.5
α_2AP (U/ml)	0.9	0.8
PAI_1 (U/ml)	6.4	5.4[a, b]

TPA, tissue plasminogen activator; α_2AP, α_2-antiplasmin; PAI_1, plasminogen activator inhibitor.
[a] Values indistinguishable from the adult.
[b] Values different from the full-term infant.

newborns. Second, plasminogen, like fibrinogen, has a fetal form. Fetal plasminogen exists in two glycoforms, but with increased amounts of mannose and sialic acid. There probably is decreased enzymatic activity of 'fetal plasmin' as well as decreased binding to cellular receptors for fetal plasminogen. The discrepancy between newborn and cord plasma concentrations of t-PA and PAI_1 can be explained by enhanced release of t-PA and PAI_1 from the endothelium shortly after birth. Further evidence for activation of the fibrinolytic system at birth comes from studies that reported shorter whole-blood clotting times, shorter euglobulin lysis times, and greater plasma concentrations of the B15-42 fibrin-related peptides than in adults. Although the fibrinolytic system is activated at birth, the ability of cord plasma to generate plasmin *in vitro* in response to stimulation with a thrombolytic agent is decreased compared with adults. The latter probably reflects low plasma concentrations of plasminogen in newborns. This reduced ability to generate plasmin impairs the overall ability of cord plasma to lyse fibrin clots. Increasing plasma concentrations of plasminogen, either with purified plasminogen or with plasma supplementation, enhances the fibrinolytic capacity of cord plasma.

The fibrinolytic system has now been studied throughout childhood (Fig. 12.13). Plasma concentrations of plasminogen and α_2AP are similar to adult values by early childhood. Somewhat unexpectedly, physiological plasma concentrations of t-PA are decreased and concentrations of PAI_1 increased throughout childhood compared with adults (Fig. 12.13). In teenage girls under basal conditions, fibrinolysis is suppressed as evidenced by lower t-PA and higher PAI_1 concentrations. Furthermore, the fibrinolytic capacity assessed by venous occlusion in these same girls was significantly poorer than in older women, suggesting not only that the fibrinolytic system probably does not provide a mechanism to lower the risk of *thromboembolic complications* in children, but also that large vessel thrombi, once formed, may not be lysed

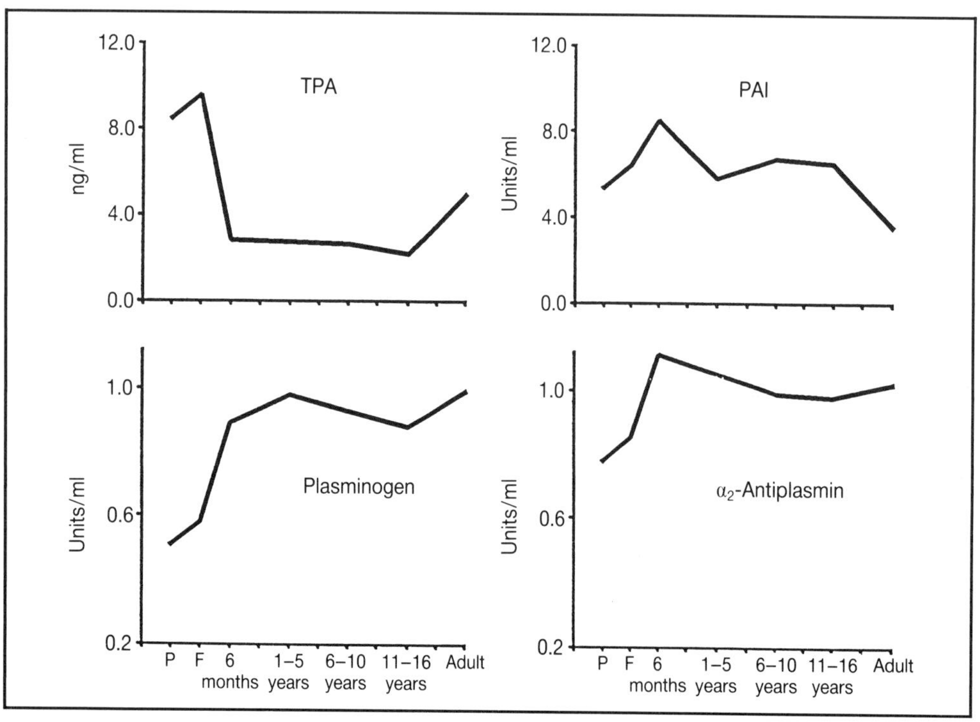

Fig. 12.13. Plasma concentrations of the components of the fibrinolytic system: tissue plasminogen activator (TPA), plasminogen activator inhibitor (PAI), plasminogen and α_2-antiplasmin in healthy premature infants on day 1 of life (P), in healthy term infants on day 1 (F) and at 6 months of life, during childhood (ages 1–5, 6–10, 11–16 years), and in adults.

as effectively in children as in adults. The latter will be important to determine in long-term follow-up studies of children with large vessel thrombotic complications.

Physiology of platelets

General

Platelets are disc-shaped cells produced by megakaryocytes in the bone marrow (see Fig. 12.1) and released into the circulation. Platelet counts in adult blood range between 150 000 and 400 000 $\times$ 10^9/liter with mean platelet volumes of 7–9 fl. Platelet counts in newborns are not different from adults, although the average count in premature infants is slightly lower than for full-term infants. Platelet counts in fetal blood between 18 and 30 weeks of gestation also fall within the adult range with a mean of 250 $\times$ 10^9/liter. Mean platelet volumes in full-term and premature infants are similar to adults. The life span of platelets is approximately 7–10 days in adults, at which time platelets are removed from the circulation by macrophages in the reticuloendothelial system. Platelet survival has not been measured in healthy infants. However, platelet survival measured with indium oxide-labeled adult rabbit platelets was similar for adult and newborn rabbits. Platelet survival in thrombocytopenic infants is shorter than in adults, the least thrombocytopenic infants having the longest survivals, with some in the normal adult range. Together these studies suggest that platelet survival in newborns probably does not differ significantly from adults.

Newborn platelet function has been studied extensively, and there are some well documented differences compared with adults. However, because of the sample volume required to perform platelet function studies, most have been performed on cord platelets rather than platelets directly from newborns. Because cord and newborn platelets may have some differences in function, they are designated separately in this review. Although studies agree that cord platelets function differently from adult platelets, there is not always uniform agreement on the details of the differences. Differences in the timing and method of collection, different sources (newborn vs cord), and differing methods of measuring platelet function all contribute to apparently conflicting reports.

Adhesion and aggregation

Under normal circumstances platelets circulate as disc-shaped structures that do not adhere to vessel walls or to other cells. When the endothelial lining of blood vessels is damaged or removed, platelets adhere to subendothelial layers, undergo shape change, spread over the surface, and bind to each other. Adhesion initiates the secretion of platelet granule contents that include ADP and adhesive proteins such as vWF and fibrinogen. These substances promote both adhesion and formation of aggregates. Platelets also participate in coagulation by providing a lipoprotein surface on which the soluble coagulation factor complexes can form, resulting in the generation of thrombin and formation of fibrin. As discussed above, thrombin itself is a potent stimulus of platelet aggregation.

The process of platelet adhesion involves a specific component of the platelet membrane, glycoprotein Ib, and an adhesive protein, vWF. Glycoprotein Ib is present on fetal platelet membranes in adult amounts. vWF is secreted by endothelial cells and platelets, and is present in both the subendothelium and plasma. Plasma concentrations of vWF are greater in newborns than in adults. In addition, the high molecular weight multimers of vWF are present in increased concentrations in newborns, thereby promoting vWF platelet adherence. The latter is reflected by the enhanced platelet agglutination response of cord platelets to low concentrations of ristocetin (Fig. 12.12). *In vitro* measurement of cord platelet adhesion has not produced consistent results.

Following activation of platelets, glycoproteins IIb and IIIa come together on the platelet surface to form a complex. The glycoprotein IIa/IIIb complex forms a binding site for fibrinogen, which binds adjacent platelets together in a process called platelet aggregation. The IIa/IIIb platelet glycoproteins are present on fetal platelet membranes from early gestation. The response of cord platelets to a variety of agonists, including ADP, epinephrine, collagen, thrombin, and arachidonic acid, has been variable, with some observations more consistent than others. Cord platelet aggregation in response to epinephrine is markedly impaired due to decreased numbers of α-adrenergic receptors. This may be due to delayed maturation of these receptors or to occupation by catecholamines that are released during the birth process. Of the other agonists, decreased cord platelet aggregation to collagen is the most consistent defect.

Normal aggregation is dependent on secretion of platelet granule contents. The decreased aggregation of cord platelets in response to collagen implies the presence of either a storage pool deficiency or an abnormality in secretion. Cord platelets have been examined for the presence of secretory granules and defects in release mechanisms. Electron microscopy studies have demonstrated normal numbers of granules; however, serotonin and ADP, which are stored in dense granules, are present at concentrations less than 50 percent of adult values. Cord platelets, however, can bind and concentrate exogenous ADP and serotonin in their granules normally. Thus a classic storage pool deficiency does not appear to be present.

Platelet secretion is a process whereby platelet granules form a cluster, then fuse with the membranes of other granules or the open connected canalicular system. The clustering of granules depends on the interaction of actin and myosin filaments, which in turn depends on Ca^{2+}/calmodulin activation of myosin light-chain kinase. The fusion of granules depends on protein kinase C. Studies of activation pathways leading to release have not identified specific abnormalities in cord platelets. Inositol phosphate production and protein phosphorylation are normal, as are production of arachidonic acid and its metabolites. In fact, cord platelets release more arachidonic acid than adult platelets in response to stimulation by thrombin. The latter may be due to platelet membranes made more reactive by low levels of vitamin E. Agonist receptors, with the exception of the α-adrenergic receptor discussed previously, do not appear to be decreased in number. Despite a poor response to collagen stimulation, cord platelets have normal amounts of the collagen receptor glycoprotein Ia/IIa present on platelet membranes. Coupling of agonist receptors to phospholipases may be the site of this transient activation defect.

A few studies have assessed platelet aggregation using newborn platelets obtained during the first few days of life; other studies have evaluated older neonates. In one study, abnormal platelet aggregation to ADP (decreased primary wave and absent secondary wave) was observed in cord platelet-rich plasma. However, improved platelet aggregation was seen in newborn platelets drawn 2 hours after birth, with normalization of platelet aggregation at 48 hours.

Although earlier studies suggested abnormalities in clot contraction, recent quantitative studies have shown no difference between adult and cord platelets. Thus both fibrinogen receptors and contractile cytoskeletons are functioning normally.

Bleeding time

Currently, bleeding time is the best *in vivo* test of platelet interaction with the vessel wall. This is particularly true for newborns, in whom platelet aggregation studies frequently are not feasible. Recently, automated devices modified for newborns and children have become available and the methodology for measuring bleeding times standardized. Bleeding times in infants during the first week of life are significantly shorter than in adults. Several mechanisms probably contribute to this enhanced platelet/vessel wall interaction, including: higher plasma concentrations of vWF in newborns; enhanced function of vWF due to increased amounts of high molecular weight, active multimers; large red cells; and high hematocrits. The significance of mild platelet aggregation defects in cord compared with adult platelets is uncertain, as bleeding times in newborns are even shorter than in adults. Throughout the rest of childhood, bleeding times are prolonged compared with adults for reasons that are not apparent. Platelet aggregation studies are similar in children compared with adults. Some evidence indicates that the vessel wall undergoes an aging process that likely begins in early life.

Activation during birth process

There is strong evidence that platelets are activated during the birth process. Cord plasma concentrations of thromboxane B_2, thromboglobulin, and platelet factor 4 are increased. Consistent with these observations, granular content of cord platelets is decreased and epinephrine receptor availability on platelets is reduced, perhaps secondary to occupation. The mechanisms of activation are likely multifactorial and include thermal changes, hypoxia, acidosis, adrenergic stimulation, and thrombogenic effects of amniotic fluid.

Conclusions

The physiological development of hemostasis in humans is a dynamic process that assumes many forms depending

upon the age of the subject. Hemostasis evolves from a relatively immature form in early fetal life to a mature adult form. In healthy fetuses, infants, and children, appropriate hemostasis is achieved and neither hemorrhagic nor thrombotic complications occur. Thus the hemostatic systems at these times of life must be considered physiological, not pathological variations of the adult system. Indeed, convincing evidence demonstrates that *thrombotic complications* occur far less frequently in children than in adults, suggesting that there are physiological advantages of the hemostatic system in the young. Detailed studies of the hemostatic system have provided evidence that an enhanced regulation of thrombin in the young is at least one mechanism contributing to this observation. Prolonged bleeding times in childhood suggest that there may be important differences in vessel wall function that contribute to protection from thrombotic complications. Concentrations of vessel wall glycosaminoglycans vary with age, perhaps affecting the antithrombotic potential in the young. Because the fibrinolytic system is suppressed in the young, it seems unlikely that the regulation of plasmin contributes to the decreased risk of thrombotic complications in the young. However, one has to be concerned that when large vessel thrombi occur in children, thrombolysis of the clot may not be as effective as in adults. Developmental aspects of hemostasis are important because they influence the clinical presentation of hemostatic problems and the selection of therapeutic options for pediatric patients.

Selected reading

Aballi AJ, de Lamerens S. Coagulation changes in the neonatal period and in early infancy. *Pediatr Clin North Am* 1962; **9**: 785.

Andrew M. Platelets in newborns: physiology and pathology. In Luban N, ed. *Transfusion sciences*. Vol. 12(4): 2. Elmsford, NY: Pergamon Press, 1991: 207.

Andrew M, Paes B, Johnston M. Development of the hemostatic system in the neonate and young infant. Clinical Research Update. *Am J Pediatr Hematol Oncol* 1990; **12**: 95.

Corrigan JJ, Sleeth JJ, Jeter M, Lox CD. Newborn's fibrinolytic mechanism: components and plasmin generation. *Am J Hematol* 1989; **32**: 273.

Hathaway W, Corrigan J. Report of the scientific and standardization subcommittee on neonatal hemostasis. *Thromb Haemostas* 1991; **65**: 323.

Schmidt B, Mitchell L, Ofosu FA, Andrew M. Alpha-2-macroglobulin is an important progressive inhibitor of thrombin in neonatal and infant plasma. *Thromb Haemostas* 1989; **62**: 1077.

13 ◆ *The immune system*

Editor: Arthur J Ammann

A. Development of Immunity

H D Ochs

Ontogeny of T-cell immunity

T-cell development in the thymus

Several lines of evidence support the importance of a thymus for T-lymphocyte development. Neonatal thymectomy in the mouse results in long-lasting impairment of cell-mediated immunity by preventing the appearance of T cells in peripheral lymphoid organs. Similarly, T cells fail to develop in *congenital athymia*, e.g. in human infants with *DiGeorge syndrome*. The thymus originates from epithelial rudiments derived from the third and fourth pharyngeal pouches. In man, this outgrowth occurs between 6 and 7 weeks of gestation, and the first lymphocytes appear in the thymus between 9 and 10 weeks of gestation. The concept of the thymus being the primary lymphoid organ of T-cell maturation and selection, from which mature T-lineage cells emigrate to colonize the periphery, first developed by studying mice, has to a large extent been confirmed in humans by phenotypic and functional studies of human fetal tissues.

Phenotypic analysis of immune cells has become possible primarily through the use of monoclonal antibodies, which specifically identify functional categories of cells, such as T cells, B cells, and natural killer (NK) cells, as well as cell populations that vary in degrees of maturity. For convenience and organizational reasons, a uniform designation system has been developed to identify these cells which are defined by the reaction of cell-surface receptors or ligands with specific monoclonal antibodies as cluster of differentiation (CD). Once defined by a monoclonal antibody, specific functions can be assigned to different cell types. The cells entering the human thymus between 7 and 9 weeks of gestation express on their surface CD7 and CD45, a protein tyrosine phosphatase, but lack the other markers characteristic of mature T cells. Soon thereafter, they begin to express CD3, a component of the T-cell receptor (TCR) complex, and CD2, a molecule involved in cell adhesion and T-cell activation. By 12 weeks, cells expressing high levels of TCR–CD3 complex can be readily identified. The major functional subdivision of T cells into T helper cells ($CD4^+$) and T suppressor cells ($CD8^+$) is initiated in the thymus. T helper cells are those cells which assist B cells in the formation of antibody, whereas T suppressor cells suppress the antibody formation by B cells. Thymocytes within the human fetal thymus show a rapid progression and maturation through initial stages involving $CD4^-$, $CD8^-$ (double negative) to $CD4^+$, $CD8^+$ (double positive) and, finally, to $CD4^+$ and $CD8^+$ cells, which are mutually exclusive (single positive). During the maturation process, extensive selection, both positive and negative, takes place. Studies of fetal mouse thymus suggest that T-cell maturation beyond the double positive stage of the thymus requires interaction of TCR with self-major histocompatibility complex (MHC) molecules, probably in association with self-peptides, resulting in a subset of thymocytes with significant binding affinity for MHC molecules. Through this process a post-thymic T-cell repertoire with self-restriction is generated. The concept of negative selection is based on the observation that most thymocytes die *in situ*, and on numerous reports describing direct thymus deletion of autoreactive clones in the mouse. It is hypothesized that this process also occurs in the human, mainly at the immature double positive stage.

Following maturation, the rate of T-cell export from the human fetal thymus increases rapidly. $CD3^+$ cells can be detected in fetal blood by 12 weeks of gestation, and at 14 weeks 20–30 percent of peripheral blood lymphocytes are $CD3^+$, expressing either CD4 or CD8, but not both; almost all express CD45RA, an isoform of CD45 associated with 'naive' T cells (cells not yet stimulated by antigen). Between 12 and 14 weeks of gestation, the development of the thymus is largely completed and, except for size, is similar to that of the newborn and infant in biological responsiveness.

Phenotypes of post-thymic T cells
(Table 13.1)

Following emigration from the thymus, mature T lymphocytes, consisting mainly of $CD4^+$ and $CD8^+$ cells,

Table 13.1. Cell markers characteristic for T and B lymphocytes

Antigen	Distribution
CD1 a,b,c	Thymocytes, dendritic cells, early B (CD1c)
CD2	T, (NK), [*SRBC-receptor*]
CD3	T
CD7	T, (NK)
CD28	T, (plasma cells)
CD4	T subset (ligand for MHC class II)
CD8	T subset (ligand for MHC class I)
CD29	T subset (β_1-integrin subunit)
CDw60	T subset
CD19	B (follicular dendritic cells)
CD20	B
CD21	B (CR2 = C3d receptor; EBV receptor)
CD22	B
CD23	B, low affinity Fcε receptor
CD24	B (granulocytes)
CD37	B
CD39	B (follicular dendritic cells, macrophages)
CD40	B (follicular dendritic cells)
CD72	B
CD77	B, activated
CD5	T, B subset
CD6	T, B subset
CD45	T, B and other hematopoietically derived cells (human leukocyte common antigen)
CD45RA (205/220 kDa)	T, B (subset naive), recognized by mAb 2H4
CD45RO (180 kDa)	T, B (activated, memory), recognized by mAb UCHL1

take up residence in secondary lymphoid organs, where they interact with antigen-presenting cells and B lymphocytes. T cells recognize specific antigen with the TCR, whose structure has similarities to immunoglobulins (Igs). Specific protein antigen can be recognized by TCR only if presented in the form of small peptides closely associated with MHC molecules on the surface of antigen-presenting cells.

Exposure to specific antigen results in T-cell activation and generation of memory T cells. This process is associated with changes in the expression of isoforms of the common leukocyte antigen, CD45, a protein tyrosine phosphatase. The CD45 antigen molecule can exist in at least five isoforms. However, two major subsets of T cells can be identified: CD45RA$^+$ and CD45RO. The expression of CD45RA and CD45RO in human T lymphocytes is in most instances mutually exclusive, each representing approximately 50 percent of peripheral blood T cells in the adult. Following mitogen stimulation *in vitro*, individual CD4$^+$ or CD8$^+$, CD45RA$^+$ T cells lose surface expression of CD45RA and express CD45RO antigen. Of interest, cord blood T cells consist almost exclusively of CD45RA$^+$ cells, which upon activation *in vitro* with PHA switch to the CD45RO phenotype. It is generally accepted that naive T cells lose CD45RA and gain CD45RO upon activation by specific antigen, and that a portion of the CD45RO cells become long-lived memory T cells. CD45RA$^+$ cells selectively produce interleukin-2 (IL-2) following stimulation by mitogens. In contrast, CD45RO$^+$ cells produce large amounts of IL-2, as well as IL-4 and interferon-γ (IFN-γ) after similar stimulation. Thus, there appears to be a clear qualitative difference between unprimed and primed T cells: antigenically naive cells can respond to activation by IL-2 synthesis and proliferation but, unlike antigenically experienced cells, cannot secrete the other effector lymphokines necessary for mature immune responses.

Other surface molecules preferentially expressed on memory T cells include adhesion molecules or integrins and their specific ligands. These receptor/ligand pairs ensure tight binding between lymphocyte subsets and antigen-presenting cells, and between cells and extracellular matrix, allowing a more intense response to activation signals. Many adhesion molecules have been identified and include lymphocyte function-associated antigen 1 (LFA-1) and very late antigen 4 (VLA-4), and ligands ICAM-1 and VCAM-1, respectively.

Ontogeny of B-cell immunity

B-cell development in the fetus

In humans, early B-cell development occurs in the fetal liver and bone marrow. Pre-B cells exhibiting cytoplasmic μ chains, the precursor for immunoglobulin M (IgM), are first recognized in the human liver by 7–8 weeks of gestation. Between 11 and 16 weeks, pre-B cells constitute 1–4 percent of nucleated liver cells and are twice as numerous as surface IgM+ B cells. As the fetus grows older, both pre-B cells and surface IgM+ B cells shift from liver to bone marrow, where pre-B cells persist throughout adult life. The first step in B-cell differentiation (Fig. 13.1) is Ig gene rearrangement. Following transcription of μ heavy chains, the cell appears morphologically as a pre-B cell. Subsequent rearrangement of light chains results in surface IgM+ B lymphocytes. Up to this point, B-cell development is antigen independent and is presumably controlled by stromal reticular cells, which produce B-cell-active cytokines. A large proportion of pre-B cells and early B cells appears to be programmed for death, possibly due to faulty or abortive rearrangements. Successful rearrangement leads to surface IgM expression and release of B cells from the bone marrow into the periphery and into secondary lymphoid organs. Negative selection, both before and after export from the bone marrow, may play a major role in the deletion of autoreactive B-cell populations. The surviving cells in adult humans form a stable, long-lived population of B cells and are submitted to selective forces determined by antigen exposure. Surface IgM serves as antigen receptor and, if triggered by antigen, initiates antigen-specific clonal expansion.

Human Ig genes and class switching

Ig molecules consist of two pairs of heavy and light polypeptide chains and are coded for by three gene families. The gene for the heavy chain is on chromosome 14; the gene for the κ light chain is on chromosome 2, and the gene for the λ light chain on chromosome 22. Each of these genes contains a variable (wherein the

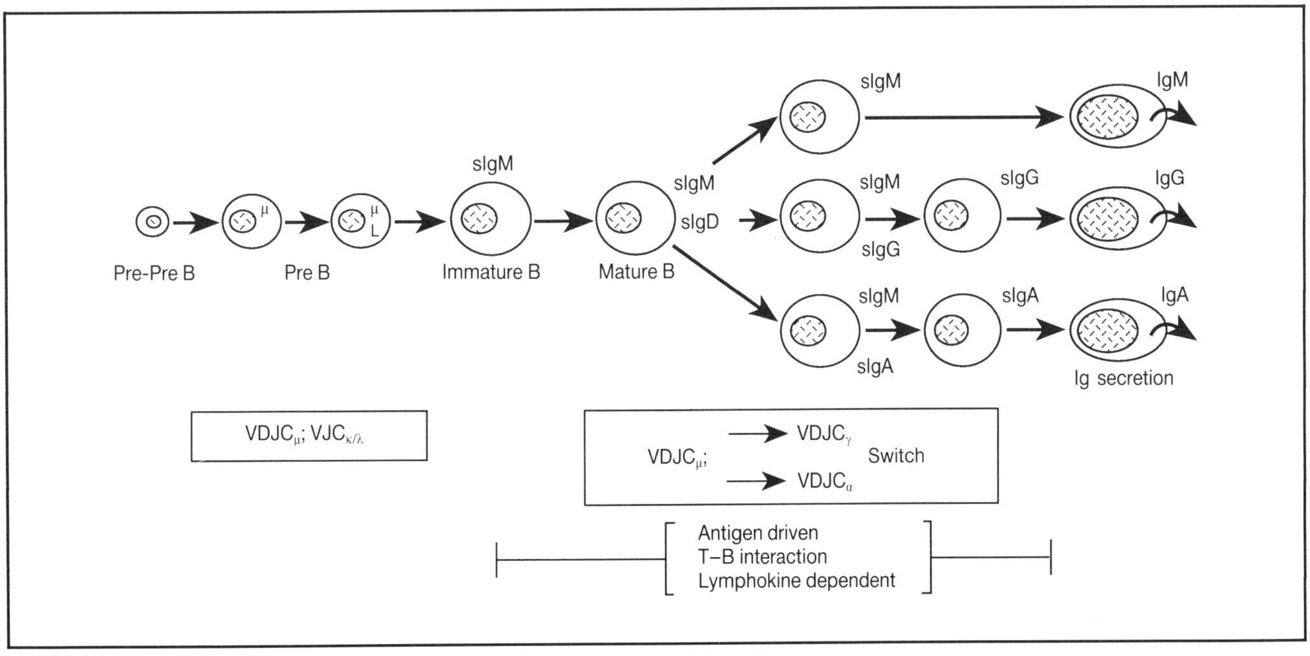

Fig. 13.1. Early (antigen-independent) and late (antigen-dependent) stages of B-cell development (see text for abbreviations).

capacity for antibody diversity resides) and a constant (C) gene region. The heavy (H) chain locus consists of multiple copies of V_H (variable), D_H (diversity) and J_H (joining) genes. The VDJ region is linked to a cluster of C_H constant genes that encode the different heavy-chain classes (μ, δ, γ3, γ1, α1, γ2, γ4, ε, α2). Each heavy-chain class defines an Ig class with distinct biological function such as half-life, passage across the placenta, and complement fixation. The two light-chain gene loci contain only V_L and J_L.

Class (isotype) switching

(see also Section 13B, p. 669)

The first heavy chain expressed during B-cell differentiation is μ, resulting in a IgM^+ B cell. Isotype switching can occur during subsequent B-cell differentiation and requires exposure to antigen and interaction with T lymphocytes. Details of the switch mechanism are not well understood, but there is evidence suggesting that T-cell-derived cytokines (lymphokines) influence the expression of different isotypes. For example, IL-4 induces the expression of IgE, and IFN-γ suppresses expression of IgE.

The antibody response

Only those B cells displaying Ig receptors that bind specific antigen with certain threshold affinity become stimulated. After antigen exposure and surface Ig expression, B cells must encounter T cells displaying receptors for the same antigen, and interact with each other through direct cell-to-cell contact. The chances of encounter are best in the secondary lymphoid organs. After seeing the right antigen, B lymphocytes are activated by growth and differentiation signals from T helper cells, and begin to proliferate for as long as antigen and T help are present. Some of the progeny develop into memory cells, which stop dividing and enter a resting phase until reactivated by the specific antigen. These memory B cells respond to a secondary antigenic challenge more rapidly than the unstimulated B cells. Other B cells differentiate into plasma cells that secrete large quantities of antibodies until they die. The first exposure to new antigen results in a predominantly IgM response, while the second exposure to the same antigen elicits a rapid increase in antibody concentration and a long persistence of IgG antibody. Secondary responses persist for many months or years, possibly due to continuous stimulation by antigen stored and processed by follicular dendritic cells or Langerhans cells. A typical secondary response requires T–B-cell interaction and is supported by adhesion molecules and complement activation.

Antibody production is a consequence of a series of reactions highly dependent on cellular interaction. Antigen binding to membrane Ig receptors of B cells causes crosslinking of the receptor and release of intracellular Ca^{2+} via the phosphoinositol system. The membrane Ig mediated activation of B cells may render B cells ready for the reception of signals from T helper cells. The formation of stable T helper cell–B cell conjugates is an important part of growth and differentiation. The stability of this conjugate is enhanced by the binding of LFA-1 to its ligand, ICAM-1 (and other adhesion molecule/ligand pairs), CD4 to the class II proteins, and TCR recognition of the class II–antigen complex. Following this interactive process, B cells increase RNA synthesis, resulting in B-cell competence for stimulation by T-cell-derived lymphokines such as IL-4 and IFN-γ.

Selected reading

Aspinall R, Kampinga J, van den Bogaerde J. T cell development in the fetus and the invariant series hypothesis. *Immunol Today* 1991; **12**: 7.

Lawton AR. B cell development. In Polin RA, Fox WW, eds. *Fetal and neonatal physiology*. Vol. II. Philadelphia: WB Saunders Company, 1992: 1432.

Mackay CR. T cell memory: the connection between function, phenotype and migration pathways. *Immunol Today* 1991; **12**: 189.

McDuffie M, Hayward AR. T cell development. In Polin RA, Fox WW, eds. *Fetal and neonatal physiology*. Vol. II. Philadelphia: WB Saunders Company, 1992: 1427.

Noelle RJ, Snow EC. Cognate interactions between helper T cells and B cells. *Immunol Today* 1990; **11**: 361.

Vitetta ES, Berton MT, Burger C, *et al*. Memory B and T cells. *Annu Rev Immunol* 1991; **9**: 193.

B. Protective Immunity

S K Burchett

Protective immunity is either actively or passively acquired. Both mechanisms of protection are tailored to specific foreign microbial agents or antigens and involve specific antibody and cellular responses. When a unique antigen is presented to the immune system, through gene rearrangement B cells produce antibody specific to that antigen, and T cells are programmed to modulate a series of cell–cell interactions that either amplify (help) or hamper (suppress) the immune system or act directly against cells targeted for destruction by the invading antigen. These maturational changes resulting in specificity of both the B-cell and T-cell arms of the immune response are orchestrated by soluble molecules called cytokines, which act as intercellular messengers to provide a means of communication.

Active immunity

B lymphocytes and antibody

B cells mediate humoral immunity by producing specific antibodies (immunoglobulins [Igs]) in response to a foreign protein or carbohydrate antigen (pathogen or toxin). Maturation of B cells progresses from an antigen-independent phase, when pre-B cells mature to B lymphocytes, to an antigen-dependent phase, when B lymphocytes mature to antibody-producing plasma cells. Ig isotypes are IgM, IgG_1, IgG_2, IgG_3, IgG_4, IgA_1, IgA_2, IgE, and IgD, each of which has a different biological mode of action. In order to generate a population of B cells with unique antibody receptors, a cascade of gene rearrangements of the Ig variable region encodes for antibody specificity and polyclonal proliferation occurs (see Section 13A, p. 667).

Isotype switching

B lymphocytes can switch Ig subclass production, but these antibodies will still retain the original antigen-binding specificity. The switch occurs within the heavy chain of IgM by deleting DNA sequences in the switch region. The new gene segment codes for the heavy chain of a different isotype, and the cell then makes only the new Ig isotype. B cells are stimulated to proliferate when the specific antigen to which the surface-bound antibody was made is presented, and clonal expansion ensues with production of additional antibody. Maturation of B cells to plasma cells allows for 'mass production' of this specific antibody, which is then secreted. This latter process is regulated by antigen/pathogen, interaction with T cells, monocytes, and complement.

Ig function

IgG constitutes 75 percent of total adult serum Ig. Its major mechanism of action is to bind to antigen and fix complement, which establishes a cascade of events resulting in destruction of the antigen. The constant region of the heavy chain determines complement fixation, placental transport, and binding to Fc receptors.

IgM fixes complement more efficiently than IgG and is the earliest Ig produced in natural infections. IgM, a pentamer of approximately 900 kDa, is too large to cross the placenta.

IgA is a class of immunoglobulin found in serum and in secretions (tears, saliva, nasal mucosa, bronchial, prostatic, vaginal, and intestinal). Secretory IgA probably plays a major role in protection from certain bacteria and possible viruses whose portal of entry is through mucous membranes. It likely inhibits bacterial adherence to mucosal surfaces and may neutralize viruses. Secretory IgA is composed of two IgA molecules joined by a J segment and a secretory component (produced from mucosal epithelial cells). Breast-feeding provides secretory IgA to the infant, which may provide a local gastro-intestinal barrier but is not absorbed. Infant concentrations are only 20 percent of adult concentrations by 1 year of age unless the immune system had a particular antigenic stimulus. The infant or even fetus has a marked capacity for IgA production if stimulated. In fact, increased neonatal blood concentrations often indicate congenital infection.

IgD is an Ig found in the circulation in small quantities. Its function is not well defined.

Passive immunity

The fetus is usually well protected in the intrauterine environment by the maternal defense system. However, the fetal/infant Ig production capacity matures gradually. Adult Ig concentrations are not attained for IgM, IgG, and IgA until 1 year, 6 years and 13 years, respectively. This slow rise in IgG produced by the infant reflects intrinsic B-cell development and the delayed inducibility, in infants, to switch from IgM to IgG and IgA production. Responsiveness to different kinds of antigens is also sequentially developed. Responses to most protein antigens require T-cell help and are inducible in the newborn interval. However, responses to bacterial polysaccharide antigens, which are essentially T cell independent, are usually mediated through IgG_2, which does not reach adult serum concentrations until 10 years of age. Bacteria with polysaccharide capsular coats can be major pathogens of infancy and childhood, especially in the first 2 years of life when the immune system is naive to foreign antigens.

During the interval of greatest host vulnerability (i.e. early infancy), passive transfer of maternal IgG across the placenta to the fetus transiently provides the newborn with antibody to a wide variety of antigens (potential pathogens). Igs of the IgG class are the only antibodies that cross the placenta. The half-life is approximately 1 month in the infant's circulation, so that concentrations of specific maternal antibody in the infant are low or absent by about 1 year of age. For passively acquired antibody to be sufficient to ablate disease to which the infant is exposed, the concentration of antibody must be adequate to result in biological activity. However, killing of the pathogen depends not only on IgG concentrations but also on other factors available to the neonate (cellular immunity, cytokines). IgG begins to cross the placenta to the fetus at 8 weeks of gestation, but transport remains low until about 20 weeks. At delivery of a term infant, neonatal IgG is equal to or slightly greater than maternal IgG. A premature infant will have low titers of maternal Ig, as will infants born to mothers who have acquired an infection late in pregnancy such that isotype switching to IgG had not been in place long enough to provide adequate IgG concentrations. An example of how an understanding of the passive immune system has resulted in a world health policy that has markedly reduced a leading cause of death in newborns is that of *tetanus*. Infants delivered in unsanitary circumstances can be exposed to the organism causing tetanus, contract the infection, and die. Routine health care practice in many developing countries, where these delivery conditions exist, includes maternal immunization against tetanus at 6 months of pregnancy. The maternal immune system responds by producing high titers of antibody, which crosses the placenta, and protects the newborn if exposed to tetanus.

T lymphocytes

T lymphocytes develop in the thymus and are subsequently distributed to the peripheral immune system to recognize antigens and pathogens with a resultant cascade of effects (see Section 13A, p. 665). When stimulated, T cells replicate and/or participate in one of three functions: (1) help, by stimulating the responses of other cells in the immune system; (2) suppression, by inhibiting the responses of other cells in the immune system; or (3) cytotoxic activity, by directly killing target cells.

Thymic development

T-cell lymphocytes develop in the microenvironment of the thymus. As the thymocytes move from the cortex to the medulla, they undergo a sequence of maturational processes such that many surface markers change (see Section 13A, p. 665). The resultant, functional circulating T lymphocytes can be grouped into two predominant phenotypes with common markers, yet differentiated by the presence of $CD4^+$ or $CD8^+$. $CD4^+$ cells constitute approximately 65 percent of peripheral T cells, and $CD8^+$ cells are approximately 35 percent. T cells are found in the peripheral blood and in secondary lymphoid tissue such as the spleen and peripheral lymph nodes.

T-cell-surface receptor

The T-cell-surface receptor (TCR) consists of an α and a β chain (each of which contains variable and constant domains); antigen binds through the variable regions. The β chain variable region is produced by sequential gene rearrangement of diversity (D), joining (J), and variable (V) gene segments to form a VDJ gene. This joins to the constant region and codes for β chain. The α chain is synthesized in much the same way. Sometimes cells will express γ-δ heterodimer rather than α-β. Akin to Igs, a given T cell expresses only one α-β or γ-δ surface receptor, thereby defining specificity. TCR complexes with CD3 before activation of the T-cell cascade. The CD3 complex acts in signal transduction to activate T cells when antigen binds. The T-cell repertoire for antigen response is almost as great as the B-cell repertoire. This process is quite similar to the rearrangement that takes place with Ig production. In fact, the TCR and Igs likely evolved from the same supergene family.

T-cell activation

T lymphocytes predominantly recognize antigen in the context of presentation with surface-associated proteins of the major histocompatibility complex (MHC). This dual recognition of antigen and MHC initiates both the effects of cytotoxic effector T cells and immunoregulatory T cells. The latter pathway is important in activating B cells and Ig production. Help is provided by $CD4^+$ cells after interacting with antigen and MHC class II molecules. Suppression/cytotoxicity is effected by $CD8^+$ cells in response to antigen (such as virus or tumor) in association with MHC class I antigens. Depending on surface molecule production, these T lymphocytes secrete cytokines after stimulation by antigens. Cytokines produced include interleukin-2 (IL-2), interferon-γ (IFN-γ), lymphotoxin, and granulocyte macrophage-colony stimulating factor (GM-CSF).

Resting T cells do not express IL-2 receptor (IL-2R). However, when the TCR is triggered by antigen and MHC binding, IL-2 receptors are then produced within hours. IL-2 binds to IL-2 receptors, and cell proliferation results. If there is not continued antigenic stimulation, the number of IL-2 receptors is reduced. Conversely, for continuation of the T-cell activation process, IL-1 (a macrophage product) is necessary.

T-cell function

T-cell function is often defined best when function is absent. This can result from a system that has not yet developed but has all of the appropriate machinery to develop adequately, or from a congenital absence of function. Occasionally disease will result in an acquired lack of function.

T-cell cytotoxicity results in resistance to viral infection and tumors. After activation, these T cells adhere to their target and release proteins much like complement, which lyse the target cell. Immature neonatal cells do not lyse targets as effectively as adult cells, which may lead to poor neonatal primary response to viral infections.

Specific cellular immunity is determined by lymphocyte proliferation or IFN-γ production, is essentially absent at birth, and is slow to respond in infants infected at birth with a pathogen that is recognized primarily by the T-cell pathway. For example, in infant herpes simplex virus infection, lymphocyte proliferation and IFN-γ production to HSV can be delayed for more than 8 weeks after infection. This delay in T-cell activation and response may well predispose infants to more severe disease.

There are many examples of congenital defects in which the T-cell activation process is dysfunctional, resulting in disease. Probably the best studied disease that has elucidated much of our understanding of the function of T cells derives from HIV-infected patients. HIV infects $CD4^+$ T cells by binding to CD4 receptor and replicates in activated $CD4^+$ T cells. In persons infected with the human immunodeficiency virus (HIV), the lack of an intact, functioning T-cell defense system is well appreciated as the *acquired immune deficiency syndrome (AIDS)* ensues, and a variety of opportunistic infections results. Persons with HIV may have recurrent, severe episodes of opportunistic infections such as herpes simplex virus, fungal infections, or parasitic infections such as *toxoplasmosis*. These manifestations exemplify the importance of immune memory to previously experienced pathogens and the consequences when memory is no longer adequate as well as the poor Ig response when T-cell help is no longer adequate. Understanding of the T-cell activation process has provided potential strategies for therapeutic intervention in AIDS.

Cytokines

Cells in the immune system are able to secrete a variety of molecules that can act as communication tools such that direct cell–cell contact is not necessary to effect cellular responses. Molecules produced by lymphocytes are called lymphokines, and those produced by monocytes/macrophages are monokines. Together these are called cytokines. These cytokines are involved in two basic processes: cell proliferation and directed maturation as seen in the immune response. Effects can be stimulatory or inhibitory and can act on a variety of cell types depending upon whether cytokine receptors are present. Cytokines are involved in regulation of Ig class switching at the level of gene rearrangement and are involved in activation of T cells. Often these messengers are produced in response to activation of the immune system. Although the production and release of cytokines may be triggered by antigen, the composition of the cytokine is not related to the molecular composition of the antigen. Thus these are relatively nonspecific messengers. They may act locally where they are produced, act on the cell that secreted them, or act at distant sites, much as hormones generating systemic effects. Improper control of cytokines may result in excessive or inadequate production and subsequent disease.

Growth factors

Many cytokines act as growth factors and may be called colony stimulating factors (CSFs) when they augment production of a particular cell lineage. For example, CSF-1 has relative specificity for macrophages and has effects on differentiated macrophages, but may also act to induce granulocyte production. G-CSF (granulocyte-CSF) classically acts on granulocytes but can also induce pre-B cells. The cytokine growth factors neither have specificity of action on a particular cell lineage nor act at a single level of differentiation or maturation.

To have an effect on cell growth, growth factors must bind to a surface receptor. Thus while the cytokines themselves are not completely lineage specific, some specificity is derived from the presence or absence of certain classes of surface receptors. These classes of receptors suggest certain families of receptors. For example, one class lacks tyrosine kinase activity and is unique in the extracellular binding domain. This class includes GM-CSF, IL-2, IL-6, and IL-7. Another family has tyrosine kinase activity and is in the cytoplasmic domain. This class includes CSF-1.

Growth factors involved in the immune process can be grouped by cell of production and cell of action. T cells produce GM-CSF, IL-2, IL-3, IL-4, and IL-5. GM-CSF is active in stimulating granulocytes to participate in host defense by stimulating phagocytosis and priming for other defense mechanisms such as chemotaxis. Inappropriate control allows for hyperstimulation of the granulocyte cell line and can result in leukemia. IL-3 is a rather non-specific growth factor and augments proliferation of monocytes/macrophages and may enhance Ig responses to T-cell-dependent antigens.

Interleukins

The distinction between cytokine growth factors and ILs (i.e. intercellular messengers) is often nebulous. However, if one considers ILs that are released in response to antigen, relevance to the immune response becomes clearer.

IL-2 is a well studied cytokine because it is pivotal in the immune response. The resting T cell does not express surface receptors for IL-2 until the immune process has been initiated by antigen. Binding of IL-2 to IL-2 receptor in the context of TCR/CD3 allows for T-cell clonal expansion to a specific antigen. In addition, IL-2 likely plays a part in T-cell maturation. It enhances cytotoxic cell activity against tumor cells independent of the MHC, and is critical to clonal expansion of cytotoxic T cells. The action of IL-4 on B cells is similar to that of IL-2 on T cells. IL-4 activates maturation of the resting B cell to a proliferating B cell in the presence of antigen.

Interferon-γ is also produced by activated T cells. It has a variety of effects in the immune system including augmentation of B-cell-stimulating cytokines and increasing antibody synthesis.

IL-1 is produced by many cells including T and B lymphocytes. It is induced by antigens and toxins and during the immune response activates synthesis of other cytokines and directly activates the T cell. IL-1 has many systemic effects, some often deleterious, including induction of fever, synthesis of acute phase proteins, and the release of ACTH and cortisol. Effects on endothelial cells can lead to hypotension and shock (by stimulating NO synthesis; see p. 469), an effect shared by another cytokine, tumor necrosis factor.

Decreased production of cytokines has been observed in some disease states. Cells may lack the innate ability to produce cytokines or their receptors, and disease results, or disease may cause inadequate production or activity of cytokines. An example of the former is found in neonatal T cells. Although these cells synthesize IL-2 and IL-2 receptor and production of most lymphokines is adequate, little IFN-γ is produced. In response to specific antigenic stimulation such as herpes simplex virus infection, neonatal T cells can produce IFN-γ, but this capacity develops far into the course of illness. This lack of IFN-γ may be responsible for the inability of neonates to curtail herpes simplex virus effectively, which often results in severe morbidity or even death.

An example of disease causing inadequate cytokine production comes from infectious HIV, which ultimately leads to AIDS. Cells from HIV-infected persons produce decreased amounts of IL-2. HIV likely down-regulates the production of IL-2 or IL-2 receptor, resulting in inadequate T-cell immunity to a variety of opportunistic infections such as fungal, viral, and parasitic infections. As HIV infection progresses, T-cell number decreases, less help is offered to B cells, and severe bacterial infections can also ensue.

Aberrations in the ability to produce many cytokines or to respond to cytokines provide an excellent, albeit unfortunate example of the intricate communication between both the B-cell and T-cell arms of the immune system and the cytokine messengers in the immune response. From basic understanding of the actions of cytokines, therapeutic strategies may well be developed such that the immune system may be maximally manipulated to produce a desired effect.

Selected reading

Blackwell TK, Alt FW. Mechanism and developmental program of immunoglobulin gene rearrangement in mammals. *Annu Rev Genet* 1989; **23**: 605.

Carding SR, Hayday AL, Bottomly K. Cytokines in T-cell development. *Immunol Today* 1991; **12**: 239.

Royer HD, Reinherz EL. T lymphocytes: ontogeny, function, and relevance to clinical disorders. *N Engl J Med* 1987; **317**: 1136.

C. Hypersensitivity Responses

D S Chudwin

Hypersensitivity responses occur when normal host immunological responses result in pathological damage to the host. These conditions are thus due to an 'overactive' immune system, in contrast to the immunodeficiencies. Gell and Coombs have classified hypersensitivity responses into four classes based on pathophysiological mechanisms.

Type 1 hypersensitivity (anaphylactic)

Type 1 hypersensitivity occurs when an IgE-mediated immune response results in inflammation due to an allergic reaction. Basophils and mast cells have IgE molecules tightly bound to receptors on their surfaces. Crosslinking of IgE molecules by an antigen, such as ragweed pollen, activates these cells which then release both preformed and newly synthesized chemical mediators. Preformed mediators include histamine, heparin, and neutrophil and eosinophil chemotactic factors. Newly synthesized mediators include cyclooxygenase regulated arachidonic acid metabolites, such as prostaglandin (PG) D_2 and the thromboxanes, lipoxygenase-mediated arachidonic acid metabolites, the leukotrienes (LTs), and platelet activating factor (PAF).

The mediators released by mast cells and basophils have important inflammatory actions. Vasoactive mediators include histamine, LTC_4, PGD_2, PAF and adenosine. Mediators with chemotactic activity for neutrophils include LTB_4, PAF and high molecular weight neutrophil chemotactic factor, and for eosinophils, PAF and eosinophil chemotactic factor A. Mediators with enzymatic activity include proteases (tryptase, chymase) and lysosomal hydrolases. The release of these mediators produces both an immediate allergic response and a late phase allergic response.

The immediate allergic response occurs within minutes and is characterized by edema, erythema, itching and mucus production. A clinical example is *anaphylaxis*. Anaphylaxis can be triggered by medications (e.g. penicillin or iodinated contrast media), venomous insect stings, food (e.g. peanuts or fish) or by idiopathic causes. Patients with anaphylaxis develop itching, hives, nausea, dyspnea and hypotension in the early stages. This may progress to angioedema, wheezing, cardiac arrhythmias and shock in more severe cases. Treatment includes epinephrine, intravenous fluids, antihistamines, corticosteroids and treatment for specific organ damage.

Another example of the immediate allergic response is *allergic rhinitis* which is caused by exposure to either seasonal or perennial allergens. Seasonal allergens include grass, tree and weed pollens, as well as mold spores. Perennial allergens include dust mites, cockroaches and animal danders.

Urticaria (hives) are raised, red, itchy welts, while angioedema is swelling of the deep tissues, often noticeably of the eyes, lips or throat. Patients may have urticaria, angioedema or both. The causes of urticaria are many. Immunological factors include allergic reactions via IgE or complement activation due to immune complexes. Non-immunological factors include nonspecific histamine release due to drugs (e.g. opiates) or certain foods (e.g. strawberries, some fish). Hormonal factors include pregnancy and hyperthyroidism. The physical urticarias result from mast cell sensitivity to factors such as cold temperatures, pressure or cholinergic stimulation. All of these processes lead to release of mediators by skin mast cells with resulting hives. Treatment consists of avoidance of triggering factors, antihistamines and corticosteroids.

The late phase allergic response occurs hours after antigen exposure. The first step is the ingress of eosinophils, neutrophils and mononuclear cells to the site of the allergic reaction in response to chemotactic factors. Eosinophils release granular contents, including major basic protein which can damage epithelial cells. Neutrophils release enzymes, while mononuclear cells produce histamine releasing factors. There also is damage to nerve endings which can make them more sensitive. In the lungs, the late phase response is characterized by delayed onset of wheezing and airway obstruction, hours after allergen exposure.

Asthma is a classic example of both the immediate and late phase allergic responses and is characterized by reversible airway obstruction (particularly small airways), airway inflammation, and bronchial hyperresponsiveness to a variety of stimuli. Symptoms often are worse at night and in response to certain triggers, including allergen exposure, exercise, cold air, smoke, medications (aspirin and other nonsteroidal anti-inflammatory drugs) and infections (viruses, *Mycoplasma, Chlamydia*). In many patients, allergic reactions in the lungs may initiate inflammation. The lungs then become responsive to nonspecific stimuli such as exercise or cold air. The pathological findings of asthma include bronchial smooth muscle constriction, mucosal edema, mucus plugging, inflammatory infiltrates and epithelial injury.

Type 2 hypersensitivity (cytotoxic)

Type 2 hypersensitivity takes place when antibodies are directed against cells or tissues in the body. Binding of antibody to the cells leads to complement activation and either cell lysis or damage. Complement activation (see Section 13E) occurs via the classic pathway when IgG or IgM molecules are deposited on a surface. C1, C4, and C2 form a C3 convertase which splits C3. Splitting of C4 leads to activation of the terminal complement components C5 through C9 which can lyse certain cells by forming a pore-like structure through the cell membrane.

Red blood cell *transfusion reactions* are an example of cytotoxic hypersensitivity. The ABO antigen system comprises one of the major blood groups. Allelic genes A, B and O code for transferases which put either galactose (group B), *N*-acetylgalactosamine (group A), or fucose (group O) at the end of a carbohydrate found on the red blood cell surface. Individuals with B blood group recognize group A red cells as foreign and have anti-A antibodies in their plasma. Similarly, people with A blood group have anti-B antibodies, those with group O have both anti-A and anti-B antibodies, while the few individuals with group AB have no plasma antibodies. Transfusion of red blood cells that have not been properly matched may produce a transfusion reaction. For example, if a patient with A blood group receives red blood cells of type B, then anti-B antibodies will attach to the transfused red blood cells and activate complement. This will lyse the red cells and produce intravascular hemolysis. Symptoms include chills, chest and back pain, hypotension and, in severe cases, acute renal failure.

Other examples of type 2 hypersensitivity are disorders in which antibodies are directed against basement membranes. In *Goodpasture syndrome*, patients develop glomerulonephritis and pulmonary hemorrhage. In the skin disease *bullous pemphigoid*, antibodies against the skin basement membrane are found. These IgG antibodies activate complement, and the disease can be passively transferred with these antibodies.

Type 3 hypersensitivity (immune complex)

Soluble antigen–antibody complexes are responsible for type 3 immune complex hypersensitivity. Immune complexes activate complement, initiating an inflammatory response. Deposition of immune complexes in the kidneys causes glomerulonephritis; in the skin, urticaria; and in blood vessels, vasculitis. The size of the immune complexes, the relative antigen/antibody ratio, and their ability to activate complement all affect the degree of tissue damage.

Serum sickness is the classic example of type 3 hypersensitivity. Following administration of a foreign protein (e.g. antitoxin derived from another species) or drug (e.g. penicillin or sulfa drugs), antibodies develop to the foreign substance. After 1–2 weeks, fever, arthritis, urticaria, and lymphadenopathy develop. Initially, there is antigen excess and the antigen–antibody complexes which form are soluble, diffuse into tissues such as the skin and synovium, and activate complement. As antibody production increases, the antigen–antibody complexes become less soluble and are cleared by the liver and spleen.

The *vasculitic disorders* also are due to type 3 hypersensitivity. The size of the blood vessel in which the immune complexes are deposited affects the clinical picture. Small vessel vasculitis clinically presents with palpable purpura and urticaria; syndromes include *systemic lupus erythematosus*, *dermatomyositis* and *Henoch–Schönlein purpura*. Involvement of the small and medium-sized arteries leads to organ damage, especially of the kidney and gut in *polyarteritis nodosa*. Large vessels are involved in *giant cell arteritis* (temporal arteries) or *Takayasu arteritis* (thoracic aorta and large arteries).

Type 4 hypersensitivity

In type 4 hypersensitivity, sensitized lymphocytes recognize a foreign antigen and initiate a cellular immune response. The sensitized lymphocytes become activated and release lymphokines. These expand the clone of activated cells, draw other cells into the area and promote an inflammatory response.

Delayed-type hypersensitivity skin testing (DTH ST) is a method of testing for cellular immune competence which acts by type 4 hypersensitivity. A small amount of antigen is placed intradermally and the site inspected at 48–72 hours. If the patient has previously been exposed to the antigen, an erythematous welt will develop. Antigens commonly employed include *Candida*, tetanus toxoid, mumps and tuberculin purified protein derivative (PPD). A response to one or more of these recall antigens indicates intact cellular immunity. A failure to respond to a battery of four or more antigens may indicate cellular immune dysfunction and is termed 'anergy'. Tuberculosis skin testing is based on the principle that a positive reaction indicates previous sensitization and infection.

Other examples of type 4 hypersensitivity include *organ transplant rejection*, *allergic contact dermatitis*, and *hypersensitivity pneumonitis*. In transplant rejection, lymphocytes recognize foreign histocompatibility antigens on the cell surfaces of the organ, and killer cells attack the transplant. In allergic contact dermatitis, lymphocytes in the skin recognize a variety of chemicals such as nickel, chromium, plant resins such as poison ivy, and topical medications. The clinical result is an eczematous reaction of the skin. With hypersensitivity pneumonitis, cellular sensitivity in the lung develops to organic materials such as the thermophilic actinomycetes or to chemicals such as poison ivy.

Selected reading

Ishizaka K. IgE binding factors and regulation of the IgE antibody response. *Annu Rev Immunol* 1988; **6**: 513.

Pearlman DS, Bierman CW. Allergic disorders. In Stichm ER, ed. *Immunologic disorders in infants and children*. Philadelphia: WB Saunders Company, 1989: 439.

Terr AI. Mechanisms of hypersensitivity. In Stites DP, Terr AI, eds. *Basic and clinical immunology*. 7th ed. Norwalk, CT: Appleton and Lange, 1991: 367.

D. Transplantation Immunology, Graft Rejection and Graft-versus-host Reactions

B L Hamilton

Graft rejection has frustrated surgeons since antiquity. It was known that tissues grafted between individuals died while tissues grafted from one site to another on the same patient survived. Sir Peter Medawar, working in England during World War II, was the first to demonstrate that foreign tissue grafts were rejected by immunological means. Medawar and his associates, Billingham and Brent, went on to describe transplantation tolerance, graft-versus-host reactions (GvHR), and the concept of the fetus as an allograft. Subsequent work by many investigators demonstrated T-cell responsibility for graft rejection and the role of histocompatibility antigens in rejection. Graft rejection is now recognized as one of the most complex immunological reactions known. Rejection involves numerous effector mechanisms and target antigens. Studies of graft rejection and tolerance laid the foundations for our current understanding of the molecular basis of the immune response.

All physicians need to know something of the immunobiology of graft rejection because transplantation and the problems of graft rejection are encountered in many clinical settings, including diagnosis of transplantable disease, selection of appropriate donor–recipient pairs, counseling patients who are considering a transplant, and management of patients undergoing graft rejection or on immunosuppressive drugs to prevent rejection. Perhaps the most common situation involves patients with chronic end-stage renal disease who are frequently considered for renal transplantation as an alternative to chronic hemodialysis. Burn patients are routinely grafted with skin from uninvolved areas and may be given temporary grafts from animal donors. Cardiac transplantation is used to treat some forms of congenital heart disease and severe myocarditis. Liver, heart-lung, and small bowel transplants are becoming increasingly common. Bone marrow transplantation, with its double complications of graft rejection and GvHR, is now a standard treatment for many hematological malignancies, severe aplastic anemia, and a variety of congenital disorders such as cellular immunodeficiencies, thalassemia, and certain metabolic disorders. The problem of GvHR may be present in infants with *severe combined immunodeficiency* who receive a transfusion of maternal lymphocytes across the placental barrier.

Types of grafts

The **nomenclature for grafts** has changed over the years (Table 13.2). Grafts exchanged between two individuals of the same species are called allografts; the older nomenclature for these grafts was homograft. Grafts exchanged between individuals of two different species are called xenografts; the older nomenclature was heterograft. Grafts exchanged between two individuals of the same inbred strain (or between identical twins) are called syngrafts. Grafts transferred from one site to another on the same individual are called autografts. The respective adjectives to describe these grafts are allogeneic, xenogeneic, syngeneic, and autologous. Some tissues and graft sites that are relatively resistant to rejection are referred to as privileged tissues or privileged sites. The cornea is an example of a privileged tissue. Tissues grafted to the correct anatomical site (e.g. typical skin and heart grafts)

Table. 13.2. Nomenclature of grafts

Grafts between:	Current	Adjective	Old	Adjective
Different site of same individual	Autograft	Autologous		
Same strain or identical twins	Syngrafts	Syngeneic		
Individuals of same species	Allograft	Allogeneic	Homograft	Homologous
Individuals of different species	Xenograft	Xenogeneic	Heterograft	Heterologous

are called orthotopic grafts while tissues grafted to incorrect anatomical sites (e.g. thymus to the abdominal fascial planes) are referred to as heterotopic grafts. Thus, pancreatic islet cells injected into the portal vein would lodge in the liver as a heterotopic allograft.

Antigens

Several groups of cell-surface antigens elicit graft rejection reactions. These include antigens encoded by genes of the major histocompatibility complex (MHC), non-MHC minor histocompatibility antigens, and tissue-specific antigens. Other groups of antigens such as the ABO blood group antigens may be involved in the death of organ grafts without eliciting classical rejection reactions.

MHC antigens

All vertebrate species have a gene complex that determines strong (major) allograft rejection reactions. This complex is called the major histocompatibility complex (MHC). The MHC in humans, called HLA (human leukocyte antigen), is located on the short arm of chromosome 6. The MHC of the mouse, H-2, is located on chromosome 17. The MHC is divided into several regions, each highly polymorphic. For example, the HLA complex is divided into A, B, C, and D/DR loci. Antigens encoded by the A, B, and C loci traditionally were defined by serological techniques, while the D region was defined by cell proliferation in mixed lymphocyte culture. Serological reagents are now available that identify three subregions of the D locus called DR, DQ, and DP. Multiple alleles exist for each locus: 24 A alleles, 52 B alleles, 11 C, 26 D, 20 DR, 9 DQ, and 6 DP. Any individual will carry only two alleles at the A locus (one from the paternal and one from the maternal chromosomes). The alleles expressed on the loci linked together on a single chromosome are called a haplotype. Thus, an individual carries two haplotypes.

The gene products encoded by the A, B, and C loci are called MHC class I antigens and are present on most somatic cells. Class I antigens are notably absent from spermatozoa, ova, and the preimplantation embryo. Erythrocytes do not in general express class I antigens, but do express one HLA-A antigen (A28) and three of the HLA-B antigens (B7, B8, and B17). The gene products encoded by the DR locus, referred to as MHC class II antigens, are generally expressed only on selected cell populations such as monocytes/macrophages and B cells. Class I antigens tend to elicit stronger graft rejection reactions than do the class II antigens. A third region of the HLA complex encodes some of the complement components including C2, C4, and factor B; these are referred to as MHC class III antigens. The class III antigens do not elicit graft rejection reactions, but polymorphism present in this region is frequently used to define haplotypes.

Minor histocompatibility antigens

Disparity at the MHC results in the rapid rejection of skin allografts, typically in about 12 days in mice and 17 days in humans. Studies in mice demonstrated that skin grafts exchanged between two strains of mice selected for MHC identity would be rejected in a much more chronic tempo, varying from 25 to over 250 days. About 40 loci have been identified in the genome of the mouse that elicit these weak (minor) rejection reactions. The gene products of these loci are called non-MHC (or non-H-2, or non-HLA) histocompatibility antigens. These antigens are more properly termed minor histocompatibility antigens. Minor histocompatibility antigens are responsible for the majority of rejection reactions when donor and recipient are matched for MHC antigens. It is estimated that there are approximately 100 minor histocompatibility loci in the mouse genome. Similar numbers of minor histocompatibility loci are thought to exist in the human genome, although none has been clearly identified in humans. Few of the minor histocompatibility antigens of the mouse have been identified as specific proteins. One notable exception is the H-3 antigen, identified as β_2-microglobulin, which is polymorphic in the mouse. One minor histocompatibility antigen that is encoded by a gene on the Y chromosome is termed H-Y; the H-Y antigen is responsible for eliciting the rejection of male skin grafts by the females of certain inbred strains of mice.

Tissue-specific antigens

Tissue-specific antigens may also elicit graft rejection reactions. Identifying these antigens in an outbred species such as humans is virtually impossible because of the presence of the minor histocompatibility antigens. Several tissue-specific antigens have been described in mice, such as skin-specific antigens. Tissue- and maturation-specific antigens may also be present on tumors. These tumor-specific antigens can elicit a tumor-specific rejection reaction that may contribute to the spontaneous regression of certain tumors.

Blood group antigens

(see Section 13C, p. 675)

In general, the ABO blood group antigens do not elicit cell-mediated allograft rejection reactions. Incompatibility at ABO can result in the acute death of a vascular graft (e.g. kidneys or hearts). This 'hyperacute' rejection is thought to result from an intravascular transfusion reaction to passenger red blood cells present in the allograft, and possibly to an antibody-mediated reaction to blood group antigens expressed on the allograft endothelium.

Effector mechanisms

T cells clearly are necessary for the initiation of allograft rejection reactions, although additional cell populations may contribute to the effector limb of the response. Experiments in rodents showed that allograft immunity could be transferred with cells, but not with serum, demonstrating that rejection was the result of cell-mediated immunity. The observation that T-cell-deficient animals (neonatally thymectomized or congenitally athymic nude mice) failed to reject allografts and that allograft immunity could be adoptively transferred with T cells demonstrated that rejection was mediated by T cells.

T cells are currently defined by the presence of the T-cell receptor–CD3 complex (TcR–CD3). The T-cell receptor interacts with small peptide antigens that are complexed to MHC class I (HLA-A, B, or C) or MHC class II (HLA-D/DR) antigens. This interaction, a low-affinity bond, is stabilized by several accessory molecules that interact between the T cell and the antigen-bearing cell. The CD8 and CD4 molecules specifically bind to non-polymorphic regions of MHC class I and II molecules, respectively. Thus, $CD8^+$ T cells are restricted to interactions with MHC class I-bearing cells, while $CD4^+$ T cells are restricted to interactions with MHC class II-bearing cells. Each subset includes cells that have helper, killer, and/or suppressor activity. In general, the majority of T killer cell activity is present in the $CD8^+$, MHC class I-restricted population of T cells, while the majority T helper cell activity is mediated by the $CD4^+$, MHC class II-restricted population. The latter population is also the predominant mediator of delayed type hypersensitivity (DTH) because of the array of lymphokines secreted by these cells.

Allograft rejection involves a number of cells and cellular interactions. The reaction traditionally has been divided into three limbs. The afferent limb involves the uptake and processing of antigen by macrophages, the trafficking of these cells from the graft to the regional lymph nodes, and the presentation of antigen to T helper cells. The central limb of the response involves the clonal expansion of antigen-reactive T cells and the maturation of T helper and T killer precursor cells into functional effector cells. The efferent limb involves the various effector cells and mediators that destroy the graft.

Afferent limb

Monocytes, macrophages, and dendritic cells enter a new graft from the blood or from adjacent tissues. These phagocytic cells randomly ingest damaged, dying, or dead cells from the graft. The various alloantigens (proteins, glycoprotein, etc.) are partially digested in the macrophage, and small fragments are complexed to MHC class I and class II antigens and presented to the cell surface. These antigen-presenting cells (APC) then migrate to the regional (draining) lymph nodes via the lymphatic channels. This migration will be delayed until there is an anastomosis of lymphatic channels between the graft and the surrounding normal host tissue. (Studies in animal model systems have shown that prolonged interruption of the lymphatics allows prolonged survival of allografts.) The APCs enter the subcortical areas of the lymph nodes, where they come into close contact with both $CD8^+$ and $CD4^+$ antigen-reactive T cells. The MHC-antigen/TcR interaction provides one activation signal to the T cell. The APC secretes interleukin-1 (IL-1), which provides a necessary second signal to the T cell. It is also possible that alloreactive T cells can recognize native MHC alloantigens on the surface of graft cells without APC processing. This form of antigen presentation may be mediated by donor graft macrophages and dendritic cells that can provide the IL-1 second signal. The afferent limb of the response takes 3–7 days.

Central limb

The interaction between APCs and T cells stimulates the T cells to cycle out of G_0 into G_1. A subset of T cells is activated to secrete IL-2, which then stimulates the expression of high-affinity interleukin-2 receptors (IL-2R; CD25). IL-2 has both autocrine and paracrine activity to maintain the proliferative response that results in the clonal expansion of alloreactive T cells. During the proliferative response, the T cells also mature into a variety of functional populations defined by the production of lymphokines (interferon-γ, TNF, IL-4, IL-5, etc.), cytotoxic granules, or memory cells. This process takes 5–7 days and results in the marked expansion in the number of alloreactive T cells as the cells divide every 8–12 hours. This process causes the enlargement of the draining lymph nodes (or spleen in the case of vascular grafts). The lymphoid hypertrophy is due predominantly to the increase in cellular volume of dividing 'immunoblasts' and only partially to the increase in total cell numbers. The *in vitro* correlate of the central limb of the response is the mixed lymphocyte reaction, which measures the proliferation of alloreactive T cells responding to alloantigen.

Efferent limb

As the alloreactive T cells (both $CD4^+$ and $CD8^+$) mature, they begin to migrate out of the draining lymph node and enter the general circulation via the major lymphatic channels such as the thoracic duct. The cells then circulate and enter the graft, where a variety of effector mechanisms come into play. The efferent limb of the response takes several days to complete.

Much controversy currently exists as to whether graft rejection is mediated predominantly by $CD8^+$ T killer cells (cytolytic T cells; CTL) or by $CD4^+$ T cells mediating delayed type hypersensitivity (DTH). Both subsets of T cells can be extracted from allografts undergoing rejection.

The argument in favor of a predominant contribution of $CD3^+CD8^+$ T killer cells to allograft rejection is based on the fact that this population is restricted to interactions with MHC class I-bearing cells. Because class I antigens are present on most somatic cells, while class II antigens are typically absent from these cells, it follows that only the MHC class I-restricted $CD8^+$ T cells would be the predominant cell population responsible for the destruction of the allograft. This conclusion is supported by the adoptive transfer of allograft immunity by $CD8^+$ T-cell populations. However, to ascribe graft rejection solely to this subset of T cells is overly simplistic. Non-T natural killer (NK) cells can also be extracted from grafts undergoing rejection and can mediate a local graft rejection when injected into target tissues. A subset of NK cells that express the CD8 molecule ($CD3^-CD8^+$) are thus MHC class I-restricted non-T killer cells, which probably contribute to the killing of somatic cells. Both populations cause cytolysis by inserting a complement-like molecule, perforin, into the membrane of the target cell. Perforin makes a donut-shaped structure, which forms a pore through the target cell membrane, allowing a large flux of water and solutes through the cell membrane, resulting in lysis of the target cell. Other cytotoxic molecules also appear to be involved in the process.

An ever-increasing body of literature indicates that $CD4^+$, MHC class II-restricted T cells play the predominant role in allograft rejection. This subset of T cells mediates a number of helper functions and delayed type hypersensitivity (DTH) by the production of lymphokines and interleukins. $CD4^+$ T cells can also mediate direct cytotoxic effects on class II-bearing target cells, and indirect cytotoxic effects mediated by lymphokines such as interferon-γ (IFN-γ) and tumor necrosis factor (TNF). IFN-γ has multiple effects, including the induction of MHC class II antigen expression on endothelial cells and the accumulation of macrophages in the allograft by its chemoattractant properties. The former effect makes the endothelial cells susceptible to attack by MHC class II-restricted $CD4^+$ killer T cells. TNF has both direct cytotoxic effects and participates in the activation of macrophages into aggressive killer cells. Other phagocytic cells such as neutrophils, basophils, and eosinophils also enter the graft and participate in the rejection reaction through phagocytosis and the elaboration of vasoactive peptides and proteolytic enzymes. Antibodies to alloantigens appear to play a minor role in the reaction by activating the complement cascade to opsonize cells, making them more susceptible to phagocytosis.

Hyperacute rejection

Some vascular grafts, such as kidney allografts, die within a few minutes to hours after grafting. This process is called a hyperacute rejection. Hyperacute rejection is thought to be mediated by antibodies to blood group and histocompatibility antigens that were present in the host before grafting. These antibodies could be the naturally occurring isohemagglutinin either to ABO blood group antigens or to other antigens to which the recipient had been sensitized by blood transfusions or other means before the transplant. The reaction involves antigen–antibody complexes that activate the complement and clotting cascades. The result is massive intravascular coagulation and hemostasis within the graft that results in the acute death of the graft due to lack of perfusion. Neutrophils also contribute to the death of the graft as they are attracted to the graft and release proteolytic enzymes.

Graft-versus-host reactions

A unique and complicated situation arises in the special case of bone marrow transplantation. As with other tissue grafts, bone marrow is susceptible to rejection by the recipient (host-versus-graft reaction; HvGR). In addition, bone marrow obtained by multiple needle aspirations is contaminated with a large amount of peripheral blood. As a result, 10–30 percent of the nucleated cells in the bone marrow inoculum are mature T cells, compared with the 1–2 percent T cells normally present in bone marrow. If the recipient is immunosuppressed to prevent graft rejection (e.g. *congenital immunodeficiency* or immunosuppressive preparation regimens), then the T cells in the graft will recognize the recipient as the foreign tissue. This results in the graft-versus-host reaction (GvHR).

As is the situation with organ grafts, the GvHR is initiated by mature donor T cells, mediated by a variety of effector mechanisms, and directed against several types of antigens, especially MHC and minor histocompatibility antigens. GvHR has many manifestations. The major target organs include the skin (rashes), gastrointestinal tract (diarrhea), and liver (jaundice, abnormal liver function). Other major target organs are the primary (bone marrow, thymus) and secondary (lymph nodes, spleen) lymphoid organs. The result of the GvHR against the lymphoid organs is a severe immunodeficiency syndrome that leaves the recipient highly susceptible to common and opportunistic infections. Two forms of the GvHR have been described. Acute GvHR develops in the first 1–3 months following transplant, tends to run a rapid course over a few weeks, and frequently resolves with treatment. Chronic GvHR develops later, typically about 6 months after transplant. This form of the reaction develops slowly and resolves slowly. Many of the manifestations of chronic GvHR represent tissue responses to chronic inflammation, including sclerodermatous changes in the skin, destruction of the salivary and lacrimal glands, chronic hepatitis, chronic immunodeficiency, and malabsorption.

Leukemic cells appear to be sensitive targets of the GvHR. Thus, the GvHR has an anti-leukemic effect that is called the graft-versus-leukemia reaction (GvL). The GvL is most likely due to a response to the usual MHC and non-MHC, minor histocompatibility antigens. It is also possible that at least some of the GvL is due to a response to leukemia-associated antigens. Some experimental evidence indicates that the GvHR is mediated primarily by $CD8^+$ T cells, while the GvL is mediated by $CD4^+$ T cells, but this hypothesis has not been supported by clinical experience.

The severity of the GvHR is a function of the antigenic disparity between donor and recipient and the number of T cells included in the marrow inoculum. (This is most likely true of organ grafts as well, but these effects can only be quantitated in the case of marrow transplantation, where the number of T cells infused can be calculated.) To overcome the more severe reactions, donor and recipient are routinely matched for MHC antigens. Despite MHC matching, multiple disparities exist at the non-MHC minor histocompatibility loci. To increase the number of potential donors available, bone marrow transplanters have developed international registries of individuals willing to donate bone marrow. Donor and recipient pairs are selected by best-fit matching of the MHC antigens, resulting in what is termed a 'matched unrelated donor' or MUD graft. Due to allelic differences within HLA antigens shown to be serologically identical, MUD grafts frequently (but not always) result in more severe GvHR than grafts between HLA-matched siblings.

To blunt the GvHR, bone marrow transplant recipients are given immunosuppression with methotrexate and/or cyclosporin A for approximately 100 days after transplant. In most patients, this results in minimal GvHR and the establishment of a long-term, stable chimeric state with immunological tolerance to the recipient's alloantigens. Successfully transplanted patients remain free of GvHR for many years without needing continued immunosuppression. Patients with chronic GvHR typically require long-term immunosuppressive treatment. Even chronic GvHR can resolve over time, allowing some patients to stop immunosuppressive therapy.

Control of rejection

Several strategies have been developed for the control of rejection reactions. These range from decreasing the antigenic disparity between donor and recipient to immunosuppressive drugs. The most effective methods prevent or minimize initiation of the reaction by eliminating antigenic disparity between donor and recipient or removing the T cells that initiate graft rejection. Stopping an immune response is very difficult once it is underway.

Antigen matching

Syngrafts and autografts are the most successful because no antigenic differences exist between donor and recipient to elicit the rejection reaction. The observation that the MHC antigens elicit the strongest rejection responses led to the common practice of matching donor and recipient for HLA antigens. This procedure is critically important in bone marrow transplantation, where fatal GvHR may be a consequence of mismatching, but appears less critical in many of the solid organ grafts, such as livers and hearts, where rejection of the organ is the major problem. Bone marrow donor and recipients typically are typed for HLA-A, B, C, and DR antigens by serological methods and for HLA-D antigens by cell proliferation in mixed lymphocyte cultures. In the case of cadaveric donors for solid organs, there is only time enough to serologically type for HLA-A, B, C, and DR antigens. Because each individual carries two HLA haplotypes, the probability of having a full HLA-matched sibling is 1:4. Because of the large numbers of alleles present at each HLA locus, the probability of finding a full HLA-matched donor in the population is very small. Thus, those grafts that require full HLA matches are most commonly obtained from HLA-matched siblings. Most cadaveric grafts carry one or more HLA disparities with the recipient.

Recent studies have shown that the serologically defined HLA antigens can be further subdivided into allelic variants by molecular techniques. For example, the HLA-B27 antigen has been divided into at least six alleles (B27.1, B27.2 . . . B27.6). These variants cannot be distinguished by the serological reagents currently available, but can elicit significant rejection episodes despite the serological matching. HLA antigens present in a given family are assumed to be more likely identical than HLA antigens present in unrelated families. This has led to the concept of 'phenotypically matched, but genotypically mismatched' HLA typing, when donor and recipient share serologically defined antigens, but are from unrelated families.

The major factor in selecting suitable donors for most solid organ grafts is based on ABO typing to prevent hyperacute rejections.

Immunosuppression

Multiple antigenic disparities exist between the donor and recipient despite the most rigorous HLA typing due to the minor histocompatibility antigens, which cannot be typed with currently available reagents. In addition, biologically significant antigenic disparity may exist in the MHC antigens due to allelic differences not detected by routine serological typing. Whatever the source, these various antigenic disparities are sufficient to elicit graft rejection reactions in normal graft recipients. Several techniques have been developed to blunt the rejection reaction. The common theme of these methods is to destroy the lymphocytes that mediate graft rejection.

Physical methods

One approach to the prevention of graft rejection has been to remove T cells physically. This has been attempted by cannulating the thoracic duct and removing the T cells, which necessarily traffic through it as they recirculate from the lymphoid tissues back into the circulation. This approach has met with limited success, but is not frequently used at present.

In the case of bone marrow transplants, the mature donor T cells present in the marrow inoculum can be removed by several methods. The technique used most commonly in clinical practice is to remove the mature T cells by agglutination techniques. The lectin soy bean agglutinin (SBA) is added to the cell suspension, causing mature T cells to clump together. The agglutinated T cells are separated from the marrow cells by differential centrifugation over a Ficoll-Hypaque gradient. Sheep red blood cells are then added to the cell suspension. Most of the remaining T cells form rosettes via the sheep red blood cell receptor (CD2) and are removed over Ficoll-Hypaque gradients. This procedure has been used successfully in many allogeneic bone marrow transplants to prevent the onset of GvHR.

Drugs

The most common approach to immunosuppression is to poison the T cells responding to the foreign antigens of the graft during the central limb of the rejection response. The most frequently used drugs are cycle-active compounds such as methotrexate, azathioprine, and cyclophosphamide. The most common drug currently used is cyclosporin A, which is more T-cell specific than other agents and appears to down-regulate the immune response by inhibiting interleukin production or metabolism. Recent studies indicate that other drugs such as FK506 may also be useful in preventing graft rejection. The major problem with immunosuppressive drugs is their lack of specificity. They inhibit or depress virtually all immune responses and thus leave the graft recipient more susceptible to opportunistic infections by viruses, yeasts, fungi, and other intracellular parasites. These patients may also be more susceptible to secondary malignancy due to the loss of immune surveillance of tumors.

Antilymphocyte serum and monoclonal antibodies

Serum from rabbits or goat immunized to human T cells (antilymphocyte serum; ALS) or the globulin fraction of these sera (antilymphocyte globulin; ALG) have been used for many years to treat rejection episodes and the GvHR with some success. The development of monoclonal antibody technology has made it possible to identify various populations of cells involved in the rejection reaction, sometimes with great specificity for small subsets of the various cell populations. One approach to immunosuppression, therefore, is to inject the graft recipient with monoclonal antibodies that are specific for a particular population of lymphoid cells. The monoclonal antibodies theoretically should equilibrate into the total extracellular water space of the patient and thus be able to 'seek and destroy' all of the target cell population. Destruction of the antibody-coated target cells could be mediated by several mechanisms, including complement-mediated opsonization and phagocytosis by macrophages or complement-mediated lysis, or by coupling the antibody to toxins or radioisotopes that will selectively kill the antibody-coated target cells. This approach, which has met with some success with antibodies directed to all T-cell populations (e.g. anti-CD3 or anti-CD2 antibody) or to large subsets (e.g. anti-CD4 or anti-CD8 antibody), has a great deal of promise because antibodies may be developed with sufficient specificity to eliminate only those T cells that recognize the foreign antigens of the graft and spare those T cells needed to mount an immune response to other pathogens.

One difficulty with the use of monoclonal antibodies is that they are routinely developed in mice, and therefore present the patient's immune system with a foreign (mouse) protein. The patients routinely make specific antibody to the mouse immunoglobulin and subsequently clear the injected antibody from the circulation. Monoclonal antibodies thus end up being useful for only a short period of time. Several attempts to circumvent this problem are in progress. One is to construct human immunoglobulin molecules that are the mouse idiotypes directed against the human CD antigens. This method attempts to prevent the patient making an antibody response to the anti-CD antibody. Another is to make human monoclonal antibodies that would not be immunogenic.

Monoclonal antibodies have been used to remove T cells from the donor bone marrow cells used in allogeneic bone marrow transplants, with limited success. Attempts to remove only $CD8^+$ or $CD4^+$ T cells selectively from the graft have not been as effective as removing the entire T-cell population. Some investigators have attempted to broaden the populations of lymphocytes removed by using 'cocktails' consisting of multiple monoclonal antibodies.

Prevention of graft-versus-host reactions

The graft-versus-host reaction may occur when immunocompetent T cells are transplanted into a histoincompatible recipient who is unable to reject the grafted cells because of immunodeficiency or a genetic inability to recognize the donor cells as foreign. GvHR most commonly develops as a consequence of allogeneic bone marrow transplantation, but may also develop when immunocompromised patients are transfused with blood products that contain viable lymphocytes. Lethal post-transfusion GvHR has been reported in infants with *DiGeorge syndrome*, *severe combined immunodeficiency* and in *immunocompromised patients* who have lymphomas, or leukemias, or who are on immuno-suppressive drugs. Lethal GvHR has also been reported in normal individuals given blood transfusions from HLA-matched family members (parents, siblings, or children). Most blood products can be contaminated with lymphocytes including whole blood, packed red blood cells, washed red cells, platelets, and granulocytes. Lymphocytes may also survive short-term freezing of blood products. The best way to prevent post-transfusion GvHR is to irradiate all blood products with 3000–6000 cGy (3000–6000 rad) from a cobalt-60 or cesium-137 source. It is strongly recommended that all newborn infants be given only irradiated blood products because their immune systems are immature.

Tolerance induction

Theoretically, the best approach to preventing graft rejection would be to elicit a state of immunological tolerance to the foreign antigens of the allograft. This would eliminate the need for immunosuppressive drugs or antibodies. A successful technique for tolerance induction would also eliminate the need for careful histo-compatibility matching of donor and recipient, making the pool of available graft donors for a given patient much larger than is currently possible. The concept of acquired allograft tolerance, developed by Medawar and colleagues in the 1950s, remains the ultimate goal of many transplantation immunologists. Only one technique is currently used in clinical practice.

It has been observed that recipients of renal allografts experience fewer rejection episodes if they have received multiple, unrelated blood transfusions. There is some evidence that the blood transfusions elicit the production of antibodies that interfere with (block) the cellular immune response to the graft. This process apparently results in state of partial allograft tolerance as the cellular response decreases over time. Although the precise mechanism and antigens involved in this phenomenon are not well understood, it is now routine practice to pretreat renal allograft recipients with a series of blood transfusions over several weeks before the graft.

Treatment of rejection episodes

Once the immune response to alloantigens has developed to the point of causing tissue damage, it is extraordinarily difficult to stop. The primary treatment of graft rejection episodes is high-dose steroids. Intravenous Solu-Medrol (methylprednisolone sodium succinate), at dose ranges of 6–10 mg/kg per day given every 12 hours, has effectively blunted severe rejection episodes. Less severe episodes can usually be controlled with oral steroids, such as prednisone at doses of 2–5 mg/kg per day. The mechanism of action of the steroids is not well understood, but probably includes lysis of T cells as well as stabilization of endothelial and phagocytic cell membranes to decrease inflammation and cytotoxicity. Additional pharmacological agents commonly used include cyclophosphamide, methotrexate, azathioprine, and chlorambucil. Attempts to destroy T cells with antithymocyte globulin (ATG) and monoclonal antibodies (e.g. anti-CD3) have also been used with some success. In general, mild rejection episodes can be successfully treated, but severe episodes frequently cannot be treated by these various methods, and loss of the graft results.

Selected reading

Frank MM, Fries LF. The role of complement in inflammation and phagocytosis. *Immunol Today* 1991; **12**: 322.

Hall BM. Cells mediating allograft rejection. *Transplantation* 1991; **51**: 1141.

Rosenberg AS, Munitz TI, Maniero TG, Singer A. Cellular basis of skin allograft rejection across a class I major histocompatibility barrier in mice depleted of $CD8^+$ T cells *in vivo*. *J Exp Med* 1991; **173**: 1463.

Storb R, Thomas ED. Allogeneic bone-marrow transplantation. *Immunol Rev* 1983; **71**: 77.

Trowsdale J, Ragoussis J, Campbell RD. Map of the human MHC. *Immunol Today* 1991; **12**: 443.

E. Complement and Acute Phase Proteins

A J Ammann

The complement system

The complement system may be viewed as an immunological amplification cascade. Once triggered, activated complement components interact with immunoglobulin molecules, cells of the immune system, pharmacological effectors, clotting factors and acute phase reactants. The complement system consists of 20 individual proteins forming an enzyme system in the plasma, triggered by specific events, which invoke molecular interactions on the surface of cells and result in the formation of active complement fragments as well as new molecular complexes.

Complement may be activated by two fundamentally distinct pathways—the classic complement pathway and the alternate pathway. Activation of the classic pathway occurs following binding of the first complement component (C1) to antibody molecules which have an altered Fc region as a consequence of antigen–antibody interaction. Not all immunoglobulin molecules are able to trigger complement activation, however, as the property is confined to certain IgG subclasses and IgM.

A major biological function of the classic pathway is to trigger cell lysis. This is accomplished utilizing complement components C1 through C9 with C1 acting as a recognition factor, C2 through C4 as activation factors and C5 through C9 as cell membrane attack factors.

Standard designations are utilized to identify specific complement components, the state of activation, functional units, and the origin of specific fragments. C1, C2, etc. refer to the major unactivated complement components; $\overline{C1}$, $\overline{C2}$, etc. refer to activated components; C1q, C2a, C4b, etc. refer to cleavage products of the parent molecule; $C3\overset{*}{b}$, $C5\overset{*}{b}$, etc. refer to a cleavage product with a binding site for another complement component.

Following activation, $\overline{C1}$ forms C1 esterase, an enzyme which cleaves C4 into C4a and C4b and C2 into C2a and C2b. $C4\overset{*}{b}$ and $C2\overset{*}{a}$ combine to form an enzyme called C3 convertase which binds to and cleaves C3 into C3a and C3b. These new fragments have additional biological activity. C3a behaves as an anaphylatoxin resulting in muscle contraction while C3b functions to enhance phagocytosis (opsonic activity). C3b also forms a complex with C4bC2a which cleaves C5 into C5a and C5b. C5a has considerably more potent anaphylactic activity than C3a and also has potent chemotactic activity. C5b binds to cell-surface receptors and reacts with the remaining complement components, C6 through C9, capable of perforating cell membranes and causing cell lysis.

In contrast to the classic pathway, which is activated by antigen–antibody complex, the alternate complement pathway is activated by endotoxin or zymosan produced by microbial agents, or antibody of the IgA class. Activation of the alternate pathway begins at C3. Factor B, factor D and initiating factor interact and produce an activated complex that functions as a C3 convertase. Properdin in turn stabilizes this complex and subsequently functions as a C5 convertase, triggering the remaining complement components.

The potential for serious continuous tissue damage following complement activation would be significant if it were not for a number of inactivators which interact at various stages of complement activation. These inactivators include C1q inhibitor, C1-esterase inhibitor, a C3-convertase inhibitor system consisting of six components, a membrane activation complex inhibitor (MAC) which competes with C5 through C9 for cell membrane binding sites, and serum carboxypeptidase N.

A variety of disorders are associated with abnormalities of the complement system. Deficiencies of individual complement components result in increased susceptibility to infection or autoimmune diseases. A genetic deficiency of the C1-esterase inhibitor, inherited in an autosomal recessive manner, results in a disorder termed *hereditary angioedema* associated with edema of the face, extremities, lung and gastrointestinal tract.

The complement system plays a role in many protective as well as destructive biological processes. It offers protection against infection, increases phagocytosis, amplifies the effect of antibody and produces physiological responses following infection. Excessive activation of complement may result in immune complex disease, anaphylactic-like reactions and coagulation disorders.

Because the complement system is activated by antigen–antibody complexes, plasma concentrations of individual complement components, as well as total complement activity, may be decreased in such disorders as *systemic lupus erythematosus*. Complement concentrations may therefore be useful in determining a response to treatment and in following the course of a disease.

Acute phase proteins

Several plasma proteins have been found to increase quickly following acute events such as trauma or infection. These are collectively referred to as 'acute phase proteins' and in some instances 'trauma-induced' or 'liver-produced serum glycoproteins'. C reactive protein (CRP) was the first acute phase protein to be described. The clinical value of this protein was evaluated in 1930. The collective group of acute phase proteins include CRP serum amyloid A protein, α_1-antitrypsin, orosomucoid, α_1-antichymotrypsin, fibrinogen, α_2-macroglobulin, ceruloplasmin, factor B, haptoglobin and immunoglobulins.

Following trauma, either physical or biological (such as myocardial infarction), or infection there may be the release of endotoxins, interleukins (IL) and cytokines, such as IL-1, IL-6, tumor necrosis factor (TNF) and interferons. Cytokines induce the liver to produce acute phase reactants such as CRP, which has been intensively evaluated and has been found to increase by as much as 500-fold to 1000-fold in severe bacterial infection. The biological function of CRP is to bind to microorganisms which contain phosphorylcholine in their membranes. The CRP–phosphorylcholine complex has the ability to activate the classic complement pathway which results in the deposition of C3b on the surface of the microbial agent, increasing phagocytic uptake and destruction. Since an elevated CRP is indicative of tissue damage, measuring CRP concentrations is useful in determining whether tissue damage has occurred. It is important to recognize that CRP concentrations and the erythrocyte sedimentation rate (ESR) do not always correlate. For example, both the ESR and CRP may be elevated in rheumatoid arthritis, whereas only the ESR is elevated in systemic lupus erythematosus. Many of the acute phase proteins behave similarly. α_1-Antichymotrypsin, haptoglobin and α_2-antitrypsin are elevated following acute injury and, by themselves, do not distinguish between types of injury or organ involvement. Unlike CRP, elevated concentrations of fibrinogen correlate with an elevated ESR and in fact, fibrinogen is the major determinant of the ESR.

Measurements of complement concentrations may also be used as an acute phase reactant index of tissue injury. However, the complement system is an independent immunological amplification system where total complement concentrations and concentrations of individual complement components may be paradoxically discrepant. For example, in some forms of SLE, total complement concentrations may be elevated while individual components, such as C4 or C1q are low due to immune complex formation and complement consumption (see discussion of complement above).

Although elevation of acute phase reactants is indicative of acute and sometimes chronic injury, they are not indicators of a specific disease process or organ involvement. Measurements of acute phase proteins have their greatest utility in defining general processes and can be useful, if elevated, in determining responses to treatment.

Selected reading

Dinarello CA. Cytokines: interleukin-1 and tumor necrosis factor (cachectin). In Gallin JI, Goldstein IM, Snyderman R, eds. *Inflammation: basic principles and clinical correlates*. New York: Raven Press, 1988: 195.

Frank MM, Fries LF. The role of complement in inflammation and phagocytosis. *Immunol Today* 1991; **12**: 322.

Muller-Eberhard HJ. Complement: chemistry and pathways. In Gallin JI, Goldstein IM, Snyderman R, eds. *Inflammation: basic principles and clinical correlates*. New York: Raven Press, 1988: 21.

Stewart SR, Gershwin ME. Diagnostic tests and procedures in rheumatic diseases. In *The laboratory in clinical medicine*. Philadelphia: WB Saunders Company, 1981: 565.

F. Autoimmune Disorders

A J Ammann

The immune system controls the delicate balance between the recognition of subtle alterations in antigenicity, which threaten the biological stability of the host, and alterations of 'self', which if recognized by the immune system might result in autoimmune disease. Autoimmune disorders represent an immunological reaction against 'self' antigens rather than foreign antigens. All major components of the immune system have been implicated in the pathogenesis of autoimmune disorders. Antibody immunity may be directed against specific antigens and result in specific destruction of target cells. A T-cell-mediated immune response may result in destruction of target cells by immune cells. A more generalized autoimmune disorder may result from the presence of circulating immune complexes. Finally, the complement system may amplify an existing immune reaction, resulting in enhanced destruction of target cells or organs.

The broad spectrum of autoimmune disorders may be divided into two general categories, organ-specific disorders and systemic disorders. Whether involving a single target tissue or multiple organs, each of the four major immune components—antibody-mediated immunity, cell-mediated immunity, immune complexes, and the complement system—may participate. Understanding of the various immunological mechanisms involved has been greatly enhanced as a consequence of improved diagnostic techniques. The ability to demonstrate specific antibody against target organs using sensitive assays for autoantibody has improved significantly. Antibodies may be detected as immune complexes in the circulation or in target organs by direct demonstration of antibody in histological sections of biopsy material. Cells sensitized to self antigens may be demonstrated *in vitro* by means of culturing lymphocytes in the presence of the suspected antigens. These improved techniques have resulted in earlier diagnosis of autoimmune diseases and prolonged survival for many patients due to earlier treatment interventions.

A major question relates to how autoimmune diseases occur. An early theory suggested that most self antigens were sequestered within their specific organs and therefore were not accessible to the immune system. Subsequent disruption by an event such as infection or trauma might result in the induction of autoantibody and autoimmune disease. Supporting this hypothesis was the observation that injury to cardiac muscle, such as occurs in myocardial infarction or cardiac surgery, resulted in autoantibody to cardiac muscle and in a syndrome of fever, fatigue, and autoantibody formation. However, this phenomenon was transient, and significant disruption of tissue and organs during surgery or other trauma did not always result in autoimmune phenomena. In addition, the destruction of tissue results in the release of DNA, which does not lead to antibody formation to DNA as is characteristically found in *systemic lupus erythematosus*. In fact, it is difficult experimentally to induce antibody formation to native DNA even when DNA is injected directly into animals along with potent adjuvants.

The normal immune system has both B cells and T cells capable of recognizing normal antigens. Rather than resulting in autoimmune disease, this may be a mechanism for regulating the immune reactivity of individual immune cells by maintaining a suppressive effect on those cells, which if they were to escape control, might evolve into autoreactive cells. Thus autoimmune disease might occur when the regulatory mechanisms that govern the degree of autoreactivity fail.

Which regulatory mechanism fails? Several possibilities exist, each supported by experimental evidence.

Because immune cells are normally present that recognize self antigen, a suppressor cell or antibody mechanism must down-regulate the expression of these autoreactive cells. This mechanism may be similar to that observed following immunization, where suppressor T cells are known to control the amount of antibody produced following B-cell and T-cell interaction. Studies in the autoimmune mouse model of *systemic lupus erythematosus* indicate that the appearance of disease is associated with a progressive loss of T suppressor cells with advancing age. The frequent occurrence of autoimmunity in patients with immunodeficiency disorders also suggests that abnormalities of T-cell regulation result in autoimmunity.

Polyclonal activation of B-cell immunity may also result in autoimmune manifestations. Certain antigens by themselves, such as superantigens, or antigens in association with adjuvants such as endotoxins, may result in autoantibody formation. For example, following *Epstein–Barr virus infection*, a variety of autoantibodies are found that may be the consequence of polyclonal activation of B cells by this virus. Chronic diseases such as *leprosy* are also associated with polyclonal B-cell activation and the presence of a variety of autoantibodies.

Recent theories suggest that increased expression of the major histocompatibility complex II (MHC II) antigens on cells is observed in a number of autoimmune disorders. This increased MHC II expression may enhance autoreactive T helper cells and result in increased autoantibody production. The trigger for the increased MHC II expression may be viral infection; following viral and other chronic infections, interferon-γ production increases, which in turn markedly up-regulates MHC II expression.

Genetic factors have also been implicated in autoimmune disorders. It is well recognized that certain human leukocyte antigen (HLA) specificities are associated with distinct autoimmune diseases. HLA-DR3 is found in association with *Addison disease,* HLA-DR4 in association with *rheumatoid arthritis,* and HLA-B27 in association with *ankylosing spondylitis* and *Reiter syndrome.* In the latter disorder, individuals are known to develop symptomatology following infection with certain enteric bacteria such as *Shigella* and *Campylobacter*. Following infection with these organisms, individuals who are HLA-B27 positive may develop arthritis, urethritis, and other manifestations of autoimmune disease. This provides a link between genetic factors and induction of autoimmunity by microbial agents.

Sex hormones are also known to regulate the expression of autoimmune disease. Removal of female hormones by oophorectomy or the administration of testosterone to female mice with autoimmune disease results in delayed expression of autoimmune disease or improvement in preexisting disease.

It is apparent that autoimmune diseases may evolve as a consequence of several mechanisms, which may act independently or synergistically. Most of these mechanisms are operative in infants and children, in whom the pathogenesis of autoimmune disease is similar to that of adults. An exception is the transient expression of autoimmunity in the newborn infant as a consequence of the passive transfer of autoantibody from an affected mother to the infant. A distinct disorder (*neonatal lupus erythematosus*), consisting of a rash and cardiac conduction abnormalities, occurs in association with the passive prenatal transfer to an otherwise normal infant of Ro antibodies from mothers with systemic lupus erythematosus. Usually this syndrome lasts only as long as maternal antibody persists in the infant's circulation (approximately 6 months) although the conduction abnormalities (e.g. *complete heart block*) may be permanent.

Autoimmune disorders associated with antibody-mediated immunity

The normal function of antibody-mediated immunity is to recognize a foreign antigen and control any adverse effect by the induction of specific antibodies. Once challenged, the normal immune system produces a variety of antibodies of different immunoglobulin classes. There are five major immunoglobulin types based on immunochemical differences. The biological functions of these classes vary in relation to half-life, molecular weight, ability to bind complement, ability to pass from the maternal circulation across the placenta to the infant, and ability to amplify various immunological effects. IgG, the most abundant antibody class, also has the longest half-life, passes the placenta, and fixes complement. IgM has a shorter half-life, but exists as a pentamer, and therefore is better able to bind antigen. IgA, primarily a secretory antibody, can under some circumstances bind to antigen within the systemic circulation and result in immune complex disease. IgE is the antibody class primarily responsible for acute allergic reactions and is not known to be associated with autoimmune diseases. IgD, present in very small amounts in the circulation, has no known function in the development of autoimmunity.

In most cases, autoimmune disorders are caused by IgG antibody, and less commonly by IgM or IgA. Under normal circumstances, the function of antibody is to remove an offending antigen or microorganism from the circulation and destroy it, either directly or within the reticuloendothelial system. Antibody binds directly to an antigen, which may be either a soluble antigen or a component of an invading microorganism. In the case of an invading microorganism such as a virus, the antibody may result in direct inactivation of the virus through an antibody-dependent cytotoxic mechanism. In this instance, the antibody activates cells that have on their surface receptors for the Fc portion of the antibody molecule. The same portion of the molecule may also result in attachment of antibody to macrophages and monocytes that bear Fc receptors and result in the ingestion of the antigen–antibody complex. These mechanisms are designed to inactivate abnormal antigens or antigens associated with microorganisms directly and to protect the host. If, however, the antigen in question is a component of a normal cell or organ, or an antigenic component of a normal cell, antibody destruction of self may occur.

There are many examples of autoimmune disorders associated with autoantibody formation. These may occur in infancy as a consequence of passive transfer of antibody from the mother to the fetus or at any time during infancy to adult life. The most easily understood antibody-mediated autoimmune disorders are those that involve blood elements. *Idiopathic thrombocytopenic purpura* is frequently associated with antibodies directed against platelets. This disorder may occur following a viral infection or may be associated with diseases such as *systemic lupus erythematosus*. *Transient thrombocytopenia* may be observed in infants born to mothers who have high levels of antibody directed against platelets. As might be suspected from the observation that only IgG crosses the placenta in significant amounts, the thrombocytopenia in infants may only last as long as maternal antibody is present in the circulation.

Another example of a direct effect of antibody on a blood cell is *autoimmune hemolytic anemia*. Normal red cells, when coated with autoantibody, are rapidly and efficiently removed from the blood by means of Fc receptor-mediated destruction in the reticuloendothelial system. Destruction of red cells at a rate in excess of production results in severe life-threatening anemia. The same mechanism is responsible for thrombocytopenia when the antibody is associated with platelets.

Autoantibodies may also be directed against components of the neutrophils, resulting in neutropenia and secondary infection, or against lymphocytes, resulting in lymphopenia and susceptibility to viral infection.

Although autoimmune hemolytic anemia or thrombocytopenia may occur as distinct autoimmune disorders, they often are early manifestations of systemic autoimmune diseases such as systemic lupus erythematosus.

The kidney and antibody-mediated autoimmunity

Direct destruction of the kidney (and the lung) occurs in *Goodpasture syndrome*. There is a linear deposition of IgG and complement along the basement membrane of the glomerular capillaries and in the lung and the antibody is directed to the glomerular basement membrane. Although glomerular basement membranes from various organs differ significantly biochemically and antigenically, the biochemical compositions of the basement membranes from the kidney and lung are similar, explaining why only these two organs are targets of destruction.

Endocrine organs and antibody-mediated autoimmunity

When antibody is formed against components of the thyroid, different autoimmune diseases may be observed depending on the specific activity of the autoantibody. Antibody obtained from patients with *Hashimoto disease* is cytotoxic for thyroid cells grown in culture. The antibody can be detected in the circulation and reacts with a microsomal antigen within thyroid cells.

The autoantibody that is found in *thyrotoxicosis* (*Graves disease*) may have a stimulatory rather than a destructive effect. Serum from patients with thyrotoxicosis contains a factor that stimulates the thyroid gland; this factor is an antibody, which blocks the binding of thyroid-stimulating hormone and acts in a manner similar to thyroid-stimulating hormone itself, perhaps by binding to specific receptors. This antibody may also cross the placenta and result in *neonatal thyrotoxicosis*.

Autoantibodies may also be directed toward intrinsic factor, resulting in *pernicious anemia*. Although pernicious anemia may occur as an isolated endocrine disorder, it may be associated with other autoimmune endocrine diseases such as *thyrotoxicosis*, *hypoparathyroidism*, or *Addison disease*. The latter disorder, although rare, is associated with specific antibodies to the adrenal gland. Curiously, many of the autoimmune endocrine disorders are also associated with an autosomal recessive immunodeficiency disease termed *chronic mucocutaneous candidiasis*. The relationship between a chronic fungal infection and autoimmune disease has not been elucidated.

Treatment of antibody-mediated autoimmune disease

The approach to treatment of antibody-mediated autoimmunity may vary with the specific organ involved. For example, the hypothyroidism that may be a consequence of autoantibodies directed against thyroid cells in *Hashimoto thyroiditis* is treated with thyroid replacement rather than immunosuppression because the disease is limited to the thyroid gland. In contrast, *autoimmune hemolytic anemia* or *thrombocytopenia* may require intensive immunosuppressive therapy directed toward reducing the amount of autoantibody formed as frequent red cell or platelet transfusions may not be possible. Initial treatment usually consists of steroids, which may control the disease by decreasing autoantibody formation and decreasing the destruction of sensitized red cells or platelets. Removal of the spleen, a primary organ of the reticuloendothelial system the function of which is to remove antibody-coated cells, results in diminished destruction of red blood cells or platelets and prolonged survival of cells. Symptomatic therapy may be the only treatment required in infants who have manifestations of autoimmune disease as a consequence of maternal transfer of autoantibody, as the autoimmune disease is self-limited as a consequence of the gradual loss of maternal autoantibody.

Autoimmune disorders associated with T-cell-mediated immunity

Although a direct role of autoantibody can be demonstrated experimentally and clinically in a variety of autoimmune disorders, it is more difficult to impugn a singular role for sensitized T cells in a specific autoimmune disorder. In most instances, autoimmune disorders are associated with a mononuclear cell infiltrate, which is composed of both lymphocytes and monocytes. The appearance of these cells, however, may be the result of a reaction to an initial antibody response. Several investigators have argued that the similarity of *graft-versus-host disease* to autoimmune disease suggests at least an amplification effect of T-cell immunity. Graft-versus-host disease occurs when subjects whose cellular immune systems are underdeveloped (e.g. *DiGeorge syndrome*) or have been completely suppressed, are given immunocompetent blood products or bone marrow cells from a related donor. In many instances, despite careful histocompatibility matching of donor cells, graft-versus-host reaction follows. In graft-versus-host disease, primarily T cells attack host cells, which express antigens different from that of the graft. This is associated with a mononuclear cell infiltrate and the release of cytokines such as tumor necrosis factor, lymphotoxin, and interferon-γ. The manifestations of graft-versus-host disease include pulmonary infiltrates, diffuse skin rash, diarrhea, liver disease, and kidney disease. Although the similarity in disease manifestations of graft-versus-host disease and autoimmune disease does not prove that these disorders have an identical etiology, it does permit the conclusion that a cellular immune response may be responsible for many manifestations of autoimmune disease. Indeed, treatment of autoimmune disease and graft-versus-host disease with steroids or cyclosporin A improves both diseases through a similar mechanism, reduction in cytokine production by sensitized lymphocytes.

Clinical disorders in which a direct effect of sensitized T cells has been thought to play a role in the manifestations of autoimmune disease comprise *autoimmune thyroiditis, ulcerative colitis* (in which colon cells have been shown to be selectively killed by sensitized lymphocytes *in vitro*), *pernicious anemia,* and various forms of *polymyositis.*

Autoimmune disorders associated with immune complex formation

The primary and the most frequent example of immune complex disease is *systemic lupus erythematosus.* Immunohistochemical studies of diseased tissue invariably show the deposition of immunoglobulin and the complement in a 'lumpy-bumpy' pattern characteristic of immune complexes. The immune complexes are in the form of antibody associated with antigen, which together activate the complement system. Antibody and complement are widespread and in most instances the antibody is of the IgG class and is directed towards DNA. As immune complexes form and activate complement, specific complement components are depleted in the serum. Sensitive assays for measuring the amount of circulating immune complexes are usually positive.

Although it is sometimes difficult to explain the seemingly haphazard distribution of organ involvement in different patients with systemic lupus erythematosus, some of the differences may be explained on the basis of the types of immune complexes which form, the presence of other autoantibodies, and genetic factors which may determine target organs. The two sites most frequently targeted by immune complexes are the skin and the kidney. These areas are particularly susceptible to 'trapping' immune complexes that, once deposited, can trigger a cascade of amplifying immunological events resulting in tissue damage.

Because the disease manifestations of systemic lupus erythematosus are related to circulating immune complexes, it is easy to understand why almost any organ may be affected. Unlike autoimmune disorders such as *Goodpasture syndrome*, where the autoantibody is directed against specific basement membranes, the deposition of immune complexes in various organs is a more indiscriminate event.

A diagnosis of systemic lupus erythematosus is readily established using several specific laboratory studies. The fluorescent autoantibody test is used to detect antibody in the patient's serum directed against nuclear antigens. Several different fluorescent patterns may be observed ranging from homogeneous to shaggy or speckled. These patterns are a result of various antibodies directed against antigens within the nucleus of the cell that differ in distribution. Although the ANA test is not specific for systemic lupus erythematosus, it is highly sensitive, and a diagnosis is difficult to consider if this test is negative. The laboratory test with the greatest specificity is that of antibody to DNA.

Activity of disease can be measured using assays for complement. Because the antigen–antibody complexes that circulate in systemic lupus erythematosus bind and deplete complement, assays for complement activity or complement levels may provide an important index of the severity of disease. Hemolytic complement levels or individual complement components are usually severely reduced in patients with long-standing or widespread disease. Complement measurements may also be used as an index of response to treatment. As effective therapy controls the disorder, the complement levels return toward normal and the antibody to DNA diminishes.

Autoimmune disorders possibly associated with immune complex formation

Several well defined diseases with similarities to systemic lupus erythematosus are thought to have a similar etiology and pathogenesis. *Mixed connective tissue disease* was initially described in adults who were thought to have a form of systemic lupus erythematosus. However, subsequent clinical and laboratory evaluations suggest that this is a distinct disorder with a different autoantibody profile and a different prognosis. Clinically the disorder has features of many autoimmune diseases, such as *polyarthritis, scleroderma, rheumatoid arthritis,* and *Sjögren syndrome.*

The laboratory abnormality characteristic of mixed connective tissue disease is an elevated antibody to ENA (extractable nuclear antigen or antibody to ribonucleoprotein). This autoantibody results in a speckled antinuclear antibody test. In contrast to systemic lupus erythematosus, antibody to DNA, although positive, is usually of low titer. Most patients with Sjögren syndrome have antibodies to SS-A and SS-B. The antinuclear antibody test may be positive, and low levels of antibody to DNA may be observed.

Autoimmune disorders of uncertain etiology

In attempting to classify autoimmune disorders into the three major categories of antibody-mediated, T-cell-mediated or immune complex-mediated, one encounters certain diseases and syndromes that do not have the classic laboratory findings found in the previously discussed entities. These diseases are placed in the autoimmune category because they have many clinical features that overlap with existing autoimmune diseases. However, there is a hazard in assuming that similar clinical or histopathological appearances indicate similar etiologies. Many diseases once felt to be autoimmune in nature are now known to be caused by infectious agents, or by infectious agents that trigger autoimmune reactions. One example is *Lyme arthritis.* Initially the disease was described as having clinical manifestations consisting of skin rash and arthritis, and in some instances meningoencephalitis, chorea, and cardiac abnormalities. The discovery of a treponeme-like spirochete transmitted by the tick, *Ixodes dammini*, established *Lyme arthritis*, previously presumed to be an autoimmune disease, as an infectious disease.

The long known association of *rheumatic fever* with *streptococcal infection* suggested that a normal immunological reaction to an invading microorganism might result in diseases with autoimmune manifestations. The degree of immunological reactivity of an individual to streptococcal antigens is correlated with the development of rheumatic fever manifestations. The myocardium of affected individuals can be demonstrated to have deposits of complement, IgG and IgM. These 'cross-reacting' antibodies do not distinguish between streptococcal antigens and self antigens.

A large number of *vasculitis syndromes* that have been described in the pediatric population do not have a defined infectious or autoimmune etiology. These disorders are characterized by inflammation and necrosis of blood vessels, which can involve arteries of both medium and small caliber as well as veins and capillaries. The manifestations of the different syndromes relate to the size and location of the blood vessels involved. Many of the vasculitis syndromes follow allergy or infection. In some instances, antibody and/or complement may be found deposited in the areas of vasculitis, further evidence that these are autoimmune-like disorders. The response of individual patients to steroids or immunosuppressive therapy further suggests that these drugs control an autoimmune process. Examples of these disorders are *Henoch–Schönlein purpura*, *polyarteritis nodosa* and *Wegener granulomatosis*.

The childhood autoimmune disease perhaps most difficult to understand is *juvenile rheumatoid arthritis*. The precise etiology and pathogenic mechanisms remain unknown. The disease has many features of autoimmunity including arthritis, fever, hepatosplenomegaly, skin rash, and chronicity. Although the joint symptomatology and pathology is similar to adult forms of arthritis, with few exceptions, there is no similarity in the laboratory diagnostic studies. For example, rheumatoid factor, an antibody directed to immunoglobulin G, is rarely found in juvenile rheumatoid arthritis.

Ankylosing spondylitis is a distinct form of arthritis similar to that occurring in adults. Inflammatory involvement of large joints and the spine are characteristic. The fact that the disease primarily affects males and is associated with the histocompatibility antigen HLA-B27 suggests that genetic factors are operative.

Laboratory diagnosis of autoimmune disorders

The most easily diagnosed autoimmune disorders consist of entities that have defined autoantibodies. The search for autoantibodies begins in the serum of the patient with an array of autoantibody tests designed to detect antibodies to specific organs. Autoantibody screens may include antibody to thyroid, parietal cells, hepatic cells, basement membrane, adrenal gland, liver, and parathyroid. Autoimmune diseases associated with systemic symptomatology may have antibody to DNA, rheumatoid factor, and extractable nuclear antigens and may result in detection of immune complexes or depletion of complement components.

Other autoimmune diseases are not associated with specific autoantibody production and may require a diagnosis based entirely on clinical features or on histopathological examination of the specific organ involved.

Treatment of autoimmune disease

Treatment of autoimmune disease varies in extremes. *Autoimmune thyroid disease* is treated by restoring thyroid function rather than using immunosuppression to control the autoimmune process. On the other hand, certain autoimmune diseases do not respond well to any form of treatment. For example, *Wegener granulomatosis* does not respond to mild immunosuppressive therapy and usually requires potent agents such as cyclophosphamide. Other diseases such as *scleroderma*, a progressive systemic disease involving the skin and muscle, do not respond well to any form of therapy and follow a progressive, indolent course. Diseases such as *systemic lupus erythematosus* and severe forms of *rheumatoid arthritis* are often treated with steroids, which reduce inflammatory reactions and secondarily reduce immune complex and antibody formation. The course of these diseases can be followed carefully, and the intensity of therapy regulated, by monitoring laboratory studies. A variety of other anti-inflammatory and immunosuppressive treatments have been used in the treatment of autoimmune diseases. The goal is always to control life-threatening disease manifestations without inducing secondary life-threatening drug effects. The mechanism whereby steroids and other immunosuppressive agents control autoimmune disease is not clearly understood; however, these agents are known to reduce cellular infiltrates, to diminish antibody production and the production of cytokines, and as a result, to control disease progression. The intensity of therapy must be tempered with the knowledge that while these drugs diminish inflammation, they also diminish the host response to infectious agents and malignancy. The ideal control of autoimmune disease has not yet been discovered.

Selected reading

Ammann AJ, Wara DW. Collagen vascular diseases. In Rudolph AM, Hoffman JIE, eds. *Pediatrics*. Norwalk, CT: Appleton and Lange, 1987: 411.

Fye KH, Sack KE. Rheumatic diseases. In Stites DP, Terr AI, eds. *Basic and clinical immunology*. Norwalk, CT: Appleton and Lange, 1991: 438.

Kelly WN, Harris ED, Ruddy S, Sledge CB, eds. *Textbook of rheumatology*. 3rd ed. Philadelphia: WB Saunders, 1989.

Steinberg A. Mechanisms of disordered immune regulation. In Stites DP, Terr AI, eds. *Basic and clinical immunology*. Norwalk, CT: Appleton and Lange, 1991: 432.

14 • *Renal function, fluid and electrolyte balance*

Editor: Jean E Robillard

A. Anatomical Development of the Kidney

J E Robillard

The development of the human kidney proceeds from a simple system of aglomerular tubules, the **pronephros**, through simple glomerulonephrons, the **mesonephros**, to culminate in the elaboration of the final complex glomerulonephron units found in the mature kidney, the **metanephros**.

The pronephros, sometimes referred to as the 'cervical kidney', is the first evidence of a renal excretory system in the human embryo. It appears about the middle of the third week of gestation and gives rise to about seven paired tubules, which undergo regression by degeneration by the fifth week. The pronephric structures do not differentiate into recognizable nephrons and are of no significance as a functioning excretory organ. The main role of the pronephros is that it gives rise to the pronephric duct, which persists after the pronephric tubules regress. The pronephric duct extends into the cloaca and is important in the development of the mesonephros.

The mesonephros (Fig. 14.1), which corresponds to the mature kidney of fish and amphibians, appears immediately caudal to the last of the pronephric tubules. The first mesonephric nephrons are seen around 24–25 days of gestation (middle of the fourth week). As with the pronephros, the earliest mesonephric nephrons (the more cephalic) start to degenerate during the fifth week of gestation while the more caudal nephrons are still differentiating. The formation of the mesonephric nephrons differs from the pronephric tubules in that the mesonephric nephrons arise by induction of differentiating vesicles within the solid cell mass of the nephrogenic cord (Fig. 14.1). The mesonephric glomerulus is vascularized and the tubules differentiate into a definite proximal tubule with convolutions and brush border, but they have no loop of Henle or distal tubule. Collectively, the mesonephros constitutes the first true functional glomerulonephron unit formed during renal embryogenesis. The mesonephros remains actively functional during early development of the metanephros so that for a time nephrons in both structures function simultaneously. The functional contribution of the mesonephros during fetal development, however, is minimal because it degenerates as the metanephros begins functioning.

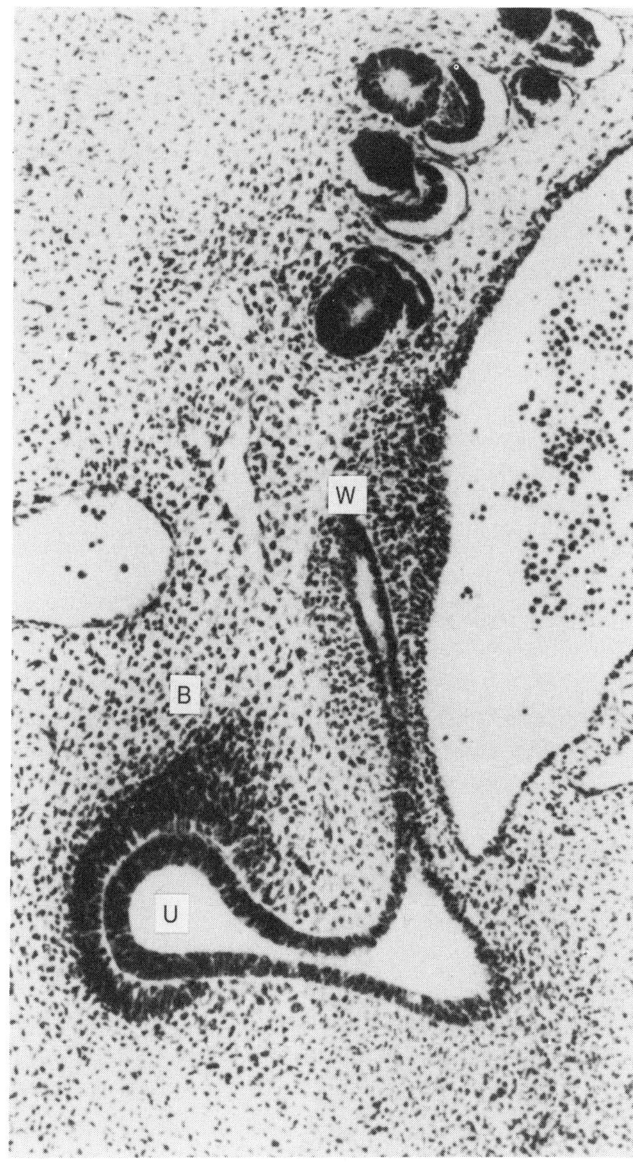

Fig. 14.1. Caudal extremity of the mesonephros from a 38-day human embryo (7 mm). U, ureteric bud; B, nephrogenic blastema; W, Wolffian duct. Magnification: x98. (From DuBois AM, 1969, with permission.)

It is recognized that the size and functional importance

of the mesonephros in various species is directly related to that of the allantois. The mesonephros and allantois are largest in species with a simple appositioned type of placenta, and are short-lived in primates, in which the placenta is highly permeable and the allantois is rudimentary. In species with a large allantoic cavity, such as the pig, rabbit, and sheep, the mesonephros has an excretory function early during development.

The main contribution of the mesonephros during embryogenesis is that it gives rise to the mesonephric duct, which induces the ureteric bud that is required for the formation of the metanephros (Fig. 14.1). The ureteric bud, which arises during the fourth week of gestation, is essential for the formation of the **urinary collecting system,** beginning with the ureter and terminating with the collecting tubules, and for the initiation of nephron formation by producing induction of the metanephric blastema (Fig. 14.1).

The metanephros or 'hind kidney' begins to develop in the human fetus early in the fifth week, and function is present by the eighth week of gestation. Before the metanephric blastema develops itself into a fully developed kidney, certain conditions need to be met. First, the undifferentiated cells of the metanephric blastema have to be committed to become nephrons well before the earliest evidence of differentiation. This process of 'nephric determination' is unique to this phase of development and never recurs in the adult animal, where all growth and regeneration involves committed epithelial cells. The second step in the development of the metanephric blastema is the progression of committed mesenchymal cells into differentiated epithelial cells under the influence of the ureteric bud, which acts as an inducer. As the ureteric bud extends dorsocranially into the nephrogenic ridges, it begins to divide and to form calyces and early divisions of the collecting ducts, and to develop into actual **nephrons** at approximately 8 weeks of gestation.

The induction of nephronic element formation starts shortly after the ureteric bud begins dividing (Fig. 14.2). Mesenchymal cells condense in a spherical mass (vesicle) located adjacent to an ampulla originating from dividing collecting ducts (ureteric bud). This spherical mass of mesenchymal cells forms an S-shaped body. Cells from one side of the S-shaped body become glomerular epithelium and cells from the other side become proximal tubules. Capillary endothelium and mesangium also arise from undifferentiated mesenchymal cells and invade the S-shaped body to form glomerular capillaries and glomerular mesangial cells.

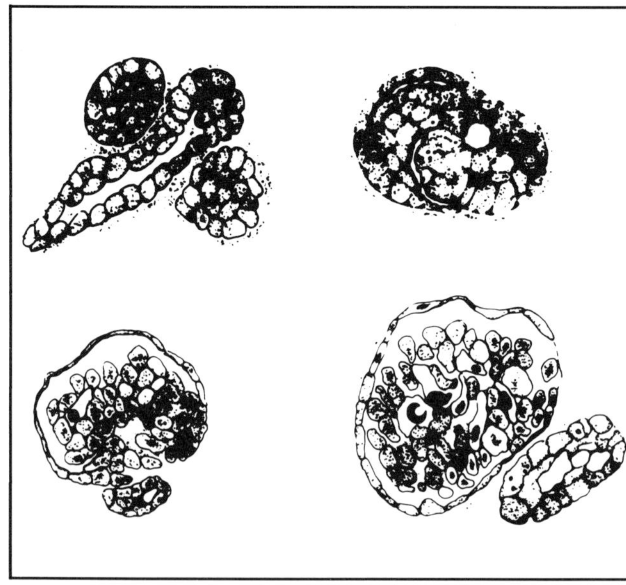

Fig. 14.2. Diagrammatic representation of the four key stages in glomerular development. Upper left: vesicles and ampulla (collecting duct). Upper right: S-shaped body. Lower left: capillary loop. Lower right: maturing glomerulus. (From Reeves WH, *et al. J Cell Biol* 1980; **85**: 735 with permission.)

The development of new nephron units proceeds in a centrifugal fashion from the center toward the periphery of the kidney until about 34 weeks of gestation, at which time approximately 800 000 nephrons have appeared in each kidney. The inner portion of the cortex, near the corticomedullary junction, contains the older glomeruli. The peripheral cortex contains the more recently formed glomeruli, the tubules of which are more shallowly placed and may remain in the cortex. This pattern of development results in a high degree of structural heterogeneity with nephron populations and nephron segments developing at different times.

Selected reading

Bacallao R, Fine FG. Molecular events in the organization of renal tubular epithelium: from nephrogenesis to regeneration. *Am J Physiol* 1989; **257**: F913.

DuBois AM. The embryonic kidney. In Rouiller C, Muller AF, eds. *The kidney: morphology, biochemistry, physiology*. Vol. 1. New York: Academic Press, 1969: 1.

McCrory WW. Embryologic development of the kidney. In McCrory WW, ed. *Developmental nephrology*. Cambridge, MA: Harvard University Press, 1972: 1.

Potter EL. Development of the kidney. In *Normal and abnormal development of the kidney*. Chicago: Year Book Medical Publishers, Inc., 1972: 3.

Reeves WH, Kanwar YS, Farguhar MG. Assembly of the glomerular filtration surface. Differentiation of anionic sites in glomerular capillaries of newborn rat kidney. *J Cell Biol* 1980; **85**: 735.

B. Renal Hemodynamics

J E Robillard

Distribution of blood flow

Whereas the kidneys of the newborn receive 15–18 percent of cardiac output, the fetal kidneys receive only 2–4 percent of the combined ventricular output during the last trimester of gestation. The proportion of cardiac output distributed to the kidneys increases to about 6 percent in the first week of life, and to approximately 15–18 percent during the first month of life. In adults, the kidneys receive between 20 and 25 percent of the cardiac output. In the fetus, renal blood flow is in the order of 1.5–2.0 ml/min per gram kidney weight. This relatively low rate of renal blood flow is associated with high renal vascular resistance and a low filtration fraction when compared with newborn animals (Fig. 14.3).

During fetal life, the intrarenal blood flow distribution is quantitatively different from that observed postnatally. Concordant with the morphological development of the kidney, which occurs from the center toward the periphery of the cortex, intrarenal blood flow distribution progresses in a centrifugal pattern (Fig. 14.4). Intrarenal distribution of glomerular perfusion rate, used as an index of intrarenal blood flow distribution, remains the same across the cortex during the last third of gestation, but the quotient between outer and inner glomerular blood flow increases significantly at birth, reflecting a shift of blood flow toward the superficial cortex. This shift in intrarenal blood flow distribution at birth is not associated with immediate changes in renal blood flow or renal vascular resistance. Only in the days following birth are significant increases in renal blood flow observed (Fig. 14.3). This intrarenal redistribution of blood flow toward the outer zone of the renal cortex may contribute to changes in glomerular and tubular function observed postnatally.

Regulation of blood flow

The increase in renal blood flow during the newborn period is probably secondary to a decrease in renal

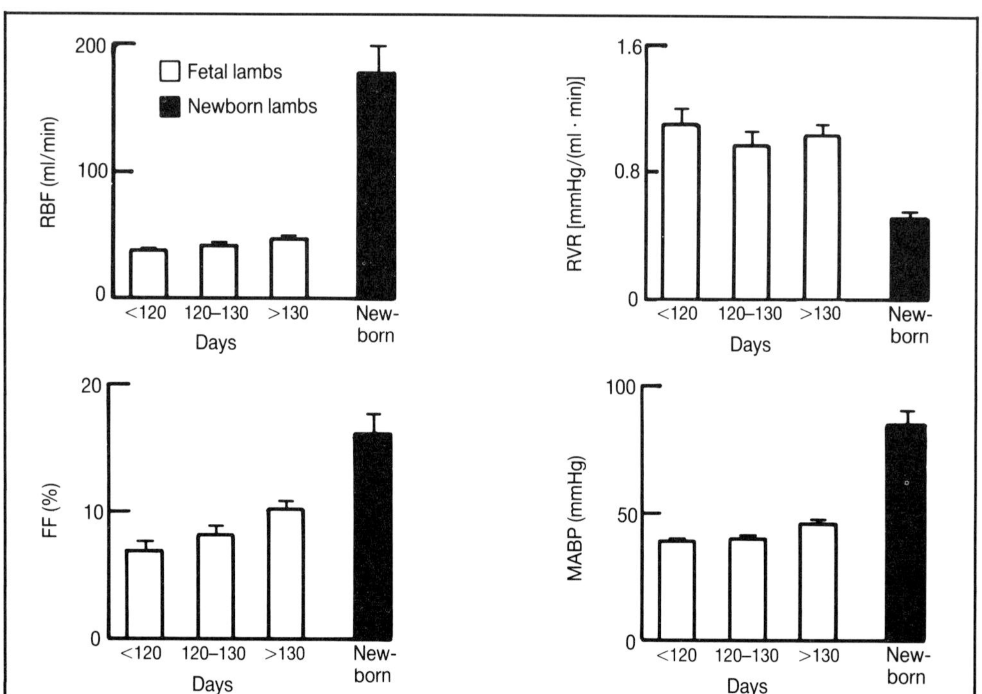

Fig. 14.3. Renal hemodynamic values in fetal and newborn sheep. The duration of gestation in sheep is 145 days. Newborn lambs were studied between 3 and 19 days postnatally. RBF, renal blood flow; RVR, renal vascular resistance; FF, filtration fraction; MABP, mean arterial blood pressure. (Adapted from Robillard JE, Nakamura KT. *Am J Physiol* 1988; **254**: F771, with permission.)

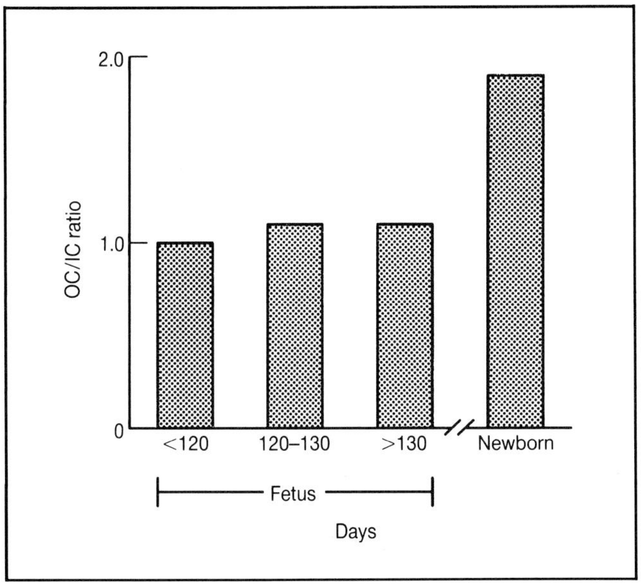

Fig. 14.4. Intrarenal blood flow distribution in fetal and newborn sheep. OC, outer cortex; IC, inner cortex. Newborn lambs were studied between 3 and 19 days postnatally. (Adapted from Robillard JE, *et al. Pediatr Res* 1981; **15**: 1248, with permission.)

vascular resistance concomitant with a rise in arterial pressure. Because the rise in arterial pressure is of lesser magnitude than the rise in renal blood flow, factors other than pressure alone are involved in the postnatal changes in renal hemodynamics.

Sympathetic nervous system

In sheep neither surgical nor pharmacological renal denervation is associated with significant changes in renal blood flow during fetal life, suggesting that renal sympathetic innervation is not an important modulator of renal hemodynamics during resting conditions prior to birth. On the other hand, renal nerves play an important role in modulating fetal renal blood flow during stressful conditions such as hypoxemia. To further clarify the role played by renal nerves in regulating renal blood flow during fetal and postnatal life, developmental differences in the renal hemodynamic response to increased efferent renal nerve activity have been investigated in fetal, newborn and adult sheep (Fig. 14.5). Renal nerve stimulation produces a decrease in renal blood flow and a rise in renal vascular resistance at all stages but the overall vasoconstrictor response to renal nerve stimulation is smaller in fetuses than in newborn and adult animals (Fig. 14.5, left panel).

In addition to its renal vasoconstrictor function, renal nerve stimulation can also produce renal vasodilatation during α-adrenoceptor blockade in fetal and newborn animals (Fig. 14.5, right panel). The ability of renal nerve stimulation to induce renal vasodilatation is particular to this developmental period, because it does not occur in adults. This renal vasodilatation, which is of greater magnitude in fetal than in newborn sheep, is independent of activation of cholinergic or dopaminergic receptors but is completely blocked by selective β_2-adrenoceptor antagonists. These results are of interest in several respects. First, they suggest that renal nerve fibers activated during renal nerve stimulation are essentially noradrenergic. Second, they provide evidence of an age-dependent neural renal vasodilator mechanism in mammals. Third, the observation that the renal vasodilatation observed during renal nerve stimulation decreases postnatally suggests that maturation of the adrenergic system is associated with a down-regulation of β-adrenoceptors in renal vessels. In favor of this

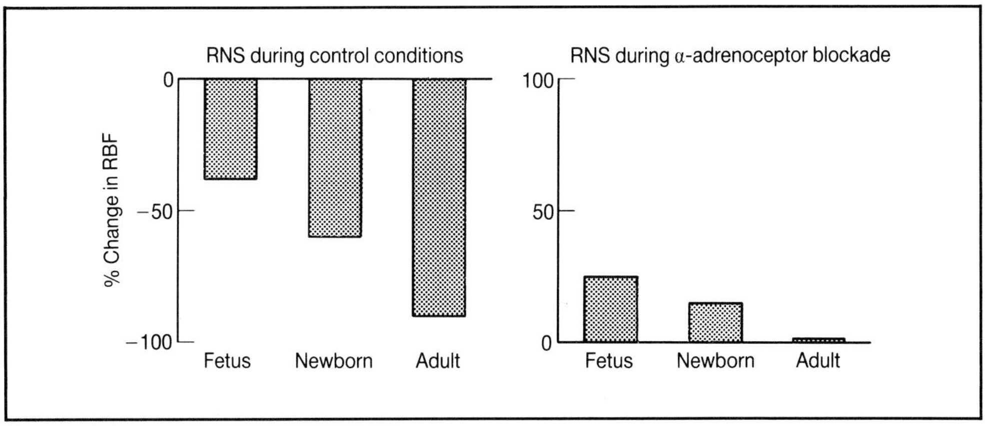

Fig. 14.5. Effect of renal nerve stimulation (RNS) on renal blood flow (RBF) during development. The effect of renal nerve stimulation at 8 Hz on renal blood flow is smaller in fetuses than in newborn lambs or adult sheep (left panel). Renal nerve stimulation during α-adrenoceptor blockade with phentolamine increases renal blood flow in fetal and newborn sheep, but not in adult sheep (right panel). (Adapted from Robillard JE, Nakamura KT. *Am J Physiol* 1988; **254**: F771, with permission.)

hypothesis is the observation in different vascular beds that β-adrenergic relaxation declines with advancing age. Furthermore, it has been demonstrated that the renal β_2-adrenoceptor is the main β-adrenoceptor subtype in the fetal kidney.

In sheep the intrarenal infusion of dopamine produces renal vasoconstriction during both fetal and postnatal life. The absence of renal vasodilatation with low dopamine doses in fetal and newborn sheep confirms results from other species demonstrating that 'α-adrenoceptor' effects of dopamine are predominant in immature animals. During α- and β-adrenergic blockade, dopamine did not increase renal blood flow in 1–2 week-old puppies, but did increase renal blood flow and glomerular filtration rate in older puppies. Similar results were observed following intravenous dopamine administration in young piglets. Intrarenal dopamine infusions during renal α- and β-adrenoceptor blockade produce similar renal vasodilatory responses in fetal, newborn, and adult sheep, suggesting that in sheep, dopamine has no age-related vasodilatory effect as previously observed in dogs and piglets.

Renin–angiotensin system

Studies of the role of the renin–angiotensin system in controlling renal hemodynamics during development have shown that the vasopressor response and the renal vasoconstrictor response to infusion of angiotensin II (AII) are less during fetal life than after birth, possibly due to a high receptor occupancy by endogenous AII early in life. Administration of AII to fetal sheep, however, increases arterial pressure, decreases umbilical flow, and decreases renal blood flow. Glomerular filtration rate remains unchanged, suggesting that AII acts primarily by increasing the tone of the efferent arteriole, as has been shown previously in adults. Studies investigating the intrarenal localization of AII-specific binding have shown that AII receptors are present in the afferent and efferent arterioles early during glomerular development, and in mesangial cells and in peritubular vessels just before birth. Immunolocalization of AII has also been found in the proximal tubule and in the thick ascending limb of Henle in fetal rats.

Atrial natriuretic factor

The renal hemodynamic response to systemic infusion of atrial natriuretic factor (ANF) differs in fetal, newborn, and adult animals. Systemic infusion of ANF to fetal and newborn animals produces a decrease in renal blood flow and a rise in renal vascular resistance, whereas no significant changes are observed in adults. This decrease in renal blood flow observed in fetal and newborn animals may be secondary to a decrease in cardiac output, as shown in adults, an increase in renal sympathetic tone and circulating catecholamines, a direct vasoconstrictor action of ANF on the fetal and neonatal vasculature, or a combination of these. Intrarenal infusion of ANF, however, causes a direct renal vasodilatation in fetal and newborn animals, suggesting that the renal vasoconstriction observed during systemic infusion of ANF is secondary to activation of compensatory mechanisms.

Eicosanoids

Prostaglandins (PGs) produced by the kidney may be involved in the regulation of renal hemodynamics and function early during development. A transient reduction in fetal renal blood flow occurs following administration of the PG inhibitors meclofenamate or indomethacin to fetal and newborn animals. Interestingly, administration of PG synthetase inhibitors to stop preterm labor in humans is associated with oligohydramnios in as many as 50 percent of cases. This oligohydramnios probably results from a decrease in fetal urine output secondary to a decrease in fetal RBF. Observations made in pregnant women given a short course of indomethacin treatment suggest that inhibition of PG synthesis leads to a significant decrease in GFR combined with low urine output in their offspring immediately after exposure. Although the alterations in renal function may be transient, one should consider prolonged treatment with PG synthetase inhibitors during pregnancy to be an important risk factor for the developing fetus.

Endothelins

Endothelins produced by endothelial cells are potent vasoconstrictors and mitogens, and are involved in the regulation of renal hemodynamics in the adult. In the fetal human kidney, specific binding sites for endothelins have been found in the cortex, medulla, and renal vessels. The presence of endothelin binding sites in the developing kidney may indicate a role for endothelin in modulating renal hemodynamics early in life and in influencing renal development.

Autoregulation of renal blood flow

The mature kidney is capable of maintaining renal blood flow relatively constant when major changes in perfusion pressure occur, a phenomenon known as autoregulation. It has been suggested that renal blood flow autoregulation is negligible at birth, but increases with postnatal development. Limited data are available on the renal autoregulatory phenomenon in the fetus. During infusion of vasopressin or AII to fetal sheep, however, no changes in renal blood flow were observed despite a moderate increase in arterial blood pressure. These data suggest that the fetus may autoregulate renal blood flow during modest increases in renal perfusion pressure.

Selected reading

Felder RA, Felder CC, Eisner GM, Jose PA. The dopamine receptor in the adult and maturing kidney. *Am J Physiol* 1989; **257**: F315.

Nakamura KT, Matherne GP, McWeeny OJ, Smith BA, Robillard JE. Renal hemodynamics and functional changes during the transition from fetal to newborn life in sheep. *Pediatr Res* 1987; **21**: 229.

Robillard JE, Nakamura KT. Neurohormonal regulation of renal function during development. *Am J Physiol* 1988; **254**: F771.

Robillard JE, Nakamura KT. Hormonal regulation of renal function during development. *Biol Neonate* 1988; **53**: 201.

Simonson MS, Dunn MJ. Endothelins: a family of regulatory peptides. State-of-the-art lecture. *Hypertension* 1991; **17**: 856.

Smith FG, Sato T, Varille VA, Robillard JE. Atrial natriuretic factor during fetal and postnatal life: a review. *J Dev Physiol* 1989; **12**: 55.

C. Glomerular Filtration

J E Robillard

In all vertebrate classes, the specialized filtration structure formed by the endothelium of the glomerular capillaries, the glomerular epithelial cells, and the basement membrane serves as an ultrafilter.

The rate at which the glomerular filtrate is formed, or glomerular filtration rate (GFR), is determined by measuring the clearance of inulin (C_{in}). C_{in} is defined as the virtual volume of plasma that is completely cleared of inulin by the kidney per unit time and is expressed as

$$C_{in} = \frac{UV}{P}$$

where U is the concentration of inulin in the urine, V is the rate of urine flow, and P is the concentration of inulin in plasma.

Glomerular filtration begins between the ninth and twelfth week of gestation in the human fetus and contributes to the formation of urine and accumulation of amniotic fluid. In fetal sheep, GFR increases by about 2.5 times during the last trimester of gestation (from 1.24 ml/min at 100 days of gestation to 3.25 ml/min at term) (Fig. 14.6), and parallels the rise in fetal body weight and kidney weight. In newborn infants delivered between 27 and 43 weeks of gestation in which GFR was measured in the first 24 hours after birth, GFR (ml/min) correlates with gestational age.

The transition from fetal to newborn life brings a sudden surge in GFR. In sheep GFR increases threefold during the first 24 hours following birth (Fig. 14.7). This rise in GFR is not associated with significant changes in total renal blood flow. Moreover, as no significant rise in arterial blood pressure is observed during the first 24 hours of postnatal life, changes in renal perfusion pressure are unlikely to contribute to the rise in GFR. On the other hand, an increase in the number of functional nephrons secondary to intrarenal redistribution of blood flow toward the outer portion of the renal cortex may contribute to the rise in GFR observed at birth.

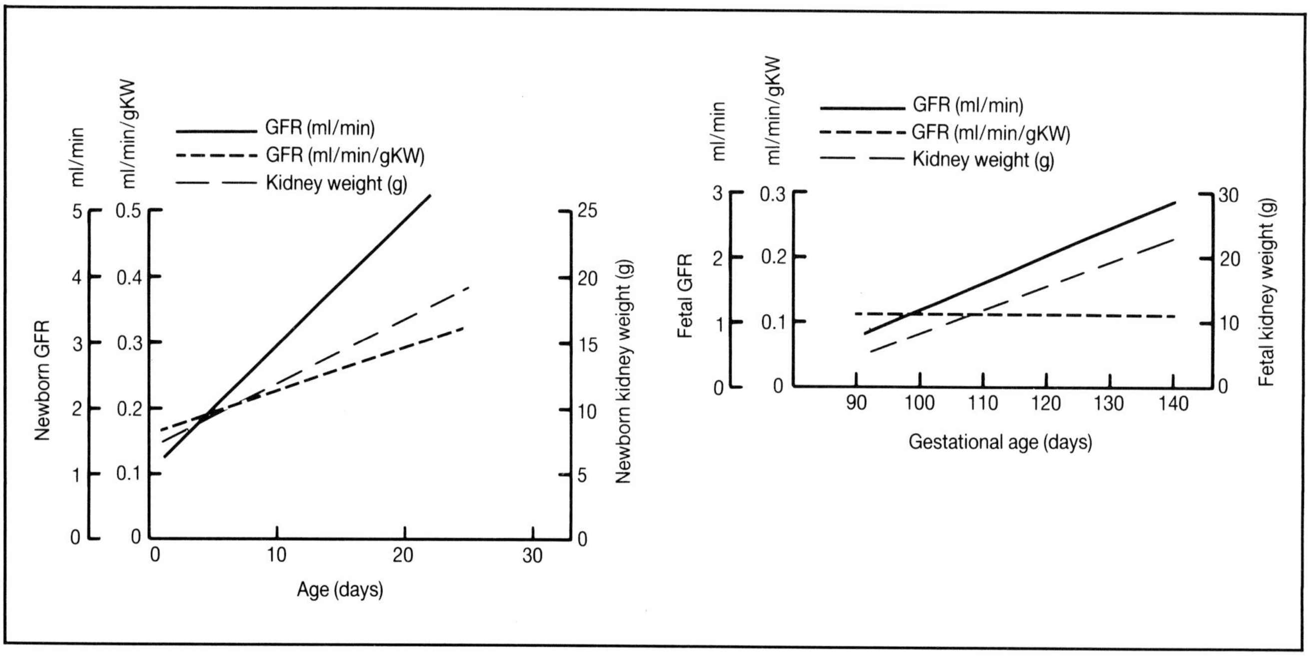

Fig. 14.6. Maturation of glomerular filtration rate (GFR) during fetal (right panel) and postnatal (left panel) life. (From Robillard JE, *et al. Am J Obstet Gynecol* 1977; **128**: 727; and Kleinman LI, Lubbe RJ. *J Physiol* 1972; **223**: 395, with permission.)

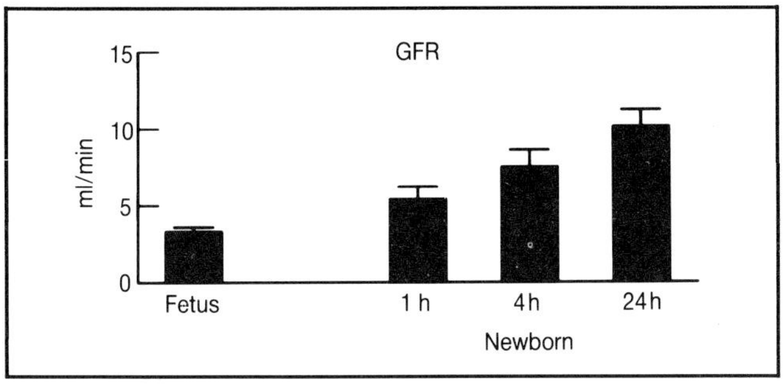

Fig. 14.7. Changes in glomerular filtration rate (GFR) during the transition from fetal to newborn life. (From Nakamura KT, *et al.* *Pediatr Res* 1987; **21**: 229, with permission.)

Regulation by vasoactive substances

It has been suggested that the changes in GFR observed postnatally may depend on changes in the concentrations of circulating vasoactive substances observed at the time of birth. At birth, plasma epinephrine and norepinephrine concentrations are elevated in human infants delivered vaginally and in lambs delivered by cesarean section, and decline slowly during the first 24 hours of postnatal life. Because the rise in GFR observed during the first day of life closely follows the decline in plasma epinephrine and norepinephrine, perhaps catecholamines influence GFR during the transition from fetal to newborn life. Based on the fact that total renal blood flow does not change immediately after birth, however, the changes observed in plasma catecholamines seem unlikely to play an important role in influencing GFR postnatally.

Because renin and angiotensin II (AII) concentrations are high at the time of birth, it has been suggested that the renin–angiotensin system may influence changes in GFR during the transition from fetal to newborn life. In support of this hypothesis, inhibition of AII synthesis with captopril tends to decrease renal blood flow and GFR during the first 24 hours of life.

Regulation by physical factors

Physical factors that effect GFR:
- glomerular surface area (S)
- effective filtration pressure (P_{UF})
- effective hydraulic permeability (k)

Changes in physical factors known to affect single nephron glomerular filtration rate (SNGFR) in the adult have been suggested to regulate the changes in SNGFR during development. Changes in glomerular surface area (S), effective filtration pressure (P_{UF}) and effective hydraulic permeability (k) are known to affect SNGFR during the newborn period. These interrelationships are expressed by the equation

$$\mathrm{GFR} = k \cdot S \cdot P_{UF}$$

These factors have not been quantified during fetal life. It appears, however, that low S, low k, and low P_{UF} may contribute to the low GFR in the fetus. In the newborn, it has been shown that the large increase in GFR (25 times) during development depends predominantly on an increase in the glomerular surface area (8 times) and, to a lesser extent, on a rise in P_{UF} (2.5 times). Changes in the hydraulic permeability of the glomerular capillary (1.3 times) contribute only minimally to the postnatal rise in GFR.

Selected reading

Guignard J-P, Torrado A, DaCunha O, Gautier E. Glomerular filtration rate in the first three weeks of life. *J Pediatr* 1975; **87**: 268.

Leake RD, Trygstad CW, Oh W. Inulin clearance in the newborn infant: relationship to gestational and postnatal age. *Pediatr Res* 1976; **10**: 759.

Robillard JE, Sessions C, Kennedy RL, Robillard LH, Smith FG, Jr. Interrelationship between glomerular filtration rate and renal transport of sodium and chloride during fetal life. *Am J Obstet Gynecol* 1977; **128**: 727.

Smith FG, Lumbers ER. Comparison of renal function in term fetal sheep and newborn lambs. *Biol Neonate* 1989; **55**: 309.

Smith FG, Robillard JE. Pathophysiology of fetal renal disease. *Semin Perinatol* 1989; **13**: 305.

Spitzer A. The developing kidney and the process of growth. In Seldin DW, Giebisch G, eds. *The kidney: physiology and pathophysiology*. New York: Raven Press, 1985: 1979.

D. Tubular Function

D1. Sodium Homeostasis

A Aperia

Regulation of Na^+ homeostasis

It is essential for the mammalian organism to maintain both arterial blood pressure and intracellular electrolyte composition within normal limits. In healthy adults, this process is so efficient–sensitive that, despite wide daily variations in salt and water intake, blood volume, blood pressure, and intracellular electrolyte composition generally are well maintained, and only large pathological losses will offset this balance.

The kidney plays an important role in this regulation. Both short- and long-term adjustments of salt and water balance are accomplished by variations in the rate of tubular reabsorption. Tubular reabsorption is under the control of renal nerves, catecholamines, and both peptide and steroid hormones. It is also regulated by hydrostatic and oncotic pressures. These physical forces in turn influence tubular and glomerular function because the glomerular filtration rate and the filtration fraction have an important influence on the hydrostatic and oncotic pressures in the peritubular capillaries and in the tubular lumen.

Ion transporters

Na^+ crosses the cell membrane via specific transporting proteins. Located in the basolateral membrane of all tubular cells, Na^+-K^+-ATPase, by transferring the energy from ATP hydrolysis to a vectorial transport of Na^+ and K^+ with a coupling ratio of 3:2, creates an electrochemical gradient across the cell membrane. Na^+-K^+-ATPase uses approximately 80 percent of all O_2 that is consumed by the kidney. The Na^+-K^+-ATPase-mediated gradient allows for a downhill transport of Na^+ from the tubular lumen into the cell via co- and counter-transporters and channels. Na^+-K^+-ATPase is an ubiquitous protein, but most of the in-transporters are selectively distributed. Some examples of Na^+ in-transporters are the Na^+-glucose and Na^+-amino acid cotransporters, which are only expressed in proximal tubular cells, and the furosemide-sensitive Na^+-K^+-Cl^- cotransporter, which is expressed in the thick ascending limb of Henle. The important Na^+-H^+ exchanger is most abundant in the proximal tubule.

As many of the Na^+ transporting proteins now are cloned, information about the transcriptional and translational regulation of these proteins is starting to emerge. Because these proteins are differentially distributed to the basolateral or apical membrane, the means by which they are directed to the appropriate side of the cell is an important developmental question.

Paracellular transport

Tubular reabsorption of salt and fluid is both transcellular and paracellular. In the proximal tubule, which is a relatively leaky epithelium, a large fraction of salt and water reabsorption occurs via the paracellular pathway. Paracellular fluxes depend on the establishment of osmotic and chemical gradients across the epithelium, which are generated by the active transcellular transport of solute. The paracellular fluxes also depend on the hydraulic conductivity of the cell junctions.

Neurotransmitters and hormones modulating Na^+ balance

Regulation of Na^+ excretion is bidirectional. Some of the best known salt-regulating factors are atrial natriuretic peptide (ANP) and dopamine, which act natriuretically, and aldosterone, angiotensin, and norepinephrine, which act antinatriuretically. Many other hormones, such as prostaglandins, bradykinin, and endothelin, also have a modulating effect on Na^+ transport in various parts of the nephron, but the mechanism(s) of action of these hormones is less well known at present. Aldosterone and ANP are both circulating factors. Aldosterone is released in response to changes in electrolyte balance. Increased circulating concentrations of aldosterone are generally an early sign of salt depletion. ANP is released from the heart in response to changes in blood volume. Recent evidence suggests that ANP is also locally produced in the kidney. Angiotensin and dopamine are formed in the kidney and act as both paracrine and autocrine factors. Dopamine is synthesized in the proximal tubular cells; the rate of synthesis is sensitive to changes in salt balance. Norepinephrine is released from nerve endings. Renal nerve activity can be influenced by many physiological factors (e.g. volume expansion will decrease renal nerve activity).

Aldosterone is a steroid hormone with an intracellular receptor that, when activated by the hormone, will cross the nuclear membrane and act as a transcriptional factor. Several lines of evidence suggest that both aldosterone and the glucocorticoid hormone can regulate the transcription of Na^+-K^+-ATPase. The effect of aldosterone differs from the effect of glucocorticoid hormone not only in that it is more specific (aldosterone receptors are selectively distributed in the distal parts of the nephron), but also in that it is age independent and also present in the mature kidney. The age-dependent effects of glucocorticoid hormone will be described under developmental aspects.

Both peptide hormones and catecholamines act on membrane receptors which, following activation, initiate a signal that is forwarded by second messengers such as cAMP, Ca^{2+}, and diacylglycerol to third messengers such as protein kinases. Eventually the activity of the Na^+ transporting protein will be altered by phosphorylation/dephosphorylation, the most common form of covalent modification of a protein. Although the physiological responses are entirely different, the principles for regulation of ion transporters via protein phosphorylation are similar in the brain and kidney.

The balance between the effect of protein kinases and the effect of phosphatases determines the basal activity of ion transporters. Hormones that act natriuretically drive the reaction in one direction, resulting in inactivation of the ion transporter, while hormones that act anti-natriuretically drive the reaction in the other direction, resulting in activation of the ion transporter. Antinatriuretic hormones often stimulate both the Na^+ in-transporters and Na^+-K^+-ATPase while natriuretic hormones often inhibit both in-transporters and Na^+-K^+-ATPase.

Developmental aspects

The infant mammalian kidney is not as efficient as the adult kidney in maintaining the volume and composition of the body fluids. Low salt intake results in negative salt balance more rapidly in the infant than in the adult. Because the newborn kidney also has a lower capacity to excrete a Na^+ load, the risk for salt and water accumulation following high salt intake is greater in the infant than in the adult.

The low capacity of the infant to vary Na^+ excretion rapidly in response to changes in salt intake does not seem to be due to a lack of regulatory factors. Most of the hormones known to be important for the regulation of Na^+ balance are appropriately released in the neonate and also in the near-term fetus.

In many cases infant renal tubule cells seem to have an altered sensitivity to hormones regulating Na^+ transport. Renal sympathetic nerves can already influence salt excretion during fetal life. In fact, high renal nerve activity might contribute to the infant's low capacity to excrete a salt load. Renal tubular cells in preterm infants and in rat pups are relatively insensitive to aldosterone due to low availability of aldosterone receptors. A blunted natriuretic response to ANP also has been reported in infants of many species and a blunted response to dopamine occurs in rat and dog pups. There is a natriuretic response to dopamine in the human infant and in rabbit pups, but the magnitude of the response in infants and adults has not been compared. Apparently the ontogeny of signal transduction systems in the renal tubular cells is quite complex. Most developmental studies on signal transduction in the kidney so far have been performed on signal pathways that are coupled to dopamine receptors. The ontogeny of the cellular response to dopamine differs in different parts of the nephrons. In the proximal tubule, the coupling of the $dopamine_1$ receptor to the adenylyl cyclase unit increases during ontogeny. The reverse appears to be the case in the medullary thick ascending limb of Henle. Protein kinase C, which might also be a third messenger of dopamine in the kidney, can phosphorylate and inactivate Na^+-K^+-ATPase. This response is blunted in the infant kidney. Yet protein kinase C activity is higher in the infant than in the adult renal cortex. From the relatively few studies conducted so far in this interesting field, one can conclude that the effect of a particular hormone on natriuresis in the infant cannot be predicted from that hormone's effect in the adult. It is tempting to speculate that in the developing kidney, signal transduction pathways are also used for growth and differentiation and that they might therefore be occupied when Na^+-regulating factors try to forward a signal.

The Na^+ transporting capacity of the infant kidney is also limited by a low number of transporting proteins. So far most determinations of available transporters are indirect and based on studies of the activity of the transporter when it is saturated with regard to substrates. In rat pups, the activities of the Na^+-K^+-ATPase Na^+-H^+ exchanger and Na^+-glucose transporter have been shown to increase significantly postnatally. The most rapid increase generally occurs during or just before the weanling period. This coincides with an upsurge in plasma concentrations of glucocorticoid hormone. Several lines of evidence suggest that the glucocorticoid hormone can act as an inducer of Na^+ transporting proteins and that, at least in case of Na^+-K^+-ATPase, this is mediated by a direct transcriptional effect on the genes of the two subunits of the enzyme. Of interest for the understanding of renal differentiation, this effect is transient and appears to be lost or attenuated in the adult kidney.

The increase in the number of transporting proteins is paralleled by an increase in the reabsorptive capacity of the tubule and also by an increase in the size of the membrane where the protein is located. If the ion transporters are prematurely induced by administration of glucocorticoid hormones, this will be followed by an increase in the functional capacity of the kidney. Observations from experimental studies indicate that the infant proximal convoluted tubule has a large hydraulic conductance and suggest that the transepithelial shunt pathway may contribute to reabsorption to a larger extent in the early postnatal period than in later life.

Clinical aspects

During the first weeks of life the preterm infant has a very low capacity to vary salt excretion and is therefore extremely sensitive to large variations in salt intake. Because the capacity to regulate body fluid tonicity is also low (see Section 14F), disturbances in serum Na^+ concentration are common. All infants have difficulties in rapidly excreting a salt load. This capacity develops gradually during the first year of life. Disturbances in salt and water balance have many adverse effects. High Na^+ and fluid intake results in blood volume expansion, which will delay closure of the ductus arteriosus and might compromise the circulation to the gut and the lungs, contributing to *necrotizing enterocolitis* and *broncho-pulmonary dysplasia*. Salt deficiency retards growth. Both hypo- and hypernatremia can lead to brain damage. The low capacity of the Na^+-H^+ exchanger predisposes to acidosis.

Healthy full-term infants generally maintain Na^+ balance well, provided they receive breast milk or a formula with corresponding electrolyte composition. If the infant has kidney disease that has led to a moderate decrease in renal function, the risk for disturbances in Na^+ balance is high. Hyponatremia and acidosis (low capacity of the Na^+-H^+ exchanger) are common in infants with moderate renal insufficiency. Like salt deficiency, acidosis will retard growth; therefore, even mild acidosis must be corrected in infants with renal insufficiency.

Selected reading

Aperia A, Celsi G. Ontogenic processes in nephron epithelia. Structure, enzymes, and function. In Seldin DW, Giebisch G, eds. *The kidney: physiology and pathophysiology*. Vol. 11, 2nd ed. New York: Raven Press Ltd, 1992: 803.

Celsi G, Nishi A, Akusjarvi G, Aperia A. Abundance of Na^+-K^+-ATPase mRNA is regulated by glucocorticoid hormones in infant rat kidneys. *Am J Physiol* 1991; **260**: F192.

Haycock GB, Aperia A. Salt and the newborn kidney. *Pediatr Nephrol* 1991; **5**: 65.

Robillard JE, Smith FG, Segar JL, *et al*. Mechanisms regulating renal sodium excretion during development. *Pediatr Nephrol* 1992; **6**: 205.

Seldin DW, Giebisch G, eds. *The kidney: physiology and pathophysiology*. Vol. 11. 2nd ed. Section 111: Renal regulation of sodium and chloride: normal. New York: Raven Press Ltd, 1992: 1807.

D2. Potassium (K^+) Handling during Development

L M Satlin

The kidney, the major route for elimination of K^+ from the body, is responsible for excretion of approximately 90 percent of the average 100 mmol K^+ ingested daily. Small obligatory extrarenal losses of K^+ occur in sweat (1–2 mmol/day) and stool (7–15 mmol/day).

In general, the rate of urinary K^+ excretion parallels dietary intake, thereby maintaining serum K^+ concentration within a narrow range of 3.5–5.0 mmol/liter. However, extreme adjustments in the K^+ excretory rate cannot be achieved as rapidly as for Na^+, nor are they as complete. Whereas urinary Na^+ virtually disappears from the urine within 3–4 days of Na^+ restriction, a minimum urinary K^+ loss of approximately 5 mmol/day persists in the K^+-restricted adult. In response to an abrupt increase in K^+ intake (oral, parenteral), urinary K^+ promptly increases, yet maximal excretory rates may not become apparent for 1–2 days.

Sites of K^+ transport in the kidney

Most of the information available regarding the renal handling of K^+ has been derived from *in vivo* micropuncture studies of segments exposed to the cortical surface (superficial nephrons) or papillary tip (juxtamedullary nephrons); segments inaccessible to micropuncture have been examined by *in vitro* microperfusion.

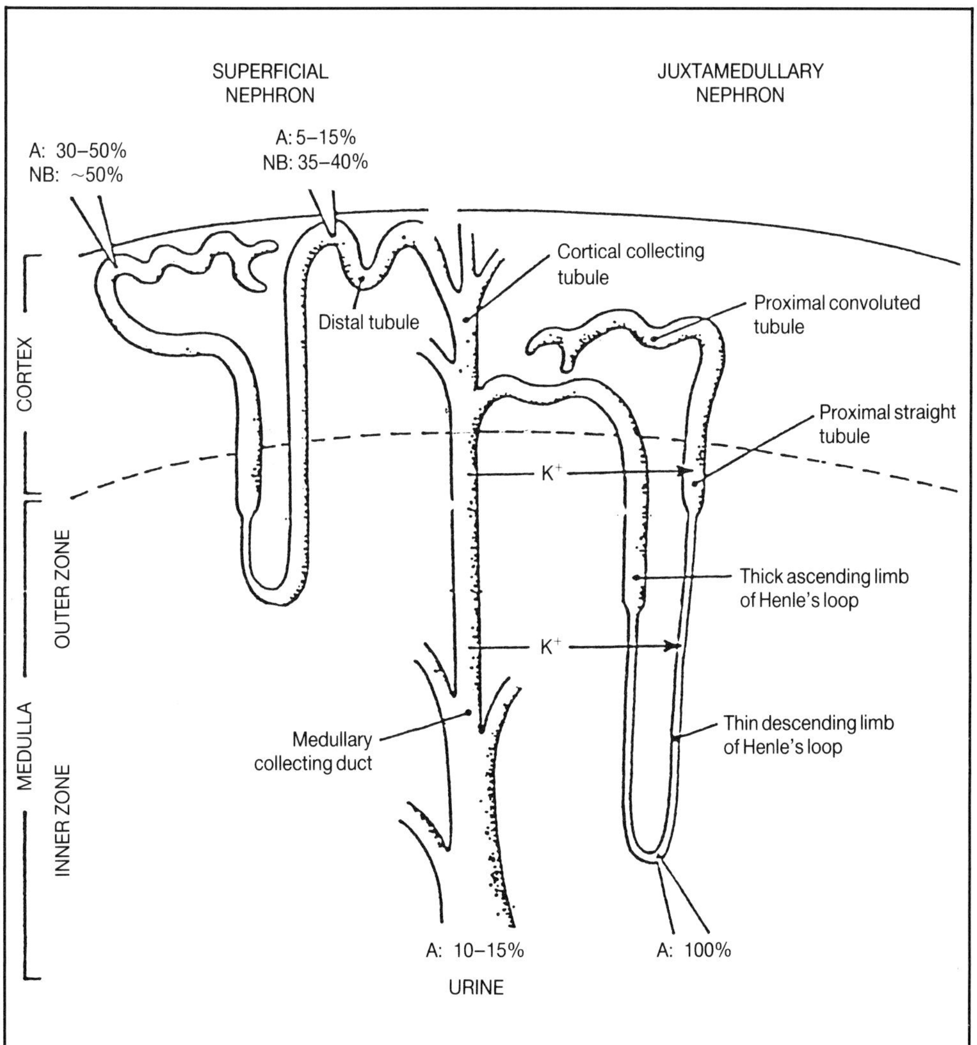

Fig. 14.8. Segmental handling of K^+ in superficial and juxtamedullary nephrons of the rat. The percentage of filtered K^+ remaining at each site is provided for the adult (A), and when known, the newborn (NB) animal. Arrows show the direction of net K^+ transport, either reabsorption or secretion. (Modified from Giebisch G *et al.* Renal transport and control of potassium excretion, In Brenner BM, Rector FC Jr, eds. *The kidney*. Philadelphia: WB Saunders, 1991: 291, with permission.)

The transport characteristics of individual nephron segments are summarized in Fig. 14.8. Filtered K^+ is reabsorbed almost entirely in proximal segments of the nephron, urinary K^+ being derived predominantly from distal K^+ secretion. Thus K^+ **balance**, at least in the adult, is maintained by renal secretion rather than reabsorption (as in the case of Na^+).

Superficial nephron

K^+ is freely filtered at the glomerulus. Approximately 50 percent of the filtered load of K^+ is reabsorbed along the initial two-thirds of the superficial proximal tubule. **Reabsorption** in this segment is passive, closely following the reabsorption of water and Na^+; thus, the concentration of K^+ in the proximal tubular fluid remains similar to that of plasma.

In the adult, 5–15 percent of the filtered load of K^+ reaches the superficial early distal tubule, indicating that significant net reabsorption of K^+ occurs in the intervening nephron segments. A major site of avid K^+ reabsorption therein is the thick ascending limb of Henle's loop which possesses a luminal electroneutral cotransporter that translocates one Na^+ and one K^+ with two Cl^- ions into the cell (Fig. 14.9a); the powerful *loop diuretics* (e.g. furosemide, ethacrynic acid) inhibit this cotransporter, resulting in Na^+ and K^+ escape into the distal tubular fluid.

Comparison of the fractional delivery of K^+ to the early distal tubule with that present in the final urine indicates that the rate of K^+ secretion along the intervening segments (late distal tubule, collecting duct) is highly variable, depending on the metabolic state and K^+ balance, but can approach 20–50 percent of the filtered load.

Juxtamedullary nephron

Analysis of the tubular fluid collected by micropuncture at the tip of the adult rat papilla indicates that the rate of K^+ delivery to the end of the descending limb of Henle's

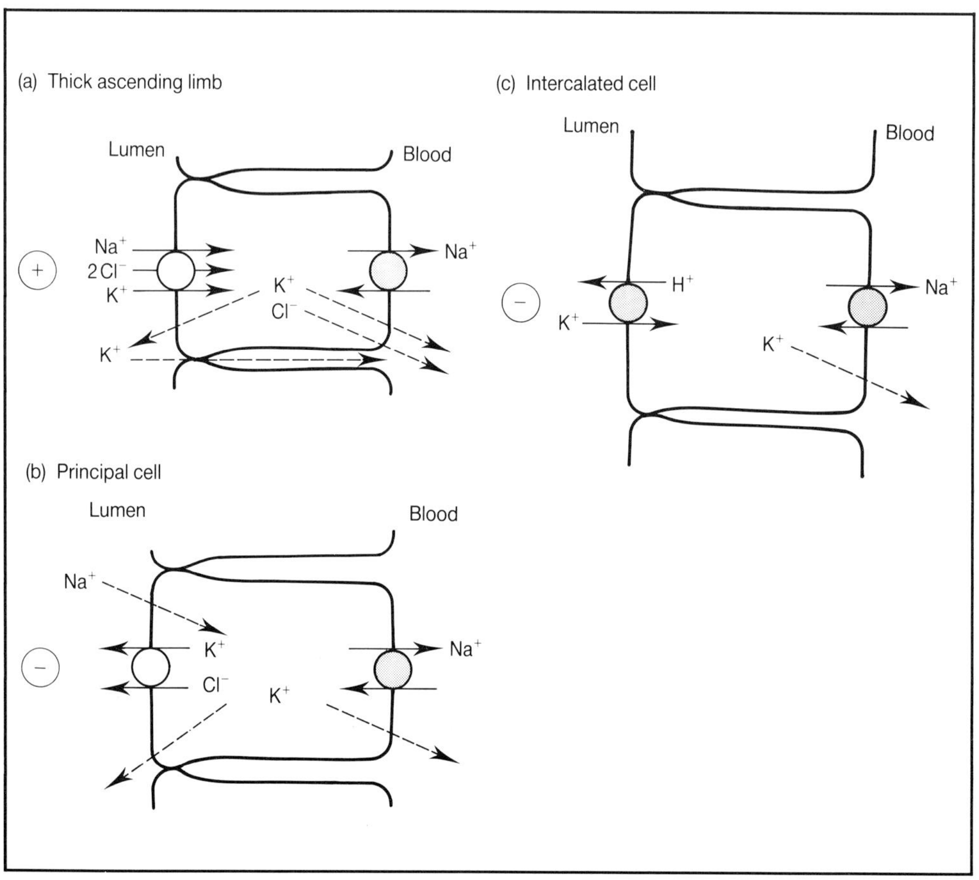

Fig. 14.9. Possible pathways of transepithelial K^+ transport in the (a) thick ascending limb, and cortical collecting duct, (b) principal cell and (c) intercalated cell. Broken arrows denote passive pathways whereas solid arrows depict active transport mechanisms. (Modified from Wright FS, Giebisch G. Regulation of K^+ excretion. In: Seldin DW, Giebisch G, eds. *The kidney*. New York: Raven Press, 1985: 1223, with permission.)

loop may exceed the filtered load. Presumably, K^+ diffuses passively from the medullary interstitium down its concentration gradient into the proximal straight tubule and thin descending limb of Henle's loop. The high concentration of K^+ in the medullary interstitial fluid is derived from reabsorption by the thick ascending limb and the outer medullary collecting duct. K^+ reabsorption by the latter segment is primarily passive, following a favorable electrochemical gradient generated by the high tubular fluid K^+ concentration leaving the cortical collecting duct and the lumen positive voltage.

The physiological role of medullary K^+ **recycling** (reabsorption by the thick ascending limb and medullary collecting duct; secretion into the proximal straight tubule and descending limb of Henle's loop) remains unclear. However, it may serve to amplify the fraction of K^+ being delivered to distal segments of the juxtamedullary nephron and may account for an increase in K^+ excretion under conditions of K^+ loading.

Distal nephron

The cortical collecting duct is the main regulatory site of K^+ secretion, capable of generating K^+ concentrations in excess of 100 mM in the luminal fluid. This segment is composed of two major cell types. The majority cell type, the **principal cell**, secretes K^+ and absorbs Na^+. The less numerous **intercalated cells**, primarily responsible for transepithelial acid–base transport, may play a role in K^+ reabsorption.

Principal cell

The model for transcellular K^+ secretion in the principal cell (Fig. 14.9b) requires the **active** cellular uptake of two K^+ ions against a large concentration gradient in exchange for the extrusion of three Na^+ ions at the basolateral membrane, a process driven by Na^+-K^+-ATPase; the unequal exchange rate creates a negative voltage within the cell. Cell K^+ then diffuses **passively** into the lumen through apical K^+-selective channels. In the presence of adequate channels, the magnitude of K^+ secretion is determined by the cell-to-lumen electrochemical gradient. The lumen negative potential difference across the cortical collecting duct, generated by apical Na^+ entry and electrogenic basolateral extrusion (via Na^+-K^+-ATPase), and high cell K^+ provide a favorable driving force for cell K^+ exit into the luminal fluid. Recent evidence suggests that a Cl^--dependent K^+ cotransporter resides on the apical membrane of this cell.

Intercalated cell

Intercalated cells, specialized for proton secretion in the medullary collecting duct, may actively absorb K^+ (Fig. 14.9c). K^+ deficiency is associated with selective hypertrophy of the apical surfaces of medullary intercalated cells and appearance of an ATP-coupled H^+-K^+ pump (which secretes protons into the urine in exchange for K^+ reabsorption) in the apical membrane of these cells in K^+-depleted animals.

Regulation of K^+ balance by the distal nephron

K^+ secretion by the cortical collecting duct depends on the interaction of various cellular, luminal, and circulating factors capable of influencing K^+ transport (Table 14.1). Factors that enhance the electrochemical driving force or apical membrane permeability to K^+ of the principal cell facilitate secretion of this cation.

Table 14.1. Factors that influence K^+ transport

Cellular
Cell K^+ concentration
Luminal
Tubular fluid flow rate
Luminal Na^+ and K^+ concentrations
Transepithelial voltage
Circulating
Acid–base balance
Aldosterone activity

Cell K^+ concentration

The chemical concentration of K^+ in the intracellular fluid ranges between 100 mmol/liter and 150 mmol/liter. K^+ activity, the effective concentration that is ionically active, appears to be substantially lower, reflecting intracellular binding of K^+ to proteins or compartmentalization of this ion within cells.

The intracellular concentration of K^+ can be altered by numerous factors, including K^+ intake. An increase in dietary K^+ results in a transient rise in plasma K^+ concentration which in turn stimulates renal K^+ excretion and adrenal release of aldosterone. At the level of the principal cell, *hyperkalemia* reduces the concentration gradient across the basolateral membrane against which the Na^+-K^+ pump must function, thereby stimulating basolateral uptake of K^+. This, in combination with an increase in transepithelial voltage, augments K^+ secretion.

Chronic K^+ loading leads to 'K^+ tolerance' in the distal nephron, an adaptation that enables the animal to survive an otherwise lethal acute K^+ load. The cellular mechanisms underlying this adaptation include increases in Na^+-K^+-ATPase activity and permeability of the apical membrane of the principal cell, modifications that together create a more favorable driving force for K^+ diffusion from cell to lumen. A similar adaptive response is seen in *chronic renal insufficiency*.

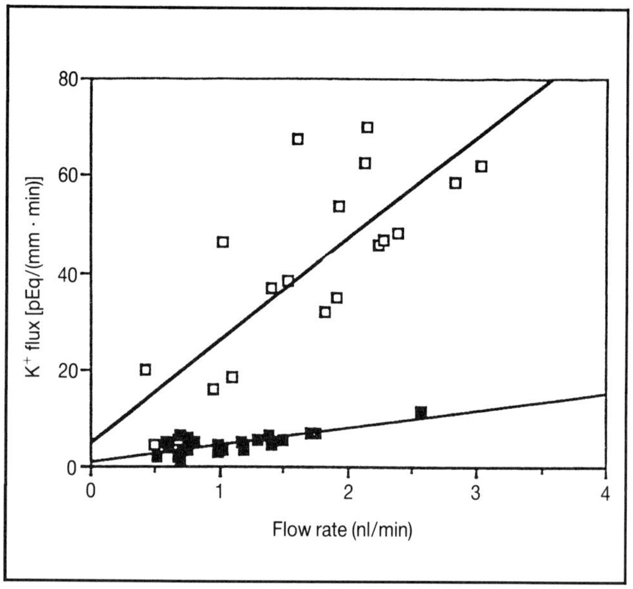

Fig. 14.10. Effect of tubular fluid flow rate on K^+ secretion (K^+ flux) in isolated perfused rabbit cortical collecting ducts. Solid squares, data from animals fed a control diet. Open squares, animals fed diet to elevate plasma aldosterone concentrations and thereby enhance K^+ secretion. (From Engbretson BG, Stoner LC. *Am J Physiol* 1987; **253**: F898, with permission.)

Rate of tubular fluid flow

K^+ secretion is strongly influenced by the rate of tubular fluid flow (Fig. 14.10) and the concentration of K^+ in the tubular fluid. At low flow rates, distal K^+ secretion results in a gradual increase in the tubular fluid K^+ concentration that opposes further K^+ secretion. As flow rate increases, the tubular fluid K^+ concentration remains constant or falls, thereby preserving or enhancing the favorable chemical gradient for the secretion of K^+. Thus *volume expansion* and *diuretics*, which increase urinary flow rate, facilitate K^+ secretion in the distal nephron.

Distal Na^+ delivery

Extracellular volume expansion and administration of diuretics (osmotic or those acting on proximal tubule or loop) promote an increase in K^+ excretion. Whereas the kaliuresis is due in part to the increase in tubular flow rate, the increased luminal Na^+ concentration reaching the cortical collecting duct can, in itself, enhance K^+ secretion. Specifically, stimulation of electrogenic Na^+ reabsorption increases the intraluminal negativity, further enhancing the electrochemical gradient favoring passive diffusion of K^+ from cell to lumen.

Luminal Na^+ concentrations exceeding 35 mmol/liter do not further influence the K^+ secretory rate; however, K^+ secretion is markedly suppressed when the tubular fluid Na^+ concentration falls below 10 mmol/liter, as might occur under conditions of maximal Na^+ retention. *In vivo* measurements of distal tubular Na^+ concentration in both adult and suckling rats generally exceed 35 mmol/liter, indicating that luminal Na^+ concentration does not regulate distal K^+ secretion under physiological conditions.

Transepithelial voltage

Because the transepithelial voltage is generated by apical Na^+ entry and electrogenic basolateral extrusion, any agent that decreases active Na^+ transport (e.g. basolateral ouabain, luminal amiloride) will reduce the lumen negative potential difference and thereby reduce K^+ secretion. A small increase in luminal electronegativity in the cortical collecting duct occurs when Na^+ delivered to that segment is accompanied by a poorly reabsorbable anion (e.g. β-hydroxybutyrate in diabetic ketacidosis, bicarbonate, or carbenicillin) instead of Cl^-; the consequent increase in K^+ movement from cell to lumen, however, may derive more from enhanced activity of the K^+-Cl^- cotransporter, stimulated by the reduction in luminal Cl^-, than from the modification in voltage.

Acid–base balance

For both respiratory and metabolic derangements, acute *alkalosis* increases, whereas acute *acidosis* reduces urinary K^+ excretion (Fig. 14.11). Although alkalosis shifts K^+ into cells and acidosis causes cells to lose K^+, principal cell K^+ concentration changes little in response to perturbations in acid–base balance. Presumably, enhanced uptake is accompanied by accelerated exit through apical pH-sensitive K^+ channels, which open in response to cell alkalinization and close with acidosis.

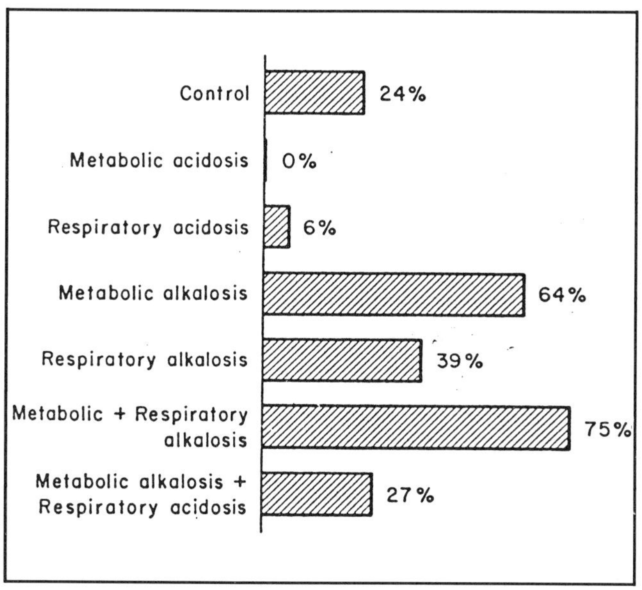

Fig. 14.11. Effect of acid–base disturbances on distal tubule K^+ secretion. Bars indicate the percentage of the amount of K^+ in glomerular filtrate present under the designated condition. (From Giebisch G, *et al*. Renal transport and control of K^+ excretion. In Brenner BM, Rector FC Jr, eds. *The kidney*. Vol. I. Philadelphia: WB Saunders, 1991, with permission.)

The effect of chronic acid–base disturbances on K^+ secretion is more complex and may be influenced by the rate of delivery of fluid to the distal nephron, modification of the glomerular filtrate (replacement of Cl^- with bicarbonate), and circulating aldosterone concentrations.

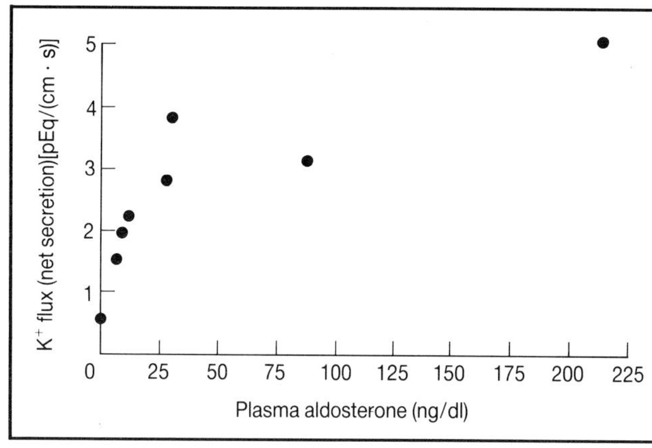

Fig. 14.12. Relationship between circulating concentrations of aldosterone and K^+ secretion (K^+ flux) in isolated perfused rabbit cortical collecting ducts. (From Schwartz GJ, Burg MB. *Am J Physiol* 1978; **235**: F583, with permission.)

Mineralocorticoid effects

Mineralocorticoids stimulate net Na^+ reabsorption and K^+ secretion in the cortical collecting duct (Figs 14.10, 14.12). Aldosterone action requires its initial binding to receptors on principal cells, followed by translocation of the hormone–receptor complex to the nucleus, where specific genes are stimulated to code for physiologically active proteins (e.g. Na^+-K^+-ATPase). Cellular effects include increases in the apical membrane permeability to Na^+ and K^+ and enhancement of basolateral Na^+-K^+-ATPase activity, the latter promoting active uptake of K^+. Stimulation of Na^+ reabsorption additionally leads to an increase in lumen negative transepithelial voltage. In sum, mineralocorticoids modulate both the electrochemical gradient and luminal membrane permeability across the distal nephron, stimulating K^+ secretion.

Prolonged administration of mineralocorticoids results in a persistent kaliuresis but only a transient phase of Na^+ retention. 'Escape' from the Na^+-retaining effects presumably follows extracellular volume expansion to a new steady state with subsequent depression in proximal or loop Na^+ reabsorption.

Developmental aspects

Overview of the renal contribution to K^+ homeostasis

Unlike adults, who are in zero balance, growing infants maintain a state of **positive** K^+ **balance**. The relative conservation of K^+ early in life is generally associated with higher plasma K^+ concentrations than in the adult (Table 14.2). The renal clearance of K^+ (C_{K^+}) in the infant is less than in the older child, even when corrected for glomerular filtration rate (C_{Cr}) (Table 14.2). Children and adults ingesting a regular diet containing Na^+ in excess of K^+ excrete urine with a Na^+-to-K^+ ratio greater than one. Although the Na^+-to-K^+ ratio of breast milk and commercial infant formulas averages 0.5, the urinary Na^+-to-K^+ ratio of the newborn is also greater than 1, consistent with significant K^+ retention.

Infants, like adults, can excrete K^+ at a rate that exceeds its filtration when given a K^+ load, indicating the capacity for net tubular secretion; however, the rate of K^+ excretion per unit body weight in response to exogenous K^+ loading is less in newborn than in older animals.

Note that the limited K^+ secretory capacity of the immature kidney becomes clinically relevant only under conditions of K^+ excess. Under normal circumstances, K^+ retention by the newborn kidney is appropriate and a requirement for growth.

Sites of K^+ transport in the kidney

Micropuncture studies indicate that approximately 50 percent of the filtered load of K^+ is reabsorbed along the initial two-thirds of the superficial proximal tubule of the suckling rat (Fig. 14.8). In contrast to the situation in the adult, up to 40 percent of the filtered load of K^+ reaches the superficial distal tubule of the newborn (Fig. 14.8), providing evidence for functional immaturity of the loop of Henle.

The capacity of the immature distal tubule and collecting duct for K^+ transport has not been well defined. Micropuncture data indicate that the mass flow of K^+ entering the tubular fluid between the late distal tubule and final urine in the newborn is less than that measured in the adult. Clearance studies in saline-expanded dogs also provide indirect evidence for a diminished capacity of the immature distal nephron to secrete K^+.

Regulation of K^+ transport in the neonate

Clearance and micropuncture studies suggest that functional immaturity of K^+ secreting segments may limit K^+ excretion at birth. Assuming that K^+ activity bears a constant relationship to concentration throughout postnatal life, cell K^+ content in the neonatal cortical collecting duct is similar to that measured in the mature segment, averaging 118 mmol/liter intracellular water. Yet Na^+-K^+-ATPase activity in neonatal segments has been reported to be only 50 percent of that measured in the mature nephron. Taken together, these findings suggest that a decreased apical membrane permeability to K^+, possibly due to a paucity of functional channels, restricts K^+ exit from principal cells; such a situation would both maintain cell K^+ concentration and limit K^+

Table 14.2. Mean plasma concentrations and renal clearance of K^+ for infants and children without significant renal disease on regular diet

Age (years)	P_{K^+} (mmol/l)	C_{cr} [ml/(min·1.73 m²)]	C_{K^+} [ml/(min·1.73 m²)]	FEK⁺ (%)	U_{Na^+/K^+}
0–4/12	5.2†‡	62†‡§	4.8†‡§	8.5†‡	1.1±1.1
5/12–1	4.9†‡	99†‡	13.5†	14.6	0.8±0.9
3–10	4.2	141	19.6	14.5	1.5±1.1
11–20	4.3	137	21.2	16.2	1.4±0.8

P_{K^+}, plasma K^+ concentration; C_{cr}, glomerular filtration rate (calculated as renal excretion/plasma level); C_{K^+}, renal clearance of K^+ (calculated as renal excretion/plasma level); FEK⁺, fractional excretion of K^+; U_{Na^+/K^+}, urinary Na^+/K^+ ratio. † $P<0.05$ versus 11–20 years. ‡ $P<0.05$ versus 3–10 years. § $P<0.05$ versus 5/12–1 year. (From Satlin LM, Schwartz GJ. Metabolism of potassium. In Ichikawa I, ed. *Pediatric textbook of fluids and electrolytes*. Baltimore: Williams and Wilkins, 1990: 90, with permission.)

movement from cell to lumen. Whereas the 'chemical' component of the electrochemical gradient driving K^+ secretion appears to remain constant during postnatal life, the 'electrical' component has not been rigorously examined.

Ultrastructural analysis of the neonatal cortical collecting duct indicates that principal cells appear morphologically immature; the cells possess few organelles, simple apical and basolateral surfaces, and occasional areas of glycogen deposition. In contrast, the mature principal cell is devoid of glycogen and possesses more mitochondria, organelles, and basolateral infoldings.

Additional factors that may limit K^+ secretion early in life include the low distal flow rates characteristic of the newborn and the unresponsiveness of the immature nephron to mineralocorticoid stimulation.

Distal tubular flow rates are low in newborn animals, even when appropriate correction is made for the small tubular size. Low flow rates in the cortical collecting duct may lead to higher concentrations of K^+ in the tubular fluid, creating a less favorable cell-to-lumen concentration gradient, thereby limiting K^+ secretion. The postnatal surge in superficial single nephron glomerular filtration rate that occurs in maturing animals at about 3–4 weeks of postnatal life should increase fluid delivery into the cortical collecting duct and promote K^+ secretion.

Plasma aldosterone concentrations in the newborn are higher than in the adult, yet clearance studies demonstrate a relative insensitivity of the immature kidney to this hormone. The density of aldosterone binding sites and receptor affinity appear to be similar in mature and immature rats, suggesting that the early hyposensitivity to aldosterone represents a postreceptor phenomenon.

In summary, those factors that may limit urinary K^+ secretion in the neonate include, at the level of the cortical collecting duct, an unfavorable electrochemical gradient or limited principal cell membrane permeability to K^+ and/or Na^+, low tubular fluid flow rates, or increased paracellular backleak. Alternatively, enhanced K^+ absorption by intercalated cell-rich distal nephron segments (e.g. outer medullary collecting duct) may further reduce net urinary K^+.

Selected reading

Giebisch G, Malnic G, Berliner RW. Renal transport and control of K^+ excretion. In Brenner BM, Rector FC Jr, eds. *The kidney*. Vol. I. Philadelphia: WB Saunders, 1991: 283.

Satlin LM. Maturation of renal K^+ transport. *Pediatr Nephrol* 1991; **5**: 260.

Satlin LM, Schwartz GJ. Renal regulation of K^+ homeostasis. In Edelmann CM Jr, ed. *Pediatric kidney diseases*. Boston: Little, Brown and Company, 1992: 127.

D3. Renal Calcium and Phosphorus Homeostasis

A Haramati and S E Mulroney

Calcium

Urinary Ca^{2+} excretion is low in the first few months of life in both preterm and term infants, and rises progressively over the next several weeks. By 3 months of age, urinary Ca^{2+} excretion, normalized by body surface area, is comparable to that in adults. Other than providing a general description of Ca^{2+} handling by the infant, few studies have specifically examined the renal regulation of Ca^{2+} homeostasis during development. Therefore, the basic principles described below are largely derived from studies in adults. Nevertheless, it is clear that the regulation of Ca^{2+} homeostasis involves two important elements: first, maintenance of positive Ca^{2+} balance, meaning that Ca^{2+} output (excretion) is less than Ca^{2+} input (dietary intake) so that sufficient Ca^{2+} is provided for the growing tissues; and second, maintenance of plasma Ca^{2+} concentration within a narrow range, which serves to minimize changes in the electrochemical Ca^{2+} gradient across cell membranes that could greatly affect cell function. These processes occur through the coordinated action of several hormonal systems, principally parathyroid hormone (PTH), calcitonin, and vitamin D, acting on bone, gastrointestinal tract, and the kidney.

More than 98 percent of total body Ca^{2+} is contained in the skeleton, one-third of which is readily exchangeable with the extracellular fluid. Of the Ca^{2+} circulating in plasma, approximately one-half exists in the free, ionized form, another 10 percent is complexed to various anions such as phosphate, bicarbonate, citrate, and sulfate, and the rest represents Ca^{2+} that is bound to protein (primarily albumin).

The homeostatic regulation of Ca^{2+} balance occurs largely at the level of the intestine, where adjustments in the rate of Ca^{2+} absorption control the influx of Ca^{2+} into the extracellular pool. The role of the kidneys in Ca^{2+} homeostasis is to reabsorb essentially all (98 percent) of the filtered Ca^{2+} and to limit urinary Ca^{2+} losses. Consequently, the kidney functions as an important contributor, rather than a primary regulator of Ca^{2+} balance.

Tubular handling of calcium

Approximately 60 percent of the total plasma Ca^{2+} (representing the ionized and complexed forms) is filtered at the glomerulus. However, only 2 percent of the filtered Ca^{2+} load is normally excreted in the urine. The bulk of tubular Ca^{2+} reabsorption (50–60 percent) occurs in the proximal tubule (both proximal convoluted and proximal straight segments) by a process that is linked to Na^+ reabsorption. This involves mostly passive Ca^{2+} diffusion, occurring via the paracellular pathway, although there is evidence for a small, active transport component as well.

In the loop of Henle, the thin descending and ascending limbs are reportedly impermeable to Ca^{2+}. The thick ascending limb, however, is a significant site where about 20 percent of the filtered Ca^{2+} load is reabsorbed. The transport of Na^+, K^+, and Cl^- in this segment, via a Na^+-K^+-$2Cl^-$ carrier, results in a lumen-positive trans-epithelial potential difference. This, together with the high permeability of this segment to Ca^{2+}, drives the passive, paracellular reabsorption of Ca^{2+}. In addition, Ca^{2+} is reabsorbed actively, particularly in the cortical thick ascending limb, by a transport system that is stimulated by PTH.

The distal convoluted tubule and the cortical collecting tubule are nephron segments that actively transport Ca^{2+} and are PTH dependent. These sites combine to reabsorb efficiently 10–15 percent of the filtered Ca^{2+}, and serve to minimize loss of Ca^{2+} in the urine.

Cellular mechanisms of renal calcium transport

Renal Ca^{2+} transport occurs through several mechanisms, both transcellular and paracellular. Ca^{2+} enters the tubular cells by passive diffusion down its electrochemical concentration gradient, as well as by facilitated diffusion via Ca^{2+}-binding protein carriers. The translocation of intracellular Ca^{2+} ions to the basolateral membrane is not well defined, but appears to involve cytosolic Ca^{2+}-binding proteins and the action of mitochondria and other organelles, which 'shuttle' Ca^{2+} from the luminal to the basolateral membrane. Because of the low intracellular Ca^{2+} concentration, exit across the basolateral membrane into the extracellular fluid occurs against an electrochemical gradient and is energy-dependent, primarily through Na^+-Ca^{2+} countertransporters and Ca^{2+}-activated ATPases.

The movement of Ca^{2+} between renal epithelial cells occurs passively by diffusion, and depends upon the transepithelial electrochemical gradient and permeability characteristics of the cell membranes and tight junctions in the various nephron segments.

Factors regulating renal calcium reabsorption

PTH decreases the urinary excretion of Ca^{2+}—an action consistent with its overall function to protect against large declines in the plasma Ca^{2+} concentration. PTH stimulates bone resorption, which releases Ca^{2+} and PO_4 to the extracellular fluid. However, the effects of PTH to decrease renal Ca^{2+} excretion and increase PO_4 excretion assure that a selective elevation occurs in plasma Ca^{2+} concentrations. At the tubular level, the action of PTH to increase Ca^{2+} reabsorption in the loop of Henle and distal nephron segments is mediated by membrane receptors coupled to adenylyl cyclase and the subsequent generation of cAMP as a second messenger. The PTH receptor–adenylyl cyclase–cAMP pathway is active in the fetal and postnatal kidney, but is not as responsive as in the adult kidney.

Vitamin D plays a key role in raising the plasma Ca^{2+} concentration through stimulation of intestinal Ca^{2+} absorption. This role is particularly important in the period between weaning and puberty, when there is an increase in the activity of the renal 1α-hydroxylase, which converts 25(OH) vitamin D to its active form of $1,25(OH)_2$ vitamin D. Indeed, the renal production of $1,25(OH)_2$ vitamin D increases rapidly during this period of growth, provided sufficient amounts of the substrate (25[OH] vitamin D) are available. Whether vitamin D also contributes directly to enhancing renal Ca^{2+} reabsorption in the neonate is unknown.

Because of the dependence of Ca^{2+} reabsorption upon NaCl reabsorption in the proximal tubule and, partly, in the loop of Henle, factors that increase NaCl excretion, such as **administration of diuretics** that act at those sites, or expansion of the extracellular volume, also cause parallel increases in Ca^{2+} excretion. **Thiazide diuretics**, however, **reduce** urinary Ca^{2+} excretion. This appears to be a direct effect on distal tubule Ca^{2+} reabsorption and not a secondary effect of volume contraction.

Several other factors have been associated with altered urinary Ca^{2+} excretion. For example, *hypercalciuria* occurs during reduced PO_4 uptake and in metabolic acidosis. Should those conditions continue for a prolonged period of time, the impairment in Ca^{2+} balance will likely affect growth adversely.

Phosphorus

In the neonatal and prepubertal period, the regulation of PO_4 homeostasis is crucial to proper growth and development. As with Ca^{2+}, the neonate maintains positive balance for PO_4, as a consequence of a relatively high intake of PO_4, efficient intestinal absorption, and reduced urinary PO_4 excretion, all of which involve the integrated action of several hormonal systems. Unlike Ca^{2+}, the primary regulation of PO_4 homeostasis is at the level of the kidney, where adjustments in the rate of renal PO_4 reabsorption control the plasma PO_4 concentration and PO_4 balance.

The majority (80 percent) of total body phosphorus is present in the skeleton, the rest being in soft tissues, muscle, and extracellular fluids. Two-thirds of the phosphorus in plasma is in the form of organic phosphates (esters and phospholipids) and one-third is inorganic PO_4 (mostly orthophosphates); the latter fraction is reported as the plasma PO_4 concentration. The plasma PO_4 concentration in infants and children is 50 percent higher than that observed in adults, which is a consequence of the relatively high rate of PO_4 reabsorption by the neonatal kidney.

Tubular handling of phosphate

Approximately 90 percent of the plasma PO_4 is freely filtered at the glomerulus. Under normal conditions, adult kidneys reabsorb 75–80 percent of the filtered PO_4 load and excrete the rest. The bulk (60–70 percent) of the filtered PO_4 is reabsorbed in the proximal convoluted tubule, and the remainder (10–15 percent) is reabsorbed in the proximal straight tubule, distal convoluted tubule, and cortical collecting tubules. The latter sites become most significant during states of PO_4 conservation such as *hypoparathyroidism* and *dietary phosphate deprivation,* where complete reabsorption of the filtered PO_4 load can occur.

The neonate, with a rapid growth rate and large PO_4 requirement, normally reabsorbs about 90 percent of the filtered PO_4. The proportionally greater conservation of PO_4 involves enhanced reabsorption in the proximal convoluted tubule and in more distal segments. However, the precise sites and mechanisms of increased PO_4 transport are not known.

Another important element that may explain the renal retention of PO_4 in the neonate is nephron heterogeneity. The capacity to transport PO_4 is greater in deep (juxtamedullary) nephrons compared with superficial (cortical) nephrons. Because nephrogenesis begins in the corticomedullary region and proceeds toward the outer cortex, the relative preponderance of functioning deep nephrons in the juxtamedullary area of the immature kidney may contribute to its overall enhanced capacity for tubular PO_4 reabsorption.

Cellular mechanisms of renal phosphate transport

Transcellular PO_4 transport is a Na^+-coupled, electroneutral, secondary active process, which depends on an electrochemical gradient for Na^+ entry into the cell, generated by the Na^+-K^+-ATPase pump on the basolateral membrane of the proximal tubular cell. PO_4 enters the cell via specific Na^+-PO_4 carrier proteins on the proximal tubule brush border membrane. In the cell, PO_4 can be incorporated into various organic compounds through one of several biosynthetic pathways, or it can simply pass through the cell. The amount of PO_4 exiting the cell can vary depending on the metabolic needs of the cell. When the intracellular PO_4 pool increases, PO_4 leaves the cell passively down its concentration gradient and crosses the basolateral membrane via Na^+-independent carriers.

Evidence from animal studies indicates that proximal tubule brush-border PO_4 uptake is higher in neonates than in adults as a result of an increased velocity of PO_4 transport (V_{max}). This suggests either an increased turnover rate or an increased number of Na^+-PO_4 cotransporters in the neonatal kidney.

Factors regulating renal phosphate reabsorption

Because the rate-limiting step in renal PO_4 reabsorption is at the level of the luminal Na^+-PO_4 cotransporter, PO_4 transport is a saturable process, characterized by a transport maximum (TmPi). The TmPi, however, is not a fixed value and can be affected by hormones, dietary PO_4, and other factors, including age. Indeed, the TmPi in the neonate (corrected by body surface area or kidney mass) is relatively greater than in adults, and contributes to the elevated plasma PO_4 concentration. Thus, the high rate of renal PO_4 retention in the neonate is not a result of limited PO_4 excretion due to a relatively low GFR, but rather the result of several different factors acting in concert specifically to elevate the tubular transport of PO_4 during development.

The principal hormonal regulator of PO_4 transport is PTH. Decreased plasma Ca^{2+} concentrations stimulate PTH release, which acts to increase Ca^{2+} and reduce PO_4 reabsorption. Studies in both human infants and immature animals indicate that the response in newborns to the phosphaturic, but not the hypocalciuric, effects of PTH is reduced compared with adults. This occurs despite normal circulating concentrations of PTH postnatally and normal generation of the second messenger for PTH (cAMP). This aspect of reduced PTH responsiveness may account in part for the high renal retention of PO_4 in the young.

Another fundamental regulator of renal PO_4 transport is dietary PO_4. An increase in PO_4 intake in adults results in a rise in urinary PO_4 excretion because of a rapid decrease in TmPi. Although the neonate responds to an increase in dietary PO_4 with an appropriate reduction in TmPi, the change is much smaller. Ostensibly, this may serve to maintain PO_4 balance. However, because the TmPi remains high in the newborn fed dietary PO_4, an excessive increase in dietary PO_4 could lead to *hyperphosphatemia*, resulting in decreased plasma Ca^{2+} concentrations and secondary hyperparathyroidism. Conversely, dietary PO_4 deprivation increases renal PO_4 reabsorption, an effect that is relatively greater in the neonate compared with the adult. However, because of the very high requirements of the newborn for PO_4, a diet too low in PO_4 may lead to PO_4 depletion, *hypophosphatemia*, and reduced growth rate despite complete tubular reabsorption of filtered PO_4.

Growth hormone is also an important factor regulating renal PO_4 reabsorption, particularly during the period of rapid growth. *Growth hormone deficiency* is associated with reduced growth rate, hypophosphatemia, and

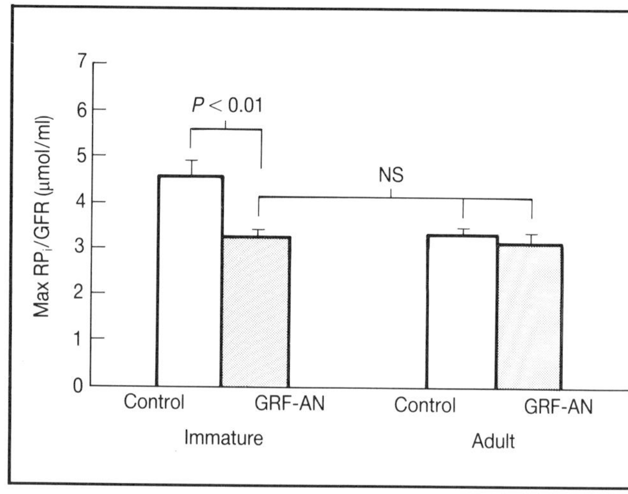

Fig. 14.13. Chronic administration of an antagonist to growth hormone releasing factor (GRF-AN), which suppresses pulsatile growth hormone release, significantly reduced the tubular capacity for PO_4 reabsorption (TmPi expressed as Max RP_i/GFR) in immature rats down to the levels seen in adult rats. GRF-AN treatment did not alter the TmPi in adult rats. Values are means ± SE. (From Haramati *et al.* *Pediatr Nephrol* 1990; **4**: 387, with permission.)

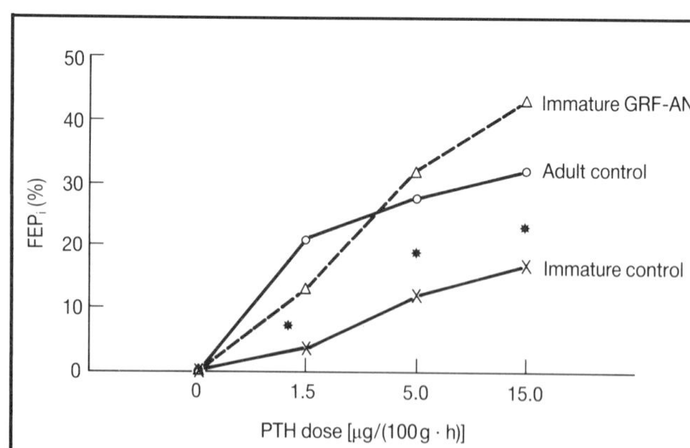

Fig. 14.14. Fractional excretion of PO_4 (FEP_i) in response to increasing doses of parathyroid hormone (PTH) in immature and adult control rats. Suppression of pulsatile growth hormone release with an antagonist to growth hormone releasing factor (GRF-AN) restored a phosphaturic effect of PTH in immature rats. (From Mulroney *et al.* *Am J Physiol* 1991; **261**: F1110, with permission.)

increased urinary PO_4 excretion, whereas the opposite has been reported with *growth hormone hypersecretion*. In a recent series of animal studies, an important link between the growth-promoting effects of growth hormone and renal PO_4 reabsorption has been established. When the pulsatile release of growth hormone was specifically suppressed in weanling rats using a synthetic antagonist to growth hormone releasing factor (GRF-AN), the growth rate was attenuated, and positive PO_4 balance was reduced due to a rapid decrease in the TmPi. Indeed, the TmPi was reduced to levels seen in adult rats. By contrast, no effect was seen on the tubular capacity to reabsorb PO_4 in the adult rats (Fig. 14.13). Suppression of growth hormone release in immature rats restored a phosphaturic response to PTH that was not different from that seen in adults (Fig. 14.14). These findings suggest that growth hormone may play a critical role in enhancing renal PO_4 reabsorption during development, and in this way assure that adequate amounts of PO_4 are provided to meet the demand for growth.

Selected reading

Haramati A, Mulroney SE, Lumpkin MD. Regulation of renal phosphate reabsorption during development: implications from a new model of growth hormone deficiency. *Pediatr Nephrol* 1990; **4**: 387.

Stewart CL, Devarajan P, Mulroney SE, Kaskel FJ, Haramati A. Transport of calcium and phosphorus. In Polin RA, Fox WW, eds. *Fetal and neonatal physiology*. Vol. II. Philadelphia: WB Saunders Company, 1992: 1223.

E. Acid–Base Regulation

D Aviles and P A Jose

The kidneys maintain normal acid–base balance by reclaiming filtered bicarbonate and by excreting the salts of non-volatile acids produced each day by cellular metabolism. This is accomplished by the urinary secretion of H^+ produced by renal tubular cells. Qualitative and quantitative differences exist between the mature and developing organism. In particular, the rate of production of non-volatile acids by an infant (2 mEq/kg per day) is twice that of the adult.

Most nephron segments can reabsorb bicarbonate, but the majority (80 percent) of filtered bicarbonate is reabsorbed in the proximal tubule. The thick ascending limb and distal convoluted tubule reabsorb 10 and 6 percent, respectively. The cortical collecting is capable of either net bicarbonate secretion or reabsorption (4 percent).

The kidney excretes the non-volatile acids produced by cellular metabolism by the excretion of titratable acids and ammonium ions (NH_4^+), resulting in the generation of new bicarbonate. As in the reclamation of filtered bicarbonate, the proximal tubule is also the major site of the formation of titratable acids and NH_4^+. Additional titratable acids are generated along the collecting ducts. After 3 days of an acid load, titratable acid production may increase two- to threefold, while NH_4^+ production may increase six- to sevenfold. Titratable acid is determined by measuring the amount of hydroxyl ions (e.g. NaOH) required to titrate the urine back to the pH of blood. Filtered PO_4 is the major component of titratable acids with some contribution from urate, creatinine, sulfate, and β-hydroxybutyrate.

The cellular mechanism involved in the secretion of H^+ is an essential step in the reabsorption of bicarbonate and formation of titratable acids. H^+ ions generated in the cell (resulting from the dissociation of H_2CO_3 into H^+ and HCO_3^-) are secreted at the luminal membrane by exchanging intracellular H^+ with luminal Na^+ and by electrogenic transport of H^+. The Na^+-H^+ exchanger (or antiporter) found in the apical membrane of the proximal tubule and thick ascending limb of Henle is responsible for most of H^+ secretion in the proximal tubule ($\approx$ 65 percent). Electrogenic transport by H^+-ATPase is responsible for the rest of H^+ secretion. H^+-ATPase is present throughout the nephron, but there is marked species variation. Two possible fates of H^+ ions secreted into the tubular lumen include: (1) reaction with filtered HCO_3^- to form H_2CO_3, and (2) reaction with HPO_4^{2-} to form $H_2PO_4^-$ (titratable acids). H_2CO_3 formed in the tubular lumen (from 1) is broken down to H_2O and CO_2 by carbonic anhydrase that is present in the brush border of proximal tubules. This is the reason why the pH of the tubular fluid in the proximal tubule does not decrease markedly; the tubular fluid pH at the late proximal convoluted tubule $\approx$ 6.7. In more distal segments of the nephron, luminal H_2CO_3 slowly forms into CO_2 and H_2O because their luminal membranes do not contain carbonic anhydrase. In the collecting ducts, the pH of tubular fluid can decrease to as low as 4.5. In the proximal tubule, the HCO_3^- remaining within the cell after the generation and secretion of H^+ is transported out of the cell at the basolateral membrane via a Cl^--HCO_3^- antiporter and a Na^+-HCO_3^- symporter.

The cortical collecting duct can reabsorb and secrete HCO_3^- at its luminal membrane. HCO_3^- reabsorption occurs as a result of H^+ secretion via the H^+-ATPase at the luminal membrane of the intercalated cell (type A). The intracellular HCO_3^- exits at the basolateral membrane via the Cl^--HCO_3^- antiporter. When the H^+-ATPase is located at the basolateral side and the Cl^--HCO_3^- antiporter is located at the luminal side, the intercalated cell of the cortical collecting duct becomes a HCO_3^- secreting cell (type B). The collecting ducts of the outer medullary also secrete H^+ via a H^+-ATPase; the collecting ducts located in the outer but not in the inner stripe of the outer medulla also reabsorb Na^+.

The other mechanism by which the kidney excretes non-volatile acids is NH_4^+ production. This occurs in the proximal tubule by conversion of glutamine to 1 mole of glutamate and 1 mole of NH_4^+ (glutamine + $H_2O \rightarrow$ glutamate + NH_4^+); glutamate thus formed is converted further to α-ketoglutarate and another mole of NH_4^+.

$$\text{Glutamate} + H_2O + NAD \rightarrow \alpha\text{-ketoglutarate} + NADH + NH_4^+$$

The metabolism of α-ketoglutarate, formed during the process of NH_4^+ production, via the Krebs cycle results in the release of 2 moles of HCO_3^-. (Two thirds of glutamine come from the plasma, and the rest comes from renal tubular metabolism.) The NH_4^+ formed is secreted into the proximal tubule and can be excreted into the urine. If NH_4^+ is not excreted in the urine, it is returned to the circulation where it is converted to urea in the liver, resulting in the generation of H^+.

$$2NH_4^+ + CO_2 \rightarrow 2H^+ + \text{urea} + H_2O$$

The $2H^+$ generated during urea formation in the liver would then neutralize the $2HCO_3^-$ generated by the proximal tubule during NH_4^+ formation. This results in zero net gain of HCO_3^-. As it turns out, under normal conditions, only 50 percent of the NH_4^+ formed is secreted in the proximal tubule and 50 percent is returned into the circulation. The NH_4^+ secreted into the proximal tubule is reabsorbed by the cells of the ascending loop of Henle to a larger extent by the Na^+-K^+(NH_4)-$2Cl^-$ transporter and to a lesser extent by voltage-driven diffusion. The mechanism of the exit of reabsorbed NH_4^+ at the basolateral membrane is unknown. In the medullary interstitium, the reabsorbed NH_4^+ splits into NH_3 and H^+. Both species are secreted into the descending limb of Henle; this countercurrent multiplier mechanism contributes to the accumulation of NH_4^+ in the medulla. The high medullary concentration of NH_3 and luminal acidification at the collecting ducts create a favorable gradient for NH_3 diffusion, and therefore secretion of NH_4^+ into the medullary collecting duct.

Urine pH, under normal conditions (and after the first 2 weeks of life in term newborns), is acidic (pH ≈ 6.1). The minimum urinary pH is about 4.5 while the maximum urinary pH is about 8.5. The net amount of acid excretion (NAE) by the kidney is the sum of ammonium excretion and titratable acids minus urine bicarbonate.

$$NAE = NH_4^+ + \text{titratable acids}$$

Under these conditions, 50 percent of NAE is contributed by NH_4^+ excretion while the other 50 percent is contributed by titratable acids. Several factors affect urinary acid excretion in the normal state. These include: distal Na^+ delivery, nature and quantity of anion delivered to the distal tubule, aldosterone, and ammoniagenesis. Reduction in distal Na^+ delivery decreases distal urinary acidification. The converse occurs; thus distal tubular acidification can be stimulated by natriuretic agents (e.g. furosemide). 'Nonreabsorbable' anions delivered to the distal tubule increase H^+ secretion (e.g. sulfates, penicillins). Aldosterone modulates renal acid production by increasing Na^+ reabsorption and creating a positive transtubular potential gradient for H^+ secretion, by stimulating the H^+ pump, and by increasing ammonia-genesis. Several factors control NH_4^+ secretion into the tubular lumen. Factors that are inversely correlated with ammonium secretion include urine pH and K^+. Factors that are positively correlated with ammonium secretion include glomerular filtration rate, capillary blood flow, and tubular flow.

Acid–base balance in the fetus is mainly dependent on maternal control mechanisms. However, the fetal kidney, at least after the second half of pregnancy, is able to acidify the urine. Growth is associated with a positive H^+ balance. Moreover, the H^+ load (sum of intake and production) is 2 mmol/kg body weight per day compared with 1 mmol/kg body weight per day in adults. In healthy preterm infants, during the first weeks of postnatal life, the **anion gap** (serum Na^+ minus serum bicarbonate and Cl^-) ranges from 15 to 22 mM, compared with values of 9–12 mM in term newborns and adults. Serum bicarbonate concentrations in preterm infants may be as low as 14 mM compared with 21–22 mM in full-term newborns. Serum bicarbonate concentrations increase with age (22 mM in infants, 24 mM in children, 28 mM in adults). The low serum bicarbonate concentration in the newborn is in part due to a lower threshold for bicarbonate. Because 75 percent of the filtered bicarbonate is reabsorbed by the proximal tubule, immaturity of proximal tubular bicarbonate reabsorption is a significant factor.

The ability of the newborn to acidify the urine and excrete an acid load is limited compared with the adult. Rapid postnatal maturity is achieved so that by 2 weeks of age, urine pH can be as low as 4.5. The ability of the newborn to excrete an acute acid load also matures rapidly and is achieved by 1–2 months of age. This is mainly due to rapid maturation of titratable acid excretion. The ability of the newborn to excrete a chronic acid load matures more slowly. This may be due to a slower maturation of ammonia production where adult levels are not attained until 2 years of life. Several conditions can increase renal tubular acidification mechanisms. Pretreatment of infants with phosphate, change of formula from breast milk to cows' milk, or increase in protein intake enhance the ability of the newborn to excrete titratable acids and ammonia.

The driving force for hydrogen ion secretion via the Na^+-H^+ antiporter is the low intracellular Na^+ concentration maintained by the basolateral Na^+-K^+-ATPase. In several animal species, Na^+-K^+-ATPase activity is lower in newborns than in adults. In the rabbit, both Na^+-H^+ antiporter and Na^+-$(HCO_3)_3$ symporter activities are also lower in fetuses and newborns than in adults. Thus, an immaturity of the transporters mediating H^+ transport may explain the decreased bicarbonate threshold in the newborn rabbit. Whether the same situation applies to other animals and human newborns remains to be determined. For example, in the young rat, the affinity of the Na^+-H^+ antiporter in the proximal tubular luminal membranes is lower, but its capacity is actually higher than those noted in adult rats. The net result is an enhanced Na^+-H^+ antiporter activity in the newborn. Under these circumstances, the short proximal convoluted tubule and decreased transport at the basolateral membrane, quantitatively decrease H^+ transport in the proximal tubule. Agents that can alter transport activity can influence the maturation of H^+ transport (e.g. glucocorticoids). The role of neurohormonal factors in the maturation of proximal tubular H^+ transport remains to be determined. In the adult, angiotensin II and α-adrenergic receptors are associated with stimulation of Na^+-H^+ antiporter activity while dopamine and parathyroid hormone are inhibitory. In the newborn, angiotensin II activity is increased, while the converse is true for dopamine. Cortical collecting duct type A and type B intercalated cells also undergo postnatal proliferation and differentiation.

In summary, urinary acidification is a highly regulated function of the kidney requiring a coordinated functioning of nephron segments with specific functions. New knowledge of the roles of different transporters have provided important insights into the cellular mechanisms of renal H^+ transport. The concept that most of H^+ secretion occurs in the proximal tubule remains true. New concepts include: titratable acid formation occurs mainly in the proximal tubule, and generation of 'new' bicarbonate due to ammoniagenesis occurs as a result of the formation of bicarbonate from α-ketoglutarate during the process of NH_4^+ production by renal tubules. Differences between the young and the adult in their ability to acidify the urine and an excrete acid load are due to the ontogeny of renal hemodynamics and transport proteins.

Selected reading

Kurtz I, Dass PD, Cramer S. The importance of renal ammonia metabolism to the whole body acid–base balance: a reanalysis of the pathophysiology of renal tubular acidosis. *Miner Electrolyte Metab* 1990; **16**: 331.

Seldin DW, Giebisch G. *The regulation of acid–base balance*. New York: Raven Press, 1989.

Wrong O. Distal renal tubular acidosis: the value of urinary pH, pCO_2, and NH_4^+ measurements. *Pediatr Nephrol* 1991; **5**: 249.

F. Regulation of Water Balance

A Aperia

Tubular water reabsorption, concentration, and dilution of urine

The bulk of filtered salt and water is reabsorbed in the proximal tubule. Approximately 20 percent of the filtrate is delivered to the loop of Henle. This fluid is still isotonic because in the leaky proximal tubule, the osmotic gradient created by the reabsorption of salt is almost immediately dissipated by water reabsorption.

In the distal part of the nephron, water and salt reabsorption are regulated by separate mechanisms. The thick ascending limb (TAL) of Henle is water impermeable and has a high capacity to transport Na^+ against a gradient. The Na^+ pump, Na^+-K^+-ATPase, is more abundant in the TAL than in most other cells. Active Na^+ reabsorption in TAL is generally considered to be the initial event in the creation of the hypertonic medullary interstitium that is a prerequisite for the process that leads to the concentration of urine. The hypertonicity of the renal medulla is potentiated by countercurrent flow in the vasa recta and the loops of Henle. It is also potentiated by recirculation of urea reabsorbed in the distal nephron. The antidiuretic hormone (ADH) acts by rendering the collecting duct cell water-permeable. In the presence of saturating concentrations of ADH, water will diffuse freely into the medullary interstitium, and the osmolality of the final urine will equal the osmolality of the inner medulla, which is 800–1200 mosmol/kg H_2O in mature kidneys. In the absence of ADH, the urine will have approximately the same osmolality as the fluid in the distal tubule, in healthy adult man approximately 60–80 mosmol/kg H_2O.

The process that leads to concentration and dilution of urine will regulate not only water balance but also the tonicity of extracellular fluids. By concentrating the urine, water will be reabsorbed in excess of Na^+ and hypertonicity will be adjusted. Dilution of urine will adjust a state of hypotonicity.

ADH, regulation of release, and mechanism of action

An increase in blood osmolality excites osmoreceptors located in the hypothalamus. This leads to a chain of events that results in the release of ADH from the pituitary gland. There are at least two types of ADH receptors, V_2 receptors, which are present in epithelial cells such as the collecting duct cells, and V_1 receptors, present in vascular smooth muscle. The V_2 receptors are coupled to a G_s-protein and stimulate adenylyl cyclase activity. The V_1 receptors stimulate phospholipase C activity. Activation of the V_1 receptors in the vessels causes vascular constriction. Activation of V_1 receptors plays an important role in the response to large blood losses. Activation of the V_2 receptors will lead to incorporation of an intracellular pool of membrane fragments containing water channels. The effect of V_2 receptors on the collecting duct is counteracted by prostaglandins.

In individuals with healthy kidneys, there is a characteristic relationship between serum levels of ADH and urine osmolality. When serum concentrations exceed 2 pg/ml, there is a sharp increase in the urine osmolality. Maximal osmolality is generally reached at serum concentrations of 8–10 pg/ml.

Developmental aspects

Most mammalian neonates have a low concentrating capacity. The human newborn rarely excretes a concentrated urine. In contrast, the capacity to dilute the urine appears to be well developed, at least in the full-term infant. The capacity to concentrate urine increases almost linearly during the first year of life. Individual variations, however, are large during this time.

Many factors contribute to the low concentrating capacity in the infant. The capacity to reabsorb Na^+ in the TAL is low due to a low content of Na^+-K^+-ATPase in the immature cells. The loop of Henle is relatively short, which will make the countercurrent system less efficient.

The urea availability is generally limited. Finally, end-organ response to ADH is blunted, probably dependent on a deficient coupling between the ADH receptor and the adenylyl cyclase unit. The capacity to release ADH appears to be well developed during the late fetal period. Circulating levels of ADH are already high during the neonatal period. It has been suggested that in the neonatal period, the main physiological role for ADH is to regulate regional vascular resistance.

Clinical aspects

The low concentrating capacity might serve a good purpose in the infant, where the water turnover needs to be very high. Low concentrating capacity, however, will render the infant much more sensitive to pathological fluid losses. *Diarrheal disease* therefore is always potentially dangerous in the infant. In the situation of dehydration, young infants are predisposed to develop hypertonic conditions because, due to the low concentrating capacity, salt can be retained more easily than fluid. The risk for hypertonic dehydration is higher in diarrhea of viral origin, where intestinal salt losses are relatively small. Preterm infants are also predisposed to develop hypertonic conditions because of the large transepithelial water losses.

Low urinary concentrating capacity can be due to lack of ADH (*central diabetes insipidus* (DI)) or to lack of responsiveness to ADH (*renal diabetes insipidus*). Renal DI can either be due to a genetic disorder of ADH receptors and/or signaling pathways coupled to the receptors or to renal disease. A transient decrease in urinary concentrating capacity can occur in pyelonephritis.

Tests of concentrating capacity

The capacity to concentrate urine can be determined with or without the administration of ADH. The osmolality of a urine sample obtained after 12 hours of food and fluid deprivation will test both central and renal mechanisms for urine concentration. The osmolality of a urine sample obtained 1–6 hours after the nasal administration of synthetic antidiuretic hormone will test the renal mechanism of urine concentration.

Fluid intake should be avoided during this test. In children about 2 years of age, the osmolality should be above 800 mosmol/kg H_2O at either test. **Caution:** in young children with diabetes insipidus 12 hours of fluid deprivation might lead to shock. The administration of ADH, if there is a free fluid intake afterwards, might lead to a condition of hypotonic volume expansion with serum Na^+ falling to 120 mmol/liter. Such a complication might result in convulsions.

Selected reading

Aperia A, Celsi G. Ontogenic processes in nephron epithelia. Structure, enzymes, and function. In Seldin DW, Giebisch G, eds. *The kidney: physiology and pathophysiology*. 2nd ed. Vol. II. New York: Raven Press Ltd, 1992: 803.

Horster MF, Gilg A, Lory P. Determinants of axial osmotic gradients in the differentiating countercurrent system. *Am J Physiol* 1984; **246**: F124.

Polácek E, Vocel J, Neugebauerová L, *et al*. The osmotic concentrating ability in healthy infants and children. *Arch Dis Child* 1965; **40**: 291 **(Gives normal values for maximal urine osmolality at different ages.)**

Seldin DW, Giebisch G, eds. *The kidney: physiology and pathophysiology*. 2nd ed. Vol. II; Section III: Water and electrolyte exchanges. New York: Raven Press Ltd, 1992: 1595.

15 ◆ *Developmental pharmacology*

Editor: *Gideon Koren*

A. Principles of Pharmacokinetics and Pharmacodynamics

D Scolnik and G Koren

In order to fully understand drug disposition in any given individual, a number of issues have to be addressed. First there is the problem of compliance, i.e. whether the drug has been taken as prescribed, erratically, or not at all. Thereafter, a knowledge of pharmacokinetics including drug absorption, distribution, metabolism, and elimination is necessary. Finally, the possibility of drug–drug interactions and of other factors, e.g. disease state influencing the actual mode of action of the drug, at a molecular and receptor level (pharmacodynamics), must be considered. In the following sections we describe central pharmacokinetic and pharmacodynamic principles that are important for understanding drug effects during development.

General principles

Compliance

It is essential to quantify **compliance** in any assessment of drug efficacy; otherwise, a potentially efficacious drug will be said erroneously to lack any clinical effect. Four principal methods are used to assess compliance.

Pill count

Although this method does not reveal when and how a drug was taken, and can easily be manipulated by the patient (or the patient's care givers), it has proven very useful when a 'count' revealing low use concurs with lack of effect.

Diary card

This method relies on patients' honesty, and it has been shown that many patients fill in details as they perceive the doctor would wish them to, thereby introducing a new source of bias.

Patient interview

This is subject to serious bias from both inaccurate and selective recall of positive and negative events.

MEMS

The 'medication event monitoring system' consists of a computerized chip in the cap of the medication bottle, which records the date and time every time the bottle is opened. This enables accurate correlation between adverse or favorable drug events and timing of doses.

Absorption

After a drug has been administered, it must be absorbed in order to have any effect. The rate and extent of **absorption** obviously depend upon the route of administration, whether it be gastrointestinal, intramuscular, percutaneous, intrathecal, or endotracheal.

The **rate** of absorption is especially pertinent when drug effect is proportional to peak concentrations obtained, as is thought to be the case with some antibiotics, or when adverse effects occur at high drug levels, such as with nifedipine. Rate of absorption is also important when the desired effect has to be achieved without delay, e.g. pain relief with acetaminophen or nitroglycerin.

Intravenous administration is considered to provide 100 percent bioavailability of drug. Oral **bioavailability** is a measure of the **extent** of absorption and is exemplified by the following formula for oral drug administration (see below):

$$\text{Oral bioavailability} = \frac{\text{area under the curve from oral administration}}{\text{area under the curve from intravenous administration}}$$

The area under the curve refers to a graphical representation of drug concentration versus time. Many factors can affect oral bioavailability including vomiting, malabsorption, and changes in gastric pH. Low oral bioavailability can also be the result of the **first-pass effect**, even after complete absorption. This is a reflection of the amount of drug that is metabolized in the liver after absorption into the portal venous system and before reaching the systemic circulation. Saturation of intestinal absorption has also been demonstrated for some drugs and results in dose-dependent oral bioavailability.

Distribution

After absorption a drug must be distributed to its site of action in order to exert an effect. The commonest measure of this is a drug's **volume of distribution** (V_d), the hypothetical blood volume that would be needed to account for the concentration of the drug in the blood assuming that the whole dose remained intravascular. It reflects how much of the drug remains in the blood after distribution is completed and is based on plasma concentration.

$$\text{Volume of distribution} = \frac{\text{total amount of drug in body}}{\text{concentration of drug in plasma}}$$

Factors that influence drug distribution are as follows.

Chemical characteristics

Lipid-soluble drugs cross membranes more easily than hydrophilic ones, and a drug's pK_a (pH at which 50 percent ionization occurs) often determines its movement as well. Some drugs have an affinity for certain tissues, e.g. aminoglycosides accumulate in renal tissue, possibly accounting for selective efficacy and toxicity.

Method of administration

High peak serum concentrations can facilitate entry of a drug into a tissue that is otherwise relatively impermeable when only low serum concentrations are achieved.

Protein and tissue binding

High levels of protein binding result in lower levels of free drug being available at the drug's site of action. Acidic drugs are usually bound to albumin and basic ones to α_1-glycoproteins, lipoproteins, and gammaglobulins. Additional drug therapy or derangements in blood chemistry, especially changes in pH, can lead to saturation of, and displacement from, binding sites.

Perfusion

Poor perfusion of a tissue or organ decreases the amount of drug reaching its site of action.

Metabolism and elimination

Most drugs are eliminated from the body via hepatic or renal routes. Hepatic metabolism usually serves to make more polar compounds, which can then be eliminated more efficiently through the bile or by the kidneys. **Phase one** (non-synthetic) hepatic reactions involve oxidation, reduction, or hydrolysis, while **phase two** (synthetic) reactions involve conjugation of new moieties to the drug molecule. In the kidney drugs can be filtered, with varying amounts of subsequent tubular reabsorption or secretion.

The **elimination constant** (K_e) is used to characterize drug elimination pattern and represents the fraction of drug eliminated per unit time. If a constant **proportion** of drug is eliminated per unit time, irrespective of drug levels, **first-order kinetics** are said to apply. **Zero-order kinetics** infer that the same **amount** of drug (not the same proportion) is eliminated per unit time. **Half-life** ($t_{1/2}$) is more useful than K_e clinically. It is commonly used to tailor optimal dosing interval (see below):

$$\text{Dose interval} = 1.44 \times \text{half-life} \times \ln \frac{\text{maximum desired concentration}}{\text{minimum desired concentration}}$$

where ln = natural logarithm. The half-life is also used to derive the clearance, which is the volume of blood totally cleared of a drug per unit time:

$$\text{Clearance} = 0.693 \times \frac{\text{Volume of distribution}}{\text{half-life}}$$

Compartmental models are mathematical attempts to explain drug concentrations obtained after drug dosing. They reflect the balance between absorption, distribution, metabolism, and the redistribution that can occur when, for instance, a drug is released from tissue binding in response to falling plasma concentrations.

Mention will be made of one final formula that is frequently used. It describes the first-order kinetic behavior of drugs in mathematical terms:

$$\text{Concentration at time } t' = \text{concentration at time } 0 \times (2.718)^{-Kt}$$

where K = rate constant and t = the time between samples 0 and t'.

Developmental perspectives

Children handle drugs differently than adults, as has been evidenced by the occurrence of the *gray baby syndrome* due to slow metabolism of chloramphenicol in young children, and *kernicterus* with sulfa therapy in jaundiced young infants. For some drugs such as morphine, theophylline and digoxin, the doses that are needed for clinical effect are highest between 6 and 12 months of life. For other drugs such as sedatives, alcohol, and amphetamines, unusual effects are seen in children. Sedatives can cause *hyperactivity*, amphetamines are used to treat hyperactivity, and alcohol can cause fatal *hypoglycemia* even in low doses in children. For many drugs, such as psychotropics, sedatives, and analgesics, estimation of pharmacological response necessitates valid patient reporting, which is impossible to obtain from infants and young children. This reality has led to suboptimal pain therapy in young children who, on average, receive only a fraction of the adult dose per kilogram, despite apparently equivalent levels of pain. There is, moreover, a relative lack of knowledge about drug pharmacokinetics in children because such information is far more difficult to gather in children than in adults due to ethical and technical considerations. The burgeoning of neonatal intensive care units has reversed this situation somewhat in the sphere of neonatology.

Absorption

Oral

Absorption of a drug after oral intake depends largely on gastric pH and emptying time.

Gastric pH

At birth gastric pH is ± 7.0 due to the presence of amniotic fluid, but within a few hours, acid secretion reduces it to pH 1.5–3.0. Milk then increases the pH to ± 7.0 for the next 24 hours, and there is a relative achlorhydria for the ensuing 10–15 days. The decrease in pH does not occur in the preterm infant. By age 3 years the child has achieved adult acid-producing capacity.

These changes contribute to the high levels that acid-labile drugs such as penicillin achieve in neonates, although decreased elimination could also play a part. Because acidic drugs such as nalidixic acid are better absorbed in the un-ionized form, the increased pH found in neonates increases the proportion of ionized drug and thereby decreases absorption.

Gastric emptying

In preterm infants gastric emptying is slow and linear, whereas in later life there is an initial rapid phase followed by an exponentially slower phase. Gastric emptying remains relatively slow for the first 6 months of life.

Although this slower gastric emptying may be thought to increase drug absorption, this is not the case for several drugs such as amoxycillin, chloramphenicol, cephalosporins, and rifampicin. But in many cases absorption approaches, and even surpasses, adult absorption by the age of 3 months.

Intramuscular

The bioavailability of a drug after intramuscular injection depends on the area that is infiltrated, the rate of penetration of the capillary membrane, and other pathological states affecting these parameters such as fever, hypovolemia, hypoperfusion, and hypoxemia. The rate of penetration of the capillary membrane is in turn dependent upon the ionization, lipid solubility, and osmolality of the drug; highly lipid-soluble drugs such as diazepam and chlordiazepoxide are less effectively and less rapidly absorbed, while water-soluble drugs such as phenobarbital are more readily absorbed. Neonates are much more prone to vasomotor instability and have decreased muscle mass and subcutaneous fat and increased body water, all leading to further variability in drug absorption after intramuscular injection.

The net effect of this is that some drugs, such as aminoglycosides and ampicillin, take the same time to peak after intramuscular injection in children as in adults, while others, such as benzylpenicillin, diazepam, and digoxin, undergo decreased or erratic absorption.

Percutaneous

Percutaneous absorption is dependent upon the thickness of the stratum corneum of the epidermis, which is decreased in the neonate, and the degree of hydration, which is increased in the neonate. Thus the net effect is that neonates have increased percutaneous absorption, as has unfortunately been found with the cases of *toxicity* due to hexachlorophene, salicylic acid, and boric acid applied to the skin.

Distribution

The amount of body water and its distribution as well as the degree of protein binding change throughout childhood, thereby influencing drug distribution. The proportion of blood reaching a given organ also varies with age. Thus increased cerebral perfusion may account for the increased *toxicity* seen in young children with diazepam, clonazepam, phenobarbital, phenytoin, and theophylline.

Protein binding

In the newborn there is relatively less albumin than in the adult, and much of it is fetal albumin, which has a decreased affinity for drugs. There are also decreased amounts of globulins and a relative acidemia and hypoxemia; in addition, maternal drugs as well as endogenous substances such as bilirubin and free fatty acids are found in increased amounts. Highly acidic drugs may displace bilirubin from plasma protein binding sites, increasing the risk of *kernicterus*. Diminished protein binding persists until normal adult levels are reached by approximately the third year of life for acidic drugs, and the seventh to twelfth year of life for basic ones. Although the increased free fraction of drugs could be expected to result in increased drug clearance, this is not the case as there is still a relative immaturity of the drug handling capacity of the nephron and hepatocyte in neonates.

Body water

The water content of the newborn is up to 75 percent, 40 percent of which is extracellular. In the adult the figures are 40 and 20 percent, respectively. Thus there is an increased volume of distribution of water-soluble drugs in neonates, resulting in lower peak drug concentrations, although the mean steady-state serum concentration is independent of the volume of distribution.

$$\text{Steady-state concentration} = \frac{\text{dose}}{\text{clearance}}$$

Elimination

Hepatic

Most hepatic metabolic functions are present at birth even in the preterm infant, but they are slower than in later life. The maturation rate of these functions varies for each enzyme complex, and some can be induced pre- and postnatally at a greater rate and to a larger extent than in adults. Because

$$\text{Drug half-life} = 0.693 \times \frac{\text{volume of distribution}}{\text{clearance}}$$

therapeutic and toxic concentrations can be achieved with lower doses, and longer dosing intervals are necessitated. The metabolism of low hepatic extraction drugs is reduced to a greater extent than that of high-extraction drugs. Hydroxylation and glucuronidation are the functions most modified after birth. Other factors that may lead to decreased drug metabolism in the newborn are maternal endogenous inhibitors, diminished liver blood flow, and relative hypoxemia. Adult doses of chloramphenicol, given to the neonate, accumulate due to decreased phase two hepatic elimination, and may lead to *shock* and *death*.

In the neonate the phase one functions of cytochrome P450 and NADPH cytochrome *c* reductase are approximately half of adult levels. Mildly depressed dealkylation and markedly depressed hydroxylation rates have been shown for many drugs. Esterase function reaches adult levels by 10–12 months. Phase one functions can increase 10–20-fold in 5 or 6 days in the neonate, and this possibility must be borne in mind when planning dosing schedules. The rates of phase two reactions generally reach adult levels by 18–24 months of age. The metabolic rate of hepatic microsomal drug metabolizing enzymes is markedly elevated for the first 2 years of life, after which it gradually decreases. At puberty there is a further sharp decrease to adult levels, presumably under hormonal control.

Renal

Many drugs such as penicillins, digoxin, and methotrexate are eliminated unchanged by the kidneys. Some are only filtered, and others are reabsorbed and/or secreted by the tubules—functions that can sometimes be induced. Because even drugs that are hepatically metabolized are subsequently excreted in the kidneys, diminished renal function can lead to accumulation of drugs and/or their metabolites.

The preterm infant has fewer glomeruli than a baby born at term, and even in the term infant glomerular, and especially tubular, function is immature. In time there is lengthening and maturation of the tubule, increased renal blood flow, improvement in filtration coefficient, and use of more superficial nephrons, and adult functional levels are reached by 6–12 months. Clearance, corrected for body weight, of some drugs such as digoxin and aminoglycosides, may be up to 30 times slower in the preterm infant than in adults. Although neonates may have higher serum concentrations of aminoglycosides, they experience less tubular reabsorption and accumulation secondary to relatively low glomerular filtration rate. Low urinary pH can lead to diminished reabsorption of weak bases and increased absorption of weakly acidic compounds. Lowered tubular secretion has been shown for penicillins and sulfonamides. The preterm infant therefore usually needs either decreased drug dosages or increased dosage intervals in many cases.

Pharmacodynamic considerations

Maturation processes of target cells or receptors are evident for many drugs. As an example, immature animals need more digoxin than mature animals in order to obtain the desired clinical effect; similar experience has been accumulated with this drug in humans. This phenomenon can be partially explained by the higher density of the pharmacological receptors for digoxin in the neonate than in the older individual. In the future researchers will have to be much more attuned to finding methods of measuring pharmacodynamic effect in the neonatal and pediatric age group.

Pathophysiology

Disease can alter drug disposition by affecting absorption, distribution, or metabolism and excretion.

Absorption

Intestinal absorption of drugs can be affected by malabsorption syndromes, e.g. decreased rate and extent of absorption is found in *celiac disease* and *cystic fibrosis*. Peak and steady-state concentrations are thereby reduced, although in some cases increased mucous membrane permeability or luminal pH seem to account for increased peak concentrations. In *cystic fibrosis* and *protein-calorie malnutrition*, low pancreatic enzyme levels cause decreased bioavailability of drugs requiring hydrolysis for absorption. *Diarrhea* by itself decreases transit time, alters gut mucosa, and is associated with dehydration. *Protein-calorie malnutrition* and *Crohn disease* are associated with increased transit times. In *Crohn disease* there is also thickening of the bowel wall and decreased surface area for absorption if bowel resection has been performed. *Pyloric stenosis* is associated with secondary achlorhydria and delayed gastric emptying. Salicylate absorption has been shown to be diminished in the acute phase of *Kawasaki disease*, even though this is not the case with other febrile illnesses. Finally, drugs absorbed through formation of micelles could be affected by liver diseases, producing decreased levels of bile acids.

Extraintestinal diseases can also affect bowel absorption. For example, *cardiac failure* is thought to diminish absorption by inducing mucosal edema and because increased sympathetic tone diminishes splanchnic blood flow. Aberrations in thyroid function may affect transit time. Drug–drug interactions can occur; for example, antacids alter tetracycline solubility and may even chelate it.

Distribution

An important determinant of drug distribution is the fraction of drug that is unbound in the serum. This in turn is proportional to plasma protein, especially albumin, concentrations. A greater unbound fraction, as may occur with true hypoproteinemia or *dilutional hypoproteinemia*, will allow more drug to distribute to peripheral compartments, increasing the drug's volume of distribution. More drug will then be available for clinical effect, metabolism, and excretion and this may require adjustments in dosing.

Many diseases lead to hypoproteinemia through decreased availability (*malabsorption syndromes*), decreased synthesis (*hepatic disease*), and increased losses (*nephrotic syndrome*) of proteins. Diseases associated with water retention, such as *cardiac, renal, and hepatic failure*, will also lead to low serum protein concentrations. *Uremia and hyperbilirubinemia* can cause displacement of drugs from protein binding sites.

Metabolism and elimination

Because the major sites for drug metabolism and elimination are the liver and the kidney, diseases affecting these organs will cause alterations in the pharmacokinetics of drugs. In the neonate the more common hepatic diseases encountered include viral infections such as *herpes-, ECHO-, and adenoviruses*, bacterial *sepsis*, inborn errors of metabolism such as *galactosemia, hereditary fructose intolerance*, *α_1-antitrypsin deficiency*, and *tyrosinemia*, *congestive cardiac failure*, and *fatty liver* secondary to hyperalimentation. Later in life *viral hepatitides*, *graft-versus-host disease*, *cystic fibrosis*, and *intoxications* are common. Other conditions include *protein-calorie malnutrition*, *hepatic cirrhosis*, and *biliary tree obstruction*, and poor hepatic blood flow secondary to *cardiac failure*.

The more completely a drug is excreted in the kidney, the more decreased renal function will diminish excretion and lead to drug retention. Lists of drugs of which the doses need to be altered at different levels of renal impairment are available. Slowed renal excretion has been shown for penicillin and chloramphenicol in *protein-calorie malnutrition*, and in *burn patients* increased glomerular filtration rates and decreased half-life have been demonstrated for several aminoglycosides.

In *cystic fibrosis* lower serum concentrations, larger volumes of distribution, and more rapid total body clearance of many drugs have been demonstrated, e.g. aminoglycosides, co-trimoxazole, ceftazidime, cloxacillin and methicillin. Although the mechanisms for these changes are unclear, there is evidence for enhanced elimination of drugs at both hepatic and renal levels.

B. Perinatal Toxicology

D Matsui and G Koren

Despite heightened awareness of the potential harmful effects to the fetus of *in utero* exposure to drugs and chemicals, their use during pregnancy remains common, and often unavoidable. According to various studies, 40–90 percent of women consume one or more medications during pregnancy.

The prescribing of medication during pregnancy must include consideration of the alterations in pharmacokinetics and drug handling that arise as a result of maternal physiological changes. In general, during pregnancy the elimination rate of agents excreted by the kidney, e.g. *digoxin*, increases. Changes in hepatic elimination patterns are less consistent, although the possibility of increased hepatic clearance does exist with some drugs such as *clindamycin*. The volume of distribution may be altered by changes in various fluid and tissue compartments. In addition, the protein binding of several *anticonvulsant medications* has been demonstrated to be decreased. Overall, the changes in drug disposition that occur during pregnancy tend to result in lower serum drug concentrations.

Placental transport is established at about the fifth week of fetal life with almost all drugs crossing to some extent.

Fetal and perinatal effects that will be discussed include *teratogenicity*, *direct drug toxicity or effect*, and *neonatal drug withdrawal*.

Human teratogens (see p. 123)

The *thalidomide* tragedy of the late 1950s highlighted the possibility of drug-induced birth defects. However, overemphasis of the teratogenic potential of medications too often results in unnecessary anxiety due to unrealistic perceptions of the risk. Fortunately, only a few drugs have been proven to be teratogenic in humans, and the vast majority probably do not pose a reproductive hazard when used in therapeutic amounts. An important issue to address when counseling women on teratogenic risks is the baseline risk of major malformations of around 3 percent. Table 15.1 lists some of the drugs and chemicals that have been proven to be teratogenic in humans.

Assessing the teratogenic potential of a drug in humans involves the analysis of case reports as well as retrospective and prospective studies. Often all available information has been gathered in animals. Animal data must be interpreted with caution as the drugs are often administered in doses and by routes that are not applicable to humans. Given the differences between various animal species it is not difficult to appreciate the reluctance to extrapolate such data to man. However, almost all known human teratogens have been shown to cause similar effects in animals.

Time of exposure is an important factor to consider. Although it is commonly stated that the fetus is at greatest risk during the first trimester, some agents may have effects later in pregnancy, for example those that affect the developing brain. During the first 2 weeks of pregnancy, the 'all-or-none' period, injuries to the embryo are likely to result in death of the conceptus or in repair and recovery. Vulnerability to teratogenic insult is greatest when the target organ is developing. For example, the neural tube closes during the fourth week of embryonic development; therefore, if an agent is to be

Table 15.1. Known teratogens

Drug	Typical manifestations
Alcohol	Fetal alcohol syndrome (facial features and mental retardation)
Isotretinoin	Skeletal, ear, cardiovascular, and central nervous system malformations
Phenytoin	Fetal hydantoin syndrome (facial features, hypoplastic digits, and mental retardation)
Thalidomide	Limb anomalies
Valproic acid	Meningomyelocele
Warfarin	Fetal warfarin syndrome (nasal hypoplasia and stippled epiphyses)

associated with the induction of a *neural tube defect* in the offspring, exposure must have occurred around that time.

The **dose** of the teratogenic agent may also play a key role. The risk of *fetal alcohol syndrome* has been proven only in chronic alcoholic women consuming at least 2 g alcohol/kg per day (equivalent to six to seven alcoholic drinks per day). Occupational exposure to most *organic solvents*, provided appropriate precautions are taken, has not been shown to pose an increased fetal risk in humans; however, more extensive use, such as during substance abuse, has been shown to cause damage to the developing brain. Similarly, the adverse effect of *methyl mercury* on the fetal brain has been documented only above a certain threshold.

Not all *in utero* exposures to teratogenic drugs result in malformations. Manifestation of the insult may depend on other factors such as genetic susceptibility. Variations in enzyme activity may be important when a toxic metabolite rather than the parent compound is the teratogenic agent. For example, it has recently been documented that fetuses suffering from *fetal hydantoin syndrome* are less likely to be able to detoxify a toxic intermediate of this anti-epileptic drug. Consideration of the underlying maternal disorder is also required as many illnesses may adversely affect fetal wellbeing.

Direct drug toxicity or effect

Most drugs cross the placenta and as a result may exert potential pharmacological and toxicological effects on the fetus. For example, indomethacin, when administered to the mother to inhibit preterm labor, may have adverse secondary effects on the fetal circulation, such as ductus arteriosus constriction. With prolonged use during pregnancy, the probability exists of developing *persistent pulmonary hypertension syndrome of the newborn*. Only very large molecules such as *heparin* and *insulin* do not cross the placental barrier in appreciable amounts. When maternal drug use occurs around the time of delivery, the newborn may experience prolonged effects due to slower neonatal drug elimination. In most instances such effects can be explained by the known actions of the drug in older individuals.

The use of β-antagonists (such as propranolol) late in pregnancy provides a typical illustration of this phenomenon. A proportion of neonates born in this situation will demonstrate transient symptoms and signs of β-blockade (bradycardia, hypotension, and hypoglycemia). Examples of direct drug toxicity are listed in Table 15.2.

Recently, in addition to the study of the toxic effects noted shortly after birth, more attention is being paid to the potential long-term effects of *in utero* drug and chemical exposure on the offspring's subsequent development and behavior. For example, there is much interest in studies to determine the long-term sequelae of *in utero cocaine* exposure. The delayed appearance of cancer is another potential concern with such drugs as *phenytoin*.

Drug withdrawal syndromes

With chronic use of certain drugs during pregnancy, especially frequent and high dose use late in gestation, dependence may develop in the fetus (as well as in the mother). After birth, when the supply of drug from the mother is no longer available, the neonate may manifest symptoms and signs of drug withdrawal.

Table 15.2. Fetal toxicity of drugs

Drug	Toxic effect
Aspirin, indomethacin, ibuprofen	? Premature closure or constriction of ductus arteriosus Abnormal hemostasis
Captopril, enalapril	Anuria/oliguria
Lithium	Hypotonia, cyanosis, bradycardia
Meperidine	Respiratory depression
Propylthiouracil	Hypothyroidism (goiter)
Streptomycin	Ototoxicity
Tetracycline	Yellow discoloration of teeth

The classic *neonatal withdrawal syndrome* is precipitated by *opioids*, the manifestations of which include irritability, tremors, hypertonicity, vomiting, high-pitched cry, respiratory distress, diarrhea, fever, and convulsions. Feeding difficulties and poor weight gain are not uncommon.

Not surprisingly, neonatal withdrawal has been described after maternal use of other classes of drugs including *alcohol*, *barbiturates*, and *benzodiazepines*. In some instances it is difficult to determine whether symptoms noted in the neonatal period are the result of drug intoxication or drug withdrawal. Such confusion exists with *cocaine* and *tricyclic antidepressants,* which exert toxic effects overlapping the typical withdrawal syndrome.

The clinical picture, including the time of onset and duration of symptoms, depends on the particular drug involved and the pattern of drug use during pregnancy (amount of dose, length of exposure, and time of last dose). For drugs with a relatively long elimination half-life (e.g. *methadone*) the withdrawal syndrome will become apparent much longer after that of drugs with a short half-life (e.g. *morphine*).

C. Drug Transfer into Human Milk

D Matsui and G Koren

Breast-feeding is widely encouraged by pediatricians and other physicians due to many advantages to both the infant and mother. Despite the possibility of exposure of the infant to drugs and chemicals transferred via breast milk, a general recommendation to discontinue nursing while taking medications is not needed. Consideration of the determinants of drug transfer into milk and the clinical relevance of a specific drug's transfer will provide assistance in guiding the breast-feeding mother.

Mechanisms and determinants of drug transfer in milk

To be present in human breast milk, drugs must reach the maternal circulation and then pass into breast milk. Thus, they must traverse a number of lipoprotein membranes, a process that occurs mainly by passive diffusion. Such transfer involves only the free fraction that is not bound to plasma proteins; therefore, drugs that are highly protein bound are less likely to enter breast milk. High lipid solubility favors passage into breast milk. The pK_a and degree of ionization of the drug in question are also important factors to consider. Weak bases, more likely to be nonionized in the maternal circulation, tend to pass into breast milk to a greater extent. Once reaching the milk, a more acidic environment, the weak bases will be ionized. This 'ion trapping' will create a gradient toward passage of the drug into breast milk. For most drugs, molecular weight is not an impediment to entrance into breast milk. As metabolites are generally more polar, they are less likely to be transferred into breast milk than their parent drug. Breast milk factors may also play a role. For example, composition of milk is not uniform (preterm vs term, foremilk vs hindmilk, etc.).

Estimation of the drug dose delivered via breast milk may be made using the following formula:

$$\text{Dose [mg/(kg·day)]} = Css \times \text{M/P ratio} \times \text{milk volume}$$

where Css = maternal steady-state serum drug concentration, M/P ratio = milk/plasma ratio, and average milk volume = 150 ml/kg of infant's body weight per day.

Clinical relevance of drug transfer into milk

Almost all maternally ingested drugs pass into the breast milk, usually in amounts less than 2 percent of the maternal dose; however, this drug transfer in many cases is not clinically significant due to the small dose offered via this route to the suckling infant.

In addition to potential adverse effects to the nursing infant, maternal ingestion of medication may influence the process of lactation to increase or decrease milk yield. For example, *bromocriptine*, a dopamine agonist, may suppress lactation.

Once the infant is fed the drug-containing breast milk, oral bioavailability, distribution, metabolism, and elimination of the drug by the infant must be considered. For example, reduced neonatal metabolism, due to decreased liver enzyme activity, and decreased neonatal renal excretion (lower glomerular filtration rate) may lead to accumulation of drug in the infant.

Drug effects in the breast-fed infant may be dose-related or idiosyncratic. Much of the information available to date has been gathered from single case reports. Studies are often conducted following a single dose, a somewhat unrealistic situation given that in practice most drugs are taken in repeated doses. Thus data gathered under such circumstances may not reflect the true picture.

To date, few drugs are absolutely contraindicated during breast-feeding (Table 15.3).

With most drugs a decision regarding breast-feeding must be reached based on a limited amount of information. Reluctance to encourage continuation of breast-feeding may arise if the inherent pharmacological action of the drug suggests that a toxic effect may occur (e.g. *cytotoxic drugs*) or if adverse effects have previously been noted in nursing infants. Experience with the direct use of the drug in infants for therapy may provide some reassurance.

Table 15.3. Drugs contraindicated during breast-feeding

Bromocriptine
Cimetidine, ranitidine
Cocaine
Cyclophosphamide
Cyclosporin
Doxorubicin
Ergotamine
Gold salts
Lithium
Methimazole
Methotrexate
Phencyclidine
Phenindione
Potassium iodide

General recommendations include use of the lowest dose of drug necessary to achieve a therapeutic effect in the mother, nursing just before drug ingestion ('trough'), observation of the infant for unusual signs or symptoms suggestive of an adverse effect, and measurement of the breast milk and/or infant's serum drug concentration(s). Fortunately, in most situations, breast-feeding may continue without major consequences in the presence of maternally ingested drugs.

Selected reading

American Academy of Pediatrics. Transfer of drugs and other chemicals into human milk. *Pediatrics* 1989; **84**: 924.

Bennett PN, ed. *Drugs and human lactation.* Amsterdam: Elsevier Science Publishers B.V., 1988: 16.

Briggs GG, Freeman RK, Yaffe SJ. *Drugs in pregnancy and lactation.* Baltimore: Williams and Wilkins, 1990: xi.

Koren G, ed. *Maternal–fetal toxicology.* New York: Marcel Dekker Inc., 1990: v.

Koren G, Prober CG, Gold R. *Antimicrobial therapy in infants and children.* New York and Basel: Marcel Dekker Inc., 1988: 3.

Schardein JL. *Chemically induced birth defects.* New York: Marcel Dekker Inc., 1985: 1.

Index